TEXTBOOK of
MEDICAL PSYCHIATRY

TEXTBOOK of
MEDICAL PSYCHIATRY

EDITED BY

Paul Summergrad, M.D.
David A. Silbersweig, M.D.
Philip R. Muskin, M.D., M.A.
John Querques, M.D.

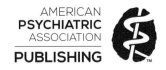

AMERICAN
PSYCHIATRIC
ASSOCIATION
PUBLISHING

If you wish to buy 50 or more copies of the same title, please go to www.appi.org/specialdiscounts for more information.

Copyright © 2020 American Psychiatric Association Publishing

ALL RIGHTS RESERVED

First Edition

Manufactured in the United States of America on acid-free paper
24 23 22 21 20   5 4 3 2 1

American Psychiatric Association Publishing
800 Maine Avenue SW
Suite 900
Washington, DC 20024-2812
www.appi.org

Library of Congress Cataloging-in-Publication Data
Names: Summergrad, Paul, editor. | Silbersweig, David, editor. | Muskin, Philip R., editor. | Querques, John, 1970– editor. | American Psychiatric Association Publishing, issuing body.
Title: Textbook of medical psychiatry / edited by Paul Summergrad, David A. Silbersweig, Philip R. Muskin, John Querques.
Description: First edition. | Washington, DC : American Psychiatric Association Publishing, [2020] | Includes bibliographical references and index. | Summary: "The Textbook of Medical Psychiatry focuses on medical disorders that can directly cause or affect the clinical presentation and course of psychiatric disorders. Clinicians who work primarily in psychiatric settings, as well as those who practice in medical settings but who have patients with co-occurring medical and psychiatric illnesses or symptoms, can benefit from a careful consideration of the medical causes of psychiatric illnesses. The editors, authorities in the field, have taken great care both in selecting the book's contributors, who are content and clinical experts, and in structuring the book for maximum learning and usefulness. The first section presents a review of approaches to diagnosis, including medical, neurological, imaging, and laboratory examination and testing. The second section provides a tour of medical disorders that can cause psychiatric symptoms or disorders, organized by medical disease category. The third section adopts the same format as the second, offering a review of psychiatric disorders that can be caused or exacerbated by medical disorders, organized by psychiatric disorder types. The final section contains chapters on conditions that fall at the boundary between medicine and psychiatry. Even veteran clinicians may find it challenging to diagnose and treat patients who have co-occurring medical and psychiatric disorders or symptoms. The comprehensive knowledge base and clinical wisdom contained in the Textbook of Medical Psychiatry makes it the go-to resource for evaluating and managing these difficult cases"—Provided by publisher.
Identifiers: LCCN 2019055530 (print) | LCCN 2019055531 (ebook) | ISBN 9781615370801 (hardcover ; alk. paper) | ISBN 9781615372829 (ebook)
Subjects: MESH: Mental Disorders | Comorbidity
Classification: LCC RC467 (print) | LCC RC467 (ebook) | NLM WM 140 | DDC 616.89—dc23
LC record available at https://lccn.loc.gov/2019055530
LC ebook record available at https://lccn.loc.gov/2019055531

British Library Cataloguing in Publication Data
A CIP record is available from the British Library.

Dedications

For Randy, Sophie, and Michael—For all the many reasons why.

Paul Summergrad

For Emily Stern, my partner in all things, with love and respect.

David A. Silbersweig

For Catherine, Matthew, and Marlene, who are my inspirations, and for Cecilia, who has wonderfully changed the direction of my life.

Philip R. Muskin

For Mom and Dad, with love.

John Querques

Contents

Contributors xiii

Foreword xxi
Professor Sir Simon Wessely

Introduction: The Importance of
Medical–Psychiatric Illness xxv
Paul Summergrad, M.D.
David A. Silbersweig, M.D.
Philip R. Muskin, M.D., M.A.
John Querques, M.D.

PART I
Approach to the Patient

1 An Internist's Approach to the
Neuropsychiatric Patient 3
Joseph Rencic, M.D.
Deeb Salem, M.D.

2 The Neurological Examination for
Neuropsychiatric Assessment 15
Sheldon Benjamin, M.D.
Margo D. Lauterbach, M.D.

3 The Bedside Cognitive Examination
in Medical Psychiatry 31
Sean P. Glass, M.D.

4 Neuroimaging, Electroencephalography, and Lumbar Puncture in Medical Psychiatry 51

Daniel Talmasov, M.D.

Joshua P. Klein, M.D., Ph.D.

5 Toxicological Exposures and Nutritional Deficiencies in the Psychiatric Patient 85

Mira Zein, M.D., M.P.H.

Sharmin Khan, M.D.

Jaswinder Legha, M.D., M.P.H.

Lloyd Wasserman, M.D.

PART II
Psychiatric Considerations in Medical Disorders

6 Cardiovascular Disease 175

Peter A. Shapiro, M.D.

7 Endocrine Disorders and Their Psychiatric Manifestations 193

Jane P. Gagliardi, M.D., M.H.S., FACP, DFAPA

8 Inflammatory Diseases and Their Psychiatric Manifestations 229

Rolando L. Gonzalez, M.D.

Charles B. Nemeroff, M.D., Ph.D.

9 Infectious Diseases and Their Psychiatric Manifestations 265

Oliver Freudenreich, M.D.

Kevin M. Donnelly-Boylen, M.D.

Rajesh T. Gandhi, M.D.

10 Gastroenterological Disease in Patients
With Psychiatric Disorders 289

    Ash Nadkarni, M.D.
    David A. Silbersweig, M.D.

11 Renal Disease in Patients With Psychiatric
Illness 319

    Lily Chan, M.D.
    J. Michael Bostwick, M.D.

12 Neurological Conditions and Their Psychiatric
Manifestations 339

    Barry S. Fogel, M.D.
    Gaston C. Baslet, M.D.
    Laura T. Safar, M.D.
    Geoffrey S. Raynor, M.D.
    David A. Silbersweig, M.D.

13 Cancer: Psychiatric Care of the
Oncology Patient 397

    Carlos G. Fernandez-Robles, M.D., M.B.A.
    Sean P. Glass, M.D.

14 Dermatology: Psychiatric Considerations
in the Medical Setting 419

    Katherine Taylor, M.D.
    Janna Gordon-Elliott, M.D.
    Philip R. Muskin, M.D., M.A.

15 Women's Mental Health and Reproductive
Psychiatry 447

    Marcela Almeida, M.D.
    Kara Brown, M.D.
    Leena Mittal, M.D.
    Margo Nathan, M.D.
    Hadine Joffe, M.D., M.Sc.

PART III
Medical Considerations in Psychiatric Disorders

16 Neurodevelopmental Disorders 481

Aaron Hauptman, M.D.
Sheldon Benjamin, M.D.

17 Psychotic Disorders Due to Medical Illnesses 499

Hannah E. Brown, M.D.
Shibani Mukerji, M.D., Ph.D.
Oliver Freudenreich, M.D.

18 Catatonia in the Medically Ill Patient 523

Scott R. Beach, M.D.
Gregory L. Fricchione, M.D.

19 Mood Disorders Due to Medical Illnesses 541

Sivan Mauer, M.D., M.S.
John Querques, M.D.
Paul Summergrad, M.D.

20 Anxiety and Related Disorders: Manifestations
in the General Medical Setting 563

Charles Hebert, M.D.
David Banayan, M.D., M.Sc., FRCPC
Fernando Espi-Forcen, M.D., Ph.D.
Kathryn Perticone, A.P.N., M.S.W.
Sameera Guttikonda, M.D.
Mark Pollack, M.D.

21 Substance Use Disorders in the Medical Setting . . 587

Samata R. Sharma, M.D.
Saria El Haddad, M.D.
Joji Suzuki, M.D.

22 Neurocognitive Disorders 629

Flannery Merideth, M.D.
Ipsit V. Vahia, M.D.
Dilip V. Jeste, M.D.

PART IV
Conditions and Syndromes
at the Medical–Psychiatric Boundary

23 Chronic Pain 651

Robert M. McCarron, D.O.
Samir J. Sheth, M.D.
Charles De Mesa, D.O., M.P.H.
Michelle Burke Parish, Ph.D., M.A.

24 Insomnia 663

Karl Doghramji, M.D.

25 Somatic Symptom and Related Disorders 677

Anna L. Dickerman, M.D.
Philip R. Muskin, M.D., M.A.

Index 697

Contributors

Marcela Almeida, M.D.
Instructor of Psychiatry, Harvard Medical School; Attending Physician, Department of Psychiatry, Brigham and Women's Hospital, Boston, Massachusetts

David Banayan, M.D., M.Sc., FRCPC
Assistant Professor of Psychiatry and Behavioral Sciences, Department of Psychiatry and Behavioral Sciences, Rush University Medical Center, Chicago, Illinois

Gaston C. Baslet, M.D.
Director, Division of Neuropsychiatry, Brigham and Women's Hospital; Assistant Professor of Psychiatry, Harvard Medical School, Boston, Massachusetts

Scott R. Beach, M.D.
Program Director, MGH/McLean Adult Psychiatry Residency, Massachusetts General Hospital; Assistant Professor of Psychiatry, Harvard Medical School, Boston, Massachusetts

Sheldon Benjamin, M.D.
Interim Chair of Psychiatry, Director of Neuropsychiatry, and Professor of Psychiatry and Neurology, University of Massachusetts Medical School, Worcester, Massachusetts

J. Michael Bostwick, M.D.
Professor of Psychiatry, Mayo Clinic College of Medicine, Rochester, Minnesota

Hannah E. Brown, M.D.
Director, Wellness and Recovery After Psychosis Program, Boston Medical Center; Assistant Professor of Psychiatry, Boston University School of Medicine, Boston, Massachusetts

Kara Brown, M.D.
Attending Psychiatrist, Veterans Affairs, New Orleans, Louisiana

Michelle Burke Parish, Ph.D., M.A.
Director of Research, Train New Trainers Primary Care Psychiatry Fellowship, Department of Psychiatry and Behavioral Sciences, University of California, Davis, California

Lily Chan, M.D.
Psychiatry Resident, Cambridge Health Alliance/Harvard Medical School, Cambridge, Massachusetts

Charles De Mesa, D.O., M.P.H.
Associate Professor and Director, Pain Medicine Fellowship, Division of Pain Medicine, University of California, Davis School of Medicine, Davis, California

Anna L. Dickerman, M.D.
Assistant Professor of Psychiatry, Weill Cornell Medical College, and Chief, Psychiatry Consultation-Liaison Service, New York–Presbyterian Hospital/Weill Cornell Medicine, New York, New York

Karl Doghramji, M.D.
Professor of Psychiatry, Neurology, and Medicine; Medical Director, Jefferson Sleep Disorders Center; and Program Director, Fellowship in Sleep Medicine, Thomas Jefferson University, Philadelphia, Pennsylvania

Kevin M. Donnelly-Boylen, M.D.
Associate Director, Psychiatric Consultation and Liaison Service, Boston Medical Center; Instructor of Psychiatry, Boston University School of Medicine, Boston, Massachusetts

Saria El Haddad, M.D.
Director of Partial Hospitalization, Dual Diagnosis, Department of Psychiatry, Brigham and Women's Hospital, Boston, Massachusetts

Fernando Espi-Forcen, M.D., Ph.D.
Assistant Professor of Psychiatry and Behavioral Sciences, Department of Psychiatry and Behavioral Sciences, Rush University Medical Center, Chicago, Illinois

Carlos G. Fernandez-Robles, M.D., M.B.A.
Clinical Director, Center for Psychiatric Oncology and Behavioral Sciences; Associate Director, Somatic Therapies Service; and Psychiatrist, The Avery D. Weisman, M.D., Psychiatry Consultation Service, Massachusetts General Hospital; Assistant Professor of Psychiatry, Harvard Medical School, Boston, Massachusetts

Barry S. Fogel, M.D.
Professor of Psychiatry, Harvard Medical School; Associate Neurologist and Senior Psychiatrist, Center for Brain/Mind Medicine, Brigham and Women's Hospital, Boston, Massachusetts

Oliver Freudenreich, M.D.
Co-Director, MGH Schizophrenia Clinical and Research Program, Massachusetts General Hospital; and Associate Professor of Psychiatry, Harvard Medical School, Boston, Massachusetts

Gregory L. Fricchione, M.D.
Director, Benson-Henry Institute for Mind Body Medicine, Massachusetts General Hospital; Professor of Psychiatry, Harvard Medical School, Boston, Massachusetts

Jane P. Gagliardi, M.D., M.H.S., FACP, DFAPA
Associate Professor of Psychiatry and Behavioral Sciences, Associate Professor of Medicine, Vice Chair for Education, Psychiatry and Behavioral Sciences, and Interim Director, Combined Residency Training Program in Internal Medicine–Psychiatry, Duke University School of Medicine, Durham, North Carolina

Rajesh T. Gandhi, M.D.
Director, HIV Clinical Services and Education, Massachusetts General Hospital; and Professor of Medicine, Harvard Medical School, Boston, Massachusetts

Sean P. Glass, M.D.
Psychiatrist, Northwest Permanente, Portland, Oregon

Rolando L. Gonzalez, M.D.
Clinical Assistant Professor of Psychiatry, University of Wisconsin School of Medicine and Public Health, Madison, Wisconsin

Janna Gordon-Elliott, M.D.
Assistant Professor of Clinical Psychiatry, Department of Psychiatry, New York–Presbyterian/Weill Cornell Medical Center, New York, New York

Sameera Guttikonda, M.D.
Chair, Consultation-Liaison Division, Department of Psychiatry, John H. Stroger Jr. Hospital, Cook County Health, Department of Psychiatry, Rush University Medical Center, Chicago, Illinois

Aaron Hauptman, M.D.
Instructor of Psychiatry, Boston Children's Hospital, Brigham and Women's Hospital, Boston, Massachusetts

Charles Hebert, M.D.
Chief, Section of Psychiatry and Medicine; Director, Psychiatric Consultation Liaison Service; Associate Professor of Internal Medicine and of Psychiatry and Behavioral Sciences, Department of Psychiatry and Behavioral Sciences, Rush University Medical Center, Chicago, Illinois

Dilip V. Jeste, M.D.
Senior Associate Dean for Healthy Aging and Senior Care; Estelle and Edgar Levi Memorial Chair in Aging, University of California, San Diego

Hadine Joffe, M.D., M.Sc.
Executive Director, Mary Horrigan Connors Center for Women's Health and Gender Biology; Paula A. Johnson Associate Professor of Psychiatry in the Field of Women's Health, Harvard Medical School; Vice Chair for Research, Department of Psychiatry, Brigham and Women's Hospital; and Director of Psycho-Oncology Research, Department of Psychosocial Oncology and Palliative Care, Dana-Farber Cancer Institute, Boston, Massachusetts

Sharmin Khan, M.D.
Clinical Assistant Professor, Department of Medicine, New York University Langone Health, New York, New York

Joshua P. Klein, M.D., Ph.D.
Associate Professor of Neurology and Radiology, Harvard Medical School, and Vice Chair for Clinical Affairs, Department of Neurology, Brigham and Women's Hospital, Boston, Massachusetts

Margo D. Lauterbach, M.D.
Director, Concussion Clinic, Neuropsychiatry Program, Sheppard Pratt Health System, Baltimore, Maryland

Jaswinder Legha, M.D., M.P.H.
Clinical Assistant Professor, Department of Medicine, New York University Langone Health, New York, New York

Sivan Mauer, M.D., M.S.
Clinical Instructor, Psychiatry, Tufts University School of Medicine, Mood Disorders Program, Tufts Medical Center, Boston, Massachusetts

Robert M. McCarron, D.O.
Professor and Vice Chair, Department of Psychiatry and Behavioral Medicine, and Co-Director, Train New Trainers Primary Care Psychiatry Fellowship, University of California, Irvine School of Medicine, Irvine, California

Flannery Merideth, M.D.
Clinical Fellow, Consultation-Liaison Psychiatry, Massachusetts General Hospital, Boston, Massachusetts

Leena Mittal, M.D.
Instructor in Psychiatry, Harvard Medical School; Attending Psychiatrist, Department of Psychiatry, Brigham and Women's Hospital, Boston, Massachusetts

Shibani Mukerji, M.D., Ph.D.
Associate Director, Neuro-Infectious Disease Unit; and Assistant Professor in Neurology, Harvard Medical School, Boston, Massachusetts

Philip R. Muskin, M.D., M.A.
Professor of Psychiatry and Senior Consultant in Consultation-Liaison Psychiatry, Columbia University Medical Center, Department of Psychiatry, Columbia University Vagelos College of Physicians and Surgeons, New York, New York

Ash Nadkarni, M.D.
Instructor, Harvard Medical School; Associate Psychiatrist and Director, Digital Integrated Care, Department of Psychiatry, Brigham and Women's Hospital, Boston, Massachusetts

Margo Nathan, M.D.
Instructor in Psychiatry, Department of Psychiatry, Brigham and Women's Hospital, Boston, Massachusetts

Charles B. Nemeroff, M.D., Ph.D.
Professor and Acting Chair of Psychiatry; Associate Chair for Research, Mulva Clinic for the Neurosciences; Director, Institute of Early Life Adversity Research; Dell Medical School, The University of Texas at Austin

Kathryn Perticone, A.P.N., M.S.W.
Assistant Professor of Psychiatry and Behavioral Sciences, Department of Psychiatry and Behavioral Sciences, Rush University Medical Center, Chicago, Illinois

Mark Pollack, M.D.
Grainger Professor and Chairman, Department of Psychiatry and Behavioral Sciences, Rush University Medical Center, Chicago, Illinois

John Querques, M.D.
Vice Chairman for Hospital Services, Department of Psychiatry, Tufts Medical Center; Associate Professor of Psychiatry, Tufts University School of Medicine, Boston, Massachusetts

Geoffrey S. Raynor, M.D.
Neuropsychiatry and Behavioral Neurology Fellow, Division of Cognitive and Behavioral Neurology, Brigham and Women's Hospital, Boston, Massachusetts

Joseph Rencic, M.D.
Associate Professor, Department of Medicine; Director of Clinical Reasoning Education, Boston University School of Medicine, Boston, Massachusetts

Laura T. Safar, M.D.
Assistant Professor of Psychiatry, Harvard Medical School; Associate Neuropsychiatrist, Brigham and Women's Hospital; Director, MS Neuropsychiatry, Department of Psychiatry, Center for Brain/Mind Medicine, Boston, Massachusetts

Deeb Salem, M.D.
Physician-in-Chief, Department of Medicine; Sheldon M. Wolff Professor and Chairman, Department of Medicine, Tufts University School of Medicine, Boston, Massachusetts

Peter A. Shapiro, M.D.
Professor of Psychiatry at Columbia University Irving Medical Center, Columbia University Vagelos College of Physicians and Surgeons; Director, Consultation-Liaison Psychiatry Service, New York–Presbyterian Hospital, Columbia University Irving Medical Center, New York, New York

Samata R. Sharma, M.D.
Director of Addiction Consult Psychiatry, Department of Psychiatry, Brigham and Women's Hospital, Boston, Massachusetts

Samir J. Sheth, M.D.
Assistant Professor, Pain Medicine, Director of Neuromodulation, and Director of Student and Resident Training, Department of Anesthesiology and Pain Medicine, University of California, Davis School of Medicine, Davis, California

David A. Silbersweig, M.D.
Stanley Cobb Professor of Psychiatry, Harvard Medical School, Boston, Massachusetts; and Chairman, Department of Psychiatry, and Co-Director, Center for the Neurosciences, Brigham and Women's Hospital, Boston, Massachusetts

Paul Summergrad, M.D.
Dr. Frances S. Arkin Professor and Chairman of the Department of Psychiatry, and Professor of Psychiatry and Medicine, Tufts University School of Medicine; and Psychiatrist-in-Chief, Tufts Medical Center, Boston, Massachusetts

Joji Suzuki, M.D.
Director, Division of Addiction Psychiatry, Department of Psychiatry, Brigham and Women's Hospital, Boston, Massachusetts

Daniel Talmasov, M.D.
Resident in Psychiatry, Brigham and Women's Hospital and Harvard Medical School, Boston, Massachusetts; and Resident in Neurology, New York University School of Medicine, New York, New York

Katherine Taylor, M.D.
Assistant Professor of Clinical Psychiatry, New York University (NYU) School of Medicine, NYU Langone Health Perlmutter Cancer Center, New York, New York

Ipsit V. Vahia, M.D.
Medical Director, Geriatric Psychiatry Outpatient Programs, McLean Hospital, Belmont, Massachusetts

Lloyd Wasserman, M.D.
Clinical Assistant Professor, Department of Medicine, New York University Langone Health, New York, New York

Professor Sir Simon Wessely, M.A., B.M., B.Ch., M.Sc., M.D., FRCP, FRCPsych, FMedSci
Regius Professor of Psychiatry, Institute of Psychiatry, Psychology & Neuroscience, King's College London; President, Royal Society of Medicine; Past President, Royal College of Psychiatrists

Mira Zein, M.D., M.P.H.
Clinical Assistant Professor, Department of Psychiatry and Behavioral Sciences, Stanford University Medical Center, Stanford, California

Disclosure of Interests

The following contributors to this textbook have indicated a financial interest in or other affiliation with a commercial supporter, manufacturer of a commercial product, and/or provider of a commercial service as listed below:

Margo D. Lauterbach, M.D.   *Equity Interest:* One-third owner of Brain Educators LLC, publishers of The Brain Card®.

Charles B. Nemeroff, M.D., Ph.D.   *Research Grants:* National Institutes of Health (NIH), Stanley Medical Research Institute; *Consultant:* Bracket (Clintara), Fortress Biotech, Gerson Lehrman Group (GLG) Healthcare and Biomedical Council, Janssen Research and Development LLC, Magstim Inc, Prismic Pharmaceuticals, Sumitomo Dainippon Pharma, Sunovion Pharmaceuticals Inc, Taisho Pharmaceutical Inc, Takeda, Total Pain Solutions (TPS), and Xhale; *Stock Holdings:* Abbvie, OPKO Health Inc, Antares, Bracket Intermediate Holding Corp, Celgene, Network Life Sciences Inc, Seattle Genetics, and Xhale; *Scientific Advisory Board:* American Foundation for Suicide Prevention (AFSP), Anxiety Disorders Association of America (ADAA), Bracket (Clintara), Brain and Behavior Research Foundation (BBRF) (formerly named National Alliance for Research on Schizophrenia and Depression [NARSAD]), Laureate Institute for Brain Research Inc, RiverMend Health LLC, Skyland Trail, and Xhale; *Board of Directors:* ADAA, AFSP, and Gratitude America; *Income or Equity ($10,000 or more):* American Psychiatric Publishing, Bracket (Clintara), CME Outfitters, Takeda, and Xhale; *Patents:* U.S. 6,375,990B1 (method and devices for transdermal delivery of lithium) and U.S. 7,148,027B2 (method of assessing antidepressant drug therapy via transport inhibition of monoamine neurotransmitters by ex vivo assay).

Peter A. Shapiro, M.D.   Dr. Shapiro affirms that he has no financial conflicts of interest to disclose. Supported in part by the Nathaniel Wharton Fund, New York.

Paul Summergrad, M.D.   *Nonpromotional Speaking:* CME Outfitters Inc, Lundbeck Foundation; *Consultant:* Compass Pathways, Mental Health Data Services, Pear Therapeutics; *Stock or Stock Options:* Karuna Therapeutics, Mental Health Data Services, Pear Therapeutics, Quartet Health; *Royalties:* American Psychiatric Association Publishing, Harvard University Press, Springer Publishing Company.

The following contributors stated that they had no competing interests during the year preceding manuscript submission:

Rolando L. Gonzalez, M.D.; Janna Gordon-Elliott, M.D.; Philip R. Muskin, M.D., M.A.; John Querques, M.D.; Joseph Rencic, M.D.; Peter A. Shapiro, M.D.; David A. Silbersweig, M.D.; Joji Suzuki, M.D.

Foreword

I am sure many of the readers of this textbook will have been to London at some stage in their lives, and no doubt seen all the wonderful sights. But unless you were there on medical business, it is unlikely that you visited the part of London known as Denmark Hill, once voted London's ugliest hill. If you had, you would have visited the embodiment of Cartesian dualism, caught here in all its splendor in what my generation still call a map.

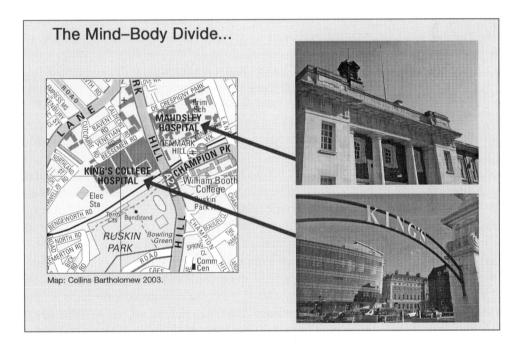

The Mind–Body Divide...

Map: Collins Bartholomew 2003.

What would you be looking at? As you walked down the hill, you would notice on your right the front of the Maudsley Hospital—which opened in 1916 for shell-shocked soldiers, before becoming a civilian mental hospital once the war was over—the first in Britain to see outpatients. For over a hundred years, it has been one of the few "brand names" in the world of psychiatry. If you looked to your left, you would see King's College Hospital. Named after King Edward VII, it is of the same vintage as the Maudsley—a large general hospital, with a busy emergency department and even a helipad on the roof, on which helicopters land with seriously injured people from all over South London, creating a din that brings all other business to a temporary halt.

You might think that because of the close proximity of these two huge and distinguished institutions, they would be umbilically linked at every level. But you would be wrong. When I started working in Denmark Hill, my interest in general hospital psychiatry combined with a wish to develop a career in academic psychiatry meant that I had a presence on both sides of the road—clinically in the general hospital, but academically over in the Maudsley—or the Institute of Psychiatry, as its research hub was called. My boss, Robin Murray, also had a foot in both camps, being both Professor of Psychological Medicine at the King's College Medical School, on the left side of the road, and also Dean of Psychiatry at the Maudsley Hospital, on the right. And I think that was it. Of the more than 5,000 people who worked at the two sites, just the two of us braved the traffic to cross Denmark Hill on a regular basis. Things got a bit better—well, safer—when the local council finally invested in a pedestrian traffic light, making the passage across Denmark Hill a little less hazardous, but still only a handful of physicians followed our footsteps.

Things are different now. There is a reasonably flourishing colony of mental health professionals who work in the A and E (accident and emergency services) at King's or who are scattered about the wards and clinics. There is a larger group of researchers who have shifted across the road, attracted by the new neuroscience building or the space in some of the labs that are dotted around King's. Traffic the other way, I have to say, remains slower—our colleagues in general medicine still seem reluctant to set foot on the psychiatric side of the street, preferring that we move our patients the hundred yards or so over to them. Academic collaborations have developed in many areas, but clinical links less so. We psychiatrists go to Grand Rounds at King's, but only the neurologists are regularly encountered at the clinical meetings in the Maudsley.

It is a pity that more of my colleagues were not exposed to a book like this one early in their careers. If they had been, I think that the now-increasing numbers of health professionals prepared to brave the traffic and cross Denmark Hill in either direction would have become a stampede. Because—as so beautifully shown—those patients who end up with "medical" disorders on the King's side of the road are very likely to also experience a range of "mental" problems, either neuropsychiatric symptoms specific to their illness or more general reactions to having a serious physical illness. One of my psychiatric colleagues, Anthony David, who teaches medical students on the King's side of the road, often asks his students to find a patient willing to come along to his teaching session, so that he can teach the students the fundamentals of psychiatry. The students panic—What kind of patient does he mean? From where? He merely smiles, says it really doesn't matter: Find anyone on any ward, in any clinic, or even in any of the coffee bars that patients frequent. Just bring them along. And invariably, as he starts to talk to the patient with the students watching, there is something that can be learned about the mind from anyone on the "physical" side of the road.

And it works both ways. One of the criticisms that can be leveled against psychiatrists is the often-poor physical health of the patients on our side of the road. It remains a scandal that a person with a major mental illness will have, on average, a life expectancy that is 15 years shorter than the life expectancy of a person without such an illness. We pay insufficient attention to the role that physical illness plays in the mental illnesses we study, nor are we doing anything like as much as we should in treating the consequences of the lifestyles that so many of our patents are forced to adopt—or the consequences of the treatments that we give them.

And then there are the vast numbers of patients who are found in the middle of Denmark Hill. Before you turn pale, I should clarify that I am referring metaphorically to those patients who are not comfortable, and occasionally not welcomed, on either side of the road—those with disorders that do not fall easily into one camp or the other; patients with chronic pain, for example, or with unexplained symptoms and syndromes that are hard to classify and sometimes even harder to manage. All too often, physicians tell these patients that there is nothing wrong with them and send them across the road, only for psychiatrists to swiftly turn them back, saying that no formal mental illness is present. Such patients are left languishing in the "no man's land" that lies between King's and the Maudsley. And some patients even prefer it that way, so great is the stigma of being seen on the "wrong" side of the road; it is not until they meet either a general or a family medicine doctor who is comfortable with both sides of the road—or, alternatively, find a very skillful physician or psychiatrist who is able to navigate these sometimes-choppy waters—that they receive any care at all.

So what is the solution? We could perhaps merge the two sides of the road, declare Denmark Hill traffic-free, remove the portals, and ensure that the signposts—and, of course, the standards used in the buildings and architecture—are uniform. But failing that, the best solution would be for everyone who works on either side of the Cartesian Divide that is Denmark Hill—a Divide that is just as pervasive in the United States as it is in the United Kingdom—to read this book.

Professor Sir Simon Wessely
Regius Chair of Psychiatry, King's College London
President, Royal Society of Medicine
Past President, Royal College of Psychiatrists

Introduction

The Importance of
Medical–Psychiatric Illness

Paul Summergrad, M.D.

David A. Silbersweig, M.D.

Philip R. Muskin, M.D., M.A.

John Querques, M.D.

This is a book for a wide range of clinicians—psychiatrists, internists, and neurologists, among others. Clinicians who work primarily in psychiatric settings, as well as those who practice in medical settings but have patients with co-occurring medical and psychiatric illnesses or symptoms, can benefit from a careful consideration of the medical causes of psychiatric illnesses. They may be challenged in such circumstances to accurately assess the cause of their patients' psychiatric or medical presentations or may find it difficult to manage care for complex patients.

There are many reasons why attention to the comorbidity of medical and psychiatric illness is important in both general and specialty medical care. Psychiatric illness and medical illness are both common, as is their co-occurrence (Druss and Walker 2011). Combined medical and psychiatric illness has significant effects on years of life lost to disability, early mortality, and the total cost of medical care (Melek et al. 2014; Walker et al. 2015). Psychiatric illnesses affect the course and presentation of medical disorders, and medical disorders and their treatments can complicate the care of psychiatric illnesses. In this textbook we focus on the general medical conditions that directly cause psychiatric illness and the medical differential diagnosis of common psychiatric illnesses. In addition, we describe how the presentation and treatment of both psychiatric and medical disorders are modified by the presence of comorbid conditions. We also note when a single underlying pathophysiology may result in both a psychiatric and a medical phenotype.

Psychiatric Illness Is Associated With a Considerable Illness Burden

Psychiatric disorders are among the largest causes of disability in advanced industrial democracies. This stems from the fact that many psychiatric illnesses have an early onset, with many disorders beginning in childhood and adolescence, as well as the high prevalence of psychiatric illness (Murray et al. 2013). Even when low- and middle-income countries are included, psychiatric illness still has a significant and increasing burden in years of life lost to disability worldwide, with particularly a burden in younger individuals (Bloom et al. 2011).

In addition to this illness burden, patients with psychiatric illness, like their age-matched cohorts, have intercurrent general medical and neurological illness. While the rates of these comorbid illnesses vary by study and illness type, there is very robust evidence that patients with psychiatric illness, including substance abuse, experience early mortality, with life spans that are between 8 and 15 years shorter compared with age-matched control subjects (Walker et al. 2015). While a percentage of this early mortality is due to suicide or overdoses, the majority is due to increased rates of death from common medical conditions such as cardiac disease, respiratory illness, and malignancies. Metabolic syndrome may be a factor, particularly in relation to the effects of psychiatric medications, as is tobacco smoking (Schroeder and Morris 2010).

Another important reason that an understanding of the interaction between psychiatric and medical illness is useful is that the elderly population in the developed world is growing. The accrual of medical morbidity, let alone dementia, with aging will increase the incidence of medical-psychiatric comorbidity.

Patients with psychiatric illness use health services in different ways from their age-matched peers. In studies from both the United States and the United Kingdom (Dorning et al. 2015; Melek et al. 2014, 2018), patients with psychiatric illnesses were more likely than persons without mental disorders to use medical inpatient and emergency services, even for similar medical conditions, and more likely to be medically hospitalized for conditions or procedures usually treated in ambulatory care settings. In the aggregate, these patterns make the total cost of the care of patients with psychiatric illness more expensive, especially due to increased medical care utilization. A study commissioned by the American Psychiatric Association in 2014, conducted by the consulting and actuarial firm Milliman, found that the medical/surgical health care expenditures for patients who had utilized psychiatric services were two to three times higher than the expenditures for patients who did not use psychiatric services (Melek et al. 2014). In real dollar terms, the total cost of care per year was increased by $292 billion per year, driven by increased hospital-based care for medical surgical services. When Milliman repeated its study in 2017 (Melek et al. 2018), the increased cost had grown to $402 billion per year.

Regardless of their financial impact, psychiatric illnesses can affect the course of medical disorders and the way in which these disorders present in general care settings. Among the better known of these effects is the impact of major depressive disorder (MDD) on the mortality associated with a recent myocardial infarction. Numerous studies have shown higher rates of death from cardiovascular disease in patients who have MDD post–acute coronary syndromes (Lichtman et al. 2014). Of course, there are other psychiatric illnesses, including substance use, that are associated with impaired medical outcomes, including medical disorders such as liver disease, cardiomyopathy, endocarditis, and lung cancer. The impact of the current opioid epidemic and its interaction with other mental disorders and general medical mortality is highly significant (Case and Deaton 2015; Olfson et al. 2018). Lifestyle and behavioral contributions are risk factors for chronic illness, including late-life noncommunicable diseases (Murray et al. 2013).

Although we remain mindful of this broader context, in this textbook we primarily focus on a specific subsection of illnesses: medical disorders that can cause psychiatric symptoms. As young physicians, we became aware of these clinical presentations during our training. For one of us (P.S.), it was as an internal medicine resident in a busy academic medical center where a bevy of patients with delirium, agitation, hallucinations, or psychotic illness had other medical disorders that were causing their symptoms. Hepatic, metabolic, infectious, and neurological disorders were frequent. Young men with dysregulated behavior (either aggressive or overly placid) had brain injuries that were directly causative of their changed behavior. An older patient receiving high-dose intravenous steroids to prevent a transplant rejection presented in a new-onset manic state. An elderly woman with wide-based gait, incontinence, and abulic affect was found to have extensive white matter hypodensities on central nervous system imaging and a vascular depression responsive to antidepressants. Another woman thought to have a depression lacked cognitive changes or mood symptoms consistent with MDD. Her worsening weakness and motor difficulties were soon revealed as severe myasthenia gravis. For another one of us (D.A.S.), it was dual training in neurology and psychiatry that allowed the consideration of the interface between the medical and the psychiatric being mediated by brain disease. Among these clinical experiences, a considerable number involved patients with multiple sclerosis and pseudobulbar affect, epilepsy and postictal psychosis, Parkinson's disease and panic attacks, and frontotemporal dementias with personality and behavior changes. In such cases, the diagnosis, management, and discussions with the patients and their families were all informed by a convergent neuropsychiatric view that transcends the typical neurological-psychiatric distinctions.

In all of these scenarios and in countless others that occur daily in hospitals, clinics, and doctor's offices, patients present with psychiatric symptoms caused by their medical disorders. Psychiatric symptoms due to other medical conditions can be as complex and disabling as classic psychiatric illnesses whose etiology is unknown. The fact that psychiatric syndromes can be well-described sequelae of medical disorders is often unfamiliar to our patients, their families, and the general public. Because of their rarity, many of these syndromes may also be unfamiliar to physicians and other clinicians. Indeed, there is an older literature that suggests a tendency for physicians to underdiagnose medical disorders, whether causative or not, in patients with psychiatric illness (Hall et al. 1978; Koranyi 1979).

The proper and careful consideration of all of the medical issues facing patients with psychiatric symptoms is important for several reasons, but primarily because such an approach is good medical practice. The high comorbidity of psychiatric and medical disorders and the shortened longevity of patients with psychiatric illness make a comprehensive evaluation imperative—as does the importance of properly diagnosing, and thus treating, these medical causes of psychiatric symptoms.

There are other reasons for considering medical issues in patients with psychiatric symptoms. First, we tend to think of mental disorders as being mentally caused. Such a view is intrinsic to our language, which separates brain and mind and also contributes to the stigma of psychiatric illnesses, which are still too commonly thought to be due to moral failing or fault. The recognition of the medical factors, as well as what we typically think of as the biological or genetic factors, that cause these illnesses is thus important. Second, attention to these medical causes is important when considering the etiology of psychiatric syndromes that are not due to a specific medical disorder. These medical disorders can broaden our thinking about the mechanisms of psychiatric disorders whose causes are at present unknown. Inflammation, autoimmunity, and endocrine mechanisms can all point to causes of psychiatric illness that our leading pathophysiological models and science may not have considered. In some cases, these mechanisms may suggest a single underlying etiopathology that looks like a psychiatric-medical "comorbidity" but may instead represent a single disease process that manifests with medical symptoms in peripheral organ systems and with psychiatric symptoms in the brain. Neurological disorders are even more intertwined mechanistically, given the role of brain circuits in producing perception, cognition, emotion, and behavior. Here, the location of disease-induced circuit abnormalities has a significant influence on psychiatric symptomatology and informs models of neuropsychiatric disease.

In those clinical areas where there are fewer medical disorders that directly cause psychiatric illness, there are nevertheless complexities in the way in which medical or psychiatric disorders may be affected by comorbid illnesses. In some cases, this complexity may be the difficulty of assigning particular symptoms—for example, fatigue secondary to medical versus psychiatric causes. In other patients, the interaction will be the known impact of psychiatric illness on the course of a medical disorder or drug interactions that may directly affect medical or psychiatric management. Where relevant, these issues are highlighted in the chapters that follow. For many of these topics, there are not systematic or randomized data on particular conditions. Where more extensive data have been developed, we have endeavored to include them. Of course, as in any such text, not all disorders can be covered.

The Approach to the Patient

Patients present in clinical settings with specialized or chief concerns for the visit. They also bring the full range of their medical and personal histories to clinical encounters, even if these are not the focus of a particular clinical service. The specialization of medical practice, a problem decried as long ago as 1933 in the *New England Journal of Medicine* in a special issue on psychiatry (Noble 1933), risks seeing patients within the context of where they are evaluated rather than their clinical history or concerns. In many situations, such a focused perspective is beneficial to care; however, when a patient's symptoms or course are atypical, a focused perspective may risk missing other causes of illness.

These issues are, if anything, more challenging in the evaluation of psychiatric symptoms and disorders. While our diagnostic precision has improved over the past 75 years, there is a high rate of comorbidity among psychiatric diagnoses, a lack of biological or imaging markers of many illnesses, and an unfortunate tendency for patients with psychiatric illness to have other medical complaints discounted. Additionally, for many diagnoses that depend on symptom clusters to generate syndromes, symptoms may be referable to bodily functions in a nonspecific fashion. Whether we are considering fatigue, tachycardia, or breathlessness, there is a risk that potentially causative medical symptoms are discounted—or, conversely, that an endless search for medical causation can miss a more obvious psychiatric disorder.

In neurological patients, psychiatric symptoms may be due to a co-occurring psychiatric illness, a response to disability, a medication, or involvement of brain regions or circuits mediating mental or behavioral functions. A number of these factors are often relevant in a single patient presentation. Not infrequently, it is the psychiatric disturbances (more than the other neurological ones) that most affect the patient and family, as well as their living situation. For this reason, we think it is essential to approach the evaluation and care of patients with a healthy dose of humility and a recognition that whatever our specialization—psychiatrist, internist, neurologist, or other—we need to keep an open mind about the patients we evaluate. That open mind can, in some cases, include reviewing or repeating laboratory or imaging studies, performing neurological or physical examinations, or being alert to loss, stress, and other psychological factors that may influence our patients' symptoms. For many of us, good practice includes getting second opinions, additional consultations, or informal "curbside" advice from colleagues whose perspectives and expertise we trust. We likewise hope that this book can make accessible much of what we know, particularly regarding medical conditions that directly cause psychiatric disorders, and thus provide guidance when difficult clinical circumstances arise.

The Organization of This Book

The book is divided into four parts. The first part, "Approach to the Patient," focuses on the approach to the patient and special aspects of medical, neurological, and imaging/laboratory examination and testing. It includes perspectives from internists with particular training in clinical decision making on how they approach diagnostic uncertainty and from neurologists with deep clinical expertise in bedside and clinical evaluation. There are chapters that detail office-based or hospital cognitive testing and that provide an extensive overview of the uses of neuroimaging. There is also a chapter on both laboratory testing and toxicological syndromes.

The second part, "Psychiatric Considerations in Medical Disorders," is organized by medical and neurological disorders. This is a section one would consult for a patient with a known medical or neurological disorder where the clinician is considering whether concomitant psychiatric symptoms are secondary to the medical illness or if there are challenges in the management of the medical and psychiatric symptoms. Some chapters—for example, those on neurological, endocrine, and inflammatory disorders, to name three—discuss conditions that have been directly linked to psychiatric presentations. Other chapters—for example, those on cardiovascular and renal disease—have fewer such conditions but include illnesses that have high co-occurrence with psychiatric disorders. There are often complex diagnostic and management issues that will bring patients with medical-psychiatric comorbidity to clinical attention.

The third part, "Medical Considerations in Psychiatric Disorders," is organized from the perspective of psychiatric conditions. This section focuses on the major diagnostic categories and clinical presentations of psychiatric illness. Here the focus is on known medical causes of each domain of psychiatric illness, and this section can be consulted by clinicians when caring for a patient with a previously identified psychiatric presentation where there has been an increasing suspicion of a medical or neurological cause. This suspicion can occur when patients have atypical presentations, histories of traumatic brain injury or other neurological insult, or unexpected medical or neurological symptoms or findings or when patients fail to respond as expected to standard psychiatric care. Dementia and delirium, which in DSM-5 are categorized as Neurocognitive Disorders (American Psychiatric Association 2013), are included in this section as well.

The final part, "Conditions and Syndromes at the Medical–Psychiatric Boundary," contains chapters on pain, insomnia, and somatic symptom and related disorders. Chronic pain and insomnia accompany many physical and mental conditions, and these chapters highlight the linkages of these symptoms to both medical and psychiatric disorders. Finally, a chapter on somatoform conditions is included. This describes a group of illnesses in which patients experience distressing bodily symptoms and functional impairment of uncertain etiology and often initially seek care for these symptoms in medical settings.

Whether patients have a known medical disorder and their clinicians are trying to assess the etiological importance of that disorder to their psychiatric symptoms, or a physician has a patient with a psychiatric presentation whose illness is atypical or nonresponsive to usual care, we hope that this text can serve as a reliable guide to what we know about these important conditions and how we may more effectively diagnose and care for our patients.

References

American Psychiatric Association: Diagnostic and Statistical Manual of Mental Disorders, 5th Edition. Arlington, VA, American Psychiatric Association, 2013

Bloom DE, Cafero ET, Jané-Llopis E, et al: The Global Economic Burden of Noncommunicable Diseases. Geneva, Switzerland, World Economic Forum, 2011

Case A, Deaton A: Rising morbidity and mortality in midlife among white non-Hispanic Americans in the 21st century. Proc Natl Acad Sci USA 112(49):15078–15083, 2015 26575631

Dorning H, Davies A, Blunt I: Focus on: people with mental ill health and hospital use. Nuffield Trust QualityWatch, Oct 10, 2015. Available at: https://www.nuffieldtrust.org.uk/research/focus-on-people-with-mental-ill-health-and-hospital-use. Accessed August 17, 2019.

Druss BG, Walker ER: Mental Disorders and Medical Comorbidity. Research Synthesis Report No 21. Princeton, NJ, Robert Wood Johnson Foundation, 2011

Hall RCW, Popkin MK, Devaul RA, et al: Physical illness presenting as psychiatric disease. Arch Gen Psychiatry 35(11):1315–1320, 1978 568461

Koranyi EK: Morbidity and rate of undiagnosed physical illnesses in a psychiatric clinic population. Arch Gen Psychiatry 36(4):414–419, 1979 426608

Lichtman JH, Froelicher ES, Blumenthal JA, et al: Depression as a risk factor for poor prognosis among patients with acute coronary syndrome: systematic review and recommendations. A scientific statement from the American Heart Association. Circulation 129(12):1350–1369, 2014 24566200

Melek SP, Norris DT, Paulus J: Economic Impact of Integrated Medical-Behavioral Healthcare: Implications for Psychiatry. Milliman American Psychiatric Association Report. Denver, CO, Milliman, 2014

Melek SP, Norris DT, Paulus J, et al: Potential Economic Impact of Integrated Medical-Behavioral Healthcare. Denver, CO, Milliman, 2018

Murray CJL, Atkinson C, Bhalla K, et al: The state of US health, 1990–2010: burden of diseases, injuries, and risk factors. JAMA 310(6):591–608, 2013 23842577

Noble RA: Psychiatry today. N Engl J Med 208(21):1086–1091, 1933. Available at: https://www.nejm.org/toc/nejm/208/21. Accessed June 2, 2019.

Olfson M, Crystal S, Wall M, et al: Causes of death after nonfatal opioid overdose. JAMA Psychiatry 75(8):820–827, 2018 29926090

Schroeder SA, Morris CD: Confronting a neglected epidemic: tobacco cessation for persons with mental illnesses and substance abuse problems. Annu Rev Public Health 31:297–314, 2010 20001818

Walker ER, McGee RE, Druss BG: Mortality in mental disorders and global disease burden implications: a systematic review and meta-analysis. JAMA Psychiatry 72(4):334–341, 2015 25671328

PART I

Approach to the Patient

An Internist's Approach to the Neuropsychiatric Patient

Joseph Rencic, M.D.
Deeb Salem, M.D.

Mr. A reported that he had experienced sudden onset of visual hallucinations 1 month earlier. He described the visual hallucinations as a face covered with a white mask that appeared in front of him from time to time. He reported that the face also talked to him and that he heard a male voice telling him that he would be harmed. He reported that he felt that his house was possessed by demons and that they were coming to get him.

Mahmood et al. 2005

Stories abound regarding patients with psychiatric symptoms resulting from treatable medical disorders (e.g., thyrotoxicosis) who are miscategorized as having primary psychiatric disorders. These errors in diagnosis are made by internists and psychiatrists alike. Such diagnostic errors are often multifactorial. Overconfidence or inability to recognize one's knowledge deficit likely plays an important role (Meyer et al. 2013). Both internists and psychiatrists can learn from each other's approaches to diagnosis, but for the purposes of this chapter, we focus on an internist's approach to patient evaluation, drawing upon recent literature on the cognitive psychology of clinical reasoning, which provides an evidence-based theoretical approach for clinical decision making in general.

What Is Diagnosis?

Diagnosis traditionally has been viewed as an analytic reasoning process akin to the scientific method. Early clinical observations or patient complaints trigger hypotheses. A clinician tests these hypotheses by obtaining additional historical and physical examination data to determine the merits of the competing hypotheses. The physician synthesizes the relevant data to create a composite of the patient's clinical findings, called a *problem representation* (Bowen 2006). A clinician finds the best match for this problem representation from the mental representations of diseases that he or she has developed through experience and study. If no diagnosis reaches a probability of disease above which the clinician believes that the benefits of treatment outweigh the risks of further testing (i.e., threshold to treat), the clinician obtains additional collateral history and laboratory or radiological data until the data reach the threshold to treat.

Cognitive Psychology Approaches to Diagnosis

The cognitive psychology literature indicates that the analytic reasoning approach of the scientific method is only one of two possible pathways to diagnosis. Kahneman (2009) referred to these two pathways as slow (i.e., analytic reasoning) and fast thinking (i.e., nonanalytic or intuitive reasoning; Kahneman 2009). Nonanalytic clinical reasoning typically occurs through rapid, unconscious pattern recognition, with the diagnosis emerging before the scientific method can be applied. For example, when a clinician sees a patient's skin covered with "dew drops on a rose petal" in a dermatomal distribution, the diagnosis of shingles immediately comes to mind. In such cases, the scientific method is set aside because of experience, diagnostic confidence, and efficiency. When no obvious pattern is recognized, a clinician typically combines nonanalytic and analytic reasoning, with certain patterns triggering a nonanalytic differential diagnosis followed by an analytic consideration of each of the potential diagnoses.

A Theory of Nonanalytic Reasoning

Nonanalytic reasoning is a black box; an observer can infer its nature only through the statements and decisions of the observee. However, even direct questioning about a doctor's clinical reasoning will provide insight only into conscious cognitive processes, whereas subconscious processes (e.g., implicit biases) will remain obscure to both observer and observee. Based on psychological research, script theory has emerged as a conceptual framework that can help explain some of the observed phenomena of nonanalytic reasoning. *Scripts* have been defined as

> (1) high-level, precompiled, conceptual knowledge structures, which are (2) stored in long-term memory, which (3) represent general (stereotyped) event sequences, in which (4) the individual events are interconnected by temporal and often also causal or hierarchical relationships, that (5) can be activated as integral wholes in appropriate

contexts, that (6) contain variables and slots that can be filled with information present in the actual situation, retrieved from memory, or inferred from the context, and that (7) develop as a consequence of routinely performed activities or viewing such activities being performed; in other words, through direct or vicarious experience. (Custers 2015, p. 457)

For example, a restaurant script includes waiting to be seated, ordering drinks and then your meal, tipping the waiter, and so on. One follows this routine or script without thinking. Script theory was transferred to the diagnostic literature through the term *illness scripts* (Clancey 1983). Illness scripts describe clinicians' mental representations of "the stories of diseases": their clinical findings, associated risk factors, and pathophysiology. For example, a psychiatrist may rapidly recognize the script or pattern of a depressive disorder in a sad, anhedonic patient with a flat affect and a family history of depression. Each clinician has idiosyncratic illness scripts for a given disease based on experience and "book knowledge." Illness script theory provides valuable insights into nonanalytic rapid diagnostic reasoning.

Accurate, comprehensive knowledge of illness scripts distinguishes expert and experienced clinicians from novices (Elstein et al. 1978). This knowledge forms the basis for heuristics (i.e., mental "rules of thumb") and pattern recognition, in which a clinician will mentally try to match a patient's presenting clinical findings with the appropriate illness script. Given the complexity of medical diagnosis, the accuracy of diagnostic reasoning is remarkable, and errors occur because of bias or misapplication of heuristics. The literature describes more than 30 different types of heuristics and biases (e.g., availability, representativeness), but the specifics are less important than the recognition that a clinician should seek ways to minimize these errors. The most common suggested "antidote" to nonanalytic reasoning–based diagnostic errors is for a clinician to force a "double-check" of the diagnosis with analytic reasoning, via a *cognitive forcing strategy*. For example, a clinician feels confident or certain about a diagnosis of major depressive disorder but chooses to review the medical differential diagnosis of depression and orders a thyroid-stimulating hormone level test to evaluate for hypothyroidism. The notion of a double-check on nonanalytic reasoning leads directly to a consideration of analytic reasoning. Given the tendency of many clinicians to discount medical causes of psychiatric symptoms and, conversely, psychiatric causes of general medical symptoms, an awareness of the limitations of implicit scripts is particularly important in this area.

Traditions of Medical Analytic Reasoning

Six traditions of medical analytic reasoning have been described: anatomic, pathophysiological, descriptive, criteria-based, probabilistic, and biopsychosocial (Richardson 2007). *Anatomic* analytic reasoning is based on finding pathology consistent with a given disease in a relevant specimen. *Pathophysiological*, or causal, analytic reasoning emphasizes coherence of the pathophysiological findings with the most likely diagnosis. *Descriptive* analytic reasoning is an explicit, conscious process of matching a patient's presenting clinical findings with typical or atypical descriptions of a given disease. *Criteria-based* analytic reasoning extends descriptive reasoning by using explicit criteria with a scoring system for determining a diagnosis within a taxonomy.

These latter two models—descriptive and criterion-based—are forms of reasoning closest to the current diagnostic model in DSM-5 (American Psychiatric Association 2013) and in clinical psychiatry, where we have, at present, a more limited number of anatomic or pathophysiological models. *Probabilistic* (i.e., Bayesian) analytic reasoning focuses on revising probability estimates of diseases based on clinical findings, using prediction rules or likelihood ratios when available, until the threshold to treat has been reached. Finally, *biopsychosocial* analytic reasoning—an approach that has been explicitly used in clinical psychiatry since the classic writings of George Engel (1977)—is a holistic process that focuses not only on a biological diagnosis but also on psychological and social aspects of a case to apprehend the causes and the patient's experience of an illness.

Although anatomic analytic reasoning sets the gold standard, for some diagnoses the risks of a pathological approach outweigh the benefits. For example, a biopsy may entail a significant probability of morbidity or mortality or may lack adequate sensitivity (i.e., too many false-negative results) or specificity (i.e., too many false-positive results). In these cases, internists fall back on the other traditions, and diagnosis becomes a probabilistic science to an even greater degree. A clinician must infer the diagnosis by seeking the disease that best explains the clinical findings within a given context (Lipton 2000).

Neuropsychiatric Diagnosis

If one considers psychiatry in the context of the six traditional approaches to medical analytic reasoning, it can be said that descriptive reasoning served as the primary approach to diagnosis until the period of neuroanatomic and infectious disease–related investigation in the late nineteenth century (e.g., the work of psychiatrists Alois Alzheimer and Solomon Carter Fuller in dementia-related illness), when classification schemes emerged for the purpose of collecting census data on mental illness. These classification efforts began with the 1952 publication of DSM-I but were more fully realized with the 1980 publication of DSM-III, which ushered in an emphasis on criteria-based diagnosis in psychiatry (American Psychiatric Association 1952, 1980). The predominance of this analytic tradition in psychiatry, in the philosophical sense, stems from the limited pathophysiological knowledge of psychiatric conditions, the lack of "objective" gold standards for the diagnosis of most conditions (Kapur et al. 2012), and the historic tendency for diagnoses with clearer pathophysiology or etiologies (e.g., the psychoses associated with tertiary syphilis) to be subsumed by other branches of medical practice. In addition, many of the descriptive criteria for psychiatric illnesses include physical symptoms but are not normed in populations that are medically ill or complex. Such an approach is not limited to psychiatry. For example, the American College of Rheumatology has created a set of diagnostic criteria (i.e., American College of Rheumatology–endorsed criteria for rheumatic diseases) for diseases within the subspecialty's purview, because rheumatologists face the same diagnostic challenges that psychiatrists do (American College of Rheumatology 2017).

Psychiatric diagnosis, especially when dependent on experience-based implicit scripts, is even more difficult if we consider the behavioral disturbances of some psychiatric illnesses, such as those that occur with somatic symptom disorder and some personality disorders. The emotional intensity of some forms of psychiatric illness, sometimes described with the terms *transference* and *countertransference*, can create diagnostic and management issues that can be quite complex in both psychiatric and general medical practice (Groves 1978; Kahana and Bibring 1964). Cognitive psychologists refer to the negative influence that these emotional phenomena can have on diagnostic accuracy as *affective bias* (Croskerry 2005). Objectivity and emotional neutrality toward patients are often considered best practices in medical diagnosis. Yet the emotions that patients engender in psychiatrists and other physicians can serve as key guides to clinical care and as clues that increase or decrease the likelihood of accurate identification of a disease. These emotional responses are idiosyncratic, and each physician, based on his or her own experiences over years of practice, will have different opinions about the value of these responses in aiding the diagnostic process. Thus, affective bias can be a double-edged sword in neuropsychiatric diagnosis.

The Challenge of Medical Causes of Psychiatric Illness

As if neuropsychiatric diagnosis were not difficult enough, medical disorders that can present as psychiatric illness compound the challenge. Clinicians must distinguish among three possibilities: 1) a primary medical disease with psychiatric symptoms not related to a known psychiatric disease, 2) a primary psychiatric disease with physical symptoms not caused by a known medical disease, or 3) primary medical and psychiatric diseases in which physical and mental symptoms are caused or exacerbated by both diseases (Figure 1–1). The incidence of medical misdiagnosis in patients with psychiatric symptoms (i.e., a psychiatrist or nonpsychiatrist physician diagnosing a primary psychiatric disease when the cause is a medical disorder) is controversial, with estimates ranging dramatically (from 19% to 80%) across studies of varying methodological rigor (Carlson et al. 1981; Hall et al. 1978, 1981; Han et al. 2009; Koranyi 1979; Olshaker et al. 1997; Riba and Hale 1990; Summers et al. 1981; Zun et al. 1996).

Regardless of the incidence of misdiagnosis, improving diagnostic accuracy is desirable, given the potential for reduced morbidity through appropriate treatment of medical disorders or for more effective care of both medical and psychiatric disorders when they co-occur.

The causes of these errors are multifactorial. A lack of skill and practice in both medical history taking and physical examination performance may increase the risk for diagnostic error. In one study, 32% (24/73) of faculty and private practice psychiatrists reported that they felt less than competent to perform a basic medical examination (McIntyre and Romano 1977). Frequent performance of an initial physical examination for inpatients and outpatients was reported by only 13% (10/73) and 8% (6/73) of these psychiatrists, respectively, although these percentages likely vary significantly depending on the setting (i.e., inpatient vs. ambulatory) and on how recently psychiatrists were trained. Regardless of setting, failure to perform an initial intake physical examination increases the risk for error due to nonanalytic bias. The availability heuristic ("Common things are common") and the representativeness heuristic ("If it looks, quacks, and waddles like a duck, then it's a duck") are powerful

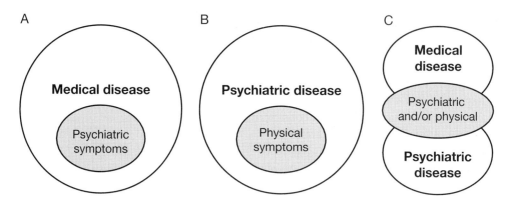

FIGURE 1–1.   Diagnostic possibilities for mixed physical and psychiatric symptomatology.
(A) Primary medical disease that causes psychiatric symptoms not related to any coexisting psychiatric disease. **(B)** Primary psychiatric disease that causes physical symptoms not related to any coexisting medical disease. **(C)** Primary medical and psychiatric diseases in which physical and/or psychiatric symptoms are caused or exacerbated by both diseases.

diagnostic strategies that can lead psychiatrists or other physicians astray when they are dealing with medically confusing presentations. In addition, confirmation bias (i.e., overvaluing data that support one's leading hypothesis and undervaluing data that do not) can lead a clinician to ignore or even fail to collect data relevant to a possible medical diagnosis.

Strategies for Minimizing Medical Misdiagnosis

Improving psychiatrists' and other physicians' knowledge about medical disorders that present psychiatrically and promoting development of clinical skills are obvious ways to reduce diagnostic error. This approach requires significant changes in physician awareness of the causes of these types of medical disorders, exposure to complex cases within residency training, and postgraduate professional development. Because medical students learn about medical and psychiatric illnesses in a siloed way, they may find it difficult to develop medical diagnostic hypotheses for psychiatric problems. Overcoming this cognitive bias is essential in clinical training. Knowing the contexts within which errors are most likely to occur and understanding the cognitive psychology literature may increase clinicians' suspicion for medical causes of psychiatric symptoms. Although some have advocated routine use of comprehensive examinations and extensive laboratory testing to rule out medical diagnoses, little evidence exists to support either the diagnostic utility or the cost-effectiveness of such a strategy. A targeted approach seems more appropriate, given the low yield of comprehensive laboratory testing.

An extensive literature review conducted by the American Association for Emergency Psychiatry (AAEP) Task Force on Medical Clearance of Adult Psychiatric Patients (Anderson et al. 2017) yielded a list of patient characteristics suggesting higher risk both for medical mimics of psychiatric disease and for coexisting medical illness (Table 1–1; Wilson et al. 2017). Patients with psychiatric presentations who have any of these risk factors should receive a comprehensive medical examination.

TABLE 1–1. **Checklist of risk factors[a] suggesting the need for a comprehensive medical examination to identify potential medical causes of psychiatric symptoms**

New-onset psychiatric symptoms after age 45 years or new onset of psychotic illness at any age

Advanced age (≥65 years)

Abnormal vital signs

Cognitive deficits (decreased level of awareness)

Delirium, severe agitation, or visual hallucinations

Focal neurological findings

Evidence of head injury

Evidence of toxic ingestion

---

[a]Any one of these findings would merit a comprehensive medical examination.

Source. Adapted from recommendation 2 (p. 643) in Wilson MP, Nordstrom K, Anderson EL, et al.: "American Association for Emergency Psychiatry Task Force on Medical Clearance of Adult Psychiatric Patients. Part II: Controversies Over Medical Assessment, and Consensus Recommendations." *The Western Journal of Emergency Medicine* 18(4):640–646, 2017.

Approaching from a different angle the dilemma posed by mixed physical and psychiatric symptoms, Shah et al. (2012) developed a screening algorithm designed to identify patients with psychiatric manifestations of a medical disease who could be directly referred for psychiatric evaluation without further medical workup or laboratory testing. This algorithm consisted of five criteria, all of which needed to be met for "medical clearance" and discharge to a psychiatric receiving facility:

1. Stable vital signs
2. A psychiatric history or age older than 30 years
3. No evidence of an acute medical condition
4. Alertness and full orientation or a Mini-Mental State Examination score higher than 23
5. No visual hallucinations

In a retrospective chart review of 485 emergency department patients who were believed to have a primary psychiatric disorder, only 1.2% of the patients who met all five of these "medical clearance" criteria prior to transfer to psychiatric care required further medical evaluation (Shah et al. 2012). Despite the circularity existing in the criteria (i.e., no evidence of an acute medical condition), their excellent negative predictive value suggests that clinicians could use them effectively to rule out medical complexity. Although the screening algorithm of Shah et al. (2012) has yet to be prospectively validated, its five "medical clearance" criteria may—together with additional risk factor criteria derived from the AAEP Task Force recommendations (Wilson et al. 2017)—yield a reasonably accurate patient risk profile that can help both psychiatric and nonpsychiatric clinicians decide whether to perform additional laboratory testing across various settings.

In addition to the risk factor checklist (see Table 1–1), the cognitive psychology literature describes cognitive forcing strategies as another means of improving diagnostic accuracy and reducing error. A cognitive forcing strategy (CFS) is a reasoning approach in which the clinician "forces" him- or herself to use analytic reasoning before making a final diagnosis, even when it seems unnecessary. In terms of the best strategy, a recent meta-analysis found that a reflection-based CFS focused on verification of an initial diagnostic hypothesis, through either a protocol or a differential diagnosis checklist, improved accuracy on paper- or Web-based clinical vignettes, whereas a reflection-based CFS focused on general reflection (e.g., "Reconsider your diagnosis") or cognitive "debiasing" (e.g., metacognitive self-reminders to "Be aware of your biases") did not (Norman et al. 2017). A typical diagnostic verification CFS protocol is presented in Table 1–2 (Mamede et al. 2008). In two studies in which internal medicine residents used a diagnostic verification protocol to check their initial diagnoses in paper-based simulated diagnostic problems, investigators found that this type of CFS protocol increased diagnostic accuracy by up to 40% (Mamede et al. 2008, 2010). This improvement occurred primarily with difficult cases, when initial diagnostic accuracy was less than 50% (Mamede and Schmidt 2017).

A Theory-Based Diagnostic Strategy to Reduce Medical Misdiagnosis

On the basis of the literature reviewed in the previous section, we suggest a best-practice strategy for reducing medical misdiagnosis in psychiatry and medicine. Initially, a clinician can use the "medical clearance" criteria of Shah et al. (2012) (see previous section, "Strategies for Minimizing Medical Misdiagnosis") to determine the need for a comprehensive medical evaluation in settings other than emergency departments and inpatient units (in which a comprehensive medical examination is standard practice). If a nonpsychiatrist performs the initial evaluation and the patient meets all five of the Shah et al. (2012) criteria as assessed by this physician, then the patient can be considered "medically cleared" and the psychiatrist can focus attention on psychiatric diagnoses, assuming that the medical evaluation is considered adequate (i.e., no evidence of an acute medical condition). If the psychiatrist feels competent to perform the initial evaluation and the patient does not meet all five criteria, then the psychiatrist may choose either to perform a comprehensive medical examination him- or herself (if he or she is comfortable with those clinical skills) or to request a medical consultation. If the psychiatrist chooses to conduct the examination him- or herself, a diagnostic verification CFS should be used with some type of clinical decision support (e.g., a checklist of common medical masqueraders) for every encounter, because clinicians often "don't know when they don't know" (Meyer at al. 2013). For example, in one study that examined the relationship between physicians' diagnostic accuracy and their confidence (rated on a scale of 1 to 10) in that accuracy (Meyer at al. 2013), internists' self-rated confidence remained similar regardless of the accuracy of their diagnoses (confidence ratings of 7.2 and 6.4 for diagnostic accuracies of 55% and 5%, respectively). Both overconfidence and cognitive "miserliness" (i.e., the tendency of the brain to minimize its effort [Stanovich 2018]) make the use of diagnostic verification CFS protocols challenging to implement for individual clinicians. Incorporation of such protocols into the electronic medical record—or into clinical decision support systems that generate differential diagnosis checklists highlighting medical presentations for common psychiatric problems—could facilitate their use. Finally, psychiatrists, like all physicians, need to be prepared to question even established diagnoses

TABLE 1–2.	Example of a typical protocol for a diagnostic verification cognitive forcing strategy

1. Choose a diagnosis based on your intuition or "gut feeling."

2. List the findings in the case presentation that support this diagnosis, the findings that speak against it, and the findings that would be expected to be present if this diagnosis were true but that were not obtained in your patient evaluation.

3. List alternative diagnoses as if your initial intuitive diagnosis had been proven to be incorrect and proceed with the same analysis for each alternative psychiatric *and* medical diagnosis.

4. Draw a conclusion about the most likely diagnosis for the case.

Source. Adapted from "Reflection for the verification of diagnostic hypothesis" subsection (p. 20) in Mamede and Schmidt 2017

when patients fail to respond as expected or their clinical course is atypical. Obtaining a second opinion from a colleague in the same or another specialty can be important. This is especially true when the patient has an acute onset of new illness, subtle neurological signs, an atypical presentation, or an unexpected response to treatment. For all physicians, maintaining clinical humility, being aware of the high rate of error in all medical diagnostic processes, and appreciating the complexity of clinical decision making are important.

The following case examples illustrate the recommended approach:

Case 1

A 22-year-old woman presented with acute psychosis (of 2 weeks' duration), associated with persecutory delusions, aggression, and visual and auditory hallucinations; she also had experienced a single focal seizure of her right hand 1 week before the symptoms began (Kukreti et al. 2015). This patient has visual hallucinations, which (according to the risk factor checklist in Table 1–1) would necessitate a comprehensive medical evaluation that can be performed by a psychiatrist or a consultant. Her physical examination was normal. Laboratory testing showed a lymphocytic pleocytosis. Testing for herpes simplex virus was negative; brain magnetic resonance imaging (MRI) and electroencephalogram (EEG) findings were normal. She was discharged on antipsychotic and antiseizure medications but returned 1 week later with a recurrent focal seizure. At this point, a careful analytic approach or a checklist of diagnoses that cause acute psychosis and seizures with normal MRI and EEG findings could help to rule out "can't miss" diagnoses. The health professionals caring for the patient recognized the possibility of N-methyl-D-aspartate receptor (NMDAR) antibody-mediated encephalitis. NMDAR antibody testing was positive, confirming the diagnosis, and led to effective treatment with plasmapheresis and corticosteroids.

This case illustrates the potential value of a careful assessment of risk factors (as described in Table 1–1) to reduce the risk of medical misdiagnosis.

Case 2

A 38-year-old woman presented with depression and unremarkable physical examination findings (Marian et al. 2009). She was initially treated with fluoxetine without significant improvement over a 2-month period. She returned to the clinic but now presented with palpitations, a fine hand tremor, subtle exophthalmos, and mild weight loss. Abnormal physical examination findings led to the diagnosis of hyperthyroidism-associated depression.

This case illustrates the atypical presentations of thyroid-related disorders and the importance of thyroid screening—with the relatively inexpensive thyroid-stimulating hormone level test—for most, if not all, patients with psychiatric presentations.

Conclusion

Neuropsychiatric diagnosis is a particularly challenging task because of a relative paucity of definitive, "objective" signs or laboratory findings for many psychiatric illnesses. Diagnostic cognitive strategies in psychiatry, descriptive and criterion-based, also tend to be normed so as not to consider the role of other medical disorders as causes of psychiatric presentations. Although future research is likely to identify valuable diagnostic biomarkers, psychiatrists need strategies that they can use now to reduce the risk of medical misdiagnosis.

In this chapter, we provided two suggested strategies—a risk factor checklist (see Table 1–1) and a diagnostic verification CFS protocol (see Table 1–2)—for reducing error and enhancing accuracy in the diagnosis of medical symptoms presenting as psychiatric illness. Although some evidence supports these strategies, future research is needed to confirm their utility.

References

American College of Rheumatology: ACR-Endorsed Criteria for Rheumatic Diseases. Atlanta, GA, American College of Rheumatology, 2017. Available at: https://www.rheumatology.org/Practice-Quality/Clinical-Support/Criteria/ACR-Endorsed-Criteria. Accessed May 5, 2017.

American Psychiatric Association: Diagnostic and Statistical Manual: Mental Disorders. Washington, DC, American Psychiatric Association, 1952

American Psychiatric Association: Diagnostic and Statistical Manual of Mental Disorders, 3rd Edition. Washington, DC, American Psychiatric Association, 1980

American Psychiatric Association: Diagnostic and Statistical Manual of Mental Disorders, 5th Edition. Arlington, VA, American Psychiatric Association, 2013

Anderson EL, Nordstrom K, Wilson MP, et al: American Association for Emergency Psychiatry Task Force on Medical Clearance of Adults, I: introduction, review and evidence-based guidelines. West J Emerg Med 18(2):235–242, 2017 28210358

Bowen JL: Educational strategies to promote clinical diagnostic reasoning. N Engl J Med 355(21):2217–2225, 2006 17124019

Carlson RJ, Nayar N, Suh M: Physical disorders among emergency psychiatric patients. Can J Psychiatry 26(1):65–67, 1981 7471036

Clancey WJ: The epistemology of a rule-based expert system: a framework for explanation. Artificial Intelligence 20(3):215–251, 1983. Available at: https://www.sciencedirect.com/science/article/abs/pii/0004370283900085. Accessed May 10, 2019.

Croskerry P: Diagnostic failure: a cognitive and affective approach, in Advances in Patient Safety: From Research to Implementation, Vol 2: Concepts and Methodology. Edited by Henriksen K, Battles JB, Marks ES, et al. Rockville, MD, Agency for Healthcare Research and Quality, 2005, pp 241–254. Available on PubMed at: https://www.ncbi.nlm.nih.gov/books/NBK20487/. Accessed May 11, 2019. Bookshelf ID: NBK20487; PMID: 21249816

Custers EJ: Thirty years of illness scripts: theoretical origins and practical applications. Med Teach 37(5):457–462, 2015 25180878

Elstein AS, Shulman LS, Sprafka SA: An Analysis of Clinical Reasoning. Cambridge, MA, Harvard University Press, 1978

Engel GL: The need for a new medical model: a challenge for biomedicine. Science 196(4286):129–136, 1977 847460

Groves JE: Taking care of the hateful patient. N Engl J Med 298(16):883–887, 1978 634331

Hall RCW, Popkin MK, Devaul RA, et al: Physical illness presenting as psychiatric disease. Arch Gen Psychiatry 35(11):1315–1320, 1978 568461

Hall RCW, Gardner ER, Popkin MK, et al: Unrecognized physical illness prompting psychiatric admission: a prospective study. Am J Psychiatry 138(5):629–635, 1981 7235058

Han JH, Zimmerman EE, Cutler N, et al: Delirium in older emergency department patients: recognition, risk factors, and psychomotor subtypes. Acad Emerg Med 16(3):193–200, 2009 19154565

Kahana RJ, Bibring G: Personality types in medical management, in Psychiatry and Medical Practice in a General Hospital. Edited by Zinberg NE. New York, International Universities Press, 1964, pp 108–123

Kahneman D: Thinking Fast and Slow. New York, Farrar, Straus, & Giroux, 2009

Kapur S, Phillips AG, Insel TR: Why has it taken so long for biological psychiatry to develop clinical tests and what to do about it? Mol Psychiatry 17(12):1174–1179, 2012 22869033

Koranyi EK: Morbidity and rate of undiagnosed physical illnesses in a psychiatric clinic population. Arch Gen Psychiatry 36(4):414–419, 1979 426608

Kukreti P, Garg A, Bhirud L: Autoimmune encephalitis masquerading as psychosis: diagnostic and therapeutic challenge. International Journal of Nutrition, Pharmacology, Neurological Diseases 5(3):108–109, 2015. Available at: http://www.ijnpnd.com/text.asp?2015/5/3/108/158373. Accessed May 10, 2019.

Lipton P: Inference to the best explanation, in A Companion to the Philosophy of Science. Edited by Newton-Smith WH. Malden, MA, Blackwell, 2000, pp 184–193

Mahmood A, Ashton AK, Hina FH: Psychotic symptoms with underlying Graves disease: a case report. Prim Care Companion J Clin Psychiatry 7(6):311–312, 2005 16498497

Mamede S, Schmidt HG: Reflection in medical diagnosis: a literature review. Health Professions Education 3(1):15–25, 2017. Available at: https://www.sciencedirect.com/science/article/pii/S2452301117300081. Accessed July 10, 2019.

Mamede S, Schmidt HG, Penaforte JC: Effects of reflective practice on the accuracy of medical diagnoses. Med Educ 42(5):468–475, 2008 18412886

Mamede S, van Gog T, van den Berge K, et al: Effect of availability bias and reflective reasoning on diagnostic accuracy among internal medicine residents. JAMA 304(11):1198–1203, 2010 20841533

Marian G, Nica EA, Ionescu BE, et al: Hyperthyroidism—cause of depression and psychosis: a case report. J Med Life 2(4):440–442, 2009 20108759

McIntyre JS, Romano J: Is there a stethoscope in the house (and is it used)? Arch Gen Psychiatry 34(10):1147–1151, 1977 911214

Meyer AN, Payne VL, Meeks DW, et al: Physicians' diagnostic accuracy, confidence, and resource requests: a vignette study. JAMA Intern Med 173(21):1952–1958, 2013 23979070

Norman GR, Monteiro SD, Sherbino J, et al: The causes of errors in clinical reasoning: cognitive biases, knowledge deficits, and dual process thinking. Acad Med 92(1):23–30, 2017 27782919

Olshaker JS, Browne B, Jerrard DA, et al: Medical clearance and screening of psychiatric patients in the emergency department. Acad Emerg Med 4(2):124–128, 1997 9043539

Riba M, Hale M: Medical clearance: fact or fiction in the hospital emergency room. Psychosomatics 31(4):400–404, 1990 2247567

Richardson WS: We should overcome the barriers to evidence-based clinical diagnosis! J Clin Epidemiol 60(3):217–227, 2007 17292015

Shah SJ, Fiorito M, McNamara RM: A screening tool to medically clear psychiatric patients in the emergency department. J Emerg Med 43(5):871–875, 2012 20347248

Stanovich KE: Miserliness in human cognition: the interaction of detection, override and mind-ware. Thinking & Reasoning 24(4):423–444, 2018. Available at: https://www.tandfonline.com/doi/full/10.1080/13546783.2018.1459314. Accessed October 1, 2019.

Summers WK, Munoz RA, Read MR, et al: The psychiatric physical examination—part II: findings in 75 unselected psychiatric patients. J Clin Psychiatry 42(3):99–102, 1981 7204358

Wilson MP, Nordstrom K, Anderson EL, et al: American Association for Emergency Psychiatry Task Force on Medical Clearance of Adults, II: controversies over medical assessment, and consensus recommendations. West J Emerg Med 18(4):640–646, 2017 28611885

Zun LS, Leikin JB, Stotland NL, et al: A tool for the emergency medicine evaluation of psychiatric patients. Am J Emerg Med 14(3):329–333, 1996 8639216

CHAPTER 2

The Neurological Examination for Neuropsychiatric Assessment

Sheldon Benjamin, M.D.

Margo D. Lauterbach, M.D.

The neuropsychiatric consultant begins planning the approach to the neurological examination from the moment the consultation request is received. The standard neurological examination is adapted to fit the consultation question, the patient's age and ability to cooperate, and the time available. The examiner may wish to adapt the examination further for patients with acute deterioration, intellectual disability, dementia, or high intelligence or for the purposes of risk assessment, rehabilitation planning, or forensic evaluation. The consultant will have formed diagnostic hypotheses from the outset. The examination is a dynamic process, continuously modified to refine hypotheses so as to facilitate neuropsychiatric formulation and treatment planning. While examining the patient, the clinician is mentally planning for diagnostic testing to confirm or refute these hypotheses.

The examiner should give thought to the basic neuropsychiatric examination toolkit. We prefer the items listed in Table 2–1. It is also helpful for the examiner to have a set of rating scales readily available. Examples of scales we find helpful are listed in Table 2–2.

General Physical Examination

The general physical examination involves observation for aspects of the patient's presentation that might serve as clues to diagnosis, including dysmorphic features,

TABLE 2–1.   **Basic neuropsychiatric examination toolkit**

Neurological toolkit

Disposable gloves

Digital pulse oximeter

Stethoscope

Sphygmomanometer (automated variety will record data)

Small flashlight with adjustable intensity

Fundoscope with panoptic head (to facilitate easy viewing)

Scented lip balm (for testing olfaction)

Snellen card (for testing visual acuity)

Optokinetic nystagmus (OKN) strip

Tongue depressors (wrapped)

Wooden applicator sticks (wrapped)

Disposable cup (for testing swallow)

Measuring tape

Reflex hammer

128 Hz and 256 Hz tuning forks

Two-point discriminator or note card with prepunched points (for testing of two-point discrimination)

Coin, paper clip, key (for stereognosis testing)

Optional: Sparking wheel toy (for testing of eye movements in less cooperative patients)

Cognitive toolkit

Clipboard

Plain white paper

Pencil and fine felt-tip pen (bleeds when patient's hand remains in one position)

Copies of any standard rating scales needed (also see Table 2–2)

Copies of bedside cognitive testing stimuli

Some helpful smartphone/tablet applications

OKN Strips

PseudoChromatic ColorTest

Digital Finger Tapping Test

Face2Gene (for identification of dysmorphic facies)

Neuropsychiatric examination pocket reference

The Brain Card® (Benjamin and Lauterbach 2016)

cutaneous signs, and general body habitus, in addition to the usual components such as cardiopulmonary auscultation.

Certain dysmorphic features increase the likelihood of the presence of abnormal brain development. For example, midline defects such as hypertelorism, which is present in several congenital syndromes, may prompt an examiner to consider partial agenesis of the corpus callosum. Microcephaly or macrocephaly often runs in families; thus, a family history of head size must be obtained before assuming abnormal brain development. Absent a family history of large head size, the thresholds for macro-

TABLE 2–2.	Useful rating scales for bedside neurological assessment

Abnormal Involuntary Movement Scale (Munetz and Benjamin 1988)

Blessed Dementia Index (Blessed et al. 1968)

Bush-Francis Catatonia Rating Scale (Bush et al. 1996)

Dementia Severity Rating Scale (Hughes et al. 1982)

Epworth Sleepiness Scale (Johns 1991)

Expanded Disability Status Scale (Kurtzke 1983)

Frontal Assessment Battery (Dubois et al. 2000)

Glasgow Coma Scale (Teasdale and Jennett 1974)

Montreal Cognitive Assessment (Nasreddine et al. 2005)

Neuropsychiatric Inventory (Cummings 1997)

Overt Aggression Scale (Yudofsky et al. 1986)

Patient Health Questionnaire—9 (Kroenke et al. 2001)

Rancho Los Amigos Rating Scale (Gouvier et al. 1987)

Unified Parkinson's Disease Rating Scale (Goetz et al. 2008)

Unified Dystonia Rating Scale (Comella et al. 2003)

cephaly are 58.4 cm in males and 57.5 cm in females. Areas to examine for commonly observed dysmorphic features are listed in Table 2–3. Phenotyping applications are available from Face2Gene.com to assist in identifying dysmorphic syndromes. At a minimum, the examiner should be able to recognize the typical physiognomies of Down, fragile X, velocardiofacial, and fetal alcohol syndromes (see also Chapter 16, "Neurodevelopmental Disorders").

The clinician must take special note of cutaneous signs in the general physical examination, because the skin and nervous system share a common embryonic ectodermal origin. Neurocutaneous syndromes may be associated with normal development, typically in the carrier state; or they may be associated with seizures, behavior changes, and intellectual disability in the fully expressed syndrome. The most common neurocutaneous signs are listed in Table 2–4.

The general physical examination also can give clues to the presence of diabetes, cardiovascular disease, or heavy cigarette smoking, any of which can increase the risk for vascular dementia. Excessive neck circumference, when combined with snoring, an enlarged upper torso, and small oropharyngeal opening, suggests the possibility of obstructive sleep apnea. Auscultation for carotid bruits is commonly done during neurological examination; however, bruits detected during carotid auscultation are often not predictive of critical stenosis when followed up with an ultrasound evaluation.

Neurodevelopmental Signs (Soft Signs)

Neurodevelopmental signs (Table 2–5), often referred to as *neurological soft signs,* may be found on examination in people with schizophrenia, bipolar disorder, substance use disorders, obsessive-compulsive disorder, antisocial personality disorder, or neurodevelopmental disorders. Neurological soft signs tend to decrease in adolescence and young adulthood. They are more suggestive of an immature nervous sys-

TABLE 2–3.	**Dysmorphic features**
Stature	Mouth and lips
Hair growth pattern	Teeth
Ear structure, placement, and size	Hand size
Nose structure and size	Fingers and thumbs
Face structure and size	Nails
Philtrum	Foot structure and size

Source. Reprinted from Table 3 in Benjamin S, Lauterbach MD: "The Neurological Examination Adapted for Neuropsychiatry." *CNS Spectrums* 23(3):219–227, 2018. Copyright © 2018, Cambridge University Press. Used with permission.

TABLE 2–4.	**Cutaneous features of common neurocutaneous syndromes**
Syndrome	**Cutaneous features**
Neurofibromatosis type I	Axillary and inguinal freckling Café au lait spots (six or more ≥1 cm) Cutaneous neurofibromas Plexiform neurofibromas
Tuberous sclerosis	Hypomelanotic macules (ash-leaf spots) Shagreen patches Subungual fibromas Angiofibromas Adenoma sebaceum
Sturge-Weber syndrome	Port-wine stain in trigeminal distribution
Ataxia-telangiectasia	Telangiectasias on ears, cheeks, trunk Premature graying of hair Progeric facies Hypopigmented macules Café au lait spots

Source. Reprinted from Table 4 in Benjamin S, Lauterbach MD: "The Neurological Examination Adapted for Neuropsychiatry." *CNS Spectrums* 23(3):219–227, 2018. Copyright © 2018, Cambridge University Press. Used with permission.

tem than of localized lesions. Children with prematurity, low birth weight, or malnutrition may have neurological soft signs as well (Whitty et al. 2009). The relation of neurological soft signs to the pathophysiology of mental illness is unclear, but these signs appear to decrease as psychiatric symptoms improve (Mittal et al. 2007). The neurodevelopmental signs in Table 2–5 are divided into signs that are *nonlateralizing* (i.e., those that do not correlate with focal brain dysfunction) and those that are *potentially lateralizing* (i.e., those that may be associated with focal brain dysfunction).

Cranial Nerves

Loss of olfaction (in the absence of chronic rhinitis or chronic smoking) may be a sign of early neurodegenerative disease, white matter disease, orbitofrontal mass lesions,

TABLE 2–5.   **Neurodevelopmental signs**

Nonlateralizing signs	
Dysarthria	Dysphagia
Inability to move eyes without moving head	Nystagmus
	Slow or irregular rapid alternating movements
Clumsiness, incoordination	Bradykinesia
Drooling	Overflow/mirror movements
Ataxia	

Potentially lateralizing signs	
Dystonic posturing	Asymmetric size of face or extremities
Hemiparesis	Astereognosis
Unsustained clonus	Agraphesthesia
Asymmetric reflexes, hyperreflexia	Motor impersistence
Slow or irregular fine movement of fingers	Extinction to visual/tactile double simultaneous stimulation

or traumatic brain injury (TBI), although it also occurs in normal aging. Bedside testing of olfaction can be accomplished with scented lip balm or multiple-choice scratch-and-sniff olfactory testing cards, if available (Doty 2015).

Assessment of the optic nerve includes direct inspection (fundoscopy) as well as testing of visual acuity (by reading a Snellen card at 14 inches), testing of visual fields to confrontation, and testing of pupillary light reflexes and accommodation. Visual acuity is customarily recorded by writing the acuity numbers to the right of a capital V, with the right eye above the left, as shown in Figure 2–1A. When testing fields to confrontation by moving a wiggling finger in from the periphery in each quadrant, extinction to double simultaneous stimulation is assessed by simultaneously wiggling the fingers in both of the upper or lower quadrants. Pupillary light reflexes are tested by shining a flashlight obliquely, first at one pupil and then at the other, with the patient staring straight ahead into the distance, and observing for direct and consensual pupillary responses. An afferent pupillary defect will cause the abnormal pupil to dilate when the light swings over it in the swinging flashlight test. While shining a light on both pupils simultaneously, the clinician should note whether the light aligns at the same "o'clock" on both pupils. Misalignment indicates dysconjugate gaze. Rather than just recording "PERRLA" (i.e., **p**upils **e**qual, **r**ound, **r**eactive to **l**ight, **a**ccommodation), recording the pupillary diameters is helpful for later comparison. This is customarily done by writing the number of millimeters of pupillary diameter to the right of the letter *P* instead of the *E* in PERRLA. The right pupillary diameter is recorded above the left, as shown in Figure 2–1B.

Ocular motility is tested by having the patient follow a stimulus and move the eyes to command, and by observing the patient's eye movement while the examiner moves the patient's head vertically and horizontally. The patient is instructed to follow the examiner's finger with his or her eyes while the examiner moves a forefinger in an "H" pattern in order to test the extraocular muscles in isolation. Saccadic intrusions (also called square-wave jerks) during pursuit testing may indicate cerebellar dysfunction. Saccadic intrusions also can be present in Parkinson's disease, progressive supranuclear palsy (PSP), and schizophrenia.

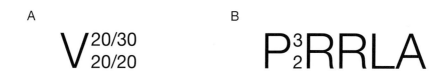

FIGURE 2–1.   Customary recording format for visual examination.

(**A**) Visual acuity, recorded with OD above OS. (**B**) Pupillary diameter, recorded with OD above OS. OD=oculus dexter (right eye); OS=oculus sinister (left eye).

Supranuclear control of gaze is tested by directing the patient to look up and down, and then left and right. Gaze-evoked nystagmus may indicate medication toxicity, metabolic problems, or abnormalities of the brain stem or cerebellum. The vestibulo-ocular reflex (doll's eyes phenomenon) is assessed by moving the patient's head vertically and horizontally and observing whether compensatory eye movements are present. Supranuclear weakness of vertical gaze with preservation of doll's eyes may be seen in PSP, a disease that occurs most frequently in late middle age. This sign also may be seen in children or young adults with Niemann-Pick type C disease. Optokinetic nystagmus (OKN) may be elicited with a wide-striped cloth, an OKN drum, or the *OKN Strips* smartphone/tablet application. The patient is asked to watch the stripes or to count them as they go by. Failure to direct the eyes to the approaching target suggests frontal pathology, whereas failure to pursue the target is indicative of more posterior pathology. The antisaccade task requires the patient to direct his or her gaze in a direction opposite to the movement of the examiner's finger, thus providing information about independent versus stimulus-bound behavior (an indicator of prefrontal function). Prolonged visual fixation can be indicative of a "visual grasp" observed in posterior cortical atrophy and in some cases of Alzheimer's disease.

Ptosis should be described by its position in relation to the pupil (e.g., "ptosis to mid-pupil"). The fatigue phenomenon, in which sustained upgaze induces ptosis or diplopia, is seen in myasthenic syndromes. Internuclear ophthalmoplegia, often seen in demyelinating disease and occasionally in vascular lesions of the medial longitudinal fasciculus, manifests as horizontal diplopia when the patient is looking away from the side with the lesion. To test for internuclear ophthalmoplegia, the examiner stands with hands laterally outstretched and instructs the patient to look quickly from one hand to the other when the examiner snaps his or her fingers. If internuclear ophthalmoplegia is present, the patient's ipsilateral eye will be unable to adduct, and the contralateral eye will develop nystagmus.

Facial sensation is assessed by light touch and sharp stimulus touch (not in a stroking motion) in each of the three trigeminal areas—V1, V2, and V3. The afferent arc of the corneal reflex is ophthalmic (V1), the "nasal tickle" is maxillary (V2), and the jaw jerk is mandibular (V3). An exaggerated jaw jerk is an indicator of upper motor neuron dysfunction. Trigeminal motor function is tested by palpation of the temporalis and masseter muscles while the patient clenches the jaw and moves the jaw horizontally. Facial strength is tested by asking the patient to raise his or her eyebrows (upper face strength may also be observed during upward gaze to command), shut his or her eyes tightly, and puff out his or her cheeks, as well as by eliciting both a smile to command and a spontaneous (limbic) smile. A spontaneous smile is evoked either by saying something humorous to the patient or by asking the patient if he or she happens to know any jokes. An asymmetric spontaneous smile paired with a symmetrical smile to command has been associated with lateralized limbic, basal ganglia, or supplementary motor area pathology, all of which are areas of neuropsychiatric interest (Hopf et al. 1992).

Hearing may be tested at the bedside by whispering into each of the patient's ears or by finger rubbing. To differentiate conductive from sensorineural loss in a patient with lateralized hearing deficit, the examiner uses the Weber test, in which the sound of a 256-Hz tuning fork applied to the top of the patient's head is experienced as louder on the defective side if the loss is conductive in nature. If the patient reports hearing loss on one side, the Rinné test is occasionally helpful. The examiner places the stem of a 512-Hz tuning fork on the mastoid process of the reportedly defective ear and moves the prongs of the tuning fork to just next to the ear as soon as the patient reports that the sound has stopped. If the patient can now hear the sound, a conductive hearing loss may be present. Ear wax buildup is a common cause of conductive hearing loss.

Dysarthria patterns can be noted by having the patient repeat the phonemes "pa," "ta," and "ka" individually and then in succession: "pa-ta-ka." This task tests sounds emphasizing labial, lingual, and guttural vocal muscles, respectively. Cerebellar dysfunction can manifest as scanning speech, characterized by an inability to maintain consistent volume and pitch when asked to utter a prolonged "ahh."

The gag reflex does not correlate well with dysphagia. A better way to assess for dysphagia is to ask the patient to swallow a tumblerful of water without pause. Dysphagia is common in neuromuscular disease, tardive dyskinesia, and parkinsonism and can be a significant cause of morbidity in psychiatric patients.

The spinal accessory nerve is assessed by shoulder shrug and lateral head turning against resistance. Unilateral lower motor neuron hypoglossal dysfunction (occasionally seen after carotid endarterectomy, after neck surgeries, or with mass lesions) manifests as deviation of the tongue toward the lesion when at rest in the mouth and contralaterally on protrusion. The lesion may be associated with fasciculations and lateralized atrophy. Bulbar amyotrophic lateral sclerosis causes upper motor neuron (contralateral) tongue weakness.

Pseudobulbar palsy is so named because bilateral corticobulbar tract lesions produce cranial nerve nuclear dysfunction. Components of pseudobulbar palsy include affective lability, dysphagia, dysarthria, increased jaw jerk, and hyperactive gag reflex (hyperactive gag reflex also may be seen in the absence of pathology). The affective lability is sometimes referred to as pseudobulbar affect, emotional incontinence, or pathological laughing and crying. Pseudobulbar palsy is frequently seen in amyotrophic lateral sclerosis, demyelinating disease, stroke, PSP, and TBI.

Motor Examination and Reflexes

All four limbs should be examined for muscle bulk, tone, and strength against resistance. After testing the deep tendon reflexes, the examiner should elicit pathological reflexes. The plantar reflex is best elicited by slowly stroking the lateral sole of the foot with a moderately sharp, disposable stimulus (e.g., flat end of an applicator stick), turning medially at the ball of the foot. An upgoing great toe with fanning of the other toes is called the Babinski reflex. If the response is equivocal, the examiner can test for signs to elicit great toe dorsiflexion via Gordon's sign (squeeze the calf muscle), Chaddock reflex (stroke the lateral malleolus with a sharp stimulus), Gonda's sign (flick another toe downward), or Oppenheim's sign (stroke the tibia between two knuckles of the hand). Positive responses indicate upper motor neuron dysfunction.

Primitive reflexes include the glabellar tap; forced grasping; and palmomental, snout, and suck reflexes. Parkinson's disease or diffuse frontal dysfunction can lead to a positive glabellar tap (also known as Meyerson's sign), in which an eyeblink persists for five or more light finger taps over the glabellar region. Upward stroking across the palm results in the patient grasping the examiner's fingers more tightly as the examiner attempts to withdraw in the forced grasping or grasp response. Although associated with contralateral medial prefrontal and supplementary motor area dysfunction, unilateral damage sometimes may produce bilateral grasping (De Renzi and Barbieri 1992). A similar sign of frontal dysfunction can be elicited by stroking the sole of the seated patient's foot with the side of the reflex hammer and then placing the hammer in front of the foot. A forced foot grasp or groping response—in which the toes curl as if to grasp the hammer, with foot extension toward the object in front of it—can be seen with frontal dysfunction (Fradis and Botez 1958). The palmomental reflex, elicited by stroking the thenar eminence while observing for ipsilateral mentalis muscle contraction, is less specific than forced grasping and can be seen in individuals with normal and abnormal brains (Owen and Mulley 2002). Primitive oral reflexes include the snout and suck reflexes, both of which are nonspecific indicators of brain dysfunction. The snout response is elicited by tapping the philtrum, and the suck response is elicited by touching an object to the lips. *Gegenhalten* rigidity (oppositional paratonia) refers to the involuntary resistance to passive movement seen in advanced dementia.

Coordination

Incoordination typically results from cerebellar dysfunction. Ataxia refers to uncoordinated irregular movements that can affect speech, eye movements, swallowing, limb motion, balance, and posture. Dysdiadochokinesia denotes an inability to alternate movements rapidly. In the upper extremities, it takes the form of inability to rapidly alternate tapping the palm and back of the hand on the thigh. In the lower extremities, it manifests by irregular heel tapping. Dysmetria (the inability to control movements of the hand, arm, leg, or eyes, resulting in over- or undershoot) is tested by finger-to-nose or heel-to-shin testing that reveals movement deterioration as the target is approached and by ocular pursuit testing (Bodranghien et al. 2016). Patients with cerebellar lesions also may show hypotonia, "past-pointing" (missing the target on finger-to-nose testing), and decreased checking responses during reflex testing or when the examiner pushes down and releases the patient's outstretched arms. The patient may have difficulty closely following the examiner's moving finger without touching it and sustaining a long vocal "ahhh" without scanning.

Sensation

The sensory examination involves testing of three major sensory systems—exteroceptive, proprioceptive, and cortical—to detect patterns of sensory loss, such as dermatomal or radicular (nerve root distribution), neuropathic (distal stocking-glove distribution), or myelopathic patterns at an identifiable level of distribution. Large-fiber and dorsal column systems are examined by testing joint position sense (also called proprioception) to assess for the presence of Romberg's sign, and vibration sense with a 128-Hz tuning fork (see "Gait and Balance" subsection later in this chapter). Small-fiber and spinothalamic tract dysfunction are detected through testing of pain and temperature sensation, comparing side to side and proximal to distal areas.

The primary sensory examination is supplemented with cortical sensory testing for parietal dysfunction via graphesthesia, stereognosis, two-point discrimination, and double simultaneous stimulation. With the eyes closed, the patient is asked to identify numbers traced on the palm (graphesthesia) or objects placed in the hand (stereognosis). Callosal dysfunction can cause an inability to name objects placed in the left hand, with preserved ability in the right hand. A two-point discriminator tool can be used to assess the minimum distance between two points at which the points are perceived as separate to test tactile spatial perception. Alternatively, a notecard with pinholes placed 5 mm, 7 mm, and 10 mm apart can be used. Double simultaneous stimulation tests the tactile, visual, and auditory systems to identify hemi-inattention or neglect. Somatosensory extinction of the neglected side is tested by asking the patient to identify, with eyes closed, the side of the body being touched when the examiner touches one side or both sides at once. Visual extinction is elicited by asking the patient to identify the finger that is moving when the examiner moves fingers in both hemifields simultaneously. Auditory extinction is elicited by simultaneously producing different sounds in each ear (e.g., crinkling paper vs. jingling keys) while asking the patient to identify the sounds.

Gait and Balance

If parkinsonism is suspected, the clinician should ask the patient to arise from a chair without using his or her hands. Romberg's test is used to assess the patient's ability to sustain balance by using proprioception and vestibular function when visual cues are removed by standing with eyes closed, feet together, and arms outstretched. This test also affords an opportunity to observe the patient for signs of motor impersistence (e.g., the patient needs continual reminding to carry out all three commands at once). Motor impersistence has been associated with right frontal dysfunction (Kertesz and Hooper 1982). The examiner can evaluate for postural instability by performing the "pull test" (propulsion and retropulsion), which involves pulling the patient's shoulders sharply while standing in front of or behind the patient. Gait examination focuses on gait initiation, balance, stride length, speed, step height, arm swing, turning, and use of any ambulation appliances. The patient is asked to first walk normally and then to walk on heels, on toes, and on an imaginary straight line (walking heel to toe [i.e., tandem walking]). "Stressed" gait is assessed by having the patient walk on the lateral surfaces of the feet to elicit abnormal hemidystonic upper-extremity posturing.

The typical gait examination in parkinsonism reveals short-stepped "marche à petits pas" gait with forward-flexed, stooping posture; decreased arm swing; and "en bloc" turning. The pull test is frequently positive for retropulsion. Patients with severe parkinsonism may develop camptocormia or bent spine syndrome. Patients with cerebellar ataxia have a wide-based, staggering gait and are usually unable to tandem walk. Sensory ataxia also manifests with a wide-based gait, but with high steppage and a positive Romberg's test result. Patients with paraparetic gait have stiff legs that "scissor" around each other, whereas hemiparetic gait affects one leg that is stiff and circumducts. Apraxia of gait includes difficulty with initiation and the appearance of the feet being stuck to the floor—yet the patient can typically step over lines on the floor and, when lying prone, can "bicycle" with legs in the air.

Involuntary Movements

Abnormal involuntary movements may be described as hyperkinetic or hypokinetic. Hyperkinetic movements include tremor, choreoathetosis, dystonia, hemiballismus, myoclonus, asterixis, tics, stereotypies, overflow, and mirror movements and occur in toxic states, delirium, neurodegenerative extrapyramidal disorders, focal lesions, metabolic disorders, and tardive dyskinetic syndromes as well as attention-deficit/hyperactivity disorder and mania. Examination for tremor includes observation of the extremities while seated and while standing at rest, with arms outstretched, and with extremity movement. A tremor can occur primarily at rest (e.g., parkinsonian tremor) or primarily with movement (i.e., action tremor). Action tremors may be postural (involved part against gravity) or intentional (cerebellar), or they may occur with any movement. Table 2–6 describes common forms of tremor.

Tics are abrupt, jerky, repetitive movements involving discrete muscle groups. Tics tend to mimic normal coordinated movements, varying in intensity and lacking rhythmicity. Motor and vocal tics may be classified as simple or complex; they occur in individuals with chronic tic disorder, Gilles de la Tourette syndrome, or obsessive-compulsive disorder (OCD) and can also occur in first-degree relatives of people with OCD or Tourette syndrome. Tics can be exacerbated by stimulant treatment and alleviated by treatment with anxiolytics, dopamine antagonists, or selective serotonin reuptake inhibitors (SSRIs).

Choreoathetoid movements are quick, "irregularly irregular" choreic contractions that flow from one muscle group to another in a dancelike fashion, combined with slow, twisting or writhing athetoid movements. They can be quantified and serially assessed by means of the Abnormal Involuntary Movement Scale (Munetz and Benjamin 1988). The examiner should first observe the seated patient carefully for any adventitious movements, which can be an early sign of a choreoathetoid movement disorder. The patient is then directed to perform a series of distraction maneuvers while the examiner continues to observe for any abnormal movements of the face, trunk, arms, and legs throughout each task. The patient is asked to hold the arms outstretched and to perform mouth opening, tongue protrusion, fine finger movements,

TABLE 2–6.   **Common forms of tremor and their characteristics**

Type	Characteristics
Essential tremor	Most common tremor Autosomal dominant Bilateral Progressive Action tremor, usually postural Affects limbs, head and neck, voice
Parkinsonian tremor	Asymmetric, resting 4–6 Hz "pill-rolling" tremor, but also occurs with action Decreases with voluntary movement Progresses to forearm pronation/supination Patient may show "reentrant tremor" after holding arms outstretched
Physiological tremor	Low amplitude, high frequency Exacerbated by anxiety, stimulants, medical conditions, fatigue
Tremor due to toxic or metabolic condition	Drug toxicity Hepatic encephalopathy (asterixis) Hypocalcemia, hypoglycemia Hyponatremia, hypomagnesemia Hyperthyroidism, hyperparathyroidism B_{12} deficiency
Cerebellar tremor	Low-frequency, disabling, slow ipsilateral intention or postural tremor (can be coarse)
Psychogenic tremor	Abrupt onset, spontaneous remission Changing characteristics Extinction with distraction Absence of other neurological signs Clinical inconsistency History of other functional conditions
Wilson's disease tremor	Rare, autosomal-recessive condition of adolescents or young adults Coarse "wing-beating" tremor

standing, and walking. Signs of dyskinesia include the bonbon sign (exploratory tongue movement with mouth closed); glottal movement; piano-playing fingers with hands outstretched; and head, neck, and trunk movements. Sudden inhalation while speaking or eating suggests diaphragmatic dyskinesia and is associated with risk of aspiration. Choreoathetosis may be a result of acute drug toxicity, a tardive drug effect, stroke, or a neurodegenerative disorder (e.g., Huntington's disease).

Dystonias are involuntary, repetitive, twisting muscle spasms and may be focal, segmental, or whole body. Common sites are the neck, eyelids, jaw, tongue, vocal cords, and extremities. Dystonias often occur during a specific action, and they may be primary, secondary to drug treatment, or psychogenic in nature. Dystonias may be associated with a sensory trick (*geste antagoniste*)—a particular physical position of the body or a light touch to a place on the body that temporarily interrupts the dystonic spasm. Causes of dystonia include acute or tardive drug effects, TBI, stroke, extrapyramidal disorders, hypoxemia, and carbon monoxide poisoning.

Hypokinesis can be seen in depression, delirium, catatonia, parkinsonism, and some dementias. Parkinson's disease is defined by the triad of akinesia, rigidity, and resting tremor. "Parkinson plus" syndromes involve a core syndrome of progressive akinetic rigidity either alone or in combination with 1) autonomic instability, gait apraxia, or ataxia (multisystem atrophy); 2) supranuclear gaze palsy (PSP); 3) alien hand syndrome or apraxia (corticobasal degeneration); or 4) early psychotic symptoms (Lewy body dementia). The applause sign, in which a patient has difficulty discontinuing hand clapping when told to clap hands three times, occurs in PSP (Dubois et al. 2000).

Catatonia and the catatonic syndrome may be either hyperactive or hypoactive. Components of the syndrome are listed in Table 2–7. Catatonia requires a medical workup and acute treatment and can constitute a medical emergency in its more severe forms (see also Chapter 18, "Catatonia in the Medically Ill Patient").

Demyelinating Disease

Patients with vague or difficult-to-explain symptoms are frequently evaluated for possible demyelinating disease. In some cases, the diagnosis of demyelinating disease is unnecessarily delayed for months or years because physicians view patient presentations as psychosomatic. The presence of deficits at multiple levels of the nervous system combined with a history of neurological symptoms occurring at different times without other explanation is most consistent with multiple sclerosis. The most common presentations of multiple sclerosis are listed in Table 2–8.

Embellishment and Malingering

Neuropsychiatrists are often called on to examine people who may be embellishing symptoms or malingering for secondary gain. Performing the neurological examination as quickly as possible will reduce the likelihood of embellishment. Building redundancy into the bedside neurological examination will also help. Several bedside techniques can be useful for detecting feigning of symptoms. When a person complains of a field cut or tunnel vision, visual field testing at different distances (30 cm, 1 m, and 5 m) may reveal symptom embellishment, because visual fields should expand with distance and not remain restricted like a tunnel. Sensory testing that precisely splits the midline in the form of anesthesia to pinprick and skin sensation to vibration is not consistent with neurogenic deficits. Hoover's sign is elicited when a supine patient fails to press down on the examiner's hand with the heel of the normal leg during attempted straight leg raising of the allegedly hemiparetic leg. Feigned hemianesthesia may be detected if the patient holds hands outstretched with thumbs facing downward, then clasps and interdigitates the hands and rotates them upward before assessing primary sensation.

TABLE 2–7.   Catatonic signs and symptoms from the Bush-Francis Catatonia Rating Scale

Excitement	Waxy flexibility
Immobility/stupor	Withdrawal
Mutism	Impulsivity
Staring	Automatic obedience
Posturing/catalepsy	*Mitgehen* (facilitatory paratonia)
Grimacing	*Gegenhalten* (oppositional paratonia)
Echopraxia/echolalia	Ambitendency
Stereotypy	Grasp reflex
Mannerisms	Perseveration
Verbigeration	Combativeness
Rigidity	Autonomic abnormality
Negativism	

Source.   Bush et al. 1996.

TABLE 2–8.   Common presentations of multiple sclerosis

Common presenting complaints
  Weakness and paresthesias
  Sensory loss
  Diplopia
  Ataxia
  Vertigo
  Bladder dysfunction
  Cognitive dysfunction
  Depression
  Fatigue
  Sexual dysfunction

Visual signs and symptoms
  Diplopia
  Optic neuritis (transient unilateral visual loss with painful eye movement)
  Afferent pupillary defect
  Internuclear ophthalmoplegia
  Scotoma

Spinal cord signs
  Spastic paraparesis
  Incontinence
  Impotence
  Impaired gait
  Lhermitte's sign

Sensory signs
  Hypoalgesia
  Paresthesia
  Dysesthesia, pain

Cerebellar signs
  Dysdiadochokinesia
  Charcot's triad: nystagmus, intention tremor, scanning speech

Cognitive signs
  Decreased attention
  Decreased memory
  Decreased processing speed

TABLE 2–9.   **Neuropsychiatric emergencies**

Condition	Associated signs and symptoms
Catatonia	See Table 2–7
Autoimmune limbic encephalitis	Viral-like prodrome; progressive confusion; short-term memory loss (over days to months); psychosis; irritability and personality change; sleep disturbance; CSF pleocytosis; ± complex partial seizures; ± EEG/MRI evidence of limbic abnormality; ± antineuronal surface antibodies; increased risks of teratoma, testicular, and other tumors
Delirium/encephalopathy	Relatively rapid onset of symptoms; fluctuating arousal, attention, and awareness; transient cognitive deficits; perceptual changes; disturbed sleep-wake cycle; emotional instability; psychomotor disturbance (hypoactive, mixed, or hyperactive with agitation, restlessness, carphologia [i.e., "lint-picking" movements])
Herpes encephalitis	Fever, delirium, seizures, headache, aphasia, altered consciousness, nuchal rigidity, CSF pleocytosis, temporal lobe CT hypodensities, T2 MRI hyperintensities
Neuroleptic malignant syndrome	Rigidity, autonomic instability, confusion, elevated creatine kinase
Status epilepticus	Intermittent, semirhythmic, involuntary twitching involving a discrete subset of muscles, usually face and ipsilateral distal hand (partial), or long-lasting stupor, staring, or unresponsiveness (complex)
Serotonin syndrome	Fever, agitation, hypomania, tremor, rigidity, myoclonus, vomiting, diarrhea, autonomic instability

Note.   CSF=cerebrospinal fluid; CT=computed tomography; EEG=electroencephalogram; MRI= magnetic resonance imaging.

Neuropsychiatric Emergencies

The examiner must always be on the alert for neuropsychiatric emergencies that require rapid diagnosis and therapeutic intervention. Examples of such conditions are listed in Table 2–9.

Neuropsychiatric Formulation

The neuropsychiatric formulation includes a summary of the neuropsychiatric signs and symptoms; localization of deficits to the appropriate level of the nervous system (i.e., peripheral nerve or muscle, spinal cord, brain stem, cerebellum, limbic system, basal ganglia, subcortical white matter, cortex, or multiple lesions) and lateralization of involved network(s); a differential diagnosis, including causes of acquired dysfunction, developmental and psychosocial contributions, and contributions from comorbid neurological and psychiatric conditions; a cognitive hypothesis for the particular neuropsychiatric symptoms (see also Chapter 3, "The Bedside Cognitive Examination in Medical Psychiatry"); an inventory of potentially reversible symptoms (matched to neurodiagnostic investigations and treatments); a prognosis; and a rehabilitation plan. Having performed a careful neurological examination, the clinician will be able to ensure that any neurodiagnostic studies ordered are aimed at confirming well-structured diagnostic hypotheses.

Conclusion

A detailed neurological examination, adapted to the patient's age and ability to cooperate, the time available, and the particular purpose of the consultation, is essential to neuropsychiatric assessment. The examination proceeds from a diagnostic hypothesis; includes a general physical examination as well as cranial nerve, motor, sensory, and gait examinations; and is followed by mental status and bedside cognitive examinations, any applicable rating scales, and ancillary laboratory and neurodiagnostic testing where appropriate. These examination data are then used as a scaffolding on which to build a neuropsychiatric formulation to guide treatment planning and prognostic assessment.

References

Benjamin S, Lauterbach M: The Brain Card®, 3rd Edition. Boston, MA, Brain Educators LLC, 2016

Benjamin S, Lauterbach MD: The neurological examination adapted for neuropsychiatry. CNS Spectr 23(3):219–227, 2018 29789033

Blessed G, Tomlinson BE, Roth M: The association between quantitative measures of dementia and of senile change in the cerebral grey matter of elderly subjects. Br J Psychiatry 114(512):797–811, 1968 5662937

Bodranghien F, Bastian A, Casali C, et al: Consensus paper: revisiting the symptoms and signs of cerebellar syndrome. Cerebellum 15(3):369–391, 2016 26105056

Bush G, Fink M, Petrides G, et al: Catatonia, I: rating scale and standardized examination. Acta Psychiatr Scand 93(2):129–136, 1996 8686483

Comella CL, Leurgans S, Wuu J, et al: Rating scales for dystonia: a multicenter assessment. Mov Disord 18(3):303–312, 2003 12621634

Cummings JL: The Neuropsychiatric Inventory: assessing psychopathology in dementia patients. Neurology 48 (5 suppl 6):S10–S16, 1997 9153155

De Renzi E, Barbieri C: The incidence of the grasp reflex following hemispheric lesion and its relation to frontal damage. Brain 115(pt 1):293–313, 1992 1559160

Doty RL: Olfactory dysfunction and its measurement in the clinic. World J Otorhinolaryngol Head Neck Surg 1(1):28–33, 2015 29204537

Dubois B, Slachevsky A, Litvan I, et al: The FAB: a Frontal Assessment Battery at bedside. Neurology 55(11):1621–1626, 2000 11113214

Fradis A, Botez M: The groping phenomena of the foot. Brain 81(2):218–230, 1958 13572692

Goetz CG, Tilley BC, Shaftman SR, et al: Movement Disorder Society-sponsored revision of the Unified Parkinson's Disease Rating Scale (MDS-UPDRS): scale presentation and clinimetric testing results. Mov Disord 23(15):2129–2170, 2008 19025984

Gouvier WD, Blanton PD, LaPorte KK, et al: Reliability and validity of the Disability Rating Scale and the Levels of Cognitive Functioning Scale in monitoring recovery from severe head injury. Arch Phys Med Rehabil 68(2):94–97, 1987 3813863

Hopf HC, Müller-Forell W, Hopf NJ: Localization of emotional and volitional facial paresis. Neurology 42(10):1918–1923, 1992 1407573

Hughes CP, Berg L, Danziger WL, et al: A new clinical scale for the staging of dementia. Br J Psychiatry 140:566–572, 1982 7104545

Johns MW: A new method for measuring daytime sleepiness: the Epworth sleepiness scale. Sleep 14(6):540–545, 1991 1798888

Kertesz A, Hooper P: Praxis and language: the extent and variety of apraxia in aphasia. Neuropsychologia 20(3):275–286, 1982 7121795

Kroenke K, Spitzer RL, Williams JB: The PHQ-9: validity of a brief depression severity measure. J Gen Intern Med 16(9):606–613, 2001 11556941

Kurtzke JF: Rating neurologic impairment in multiple sclerosis: an Expanded Disability Status Scale (EDSS). Neurology 33(11):1444–1452, 1983 6685237

Mittal VA, Hasenkamp W, Sanfilipo M, et al: Relation of neurological soft signs to psychiatric symptoms in schizophrenia. Schizophr Res 94(1–3):37–44, 2007 17543502

Munetz MR, Benjamin S: How to examine patients using the Abnormal Involuntary Movement Scale. Hosp Community Psychiatry 39(11):1172–1177, 1988 2906320

Nasreddine ZS, Phillips NA, Bédirian V, et al: The Montreal Cognitive Assessment, MoCA: a brief screening tool for mild cognitive impairment. J Am Geriatr Soc 53(4):695–699, 2005 15817019

Owen G, Mulley GP: The palmomental reflex: a useful clinical sign? J Neurol Neurosurg Psychiatry 73(2):113–115, 2002 12122165

Teasdale G, Jennett B: Assessment of coma and impaired consciousness: a practical scale. Lancet 2(7872):81–84, 1974 4136544

Whitty PF, Owoeye O, Waddington JL: Neurological signs and involuntary movements in schizophrenia: intrinsic to and informative on systems pathobiology. Schizophr Bull 35(2):415–424, 2009 18791074

Yudofsky SC, Silver JM, Jackson W, et al: The Overt Aggression Scale for the objective rating of verbal and physical aggression. Am J Psychiatry 143(1):35–39, 1986 3942284

CHAPTER 3

The Bedside Cognitive Examination in Medical Psychiatry

Sean P. Glass, M.D.

The bedside cognitive examination is best approached in a systematic and structured manner. Although the history and mental status examination provide critical information pertaining to cognitive functions, the use of specific and structured tests is vital in accurately assessing, diagnosing, and monitoring neurodegenerative and other clinical conditions. Cognitive testing can be performed by using validated tests of global function that include assessments of various cognitive domains in the same test. Testing also can be approached by individually examining cognitive functions. Regardless of approach, it is important to appreciate the interconnectedness and hierarchical nature of cognitive functions and the underlying brain networks that constitute them. To varying degrees, certain cognitive functions require other functions to be intact.

Some of the major goals of the cognitive examination include helping to clarify which cognitive functions are abnormal, determining the extent of dysfunction, aiding in making a specific diagnosis (i.e., certain patterns of dysfunction may point to one diagnosis over another), determining the functional limitations caused by cognitive dysfunction, and monitoring progress or decline by repeating testing over time. Testing may detect important clinical and functional findings that provide a basis for formal neuropsychological testing, neuroimaging, or electroencephalography. Moreover, bedside cognitive examinations may be a crucial starting point for referral for additional psychiatric, neurological, or medical care or for referral to an occupational or physical therapist.

Hierarchy of Cognitive Function

Foundational cognitive functions are necessary for "higher-order" ones. The most fundamental of these is *arousal* (synonymous with *consciousness* or *wakefulness*). Put simply, if a patient is not awake and alert, further testing may be impossible. *Attention* and *working memory* also are instrumental. Patients who are highly distracted by exteroceptive or interoceptive stimuli and who therefore cannot hold on to information long enough for adequate processing (i.e., who have deficits in attention or working memory) cannot participate reliably in cognitive testing. Similarly, certain types of aphasias may preclude global cognitive assessment if patients are unable to comprehend questions and instructions or if they are unable to produce a clear verbal or written response. Depression, anxiety, and apathy all may prevent cognitive testing because of their broad adverse influence on cognitive functions. Given that primary sensory and motor functions are necessary for the intact functioning of certain cognitive domains, cognitive assessment also includes a neurological examination. Isolating a given cognitive function with a singular bedside test in "pure" form is difficult.

Tests of Global Functions

Instruments for global cognitive assessment include the Montreal Cognitive Assessment (MoCA; Nasreddine et al. 2005), the Mini-Mental State Examination (MMSE; Folstein et al. 1975), and Addenbrooke's Cognitive Examination–Revised (ACE-R; Mioshi et al. 2006). These standardized bedside global screening tools provide a numerical score that can be tracked and monitored over time, hence providing information about stage of illness. They are generally easy to administer, can be completed relatively quickly, and include normative data to which the social, demographic, and medical features of a given patient can be compared. Although no single test includes all of the elements needed for a thorough bedside cognitive examination, other assessments that focus on a distinct cognitive domain (e.g., executive function) or brain region (e.g., the frontal lobes) can be added for a more comprehensive analysis. For example, the MMSE, which is weighted heavily in the verbal domain, lacks formal tests of executive function and working memory. An updated version of the MMSE, the Modified Mini-Mental State Examination (Teng and Chui 1987), assesses executive functions and other tasks. The Frontal Assessment Battery (Dubois et al. 2000) or individual tests of executive function and sustained attention, such as the Trail Making Test (Reitan 1958), can be added to general screening examinations that are less weighted in these areas. The MoCA includes analyses of attention, memory, visuospatial function, language function, and abstraction and is more sensitive than the MMSE to the presence of mild cognitive impairment (Ismail et al. 2010; Nasreddine et al. 2005); it takes approximately 10 minutes to administer and is widely used in various clinical settings. The ACE-R takes approximately 15 minutes to administer and assesses attention/orientation, memory, verbal fluency, language, and visuospatial abilities (Hodges 2007a; Ismail et al. 2010; Mioshi et al. 2006).

Various factors need to be considered when selecting a particular global cognitive test. Clinician experience, time constraints, patient educational and cultural factors, and a working knowledge of the inherent limitations of any test are all necessary considerations for proper test selection and accurate test interpretation. Strauss et al. (2006) have compiled normative data for many of the tests discussed in this chapter, including guidance on test selection and interpretation. Precise testing protocols should be followed for each test, because improper administration will likely confound the clinical picture and lead to inaccurate diagnoses or treatments. Instructions for many tests are available online.

Quick Screens and Tests

Although tests of global function along with individual tests and batteries of additional cognitive domains are most often recommended for general neurocognitive screening, in some situations, more focused testing may be indicated. Examples of situations requiring a more focused approach include those involving more restrictive time constraints or the screening of patients in whom there may be a lower pretest probability of uncovering any major cognitive difficulties.

The Mini-Cog takes approximately 3 minutes to administer, has high sensitivity (99%) and specificity (93%) in dementia screening, and is not confounded by language or cultural factors (Borson et al. 2000). It consists of a three-word registration trial, verbal recall, and a clock-drawing task. It is scored from zero to five, and a cutoff score of less than four may indicate the need for further cognitive testing.

Clock drawing is a versatile and useful tool that tests various cognitive domains. Normal clock drawing depends on unimpaired processes extending across multiple cognitive domains and neural networks, including visuospatial processing, executive functions, language comprehension, sustained attention, working memory, motor functions, and semantic memory. This task is included in many commonly used standard tests of global function, including the MoCA, the MMSE, the ACE-R, and the Mini-Cog. Common types of clock-drawing errors may point to deficits in specific neural networks and cognitive domains. Common errors include writing deficits, stimulus-bound responses, conceptual difficulties, spatial or planning deficits, and perseveration (Eknoyan et al. 2012). Multiple schemes for administration and scoring are available. The standard clock-drawing test involves a predrawn circle approximately 10 cm in diameter. The patient is asked to fill in the numbers and to "set the time to 10 past 11" (Shulman 2000). An executive clock-drawing task (CLOX; Royall et al. 1998) was designed to differentiate frontal/executive function problems from parietal/visuospatial problems (Royall 2000). In the CLOX, patients are first asked to draw a clock freehand. If they are unable to do this accurately, they are asked to copy a completed clock. Frontal/executive impairment is more likely when patients cannot accurately draw a freehand clock, because this task requires intact planning, organization, response inhibition, working memory, and other executive functions. Difficulties with semantic memory also may be identified when patients are asked to draw a clock without further instructions (as opposed to copying a clock). Visuospatial/parietal lobe deficits may appear on freehand or copied clocks. Various scoring criteria are available for clock-drawing tests (Mendez et al. 1992; Morris et al. 1989), but a qualitative assessment of results is often sufficient.

A quick comprehensive cognitive screen may include the following elements: assessment of orientation to location, situation, time, and date; bedside tests of attention and verbal recall; a clock-drawing task; and a screening neurological examination.

Tests of Individual Cognitive Domains

Arousal/Consciousness/Wakefulness

The terms *arousal, consciousness,* and *wakefulness* are used synonymously to denote whether a patient is fully awake and alert and, if not, the stimulus required to elicit a response (e.g., loud voice, pressure applied to the nail bed or sternum). Arousal and the sleep-wake cycle are heavily mediated by the brain stem, the hypothalamus, and thalamic projections to diffuse areas of the cerebral cortex (Benarroch 2008; Mesulam 2000; Saper et al. 2005). In cases of decreased arousal, notation of the patient's behavioral response to the applied stimulus and its duration is critical. Descriptors for decreased level of arousal include somnolence (or lethargy), obtundation, stupor, and coma (Posner et al. 2007). *Somnolence,* or *lethargy,* denotes a "sleepy" patient who may sleep without stimulation but who also may awaken and participate in an interview without further stimulation. *Obtundation* refers to mild to moderate drowsiness that is less easily overcome by stimulation. *Stupor* indicates a more marked state of decreased arousal and sleepiness that can be overcome only by a forceful stimulus, which needs to be maintained or frequently repeated. *Coma* denotes no spontaneous or provoked wakefulness. The comatose patient is unresponsive even to vigorous stimuli.

The Glasgow Coma Scale (GCS; Table 3–1) quantifies a patient's level of consciousness that occurs spontaneously, in response to voice, and in response to painful stimuli (Teasdale and Jennett 1974; Teasdale et al. 2014). Three types of behavioral responses are noted: verbal, motor, and eye opening. The GCS is scored on a scale of 3–15; scores of 3–8 usually denote coma.

Hyperarousal may be seen in certain neuropsychiatric conditions, including hyperactive delirium and mania. The clinician may observe excessive eye or motor movements, increased verbal output, and hyperkinetic movements; behavior, speech, and motor production may be nonpurposeful.

Inquiry into a patient's sleep patterns is a crucial part of any neuropsychiatric examination, because sleep abnormalities may powerfully and negatively affect cognition in virtually any realm. Asking about sleep habits and patterns—including the time it takes to fall asleep, the duration of sleep, the quality of sleep, and whether any distressing sensations, worries, or nightmares occur—adds vital information to the overall cognitive examination. Obstructive sleep apnea is known to affect multiple cognitive domains adversely, and its treatment has been shown to improve these functions (Beebe and Gozal 2002; Canessa et al. 2011). The Epworth Sleepiness Scale is a quick, easily administered, and effective screening tool for obstructive sleep apnea that can be used in the office or at the bedside (Johns 1991).

Orientation

Attention and memory (working, visuospatial, and declarative) are necessary for orientation to place, time, and setting (including contextual information such as the rea-

TABLE 3–1.	Glasgow Coma Scale	
Eye opening	4—Spontaneous	
	3—To sound	
	2—To pressure	
	1—No response	
Verbal response	5—Oriented to time, place, person	
	4—Confused	
	3—Inappropriate words	
	2—Incomprehensible sounds	
	1—No response	
Motor response	6—Obeys commands	
	5—Moves to localized pressure	
	4—Flexion withdrawal from pressure (normal flexion)	
	3—Decorticate flexion (abnormal flexion)	
	2—Decerebrate extension	
	1—No response	

Source. Teasdale and Jennett 1974.

son for the office visit or hospital admission). Testing of place orientation includes questions about country, state, city, street, building, floor, and room. Testing of time orientation involves queries about time of day, date, day of week, month, season, and year. Time orientation is typically more impaired than place orientation earlier in most neurodegenerative processes except for some cases of semantic dementia, in which patients have naming (semantic) deficits. Disorientation to person likely indicates very advanced dementia, a psychogenic condition, or malingering.

Processing Speed

Processing speed relies on arousal, motivation, the motor system, and executive functions. Qualitative evaluation of how long it takes a patient to perform a given task usually indicates a normal or an abnormal performance; performance norms, which are available for many tests, can facilitate more precise analysis (Strauss et al. 2006).

Attention

Attention refers to the selection of certain targeted information and the simultaneous ignoring of extraneous information. *Concentration* and *focus* are synonymous terms. *Vigilance* refers to the unabated continuation of attentional processes over time; it also refers to the selection of salient, emotionally meaningful stimuli. Arousal, wakefulness, working memory, and executive functions are critical to the attentional matrix. Depending on its subtype (e.g., vigilance, threat, spatial, and verbal), attention is represented in various circuits, including the frontal lobes, the parietal lobes, the amygdala, and the insula, and their subcortical connections in the brain stem, basal ganglia, and thalamus. Pain, anxiety, mood changes, hallucinations, and internally generated stimuli (e.g., hunger) may result in subjective attentional complaints or objective findings of inattention. In this sense, patients may attend to salient stimuli or be distracted by them in ways that interfere with higher-order attentional processes. External distractors in the environment, such as noises and movement, may likewise negatively affect the patient's ability to focus and sustain attention. Care should be taken to ensure that confounding distractors are minimized or are at least taken into account when assessing attentive abilities.

The interdependency among attention, working memory, and executive functions can result in clinical phenomena or test results that are difficult to "pin" to a single cognitive domain. Although attention is still somewhat dependent on these other cognitive domains, certain bedside tests of selective and sustained attention more accurately isolate this specific cognitive domain. These tests include recitation of the months of the year backward (Meagher et al. 2015), verbal or digit vigilance tasks (Strauss et al. 2006), the Trail Making Test (Reitan 1958; Tombaugh 2004), and the verbal Trail Making Test (Ricker and Axelrod 1994).

The months of the year backward test starts by asking patients to recite the months of the year forward. Successful completion indicates that the patient is adequately engaged and can understand simple commands. The patient is then asked to recite the months of the year backward, starting with December. Cognitively intact patients typically complete the test in 20 seconds without any errors (Meagher et al. 2015). The upper time limit for test completion increases with age, with lower educational achievement, and in the presence of cognitive impairment (e.g., delirium or various types of dementia).

Trail-making tasks are divided into numbers only (Trail Making Test Part A) and alternating number-letter combinations (Trail Making Test Part B). In the written version of the Trail Making Test Part A, patients are given a pen and a worksheet containing 25 circled numbers and are asked to connect the numbers in sequential order without lifting the pen off the page. In the verbal version of Part A, patients are asked to count from 1 to 25 as quickly as possible. The verbal version relies heavily on language functions, but normal performance also denotes normal sustained attention. In the written version of the Trail Making Test Part B, patients are asked to connect alternating number-letter pairs (e.g., 1-A, 2-B) progressively up to 13-M. Part B relies on intact sustained attention but also relies on intact executive functions and working memory. Approximately 98% of younger patients without significant medical comorbidities are able to complete Part A in less than 11 seconds and Part B in less than 64 seconds (Ruchinskas 2003).

For visual and spatial attention, the line bisection task (Reuter-Lorenz and Posner 1990) is helpful for assessing equal attention to right- and left-sided aspects of external space. Cancellation tasks require that patients effectively scan through randomly oriented stimuli (e.g., letters, numbers, shapes) and mark off a specific stimulus (e.g., the letter *A*). This task tests for spatial, selective, and sustained attention while also screening for possible visual field deficits (Mesulam 2000; Weintraub 2000). Approximately 98% of healthy adults complete the random symbol cancellation task in less than 90 seconds with fewer than two errors of omission per hemifield (Lowery et al. 2004). Most healthy older adults complete the task in less than 3 minutes without more than two errors of omission in each hemifield (Weintraub 2000).

Certain performance parameters and clues that arise during testing may help distinguish the nature of any deficits present. For tests of attention, these include errors of omission (leaving out a response), errors of commission (adding an extraneous response), perseverative responses or behaviors, impulsive or disinhibited behaviors, "zoning out" (losing focus) during tests of sustained attention, and requiring excessive time to initiate and complete testing. For tests involving spatial attention (e.g., cancellation tasks), these same parameters are noted, along with the strategy used to complete the task (e.g., whether the patient approaches the task in a purposeful and coherent or random and disorganized manner) and the presence of visual field deficits or spatial neglect. Official guidelines are available for test procedures, norms, and interpretation of results (Strauss et al. 2006).

Working Memory

Working memory is a process by which visuospatial, auditory, or verbal information is held "online" temporarily for the purpose of manipulating stored information to guide goal-specific decisions. Information in working memory is continually updated; a key function of this process is the adequate use, allocation, or forgetting of the seemingly immeasurable amount of information that is being processed by the brain at any given moment. Working memory may be likened to a "sketch pad" or "whiteboard"—or to random access memory (RAM) in computers—for mental contents. Working memory also can be viewed as a here-and-now mechanism of attention and memory systems, to which it is intimately linked. Its capacity is limited, and an oft-cited example of this capacity limit is the "magical number seven rule" (e.g., telephone numbers contain only seven digits) (Miller 1956). Working memory is not short-term memory, which is a cognitive process more aligned with recall of recently learned information. Working memory appears to involve integrated and overlapping processing that, in Baddeley's multicomponent model, consists of a "central executive" control mechanism centered in the frontal lobes, a "visuospatial sketch pad" that relies heavily on parietal lobe function, a "phonological loop" (for auditory rehearsal of information) centered in the temporal cortices, and an "episodic buffer" (bringing memory systems online) that calls on medial temporal lobe circuitry (Baddeley 2000; Baddeley and Hitch 1974).

Commonly used tests of working memory include serially counting backward by 7 from 100, spelling "world" backward, and registering verbal (or spatial) items for later recall or recognition. These tests also rely on intact processing in attention and executive function domains. Thus, a poor performance may not indicate whether the primary culprit is in the domain of working memory, executive functions, or attention. A more straightforward test of working memory is digit span (Strauss et al. 2006; Wechsler 1955). In forward digit span, digits are read aloud to the patient in a monotone fashion at a rate of one per second, and the patient attempts to recall the digits in the order they appeared. One digit is added with each successful repetition (or after two successful repetitions with the same number of digits), and this process is continued until the patient fails to repeat the correct number and order of digits. The average forward digit span for most adults is three to seven and shows age-related decline (Bopp and Verhaeghen 2005; Strauss et al. 2006). Similar tests that use letters or shapes are also available.

Backward digit span is a more complicated version of digit span (and also relies on intact executive functions) and should be tested after completion of forward digit span. Here, numbers are read aloud as in the forward digit span, and patients are asked to repeat them in reverse order (e.g., the examiner reads "2, 7, 5," and the patient repeats "5, 7, 2"). The average backward digit span for most adults is four to six, and this span, as with forward digit span, tends to decrease with age (Bopp and Verhaeghen 2005; Strauss et al. 2006).

Language

Voice, speech, and language are related yet divisible functions subserved by different neurobiological mechanisms. *Voice* refers to the sounds produced during speech output (caused by vibration of the vocal cords); *speech* refers to the coordination of muscular processes responsible for the articulation of words and sentences. *Language* refers to communication of thoughts and experiences through the use of various symbols, including speech, sign language, music, reading, and writing. Classically, the bedside evaluation of language has been strongly influenced by the aphasia syndromes seen in stroke patients. These syndromes were traditionally linked to major hubs in the left hemisphere (e.g., Broca's area, Wernicke's area, the arcuate fasciculus). The different aphasia syndromes are deduced by examining fluency (referring to speech articulation), comprehension, naming, and repetition. The mechanisms underlying language processing and production are now understood to involve wide-ranging interrelated networks in cortical and subcortical areas (Hillis 2007).

A confluence of various cognitive processes is responsible for normal language function: semantic representation, visual and phonological representations, motor planning, programming, and language production (Hillis 2007). Lexical, or syntactic, rules, which are dissociated from phonological or semantic processes, also are represented in language-processing schemas (Dell and O'Seaghdha 1992; Hillis 2007). Dual-stream language-processing networks consisting of dorsal and ventral streams with interconnections by major subcortical white matter tracts have gained credence in recent years as an explanatory model for language function (Dick et al. 2014). The dorsal stream consists of frontal, temporal, and parietal hubs interconnected through the superior longitudinal fasciculus and arcuate fasciculus. This stream is thought to map sounds to motor representations and syntax processing. The ventral stream involves the uncinate fasciculus, inferior longitudinal fasciculus, inferior fronto-occipital fasciculus, extreme capsule, and middle longitudinal fasciculus (semantic networks) and maps sounds to meaning. Corticobulbar tracts, subserving speech functions, and cortico-cerebello-cortical loops have been identified as vital components of language and speech functions. Naming ability, which is represented in diffuse areas in the brain, involves the following basic components, which are organized temporally: processing and recognition of an external stimulus, semantic processing of that stimulus, selection of an abstract representation (lexical access), and output of the stimulus's name (Gleichgerrcht et al. 2015).

Language assessment is performed largely while taking the history. The processes of articulation, cadence, tone, grammar, syntax, word choice, naming, and word-finding abilities all can be noticed during the interview before more specific examination begins. Intact language comprehension may be assumed if patients answer questions appropriately; vague or seemingly inaccurate responses require more detailed assessment.

Language comprehension is assessed in a stepwise manner starting with asking patients simple yes-or-no and true-or-false questions and then increasingly more complex questions. This method mitigates the overlapping influences of working memory, sustained attention, executive functions, semantic memory, and other processes that overlap with language comprehension. Examples of language comprehension questions include "Do pigs fly?" "Do you put your coat on before your shirt?" and "A lion was eaten by a tiger; who survived?" The examiner should ask multiple questions, because patients have a 50% chance of answering these correctly. The written instruction on the MMSE ("close your eyes") tests language comprehension. The "three-step command" on the MMSE ("Take this paper with your left/right hand, fold it in half, and hand it back to me") and similar tests rely heavily on executive functions, praxis, and other functions that degrade their specificity for language comprehension.

Assessment of fluency includes paying attention to phrase length, pauses, word-finding difficulty, and agrammatism (characterized by an inability to construct a grammatical or an intelligible sentence while retaining the ability to speak single words). Both verbal and written language are assessed, the latter by asking the patient to write a sentence (as on the MMSE) or a paragraph. Fluent speech generally consists of phrases with more than eight words with few or no word-finding difficulties, pauses, or agrammatisms (Arciniegas 2013). Tests of verbal fluency on global cognitive tests such as the MoCA require a patient to name as many words as possible from a given category—which can be phonetic (e.g., words starting with the letter *P*) or semantic (e.g., the category *animals*)—within a specified time frame. This task predominantly tests executive control of language but also relies heavily on semantic memory, working memory, and sustained attention. Although fluency tests do not require a patient to speak in full sentences, screening for agrammatism, paraphasia, neologism, and other lexical and semantic difficulties is still possible during semantic and phonetic word-generation tests.

Word-finding difficulty during normal conversation can be influenced by inattention, defective executive search strategies, semantic memory deficits, and deficits in recognition memory in multiple sensory domains. Confrontational naming is assessed by asking patients to name an object chosen by the examiner and then to list as many subcomponents of that object as possible. For example, a person may be asked to name a watch and then to list its subcomponents (e.g., face, hands, crystal, stem, band) as the examiner points to them. Word and sentence repetition should include increasingly complex examples, starting with two-syllable words and building up to polysyllabic words and then sentences. Asking patients to repeat polysyllabic words also screens for articulation problems. This task can be combined with having patients provide definitions of the repeated words to screen simultaneously for semantic deficits. Asking patients to repeat sentences (as on the MoCA) relies also on auditory-verbal working memory. Table 3–2 lists commonly encountered language disturbances. Table 3–3 lists common language disturbances seen in aphasia syndromes.

Prosody

Prosody refers to the paralinguistic confluence of language with affect, whereby emotion is imparted onto propositional language (Ross 2000). Melody, pauses, intonation, accents, and stresses modify verbal communication to convey meaning, as do gestures conveyed by body language. The ability to comprehend and express prosodic

TABLE 3–2.   **Commonly encountered language abnormalities**

Abnormality	Definition
Semantic paraphasia	Substituting a semantically related word for the intended word
Phonemic paraphasia	Phonemic substitution or transposition; results in mispronouncing the intended word
Neologism	Creation of a novel, often meaningless word
Circumlocution	Talking "around" a word or concept
Echolalia	Meaningless repetition of the examiner's words or phrases
Palilalia	Repetition of one's own spoken words
Clanging (clang associations)	Rhyming words

TABLE 3–3.   **Aphasia syndromes**

Aphasia type	Fluency	Repetition	Comprehension	Naming
Broca's	Impaired	Impaired	Intact	Impaired
Wernicke's	Intact	Impaired	Impaired	Impaired
Conduction	Intact	Impaired	Intact	Impaired
Transcortical motor	Impaired	Intact	Intact	Impaired
Transcortical sensory	Intact	Intact	Impaired	Impaired
Mixed transcortical	Impaired	Intact	Intact	Impaired
Global	Impaired	Impaired	Impaired	Impaired

elements is based in right hemispheric prosody networks, which crudely mirror receptive and expressive language-processing networks in the left hemisphere (Mesulam 2000; Ross 2000). Aprosody may be caused by deficits in comprehension, repetition, and production or expression of speech.

Testing of prosody begins with observation of a patient's spontaneous body language and the affective qualities of verbal output during the interview. If dysprosodic or aprosodic features are detected during the initial observation, more formal testing should follow. Patients are asked to repeat a sentence that is devoid of personal meaning (e.g., "That is a car") while trying to express different emotions. Both positive and negative emotions should be tested; anger or irritability, anxiousness, excitement, and happiness usually suffice as good screening tests for aprosodia. Receptive aprosodia can be tested by having the patient face away while the examiner speaks sentences colored with different emotions; the patient is asked to identify the emotions expressed. Repetition aprosodia can be assessed by asking a patient to mimic the examiner's gestures and speech patterns of words and sentences that are infused with different emotions.

Memory

Memory for autobiographical events can be divided temporally into immediate (seconds), recent (minutes to days), and remote (months to years) (Filley 2011). The autobiographical memory system is primarily dependent on hippocampal-mediated circuitry and includes vital contributions from the prefrontal cortex and limbic structures, including the anterior cingulate cortex, the anterior nucleus of the thalamus, and the hypothalamic mammillary bodies as part of the Papez circuit (Dickerson and Eichenbaum 2010; Mesulam 2000; Papez 1937; Squire 2004). The successful operation of memory processes starts with intact attention and working memory, which are mediated by interactions between the frontal and parietal lobes.

Patients with dysfunctional working memory, attention, and executive functions cannot learn (encode) new information and later store it or execute a practical search strategy for specific memories. Testing these processes is crucial in determining whether a "memory system" is to blame for faulty learning or for poor retrieval of previously learned information. Verbal or visual memory can be investigated by examining registration (an immediate here-and-now process dependent on working memory and attention) and, after a delay, either spontaneous recall (the ability to remember items without cuing) or recall with external cues (semantic or recognition cues are used if spontaneous recall is impaired). Normal registration and normal spontaneous recall after a specified temporal delay (typically 5, 15, and 30 minutes) indicate an intact episodic memory system. Inability to recall information spontaneously that is later correctly recalled with the aid of semantic cues (e.g., an associated word) or recognition cues (e.g., multiple choices or a picture) indicates compromised executive (prefrontal) control of memory retrieval and not necessarily defective medial temporal- or hippocampal-mediated encoding processes. Intact registration with failure to recall with cues indicates impaired new learning and possible pathology in the episodic memory system (Arciniegas 2013).

The number of items to be recalled during verbal or visual recall can greatly influence accurate interpretation of memory abilities. Whereas the MMSE tests three words, the MoCA tests five (and provides opportunities for cuing, but points are not given for correct recall with cuing), and the ACE-R tests seven items (a name and an address). For patients with higher educational attainment and higher premorbid functioning, remembering three words may be quite easy, and despite having mild to moderate memory dysfunction, they may obtain a perfect score.

Defective anterograde memory (impaired learning after injury or disease onset) and defective retrograde memory (inability to remember personal events that occurred before injury or disease onset) need to be distinguished. When asking a patient about recent or remote events, it is important to be wary of responses that are overly generic or "overlearned" (i.e., relating to knowledge that may have been acquired very early in life). It may be easy to overlook the presence of actual memory deficits when a patient provides generic responses whose accuracy is difficult to prove (e.g., having a good time with family on Thanksgiving is plausible but may not accurately reflect actual events). Moreover, clinicians should be vigilant for confabulation or attempts to change the subject, which may indicate intact insight into the presence of actual memory deficits. These phenomena may be circumvented by asking about (and remaining persistently focused on) *specific* details surrounding recent and important events such as birthdays, promotions, graduations, and other occasions.

Different neurodegenerative disorders may be distinguished by the patient's performance on bedside tests of memory (even though full neuropsychological testing, imaging, and other evaluations are still indicated). Patients with frontal or frontotemporal pathology (as in frontotemporal dementia) may show more difficulty with registration, attention, and executive control of memory recall (poor spontaneous recall with intact recall when aided by semantic or recognition cues). Patients with Alzheimer's disease typically show the opposite pattern (i.e., poor recall despite cues) earlier in the disease course (Budson and Price 2005). Patients with Lewy body dementia may show difficulty in registering and encoding information on multiple trials, whereas those with Alzheimer's disease will show improvement in registration and encoding on subsequent trials (Sajjadi and Nestor 2016).

Episodic memory dysfunction, in which memory returns to a previous baseline state between episodes, needs to be distinguished from the progressively worsening memory dysfunction that occurs with neurodegenerative processes. Examples of disorders manifesting episodic memory dysfunction include transient global amnesia, epilepsy (transient epileptic amnesia), dissociative states, and psychogenic amnesia (in which loss of personal identity or other information also may occur).

Anxiety, depression, vigilance for perceived or expected deficits, limited ability to participate in testing, volitional deceit, confabulation, and distraction by anxiety-provoking memories or stimuli all may complicate memory testing.

Semantic Memory

Semantic memory denotes the acquired knowledge of facts, concepts, and objects. This type of memory consists of generalized knowledge about the world that becomes stripped of any reference to personal experience. For example, most Americans would know that George Washington was the first president of the United States regardless of what situation or location they were in. Neurobiological models of semantic memory processing are complex and have grown in recent years. One model includes the diffuse participation of multiple networks with key semantic convergence zones ("hubs") in the anterior temporal and inferior parietal lobes (Binder and Desai 2011). Semantic processing equates with detailed sensory information and autobiographical information becoming increasingly abstract, distinct from medial temporal (hippocampal) regions, and "amodal," meaning that information stored in anterior temporal or inferior parietal lobes is independent of context.

Semantic processing is linked with sensory and motor processing, episodic memory, language functions, and executive function control mechanisms. Certain strategies may help isolate semantic functioning at the bedside. As with the other domain-specific cognitive functions, deficits in sensory or motor processing, working memory, and other integral components may either mask or expose a semantic-processing deficit that may be more accurately attributable to other cognitive domains. Semantic deficits may appear to be the result of language-processing problems, such as anomia or word-finding problems, whereas naming problems do not necessarily suggest semantic deficits (Sajjadi and Nestor 2016). Patients with semantic dementia may be able to name basic objects (i.e., "overlearned" words). It is more helpful to ask patients to identify objects that are less commonly used or encountered but not rare or exceptional. Office- or bedside-based examples of such objects would include staplers, stethoscopes, and paper clips (Sajjadi and Nestor 2016). Patients should be asked questions about items they cannot name. If a patient is unable to come up with the word for an object (naming vs. word-retrieval vs. semantic deficit), he or she can be asked further questions about the object, such as to describe what it is or what it does. For instance, if a patient is unable to name a stethoscope but can tell the examiner that doctors use it to listen to the chest, then the problem is likely a naming or word-retrieval error, because patients with deficits in semantic memory would not be able to provide such information (Sajjadi and Nestor 2016). The provision of correct responses after cuing with word stems or multiple choices would also help in distinguishing semantic deficits from language-processing problems. The ACE-R offers another way of testing semantic memory: providing a patient with a description of an object and asking him or her to name it (e.g., asking a patient to point to the object with "a nautical connection" [anchor]).

Visuospatial Ability

Examination of visuospatial ability may identify deficits in any of its subdomains: construction of shapes in two or three dimensions, spatial attention and awareness, hemifield neglect or inattention, self-other spatial relationships, and navigation of extrapersonal space. Overlapping neural networks with a major hub in the inferior right parietal lobule give rise to visuospatial cognitive abilities (Mesulam 2000).

The visuospatial examination begins with observation of the patient's appearance and of whether clothing, facial hair, and other features appear symmetrical. The line bisection task or symbol, letter, or number cancellation tasks may reveal hemineglect, difficulties with left-right discrimination, or visual field defects. Sustained attention and working memory are other critical aspects underlying successful performance of these tasks. Extinction to double-simultaneous stimulation may show spatial inattention or neglect if the basic sensory functions are intact. Patients may report the presence of the stimulus when it is applied unilaterally to the abnormal (affected) side but fail to recognize the stimuli when they are presented simultaneously on both sides. Asking the patient to identify the examiner's right or left hand or giving the patient a "cross-body command" (e.g., "touch your right ear with your left thumb") may identify difficulties with left-right discrimination if language, attention, praxis, sensory, and motor functions are intact. Having the patient copy a two-dimensional object such as overlapping pentagons (as on the MMSE), or a three-dimensional object such as a cube or cylinder (as on the MoCA), could reveal difficulties with spatial awareness or construction, with right parietal lobe involvement.

Visual and spatial memory can be assessed by first showing a patient three objects and asking him or her to identify them, then hiding the objects (preferably in random areas in the room representing a wide angle in the visual field), and finally asking the patient to name the objects and identify where they were hidden. Both visual clues (pointing) and semantic or multiple-choice clues can be used.

In the three-words/three-shapes test, patients are asked to copy three objects (Weintraub et al. 2000). They are then asked to draw the objects from memory after delays of various lengths—most often 5, 15, and 30 minutes. Verbal and visual memory are assessed by asking patients to recall the objects they were shown (and drew).

Praxis

Praxis refers to the performance of skilled learned movements. An inability to carry out these movements can be attributed to apraxia or dyspraxia if language networks, attention, and basic motor and sensory functions are intact. Praxis should be tested in patients who have actual or suspected neurodegenerative processes, especially patients with early involvement of the parietal lobes, such as corticobasal syndrome and Alzheimer's dementia. If dyspraxia or apraxia is evident, it is important to confirm that language comprehension and basic motor tracts do not significantly confound the clinical picture. Liepmann (1913) described three major subtypes of apraxia: limb-kinetic, ideomotor, and ideational.

Limb-kinetic (or melokinetic) apraxia refers to disturbances in fine motor control (such as inaccurate or awkward movements). It is identified through observation of spontaneous fine motor skills and by asking the patient to pantomime fine motor movements, such as finger tapping or buttoning a shirt.

Ideomotor apraxia denotes an inability to execute a motor sequence in response to questioning or command while the ability to perform these movements spontaneously remains intact. Patients are asked to carry out routine movement sequences involving buccal, limb, or axial musculature. Common commands include combing hair, brushing teeth, lighting a match and blowing it out, throwing a ball, catching a ball, and using scissors. Problems with semantic memory, executive functions, working memory, attention, and basic sensory and motor skills may confound performance on these tasks. A more useful screen for ideomotor apraxia may be to have the patient imitate meaningless gestures that do not rely heavily on semantic memory or other cognitive processes (Sajjadi and Nestor 2016).

Ideational apraxia signifies an inability to carry out sequential movements with objects despite an intact ability to perform the individual steps. The three-step motor command on the MMSE (see "Language" in the section "Tests of Individual Cognitive Domains") is a common example. This and similar tests also rely very heavily on intact executive functions, language comprehension, working memory, sustained attention, and basic motor pathways.

Gnosis

Recognition of objects in various sensory realms results from the successful integration of intact sensory processing with accurate object recognition from memory stores. Teuber's early elegant definition of *agnosia* as "a percept stripped of its meanings" indicates that this condition occurs when otherwise normal sensory processing is disconnected from recognition schemas (Milner and Teuber 1968). Mechanistically, agnosia in specific sensory realms can be thought of as a disconnect between a normal sensory percept and its representation in memory stores or language networks because of a failure in activation of higher-order, transmodal areas (associative agnosia) (Mesulam 2000). Agnosia can be more confidently suspected when the patient does not have any concurrent deficits in the specific sensory realm in which agnosia is suspected and when the error in recognition cannot be explained by deficits in language, attention, semantic memory, or other functions.

Agnosia is likely when a patient fails to identify an object in one domain but identifies it in others. For instance, a patient with astereognosia would not recognize a paper clip placed in his hand but would be able to recognize it if he could see it. Anomia is likely when a patient fails to identify an object in multiple domains.

Calculation

The ability to perform mathematical calculations accurately relies on intact functioning of working memory, sustained attention, visuospatial processes (as in the case of written operations), executive functions, and other state and channel functions. Also necessary are proper serial and parallel processing of sensory information, goal selection, performance monitoring, freedom from distraction, and comparison of outcomes with what would be expected from prior knowledge or memory stores (i.e., fact checking), among other processes. Furthermore, consideration of developmental, educational, and vocational achievement is paramount; one would expect radically different outcomes in an individual with a lifelong developmental or acquired learning disability compared with a mathematician. In the latter case, assessment of basic functions is quite likely to reveal exceptional performance despite severe cognitive dysfunction, because basic operations would be overlearned and very well represented across cognitive networks. Patients with damage to the left angular gyrus, situated in the inferior parietal lobule, may develop acalculia in isolation or as part of Gerstmann's syndrome (along with any combination of anomia, alexia, agraphia, finger agnosia, and left-right disorientation) (Ardila and Rosselli 2002; Gerstmann 1940; Weintraub 2000). An isolated left parietal lesion may be responsible in patients whose language, visuospatial ability, executive functions, attention, and other processes are intact but who have isolated difficulties with calculation ("antiarithmetria").

Testing of calculation in the office or at the bedside consists of asking the patient to perform basic verbal and written arithmetic problems and simple problem-solving tasks involving calculation (e.g., "How much would you have left over if you had $7 and bought four apples for $3.27?").

Executive Function

Executive function is a wide-ranging term encompassing control and regulatory processes that are largely dependent on the dorsolateral prefrontal cortex and associated cortical and subcortical connections (Cummings 1993; Mesulam 2000). Executive functions (Table 3–4) are intimately linked with other cognitive domains and can be thought of as a set of superordinate or metacognitive control mechanisms that regulate more basic cognitive functions, including language, motor responses, attention, memory, and visuospatial function. Many domains may be included under this umbrella term: planning, organization, inhibiting automatic responses, problem solving, mental flexibility, set shifting, abstraction, motor sequencing, temporal order judgments, error detection, error correction, and pattern recognition (Chan et al. 2008; Hodges 2007b). Executive functions enable an individual to perform a desired action in the face of many possible choices, including prepotent impulses and maladaptive reactions. Executive functions help guide appropriate and effective behavior by allowing for adequate modification and freedom from distracting influences and impulsive or habitual responses when not contextually appropriate (Hodges 2007b). Executive functions can be tested either individually or as a group (as in the Frontal Assessment Battery). Executive functions and their associated bedside tests are shown in Table 3–4.

TABLE 3–4.   Executive functions and bedside tests

Executive functions	Tests	Abnormal findings
Environmental autonomy	Prehension behavior: patient places hands palms up, examiner extends his or her hand and says, "Do not take my hand"	Stimulus-bound behavior (patient grabs examiner's hand)
Set shifting and response inhibition	Verbal Trail Making Test Part B (e.g., "1-A, 2-B, 3-C, 4-D")	Incorrect sequencing, perseveration of a number or letter, slow speed
	Written alternating sequences (the patient copies alternating cursive *m* and *n* sequences; alternating triangles and squares)	Perseveration of a single shape, perseveration of the sequence beyond the edge of the page, difficulty replicating patterns
	Sensitivity to interference ("Tap twice when I tap once" and "Tap once when I tap twice"), followed by the go/no-go test (inhibitory control) ("Tap once when I tap once" and "Do not tap when I tap twice")	Stimulus-bound behavior, perseveration, mimicking the examiner (echopraxia)
Complex motor sequencing	Luria three-step test: patient repeats a fist-edge-palm motor sequence for multiple repetitions after the examiner demonstrates three repetitions	Poor planning, hesitation, sequencing errors, perseveration of same hand position, slow speed
Abstraction	Similarities: "How are a banana and an orange similar?"	Concrete interpretations ("They both have peels")
	Proverb interpretation: "People in glass houses shouldn't throw stones"	Concrete interpretations ("Stones will break the glass")
	Cognitive estimations: "What is the length of an average man's spine?"	Grossly erroneous estimation ("6 feet")
Frontal Assessment Battery	Similarities Lexical fluency Complex motor sequencing Sensitivity to interference and inhibitory control Environmental autonomy	Difficulties in each domain as noted earlier

Conclusion

Various cognitive domains and their underlying brain networks are related to one another with various degrees of influence and are arranged in a hierarchical fashion. Global functions such as arousal, attention, and mood are required for the correct operation of most cognitive tasks. Tests composed of various cognitive tasks, such as the MMSE and MoCA, are often sufficient for adequate screening. These tests should be supplemented by other tests that further explore certain cognitive domains (when needed). The bedside cognitive examination may yield vital clinical information that assists the examiner in formulating a more accurate diagnosis, in ordering appropriate tests, and in referring patients to colleagues when necessary.

References

Arciniegas DB: Mental status examination, in Behavioral Neurology and Neuropsychiatry. Edited by Arciniegas DB, Anderson CA, Filley CM. Cambridge, UK, Cambridge University Press, 2013, pp 344–393

Ardila A, Rosselli M: Acalculia and dyscalculia. Neuropsychol Rev 12(4):179–231, 2002 12539968

Baddeley A: The episodic buffer: a new component of working memory? Trends Cogn Sci 4(11):417–423, 2000 11058819

Baddeley A, Hitch G: Working memory, in The Psychology of Learning and Motivation: Advances in Research and Theory, Vol 8. Edited by Bower GH. New York, Academic Press, 1974, pp 47–89

Beebe DW, Gozal D: Obstructive sleep apnea and the prefrontal cortex: towards a comprehensive model linking nocturnal upper airway obstruction to daytime cognitive and behavioral deficits. J Sleep Res 11(1):1–16, 2002 11869421

Benarroch EE: The midline and intralaminar thalamic nuclei: anatomic and functional specificity and implications in neurologic disease. Neurology 71(12):944–949, 2008 18794498

Binder JR, Desai RH: The neurobiology of semantic memory. Trends Cogn Sci 15(11):527–536, 2011 22001867

Bopp KL, Verhaeghen P: Aging and verbal memory span: a meta-analysis. J Gerontol B Psychol Sci Soc Sci 60(5):223–233, 2005 16131616

Borson S, Scanlan J, Brush M, et al: The Mini-Cog: a cognitive "vital signs" measure for dementia screening in multi-lingual elderly. Int J Geriatr Psychiatry 15(11):1021–1027, 2000 11113982

Budson AE, Price BH: Memory dysfunction. N Engl J Med 352(7):692–699, 2005 15716563

Canessa N, Castronovo V, Cappa SF, et al: Obstructive sleep apnea: brain structural changes and neurocognitive function before and after treatment. Am J Respir Crit Care Med 183(10):1419–1426, 2011 21037021

Chan RC, Shum D, Toulopoulou T, et al: Assessment of executive functions: review of instruments and identification of critical issues. Arch Clin Neuropsychol 23(2):201–216, 2008 18096360

Cummings JL: Frontal-subcortical circuits and human behavior. Arch Neurol 50(8):873–880, 1993 8352676

Dell GS, O'Seaghdha PG: Stages of lexical access in language production. Cognition 42(1–3):287–314, 1992 1582160

Dick AS, Bernal B, Tremblay P: The language connectome: new pathways, new concepts. Neuroscientist 20(5):453–467, 2014 24342910

Dickerson BC, Eichenbaum H: The episodic memory system: neurocircuitry and disorders. Neuropsychopharmacology 35(1):86–104, 2010 19776728

Dubois B, Slachevsky A, Litvan I, et al: The FAB: a frontal assessment battery at bedside. Neurology 55(11):1621–1626, 2000 11113214

Eknoyan D, Hurley RA, Taber KH: The clock drawing task: common errors and functional neuroanatomy. J Neuropsychiatry Clin Neurosci 24(3):260–265, 2012 23037640

Filley CM: Memory disorders, in Neurobehavioral Anatomy, 3rd Edition. Boulder, University Press of Colorado, 2011, pp 63–74

Folstein MF, Folstein SE, McHugh PR: "Mini-mental state": a practical method for grading the cognitive state of patients for the clinician. J Psychiatr Res 12(3):189–198, 1975 1202204

Gerstmann J: Syndrome of finger agnosia, disorientation for right and left, agraphia and acalculia: local diagnostic value. Archives of Neurology and Psychiatry 44(2):398–408, 1940

Gleichgerrcht E, Fridriksson J, Bonilha L: Neuroanatomical foundations of naming impairments across different neurologic conditions. Neurology 85(3):284–292, 2015 26115732

Hillis AE: Aphasia: progress in the last quarter of a century. Neurology 69(2):200–213, 2007 17620554

Hodges JR: The Addenbrooke's Cognitive Examination—Revised and supplementary test suggestions, in Cognitive Assessment For Clinicians, 2nd Edition. New York, Oxford University Press, 2007a, pp 155–184

Hodges JR: Distributed cognitive functions, in Cognitive Assessment for Clinicians, 2nd Edition. New York, Oxford University Press, 2007b, pp 1–29

Ismail Z, Rajji TK, Shulman KI: Brief cognitive screening instruments: an update. Int J Geriatr Psychiatry 25(2):111–120, 2010 19582756

Johns MW: A new method for measuring daytime sleepiness: the Epworth sleepiness scale. Sleep 14(6):540–545, 1991 1798888

Liepmann H: Motor aphasia, anarthria, and apraxia, in Transactions of the 17th International Congress of Medicine, Section XI, Part II. London, Henry Frowde, 1913, pp 97–106

Lowery N, Ragland JD, Gur RC: Normative data for the symbol cancellation test in young healthy adults. Appl Neuropsychol 11(4):218–221, 2004 15673495

Meagher J, Leonard M, Donoghue L, et al: Months backward test: a review of its use in clinical studies. World J Psychiatry 5(3):305–314, 2015 26425444

Mendez MF, Ala T, Underwood KL: Development of scoring criteria for the clock drawing task in Alzheimer's disease. J Am Geriatr Soc 40(11):1095–1099, 1992 1401692

Mesulam M-M: Behavioral neuroanatomy: large-scale networks, association cortex, frontal syndromes, the limbic system, and hemispheric specializations, in Principles of Behavioral and Cognitive Neurology, 2nd Edition. Edited by Mesulam M-M. New York, Oxford University Press, 2000, pp 1–120

Miller GA: The magical number seven plus or minus two: some limits on our capacity for processing information. Psychol Rev 63(2):81–97, 1956 13310704

Milner B, Teuber HL: Alteration of perception and memory in man, in Analysis of Behavioral Change. Edited by Weiskrantz L. New York, Harper & Row, 1968, pp 268–375

Mioshi E, Dawson K, Mitchell J, et al: The Addenbrooke's Cognitive Examination Revised (ACE-R): a brief cognitive test battery for dementia screening. Int J Geriatr Psychiatry 21(11):1078–1085, 2006 16977673

Morris JC, Heyman A, Mohs RC, et al: The Consortium to Establish a Registry for Alzheimer's Disease (CERAD), I: Clinical and neuropsychological assessment of Alzheimer's disease. Neurology 39(9):1159–1165, 1989 2771064

Nasreddine ZS, Phillips NA, Bédirian V, et al: The Montreal Cognitive Assessment, MoCA: a brief screening tool for mild cognitive impairment. J Am Geriatr Soc 53(4):695–699, 2005 15817019

Papez JW: A proposed mechanism of emotion. Arch Neurol Psychiatry 38(4):725–743, 1937

Posner JB, Saper CB, Schiff ND, Plum F: Pathophysiology of signs and symptoms of coma: definitions, in Plum and Posner's Diagnosis of Stupor and Coma (Contemporary Neurology Series), 4th Edition. New York, Oxford University Press, 2007, pp 5–9

Reitan RM: Validity of the Trail Making Test as an indicator of organic brain damage. Perceptual and Motor Skills 8:271–276, 1958. Available at: https://journals.sagepub.com/doi/10.2466/pms.1958.8.3.271. Accessed May 18, 2019.

Reuter-Lorenz PA, Posner MI: Components of neglect from right-hemisphere damage: an analysis of line bisection. Neuropsychologia 28(4):327–333, 1990 2342639

Ricker JH, Axelrod BN: Analysis of an oral paradigm for the Trail Making Test. Assessment 1(1):47–52, 1994 9463499

Ross ED: Affective prosody and the aprosodias, in Principles of Behavioral and Cognitive Neurology, 2nd Edition. Edited by Mesulam M-M. New York, Oxford University Press, 2000, pp 316–331

Royall DR: Executive cognitive impairment: a novel perspective on dementia. Neuroepidemiology 19(6):293–299, 2000 11060503

Royall DR, Cordes JA, Polk M: CLOX: an executive clock drawing task. J Neurol Neurosurg Psychiatry 64(5):588–594, 1998 9598672

Ruchinskas RA: Limitations of the Oral Trail Making Test in a mixed sample of older individuals. Clin Neuropsychol 17(2):137–142, 2003 13680420

Sajjadi SA, Nestor PJ: Bedside assessment of cognition, in Oxford Textbook of Cognitive Neurology and Dementia. Edited by Husain M, Schott JM. New York, Oxford University Press, 2016, pp 105–112

Saper CB, Scammell TE, Lu J: Hypothalamic regulation of sleep and circadian rhythms. Nature 437(7063):1257–1263, 2005 16251950

Shulman KI: Clock-drawing: is it the ideal cognitive screening test? Int J Geriatr Psychiatry 15(6):548–561, 2000 10861923

Squire LR: Memory systems of the brain: a brief history and current perspective. Neurobiol Learn Mem 82(3):171–177, 2004 15464402

Strauss E, Sherman EM, Spreen O: A Compendium of Neuropsychological Tests: Administration, Norms, and Commentary, 3rd Edition. New York, Oxford University Press, 2006

Teasdale G, Jennett B: Assessment of coma and impaired consciousness: a practical scale. Lancet 2(7872):81–84, 1974 4136544

Teasdale G, Maas A, Lecky F, et al: The Glasgow Coma Scale at 40 years: standing the test of time. Lancet Neurol 13(8):844–854, 2014 25030516

Teng EL, Chui HC: The Modified Mini-Mental State (3MS) Examination. J Clin Psychiatry 48(8):314–318, 1987 3611032

Tombaugh TN: Trail Making Test A and B: normative data stratified by age and education. Arch Clin Neuropsychol 19(2):203–214, 2004 15010086

Wechsler D: Manual for the Wechsler Adult Intelligence Scale. New York, Psychological Corporation, 1955

Weintraub S: Neuropsychological assessment of mental state, in Principles of Behavioral and Cognitive Neurology, 2nd Edition. Edited by Mesulam M-M. New York, Oxford University Press, 2000, pp 121–173

Weintraub S, Peavy GM, O'Connor M, et al: Three words three shapes: a clinical test of memory. J Clin Exp Neuropsychol 22(2):267–278, 2000 10779840

Neuroimaging, Electroencephalography, and Lumbar Puncture in Medical Psychiatry

Daniel Talmasov, M.D.

Joshua P. Klein, M.D., Ph.D.

A number of diagnostic testing modalities are available to medical psychiatrists and other clinicians for evaluating potential medical or neurological causes of neuropsychiatric symptoms. These include neuroimaging; electroencephalography (EEG); and laboratory studies of cerebrospinal fluid (CSF), serum, and urine. In this chapter, we discuss the uses of neuroimaging, EEG, and lumbar puncture as part of the medical psychiatry workup (Table 4–1); serological and urine testing are discussed elsewhere in this book (see Chapter 5, "Toxicological Exposures and Nutritional Deficiencies in the Psychiatric Patient," and Chapter 9, "Infectious Diseases and Their Psychiatric Manifestations"). No pathognomonic findings on diagnostic testing have yet been identified for primary psychiatric disorders, so these modalities are used almost exclusively in ruling out medical illness or structural neurological lesions as causes of neuropsychiatric symptoms. We provide an overview of three categories of diagnostic techniques—structural and functional neuroimaging, EEG, and lumbar puncture—and discuss their indications, advantages, limitations, and clinical applications, with an emphasis on applications for evaluating conditions with a neuropsychiatric presentation.

The authors thank Daniel S. Weisholtz for his generous contribution of electroencephalographic tracings and his critical review of the electroencephalography section of the chapter.

TABLE 4–1.   Examples of indications for neurodiagnostic testing in medical psychiatry

Indication	Test	Diagnostic utility
Insidious-onset cognitive or behavioral impairment in an elderly patient	Structural MRI	Evaluation for possible dementia
Altered mentation with new focal neurological signs or symptoms	Structural MRI with contrast	Evaluation for possible intracranial mass lesion or stroke
New-onset psychotic symptoms (with or without catatonia or seizures) in a patient with known malignancy	Lumbar puncture with autoimmune antibody panel; MRI to evaluate for temporal lobe enhancement	Evaluation for possible limbic encephalitis (can also be idiopathic, without known malignancy)
New encephalitis with somnolence or agitation (with or without focal or generalized seizures)	Lumbar puncture with HSV PCR; MRI to evaluate for temporal lobe enhancement	Evaluation for possible herpes simplex encephalitis
Altered mentation with headache and fever	Lumbar puncture with cell count and differential	Evaluation for possible meningitis
Episodic changes in mentation or behavior	EEG (short-term or continuous monitoring; can be accompanied by video monitoring)	Evaluation for possible epileptic seizures
Periodic seizure-like motor activity that fails to respond to antiepileptic drugs	EEG accompanied by video monitoring	Evaluation for possible refractory seizures (versus psychogenic motor activity)
Fluctuating mental status changes marked by inattention, raising concern for delirium	EEG	Evaluation for possible encephalopathy (alpha slowing, appearance of theta/delta waves, or triphasic waveforms)

Note.   EEG=electroencephalography; HSV=herpes simplex virus; MRI=magnetic resonance imaging; PCR=polymerase chain reaction.

Neuroimaging

Structural Neuroimaging Modalities

Various neuroimaging modalities have proliferated in recent decades for the study of both the structure and the function of the human nervous system in vivo. Pathognomonic neuroimaging findings have not yet been identified for primary psychiatric disorders such as schizophrenia, bipolar disorder, and depression despite significant research over the past several decades. The structural imaging modalities of computed tomography (CT) and magnetic resonance imaging (MRI) are therefore used in the medical psychiatry patient population almost exclusively to rule out underlying structural brain lesions that secondarily produce neuropsychiatric symptoms (Table 4–2).

A general approach to neuroimaging involves an assessment of brain volume (normal, increased, decreased) and signal (normal, increased, decreased) (Figure 4–1). Different pathophysiological processes can produce focal, multifocal, or diffuse changes in brain volume and signal. Most acute or subacute processes are associated with an increase in volume of the affected tissue, whereas chronic processes (e.g., neurodegeneration, gliosis, scarring) are associated with a reduction in volume of the affected tissue. With loss of brain parenchyma, *ex vacuo* enlargement of the ventricles and cortical sulci typically occurs; this enlargement can be focal or diffuse, depending on the underlying process.

Computed Tomography

Background and history. Developed in the 1970s, CT combined X-ray technology used in medical practice since the late nineteenth century with then-emerging computerized image reconstruction methods, leading to a revolution in clinical imaging. X rays penetrate objects of lesser density more readily than they penetrate objects of greater density (i.e., *radiodense* materials). Denser materials are thus said to have greater X-ray attenuation. Clinically, the media through which X rays pass, in order of increasing X-ray attenuation (and thus decreasing *radiopenetrance*), are air, lipid, fluid, soft tissue, bone, and metal. On imaging, materials through which X rays pass most easily (e.g., air) appear black, whereas radiodense objects appear white (i.e., bone, metal). In CT, X rays emitted from sources arranged circumferentially around a patient pass through the patient's tissues, and the resulting beams (attenuated differentially by tissues of varying radiodensity) are recorded. CT images are subsequently digitally reconstructed, allowing for the viewing of structures from different angles and along different planes (e.g., sagittal, coronal, or transverse). CT is most effective in distinguishing structures with distinct radiodensities (e.g., air, fluid, soft tissue, bone, and metal). Thus, CT readily identifies differences among brain tissue (which appears gray), CSF (black), and skull (white) but has poorer resolution for structural detail within materials of nearly consistent density (e.g., there is only a subtle difference between gray matter [slightly more hyperdense] and white matter [slightly less hyperdense]). For greater resolution of nearly isodense structures such as gray and white matter, MRI is the preferred modality.

TABLE 4–2. Structural neuroimaging modalities and their advantages and limitations

Modality	Utility	Limitations
Computed tomography (CT)	Allows rapid assessment; is appropriate for emergency settings Is effective in identifying acute hemorrhage, masses, herniation, atrophy	In comparison with MRI, has poor resolution for distinguishing structures with differing tissue densities (normal brain, tumor, inflammatory/infectious process) Exposes patients to ionizing radiation
CT with iodinated contrast	Can identify pathology disruptive to blood-brain barrier (e.g., tumor, infection, inflammation)	Nephrotoxic; should not be given if estimated glomerular filtration rate <60 mL/min/1.73 m^2; should not be given with nephrotoxic drugs
Magnetic resonance imaging (MRI)	Sensitivity to distribution of water molecules allows for excellent resolution of intracranial structures Does not expose patients to ionizing radiation	MRI scanners can trigger claustrophobia Noise/volume may be disturbing to patients Require longer scanning times compared with CT
T1	Reflects brain appearance most closely, with gray matter darker than white matter; effective for overall evaluation of neuroanatomy	
T2	Darker appearance of white matter compared with T1 facilitates visual identification of abnormal lesions as hyperintensities over a dark background	
T2-weighted fluid-attenuated inversion recovery	Muted signal from cerebrospinal fluid (which appears black instead of white [as on T2]) allows for easier identification of periventricular and cortical lesions	
Diffusion-weighted imaging	Visualization of regions of increased anisotropy (limited directional freedom for water diffusion) facilitates identification of lesions (e.g., acute ischemic infarction)	

TABLE 4–2. Structural neuroimaging modalities and their advantages and limitations *(continued)*		
Modality	**Utility**	**Limitations**
Magnetic resonance imaging (MRI) *(continued)*		
Susceptibility-weighted imaging	Sensitive to blood and blood products; useful for identification of bleed, especially small hemorrhages or diffuse microhemorrhages (e.g., in hypertensive vasculopathy and cerebral amyloid angiopathy)	
MRI with gadolinium contrast	Identifies pathology disruptive to blood-brain barrier (e.g., tumor, infection, inflammatory change)	Chance of nephrotoxic systemic fibrosis

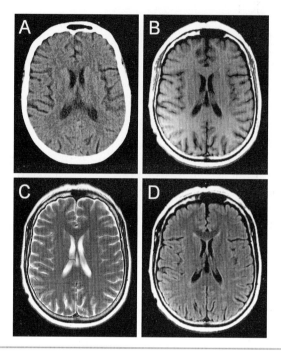

FIGURE 4–1.   Imaging of a normal adult brain.

(A) Unenhanced axial computed tomography (CT); (B) T1-weighted magnetic resonance imaging (MRI); (C) T2-weighted MRI; and (D) T2-weighted fluid-attenuated inversion recovery (T2-FLAIR) images are shown. Gray matter appears brighter than white matter on CT and T2-weighted images and darker than white matter on T1-weighted images. Cerebrospinal fluid in the ventricles and sulcal spaces appears brighter than the brain on T2-weighted images and darker than the brain on CT, T1, and T2-FLAIR images.

Source.   Provided by author Joshua P. Klein, M.D., Ph.D., Department of Neurology, Brigham and Women's Hospital and Harvard Medical School, Boston, Massachusetts.

Clinical applications.   In its applications to neuroimaging, CT is diagnostically effective when pathology can be readily identified by either 1) aberrant signal of differing radiodensity (e.g., fluid in an acute hemorrhage or pathological calcification) compared with normal brain or 2) aberrant swelling or atrophy caused by an underlying disease process. In clinical practice, the most common indication for use of CT in medical psychiatry is for the emergent evaluation of an acute to subacute mental status change in the emergency department, most often to rule out an intracranial hemorrhage. Intracranial bleeding, a cause of particular concern in the elderly and in patients receiving anticoagulation, can manifest solely as a change in mental status (e.g., a decrease in awareness or orientation compared with baseline) or together with other neurological examination findings. In the emergency department, CT is the most time-effective and safe method to evaluate for intracranial hemorrhage and should be performed promptly in patients with unexplained mental status changes, especially following known or suspected head trauma. CT also may be used for identifying ischemic stroke, but it is less sensitive for detection of acute ischemic (embolic) stroke compared with MRI and better able to detect chronic (old) postischemic structural changes.

Use of iodinated contrast: evaluation of neoplastic, infectious, and inflammatory processes.   CT is poorly suited to identifying and differentiating other intracranial pathologies, such as abscesses, neoplasms, or inflammatory processes. These pathologies are much better visualized on CT if intravenous contrast (most commonly, an iodinated contrast medium) is used. Intravenous contrast involves introduction of a radiodense signal into the bloodstream. In the absence of intracranial pathology, an intact blood-brain barrier effectively prevents intravenous contrast from infiltrating brain parenchyma; in the presence of significant intracranial pathology that compromises the blood-brain barrier (e.g., inflammation, vascularized neoplasm, intracranial abscess), the presence of a radiodense signal in the brain parenchymal region on images obtained after the administration of contrast indicates that the blood-brain barrier is disrupted. MRI offers a significantly higher resolution for the evaluation of such pathological changes and should be performed as a follow-up test after an abnormal CT result. Iodinated contrast should be avoided in patients with renal dysfunction or known contrast allergies and in pregnant patients, and special care should be given when considering use of iodinated contrast in patients with diabetes mellitus because of an increased risk for contrast-induced nephropathy (American College of Radiology 2007, 2008).

Magnetic Resonance Imaging

Background and history.   Since its introduction into clinical practice in the early 1980s, MRI has become the modality of choice for the neuroimaging of intracranial pathology because it offers higher-resolution imaging of brain tissue compared with CT and does not expose patients to ionizing radiation, but rather exploits the magnetic properties of molecules to generate images. MRI evolved out of nuclear magnetic resonance spectroscopy (MRS), a technique developed by chemists to study the structural properties of atoms and molecules in the late 1940s. Exploiting the electrical dipoles inherent to isotopes with odd numbers of protons in their atomic nuclei, MRI scanners expose a patient to a powerful static magnetic field, causing the axis along which atomic nuclei naturally spin to align longitudinally with the direction of the imposed magnetic field vector. Subsequently, an electromagnetic coil on the magnetic resonance scanner emits a radiofrequency (RF) pulse of electromagnetic radiation, which disrupts the alignment of these nuclei, causing them to disalign their axes from the vector imposed by the static magnetic field. When the RF pulse ceases, these nuclei realign themselves with the magnetic field, and the energy absorbed in changing their alignment is re-emitted by the same nuclei as an independent RF signal. This signal is detected by electromagnetic coils and subsequently recorded by the magnetic resonance scanner's computer, which assembles these signals into matrices that can be digitally reconstructed and viewed as images on a screen. MRI offers significantly greater resolution for the evaluation of soft tissues compared with CT.

Because MRI technology uses powerful magnetic fields, certain safety precautions should be taken. Patients should be screened for a history of implanted metals or foreign bodies.

Reasons for the effectiveness of MRI in neuroimaging.   MRI is able to provide superior resolution of neural structures because magnetic fields apply to atoms with odd-numbered nuclei, of which the most vastly abundant is hydrogen, present in great quantities in the body's water molecules. Thus, MRI provides a visual representation of bodily hydrogen, found largely in water, influenced by the local microenvironment of the hydrogen atoms in question (e.g., whether they exist as part of free water or as part of water bound by other macromolecules). Because of its sensitivity to water content, tissues, and the local microenvironment of water, MRI is extremely effective in providing high-resolution data on tissues. MRI can readily distinguish between gray and white matter, delineate the structural detail of brain parenchyma, and identify pathological changes such as those caused by neoplasia, infection, inflammation, or stroke, which are accompanied by increases in local free water content (edema).

T1- versus T2-weighted sequences and T2-weighted fluid-attenuated inversion recovery.   In order to visualize different aspects of tissue structure (e.g., gray vs. white matter), MRI scanners use different RF pulse sequences by modulating two variables: the length of time the RF pulse is emitted and the length of time allotted for data acquisition after emission of the RF pulse. The two standard RF pulse sequences in all MRI studies are referred to as T1- and T2-weighted sequences.

T1-weighted sequences use shorter RF pulses and shorter subsequent data acquisition windows compared with T2-weighted sequences. The shorter pulses used in T1 imaging tend to highlight hydrogen atoms in more hydrophobic, lipid-heavy environments; thus, fat appears white (*hyperintense*), and CSF appears dark (*hypointense*). In T1-weighted imaging, gray matter appears darker, and white matter (containing more lipid in myelin) appears lighter, similar to their relation on pathological examination (i.e., gray matter appears gray, and white matter appears white). For these reasons, T1-weighted imaging is often viewed first to evaluate neuroanatomic structure grossly.

T2-weighted sequences use longer RF pulses and allow for longer collection time, highlighting environments of higher water content; thus, CSF appears white, lipid appears dark, and gray matter appears more hyperintense than white matter (i.e., gray matter appears white, and white matter appears gray). T2-weighted sequences can be a very effective tool in evaluating brain parenchyma (in particular, the white matter) for signs of focal pathology because the tissue appears generally darker than it does on T1-weighted imaging, with areas of elevated water content (a marker for inflammation, stroke, and infection) appearing white against a dark background.

T2-weighted fluid-attenuated inversion recovery (T2-FLAIR) is a type of T2-weighted RF sequence that yields images similar to T2 images, but the intensity of free fluid is attenuated by the addition of an extra RF pulse; thus, CSF appears dark (rather than white as it does on standard T2-weighted sequences) (see Figure 4–1). This sequence visually facilitates the identification of focal pathology, because areas of pathological edema will appear bright against dark brain parenchyma. Because normal CSF will no longer have a bright signal, the T2-FLAIR sequence is especially useful for evaluation of lesions proximal to CSF spaces (e.g., periventricular or cortical lesions).

Diffusion-weighted imaging.   Diffusion-weighted imaging is an MRI sequence that measures and visualizes the degree to which water molecules are able to diffuse freely in their local environment. *Anisotropy* (Greek: *anisos,* unequal; *tropos,* turn) is a term that describes the behavior of water molecules that are unable to diffuse freely in all directions and are limited by their local microenvironment to diffusing along a particular vector preferentially (e.g., longitudinally along white matter tracts). Visualizing the anisotropic diffusion of water is clinically useful because many pathological changes—including acute infarction (with associated cytotoxic cellular edema), abscesses, and hypercellular tumors—are accompanied by limitations to the free diffusion of water.

Susceptibility-weighted imaging and gradient echo. Susceptibility-weighted imaging and the older gradient echo sequence are modalities that detect the presence of blood and its breakdown products and can offer information complementary to standard MRI techniques. Their sensitivity to hemorrhage can be useful in the evaluation of focal bleeding, as in sequelae of traumatic brain injury, or diffuse microhemorrhage, as seen in cerebral amyloid angiopathy. These sequences are particularly helpful in detecting the presence of microhemorrhages that are too small to be detected on other sequences. Visualization of microhemorrhages is possible because of an artifact inherent in these sequences called *blooming*, which makes the lesion appear slightly larger than its actual size.

Use of gadolinium contrast. Similar to the use of iodinated contrast in CT to identify pathology when the blood-brain barrier is compromised, the paramagnetic metal gadolinium, which reduces the time required for proton relaxation in tissues and provides a strong magnetic resonance signal on T1-weighted sequences, is used as a contrast agent in MRI. As with iodinated CT, gadolinium contrast should be avoided in patients with renal dysfunction or known contrast allergies and in pregnant patients (American College of Radiology 2007; Kanal et al. 2007).

Stress associated with MRI scanning: considerations for the psychiatric population. Clinicians should be aware that undergoing MRI can be uncomfortable or anxiety provoking for many patients because of a combination of physical enclosure, significant noise, and significant scanning time over which the patient is exposed to these factors. This consideration can be especially important in psychiatric populations whose concerns about potential discomfort during the scanning protocol may limit adherence and prevent patients from undergoing diagnostic tests important to their medical and psychiatric care. MRI scanners can precipitate claustrophobia, because traditional scanners enclose at least part of the patient's body circumferentially as the scan is taking place. Noise also is a frequently cited complaint among patients undergoing MRI; mechanical forces acting on gradient coils (electromagnets involved in a component of magnetic resonance scanning) create a lot of noise, which some patients, especially those affected by anxiety, hyperarousal, or paranoia, may find distressing. Patients may be offered earplugs to offset this discomfort.

Furthermore, MRI protocols, which rely on the use of several RF pulse sequences and corresponding tissue relaxation times for data collection, require significantly more scanning time compared with CT. A routine CT can be obtained in a matter of minutes, whereas MRI scan time can exceed 30 minutes depending on the number of sequences obtained and contrast use.

Clinicians are advised to be sensitive to the comfort of psychiatric patients undergoing MRI, in order to maximize patient adherence to imaging protocols. In addition to provision of support and reassurance, administration of a low dose of an anxiolytic (e.g., lorazepam) before MRI may be indicated in some cases.

Cerebral Angiography

The cerebral vasculature can be imaged with contrast-based CT and MRI techniques. If images are acquired while the contrast agent is passing through the arteries, an arteriogram is produced. Likewise, if images are acquired while the contrast agent is passing through the venous structures, a venogram is produced. These images are use-

ful for characterizing cerebrovascular disease, including vascular stenoses or occlu-
sions, aneurysms, and other vascular malformations. Angiography obtained via cath-
eter-based arterial injections of contrast provides the highest-resolution images of the
vasculature but is a more invasive procedure than intravenous contrast injection.

Functional Neuroimaging Modalities

Advances in magnetic resonance, radiochemistry, and nuclear imaging technologies
have led to the emergence of imaging techniques capable of providing data on aspects
of brain activity (Table 4–3), by exploiting the sensitivity of imaging techniques to
markers of brain metabolism (e.g., blood oxygenation levels; the activity of biologically relevant molecules).

Functional Magnetic Resonance Imaging

Functional MRI (fMRI) refers to an MRI technique pioneered by Seiji Ogawa and colleagues in the early 1990s (Ogawa et al. 1990) in which a magnetic resonance signal
sensitive to changes in blood oxygenation is used as an indirect measure of neural activity. fMRI detects local effects on spin alignment in hydrogen nuclei caused by
changing oxygenation states in hemoglobin molecules (a blood-oxygen-level dependent, or BOLD, signal). fMRI techniques have been applied across task-based and
task-free paradigms. Task-based fMRI involves the monitoring of activity-related
changes in the BOLD signal as a patient engages in a cognitive, motor, or visual task,
whereas task-free (or "resting") fMRI attempts to determine neuroanatomical patterns of synchronous activity (endogenous networks) in the absence of an explicit
task. Clinically, fMRI has been used for functional mapping as part of neurosurgical
planning (e.g., using language-based tasks to determine the laterality of language in
a neurosurgical patient undergoing resection). Although fMRI techniques have been
applied extensively across psychological and neuropsychiatric research, fMRI has yet
to be translated into clinical diagnostic or therapeutic use in psychiatry.

Positron Emission Tomography

Positron emission tomography (PET) is a form of molecular neuroimaging that exploits signals emitted by radioactive constituents that are incorporated into biologically active molecules of interest (e.g., glucose, oxygen, or neurotransmitters) by using
a particle accelerator called a cyclotron. These molecules are designated PET *ligands* or
tracers and are injected intravenously. By measuring gamma radiation released as pos-
itrons are spontaneously emitted from PET ligands, images are generated that show
the precise localization of these particular molecules of interest. The localization of
PET ligands in neuroimaging applications depends on cerebral perfusion providing
the brain a supply of the ligand and the rate at which the ligand is taken up and used
biologically.

   PET imaging renders a three-dimensional representation of ligand distribution
that is usually shown as spatially superimposed on structural neuroimaging obtained
simultaneously to characterize underlying neuroanatomy. PET imaging is most often
accompanied by structural CT (PET/CT). PET/MRI technology is available at greater
cost at some medical centers but is not yet in routine clinical use and may be considered in cases when high soft-tissue contrast (e.g., grading of gliomas, evaluation of

TABLE 4–3.	Functional neuroimaging modalities
Modality	**Mechanism and utility**
Functional magnetic resonance imaging	Approximates regional brain activity by exploiting local effects of hemoglobin deoxygenation on spin alignment in the hydrogen nuclei of water molecules, generating a blood-oxygen-level dependent signal
Positron emission tomography	Visualizes activity and localization of an intravenously introduced biologically active molecule (e.g., glucose or specific neurotransmitter), termed a *radiotracer* or *radioligand*
Magnetic resonance spectroscopy	Detects the presence of biologically active molecules
Single-photon emission computed tomography	Visualizes distribution of a radiotracer using a gamma-sensitive camera

Alzheimer's disease) or lower radiation exposure (e.g., pediatric populations) is desired (Nensa et al. 2014).

A PET tracer in common use is ^{18}F-fluorodeoxyglucose (FDG), which is sensitive to glucose uptake in tissues and can be used in neuroimaging to study the uptake of glucose by neuronal and glial tissues as an estimation of regional patterns of neural activity. Thus, FDG-PET will reveal hypermetabolism in active areas and networks in healthy patients and, conversely, hypometabolism in patients with corresponding pathology (e.g., neurodegeneration in dementia). Other notable tracers in clinical use for neuroimaging applications include ^{18}F-fluorodopa (F-DOPA), a DOPA-based biomarker used in the diagnostic assessment of Parkinson's disease, and a range of tracers designed to bind to amyloid-β plaques used in the evaluation of suspected Alzheimer's disease. Additionally, tracers are being developed to assess immune system activation in diseases such as multiple sclerosis (Singhal et al. 2017).

Several PET tracers corresponding to important signaling molecules pertinent to psychiatry have been introduced, including serotonin, dopamine, and opioid-based ligands; these have seen numerous applications in psychiatric research, including drug development and pharmacokinetic studies, but are not yet common in clinical use. The availability and cost of use of medical cyclotrons can be a limiting factor for the production of less common PET tracers, such as ligands for specific neurotransmitters, whereas common ligands, such as FDG, are more readily available from radiopharmaceutical distributors.

Magnetic Resonance Spectroscopy

Whereas standard MRI exploits the magnetic properties of odd-numbered nuclei to generate a neuroanatomically accurate visual representation of the brain's hydrogen, MRS exploits this same technology to study a wide range of biologically and metabolically significant molecules with odd-numbered nuclei. MRS produces a waveform with multiple peaks along the x axis. Each peak distinguishes the presence of a chemically unique species of odd-numbered nuclei (made unique on the basis of its position within a molecule and the relative degree of electron shielding in its orbit), whereas the area under the peak represents the relative quantity of that species. MRS has been used in research applications to study both endogenous cerebral metabolites and the metabolites of psychotropic compounds such as lithium and fluorinated polycyclic drugs (e.g., fluoxetine, paroxetine, fluvoxamine) (Lyoo and Renshaw 2000). Hydrogen-1 MRS can be used to study several important cerebral metabolites, such as choline, creatine, N-acetyl aspartate, lactate, myoinositol, glutamate, glutamine, and glycine (Castillo et al. 1996). Clinical applications of hydrogen-1 MRS include tumor imaging, identification of intracerebral radiation injury, and evaluation of neurodegenerative disease (Castillo et al. 1996).

MRS can delineate regional differences in cerebral metabolite levels by employing voxel-based (spatially specific) calculations, allowing for some discrimination among different neuroanatomical regions. Notably, MRS is limited by poorer resolution compared with PET technology in molecular neuroimaging, but it has the advantages of not requiring radiotracer compounds, being compatible with many available 1.5 Tesla magnetic resonance scanners, and not exposing patients to ionizing radiation.

Single-Photon Emission Computed Tomography

Single-photon emission computed tomography (SPECT) is an imaging technique sensitive to cerebral blood flow that is dependent on the inhalation or injection of radiopharmaceutical compounds whose localization can be detected with a gamma-sensitive camera. SPECT radioligands consist of radioactive isotopes attached to a lipophilic molecule, allowing the tracer to cross the blood-brain barrier readily into the cerebral vasculature, diffusing into cells in a perfusion-dependent manner. The most commonly used SPECT radiotracer in neuroimaging is technetium-99m (^{99m}Tc). SPECT has no currently accepted use in the evaluation of primary psychiatric disorders and is more commonly used in other organs than in neuroimaging but may be useful in assessment of stroke and traumatic brain injury. SPECT also plays a role in the evaluation of neurodegenerative disease.

Neuroimaging Findings in Dementia and Cognitive Disorders

In 2010, dementia affected 36.5 million people worldwide; its prevalence is projected to double every 20 years (Prince et al. 2013). Currently, the diagnosis of all neurocognitive disorders—including mild cognitive impairment (MCI) as well as dementia due to Alzheimer's disease, frontotemporal lobar degeneration, cerebrovascular disease, or Lewy body disease—remains largely clinical. However, both structural and functional neuroimaging may be useful in assessing patients when the clinician has high clinical suspicion for neurocognitive decline and in identifying the subtype of dementing illness (Mortimer et al. 2013; Scheltens et al. 2016). Normal aging is associated with a generalized decline in cortical volume and a concurrent proportional increase in ventricular volume, as well as with development of nonspecific lesions in the periventricular and subcortical white matter. More significant cerebral atrophy, or extensive white matter abnormalities, associated with a decline in cognitive functioning can be a sign of age-associated neurodegenerative illness (dementia) (Table 4–4). Intellectual abilities in several dissociable cognitive domains may be differentially affected in such illnesses, such as executive functioning (impulse control, working memory, attention, and cognitive flexibility) in frontotemporal lobar degeneration or short-term memory in Alzheimer's disease.

In some cases, neuroimaging will reveal brain changes that correlate with specific types of dementing illness (Figure 4–2), and clinical deficits will reflect impairment in cognitive domains associated with these disorders. Such findings, when complemented by history, clinical examination, and results of formal neuropsychological testing, may be useful in the diagnosis of specific neurocognitive disorders. In other cases, patients will have MCI—that is, a decline in cognitive ability out of proportion to age and education but without significant impairment in day-to-day functioning. Such cases may be marked by medial temporal lobe degeneration or may show no significant changes on neuroimaging. In the later stages of various disorders, more diffuse atrophy will be present on imaging, often reflecting advanced or wide-ranging cognitive deficits. Generally, it is advisable that any patient presenting with cognitive impairment undergo structural imaging at least once to rule out potentially reversible causes of cognitive dysfunction, such as a subdural hematoma or mass lesion.

Mild Cognitive Impairment

The term *MCI* (mild neurocognitive disorder in DSM-5; American Psychiatric Association 2013) does not denote a specific pathological entity but rather signifies a range of clinical presentations in which a patient develops nonimpairing cognitive limitations (as assessed by quantitative test performance that is below normal values for the patient's age and educational level). MCI may subsequently develop into a major neurocognitive disorder—most commonly, Alzheimer's disease (particularly the amnestic subtype of MCI), but potentially several other distinct dementing illnesses. According to longitudinal neuroimaging studies of dementing illness, the most common MRI finding in patients with MCI is a decrease in medial temporal lobe volume, including the amygdala, anterior hippocampus, fusiform gyrus, and entorhinal cortex (McDonald et al. 2009; Whitwell et al. 2007).

Alzheimer's Disease

Alzheimer's disease is defined pathologically by the abnormal accumulation of two proteins, extracellular amyloid-β plaques and intraneuronal tau peptide tangles. Epidemiologically, Alzheimer's disease is the most common cause of dementia, accounting for 54% of all cases in individuals older than 65 years, according to a European analysis (Lobo et al. 2000).

MRI findings in Alzheimer's disease.   MRI in Alzheimer's disease shows a general posterior-to-anterior progression, with atrophy heavily involving the temporal cortex and expanding with increased severity into neighboring regions, including parietal, frontal, and occipital cortices, but largely sparing sensory and motor pathways (see Table 4–4). The earliest atrophic changes in Alzheimer's disease are limited to medial temporal regions and can be present in asymptomatic individuals and in patients with MCI. As MCI progresses to more significant cognitive dysfunction in Alzheimer's disease (major neurocognitive disorder due to Alzheimer's disease in DSM-5), medial temporal atrophy often becomes more marked, a phenomenon that can be appreciated visually or with volumetric analysis. Although formal volumetric analysis of the hippocampus has been used in research settings, direct visual assessment of

TABLE 4–4. Characteristic imaging findings in dementia

Dementia type	Structural MRI	PET or SPECT imaging
Alzheimer's disease (*mild* cognitive impairment)	Early/mild Medial temporal atrophy, including amygdala, anterior hippocampus, entorhinal cortex, fusiform gyrus	Amyloid PET Positive for amyloid deposition (can also be positive in absence of cognitive impairment)
Alzheimer's disease (*major* cognitive impairment)	Moderate Temporal lobe atrophy, including medial temporal lobe, middle temporal gyrus, posterior temporal lobe, hippocampus Parietal atrophy, including inferior parietal cortex; posterior cingulate cortical atrophy progressing to anterior cingulate cortical atrophy Late/severe Diffuse atrophy including broad involvement of temporal lobe and parietal lobe, aspects of frontal and anterior occipital regions; sparing of primary sensory and motor regions	FDG-PET Temporal and parietal hypometabolism Posterior cingulate cortical hypometabolism Amyloid PET Positive for amyloid deposition
Frontotemporal dementia	Severe temporal and frontal lobe atrophy Asymmetrical pattern with greater left-sided atrophy, especially in temporal region	FDG-PET Frontal and temporal hypometabolism Asymmetrical pattern of hypometabolism Anterior cingulate and anterior temporal hypometabolism
Vascular dementia (adapted from NINDS-AIREN criteria; Román et al. 1993)	Large-vessel strokes Bilateral anterior cerebral artery Posterior cerebral artery (including bilateral paramedian thalamic lesions, inferior medial temporal lobe lesions) Association areas: Temporoparietal, temporo-occipital	

TABLE 4–4.   **Characteristic imaging findings in dementia** *(continued)*

Dementia type	Structural MRI	PET or SPECT imaging

Vascular dementia *(continued)* (adapted from NINDS-AIREN criteria; Román et al. 1993)	Watershed carotid territories
	  Superior frontal, parietal areas
	Small-vessel disease
	    Basal ganglia lacunae
	    Frontal white matter lacunar infarcts
	    Extensive periventricular white matter lesions
	    Bilateral thalamic lesions
	Diffuse disease
	  Bilateral large-vessel hemispheric strokes
	  Large-vessel lesions of the dominant hemisphere
	  Leukoencephalopathy involving at least one-fourth of total cortical white matter	

Lewy body dementia	Medial temporal atrophy; less severe than that in Alzheimer's disease General cortical atrophy	SPECT Abnormally low dopamine transporter binding in basal ganglia measured by ^{123}I-FP-CIT SPECT

Note.   FDG = ^{18}F-fluorodeoxyglucose; ^{123}I-FP-CIT = iodine-123-2β-carbometoxy-3β-(4-iodophenyl)-*N*-(3-fluoropropyl) nortropane; MRI = magnetic resonance imaging; NINDS-AIREN = National Institute of Neurological Disorders and Stroke–Association Internationale pour la Recherché et l'Enseignement en Neurosciences; PET = positron emission tomography; SPECT = single-photon emission computed tomography.

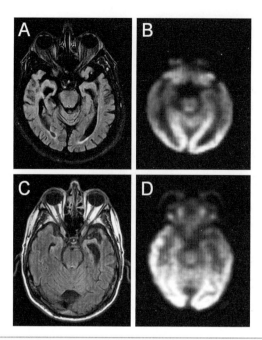

FIGURE 4–2. Characteristic imaging findings in neurodegenerative disease.

In Alzheimer's disease, symmetrical atrophy and hypometabolism of the brain occur, most notably in the temporal and parietal lobes, as seen on **(A)** axial T2-weighted fluid-attenuated inversion recovery (T2-FLAIR) magnetic resonance imaging (MRI) and **(B)** ^{18}F-fluorodeoxyglucose positron emission tomography (FDG-PET) images. In frontotemporal dementia, asymmetrical atrophy and hypometabolism occur most often in the frontal or temporal lobes. Such asymmetrical changes are noted in the left temporal lobe on **(C)** axial T2-FLAIR MRI and (D) FDG-PET images.

Source. Provided by author Joshua P. Klein, M.D., Ph.D., Department of Neurology, Brigham and Women's Hospital and Harvard Medical School, Boston, Massachusetts.

medial temporal atrophy is more commonly applied clinically. Visual rating scales of medial temporal atrophy (Scheltens et al. 1992) have been developed and shown to correlate with results on cognitive tests. As cognitive decline progresses, the picture of atrophy seen in MCI in medial temporal areas (amygdala, anterior hippocampus, fusiform gyrus, and entorhinal cortex) extends further to involve the middle temporal gyrus and posterior aspects of the temporal lobe, the entirety of the hippocampus, and the parietal cortex (Whitwell et al. 2007).

Other structural markers on MRI for worsening Alzheimer's disease include the progression of parietal atrophy from posterior cingulate cortex to anterior cingulate regions and the eventual involvement of frontal and lateral occipital areas as well (McDonald et al. 2009). The posterior occipital cortex (visual cortex), a primary sensory area, is generally spared, as are other primary sensory regions (auditory and somatosensory cortices) and the motor cortex. Lobar or asymmetrical cerebral atrophy is not typically seen in Alzheimer's disease.

FDG-PET findings in Alzheimer's disease.   The vast majority of patients affected by Alzheimer's disease will have regional cortical hypometabolism, reflecting areas affected by neurodegeneration, and these metabolic changes may precede volumetric changes seen on structural imaging scans. Thus, a normal FDG-PET scan has a high negative predictive value for the presence of a neurodegenerative disease (Perani et al. 2014).

Patterns of hypometabolism on an abnormal FDG-PET scan can be suggestive but not diagnostic of a specific pathology (see Table 4–4). Temporoparietal hypometabolic patterns are suggestive of Alzheimer's disease, whereas an anterior and asymmetrical pattern is suggestive of frontotemporal lobar degeneration (FTLD); however, a significant number of FDG-PET scans with a temporoparietal hypometabolic picture that are initially interpreted as Alzheimer's disease may later, on pathological examination, be shown to be FTLD. In such cases, careful attention to the presence of anterior cingulate and anterior temporal hypometabolism can be revealing, because these patterns are more specific and have a greater positive likelihood ratio for the diagnosis of FTLD than does temporoparietal hypometabolism for Alzheimer's disease (Womack et al. 2011).

Amyloid PET findings in Alzheimer's disease.   Tracers for compounds that serve as pathological markers, such as amyloid-β in Alzheimer's disease, have more recently been developed as diagnostic tools. Currently, three U.S. Food and Drug Administration (FDA)–approved radiotracers are commercially available for PET imaging of amyloid-β in vivo: florbetapir, florbetaben, and flutemetamol.

Although amyloid-β plaque deposition is a defining element of Alzheimer's disease pathology, the presence of cerebral amyloidosis is not by itself (i.e., in the absence of cognitive impairment) diagnostic of Alzheimer's disease, given that amyloid deposition is also associated with normal aging and with the apolipoprotein E *(APOE)* genotype (Jansen et al. 2015). Significant amyloid burden can be present even in individuals without any marked cognitive impairment, but it may be associated with increased risk for developing future cognitive impairment, with a lag time of 20–30 years (Jansen et al. 2015). Thus, a negative amyloid PET scan result can be useful in excluding Alzheimer's disease in individuals with an unknown cause of cognitive impairment, whereas positive amyloid PET findings alone are not diagnostic of Alzheimer's disease. Similarly, amyloid PET imaging should not be used to gauge the severity of dementia, because extensive amyloid deposition on PET can precede cognitive impairment, and amyloid burden is only weakly correlated with severity of cognitive impairment (Villemagne et al. 2011).

Frontotemporal Lobar Degeneration

FTLD, also known as frontotemporal dementia, denotes a range of clinically and pathologically heterogeneous processes that are characterized by the preferential degeneration of frontal and temporal lobe cortical structures (see Table 4–4). Virtually all cases of FTLD are marked by the presence of neuronal inclusion bodies containing one of three abnormal proteins: tau (a microtubule-associated protein), transactive response (TAR) DNA-binding protein 43, or fused-in sarcoma (FUS) (Whitwell and Josephs 2012). The differential anatomical deposition of these proteins and the ensuing pattern of neural atrophy define the clinicoanatomical subtype of FTLD. Recognized clinicoanatomical subtypes of FTLD include behavioral variant frontotemporal lobar dementia and primary progressive aphasia (which is further subdivided into semantic dementia, nonfluent progressive aphasia, and logopenic progressive aphasia). Like all neurocognitive diagnoses, FTLD cannot be diagnosed by imaging alone but requires clinical correlation with history and cognitive examination or neuropsycho-logical test findings.

Structural MRI findings in frontotemporal lobar degeneration.   On structural MRI, frontotemporal dementia is marked by severe frontal or temporal lobe degeneration and only mild hippocampal degeneration (see Figure 4–2). This pattern contrasts with that in Alzheimer's disease, which is marked by severe hippocampal degeneration, moderate temporal degeneration, and very limited frontal involvement until late in the disease (Boccardi et al. 2003). The hippocampus is affected in both Alzheimer's disease and FTLD, but it is more markedly affected in Alzheimer's disease, and atrophy of other nonhippocampal medial temporal lobe structures—a marker for disease severity in Alzheimer's disease—is absent or much less prominent in FTLD (Frisoni et al. 1996). Asymmetry is more marked in FTLD than in Alzheimer's disease, with worsening degeneration on the left side, especially in temporal areas (Boccardi et al. 2003).

FDG-PET findings in frontotemporal lobar degeneration.   FDG-PET in FTLD reveals an anterior pattern of cortical hypometabolism, with frontal and temporal structures being primarily affected (see Figure 4–2); this pattern is typically more asymmetrical than the hypometabolic pattern seen in Alzheimer's disease, showing a predilection for the left hemisphere (Mortimer et al. 2013; Womack et al. 2011). Temporoparietal hypometabolism on PET may indicate Alzheimer's disease but is not specific for that diagnosis; in cases with this finding, clinicians should evaluate anterior cingulate and anterior temporal hypometabolism and consider a diagnosis of FTLD if consistent with the clinical presentation (Womack et al. 2011).

Vascular Dementia

Vascular dementia (major or mild vascular neurocognitive disorder in DSM-5), a general term referring to cognitive impairment arising out of underlying vascular disease, represents a clinically and pathologically diverse entity. The National Institute of Neurological Disorders and Stroke–Association Internationale pour la Recherché et l'Enseignement en Neurosciences (NINDS-AIREN) international workgroup (Román et al. 1993) published a widely used set of diagnostic criteria for the evaluation of vascular dementia, emphasizing the importance of brain imaging to correlate clinical findings and establish a temporal relationship between the onset of cognitive deficits and cerebrovascular events. These criteria emphasize the pathological diversity that gives rise to vascular dementia, including cortical ischemic or hemorrhagic strokes, subcortical lacunar infarcts (senile leukoencephalopathic lesions), or global cerebral hypoxic-ischemic vascular events, such as in cardiac arrest. The presence of cognitive deficits must be elicited clinically and through neuropsychological testing, and the presence of cerebrovascular disease on neuroimaging is required for a diagnosis of vascular dementia (see Table 4–4).

Lewy Body Disease (Dementia With Lewy Bodies)

Lewy body dementia (major or mild neurocognitive disorder with Lewy bodies in DSM-5) accounts for 4.2% of all dementia cases diagnosed in the community and 7.2% of all dementia cases diagnosed in a secondary care setting (Vann Jones and

O'Brien 2014). Pathologically, Lewy body disease is characterized by the presence of neuronal inclusion bodies—composed primarily of α-synuclein aggregates—spread diffusely throughout the cortex. The absence or relative scarcity of amyloid plaques and neurofibrillary tangles distinguishes Lewy body disease from Alzheimer's disease (see Table 4–4).

Practically, the diagnosis of dementia secondary to Lewy body disease is based on clinical presentation and the presence of significant cognitive impairment combined with the presence of parkinsonian features or visual hallucinations. Definitive diagnostic confirmation is possible only on pathological examination. Clinicians suspecting Lewy body dementia may use neuroimaging to supplement clinical findings. On structural MRI, Lewy body disease is marked by medial temporal lobe atrophy worse than that in age-matched control subjects but less severe than that in Alzheimer's disease (Barber et al. 1999). Unlike other forms of dementia, Lewy body dementia is associated with significant degeneration of dopaminergic neurons in the nigrostriatal pathway; thus, SPECT with a ligand sensitive to dopamine transporter (DAT) activity is clinically useful (see Table 4–4). In patients with suspected Lewy body dementia, SPECT will reveal decreased DAT activity in the basal ganglia, with a sensitivity of 77.7% for detecting Lewy body disease and a specificity of 90.4% for excluding Lewy body disease (McKeith et al. 2007).

Neuroimaging Findings in Other Common Neurological Disorders

Many other neurological conditions can produce or be associated with psychiatric symptoms. Most of these conditions are acquired disorders that cause structural changes to the brain, leading to a variety of symptoms, including behavioral changes, seizures, and cognitive impairment. Figure 4–3 shows typical brain-imaging findings in a selection of such disorders. (A more detailed discussion of neurological disorders is presented in Chapter 12, "Neurological Conditions and Their Psychiatric Manifestations," in this volume.) The diagnosis of these disorders is generally suggested by the clinical history and supported by the presence of characteristic abnormalities on imaging.

Electroencephalography

History and Background

EEG is an electrophysiological technique that monitors temporal patterns of the brain's electrical activity by means of electrodes distributed across the scalp. The use of EEG for monitoring brain activity in humans was first described by Hans Berger in Germany in 1924. Notably, EEG has very high temporal resolution for electrical activity within the brain (on the order of milliseconds) but, conversely, has poor spatial resolution, an important limitation. Thus, EEG has limited utility in identifying focal neurological lesions (a role more appropriate for neuroimaging), although it can identify asymmetrical abnormalities that may warrant further investigation with neuroimaging in patients without a previous scan.

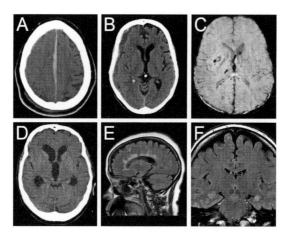

FIGURE 4–3. Characteristic imaging findings in common neurological disorders.

(A) Axial unenhanced computed tomography (CT) scan of the head shows a traumatic hyperdense subdural hematoma adjacent to the right aspect of the falx cerebri. **(B)** Axial unenhanced CT of the head in a different patient shows a right convexity mixed-density subdural fluid collection representing acute (hyperdense) and subacute (less hyperdense) blood products. In both *A* and *B*, the cerebral structures subjacent to the hematomas are compressed. **(C)** Axial susceptibility-weighted magnetic resonance imaging (MRI) scan in a patient with traumatic axonal shear injury shows multifocal punctate hypointense foci in the deep white matter on the right, along some midline structures, and along the margin of the right lateral ventricle. The punctate foci of hypointensity represent traumatic microhemorrhages. **(D)** Axial unenhanced CT in a patient with normal-pressure hydrocephalus shows ventriculosulcal disproportion. **(E)** Parasagittal T2-weighted fluid-attenuated inversion recovery (T2-FLAIR) MRI of a patient with multiple sclerosis shows multiple radially oriented T2-hyperintense periventricular lesions as well as several juxtacortical T2-hyperintense lesions. **(F)** Coronal T2-FLAIR MRI in a patient with temporal lobe epilepsy shows left hippocampal sclerosis.

Source.   Provided by author Joshua P. Klein, M.D., Ph.D., Department of Neurology, Brigham and Women's Hospital and Harvard Medical School, Boston, Massachusetts.

EEG has two chief roles in medical psychiatry: evaluation of suspected toxic or metabolic encephalopathies and evaluation of seizures as a suspected cause of episodic cognitive or behavioral abnormalities. EEG changes associated with selected conditions pertinent to the medical psychiatrist are summarized in Table 4–5. Readers interested in a more thorough treatment of basic EEG interpretation, including normal morphology and clinical findings in neurological and medical disorders, are encouraged to seek out resources such as a basic EEG atlas (Misulis 2013) or a clinical primer (Boutros et al. 2011; Marcuse et al. 2016c).

In addition to standard EEG, EEG recording with simultaneous video recording (video EEG) is becoming increasingly available in hospitals. Video EEG is diagnostically useful in cases for which the temporal correlation of EEG findings to apparent seizure semiology needs to be ascertained. This information can be especially helpful in differentiating epileptic seizures from psychogenic nonepileptic seizures (discussed later in this section; see "Electroencephalography Findings in Specific Seizure Disorders").

TABLE 4–5.   **Electroencephalography (EEG) findings pertinent to medical psychiatry**

Condition	EEG findings
Diffuse encephalopathy (e.g., hepatic encephalopathy, uremia, electrolyte disturbance, anoxia, drug intoxication)	Generalized slowing: mild slowing (7–8 Hz, upper theta range), moderate slowing (4–7 Hz, mid theta range), or severe slowing (0–4 Hz, delta range) Slowing or absence of posterior dominant rhythm Triphasic wave (also known as generalized periodic discharges with triphasic morphology)
Antipsychotic treatment (more evident with clozapine or olanzapine than with risperidone or haloperidol; absent with quetiapine)	Generalized background slowing Paroxysmal theta or delta range activity Epileptiform activity (including spikes, sharp waves, spike-and-wave complexes, and sharp-and-slow-wave complexes)
Frontal lobe epilepsy	Interictal midline theta activity; interictal epileptiform discharges over the anterior head regions
Temporal lobe epilepsy	Interictal epileptiform discharges (usually sharp waves or sharp-and-slow-wave complexes) over the anterior temporal region
Nonconvulsive status epilepticus	Absence status epilepticus: 2–3 Hz spike-and-wave discharges (Meierkord and Holtkamp 2007); can range from 0.5 Hz to 4.0 Hz for late-onset absence status epilepticus in elderly patients (Thomas et al. 1992) Simple partial status epilepticus: Focal spike-and-wave discharges or evolving rhythmic activity (Meierkord and Holtkamp 2007); note that EEG may be normal during simple partial seizures Complex partial status epilepticus: Spike-and-wave discharges or evolving rhythmic activity; more distributed than in simple partial status epilepticus (Meierkord and Holtkamp 2007)
Psychogenic nonepileptic seizures	Normal EEG
Limbic encephalitis	Focal or generalized slowing, epileptiform activity; most pronounced in temporal regions in all of 22 patients in one study of paraneoplastic limbic encephalitis (Lawn et al. 2003) Extreme delta brush: Generalized rhythmic delta-frequency activity at 1.0–2.5 Hz, with superimposed beta-frequency activity (Schmitt et al. 2012); occurs with anti-*N*-methyl-D-aspartate receptor encephalitis and is associated with more prolonged illness (Schmitt et al. 2012)

Electroencephalography Findings in Diffuse Encephalopathies

Toxic and metabolic encephalopathies are very common and should be considered in the differential diagnosis of all acute mental status changes, especially those characterized by attentional deficits, waxing and waning time course, or behavioral hyper- or hypoactivity. In patients with an acute mental status change, an abnormal EEG result can help corroborate a clinical diagnosis of encephalopathy and thus usefully steer diagnostic attention away from other causes, including primary psychiatric conditions (in which EEG tracings typically are normal).

In normally mentating adults, the waking EEG is characterized by the presence of a *posterior dominant rhythm* (PDR) in the alpha frequency range (8–13 Hz), with maximal amplitude in the occipital regions. The PDR is most evident when the individual's eyes are closed, and the amplitude attenuates with eye opening. The PDR is generally greater than 8.5 Hz in normally mentating adults (Marcuse et al. 2016b), and slowing or disappearance of the PDR may be a marker of an encephalopathic process (however, slowing also may occur with normal drowsiness, and the PDR generally disappears entirely during sleep). As encephalopathy worsens, diffuse slowing of the EEG can be seen, although the level of slowing does not always correlate directly with the level of clinical impairment. The degree to which the primary background frequency slows below the normal alpha range in adults is classified as mild slowing (7–8 Hz, upper theta range), moderate slowing (4–7 Hz, mid theta range), or severe slowing (0–4 Hz, delta range) (Marcuse et al. 2016a). Diffuse slowing should be interpreted in its clinical context; far from being pathognomonic of diffuse encephalopathy, this finding can also be seen in drowsiness, severe dementia, or postictally, among other contexts. Focal slowing should be distinguished from diffuse slowing because it suggests underlying focal pathology. Focal slowing can occur postictally or interictally in patients with focal epilepsy, or it may occur in patients with structural lesions such as masses, focal infections (e.g., herpes simplex encephalitis), or strokes.

In addition to generalized slowing in encephalopathy, triphasic waves (also known as *generalized periodic discharges with triphasic morphology*) may become evident on EEG. Triphasic waves are most often described in the context of hepatic encephalopathy but can be present in any diffuse encephalopathic process, including uremia or acute electrolyte disturbance. Triphasic waves classically consist of three phases: negative (upgoing deflection), positive (downgoing deflection), and negative (upgoing deflection), with each successive phase in the triphasic complex longer than the previous phase; these complexes typically progress at 1.5–3 Hz (Smith 2005).

Figure 4–4 shows EEG patterns in a normally mentating adult and in a series of adults with encephalopathy.

Electroencephalography Findings in Specific Seizure Disorders

EEG can be useful in the evaluation of seizures as a suspected cause of psychiatric abnormalities, especially episodic phenomena. An important limitation of EEG is that EEG is specific for seizures when ictal (seizure) activity is detected, but the lack of ictal activity on EEG does not rule out seizures. It is also important to note that EEG is less

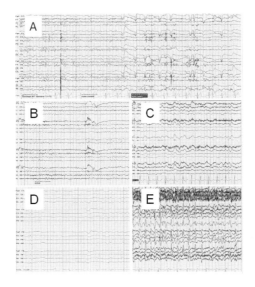

FIGURE 4–4. Electroencephalogram (EEG) patterns in a normally mentating adult and in a series of adults with encephalopathy.

(A) Normal EEG result in a patient with eyes closed, showing a posterior dominant alpha rhythm. Halfway through this tracing, the patient's eyes opened, and the posterior dominant rhythm attenuated. Varying degrees of slowing in patients with **(B)** mild, **(C)** moderate, and **(D)** severe encephalopathy. **(E)** Triphasic waves, or generalized periodic discharges with a triphasic morphology.

Source. Courtesy of Daniel S. Weisholtz, M.D., Department of Neurology, Brigham and Women's Hospital and Harvard Medical School, Boston, Massachusetts.

sensitive in detecting ictal activity in deeper brain structures as compared with in-surface structures. Additionally, evaluation of patients with EEG often relies on detection of interictal abnormalities on EEG rather than capturing seizure events directly; a seizure may not occur while an EEG is being recorded, but interictal abnormalities may be present.

Frontal lobe epilepsy (FLE), temporal lobe epilepsy (TLE), and nonconvulsive status epilepticus (NCSE) all may present with psychiatric complaints and thus should be included in the differential diagnosis of patients with behavioral, affective, or perceptual symptoms.

TLE may be characterized on EEG by interictal paroxysmal activity consisting of sharp- and slow-wave complexes, most often seen over the anterior or temporal head regions (Figure 4–5). A significant number of patients may have bilateral anterior or temporal discharges interictally, but in unilateral TLE, such discharges tend to predominate on the side of the seizure focus (Williamson et al. 1993). Temporal lobe seizures are characterized on EEG by a buildup of sharp waves or evolving rhythmic activity lateralized to the side of seizure origin and maximal (at least early on in the seizure) over the temporal head region (Williamson et al. 1993).

FLE may be missed on surface EEG because of muscle artifact and relative depth of the epileptic focus within the frontal lobe sulci. One-third of FLE patients have a normal or nonspecific EEG correlate in both ictal and interictal periods (Bagla and Skidmore 2011; Gold et al. 2016). Half of patients with FLE will have rhythmic mid-

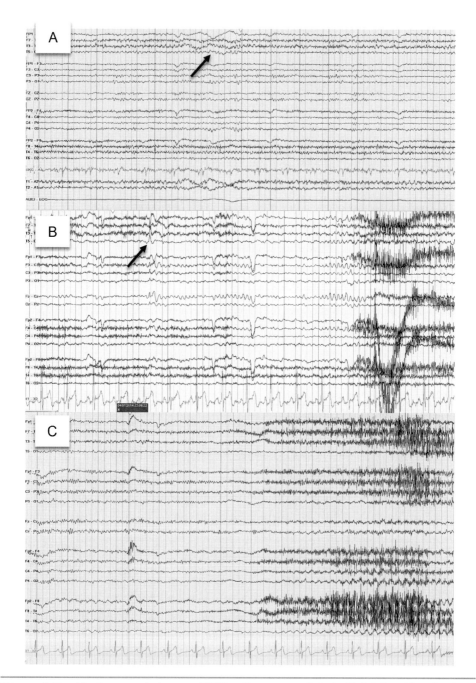

FIGURE 4–5.   Electroencephalogram (EEG) patterns associated with ictal and interictal activity in adults with temporal lobe epilepsy (TLE).

(A) Left-temporal delta waves *(arrow)* (seen in the left-sided or odd-numbered leads) in the interictal period in a patient with left temporal lobe epilepsy. **(B)** Left-temporal interictal sharp-and-slow-wave complex *(arrow)* in the interictal period in a different patient with temporal lobe epilepsy. **(C)** Patient with a right-sided temporal lobe epileptic seizure initiating approximately halfway through the tracing, seen predominantly over the right (even-numbered) hemispheric leads, with subsequent spread to the left side.

Source.   Courtesy of Daniel S. Weisholtz, M.D., Department of Neurology, Brigham and Women's Hospital and Harvard Medical School, Boston, Massachusetts.

line theta activity interictally, and many patients will have interictal epileptiform discharges, although these are often diffuse or generalized and without localizing value (Beleza and Pinho 2011; Gold et al. 2016).

NCSE refers to continuous seizure activity in the absence of frank motor signs of epilepsy; this activity presents diversely, depending on the affected brain areas. The neuropsychiatric presentations of NCSE include fluctuating levels of consciousness, disorientation, confusion, mood alterations, hallucinations (across a range of sensory modalities), and behavioral changes ranging from automatisms to behavioral disinhibition (Meierkord and Holtkamp 2007). Given its diverse presentations and the importance of prompt treatment, NCSE should be considered in the differential diagnosis for neuropsychiatric patients suspected of having metabolic encephalopathy, primary psychiatric disorders, or substance intoxication, particularly those patients with a fluctuating course, a history of frank seizures, or persistent impairments in consciousness without a known structural cause (Meierkord and Holtkamp 2007). EEG findings in NCSE reveal prolonged or recurrent seizure activity, although specific patterns may vary, depending on the seizure subtype and the localization of seizure focus (Meierkord and Holtkamp 2007; see Table 4–5 for a summary of EEG findings associated with specific forms of NCSE).

Psychogenic nonepileptic seizures (PNES), a form of functional neurological symptom disorder (conversion disorder) characterized by spells of motor or behavioral activity resembling epileptic seizures, are best diagnosed with video EEG. The absence of an EEG change in the midst of a symptomatic episode, together with signs suggestive of a psychogenic seizure (including preserved awareness during a bilateral motor event, eye closing or eye fluttering, asynchronous movements, waxing-and-waning semiology within the course of an episode), supports the diagnosis of PNES (Baslet et al. 2016). Care must be taken to avoid misdiagnosing PNES in patients experiencing epileptic seizures that might not have a clear EEG correlate, such as simple partial seizures or frontal lobe seizures (see also Chapter 25, "Somatic Symptom and Related Disorders").

Electroencephalographic Abnormalities in Patients Taking Antipsychotics

Clinicians referring patients for EEG or interpreting EEG results should be aware that patients under treatment with antipsychotic medications may have altered EEG profiles. For example, one relevant study that blindly evaluated EEG tracings in a cohort of 323 hospitalized psychiatric inpatients reported a differential risk of EEG abnormalities among antipsychotic agents, with the highest rate of abnormality with clozapine (47.1%), followed by olanzapine (38.5%), risperidone (28.0%), first-generation antipsychotics (14.5%), and quetiapine (0.0%) (Centorrino et al. 2002). These risks were amplified by hypertension, bipolarity, and older age. In the case of clozapine and olanzapine, the rate of EEG abnormalities is dose dependent (Amann et al. 2003; Leppig et al. 1989). EEG findings described in patients under antipsychotic treatment include generalized background slowing, increases in paroxysmal theta- or delta-range slowing, and epileptiform activity (including the appearance of spikes, sharp waves, spike-and-wave complexes, and sharp-and-slow-wave complexes) (Amann et al. 2003).

Electroencephalography Findings in Limbic Encephalitis

EEG findings in limbic encephalitis are presented in the section "Neuroimaging, Electroencephalography, and Lumbar Puncture in Limbic Encephalitides" later in this chapter.

Lumbar Puncture

Background

Lumbar puncture is performed in medical and neurological settings to obtain CSF for analysis, which has a diagnostic role in the workup of central nervous system (CNS) infections and neuroinflammatory illnesses (including limbic encephalitides, multiple sclerosis, and neurosarcoidosis). In the acute setting, lumbar puncture is done to evaluate for suspected meningitis in a patient presenting with acute headache.

Lumbar puncture is performed by passing a needle between two lumbar vertebrae, below the level at which the spinal cord terminates, through superficial tissues and meningeal layers into the subarachnoid space to obtain CSF, at which point a CSF opening pressure can be measured if needed to assess for intracranial hypertension. CSF is subsequently analyzed with laboratory studies as indicated, which in the case of suspected CNS infection can include cell count and differential, Gram's stain (and other bacterial and fungal stains as appropriate), glucose and protein concentrations, cytology, bacterial and fungal cultures, polymerase chain reactions (PCRs) for viral nucleic acids, and testing for specific antigens and antibodies (Table 4–6).

Psychiatrists do not routinely request lumbar puncture. CSF analysis has no accepted role in the diagnosis of primary psychiatric disorders; however, patients whose psychiatric symptoms are suspected to be associated with another medical disorder or whose clinical course appears atypical may be candidates for lumbar puncture. Psychiatrists may suggest lumbar puncture in a consultative or an inpatient setting to rule out infectious illness (e.g., meningoencephalitis) or inflammatory processes (e.g., limbic encephalitides). Contraindications to lumbar puncture include increased intracranial pressure resulting from intracranial mass lesions (in which case lumbar puncture carries a risk of uncal, transtentorial, or cerebellar tonsillar herniation due to pressure gradients), coagulopathy (bleeding diathesis), and skin infection or abscess at the puncture site.

Although lumbar puncture does not currently play a role in the evaluation of primary psychiatric disorders, biochemical changes in CSF have been observed in psychiatric conditions. Notable in this regard is a well-known Swedish study that found an association between decreased levels of the serotonin metabolite 5-hydroxyindoleacetic acid (5-HIAA) and risk of attempting suicide and also of using more violent means to attempt suicide (Åsberg et al. 1976).

TABLE 4–6. Cerebrospinal fluid (CSF) studies and their diagnostic utility

CSF study	Diagnostic utility
Cell count and differential	Red blood cell count: evaluation of subarachnoid hemorrhage (should differentiate from traumatic lumbar puncture; xanthrochromia will be present in subarachnoid hemorrhage) White blood cell count: screening for infection (leukocytosis); differential with high polymorphonuclear leukocytes suggests bacterial infection; lymphocytes suggest viral, fungal, or mycobacterial infection
Protein concentration	Elevated CSF protein: increased permeability of the blood-brain barrier
Glucose concentration	Identification of infectious pathogen Viral infection: normal glucose Bacterial, fungal, or mycobacterial infection: decreased glucose
Staining	Gram's stain: for bacterial organisms Acid-fast stain: for mycobacteria India ink: for fungal organisms
Bacterial or fungal cultures	Identification of infectious pathogen Antibiotic sensitivity testing
Polymerase chain reaction (PCR)	Diagnosis of viral central nervous system infections, including encephalitis due to herpes simplex virus 1 or 2 (HSV-1 or HSV-2 PCR) and encephalitis due to varicella zoster virus (VZV PCR) or Epstein-Barr virus (EBV PCR)
Cytology	Cytopathological evaluation of intracerebral or leptomeningeal infiltration
Oligoclonal bands	Diagnostic evaluation of multiple sclerosis and other diseases characterized by intrathecal antibody production
Angiotensin converting enzyme	Diagnostic evaluation of neurosarcoidosis (poorly sensitive)
Specific antigen	Testing for specific fungal antigens (e.g., cryptococcal and histoplasma polysaccharides)
Specific antibodies	Testing for antibodies to viral pathogens (e.g., HSV, VZV) Testing for paraneoplastic or autoimmune antibodies associated with limbic encephalitides

Lumbar Puncture in Suspected Central Nervous System Infections

Lumbar puncture plays a critical role in the diagnosis of CNS infections, which can present with altered mentation ranging from decreased arousal to confused agitation (encephalopathy), along with other symptoms based on the specific pathogen and its dissemination through nervous and meningeal systems.

Psychiatrists working in a consultative, emergency, or inpatient setting should maintain a high index of suspicion for meningitis when assessing altered mental status, because untreated meningitis can be lethal within a very short time. Meningitis manifests with headache together with fever, nuchal rigidity, and altered mental status and should be suspected when two or more of these signs or symptoms are present. Meningitis should be considered alongside intracranial hemorrhage in a patient with headache and altered mentation. Lumbar puncture should be performed urgently if altered mentation manifests with fever or nuchal rigidity. Patients with suspected meningitis in whom lumbar puncture cannot be done in a timely fashion must be treated empirically. Of note, not all patients with meningitis experience headache, and patients with altered mental status may be unable to report reliably whether headache is present. When lumbar puncture can be performed, CSF studies can be useful in distinguishing among bacterial, viral, and fungal etiologies of meningeal and encephalitic infections (Roos 2015).

Lumbar puncture is also important in the diagnosis of infectious encephalitis to identify a causative organism. Infectious encephalitis is most often viral, with herpesviruses, including herpes simplex viruses 1 and 2 (HSV-1, HSV-2), and varicella zoster virus (VZV) being the most common. PCRs, used to amplify small amounts of viral nucleic acids present in CSF to detectable quantities, are important in the definitive diagnosis of viral encephalitis. Other causes of infectious encephalitis include enteroviruses; bacteria, including mycobacteria; and fungal organisms. CSF staining; bacterial and fungal cultures; CSF glucose levels, especially when markedly reduced in comparison with simultaneous blood glucose levels; CSF protein; and testing for specific antibodies (e.g., fungal polysaccharides) or antibodies associated with CNS infections all play a role in the workup of infectious encephalitis or meningitis (see Table 4–6).

Neuroimaging, Electroencephalography, and Lumbar Puncture in Limbic Encephalitides

Background

Limbic encephalitides are a group of inflammatory brain conditions characterized by temporolimbic inflammation, which can be driven by an increasingly well-documented range of autoimmune, paraneoplastic, or postinfectious etiologies. Limbic encephalitides manifest with diverse constellations of focal neurological and diffuse encephalopathic changes but most often have presentations involving sequelae of limbic dysfunction, including amnesia, confusion, seizures (temporal or generalized), and psychosis (Kayser and Dalmau 2011). Other prominent signs can include catatonic features, such as malignant catatonia, dyskinesias, autonomic instability, and hypoventilation requiring intubation (Kayser and Dalmau 2011). Neuroimaging, EEG, and CSF analysis all have a role in the diagnostic evaluation of limbic encephalitides (Table 4–7; Figure 4–6).

Neuroimaging

Neuroimaging can contribute to a diagnosis of limbic encephalitis, with unilateral or bilateral medial temporal lobe abnormalities being the most commonly cited finding (see Figure 4–6). In a serial MRI study of a heterogeneous group of 20 individuals with limbic encephalitis, Urbach et al. (2006) described a pattern of unilateral or bilateral medial temporal lobe swelling and hyperintensity on T2-weighted sequences. Different forms of limbic encephalitides are associated with different levels of MRI abnormalities; notably, anti–*N*-methyl-D-aspartate receptor (anti-NMDAR) encephalitis was associated with a normal initial MRI scan in more than 60% of cases in a study of 540 patients with anti-NMDAR encephalitis and available MRI data (Titulaer et al. 2013).

PET studies of patients with paraneoplastic encephalitis similarly indicate temporal lobe hypermetabolism (Basu and Alavi 2008), and mesial temporal lobe hypermetabolism has been described in autoimmune encephalitis (and appears to be more common with antibodies directed at intracellular rather than extracellular antigens) (Baumgartner et al. 2013). Whole-body PET may play an additional role in helping to confirm suspected paraneoplastic varieties of autoimmune encephalitis, because it can identify an unknown primary malignancy or metastases.

Electroencephalography

EEG is an important component of the diagnostic evaluation of suspected paraneoplastic or autoimmune encephalitis. In one study of 22 patients with paraneoplastic limbic encephalitis, all 22 patients showed EEG abnormalities (focal or generalized slowing or epileptiform activity that was most pronounced in temporal regions) (Lawn et al. 2003). In a large study that included EEG data on 482 patients with anti-NMDAR encephalitis, 90% of the patients had an abnormal EEG finding (Titulaer et al. 2013). Of note, a distinct EEG pattern termed *extreme delta brush* activity has been described in patients with anti-NMDAR encephalitis, occurring often in comatose patients, and is associated with prolonged disease (Schmitt et al. 2012).

Cerebrospinal Fluid Antibodies

CSF should be screened for antibodies associated with paraneoplastic and autoimmune encephalitides when limbic encephalitis is suspected. Although all patients with suspected limbic encephalitis should be screened for serum antibodies as well, CSF screening is important because serum testing may be negative when CSF screening is positive, or CSF may have higher antibody titers than serum; this is especially true for limbic encephalitis that is associated with antibodies expressed at the level of the cell membrane (e.g., anti-NMDAR encephalitis) (Gresa-Arribas et al. 2014).

TABLE 4–7.   Characteristic findings in limbic encephalitides

Diagnostic modality	Potential findings in limbic encephalitis
Magnetic resonance imaging	Medial temporal lobe swelling and hyperintensity on T2-weighted sequences Can appear normal in some cases
^{18}F-Fluorodeoxyglucose positron emission tomography	Temporal lobe hypermetabolism in paraneoplastic encephalitis (Basu and Alavi 2008) Mesial temporal lobe hypermetabolism; appears more commonly in autoimmune encephalitis with antibodies to intracellular antigen than with antibodies to extracellular antigen (Baumgartner et al. 2013)
Electroencephalography	Focal or generalized slowing, epileptiform activity; most pronounced in temporal regions in all of 22 patients in one study of paraneoplastic limbic encephalitis (Lawn et al. 2003) Extreme delta brush: Generalized rhythmic delta-frequency activity at 1.0–2.5 Hz, with superimposed beta-frequency activity (Schmitt et al. 2012); occurs with anti-N-methyl-D-aspartate receptor encephalitis and is associated with more prolonged illness (Schmitt et al. 2012)
Lumbar puncture	Cerebrospinal fluid antibodies: Growing roster of antibodies (to both intracellular and extracellular antigens) have been identified that are associated with paraneoplastic disease or autoimmune etiology without malignancy

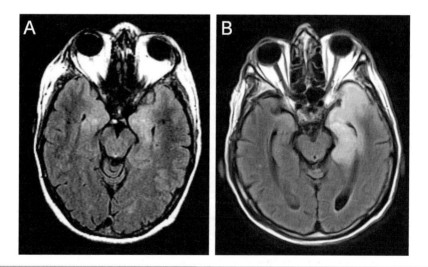

FIGURE 4–6.   Magnetic resonance imaging findings in limbic encephalitis.

Limbic encephalitis can be associated with infectious and noninfectious inflammatory etiologies. (A) A case of paraneoplastic limbic encephalitis is shown on axial T2-weighted fluid-attenuated inverse recovery magnetic resonance imaging, with abnormal symmetrical hyperintensity of medial temporal structures. This patient was found to have voltage-gated potassium channel antibodies and a thymoma. (B) Unilateral hyperintensity is seen in a different patient with herpes simplex virus 1 (HSV-1) encephalitis. *Source.*   Provided by author Joshua P. Klein, M.D., Ph.D., Department of Neurology, Brigham and Women's Hospital and Harvard Medical School, Boston, Massachusetts.

Conclusion

Neuroimaging, EEG, and lumbar puncture each play an important role in the workup of medical or neurological causes of neuropsychiatric presentations in the medical psychiatry patient population. Familiarity with the indications, clinical applications, advantages, and limitations of each diagnostic modality facilitates appropriate testing and enhances quality of care.

References

Amann BL, Pogarell O, Mergl R, et al: EEG abnormalities associated with antipsychotics: a comparison of quetiapine, olanzapine, haloperidol and healthy subjects. Hum Psychopharmacol 18(8):641–646, 2003 14696024

American College of Radiology: ACR Practice Guideline for the Use of Intravascular Contrast Media. Reston, VA, American College of Radiology, 2007

American College of Radiology: ACR Practice Guideline for Imaging Pregnant or Potentially Pregnant Adolescents and Women With Ionizing Radiation. Reston, VA, American College of Radiology, 2008

American Psychiatric Association: Diagnostic and Statistical Manual of Mental Disorders, 5th Edition. Arlington, VA, American Psychiatric Association, 2013

Åsberg M, Träskman L, Thorén P: 5-HIAA in the cerebrospinal fluid: a biochemical suicide predictor? Arch Gen Psychiatry 33(10):1193–1197, 1976 971028

Bagla R, Skidmore CT: Frontal lobe seizures. Neurologist 17(3):125–135, 2011

Barber R, Gholkar A, Scheltens P, et al: Medial temporal lobe atrophy on MRI in dementia with Lewy bodies. Neurology 52(6):1153–1158, 1999 10214736

Baslet G, Seshadri A, Bermeo-Ovalle A, et al: Psychogenic non-epileptic seizures: an updated primer. Psychosomatics 57(1):1–17, 2016 26791511

Basu S, Alavi A: Role of FDG-PET in the clinical management of paraneoplastic neurological syndrome: detection of the underlying malignancy and the brain PET-MRI correlates. Mol Imaging Biol 10(3):131–137, 2008 18297363

Baumgartner A, Rauer S, Mader I, et al: Cerebral FDG-PET and MRI findings in autoimmune limbic encephalitis: correlation with autoantibody types. J Neurol 260(11):2744–2753, 2013 23900756

Beleza P, Pinho J: Frontal lobe epilepsy. J Clin Neurosci 18(5):593–600, 2011 21349720

Boccardi M, Laakso MP, Bresciani L, et al: The MRI pattern of frontal and temporal brain atrophy in fronto-temporal dementia. Neurobiol Aging 24(1):95–103, 2003 12493555

Boutros N, Galderisi S, Pogarell O, et al: Standard Electroencephalography in Clinical Psychiatry. Chichester, UK, Wiley-Blackwell, 2011

Castillo M, Kwock L, Mukherji SK: Clinical applications of proton MR spectroscopy. AJNR Am J Neuroradiol 17(1):1–15, 1996 8770242

Centorrino F, Price BH, Tuttle M, et al: EEG abnormalities during treatment with typical and atypical antipsychotics. Am J Psychiatry 159(1):109–115, 2002 11772698

Frisoni GB, Beltramello A, Geroldi C, et al: Brain atrophy in frontotemporal dementia. J Neurol Neurosurg Psychiatry 61(2):157–165, 1996 8708683

Gold JA, Sher Y, Maldonado JR: Frontal lobe epilepsy: a primer for psychiatrists and a systematic review of psychiatric manifestations. Psychosomatics 57(5):445–464, 2016 27494984

Gresa-Arribas N, Titulaer MJ, Torrents A, et al: Antibody titres at diagnosis and during follow-up of anti-NMDA receptor encephalitis: a retrospective study. Lancet Neurol 13(2):167–177, 2014 24360484

Jansen WJ, Ossenkoppele R, Knol DL, et al: Prevalence of cerebral amyloid pathology in persons without dementia: a meta-analysis. JAMA 313(19):1924–1938, 2015 25988462

Kanal E, Barkovich AJ, Bell C, et al: ACR guidance document for safe MR practices: 2007. AJR Am J Roentgenol 188(6):1447–1474, 2007 17515363

Kayser MS, Dalmau J: The emerging link between autoimmune disorders and neuropsychiatric disease. J Neuropsychiatry Clin Neurosci 23(1):90–97, 2011 21304144

Lawn ND, Westmoreland BF, Kiely MJ, et al: Clinical, magnetic resonance imaging, and elec-troencephalographic findings in paraneoplastic limbic encephalitis. Mayo Clin Proc 78(11):1363–1368, 2003 14601695

Leppig M, Bosch B, Naber D, et al: Clozapine in the treatment of 121 out-patients. Psychophar-macology (Berl) 99 (suppl):S77–S79, 1989 2813669

Lobo A, Launer LJ, Fratiglioni L, et al: Prevalence of dementia and major subtypes in Europe: a collaborative study of population-based cohorts. Neurologic Diseases in the Elderly Re-search Group. Neurology 54 (11 suppl 5):S4–S9, 2000 10854354

Lyoo IK, Renshaw PF: Magnetic resonance spectroscopy: current and future applications in psychiatric research. Biol Psychiatry 51(3):195–207, 2000 11839362

Marcuse LV, Fields MC, Yoo J: The abnormal EEG, in Rowan's Primer of EEG, 2nd Edition. Lon-don, Elsevier, 2016a, pp 87–119

Marcuse LV, Fields MC, Yoo J: The normal adult EEG, in Rowan's Primer of EEG, 2nd Edition. London, Elsevier, 2016b, pp 39–66

Marcuse LV, Fields MC, Yoo J: Rowan's Primer of EEG, 2nd Edition. London, Elsevier, 2016c

McDonald CR, McEvoy LK, Gharapetian L, et al: Regional rates of neocortical atrophy from normal aging to early Alzheimer disease. Neurology 73(6):457–465, 2009 19667321

McKeith I, O'Brien J, Walker Z, et al: Sensitivity and specificity of dopamine transporter imag-ing with 123I-FP-CIT SPECT in dementia with Lewy bodies: a phase III, multicentre study. Lancet Neurol 6(4):305–313, 2007 17362834

Meierkord H, Holtkamp M: Non-convulsive status epilepticus in adults: clinical forms and treatment. Lancet Neurol 6(4):329–339, 2007 17362837

Misulis EK: Atlas of EEG, Seizure Semiology, and Management. New York, Oxford University Press, 2013

Mortimer AM, Likeman M, Lewis TT: Neuroimaging in dementia: a practical guide. Pract Neu-rol 13(2):92–103, 2013 23468560

Nensa F, Beiderwellen K, Heusch P, et al: Clinical applications of PET/MRI: current status and future perspectives. Diagn Interv Radiol 20(5):438–447, 2014 25010371

Ogawa S, Lee TM, Kay AR, et al: Brain magnetic resonance imaging with contrast dependent on blood oxygenation. Proc Natl Acad Sci U S A 87(24):9868–9872, 1990 2124706

Perani D, Della Rosa PA, Cerami C, et al: Validation of an optimized SPM procedure for FDG-PET in dementia diagnosis in a clinical setting. Neuroimage Clin 6:445–454, 2014 25389519

Prince M, Bryce R, Albanese E, et al: The global prevalence of dementia: a systematic review and meta-analysis. Alzheimers Dement 9(1):63–75, 2013 23305823

Román GC, Tatemichi TK, Erkinjuntti T, et al: Vascular dementia: diagnostic criteria for re-search studies. Report of the NINDS-AIREN International Workshop. Neurology 43(2):250–260, 1993 8094895

Roos KL: Bacterial infections of the central nervous system. Continuum (Minneap Minn) 21 (6 Neuroinfectious Disease):1679–1691, 2015 26633782

Scheltens P, Leys D, Barkhof F, et al: Atrophy of medial temporal lobes on MRI in "probable" Alzheimer's disease and normal ageing: diagnostic value and neuropsychological cor-relates. J Neurol Neurosurg Psychiatry 55(10):967–972, 1992 1431963

Scheltens P, Blennow K, Breteler MM, et al: Alzheimer's disease. Lancet 388(10043):505–517, 2016 26921134

Schmitt SE, Pargeon K, Frechette ES, et al: Extreme delta brush: a unique EEG pattern in adults with anti-NMDA receptor encephalitis. Neurology 79(11):1094–1100, 2012 22933737

Singhal T, Weiner HL, Bakshi R: TSPO-PET imaging to assess cerebral microglial activation in multiple sclerosis. Semin Neurol 37(5):546–557, 2017 29207414

Smith SJ: EEG in neurological conditions other than epilepsy: when does it help, what does it add? J Neurol Neurosurg Psychiatry 76 (suppl 2):ii8–ii12, 2005 15961870

Thomas P, Beaumanoir A, Genton P, et al: "De novo" absence status of late onset: report of 11 cases. Neurology 42(1):104–110, 1992 1734289

Titulaer MJ, McCracken L, Gabilondo I, et al: Treatment and prognostic factors for long-term outcome in patients with anti-NMDA receptor encephalitis: an observational cohort study. Lancet Neurol 12(2):157–165, 2013 23290630

Urbach H, Soeder BM, Jeub M, et al: Serial MRI of limbic encephalitis. Neuroradiology 48(6):380–386, 2006 16586118

Vann Jones SA, O'Brien JT: The prevalence and incidence of dementia with Lewy bodies: a systematic review of population and clinical studies. Psychol Med 44(4):673–683, 2014 23521899

Villemagne VL, Pike KE, Chételat G, et al: Longitudinal assessment of β and cognition in aging and Alzheimer disease. Ann Neurol 69(1):181–192, 2011 21280088

Whitwell JL, Josephs KA: Neuroimaging in frontotemporal lobar degeneration—predicting molecular pathology. Nat Rev Neurol 8(3):131–142, 2012 22290573

Whitwell JL, Przybelski SA, Weigand SD, et al: 3D maps from multiple MRI illustrate changing atrophy patterns as subjects progress from mild cognitive impairment to Alzheimer's disease. Brain 130(pt 7):1777–1786, 2007 17533169

Williamson PD, French JA, Thadani VM, et al: Characteristics of medial temporal lobe epilepsy, II: interictal and ictal scalp electroencephalography, neuropsychological testing, neuroimaging, surgical results, and pathology. Ann Neurol 34(6):781–787, 1993 8250526

Womack KB, Diaz-Arrastia R, Aizenstein HJ, et al: Temporoparietal hypometabolism in frontotemporal lobar degeneration and associated imaging diagnostic errors. Arch Neurol 68(3):329–337, 2011 21059987

CHAPTER 5

Toxicological Exposures and Nutritional Deficiencies in the Psychiatric Patient

Mira Zein, M.D., M.P.H.

Sharmin Khan, M.D.

Jaswinder Legha, M.D., M.P.H.

Lloyd Wasserman, M.D.

Consultants are frequently called to determine the possible contribution of psychotropic medications and other exposures to neuropsychiatric findings, other toxicities, and laboratory abnormalities. Often, physicians—including internists, emergency medicine physicians, and psychiatrists—are the first to encounter patients with neuropsychiatric symptoms, and they are faced with identifying underlying causative factors. This chapter begins with a presentation of the neuropsychiatric toxidromes caused by psychotropic medications: neuroleptic malignant syndrome (NMS), serotonin syndrome, anticholinergic toxicity, and valproate-induced hyperammonemic encephalopathy (VHE). The next section proceeds with a discussion of neuropsychiatric toxidromes caused by street drugs and environmental exposures and psychiatric findings associated with specific micronutrient deficiencies. The final section of the chapter provides an overview of selected important adverse effects of psychiatric medications, including hyponatremia, acquired long QT syndrome, drug-induced liver injury (DILI), and orthostatic hypotension. The chapter closes with an appendix table summarizing relevant laboratory investigations in a patient presenting with psychiatric symptoms.

Altered Mental Status Caused by Psychotropic Medications

Neuroleptic Malignant Syndrome

NMS is a relatively uncommon, life-threatening, idiosyncratic reaction to antipsychotic drugs and other dopamine antagonists (at therapeutic dosages) characterized by fever, altered mental status, muscle rigidity, and autonomic dysfunction. In most cases, onset usually occurs within 1–2 weeks of starting or restarting an antipsychotic drug or other dopamine antagonist. It may also be provoked by withdrawal of a dopaminergic agonist.

Epidemiology and Risk Factors

In prospective studies, NMS occurs in 0.24–13.45 out of every 1,000 patients at risk. A recent meta-analysis of available epidemiological data found an overall estimate of 0.991 cases per 1,000 people; the pooled risk from all included studies was 0.1% (Tse et al. 2015). NMS is more common in men than women, and the peak age of diagnosis is 25 years. It occurs with all antipsychotics, but the risk is greatest with high-potency first-generation agents (e.g., haloperidol) (Berman 2011; Tse et al. 2015). High doses, depot preparations, rapid dosage escalation, use of more than one antipsychotic agent, and a history of previous NMS predispose to this condition. NMS-like syndromes can occur after withdrawal of levodopa and other dopaminergic agents and during treatment with lithium, tricyclic antidepressants (TCAs), monoamine oxidase inhibitors (MAOIs), or serotonin reuptake inhibitors (Berman 2011; Tse et al. 2015).

Clinical Presentation and Diagnosis

Symptoms may appear within hours of exposure to the offending antipsychotic. Half or more of all cases develop within 1 week and 75%–96% within 30 days. Once symptoms appear, progression can be rapid and can reach peak intensity in as little as 3 days (Tse et al. 2015). The clinical course typically begins with muscle rigidity and progresses to fever and mental status changes and autonomic instability; however, the clinical presentation can be heterogeneous. Muscle rigidity ranges from generalized to symmetrical with variations in increased tone (at extremes causing opisthotonus). Focal increases of tone can occur as part of extrapyramidal findings, trismus, blepharospasm, and oculogyric crisis (Berman 2011; Tse et al. 2015). Additional extrapyramidal symptoms that have been reported include tremor, chorea, and akinesia. Autonomic instability symptoms include labile blood pressure, heart rate changes, tachypnea, tachycardia, extreme diaphoresis, flushing, incontinence, and sialorrhea (Berman 2011; Tse et al. 2015). Other findings may include dysphagia, dyspnea, abnormal reflexes, mutism, and seizures (Berman 2011). Delirium is the most common mental status change, with manifestations including varying levels of confusion, drowsiness to alertness, and agitation. Patients can progress to severe delirium or coma (Berman 2011; Tse et al. 2015).

There is no gold standard for diagnosis of NMS, and there are several different existing sets of diagnostic criteria (Tse et al. 2015). In 2011, an international panel of experts published a scoring system validated in later studies (Table 5–1) (Gurrera et al. 2011, 2017). Given the syndromic nature of this diagnosis and the lack of a gold standard, diagnosis of NMS will depend on a thorough clinical history (including a detailed drug history), a detailed physical examination, and a comprehensive initial laboratory workup.

Typical laboratory findings include an increased white blood cell (WBC) count, increased creatine kinase (usually above 1,000 IU/L), and abnormal liver enzymes (Table 5–2). Myoglobinuria due to the muscle injury associated with the syndrome (and reflected in the increased creatinine kinase) can cause acute kidney injury. Disseminated intravascular coagulation (DIC) may result in thrombocytopenia, schistocytes, prolongation of partial thromboplastin time and prothrombin time, and increased fibrin degradation products (Tse et al. 2015).

Differential Diagnosis

Toxicological causes of syndromes similar to NMS include the serotonin syndrome; anticholinergic toxicity; lithium intoxication; central nervous system (CNS) stimulant use (particularly cocaine, amphetamine, and amphetamine-like agents); and drug-induced malignant catatonia. Nontoxicological syndromes with overlapping features include heat stroke, CNS infection, anti–*N*-methyl-D-aspartate (NMDA) receptor encephalitis, and non-drug-induced malignant catatonia. No laboratory test result is diagnostic for NMS (Berman 2011; Tse et al. 2015).

Treatment

NMS is a neurological emergency. Delay in treatment can result in serious morbidity or death. It may be prudent to treat for NMS even if there is doubt about the diagnosis (Berman 2011; Katus and Frucht 2016; Susman 2001; Tse et al. 2015).

Supportive Therapy

- Discontinue the offending dopamine antagonist immediately.
- In cases caused by withdrawal of dopamine agonists (levodopa, bromocriptine, amantadine), restart these agents immediately.
- Rule out other causes of rigidity, hyperthermia, or altered mental status.
- Aggressive IV hydration with careful monitoring is required; large insensible fluid losses may increase risk of acute kidney injury due to prerenal failure and rhabdomyolysis.
- Initiate mechanical cooling for hyperthermia. Acetaminophen and nonsteroidal anti-inflammatory drugs (NSAIDs) are usually ineffective.
- Anticholinergic agents can impair heat dissipation. Many would recommend tapering these off, but they should be tapered carefully; cholinergic rebound may exacerbate NMS.
- Anticipate common complications of NMS and institute prophylactic measures or monitoring. These complications include renal failure and DIC secondary to rhabdomyolysis; seizures; deep venous thrombosis and pulmonary embolism; respiratory failure; aspiration pneumonia; and sepsis. Other documented medical complications include cardiopulmonary failure, arrhythmias, and myocardial infarction (Berman 2011).

TABLE 5–1.   Consensus criteria for neuroleptic malignant syndrome

Clinical finding	Score[a]	Comments
Administration of dopamine antagonist or withdrawal of dopamine agonist within the previous 72 hours.	20	
Temperature >100.4°F at least twice	18	Oral temperature
Rigidity	17	Rigidity may manifest as mild symmetrical nonfocal increased muscle tone on a continuum to severe lead pipe rigidity. Other extrapyramidal signs may be present as well, including tremor, cogwheel rigidity, dystonia, etc.
Change in mental status	13	
Creatine kinase ≥four times the upper limit of normal	10	
Sympathetic nervous system lability, defined by two or more of the following: SBP or DBP ≥25% above baseline ≥25 mm SBP change or ≥20 mm DBP change within the previous 24 hours Diaphoresis Urinary incontinence	10	
Hypermetabolism: Heart rate ≥25% and respiratory rate ≥50% above baseline	5	
Negative evaluation for other causes of presentation (infectious, toxic, metabolic, and neurological)	7	For example, encephalitis, sepsis, CNS stimulant toxicity, serotonin syndrome, hyperthyroidism

Note. CNS=central nervous system; DBP=diastolic blood pressure; SBP=systolic blood pressure.
[a]The cut point for a positive test is >74 points.
Source. Adapted from Gurrera et al. 2011 (Table 1, p. 1225) and Gurrera et al. 2017 (Table 1, p. 68).

TABLE 5–2. Diagnostic evaluation in neuroleptic malignant syndrome (NMS)

Laboratory/other tests	Indications
Complete blood count, PT/PTT	Assess for infection as cause of delirium and fever Monitor for DIC
Blood cultures/urine culture	Assess for infection as cause of delirium and fever
Serum iron concentration	Assess for low serum iron, which is often cited as a sensitive marker for NMS; however, limitations in study design, small sample sizes, and conflicting data make this conclusion premature. It is not clear whether serum iron, a negative acute-phase reactant, is capable of distinguishing NMS from other equally severe illnesses (Lee 1998; Rosebush and Mazurek 1991; Weller and Kornhuber 1993).
CK, urine myoglobin level, LFTs, calcium and phosphate levels, BUN, and creatinine	Assess for rhabdomyolysis (with associated electrolyte abnormalities and acute kidney injury) caused by NMS rigidity and hyperthermia
Arterial blood gas, serum sodium, serum chloride, serum bicarbonate (total CO_2)	Assess for respiratory failure from hypoventilation caused by rigidity, aspiration, or adverse effects of therapeutic agents Assess for anion gap acidosis caused by complications of NMS or other agents contributing to delirium and hyperthermia
CSF evaluation: Cell count, protein, glucose, bacteriology; HSV PCR, immunoglobulin G anti-GluN1 antibodies (for anti-NMDAR receptor encephalitis)	Assess for CNS infection or autoimmune encephalitis as cause of presentation
Electrocardiogram	Assess for cardiovascular complications Screen for electrocardiographic signs of coingestants
Serum or urine toxicological screening (cocaine, amphetamines, phencyclidine, opiates, benzodiazepine)	Assess for substance intoxication as cause of delirium or fever (MDMA, cocaine, amphetamine, and PCP intoxication can produce hyperthermia, altered mental status, and autonomic dysfunction)

Note. BUN=blood urea nitrogen; CNS=central nervous system; CK=creatine kinase; CSF=cerebrospinal fluid; DIC=disseminated intravascular coagulation; HSV=herpes simplex virus; LFTs=liver function tests; MDMA=3,4-methylenedioxy-methamphetamine; NMDAR=N-methyl-D-aspartate receptor; PCP=phencyclidine; PCR=polymerase chain reaction; PT=prothrombin time; PTT=partial thromboplastin time.

Source. Data from Berman 2011; Tse et al. 2015.

Pharmacological Therapy

There is disagreement about the role of pharmacological therapy in the treatment of NMS. Use of dantrolene, bromocriptine, benzodiazepines, or other dopaminergic agents is recommended by some. Almost all available data regarding use of these agents are based on reviews of case reports or small series, without any randomized controlled trials. Data regarding benefits and harms of dantrolene are mixed. For patients with severe NMS or for those who fail to improve with supportive measures, it is reasonable to try the agents described in Table 5–3. In cases that do not respond to standard medical care, electroconvulsive therapy is often effective (Katus and Frucht 2016).

Rechallenging with dopamine antagonists.   Risk of recurrent NMS is reduced if antipsychotic drugs or other dopamine antagonists are not restarted until 2 weeks after the resolution of NMS (6 weeks for long-acting injectable antipsychotics). These medications should be introduced with slow dose titration and careful monitoring (Susman 2001; Tse et al. 2015). An antipsychotic different from the one originally associated with development of the syndrome should be chosen. High-potency first-generation antipsychotics should be avoided.

Course and Prognosis

Most NMS cases resolve within 2 weeks after discontinuing antidopaminergic agents, unless complications occur (Tse et al. 2015). The mortality rate, which was up to 27.7% prior to the 1980s, declined to 5.6%–8.6% after the year 2000 (Katus and Frucht 2016; Modi et al. 2016). The use of second-generation antipsychotics, which have approximately 3% NMS-specific mortality, may account for much of this mortality reduction (Modi et al. 2016). Surviving patients may have residual catatonia or parkinsonism as well as significant morbidity secondary to renal or cardiopulmonary complications (Modi et al. 2016; Tse et al. 2015).

Serotonin Syndrome

Serotonin syndrome is a condition that is most commonly caused by the combination of two or more 5-hydroxytryptamine (5-HT [serotonin]) agonists, although it can happen following a single 5-HT agonist in overdose or at therapeutic dosages (Boyer and Shannon 2005; Iqbal et al. 2012). Severe toxicity, characterized by hyperthermia and increased muscle tone/rigidity, usually mainly occurs when a combination of two or more drugs that act on serotonin have been taken at therapeutic or toxic doses. Combinations of a serotonergic drug and MAOIs often result in serotonin syndrome. Moderate toxicity has been reported with an overdose of a single drug and occasionally from increasing therapeutic doses. Incidence is difficult to assess, but in large case series of overdoses, moderate serotonin toxicity occurred in 14%–16% of poisonings with selective serotonin reuptake inhibitors (SSRIs) and 19%–29% of venlafaxine overdoses (Iqbal et al. 2012).

Many nonpsychiatric medications regulate serotonin release, reuptake, and metabolism; serotonin receptor agonists also may play a role in serotonin syndrome (Boyer and Shannon 2005; Iqbal et al. 2012). Some agents in the "Increased serotonin precursors/serotonin agonist" group in Table 5–4 are often cited as complicit in cases of serotonin syndrome, but the evidence supporting this risk is limited and problematic

TABLE 5–3. Pharmacological therapy for neuroleptic malignant syndrome (NMS)

Medication	Mechanism/Indication	Administration	Comments
Amantadine	Dopaminergic agent	By mouth or NG tube 100 mg bid to tid No IV formulation	Associated with orthostatic hypotension May exacerbate psychosis Dosage adjustment with decreased GFR
Bromocriptine	Dopaminergic agent	By mouth or NG tube only Starting dosage: 2.5 mg bid to tid May increase each dose upward by 2.5 mg every day Maximum daily dosage 45 mg/day Continue for 10 days after symptoms resolve and then taper slowly	Like other dopaminergic agents, it may exacerbate psychosis Causes orthostatic hypotension and nausea
Dantrolene	Muscle relaxant: interferes with sarcoplasmic release of calcium ions. Used to decrease rigidity (prevent rhabdomyolysis) and decrease hyperpyrexia.	Initial bolus: 1–2.5 mg/kg intravenously Dosing: 1 mg/kg intravenously every 6 hours, may increase to 2.5 mg/kg every 6 hours	Risk of death from liver failure 0.3% in those with prolonged use Risk higher in women, with dosages >300 mg/day, and with treatment >60 days Often discontinued as soon as NMS resolves to prevent hepatotoxicity
Lorazepam, other benzodiazepines	GABA effects in basal ganglia are dopaminergic. Used to treat agitation and seizures.	Wide range of dosages reported	Dosing schedule determined by agent, response, and toxicity
Carbidopa-levodopa	Dopaminergic agent	Initial dosage 25–100 mg by mouth or NG tube tid Upward dosage titration not well described for this diagnosis	May exacerbate psychosis Causes orthostatic hypotension and nausea

Note. bid=twice a day; GABA=γ-aminobutyric acid; GFR=glomerular filtration rate; NG=nasogastric; tid=three times a day.
Source. Data from Berman 2011; Katus and Frucht 2016; Susman 2001; Tse et al. 2015.

TABLE 5–4.   **Mechanisms of agents causing serotonin toxicity**

Decreased serotonin reuptake	Increased serotonin release
SSRIs, SNRIs	Fenfluramine
TCAs (mainly clomipramine and imipramine)	MDMA
	Amphetamines
Some opioids (tramadol, meperidine, fentanyl, methadone)	Methylphenidate
	Cocaine
St. John's wort	Reserpine
Dextromethorphan	Buspirone
Sibutramine	
Some antihistamines (chlorpheniramine, brompheniramine)	**Increased serotonin precursors/ serotonin agonist**
Amphetamines	L-tryptophan
MDMA	Triptans
	LSD
Reduced serotonin catabolism	
MAOIs	**Miscellaneous**
Linezolid	Lithium (possibly increases serotonin release)
Methylene blue	
Buspirone	

Note.   LSD=lysergic acid diethylamide; MAOIs=monoamine oxidase inhibitors; MDMA =3,4-methyl-enedioxymethamphetamine; SNRIs=serotonin-norepinephrine reuptake inhibitors; SSRIs=selective serotonin reuptake inhibitors; TCAs=tricyclic antidepressants.

Source.   Adapted from Gillman 2006 (Table 2, p. 1048), with data from Gillman 2010; Ng and Cameron 2010.

(except for lithium) (Sun-Edelstein et al. 2008). It is unlikely that these agents pose risk for severe, life-threatening serotonin syndrome (Sun-Edelstein et al. 2008).

Clinical Presentation and Diagnosis

Serotonin toxicity usually starts within hours of ingesting drugs that cause an increase in serotonin; more than 60% of cases begin within 6 hours, and 74% of cases begin within 24 hours (Boyer and Shannon 2005). The classic triad of clinical features is neuromuscular excitation (e.g., clonus, ocular clonus, hyperreflexia, myoclonus, rigidity), autonomic nervous system excitation (e.g., hyperthermia, tachycardia), and altered mental state (e.g., agitation, confusion). Patients often have diarrhea. Acute onset of these features should trigger a search for a toxicological explanation. Severe serotonin toxicity is a medical emergency; it may be complicated by clinically significant hyperthermia, rhabdomyolysis, DIC, and adult respiratory distress syndrome (Boyer and Shannon 2005; Iqbal et al. 2012).

There is no gold standard for diagnosis of serotonin syndrome. Different sets of clinical criteria have been formulated. The Hunter Serotonin Toxicity Criteria set (Dunkley et al. 2003) performs favorably compared with older criteria and is based on a retrospective assessment of a robust data set: prospectively collected data on more than 2,200 patients who overdosed on a serotonergic agent. The Sternbach Criteria set (Sternbach 1991) was formulated after review of 38 case reports of patients with serotonin syndrome due to combinations of serotonergic agents at therapeutic doses. Although the Sternbach criteria are based on a small number of cases, a comparison of the Sternbach criteria with the Hunter criteria may capture differences in manifestation of serotonin syndrome caused by overdose versus polypharmacy (Table 5–5).

Differential Diagnosis

Serotonin syndrome may be difficult to distinguish from NMS in patients taking both antipsychotics and serotonergic agents. Myoclonus and rigidity may occur in both syndromes, but myoclonus is more common in serotonin syndrome, and rigidity is more common in NMS (Iqbal et al. 2012; Katus and Frucht 2016). Serotonin syndrome tends to manifest with agitation, whereas patients with NMS tend to display more hypokinesis and catatonia. Serotonin syndrome may manifest with diarrhea; this presentation is not a feature of NMS. Sympathomimetic toxicity and alcohol withdrawal syndrome both share features with serotonin syndrome. Encephalitis may manifest with fever, autonomic signs, rigidity, opsoclonus, or myoclonus. Serotonin syndrome is a clinical diagnosis; there are no diagnostic laboratory tests. Laboratory testing is used mainly to rule out other diseases in the differential diagnosis and for complications of delirium, agitation, and hyperthermia, including rhabdomyolysis, DIC, renal failure, and respiratory failure (Boyer and Shannon 2005; Iqbal et al. 2012; Uddin et al. 2017) (Table 5–6).

TABLE 5–5.   **Diagnostic criteria for serotonin syndrome**

Sternbach criteria (Sternbach 1991)

Other etiologies of symptoms have been ruled out.

An antipsychotic was not started or increased in dosage before the onset of symptoms.

At least three of the following symptoms after the addition of or dosage increase of a serotonergic agent:

    Mental status changes (confusion, hypomania)

    Agitation

    Myoclonus

    Hyperreflexia

    Diaphoresis

    Shivering

    Tremor

    Diarrhea

    Incoordination

    Fever

Hunter criteria (Dunkley et al. 2003)

One of the following sets of symptoms in a patient taking a serotonergic agent:

    Spontaneous clonus

    Inducible clonus **PLUS** agitation **or** diaphoresis

    Ocular clonus **PLUS** agitation **or** diaphoresis

    Tremor **PLUS** hyperreflexia

    Hypertonia (increased motor tone) **PLUS** temperature >100.4°F (38°C) **PLUS** ocular clonus or inducible clonus

TABLE 5–6.   **Diagnostic evaluation for serotonin syndrome**

Laboratory/Other tests	Indications
Complete blood count, PT/PTT	Assess for infection as cause of delirium and high fever Monitor for DIC
Blood cultures, urine culture	Assess for infection as cause of delirium and high fever
CK, urine myoglobin level, calcium and phosphate levels, BUN, and creatinine	Assess for rhabdomyolysis (with associated electrolyte abnormalities and acute kidney injury) caused by NMS rigidity and hyperthermia
Serum and urine toxicology screen: opiates/opioids (meperidine), salicylates, acetaminophen, TCAs, amphetamines, phencyclidine, and cocaine	Assess for coingestion of any other toxic substance Assess for sympathomimetic toxicity as cause of hyperthermia and agitated delirium
Arterial blood gas, serum sodium, serum chloride, serum bicarbonate (total CO_2)	Assess for respiratory failure from hypoventilation caused by rigidity, aspiration, or adverse effects of therapeutic agents Assess for anion gap acidosis caused by complications of NMS or other agents contributing to delirium and hyperthermia
Electrocardiography	Assess for cardiovascular complications Screen for electrocardiographic signs of coingestants
CSF evaluation	Assess for CNS infection as cause of fever and altered mental status

Note.   BUN=blood urea nitrogen; CNS=central nervous system; CK=creatine kinase; CSF=cerebrospinal fluid; DIC=disseminated intravascular coagulation; NMS=neuroleptic malignant syndrome; PT=prothrombin time; PTT=partial thromboplastin time; TCAs=tricyclic antidepressants.
Source.   Data from Iqbal et al. 2012; Sun-Edelstein et al. 2008.

Treatment

Recovery from serotonin syndrome is attainable with low mortality (1%) when the following approaches are applied (Isbister et al. 2003, 2004):

Supportive therapy (Uddin et al. 2017):

- Discontinue serotonergic agents. In mild to moderate cases, improvement begins 1–3 days after stopping serotonergic drugs, but cases involving medications with long half-lives (e.g., fluoxetine, lithium) or irreversible MAOIs may resolve more slowly.
- Ensure adequate hydration.
- In moderate to severe cases, careful monitoring, in an intensive care unit or high acuity unit, of vital signs, mental status, and urine output is necessary.
- In moderate serotonin toxicity, agitation is generally the most troublesome symptom, and sedation with oral or intravenous benzodiazepines may be required.
- Treat hyperthermia with active cooling.

Pharmacological treatment:

- In addition to cooling, treat hyperthermia with sedatives to reduce muscle hyper-activity (i.e., benzodiazepines). For patients with a temperature above 41.1°C, rec-ommended treatment includes immediate sedation, paralysis, and intubation (Uddin et al. 2017).
- Cyproheptadine, an antihistamine and 5-HT$_{2A}$ antagonist, has been used to treat moderate serotonin toxicity, with doses of 8–16 mg orally up to a daily maximum of 32 mg. It does not come in parenteral form (Gillman 1999; Iqbal et al. 2012).
- For severe serotonin toxicity, intravenous chlorpromazine is the most commonly used 5-HT$_{2A}$ antagonist, but intravenous fluid loading is essential to prevent hypotension. A dose of 50–100 mg intramuscularly, up to a total of 400 mg/day, has been given. Chlorpromazine should not be routinely used if the patient is hypotensive or NMS cannot be excluded (Gillman 1999; Iqbal et al. 2012).

Anticholinergic Toxicity

Antimuscarinic drugs (e.g., benztropine, trihexyphenidyl) are commonly prescribed for the treatment of antipsychotic-induced extrapyramidal syndromes. Other anti-muscarinics that are frequently prescribed for patients with psychiatric illness in-clude first-generation antihistamines, some antipsychotic drugs, and TCAs (Table 5–7 shows levels of anticholinergic potency for these and other drugs). Some other agents cause anticholinergic effects by reducing acetylcholine synthesis; these include carbamazepine, opiates, and clonidine (Dawson and Buckley 2016). Antimuscarinic drugs are responsible for approximately 15%–20% of acute poisoning admissions and up to 40% of poisoning admissions to intensive care units (Dawson and Buckley 2016). These agents should be used cautiously in persons with prostatic hypertrophy, urinary retention, or narrow-angle glaucoma.

Clinical Presentation and Diagnosis

Anticholinergic toxidromes manifest both CNS and peripheral nervous system com-ponents. Serum levels of these drugs are not readily available; diagnosis is based on clinical findings and collateral information regarding medications, herbs, or drugs taken. Anticholinergic findings may be overshadowed by other effects of intoxicating agents, particularly those with anticholinergic and/or multiple other effects (see Ta-bles 5–7 and 5–8).

Diagnosis is based on clinical findings, but basic screening tests will be helpful in management (Table 5–9).

Management

In addition to the basic screening tests, the following management approaches for anticholinergic toxidromes are helpful.

TABLE 5–7. **Anticholinergic activity of psychotropic medications**

Drug class	Anticholinergic activity		
	High	**Moderate**	**Low**
Anticholinergic/ antiparkinsonian agents	Benztropine Trihexyphenidyl	**Amantadine**	**Amantadine**
Antidepressants			
MAOIs			Phenelzine
SSRIs	**Paroxetine**	**Paroxetine**	**Paroxetine** All other SSRIs
TCAs	Amitriptyline Amoxapine Clomipramine **Desipramine** Doxepin Imipramine Maprotiline Protriptyline	**Desipramine** Nortriptyline	
Other			Bupropion Mirtazapine Nefazodone Venlafaxine Trazodone
Antipsychotics			
First-generation agents	Chlorpromazine **Fluphenazine** **Perphenazine** **Thioridazine** Thiothixene **Trifluoperazine**	**Haloperidol** Loxapine Molindone **Perphenazine** **Prochlorperazine**	**Fluphenazine** **Haloperidol** **Perphenazine** **Prochlorperazine** **Thioridazine** **Trifluoperazine**
Second-generation agents	**Clozapine** **Olanzapine** **Quetiapine**	**Olanzapine** **Quetiapine**	Aripiprazole Asenapine **Clozapine** Iloperidone **Olanzapine** Paliperidone **Quetiapine** Risperidone Ziprasidone
Benzodiazepines	**Alprazolam** **Clorazepate**		**Alprazolam** **Clorazepate** Other benzodiazepines
Mood-stabilizing agents		**Carbamazepine** Oxcarbazepine	**Carbamazepine** Divalproex Lithium Valproic acid

TABLE 5–7. **Anticholinergic activity of psychotropic medications (continued)**

	Anticholinergic activity		
Drug class	High	Moderate	Low
Other	First-generation antihistamines (e.g., diphenhydramine, hydroxyzine, doxylamine)	Methadone	

Note. Classifications are based on clinical studies, not in vitro assessments.Agents in **bold type** were classified as having different anticholinergic potencies in different studies. MAOI=monoamine oxidase inhibitor; SSRI=selective serotonin reuptake inhibitor; TCA=tricyclic antidepressant.

Source. Adapted from Table 2 (pp. 5–9) in Salahudeen MS, Duffull SB, Nishtala PS: "Anticholinergic Burden Quantified by Anticholinergic Risk Scales and Adverse Outcomes in Older People: A Systematic Review." *BMC Geriatrics* 15:31, 2015. Copyright 2015, Salahudeen et al.; licensee BioMed Central. This article is published under license to BioMed Central Ltd. This is an Open Access article distributed under the terms of the Creative Commons Attribution License (http://creativecommons.org/licenses/by/4.0), which permits unrestricted use, distribution, and reproduction in any medium, provided the original work is properly credited.

Monitoring (Dawson and Buckley 2016; see Table 5–9):

- Depending on degree of agitation, delirium, or lethargy; risk of arrhythmia (e.g., TCA overdose, severe long QT from any agent, thioridazine overdose); and severity of hemodynamic abnormalities, consider monitoring with telemetry in a step-down unit or intensive care unit.
- Check glucose, liver function tests (LFTs), blood urea nitrogen (BUN)/creatinine, and electrolytes to assess for other causes of altered mental status.
- Monitor electrocardiogram (ECG) for findings consistent with specific overdoses.
- Check for sinus tachycardia in most anticholinergic overdoses.
- Check for a positive terminal R wave in aVR and negative terminal S wave in I or aVL in TCA overdose.
- Check for prolonged PR and QRS in TCA overdose.
- Check for QT prolongation in antipsychotic, TCA, or SSRI overdose.
- Check creatine kinase, especially in patients with seizures and/or persistent agitation.
- Monitor oxygen saturation and/or blood gases for respiratory acidosis and hypoxemia.

Nonpharmacological interventions:

- Provide low-stimulus environment and frequent reorientation.
- Support with intravenous crystalloids as appropriate for hemodynamic abnormalities, rhabdomyolysis, and inability to take by mouth.
- Treat hyperthermia with external cooling and measures for agitation.
- Monitor for urinary retention; assess need for indwelling urinary catheter.
- Monitor for abdominal distension, constipation, and obstipation due to pseudo-obstruction; assess need for nasogastric decompression with intermittent suction.

TABLE 5–8. Presentation of anticholinergic mono-intoxications by drug class

Clinical findings	Primarily anticholinergic agents (e.g., benztropine, atropine, scopolamine)[a]	First-generation antihistamines (e.g., diphenhydramine, chlorpheniramine doxylamine)[b]	Tricyclic antidepressants[c]	Antipsychotics[d]
Disturbance of consciousness	Agitation > than lethargy	Somnolence and coma as often or more often than agitation	Somnolence and coma as often or more often than agitation (unless serotonin syndrome)	Somnolence and coma; agitation uncommon
	Delirium	Delirium may occur	Prolonged delirium in recovery	
	Hallucination	Hallucination may occur	Hallucinations may occur during presentation or in recovery	Hallucinosis due to overdose not well described
Pupillary findings	Mydriasis	Mydriasis	Mydriasis	Meiosis > > mydriasis
Autonomic findings	Sinus tachycardia Hyperthermia may occur	Sinus tachycardia Hyperthermia may occur	Sinus tachycardia Hyperthermia may occur	Sinus tachycardia Hypothermia may occur
Cutaneous findings	Dry, warm skin and mucous membranes Flushing	Dry, warm skin and mucous membranes Flushing	Dry, warm skin and mucous membranes Flushing	Sialorrhea may occur Dry skin and mucous membranes may occur
Urinary abnormalities	Difficulty voiding urine Urinary retention	Difficulty voiding urine Urinary retention	Difficulty voiding urine Urinary retention	Difficulty voiding urine Urinary retention
Gastrointestinal abnormalities	Decreased bowel sounds Constipation Pseudo obstruction	Decreased bowel sounds Constipation Pseudo obstruction	Decreased bowel sounds Constipation Pseudo obstruction	Decreased bowel sounds Constipation Pseudo obstruction

TABLE 5–8. Presentation of anticholinergic mono-intoxications by drug class *(continued)*

Clinical findings	Primarily anticholinergic agents (e.g., benztropine, atropine, scopolamine)[a]	First-generation antihistamines (e.g., diphenhydramine, chlorpheniramine doxylamine)[b]	Tricyclic antidepressants[c]	Antipsychotics[d]

Findings that may overshadow anticholinergic effects	Rhabdomyolysis
	Seizures
	Respiratory depression not typical
		Rhabdomyolysis
		Seizures
		Occasional respiratory depression
			Rhabdomyolysis
			Seizures
			Respiratory depression
			
			ECG changes:
			  QT prolongation, quinidine-like effects
			
			Supraventricular tachycardias, ventricular tachycardias, torsades de pointes, heart block
			
			Hypotension
			
			Serotonin syndrome (mainly with clomipramine and imipramine)
				Rhabdomyolysis
				Seizures
				Respiratory depression
				
				ECG changes:
				  QT prolongation
				
				Arrhythmias uncommon (excluding thioridazine), although torsades de pointes may occur
				
				Hypotension
				Extrapyramidal syndromes

Note. Differences in presentation between primarily anticholinergic agent overdose and overdose with other anticholinergic agents are indicated by **bold type.**
ECG=electrocardiogram.
[a]Data from Forrester 2006; Parfitt 1947; Vallersnes et al. 2009.
[b]Data from Pragst et al. 2006.
[c]Data from Kerr et al. 2001.
[d]Data from Levine and Ruha 2012.

TABLE 5–9.   **Diagnostic evaluation for anticholinergic toxicity**

Laboratory/Other tests	Indications
Glucose	Assess for hypoglycemia as contributor to or cause of altered mental status
Acetaminophen, salicylate levels, toxicology screening tests	Exclude other coingestants as a cause and assess for other potential causes of hyperthermia and delirium
Electrocardiogram	Assess for cardiovascular complications Screen for electrocardiographic signs of coingestants
Complete blood count, PT/PTT	Assess for DIC Assess for infectious causes of fever and delirium
Blood and urine cultures	Assess for infection as cause of fever and delirium
Serum chemistry and electrolyte analysis	Obtain clues regarding potential intoxicating agents and coingestants
Creatine kinase	Rule out rhabdomyolysis associated with anticholinergic toxicity and consequent hyperthermia
Arterial blood gas analysis	Assess for acid-base abnormalities and monitor for respiratory failure
Free T_4 and TSH tests	Rule out thyroid disease as the cause of agitated delirium

Note.   DIC=disseminated intravascular coagulation; PT=prothrombin time; PTT=partial thromboplastin time; T_4=thyroxine; TSH=thyroid-stimulating hormone.

Pharmacological therapy (Table 5–10):

- Consider decontamination with activated charcoal (1 mg/kg, maximum dose 59 mg) if ingestion has occurred within the previous hour (use of charcoal at later times may be considered as anticholinergic drugs delay gastric emptying). Avoid in patients with pseudo-obstruction, those who cannot protect their airway, and patients who are not alert.
- Withdraw any medications with anticholinergic effects.
- Treat agitation with benzodiazepines and/or physostigmine.
- Serious cardiovascular effects of TCAs are not mediated by anticholinergic effects; management is not addressed in this chapter.

Valproic Acid–Induced Hyperammonemic Encephalopathy

VHE is an uncommon outcome of valproic acid (VPA) treatment; it occurs in approximately 2.5% of psychiatric patients (Lewis et al. 2012). The exact pathophysiology is unclear, but it involves carnitine depletion, indirect inhibition of the urea cycle, and increased renal glutamate uptake—all contributing to hyperammonemia (Chopra et al. 2012; Lewis et al. 2012). Elevated brain ammonia concentrations coupled with elevated concentrations of neurotoxic VPA metabolites may be responsible for inhibition of glutamine release from astrocytes and excess levels of glutamine due to excessive activation of NMDA receptors, release of glutamate, and conjugation of glutamate

TABLE 5–10. Drug therapy for anticholinergic toxicity

Medication	Dosage	Pros and cons of each agent	Adverse effects	Contraindications
Benzodiazepines	Dosages and choice of agent vary	Increased risk of intubation compared with physostigmine Improvement in agitation Prevention of seizures No improvement in delirium	Increased lethargy Increased risk of aspiration Increased risk of intubation Paradoxical worsening of delirium at high doses	
Physostigmine	Initial dose 1 mg (0.5 mg in pediatric cases) intravenously over >5 minutes Dosing protocols for subsequent dosing frequency vary between 5 minutes and 12 hours Although the T_{max} for IV physostigmine is very fast, the brain acetylcholine peak effect lags behind the T_{max} of acetylcholine. Therefore, we recommend repeating administration of physostigmine 0.5 mg intravenously every 10–30 minutes until delirium resolves or cholinergic toxicity occurs.	In certain cases may precipitate seizures and cardiac toxicity (as described in "Adverse effects" column at right) Improvement in agitation and delirium	Nausea and emesis Diaphoresis Diarrhea Seizures, particularly when infused quickly Bradycardia, heart block, and asystole, particularly in severe TCA overdose	QRS duration >100 milliseconds PR duration >200 milliseconds Mechanical bowel obstruction Mechanical urinary obstruction Heart rate <100 beats per minute in severe anticholinergic toxicity may predict asystole as a complication of treatment with physostigmine.

Note. TCA=tricyclic antidepressant; T_{max}=time to peak blood concentration.
Source. Data from Burns et al. 2000; Dawson and Buckley 2016.

and ammonium to glutamine. The excess glutamine creates an osmotic gradient that leads to astrocyte swelling and cerebral edema (Chopra et al. 2012).

Risk Factors

VHE is more likely when VPA is used in combination with phenobarbital, phenytoin, carbonic anhydrase inhibitors (e.g., acetazolamide), or carbamazepine. Case studies have reported VHE development in patients with VPA and clozapine, topiramate, or risperidone polypharmacy. Urea-cycle defects, carnitine deficiency, infection with urea-splitting bacteria, cirrhosis, and portosystemic shunts increase the risk of developing VHE (Chopra et al. 2012; Lewis et al. 2012).

Clinical Presentation and Diagnosis

VHE is characterized by impaired consciousness with confusion or lethargy, asterixis, focal or bilateral neurological signs, aggression, ataxia, gastrointestinal symptoms including nausea and vomiting, and increased seizure frequency. Behavioral changes may be mistaken for postictal effects, psychiatric disturbances, or nonconvulsive status epilepticus, and the dosage of VPA may be inappropriately increased in response. VHE should always be investigated in patients prescribed VPA with changes in behavior or level of consciousness. Untreated VHE will progress to stupor, coma, and death (Chopra et al. 2012; Lewis et al. 2012).

VHE is not consistently correlated with VPA serum levels; thus, obtaining VPA levels is useful only in the following situations: 1) for differential testing in an encephalopathy patient presenting with unknown medication history and 2) for monitoring serum levels in VPA overdose. VHE can occur acutely with initial VPA doses or can develop with chronic VPA treatment. VHE will most commonly manifest with hyperammonemia and normal LFTs; however, VHE can also occur with normal serum ammonia levels. If VPA levels are obtained, a free VPA level should be included because the free drug concentration can be elevated even if the total serum VPA is normal. Ammonia levels also should be obtained, as should levels of electrolytes, LFTs, platelets, and serum lactate. Serum and cerebrospinal fluid glutamine levels may frequently be elevated and theoretically may be used as an adjunct test, although checking of glutamine levels is usually not done in clinical practice (Chopra et al. 2012; Lewis et al. 2012).

Differential Diagnosis

The differential diagnosis of altered mental status with neurological signs is broad and includes intracerebral hemorrhage, infections of the CNS (e.g., meningitis, encephalitis), metabolic derangements (e.g., hypoglycemia, hyponatremia), and ictal and postictal states. The diagnosis of VHE is made on the basis of relevant clinical history and suggestive findings (i.e., asterixis, elevated ammonia with normal LFTs) (Table 5–11); however, if there is high clinical suspicion of the diagnosis, treatment should commence immediately (Chopra et al. 2012; Lewis et al. 2012; Verrotti et al. 2002).

Treatment

The definitive treatment of VHE is discontinuation of VPA. IV or oral carnitine has been used in several studies, with varied dosages (average of 50–100 mg/kg intravenously over 30 minutes, followed by 15 mg/kg intravenously over 10–30 minutes

TABLE 5–11. **Diagnostic evaluation for valproic acid (VPA)-induced hyperammonemic encephalopathy (VHE)**

Laboratory/Other tests	Indications
Complete blood count, urine culture, and blood cultures	Assess for infection as cause of delirium and high fever Assess for neutropenia and thrombocytopenia, which can occur with VPA use Assess for urinary infection with urea-splitting bacteria
Total and free VPA levels	In patient with unclear medication history In patient with suspected or known VPA overdose/toxicity
Ammonia levels[a]	Ammonia levels are frequently elevated in VHE; however, a normal level does not exclude the diagnosis and should not prevent treatment
Liver function tests	Rule out hepatic impairment as cause of altered mental status or assess for hepatic toxicity as VPA complication
Electrolytes	Rule out electrolyte derangements as cause of altered mental status
Urine toxicology screen	Rule out substance use/intoxication as cause of altered mental status
EEG	Rule out seizure activity. EEG findings in encephalopathy can have continuous generalized slowing, a predominance of theta and delta activity, occasional bursts of frontal intermittent rhythmic delta activity, and triphasic wave (however, EEG can also be normal).

Note. EEG=electroencephalogram.
[a]Sample should be placed on ice and brought promptly to the laboratory.
Source. Data from Chopra et al. 2012; Lewis et al. 2012.

every 4 hours until clinical improvement). Lactulose has also been used in patients with elevated ammonia levels and VHE to decrease ammonia production. The condition of patients with severe VHE should be monitored with the Glasgow Coma Scale; for less severe cases, neuropsychological tests of motor speed, visual perception, concentration, and attention are useful (Chopra et al. 2012).

Drug Exposures, Environmental Exposures, and Micronutrient Deficiencies as Causes of Psychiatric Symptoms and Syndromes

Drug Exposures: Drugs of Abuse

Illicit and prescription substances that are frequently abused and produce neuropsychiatric symptoms are discussed here; these include stimulants, cannabinoids (CBs), sedative-hypnotics, dissociative anesthetics, club drugs, and anabolic steroids. Opioids and inhaled solvents are not discussed in this section. Opioids are important, and screening should be performed in patients presenting with suspected substance use (see the appendix at the end of the chapter). Opioids cause higher rates of medical complications and death when used with other CNS depressants (Ries et al. 2015). Opioid intoxication may manifest with confusion and delirium, particularly in the elderly. Opioid withdrawal alone does not produce the type of neuropsychiatric symptoms that are confused with other psychiatric presentations. Inhaled solvents do not have psychiatric symptoms that can lead to hospital or primary care presentations.

Stimulants: Cocaine, Amphetamines, Cathinones

The acute effects of cocaine, amphetamines, and other stimulants are due mainly to increases in catecholamine neurotransmitter activity. With high-dose or repeated use, stimulant intoxication often leads to affective symptoms (e.g., anxiety, irritability, interpersonal sensitivity, hypervigilance), changes in behavior (e.g., suspiciousness, grandiosity), and general impairment in judgment. Psychotic symptoms such as paranoia and hallucinations may occur (Bramness and Rognli 2016; Harris and Batki 2000; Ries et al. 2015; Williamson et al. 1997). Patients with stimulant-induced psychoses may closely resemble those with acute schizophrenia and may be misdiagnosed as such (Ries et al. 2015). Cocaine-induced psychosis can sometimes be differentiated from a primary psychotic disorder, as these patients will have less thought disorder and fewer bizarre delusions and negative symptoms such as alogia or inattention. Stimulant-induced hallucinations may be auditory, visual, or somatosensory. Tactile hallucinations such as the sensation of something crawling under the skin (formication) are especially typical of stimulant psychosis (Bramness and Rognli 2016; Harris and Batki 2000). Hallucinations may be exacerbated by anxiety elicited by the physiological symptoms commonly associated with stimulant use, such as palpitations and hyperventilation. Table 5–12 provides a summary of relevant information regarding these agents.

Cannabinoids

The major psychological manifestations of marijuana are mediated by the interaction of delta-9-tetrahydrocannabinol (THC) with specific CB receptors on nerve cells throughout the brain. Other CBs found in marijuana (e.g., cannabidiol, cannabichromene) do not produce the typical marijuana effects associated with behavioral symptoms. Although THC is a weak partial agonist at CB receptors, synthetic CBs are potent CB receptor agonists.

The initial, usually desired, psychological effects of marijuana intoxication include relaxation, euphoria, slowed time perception, altered (often intensified) sensory perception, increased awareness of the environment, and increased appetite (Ries et al. 2015; Sachs et al. 2015). Higher doses, repeated use, or a stressful setting are associated with adverse effects (hypervigilance, anxiety, paranoia, derealization, depersonalization, panic, auditory or visual illusions or hallucinations, psychosis, delirium). Marijuana-induced psychosis differs from a primary psychotic disorder in its transient time course and more commonly manifests with derealization/depersonalization experiences and visual, rather than auditory, hallucinations. Preexisting psychopathology increases the risk of adverse events such as panic or psychosis. Table 5–13 provides a summary of relevant information regarding CBs.

TABLE 5-12. Stimulant drugs

	Cocaine	Methamphetamines	Cathinones (bath salts, khat)
Estimated number of U.S. users age 12 years and older and demographic data	4.8 million. Most cocaine use is by urban men age 15–35 years (Substance Abuse and Mental Health Services Administration 2017).	0.9 million (Substance Abuse and Mental Health Services Administration 2017). High-risk groups include residents in rural areas, people of Hispanic and Asian ethnicities, and, among male individuals, those with gay or bisexual sexual orientation.	Data are extremely limited. As of May 2011, 2,371 calls related to bath salts had been made to the American Association of Poison Control Centers (Prosser and Nelson 2012).
Onset of action	Intranasal: Within 5 minutes Intravenous: 10–60 seconds Inhalation: 3–5 seconds	Intranasal: 60–90 minutes Intravenous: 20–60 minutes Inhalation: 5–15 minutes	Intranasal: psychoactive effects after 10–20 minutes (Prosser and Nelson 2012) Oral: 30–45 minutes Intravenous: Within minutes
Duration of action	Intravenous or inhaled administration: 15–30 minutes Intranasal: 1 hour Gastrointestinal: 3 hours	Overall effects typically last 3–8 hours, residual effects up to 12 hours. Psychotic symptoms can last for weeks and even permanently after heavy chronic use due to dopamine depletion (Bramness and Rognli 2016; Williamson et al. 1997).	Oral: 2–5 hours (Prosser and Nelson 2012) Intranasal: 1–2 hours Intravenous: 30 minutes
Prevalence of psychiatric symptoms	Up to 25% of non-treatment-seeking cocaine users may experience anxiety, depression, sleep disturbance (Williamson et al. 1997). Cocaine-associated psychotic symptoms are reported by up to 80% of individuals with a cocaine use disorder (Roncero et al. 2012; Williamson et al. 1997).	Psychotic symptoms occur in up to 40% of users (Bramness and Rognli 2016).	Unclear currently

TABLE 5–12.   Stimulant drugs (continued)

	Cocaine	Methamphetamines	Cathinones (bath salts, khat)
Psychiatric symptoms of intoxication	Aggression, anxiety, delusions, hallucinations Symptoms usually remit 24–48 hours after last use (Roncero et al. 2012; Williamson et al. 1997). Hallucinations are often tactile (formication), can also be visual, auditory.	Aggression, anxiety, delusions, hallucinations	Agitation and aggression most commonly reported symptoms Anxiety, paranoia, memory loss, and aggression, in particular with MDPV[a] Hallucinations can occur, depending on cathinone type.
Psychiatric symptoms of withdrawal	Depressive symptoms occur following cessation of use: fatigue, anhedonia, impaired concentration, lethargy. These remit 1–2 weeks after last use (Coffey et al. 2000; Lago and Kosten 1994). With initial "crash," intense depressive symptoms and suicidal ideation can occur (Coffey et al. 2000; Lago and Kosten 1994).		
Diagnosis	Metabolite detected in urine 2–3 days after last use (Verstraete 2004).	Blood concentrations can be used to distinguish therapeutic use from abuse. 0.02–0.05 mg/L is typical for therapeutic use. Recreational range: 0.01–2.5 mg/L, median 0.6 mg/L Urine testing detects last use within 1–4 days (Verstraete 2004).	Not in standard drug test panels. Specific blood and urine tests for certain synthetic cathinones such as mephedrone and butylone can be ordered. Acutely intoxicated patients can present with hyponatremia. Can cause false positive methamphetamine screen
Management of psychiatric symptoms	Place in quiet, nonthreatening environment. Provide symptomatic treatment (i.e., intramuscular antipsychotic or benzodiazepine for acute agitation).		

[a]MDPV = methylenedioxypyrovalerone—a synthetic cathinone popular in the United States (Baumann et al. 2013).

TABLE 5–13.   Cannabinoids

	Marijuana	Synthetic cannabinoids (spice, molly, K2)
Estimated number of U.S. users age 12 years and older and demographic data	22.2 million current users of marijuana (Substance Abuse and Mental Health Services Administration 2017)	Limited data are available. U.S. poison centers received 2,668 calls about exposures in 2013, 3,682 calls in 2014, and 7,794 calls in 2015. In January–October 2017, there were 1,741 calls (American Association of Poison Control Centers 2017; Castaneto et al. 2014). Synthetic cannabinoid-related emergency department visits increased from 11,406 visits in 2010 to 28,531 visits in 2011(Castaneto et al. 2014).
Onset of action	Smoked: 1–10 minutes Oral: 30–120 minutes	Current limited data suggest onset within minutes of smoking (Castaneto et al. 2014).
Duration of action	Smoked: 1–4 hours; aftereffects 2–24 hours (Ries et al. 2015) Oral: 4–10 hours; aftereffects 6–24 hours (Ries et al. 2015) Due to fat solubility, heavy chronic users can experience symptoms for weeks.	Current limited data suggest duration of 2–5 hours, with most recovering in less than 24 hours (American Association of Poison Control Centers 2017).
Prevalence of psychiatric symptoms	~20% panic attacks, anxiety, paranoia, depression (Johns 2001) ~5% psychotic symptoms (Murray et al. 2016; Núñez and Gurpegui 2002)	61.9% (included neurological and psychiatric; Castaneto et al. 2014)
Psychiatric symptoms of intoxication	Hypervigilance, anxiety, paranoia, derealization and depersonalization; acute panic (associated with anxiety), illusions, or hallucinations (usually auditory or visual [Johns 2001; Murray et al. 2016])	Anxiety, disorientation, agitation, paranoia, hallucinations (Castaneto et al. 2014; Murray et al. 2016)

TABLE 5–13. **Cannabinoids** *(continued)*

	Marijuana	Synthetic cannabinoids (spice, molly, K2)
Psychiatric symptoms of withdrawal	Anxiety, craving, irritability, insomnia, appetite disturbance, dysphoria/depression (Bonnet and Preuss 2017)	Drug craving, anxiety, nightmares (from case reports; Bonnet and Preuss 2017)
Diagnosis	Urine: metabolite detected 1–4 days after occasional use, 7–10 days following heavy use, but has been detected as long as 25 days later (Verstraete 2004) Blood: metabolite detected on average up to 36 hours after use (Verstraete 2004)	Do not produce positive results for cannabis; some specific assays available for metabolites of certain synthetic cannabinoids (Ries et al. 2015) Associated laboratory abnormalities include leukocytosis, lactic acidosis, and elevated creatine kinase (Ries et al. 2015).
Management of psychiatric symptoms	Supportive	Supportive: intramuscular antipsychotic and benzodiazepine use to control acute agitation

Alcohol

Almost 88% of the U.S. population has used alcohol at least once in their lifetime. Annual U.S. alcohol-related economic costs in terms of lost productivity and health care are estimated at $223 billion. Alcohol acts on multiple receptor types throughout the brain, including γ-aminobutyric acid (GABA), glycine, acetylcholine, serotonin, and glutamate, leading to a large variety of neuropsychiatric symptoms in addition to the multiple organ systems it impacts (Ries et al. 2015). Table 5–14 provides a summary of relevant information regarding these alcohol-related problems. Management of withdrawal seizures is not discussed here.

Sedative-Hypnotics (Excluding Alcohol)

Sedative-hypnotic medications limit excitability and are anxiolytic (sedative), produce drowsiness, and facilitate sleep (hypnosis). They are among the most widely used prescription drugs in the United States. Their mechanism of action mainly involves enhancement of inhibitory effects of GABA by allosteric modulation of $GABA_A$ receptors. Drugs in this class that are commonly associated with severe withdrawal states (in addition to alcohol) include methaqualone, glutethimide, phenobarbital, and short-acting benzodiazepines such as alprazolam and triazolam (Goldfrank et al. 2015; Ries et al. 2015). Sedative drugs associated with less severe clinical withdrawal states include long-acting benzodiazepines, meprobamate, and chlordiazepoxide (Goldfrank et al. 2015; Ries et al. 2015). Table 5–15 provides a summary of relevant information regarding these agents.

Hallucinogens

Hallucinogens are a diverse group of drugs that alter and distort perception, thought, and mood without clouding the sensorium. Hallucinogens are differentiated by their chemical structures and fall into one of two categories. The indolealkylamine hallucinogens (i.e., lysergic acid diethylamide [LSD], psilocybin, N,N-dimethyltryptamine [DMT], peyote, ayahuasca) are structurally related to serotonin and act as $5\text{-}HT_{2A}$ agonists. The phenylethylamine hallucinogens (mescaline, 2,5-dimethoxy-4-methylamphetamine [DOM; also known as STP (for Serenity, Tranquility and Peace)]) are structurally related to norepinephrine. In addition, there are several unique hallucinogens, such as *Salvia divinorum*, "nutmeg," kratom, and kava kava (Goldfrank et al. 2015; Ries et al. 2015). These Schedule 1 medications are increasingly being studied for anxiety and depression in persons with a variety of conditions including end-stage cancer.

The subjective experience of hallucinogen use is influenced greatly by the expectations and personality of the user as well as the setting in which use occurs. Mood can vary from euphoria and bliss to depression, anxiety, and intense fear. Perceptions are intensified and distorted, with alterations in the sense of time, space, and body. Synesthesias (blending of senses, e.g., colors are heard and sounds seen) can occur. Cognitive function varies, although reality testing is usually preserved (Abraham et al. 1996; Katz et al. 1968; Ries et al. 2015). Table 5–16 provides a summary of relevant information regarding classic hallucinogens.

TABLE 5–14.   Alcohol

Estimated number of U.S. users age 12 years and older	138.3 million current alcohol users; 66.7 million reported binge alcohol use in past 30 days; 17.3 million heavy alcohol users (Substance Abuse and Mental Health Services Administration 2017)
Onset of action	Varies depending on fasting state, gender, age, percent alcohol volume for beverage. Average onset is 30 minutes (Mitchell et al. 2014).
Duration of action	Varies depending on BAL. On average, intermittent users clear ethanol at rates of 15–20 mg/dL (3.3–4.3 mmol/L) per hour; chronic users clear faster at rates of 25–35 mg/dL (5.4–7.6 mmol/L) per hour (Mitchell et al. 2014).
Prevalence of psychiatric symptoms	Delirium tremens: 3%–5% of patients hospitalized for alcohol withdrawal (Schuckit 2014) Alcoholic hallucinosis in withdrawal or mild perceptual changes: 25% of chronic alcohol users with withdrawal symptoms More severe hallucinations: 0.4% in general population, 4% prevalence in chronic users (Engelhard et al. 2015) Chronic: alcohol-related neurocognitive dysfunction, ~9% of users full dementia Wernicke's encephalopathy: autopsy reports with Wernicke lesions in alcohol-related deaths range from 29% to 59%.
Psychiatric symptoms of intoxication	Changes in mood, personality, and increased impulsive behavior including increased risk of violence, suicidal ideation and behavior, poor coordination, slurred speech, and agitation (Ries et al. 2015) At higher doses, alterations in cognition and level of arousal occur.
Psychiatric symptoms of withdrawal	90% of patients: mild to moderate withdrawal that peaks between 24 and 36 hours Early withdrawal signs and symptoms (6–24 hours after last use): anxiety, sleep disturbances, vivid dreams, tremor, tachycardia, diaphoresis, anorexia, nausea, and headache Hallucinosis (12–24 hours after drinking cessation, resolved in 24–48 hours): visual hallucinations frequently involving animals; tactile hallucinations, formication; and auditory hallucinations. This syndrome is not characterized by a confusional state (Engelhard et al. 2015). Delirium tremens (typically appears 72–96 hours after last use, duration average of 2–3 days): global confusion and disorientation, frequent hallucinations without insight, lack of reality testing, severe sleep-wake cycle disruption, agitation, increases in psychomotor activity. Physical symptoms can include tachycardia, nausea/vomiting, tremor, and fever (Schuckit 2014).

TABLE 5–14.	**Alcohol** *(continued)*
Diagnosis	BAL: detects alcohol use within preceding few hours. Quantitative levels can provide corroboration for clinical presentation; however, typical symptoms for a range of BALs may vary depending on a person's level of use. Heavy chronic users can have fewer symptoms at higher levels and can fall into withdrawal while still having a positive BAL (Currier et al. 2006; Ries et al. 2015). Breathalyzer testing: lower accuracy of estimating BAL; low false-positive rate (Currier et al. 2006) Urine testing: qualitative marker of recent ingestion within preceding 8 hours on average; metabolite can be detected in urine from 24 hours up to 4 days after use, depending on amount ingested. However, metabolite has risk of false-positive test result (i.e., can be positive with use of hand sanitizer, use of alcohol-containing mouthwash, glucosuria) (Currier et al. 2006; Ries et al. 2015). Liver function tests, including AST, ALT, and GGT, can provide information about recent alcohol use even with negative BAL (Ries et al. 2015).
Chronic complications of use	Chronic complications are due to a combination of neuronal toxicity from chronic use and/or malnourishment seen in chronic heavy use. Wernicke's encephalopathy and Korsakoff syndrome (see "Wernicke-Korsakoff Syndrome: Thiamine [Vitamin B₁] Deficiency" in "Micronutrient Deficiencies" section) Cognitive dysfunction and ventricular enlargement Alcoholic cerebellar degeneration: ataxia in gait and stance (can resemble acute intoxication); later progresses to incoordination and tremor in arms, dysarthria, intermittent double/blurred vision (Ries et al. 2015)
Management of psychiatric symptoms	Agitation in acute intoxication: intramuscular/oral antipsychotics (Engelhard et al. 2015; Ries et al. 2015) Uncomplicated withdrawal with mild behavioral symptoms: symptom-triggered therapy with frequent monitoring utilizing validated scale such as CIWA. Benzodiazepines such as chlordiazepoxide, diazepam, or lorazepam are more frequently used, although benzodiazepine-sparing regimens exist (Long et al. 2017). Alcoholic hallucinosis: supportive care, antipsychotic to control hallucinations (Engelhard et al. 2015; Long et al. 2017)

TABLE 5–14.   Alcohol *(continued)*

Management of psychiatric symptoms *(continued)*	Delirium tremens (Long et al. 2017):
	Provide care in an ICU or other high-acuity setting.
	Diaphoresis and other insensible losses as well as frequent inability to eat warrant careful infusion of crystalloid with renal and electrolyte monitoring.
	Perform workup to rule out medical conditions that may contribute to presentation and optimize management of comorbidities that will affect outcome.
	Administer thiamine intravenously 100 mg at least once and then orally 100 mg daily with a B complex supplement.
	Assess for Wernicke's encephalopathy and pellagra and treat as appropriate (see "Micronutrient Deficiencies" section).
	Primary pharmacotherapy is protocolized escalating doses of IV benzodiazepines in dosages high enough to achieve lightly dozing but arousable state.
	If patient is resistant to high doses of benzodiazepines, administer phenobarbital 10 mg/kg over 30 minutes. If patient will require intubation, can administer propofol (0.3–1.25 mg/kg, up to 4 mg/kg per hour, for up to 48 hours). Haldol can be used sparingly for severe delirium, but dose cautiously given effect on seizure threshold.

Note.   ALT=alanine aminotransferase; AST=aspartate aminotransferase; BAL=blood alcohol level; CIWA=Clinical Institute Withdrawal Assessment; GGT=γ-glutamyl transferase; ICU=intensive care unit.

TABLE 5–15. Sedative-hypnotics (benzodiazepines, barbiturates, sleep aids)

Estimated number of U.S. users age 12 years and older	Over the past year: misuse of sedatives: 1,531,000 (Substance Abuse and Mental Health Services Administration 2017); misuse of tranquilizers: 1,953,000 (Substance Abuse and Mental Health Services Administration 2017)
Onset of action	Varied depending on pharmacokinetic properties. The fastest-acting barbiturates and benzodiazepines have an onset within 30 seconds to several minutes after administration.
Duration of action	Varied depending on pharmacokinetics, ranging from a few hours to more than 30 hours
Prevalence of psychiatric symptoms	Benzodiazepine withdrawal syndrome reported in 30%–100% of patients over various studies. Prevalence impacted by dosage and type of benzodiazepine used (O'Brien 2005). Prolonged withdrawal occurs in 10%–15% of patients after last benzodiazepine use (Chouinard 2004).
Psychiatric symptoms of intoxication	Mild to moderate toxicity manifests with slurred speech, decreased alertness, ataxia, and poor coordination. In older adults, a paradoxical agitated confusion and even delirium may be produced. Severe stages of intoxication: stupor and coma develop.
Psychiatric symptoms of withdrawal (Chouinard 2004; Pétursson 1994; Santos and Olmedo 2017)	Short term: rebound anxiety and insomnia lasting 1–4 days after discontinuation More severe withdrawal: lasts 1–4 weeks after discontinuation Common: anxiety, insomnia, restlessness, agitation, irritability, muscle tension, and neuropsychiatric symptoms, including perceptual distortions and hypersensitivity to light, sound, and touch Less frequent: nightmares, depression Uncommon: confusion, paranoid delusions, and hallucinations A small proportion of patients after long-term sedative-hypnotic use can have prolonged withdrawal for weeks to months with irregular waxing/waning of insomnia, perceptual disturbances, sensory hypersensitivities, and anxieties.
Acute medical complications	CNS, cardiovascular, and respiratory depression, which can lead to death when combined with other CNS depressants (alcohol, opioids) or when overdose occurs with older agents (phenobarbital, chloral hydrate) (Ries et al. 2015)

TABLE 5–15.   Sedative-hypnotics (benzodiazepines, barbiturates, sleep aids) (continued)

Diagnosis	Blood: benzodiazepine screening is part of standard drug of abuse screens. Standard assays that rely on picking up oxazepam as a metabolite will not detect benzodiazepines that are not metabolized to oxazepam; these include alprazolam, clonazepam, lorazepam, midazolam, and triazolam. Sleep aid agents (i.e., zolpidem, zopiclone) are not detected by commercially available assays (Verstraete 2004) Urine: detected for up to 2 days if short acting, 5 days if intermediate acting, and up to 10 days if long acting. Phenobarbital can be detected for up to 15 days (Verstraete 2004).
Management of psychiatric symptoms	Withdrawal: similar to alcohol withdrawal, using symptom-triggered therapy versus benzodiazepine taper for withdrawal (Pétursson 1994; Santos and Olmedo 2017) Intoxication: supportive care, including high-acuity-setting management and intubation/ventilatory support in more severe cases of respiratory and CNS depression (Ries et al. 2015) Repeated doses of activated charcoal or gastrointestinal tract evacuation with orogastric tube can be used for benzodiazepines, phenobarbital, meprobamate, glutethimide (Ries et al. 2015). Flumazenil is rarely used to reverse benzodiazepine intoxication due to high risk of seizures in those physiologically dependent on benzodiazepines and in patients also administered substances that reduce seizure threshold, i.e., selective serotonin reuptake inhibitors, tricyclic antidepressants (Ries et al. 2015).

Note.   CNS=central nervous system.

TABLE 5–16. Classic hallucinogens

Estimated number of U.S. users age 12 years and older	1.2 million current users of hallucinogens; 41.5 million had used in their lifetime (Substance Abuse and Mental Health Services Administration 2017).
Onset of action	LSD: 30–40 minutes (Abraham et al. 1996; Ries et al. 2015) DMT: 30–60 seconds (smoked); 30–50 minutes (oral as ayahuasca) (Callaway et al. 1999)
Duration of action	LSD: 8–14 hours (oral) (Abraham et al. 1996) Psilocybin: 4–8 hours (oral) (Passie et al. 2002) DMT: 30–60 minutes (smoked or inhaled powder); 3–4 hours (oral as ayahuasca) (Callaway et al. 1999)
Prevalence of psychiatric symptoms	100% of users will experience some symptoms with a normal dose range. Rates of psychosis range in literature from 0.08% to 4.6%, with higher rates among patients with psychiatric comorbidities (Abraham et al. 1996). Withdrawal symptoms: ~10% of hallucinogen users (Abraham et al. 1996). HPPD: rates range in literature from 28% to 71%, depending on level of drug use, comorbid substances, and history of psychiatric illness (Halpern and Pope 2003)

Psychiatric symptoms of intoxication	Typical symptoms described (not inclusive) (Cakic et al. 2010; Katz et al. 1968):
	  Positive perceptual and affective responses: "consciousness expansion," mystical experience, sense of profound discovery, euphoria, catharsis, synesthesia
	  Negative perceptual and affective responses: Psychosomatic complaints, megalomania, suicidal ideation, impaired judgment, impulsivity, memory/cognition changes, depersonalization, odd behavior, depression, derealization, paranoid ideation, anxiety/panic, intense labile affect, dreamlike state, altered body image, hallucinations, altered time/space, increased suggestibility, illusions, detachment, indifference
	Less typical (but more likely to lead to acute medical presentation) (Abraham et al. 1996; Callaway et al. 1999; Passie et al. 2002):
	  Transient psychosis: resembles acute schizophrenia but more commonly includes visual hallucinations. Users may have insight into their drug-related psychosis.
	  "Bad trip": anxiety or panic attack, significant mood swings, experiences of depersonalization
	  Acute toxic delirium: delusions, hallucinations, agitation, confusion, paranoia, and inadvertent suicide attempts (e.g., attempts to fly). May resemble schizophrenia, but confusion, visual hallucinations, and some insight into drug-induced state help differentiate.

TABLE 5–16. Classic hallucinogens (continued)

Psychiatric symptoms of withdrawal	Fatigue, irritability, anhedonia (Ries et al. 2015)
Chronic complications of use	HPPD ("flashbacks"): episodes last a few seconds to hours. HPPD can persist for days to several months after last drug experience (can last for years in some patients). The most frequent symptoms are visual hallucinations; other symptoms include depersonalization, paresthesias, auditory trailing, and emotional lability during the flashback (Halpern and Pope 2003). Persistent psychosis: occurs primarily in patients with underlying psychotic or mood disorder. Treated as a psychotic disorder with antipsychotic medication (Abraham et al. 1996).
Diagnosis	Blood: detectable for up to 24–48 hours (LSD) (Verstraete 2004) Urine: detectable for up to 36 hours. Metabolite can be detected up to 96 hours (LSD) (Verstraete 2004).
Management of psychiatric symptoms	Intoxication including toxic delirium: supportive treatment with quiet environment and minimal sensory input, verbal reassurance ("talk down"), with oral benzodiazepines as first-line medication. Can use intramuscular lorazepam if needed (patients usually clear within 24 hours) (Ries et al. 2015). For significant agitation, high-potency antipsychotics such as haloperidol can be used; atypical antipsychotics may be used, but there is the risk of increasing psychotomimetic effects. HPPD: primarily treated with benzodiazepines to reduce distress. Risperidone is reported to worsen symptoms and is contraindicated thus far in treatment (Ries et al. 2015).

Note.   DMT=*N*-dimethyltryptamine; HPPD=hallucinogen persisting perception disorder; LSD=lysergic acid diethylamide.

MDMA and Gamma-Hydroxybutyrate

3,4-Methylenedioxymethamphetamine (MDMA) is an amphetamine analogue that is used frequently in clubs and at festivals and raves (where it is known as Ecstasy). It has also increasingly been studied in randomized trials examining its efficacy in persons with posttraumatic stress disorder. Its effects are those of a stimulant combined with a compound that increases oxytocin, prolactin, and cortisol, and it acts as a norepinephrine/epinephrine agonist as well as reuptake inhibitor. γ-Hydroxybutyrate (GHB, "liquid Ecstasy") is a naturally occurring metabolite of GABA that functions at $GABA_B$ receptors (Ries et al. 2015). Table 5–17 provides a summary of relevant information regarding these drugs.

Dissociative Anesthetics: Phencyclidine, Ketamine, Dextromethorphan

Phencyclidine (PCP) and its analogue ketamine are dissociative anesthetics (Ries et al. 2015). The main effects of PCP and ketamine are mediated by their action as noncompetitive antagonists of the NMDA-glutamate excitatory amino acid neurotransmitter receptor, although direct interaction with other neurotransmitter systems (such as dopamine) may occur at high doses (Goldfrank et al. 2015; Ries et al. 2015). In addition to NMDA antagonism, dextromethorphan has activity at the sigma receptor, which likely mediates its therapeutic effects as a cough suppressant. Ketamine has increasingly been studied as a treatment for depression, including as an acute treatment for accompanying suicidality.

Dissociative anesthetics produce a range of intoxicated states that can be grouped into three stages:

- Stage I—conscious, with psychological effects but mild or no physiological effects
- Stage II—stuporous or in a light coma, yet responsive to pain
- Stage III—comatose and unresponsive to pain.

The time course of psychological effects is highly variable and unpredictable, so even a recovering patient should be kept under observation until all symptoms have resolved (typically, at least 12 hours) (Goldfrank et al. 2015; Ries et al. 2015). Patients may move between the stages of intoxication, and the entire clinical episode may take weeks to resolve (Ries et al. 2015). Table 5–18 provides a summary of relevant information regarding PCP, ketamine, and dextromethorphan.

Hallucinogenic Plants (Including Herbs of Abuse)

Hallucinogenic plants including herbs of abuse often contain multiple psychoactive compounds; thus, patient presentations can have combinations of different symptoms (Table 5–19). They can be categorized as predominantly hallucinogenic or stimulating. Hallucinogenic plants achieve their psychotomimetic effects principally at serotonergic or cholinergic receptors. Stimulating herbs generally augment the activity of norepinephrine, dopamine, or acetylcholine (Ries et al. 2015). Thus, the manifestations and management of intoxication syndromes for this varied group of substances generally follow those for hallucinogen and stimulant intoxication.

TABLE 5–17. MDMA and GHB

	MDMA/MMDA[a]	GHB[b]
Estimated number of U.S. users age 12 years and older	18,459,000 tried over lifetime (Substance Abuse and Mental Health Services Administration 2017)	1,401,000 tried over lifetime (Substance Abuse and Mental Health Services Administration 2017)
Onset of action	Oral: within 30 minutes (Kalant 2001)	Oral: within 15 minutes (Liechti et al. 2016)
Duration of action	Intense initial effect ("rush") lasting 30–45 minutes; plateau lasting several hours (Kalant 2001)	2–4 hours (Liechti et al. 2016)
Psychiatric symptoms of intoxication	Resembles stimulants/hallucinogens: Low doses: initial increased wakefulness and energy, euphoria, increased sexual desire and satisfaction, heightened sensory perception, sociability, and increased empathy and sense of closeness to others. Plateau of less intense experience occurs, during which repetitive movement is common. Higher dose/repeated use: hyperactivity, fatigue, insomnia, anxiety, agitation, impaired decision making, flight of ideas, hallucinations, depersonalization/derealization, and bizarre or reckless behavior. Symptoms usually resolve as drug is metabolized.	Low oral doses (<20 mg/kg): relaxation, euphoria, sedation, disinhibition, sociability, and anterograde amnesia. Higher doses: somnolence, confusion, and hallucinations. Effects are prolonged and intensified when taken with other CNS depressants, such as alcohol. Patients may wake up abruptly after acute intoxication with a clear sensorium or may have a brief period of agitation and combativeness.
Acute medical complications of intoxication and withdrawal	At high doses (>200 mg), possible severe complications: 1. Hyperthermia. Presentation similar to heatstroke, sometimes with hypernatremia due to dehydration. Complications include rhabdomyolysis from high body temperature, with resulting renal failure, liver failure, and DIC. Treatment hinges on early detection, reversal of hyperthermia, close monitoring of creatinine kinase to detect rhabdomyolysis. Treat rhabdomyolysis with hydration (monitor changes in sodium if hypernatremic) and alkalinization of urine.	Cessation of chronic GHB use leads to a discrete withdrawal syndrome occurring 2–12 hours after the last dose. Significant medical withdrawal findings include tachycardia, hypertension, nystagmus, tremors, nausea, vomiting, and seizures. Autonomic instability can occur in severe withdrawal.

TABLE 5–17. **MDMA and GHB** (*continued*)

	MDMA/MMDA[a]	**GHB**[b]
Acute medical complications of intoxication and withdrawal (*continued*)	2. Acute hepatic toxicity. Varies from mild hepatitis to fulminant liver failure, exacerbated by hyperthermia. 3. Acute cardiovascular toxicity from increased catecholamines. Treat with a combination of α- and β-blocking adrenergic antagonists, use in combination with nitroglycerin or nitroprusside if needed. 4. MDMA neurotoxicity caused by hyponatremia (from loss of sodium in sweat and hemodilution from large amounts of water combined with MDMA antidiuretic effect). Can lead to seizures and intracranial fluid shifts. Treat hyponatremia initially with fluid restriction; use hypertonic saline if needed, monitoring changes in sodium level to prevent rapid correction.	
Psychiatric symptoms of withdrawal	Similar to mild form of stimulant withdrawal ("crash") with depression, anxiety, fatigue, and difficulty concentrating. Small proportion may develop recurrent depressive, psychotic, or anxiety symptoms, which require ongoing psychiatric treatment.	Psychiatric withdrawal symptoms include anxiety and restlessness. More severe withdrawal may cause delirium with hallucinations, psychosis, agitation. Mild symptoms usually resolve gradually over 1–2 weeks.
Diagnosis	History of drug intake. MDMA is not detected by routine urine or blood drug screens, but screens may be positive for amphetamines, products of MDMA metabolism. Patients with hyperthermia should have creatine kinase measured to monitor for rhabdomyolysis. Patients may present with concomitant hypernatremia and volume depletion, OR patients can present with significant hyponatremia if drinking large amounts of water.	The diagnosis of GHB intoxication is based on clinical suspicion, a history of drug intake, or analysis of uningested drug still in the possession of patient or family/friends. The signs and symptoms resemble those of any CNS depressant. GHB is not detected by routine drug toxicology assays.

TABLE 5–17. **MDMA and GHB** *(continued)*

	MDMA/MMDA[a]	GHB[b]
Management of psychiatric symptoms	Intoxication: Initial treatment is usually placement in a quiet, reassuring environment, with observation to reduce the risk of unintended self-injury. Physical restraints are contraindicated because they worsen anxiety and increase the risk of rhabdomyolysis. If severe or persisting symptoms require medication, benzodiazepines are preferred. Antipsychotics should be avoided if possible because they may increase the risk of hyperthermia and seizures. If needed (i.e., to control agitation), a high-potency antipsychotic such as haloperidol should be used. Withdrawal: Usually self-limited and does not require treatment. Prolonged withdrawal would benefit from medication/therapy according to the symptoms present.	Intoxication: Supportive at lower doses At higher doses, management of acute physical symptoms (i.e., CNS and respiratory depression, seizures, coma) No specific antidote in clinical use Role of activated charcoal is unclear, and there is no evidence for improvement of GHB recovery using physostigmine. Withdrawal: Managed with tapered dosing of a long-acting benzodiazepine Gabapentin or low-dose antipsychotics may be used if patients are unresponsive to benzodiazepines. Acute withdrawal is best done in a monitored hospital setting.

Note. CNS=central nervous system; DIC=disseminated intravascular coagulation; GHB=γ-hydroxybutyrate; MDMA=3,4-methylenedioxy-methamphetamine; MMDA=3-methoxy-4,5-methylenedioxyamphetamine.

[a]Data from Baylen and Rosenberg 2006; Goldfrank et al. 2015; Kalant 2001; Ries et al. 2015.

[b]Data from Goldfrank et al. 2015; Mason and Kerns 2002; Miotto et al. 2001; Ries et al. 2015.

TABLE 5–18. **Dissociative anesthetics**

	PCP/Ketamine[a]	DXM[b]
Estimated number of U.S. users age 12 years and older	PCP: 6,450,000 Ketamine: 3,440,000	10,088,000; misused primarily by younger adolescents

Onset of action	PCP:
	  Smoked: 2–5 minutes
	  Oral: 15–20 minutes
	Ketamine:
	  IV: Seconds
	  Intramuscular: 1–5 minutes
	  Oral: 15–20 minutes
	  Nasal: 5–10 minutes
		15–30 minutes

Duration of action	PCP:
	  Smoked and oral: 4–6 hours, aftereffects up to 48 hours
	Ketamine:
	  IV: 30–45 minutes
	  Intramuscular: 30–45 minutes
	  Oral: 60–120 minutes
	  Nasal: 45–60 minutes
		Hydrobromide form: 6 hours
		Long-acting polistirex form (in brand name Delsym): 12 hours

Prevalence of psychiatric symptoms	Over 50% of patients present with classic toxidrome of violent behavior, nystagmus, tachycardia, hypertension, anesthesia, analgesia. Can wax and wane between CNS stimulation and depression 25% of heavy PCP users experience withdrawal symptoms.	

TABLE 5–18.   Dissociative anesthetics (continued)

	PCP/Ketamine[a]	DXM[b]
Psychiatric symptoms of intoxication	Stage I: delirium, psychosis, catatonia, hypomania with euphoria, depression with lethargy. Agitated or bizarre behavior, with increased risk of violence, can occur with any of the other psychiatric symptoms. Stage II: stuporous or in a light coma, but responsive to pain Stage III: comatose and unresponsive to pain Stage II and III intoxication are medical emergencies that require treatment in a comprehensive medical setting to maintain life support functions until the drug has been eliminated from the body.	Effects divided into four plateaus: 1. Mild euphoria, auditory changes, distorted gravity perception 2. Intense euphoria and hallucinations (including closed-eye hallucinations), visual distortions 3 and 4. Increasing levels of disorientation, depersonalization, dissociative sedation, psychosis, hyperexcitability, lethargy DXM can interact with other serotonergic agents such as SSRIs, linezolid, meperidine, and tramadol to cause serotonin syndrome. OTC cough formulations commonly abused often have chlorpheniramine, which can cause signs of anticholinergic toxicity. It can also cause seizures, rhabdomyolysis, and hyperthermia.
Psychiatric symptoms of withdrawal	Depression, anxiety, irritability, hypersomnolence, diaphoresis, and tremor	Craving, dysphoria, insomnia, panic attacks, and nightmares
Diagnosis	PCP is detected on most standard urine drug screens. Detectable for 2–4 days after PCP use. Chronic users can be positive for >1 week. High doses of diphenhydramine, DXM, and venlafaxine can cause a urine specimen to test positive for PCP if tests other than gas chromatography/mass spectrometry are used.	History, signs, and symptoms Does not react with standard urine drug screens Elevated serum chloride on certain auto-analyzers can occur. It is important to check acetaminophen levels because OTC cough formulations often contain acetaminophen.

TABLE 5–18. **Dissociative anesthetics (continued)**

	PCP/Ketamine[a]	DXM[b]
Management of psychiatric symptoms	Intoxication: Stage I: supportive (quiet environment, minimize stimuli, reassuring communication) Benzodiazepines for agitation if needed (Note: At higher doses, benzodiazepines can slow PCP clearance.) For psychotic symptoms, haloperidol can be used. Withdrawal: TCAs such as desipramine may reduce the psychological symptoms of PCP discontinuation.	Supportive (quiet environment, minimize stimuli, reassuring communication) Use of benzodiazepines for agitation if needed
Management of medical complications	Stage II and III symptoms: Muscle rigidity: diazepam 2.5 mg intramuscular/IV, up to 25 mg Status epilepticus: diazepam 5–10 mg intravenously, up to 30 mg Hypertension: propranolol 1 mg intravenously every 30 minutes prn, up to 8 mg; hydralazine 5–20 mg intravenously, depending on severity Bronchospasm: aminophylline 250 mg intravenously Increase renal clearance of PCP: diuresis with furosemide 20–40 mg intravenously every 6 hours along with urine acidification with IV ascorbic acid (1.5–2 g in 500 mg saline every 6 hours prn). Monitor for metabolic acidosis with urine acidification. Removal of drug: can utilize activated charcoal	

Note. CNS=central nervous system; DXM=dextromethorphan; OTC=over the counter; PCP=phencyclidine; prn=as needed; SSRI=selective serotonin reuptake inhibitor.
[a]Data from Bey and Patel 2007; Ries et al. 2015.
[b]Data from Burns and Boyer 2013; Ries et al. 2015.

TABLE 5–19. Hallucinogenic plants and herbs of abuse

Herb/plant	Dominant category	Onset and duration of action	Standard laboratory testing	Toxicology concerns: neurobehavioral and medical complications
Salvia	Hallucinogen (acts on kappa opioid receptors)	Chewed Onset: seconds to minutes Duration: up to 1 hour Inhaled Onset: seconds Duration: 20–30 minutes	Not routinely available	May cause racing thoughts, panic attacks, vivid hallucinations and synesthesias, profound diaphoresis, nausea, and emesis
Mitragyna speciosa (kratom)	Stimulant at low doses, opioid effect at higher doses	Oral route Onset: 5–10 minutes Duration: 1 hour	Not routinely available	May cause decreased appetite and weight loss; nausea, vomiting, and/or diarrhea; increased diaphoresis; tremor; and psychosis. It may or may not cause seizures.
Myristica fragrans (nutmeg)	Hallucinogen	Oral route Onset: 1–4 hours Duration: 24–72 hours	Not routinely available	Adverse effects usually mild to moderate, including agitation, nausea, vomiting, abdominal pain, and hallucinosis Resembles anticholinergic toxicity but without meiosis
Peyote/mescaline	Hallucinogen	Oral route Onset: 30–45 minutes Duration: 6–12 hours	Not routinely available	Causes hallucinosis and can cause toxicity resembling a sympathomimetic toxidrome with tachycardia, agitation, and mydriasis Nausea and emesis occur early after intake. Psychosis and seizure may occur.

TABLE 5–19. Hallucinogenic plants and herbs of abuse *(continued)*

Herb/plant	Dominant category	Onset and duration of action	Standard laboratory testing	Toxicology concerns: neurobehavioral and medical complications
Psilocybin ("magic mushrooms")	Hallucinogen	Oral route Onset: 30–45 minutes Duration: 2–6 hours	Not routinely available	Users usually seek medical attention for "bad trips," characterized by anxiety, agitation, disorientation, or confusion. Acute psychosis may occur. Bad trips may be followed by depressed mood or paranoia for days to months. Other acute effects include nausea, muscle aches, shivering, and mydriasis. Tachycardia and hypertension may occur. Mushroom ingestion may cause abdominal pain and emesis.
Amanita muscaria (fly agaric)	Hallucinogen	Oral route Onset: 0.5–3 hours Duration: 12 hours to days; highly variable duration among users	Not routinely available	Severe toxicity: marked agitation, confusion, CNS depression, seizures, coma
Ayahuasca	Hallucinogen	Oral route Onset: 30–50 minutes Duration: 3–4 hours Smoked or inhaled Onset: seconds Duration: 20–60 minutes	Not routinely available	Serotonin toxicity, particularly when the street preparations are smoked or inhaled; often sold as dimethyltryptamine (DMT) The risk of this toxicity is very low with oral ayahuasca prepared for indigenous ritualistic use. Nausea and vomiting

TABLE 5–19. Hallucinogenic plants and herbs of abuse (continued)

Herb/plant	Dominant category	Onset and duration of action	Standard laboratory testing	Toxicology concerns: neurobehavioral and medical complications
Lysergic acid amide (LSA)—in multiple plants, including morning glory and Hawaiian baby woodrose seeds	Hallucinogen	Oral route Onset: 20–40 minutes Duration: 6–10 hours	Not routinely available	"Bad trip," characterized by dysphoria, paranoid ideas, psychosis, and agitation. Users may present with sympathomimetic toxicity: mydriasis, tachycardia, hypertension, and piloerection. Hyperthermia may occur. Serotonin syndrome is unlikely but possible; if it occurs, will probably not be severe. Toxidrome is rarely fatal.
Jimsonweed (*Datura stramonium*)—contains atropine, scopolamine, hyoscyamine	Hallucinogen (acts more as a deliriogenic agent with anticholinergic symptoms)	Oral route Onset: 30–60 minutes Duration: 1 to several days	Not routinely available	Toxic delirium is marked by pronounced anterograde amnesia, confusion, dissociation, hallucinations, delusions, and an excited, giddy affect. Anticholinergic toxicity Overdose can be lethal with fever, tachycardia, and arrhythmia. Bizarre self-injury due to significant derealization may occur.
Ephedra species (supplements with ephedra alkaloids currently banned in the United States)	Stimulant	Oral route Onset: 2–3 hours Duration: 6 hours	Tests positive for methamphetamine	The most common adverse effects are cardiovascular: hypertensive emergency, cardiomyopathy, myocardial infarction, stroke, and seizure. Impaired thermoregulation leading to heat injury It may cause psychosis, mania, severe depression, and agitation.

TABLE 5–19. Hallucinogenic plants and herbs of abuse *(continued)*

Herb/plant	Dominant category	Onset and duration of action	Standard laboratory testing	Toxicology concerns: neurobehavioral and medical complications
Yohimbine (Goldfrank et al. 2015)	Stimulant in supplements for weight loss and erectile dysfunction. May be prescribed.	Oral route Onset: 10–15 minutes Duration: 3–4 hours	Not routinely available	Abdominal pain, nausea, emesis Sympathomimetic toxicity: anxiety, agitation, tachycardia, hypertension, myocardial infarction, arrhythmia, priapism
Khat/qat (cathinones)	Stimulant	See subsection "Stimulants: Cocaine, Amphetamines, Cathinones"		
Areca nut (betel nut)	Stimulant	Onset: <1 minute Duration: 2–17 minutes	Not routinely available	Dizziness, vertigo, vomiting Cholinergic toxicity: rare, with SLUDGE syndrome Bronchospasm Tachycardia Meiosis, but mydriasis can also occur Psychosis and delirium may occur rarely, mainly with toxic dose.

Note. CNS=central nervous system; prn=when necessary; SLUDGE=salivation, lacrimation, urination, defecation, gastrointestinal distress, emesis.
Source. Data from Abraham et al. 1996; Callaway et al. 1999; Goldfrank et al. 2015; Halpern 2004; Passie et al. 2002; Ries et al. 2015.

Anabolic Steroids

Anabolic androgenic steroids (AAS) are endogenous and synthetic derivatives of the male hormone testosterone that are altered to maximize anabolic effects, minimize androgenic effects, and elude detection (Table 5–20). These alterations lead to a higher serum concentration and longer half-life than testosterone. AAS abuse differs from abuse of other illicit substances because it does not cause the same immediate surge in dopamine, although tolerance and dependence have been demonstrated. The prevalence and severity of AAS-induced psychiatric effects are unclear. Data are extremely limited and derived mostly from case reports and small cross-sectional studies (Kanayama et al. 2010; Mareck et al. 2008; Ries et al. 2015).

Heavy Metals and Related Environmental Exposures

Symptoms from heavy metal exposures depend on exposure route, dose, and chronicity, with higher acute doses more likely to cause systemic toxicity and death, and lower subacute to chronic exposures leading to medical and neurobehavioral symptoms (Bjørklund et al. 2017; Goldfrank et al. 2015; Rehman et al. 2018). Genetic disorders (e.g., Wilson's disease), age, and nutritional status in exposed individuals also play a role in level of toxicity. Heavy metal exposures are often occupationally acquired, from growing industrial, agricultural, domestic, and technological applications. Additional sources include environmental pollution (particularly in areas such as mining, foundries, and smelting) and contaminated food and pharmaceuticals due to contaminated soil, containers, and production processes. Metalloid exposures that have neurobehavioral complications are covered in Table 5–21; other metal toxicities that do not have reported neurobehavioral symptoms (i.e., chromium, bismuth, antimony) are not covered. Arsenic, cadmium, lead, and mercury cause particularly high levels of toxicity even at lower levels of exposure and are classified as human carcinogens according to the U.S. Environmental Protection Agency and the International Agency for Research on Cancer. These diagnoses should be considered when patients present with changes in behavior or in overall function and an occupational or exposure history suspicious for an elemental exposure.

Micronutrient Deficiencies

Scurvy: Ascorbic Acid (Vitamin C) Deficiency

Risk factors.   Those at risk of scurvy include persons with alcoholism and patients with gastric bypass, chronic nausea, chronic vomiting, chronic diarrhea/malabsorption, and reduced intake of vitamin C (Popovich et al. 2009). Vitamin C deficiency may occur after 4–6 weeks of a diet free of ascorbic acid (Raynaud-Simon et al. 2010). In one study, 12% of hospitalized geriatric patients were diagnosed with scurvy, with need for assistance with feeding being predictive of this diagnosis (Raynaud-Simon et al. 2010). Vitamin C deficiency increases in end-stage kidney disease and may be worsened by hemodialysis.

Clinical findings.   Apathy, irritability, and depressed mood are features of vitamin C deficiency. These symptoms may begin before the appearance of mucocutaneous findings (petechiae, ecchymoses, gingival bleeding, or follicular hyperkeratosis). Depression that clears after a few days of treatment with vitamin C is characteristic (Brown 2015).

TABLE 5–20.	**Anabolic androgenic steroids**
Estimated number of U.S. users age 12 years and older	1,084,000[a] Monitoring the Future national survey results on drug use, 1975–2018 (Miech et al. 2019): U.S. 12th graders had a statistically significant drop in lifetime steroid use, from 2.3% to 1.6%.
Routes of administration	Oral, intramuscular, topical, and transdermal patches
Prevalence of psychiatric symptoms	22% of 41 body builders had full affective syndrome; 12% displayed psychotic symptoms. Prominent irritability or hypomania: 5% of subjects
Psychiatric symptoms of intoxication/ chronic use	Hypomanic/manic symptoms: faster speech, more energy, less sleep, and more impulsive behavior Case reports have described delusions and hallucinations. Limited description of violent outbursts and verbal aggression— occurs in supraphysiological doses combined with severe abuse
Psychiatric symptoms of withdrawal	Depressive symptoms: mood swings, fatigue, restlessness, loss of appetite, sleep problems, and decreased sex drive
Diagnosis	Urine and blood tests for steroids and metabolites: Measure ratio of testosterone to epitestosterone (T:E ratio >6 indicates illicit use). Metabolites are detectable in blood for 14–28 days after intake. Detection times for various anabolic steroids vary; testing is used primarily in screening for professional sports competitions unless a patient is presenting with psychiatric symptoms and a recent history suggestive of steroid use. Anadrol (oxymetholone): 2 months Anavar (oxandrolone): 3 weeks Deca-Durabolin (nandrolone decanoate): 17–18 months Dianabol (methandrostenolone): 5–6 weeks Equipoise (boldenone undecylenate): 4–5 months Halotestin (fluoxymesterone): 2 months Masteron (drostanolone propionate): 2 weeks Nandrolone phenylpropionate: 11–12 months Omnadren: 3 months Parabolan (trenbolone hexahydrobenzylcarbonate): 4–5 months Primobolan (oral): 4–5 weeks Sustanon 250: 3 months Testosterone cypionate: 3 months Testosterone enanthate: 3 months Testosterone propionate: 2 weeks Testosterone suspension: 1–3 days Trenbolone acetate: 4–5 months Turinabol (4-chlorodehydromethyltestosterone): 11–12 months Winstrol (stanozolol): 2 months
Management of psychiatric symptoms	Intoxication: supportive care; symptoms subside with cessation of use Withdrawal depression: supportive care, selective serotonin reuptake inhibitor, refer for therapy

[a]Prevalence from 1994, the last year that the National Household Survey on Drug Abuse queried steroid use (Substance Abuse and Mental Health Data Archive 1996).
Source. Data from Kanayama et al. 2010; Mareck et al. 2008; Ries et al. 2015.

TABLE 5–21. **Presentation, diagnosis, and treatment of elemental exposures that have associated neurobehavioral sequelae**

Metal	Clinical presentation	Diagnosis	Treatment
Manganese (Mn)	"Manganese madness": visual hallucinations, behavioral changes, anxiety, and compulsive actions These symptoms subside after several weeks and are replaced by extrapyramidal abnormalities—marked bradykinesia, rigidity, postural instability, mask-like face (loss of facial expression), impaired speech, and parkinsonian gait disturbances.	Exposure: occupational history (e.g., welders, ore crushers, miners) and presentation of symptoms, ruling out drug toxicities and exposures important Laboratory diagnosis: Mn levels may not be elevated as symptoms can progress years after exposure has ceased.	Levodopa treatment helpful, may not be effective in patients without dystonia/rigidity IV chelation with edetic acid is sometimes helpful if patient is currently exposed and there are elevated Mn concentrations in blood, CSF, urine, hair or skin.
Cadmium (Cd)	Neurobehavioral complications: Acute: none Chronic: impacts children more than adults but can cause impairment in learning ability, attentional difficulties, and behavioral changes Medical complications: Acute inhalation: shortness of breath due to pneumonitis and gastrointestinal symptoms Chronic: ESRD, bone demineralization, increased breast, prostate, renal cancer risk, and motor neuron disease	Exposure: People exposed to incineration fumes of Cd products (color pigments, several alloys, polyvinyl chloride–related products). Other major sources of Cd exposure are phosphate fertilizers and drinking water. Some exposure from cigarette smoking Laboratory diagnosis: Blood Cd concentration provides more accurate estimate of recent exposures, whereas measurement of urine Cd concentration is recognized to indicate past exposure and body burden of Cd.	Remove exposure. No specific methods for treating acute or chronic Cd exposure except for supportive therapy Cd-associated osteomalacia has been treated with high-dose vitamin D.

TABLE 5–21. **Presentation, diagnosis, and treatment of elemental exposures that have associated neurobehavioral sequelae** *(continued)*

Metal	Clinical presentation	Diagnosis	Treatment
Arsenic (As)	Neurobehavioral complications: Acute: acute encephalopathy can develop and progress over several days, with delirium. Chronic psychiatric: increased anxiety and social isolation, disturbances in speech, problems with visual perception, memory problems, and reduced cognitive performance Medical complications: Acute: garlic taste, nausea/vomiting, hematemesis, watery diarrhea, QTc prolongation, torsades, cardiac arrhythmias, and shock. Encephalopathy can progress to coma, and seizures. Chronic: HTN, CVD, dermatitis, and symmetrical sensorimotor polyneuropathy	Exposure: Drinking water contaminated by industrial waste or agrochemical waste Food containing pesticides, grown in high-As soil, fossil fuel burning, and smelting Laboratory diagnosis: Hair and nails levels are the best measure of chronic exposure. Urine is the best measure of recent exposure.	Remove exposure Acute poisoning: skin decontamination if needed and cardiac and electrolyte monitoring. Limited data are available on activated charcoal. Chronic poisoning: DMSA chelation (dosing: 10 mg/kg per dose three times per day for 5 days, followed by 10 mg/kg per dose twice per day for 2 weeks)
Aluminum (Al)	Neurobehavioral complications: Acute: encephalopathy (disorientation, confusion, speech disturbances, progresses to coma) Chronic: dementia Medical complications: Acute: myoclonus and seizures Chronic: bone and muscle pain, weakness, and iron-resistant anemia	History: long-term CKD patients on hemodialysis who were treated with Al-salt-containing medications such as Al hydroxide or sucralfate OR chronic overexposure to Al in antacids Laboratory tests: Serum Al will range from mild (20 µg/L) to extremely elevated (>200 µg/L). Hypochromic, microcytic anemia that does not respond to iron replacement.	Serum levels >200 µg/L: Stop all Al-containing drugs, hemodialysis 6 times per week with high-flux membrane until serum Al drops below 200 µg/L. Then perform low-dose deferoxamine stimulation test. Serum levels 20–200 µg/L: low-dose deferoxamine stimulation test then treatment with IV deferoxamine 5 mg/kg, depending on test response

TABLE 5–21. Presentation, diagnosis, and treatment of elemental exposures that have associated neurobehavioral sequelae *(continued)*

Metal	Clinical presentation	Diagnosis	Treatment
Aluminum (Al) *(continued)*		EEG abnormalities in encephalopathy include slowing of the normal rhythm and high-voltage biphasic or triphasic spikes.	
Copper (Cu)	Neurobehavioral complications: depression, declining school/work performance, personality changes, irritability, impulsiveness, labile mood, sexual exhibitionism, delusions and hallucinations, and cognitive impairment Medical complications: acute and chronic hepatitis, cirrhosis, and acute liver failure. Neurological symptoms include dysarthria and dystonia, which are most common, cerebellar ataxia, tremor, drooling, bradykinesia, postural instability, and cogwheeling facial spasms creating "sardonic expression."	Exposures: Wilson's disease, drinking from copper-lined vessels, water source contamination, occupational copper dust exposure. Diagnosis with Wilson's disease: High urine Cu (24-hour urine Cu >100 μg/day) Low blood ceruloplasmin (<20 mg/dL) Kayser Fleischer rings on slit-lamp examination Elevated LFTs CSF levels will be increased threefold to fourfold in patients with neurological symptoms.	Chelation with D-penicillamine
Lead, organic	Neurobehavioral complications: initially nonspecific insomnia, emotional instability, and decreased appetite. Progression to encephalopathy with delusions, hallucinations, and hyperactivity. Encephalopathy can deteriorate to coma and death.	Exposure: usually in people handling or intentionally inhaling leaded gasoline Laboratory diagnosis: BLL (see below)	Limit/remove exposure. Chelation with succimer (DMSA) or CaNa₂EDTA: At BLL >80 (inpatient >100) At BLL 40–80, depends on presence of symptoms, duration of exposures, and other medical issues

TABLE 5–21. **Presentation, diagnosis, and treatment of elemental exposures that have associated neurobehavioral sequelae (continued)**

Metal	Clinical presentation	Diagnosis	Treatment
Lead, organic *(continued)*	Medical complications: initially presents with nausea, vomiting, tremor, and increased deep tendon reflexes. Liver/kidney injury can develop later.		
Lead, inorganic Children	Mild/"asymptomatic": Neurobehavioral: impaired cognitive abilities Medical: impaired fine-motor coordination/balance, impaired hearing, and impaired growth Moderate: Neurobehavioral: hyperirritable behavior, intermittent lethargy, and decreased interest in play; "difficult child" Medical: intermittent vomiting, abdominal pain, and anorexia Severe: Neurobehavioral: encephalopathy (coma, altered sensorium, bizarre behavior, and loss of developmental skills) Medical: persistent vomiting, pallor, and medical symptoms of encephalopathy (cranial nerve palsies, ataxia, papilledema, incoordination, and seizures)	Exposure: ingestion (i.e., groundwater, leaded paint, lead-containing toys) and pica due to nutritional deficiencies Laboratory diagnosis (BLL, $\mu g/dL$): ≤ 49: mild 50–70: moderate ≥ 70: severe Patients also develop progressive iron-deficiency anemia due to impairment of heme biosynthesis.	Limit/remove exposure. Asymptomatic patients, BLL >45: chelation therapy with IV $CaNa_2EDTA$ or oral penicillamine or oral succimer (DMSA) Symptomatic patients, BLL >45, or lead encephalopathy: combined chelation with IV $CaNa_2EDTA$ and dimercaprol

TABLE 5–21. **Presentation, diagnosis, and treatment of elemental exposures that have associated neurobehavioral sequelae** *(continued)*

Metal	Clinical presentation	Diagnosis	Treatment
Lead, inorganic *(continued)*			
Adults	Mild: Neurobehavioral: depressive symptoms (apathy, moodiness), fatigue, somnolence, and subtle changes in cognition Medical: adverse effects on reproduction, kidney function, bone density, HTN, and cardiovascular disease Moderate: Neurobehavioral: memory loss, decreased libido, and insomnia Medical: headache, peripheral neuropathy, metallic taste, abdominal pain, constipation, anorexia, arthritis due to saturnine gout, myalgias, weakness, and arthralgias Severe: Neurobehavioral: delirium due to encephalopathy Medical: encephalopathy (coma, seizures, obtundation, focal motor disturbances, headaches, papilledema, optic neuritis), foot and wrist drop, abdominal colic, pallor, and nephropathy	Mostly occupational exposure (paint removal, construction, foundry/mining, lead-acid battery manufacturing). Exposure also occurs with use of moonshine, leaded bullets, and some cosmetics and herbal remedies/supplements containing lead. BLL (µg/dL): Mild: 20–69[a] Moderate: 70–100 + mild anemia Severe: >100	Limit/remove exposure. Chelation with succimer or CaNa$_2$EDTA: At BLL >80 (inpatient >100) At BLL 40–80, depends on presence of symptoms, duration of exposures, and other medical issues

TABLE 5–21. Presentation, diagnosis, and treatment of elemental exposures that have associated neurobehavioral sequelae *(continued)*

Metal	Clinical presentation	Diagnosis	Treatment
Mercury (Hg), organic	Neurobehavioral complications: chronic intellectual disabilities in children (as part of Minimata disease) and poor concentration and memory from permanent neurotoxicity Medical complications: Acute: gastrointestinal symptoms, tremor, respiratory distress, and dermatitis possible Chronic: motor disturbances (ataxia, trembling), impaired vision, and other dysesthesias Minimata disease: severe exposure in children; medical symptoms include decreased visual-spatial and gross motor skills, cerebellar ataxia, physical growth stunting, dysarthria, limb deformities, hyperkinesis, hypersalivation, seizures, and strabismus.	Exposure: Hg-contaminated fish Laboratory diagnosis: Blood Hg concentration of ≥9 ng/mL indicates acute poisoning. Urinary HG excretion of ≥2 µg/24 hours may be associated with symptoms and signs of chronic mercury exposure. The correlation between the levels of Hg excretion in the urine and clinical symptoms in chronic Hg exposure is poor, as blood and urine concentrations do not reflect total body mercury content in the setting of chronic exposure.	Remove exposure CNS toxicity is resistant to treatment with chelation. Dimercaprol will mobilize Hg to the brain and should be avoided.
Mercury (Hg), inorganic salts and elemental Hg	Neurobehavioral complications: Acute: none Chronic: Neurasthenia: fatigue, depression, headaches, hypersensitivity to stimuli, psychosomatic complaints, weakness, and memory and concentration deterioration.	Exposure: Elemental: occupational (gold mining, thermometer and barometer manufacturing) Inorganic: occupational (chloralkali industries, metal refineries)	Remove exposure At blood or urine levels >100 µg/dL, treat with chelation. Unithiol (DMPS) is best studied agent; succimer (DMSA) is the U.S. equivalent. Dimercaprol or penicillamine can also be used.

TABLE 5–21.   Presentation, diagnosis, and treatment of elemental exposures that have associated neurobehavioral sequelae (continued)

Metal	Clinical presentation	Diagnosis	Treatment
Mercury (Hg), inorganic salts and elemental Hg (continued)	Neurobehavioral complications: Chronic (continued): Erethism: easy blushing and extreme shyness, anxiety, emotional lability, irritability, insomnia, anorexia, weight loss, and delirium Medical complications: Acute: severe interstitial pneumonitis (inhaled), cough, dyspnea, chest pain, severe nausea, vomiting, and diarrhea, conjunctivitis, and dermatitis Chronic: fine central intention tremor, choreoathetosis, spasmodic ballismus (severe), ataxia, concentric constriction of visual fields ("tunnel vision"), anosmia, metallic taste, burning in the mouth, nausea, loose teeth, gingivostomatitis, and hypersalivation	Laboratory diagnosis: Blood Hg concentration of ≥9 ng/mL indicates acute poisoning. Urinary HG excretion of ≥2 µg/ 24 hours may be associated with symptoms and signs of chronic mercury exposure. The correlation between the levels of Hg excretion in the urine and clinical symptoms in chronic Hg exposure is poor, as blood and urine concentrations do not reflect total body mercury content in the setting of chronic exposure.	

Note.   BLL=blood lead level; CKD=chronic kidney disease; CNS=central nervous system; CSF=cerebrospinal fluid; CVD=cerebrovascular disease; DMSA=dimercaptosuccinic acid; DMPS=2,3-dimercapto-1-propanesulfonic acid; EDTA=ethylenediaminetetraacetic acid; EEG=electroencephalogram; ESRD=end-stage renal disease; HTN=hypertension; LFT=liver function test.

[a]In chronic lead exposure, blood concentrations of lead lower than those listed may be associated with these symptoms, because blood levels do not reflect total body lead in chronic exposure.

Source.   Data from Bjørklund et al. 2017; Goldfrank et al. 2015; Rehman et al. 2018.

Diagnosis. Diagnosis of vitamin C deficiency is based upon the constellation of dietary factors, risk factors, and clinical presentation. Whole blood ascorbic acid concentration reflects only recent intake and not total stores. Serum or plasma ascorbic acid levels less than 0.3 mg/dL represent a high risk for development of scurvy if vitamin C intake does not increase. The utility of this test is limited (Sauberlich 1975).

Treatment. The optimal dose of ascorbic acid for the treatment of vitamin C deficiency has not been established. Recommendations range from ascorbic acid 100 mg orally three times a day to 250 mg orally four times a day. Critically ill patients may require intravenous infusion (Woodruff 1975).

Pellagra: Niacin (Vitamin B₃) Deficiency

Risk factors. Endemic pellagra occurs in nations where untreated corn and corn products are the main dietary staple, particularly during time of famine. Although corn and corn tortillas are dietary staples in Central and South America, pellagra is not common there, because the corn in this region is prepared in an alkaline solution, which liberates bound niacin so that it becomes bioavailable. Nonendemic pellagra occurs among individuals with alcohol abuse, malabsorption, anorexia, dietary deficiency of niacin or tryptophan, or carcinoid syndrome and those taking certain antimycobacterial or antiepileptic drugs. Dermatitis and diarrhea are frequently absent in nonendemic forms. Risk is increased by administration of other B vitamins without niacin (Delgado-Sanchez et al. 2008; Hegyi et al. 2004).

Clinical findings. Neuropsychiatric disturbances occur in approximately 40% of unselected cases with pellagra. Depression occurs in 31% of all cases and delirium in 7% (Singer 1915). In the largest observational study of psychiatric inpatients with pellagra, approximately 11% had a schizophrenia-like illness, and 12% had mania/bipolar illness. The rest were described using an archaic categorization and nosology of psychiatric illness, making characterization difficult; however, they were probably experiencing what today would be diagnosed as dementia, delirium, psychotic depression, severe depression, or psychiatric illness with focal neurological signs (Pitche 2005). Patients with acute severe cases may present with delirium, oppositional hypertonus, and coma (Pitche 2005). Pellagra usually does not manifest with all of the "three Ds": dermatitis, dementia, and diarrhea. In fact, depression and delirium are more common than dementia (Delgado-Sanchez et al. 2008; Hegyi et al. 2004). The cutaneous findings are symmetrical. There is skin thickening, scale, or erythema in a photo-distributed area, especially the arms and neckline (Delgado-Sanchez et al. 2008; Hegyi et al. 2004).

Diagnosis. Diagnosis of pellagra is based upon the constellation of dietary factors, risk factors, clinical presentation, and laboratory test results. Laboratory tests alone are imperfect markers of this deficiency state, are not usually available in a timely fashion, and are often not necessary. The most commonly used test is the ratio of urinary 1-methylnicotinamide (1-MN) to urinary creatinine. Results <1.6 mg 1-MN per gram creatinine are positive for niacin deficiency. On the basis of one small study, this test was found to be approximately 82% sensitive and 79% specific (Creeke et al. 2007).

Treatment.   Treatment for pellagra is nicotinamide or nicotinic acid 300 mg/day in divided doses. Flushing and toxicity make nicotinic acid less tolerable than nicotinamide. Treatment should not be delayed while waiting for results of laboratory testing (Hegyi et al. 2004).

Folic Acid Deficiency

Risk factors.   Dietary risk for folate deficiency occurs with poor intake of fortified grains, legumes, green leafy vegetables, and folate-containing fruits. Other risk factors include medications, including methotrexate, oral contraceptives, and antiepileptic drugs; malabsorption; prolonged lactation; alcoholism; tobacco smoking/smoke exposure; and conditions with increased folate requirements including pregnancy, inflammatory bowel disease, psoriasis, eczema, hematological malignancy, and anemia (Devalia et al. 2014; Herbert 1972; Hild 1969; Pan et al. 2017).

Clinical findings.   A borderline or low level of folate is identified in 15%–38% of adults with severe depression. Reports vary, but the rate of mood disorder among patients with frank folic acid deficiency appears high (Lazarou and Kapsou 2010). Folate deficiency results in lower response rates to antidepressants, and treatment with folic acid may increase responsiveness of women with depression to antidepressant therapy, even among those not deficient in folic acid (Taylor et al. 2004).

Diagnosis.   There are insufficient data to identify which measurement is more accurate for diagnosing folic acid deficiency: serum folate or red blood cell (RBC) folate. Serum folate measurement is less expensive, simpler to perform, and superior in the setting of coexisting vitamin B_{12} deficiency; the latter causes lower RBC uptake of folate (Farrell et al. 2013). Serum folate should be measured in a fasting sample. Concentrations greater than 4.5 ng/mL are normal, while those less than 3 ng/mL are low. Measurement of RBC folate may be helpful with indeterminate results between 3 and 4.5 ng/mL, but empiric therapy with folic acid is safe and inexpensive (Devalia et al. 2014).

Treatment.   Treatment of folic acid deficiency involves folic acid dosages of 5 mg daily for 4 months; patients with malabsorption should receive dosages as high as 15 mg daily over 4 months (Lazarou and Kapsou 2010).

Wernicke-Korsakoff Syndrome: Thiamine (Vitamin B_1) Deficiency

Risk factors.   Populations in which polished rice is a major dietary staple are at increased risk of thiamine deficiency; such outbreaks occurred historically in Thailand and in West African countries such as Gambia. In the United States, dietary fortification has led to a much lower risk of thiamine deficiency. Risk factors seen in the United States are alcoholism, chronic dialysis, chronic severe diarrhea, malabsorption syndromes (including those due to gastrointestinal surgery), increased metabolic requirements (e.g., during systemic illness), and chronic, high doses of diuretics. There are also rare genetic mutations that impact thiamine transport (Sechi and Serra 2007).

Clinical findings.   Wernicke-Korsakoff syndrome is the best-known neuropsychiatric complication of thiamine deficiency. The classic signs of Wernicke's encephalopathy are the triad of 1) encephalopathy (confusion, inattentiveness, impaired memory, and decreased level of consciousness if untreated); 2) gait ataxia; and 3) oculomotor dysfunction (i.e., nystagmus, gaze palsies). All three signs occur in only one-third of patients, with confusion as the most common symptom, followed by staggering gait, then ocular problems. Korsakoff syndrome is a late neuropsychiatric manifestation in patients who have experienced repeated Wernicke's encephalopathy, with selective anterograde and retrograde amnesia (relative preservation of long-term memory and other cognitive skills) and apathy (Sechi and Serra 2007).

Diagnostic testing.   No laboratory studies are diagnostic for Wernicke's encephalopathy, and existing tests can be difficult to order and have limited use. Treatment should be promptly initiated if there is clinical suspicion for Wernicke's encephalopathy, regardless of testing. Thiamine deficiency is best measured by erythrocyte transketolase activity (ETKA) before and after addition of thiamine pyrophosphate (TPP). Low ETKA with more than 25% stimulation establishes the diagnosis (ETKA is not a readily available test) (Whitfield et al. 2018). Serum thiamine or TPP levels can be measured with high-performance liquid chromatography; however, blood level may not accurately reflect thiamine level. Normal blood levels do not exclude Wernicke's encephalopathy (Whitfield et al. 2018). Typical magnetic resonance imaging findings in acute Wernicke's encephalopathy include hyperintensities on T2-weighted images involving the third ventricle, medial thalamus, periaqueductal area, and mammillary bodies (Jung et al. 2012).

Treatment.   Treatment of Wernicke's encephalopathy involves immediate intravenous administration of thiamine 500 mg three times daily for 2 days, and then 250 mg intravenously/intramuscularly every day for an additional 5 days in combination with other B vitamins. Thiamine should be administered before giving intravenous dextrose, because dextrose administration can worsen thiamine deficiency. Thiamine-dependent enzymes require appropriate magnesium stores; thus, patients with low or low-normal serum magnesium concentrations should receive IV magnesium supplementation. Oral supplementation with thiamine 100 mg/day should be continued after parenteral treatment. Korsakoff syndrome is usually irreversible, and patients require psychosocial support measures (Thomson et al. 2002).

Vitamin B$_{12}$ (Cobalamin) Deficiency

Risk factors (Allen 2008; Bourre 2006; Devalia et al. 2014).   Risk factors for developing vitamin B$_{12}$ deficiency include decreased dietary intake (either due to chronic malnutrition or dietary choice) and conditions/medications that decrease absorption. Dietary restrictions include a strict vegan diet or a vegetarian diet during pregnancy. An infant breastfed by a B$_{12}$-deficient mother may become B$_{12}$-deficient. Conditions that impact absorption include the following:

- Autoimmune gastrointestinal abnormalities: Malabsorption syndromes, inflammatory bowel disease, celiac disease, autoantibodies to intrinsic factor or gastric parietal cells, autoimmune metaplastic atrophic gastritis; other autoimmune disorders such as thyroid disease or vitiligo
- Surgeries: Gastrectomy/bariatric surgery, ileal resection or bypass
- Fish tapeworm infection

- Iatrogenic agents (interfere with absorption): Neomycin, metformin, proton pump inhibitors, histamine-2 receptor antagonists (cimetidine), nitrous oxide gas (used in anesthesia or recreationally)
- Rare genetic disorder: Transcobalamin II deficiency

Clinical findings.   Vitamin B_{12} deficiency usually develops over years (with the exception of nitrous oxide exposure, which causes rapid B_{12} depletion). Psychiatric findings can initially be subtle and include depressive symptoms, insomnia, forgetfulness, psychotic symptoms (i.e., delusions, hallucinations), cognitive slowing, and eventually dementia. The most common neurological finding in B_{12} deficiency is a symmetrical sensory/sensorimotor neuropathy impacting the legs more than the arms. Subacute combined deficiency of the spinal cord usually presents with paresthesias and ataxia. Loss of vibration and position sense often occurs before loss of pain and temperature sense; it can progress to severe weakness, spasticity, paraplegia, and urinary incontinence. Other sentinel signs and symptoms include a macrocytic anemia (neuropsychiatric symptoms can occur even with no anemia) and glossitis (Devalia et al. 2014; Lachner et al. 2012; Lindenbaum et al. 1988).

Diagnostic testing.   Complete blood count findings may include macrocytic anemia, mild leukopenia or thrombocytopenia, low reticulocyte count, and hypersegmented neutrophils. A mean corpuscular volume greater than 115 is more likely to be due to vitamin B_{12}/folate deficiency than other conditions. Other findings may include increased lactate dehydrogenase, increased indirect bilirubin, and low haptoglobin due to premature destruction of developing RBCs. The absence of hematological abnormalities does not rule out B_{12} deficiency.

Serum levels of B_{12} greater than 300 pg/mL suggest that deficiency is unlikely (sensitivity ~90% except in individuals with intrinsic factor antibodies); levels 200–300 pg/mL suggest that deficiency is possible; and levels less than 200 pg/mL are consistent with deficiency. Given that there are several situations that can spuriously increase or decrease B_{12} levels, methylmalonic acid and homocysteine levels are often sent for confirmation. Elevated methylmalonic acid and homocysteine suggest vitamin B_{12} deficiency (±folate deficiency); elevated homocysteine only suggests folate deficiency (Devalia et al. 2014).

Treatment.   Replenish vitamin B_{12} at 1,000–2,000 µg daily (oral) or weekly (intramuscular/subcutaneous) until level is normalized. Continue supplementation with 1,000 µg intramuscular/subcutaneous monthly or high-dose daily oral therapy (1,000 µg) for those with chronic poor absorption or dietary restriction (Devalia et al. 2014).

Vitamin D Deficiency

Risk factors.   Risk factors for vitamin D deficiency include reduced sun exposure, darkly pigmented skin, decreased intake or absorption (including gastric bypass, small bowel disease, diet, and pancreatic insufficiency), defective 1-alpha-25-hydroxylation (hypoparathyroidism, renal failure, vitamin D–dependent rickets type 1), and defective 25-hydroxylation, which occurs in cirrhosis (Holick et al. 2011).

Clinical findings.   Studies have examined the possible relationship of vitamin D deficiency to seasonal affective disorder, schizophrenia, and depression. The strongest (although limited) correlation according to cross-sectional studies and cohort studies is that people ages 65 years and older with vitamin D deficiency were more likely to have depressive disorders compared with control subjects (Parker and Brotchie 2011; Parker et al. 2017). Vitamin D deficiency results in abnormalities in calcium, phosphate, and bone metabolism that may lead to osteopenia and osteoporosis in adults and to rickets in children. Vitamin D deficiency may also cause muscle weakness due to low phosphate as well as general bone and muscle pain (Dawson-Hughes 2017; Mascarenhas and Mobarhan 2004).

Diagnostic testing. Laboratory measurements of total 25-hydroxyvitamin D concentrations less than or equal to 20 ng/mL are considered insufficient, and concentrations less than 12 ng/mL are considered deficient. Patients will also have a secondary hyperparathyroidism and may have phosphaturia and low serum phosphate (Durazo-Arvizu et al. 2010; Munns et al. 2016).

Treatment. Per the U.S. Institute of Medicine and Endocrine Society Guidelines, treat vitamin D deficiency with supplementation with ergocalciferol (D_2) or cholecalciferol (D_3). For deficient adults, treat with 50,000 IU of D_2 or D_3 once per week for 8 weeks or 6,000 IU/day to achieve a level greater than 30 ng/mL. Consider the same treatment doses for people with vitamin D concentration of 12–20 ng/mL if they are experiencing musculoskeletal symptoms or psychiatric symptoms consistent with vitamin D deficiency. Follow with maintenance of 1,500–2,000 IU/day (treatment based on supplementation for bone abnormalities and not on psychiatric symptoms). In contrast, the U.S. Preventive Services Task Force found inadequate evidence to support screening for vitamin D deficiency and supplementation in asymptomatic patients with deficiency (Holick et al. 2011; Institute of Medicine Committee to Review Dietary Reference Intakes for Vitamin D and Calcium 2011).

Zinc Deficiency

Risk factors. Inadequate dietary intake of zinc is noted to be a worldwide problem impacting poor children in developing countries. Zinc deficiency is prevalent in developing countries, especially in South Asia, Sub-Saharan Africa, and segments of Central and South America. Elsewhere, zinc deficiency is associated with diets low in animal protein and/or high in phytates and fiber. Older age, malabsorptive syndromes, alcoholism, kidney disease, cirrhosis, pregnancy, and lactation all are risk factors for zinc deficiency (Nriagu 2011).

Clinical findings. Recent meta-analyses indicate that there is a link between zinc deficiency and depression, obsessive-compulsive disorder, and panic disorder; however, the overall evidence is limited (Li et al. 2017; Swardfager et al. 2013). In one study, significantly lower levels of zinc were found in depressed patients compared with healthy patients. A large recent cross-sectional study using data from the National Health and Nutrition Examination Survey study found that zinc, iron, copper, and selenium intakes were inversely associated with depression (Swardfager et al. 2013). Zinc deficiency also manifests as impaired growth in children, hypogonadism, decreased spermatogenesis, alopecia, impaired taste, immune dysfunction, night blindness, impaired wound healing, and various skin lesions (Nriagu 2011; Prasad 2012).

Diagnostic testing.   Plasma or serum zinc concentrations obtained from a morning fasting sample are considered low if the zinc concentration is less than 70 µg/dL for women or less than 74 µg/dL for men. Plasma and serum levels may not always distinguish individuals with zinc deficiency from those who do not have zinc deficiency. Factors besides nutritional zinc intake that increase plasma zinc levels include inflammation, starvation, hemolysis, and delayed separation of red blood cells from plasma in the subject's blood sample. Eating causes an acute decrease in plasma zinc level (Hess et al. 2007; Lowe et al. 2009).

Treatment.   There are no standard guidelines for adult dosages of zinc supplements to treat zinc deficiency. One source recommends treating mild zinc deficiency with two to three times the recommended daily allowance (RDA) of elemental zinc for 6 months, and treating moderate to severe zinc deficiency with four to five times the recommended daily allowance of zinc for 6 months for adults without other significant comorbidities. RDAs for zinc are 11 mg for adult men, 8 mg for adult women, 11 mg for pregnant women, and 12 mg for lactating women (Saper and Rash 2009). Zinc supplementation at a dosage of 25–30 mg/day may be useful either as monotherapy in depression or as augmentation to antidepressant treatment (Lai et al. 2012; Ranjbar et al. 2014; Solati et al. 2015).

Other Selected Psychotropic Toxicities

Drug-Induced Electrolyte Abnormalities

Drug-Induced Hyponatremia

SSRIs and venlafaxine have the highest risk of drug-induced hyponatremia (Table 5–22) compared with other antidepressants. TCAs pose a moderate risk, and mirtazapine is associated with little or no risk. Paroxetine and sertraline may cause less hyponatremia than other SSRIs. There are insufficient data to estimate risk with duloxetine or MAOIs (De Picker et al. 2014). Recorded incidence varies widely depending on study population and definition, but second-generation antidepressants confer an increase in the risk of hospitalization with hyponatremia (relative risk, 5.5); however, the increase in absolute risk above that of control subjects is small (0.25%) (Gandhi et al. 2017). Median time to onset of hyponatremia is 13 days, with 75% of cases occurring within 4 weeks of starting therapy. Sodium returns to baseline within 28 days of discontinuing therapy (Liu et al. 1996).

Oxcarbazepine and carbamazepine are associated with the greatest risk of drug-induced hyponatremia of all psychotropic medications. In one large pharmacovigilance study, the risk of hyponatremia with oxcarbazepine was almost 18 times as great as that with SSRIs (Letmaier et al. 2012). VPA also is associated with hyponatremia (Beers et al. 2010). Antipsychotic use may be associated with hyponatremia, but the study of this association is complicated by the high prevalence of polydipsia and comorbidity contributing to hyponatremia in this population (Meulendijks et al. 2010).

Severe symptoms and signs occur with more acute and/or severe hyponatremia. Patients may present with nausea, emesis, headache, muscle cramps, lethargy, seizure, unresponsiveness, and respiratory arrest. With chronic and nonsevere hypona-

TABLE 5–22. Electrolyte abnormalities due to psychotropic medications

Electrolyte abnormality	Medication	Comments
Hypercalcemia	Lithium compounds (Meehan et al. 2018)	Mechanism: drug-induced hyperparathyroidism Hypercalcemia usually mild Reversible unless there has been long-term exposure
Hypernatremia	Lithium compounds (Goldfrank et al. 2015)	Mechanism: nephrogenic diabetes insipidus Common symptoms: polyuria and polydipsia Hypernatremia occurs only when patients are instructed to fast or are not replacing water losses because physical restraint, chemical restraint, or a pathological process prevents them from taking in sufficient water. Mostly reversible unless there has been long-term lithium exposure
Hyponatremia (De Picker et al. 2014; Letmaier et al. 2012; Liu et al. 1996; Meulendijks et al. 2010)	Oxcarbazepine, carbamazepine, valproate, SSRIs, serotonin-norepinephrine reuptake inhibitors, TCAs, antipsychotics	Due to syndrome of inappropriate antidiuretic hormone secretion Frequency with these agents from most to least: oxcarbazepine > carbamazepine > valproic acid, SSRIs and venlafaxine > TCAs > antipsychotic agents. Insufficient data regarding duloxetine. Use monitoring for polydipsia and urine studies to distinguish from psychogenic polydipsia.

Note. SSRIs=selective serotonin reuptake inhibitors; TCAs=tricyclic antidepressants.

tremia, impairment of attention and gait as well as increased falls may occur. Antidepressant- and antiepileptic-induced hyponatremia occurs due to the syndrome of inappropriate antidiuretic hormone (SIADH) or increased tubular sensitivity to antidiuretic hormone, characterized by an elevated urine osmolality (>300 mOsm/kg) and urine sodium (>40 mEq/L). Mixed causes of hyponatremia due to other medications, comorbidities, and (often occult) psychogenic polydipsia frequently occur, limiting the usefulness of urine studies in these cases. In isolated psychogenic polydipsia, the urine osmolality is usually less than 100 mOsm/kg. The treatment of hyponatremia is outside the scope of this brief review (De Picker et al. 2014; Meulendijks et al. 2010). Patients ages 65 years and older, those taking other hyponatremia-inducing medications, or those with comorbidities associated with hyponatremia should be monitored periodically for development of hyponatremia, particularly the week and month after initiation or dose adjustment (Gandhi et al. 2017).

Lithium-Induced Hypernatremia

Lithium causes nephrogenic diabetes insipidus, which clinically manifests as an impaired ability to concentrate urine. Nephrogenic diabetes insipidus occurs within 8 weeks of starting therapy and improves over 8 weeks after cessation of lithium. Prolonged exposure, especially at higher doses, may result in clinically significant, irreversible deficits that correlate with total lifetime grams of lithium consumed. Patients with diabetes insipidus who cannot keep up with ongoing water losses (e.g., because of impaired cerebral thirst regulation, restraints, or difficulty swallowing) will develop hypernatremia (see Table 5–22; Goldfrank et al. 2015).

Drug-Induced Liver Injury

DILI is the fourth leading cause of liver damage in Western countries. DILI can be classified as hepatocellular, cholestatic, or mixed, depending on the type of underlying liver injury. LFT abnormalities are common among patients taking medications for psychiatric disorders; these abnormalities may be caused by comorbidities (including alcohol abuse, viral hepatitis, and metabolic syndrome) or drug-induced liver injury. Table 5–23 provides a risk stratification of different psychotropic agents according to Roussel Uclaf Causality Assessment Method (RUCAM) criteria (Björnsson and Hoofnagle 2016).

Risk With Different Agents

Antidepressant drugs. Approximately 15% of patients prescribed TCAs and 5% of patients prescribed serotonin reuptake inhibitors will have mild asymptomatic LFT abnormalities (aspartate transaminase [AST] and alanine aminotransferase [ALT] <100 U/L; γ-glutamyl transferase <200 U/L) (Voican et al. 2014). A prospective multicenter study of psychiatric inpatients documented serious elevations of LFTs or symptomatic liver injury in 0.05% of patients taking antidepressants. These events were greatest with TCAs/tetracyclic antidepressants (0.14%), least with SSRIs (0.03%), and intermediate with others (Friedrich et al. 2016). Pharmacovigilance data from the World Health Organization suggest the U.S. Food and Drug Administration–approved antidepressants conferring the highest risk of drug-induced liver injury are nefazodone, phenelzine, imipramine, amitriptyline, duloxetine, bupropion, trazodone, tianeptine, and agomelatine. The antidepressants with the least potential for hepatotoxicity are citalopram, escitalopram, paroxetine, and fluvoxamine. All SSRIs evaluated in this study had an odds ratio for drug-induced liver injury of 1 or less (Voican et al. 2014).

Antipsychotic drugs.   Approximately one-third of patients prescribed antipsychotic drugs will have LFT abnormalities, and 4% will have transaminases greater than three times the upper limit of normal or an alkaline phosphatase greater than twice the upper limit of normal. LFT abnormalities usually occur between 1 and 6 weeks after initiation of the drug (Marwick et al. 2012). LFTs frequently normalize even if the agent is continued but normalize more often and more quickly with medication discontinuation or dosage reduction. Chlorpromazine has the highest rate of antipsychotic-induced liver injury and liver failure. It causes more cases of cholestatic injury than of hepatocellular or mixed injury (Marwick et al. 2012).

Mood-stabilizing agents.   LFT abnormalities caused by lithium are uncommon, and acute liver injury is extremely rare. Likewise, lamotrigine is associated with LFT abnormalities in only approximately 1% of patients, and significant hepatotoxicity is very rare (Au and Pockros 2013). Oxcarbazepine has been associated with fewer than three published cases of DILI. LFT abnormalities and DILI occur more frequently with valproate and carbamazepine (they are among the most common psychotropic agents to cause DILI); however, severe hepatotoxicity and liver failure are rare with both (Au and Pockros 2013). Approximately 15% of patients taking valproate have transient LFT abnormalities. True hepatotoxicity usually occurs within the first 3 months of use (Au and Pockros 2013). Approximately 61% of patients prescribed carbamazepine will experience asymptomatic and usually transient mild LFT abnormalities. These usually develop within 2 months of first taking the medication.

Prevention

Patients with preexisting liver disease have a lower reserve for avoiding future liver injury. These patients should be prescribed agents with a lower risk of hepatotoxicity. For all patients, prevention of significant liver injury requires periodic monitoring of LFTs, which should be monitored monthly for the first 2 months of therapy with the agents listed in categories A–C (see Table 5–23) and then every 6–12 months thereafter (Björnsson and Hoofnagle 2016). Consider more frequent monitoring for patients with preexisting liver disease. All patients should be periodically assessed for upper-right-quadrant pain or tenderness, nausea, vomiting, or jaundice, and appropriate laboratory and imaging assessment should be performed if these occur.

Assessment and Management

Clinical history is important in determining causative factors of liver injury, including relevant viral infections (hepatitis B virus, hepatitis C virus, and HIV), alcohol use history, potentially hepatotoxic medication, and herbal agents the patient is using. Asymptomatic patients with AST or ALT three times the upper limit or more of normal or with alkaline phosphatase more than two times the upper limit of normal should have serology sent for hepatitis B virus, hepatitis C virus, and HIV, as well as assessment of prothrombin time/international normalized ratio (INR). Alcohol use history should be obtained, and a determination of the risk of metabolic syndrome and fatty

TABLE 5–23. Risk classification for drug-induced liver injury using Roussel Uclaf Causality Assessment Method criteria

Medication class	Category A: drugs most likely to cause liver injury and known to cause liver injury (more than 50 published cases)	Category B: drugs known or highly likely to cause idiosyncratic liver injury (between 12 and 50 published cases)	Category C: drugs that probably cause liver injury, but uncommonly (4–11 published cases)	Category D: drugs that possibly, rarely cause liver injury, but reports are unconvincing (1–3 published cases)	Category E: drugs not associated with cases of possible and clinically apparent liver injury
Antipsychotics	Chlorpromazine	Clozapine Haloperidol Thioridazine	Olanzapine Quetiapine Risperidone	Molindone Ziprasidone	Paliperidone Trifluoperazine Fluphenazine Aripiprazole Iloperidone (2010[a]) Asenapine (2009[a]) Lurasidone (2010[a]) Brexpiprazole (2015[a]) Cariprazine (2015[a]) Pimavanserin (2016[a])
Antidepressants		Amitriptyline Desvenlafaxine Duloxetine Imipramine Paroxetine Sertraline Venlafaxine	Bupropion Citalopram Clomipramine Escitalopram Fluoxetine Nefazodone Mirtazapine Phenelzine Trazodone	Clomipramine Doxepin Nortriptyline Tranylcypromine	Fluvoxamine Desipramine

TABLE 5–23. Risk classification for drug-induced liver injury using Roussel Uclaf Causality Assessment Method criteria *(continued)*

Medication class	Category A: drugs most likely to cause liver injury and known to cause liver injury (more than 50 published cases)	Category B: drugs known or highly likely to cause idiosyncratic liver injury (between 12 and 50 published cases)	Category C: drugs that probably cause liver injury, but uncommonly (4–11 published cases)	Category D: drugs that possibly, rarely cause liver injury, but reports are unconvincing (1–3 published cases)	Category E: drugs not associated with cases of possible and clinically apparent liver injury
Anxiolytics				Alprazolam Chlordiazepoxide Triazolam Flurazepam	Buspirone Clorazepate Diazepam Lorazepam Midazolam Temazepam Lithium
Mood stabilizers	Carbamazepine Valproate	Lamotrigine		Oxcarbazepine	Lithium
Other			Amphetamines Atomoxetine Methylphenidate Desmethylphenidate		Benztropine Trihexyphenidyl

[a]Year of U.S. Food and Drug Administration approval. Relatively recent approval may explain the lack of postmarketing reports on liver injury (i.e., there has not been enough time to identify such effects if they exist); thus, a low risk rating may be unreliable.

Source. Data from Björnsson and Hoofnagle 2016; Livertox 2017.

liver should be made. Once other causes of elevated LFTs are ruled out, the clinician should consider dosage reduction, discontinuation, or switching the treatment agent to a lower-risk medication. Often, mild LFT abnormalities will normalize even if the agents are continued.

Circumstances under which the psychotropic agent should be discontinued include the following:

- Nausea or vomiting
- Upper-right-quadrant pain or tenderness
- Jaundice
- Indications of drug-induced hypersensitivity syndrome or drug reaction with eosinophilia and systemic symptoms (DRESS syndrome): fever, lymphadenopathy, rash or mucocutaneous syndrome, eosinophilia, or other organ involvement
- AST or ALT more than five times the upper limit of normal
- Total bilirubin >2–2.5 mg/dL
- INR >1.5 without other cause

Elevations of bilirubin or INR are indications to request assistance from a hepatologist/gastroenterologist. In rare cases of patients with fulminant hepatitis resulting from drug hepatotoxicity, liver transplantation may be lifesaving.

Drug-Induced Long QT Syndrome and Torsades De Pointes

Long QT syndrome is characterized by abnormal cardiac repolarization, prolonged electrocardiographic QT interval, and increased risk of polymorphic ventricular tachycardia and sudden cardiac death. Antipsychotic and antidepressant medications block the *hERG* channel responsible for the rapid delayed rectifier potassium current (I_{kr}), which causes increases in the QTc (QT corrected for rate) and the acquired long QT syndrome. Although drug-induced torsades de pointes (TdP) is not a frequent event, the mortality risk conferred with long-term use of antipsychotic and antidepressant agents warrants attention (Hasnain and Vieweg 2014; Salvo et al. 2016).

Risk Factors

Current data provide little evidence that QTc interval prolongation associated with use of antidepressants or antipsychotics is sufficient to predict TdP (Hasnain and Vieweg 2014). Table 5–24 provides data as of June 2019 for risk categorization of medications that induce QT prolongation and TdP based on a comprehensive review of published and reported cases. These data are publicly available online at the Arizona Center for Education and Research on Therapeutics (AZCERT) website (www.CredibleMeds.org; Woosley et al. 2019).

A meta-analysis of six observational studies utilized meta-regression to determine the odds ratios of sudden cardiac death associated with different antipsychotics (Salvo et al. 2016). The mean odds ratio of sudden cardiac death was 2.65, with more than 40% of the difference between agents explained by *hERG* blockade potency of the medication. The individual odds ratios from the meta-analysis are shown in Table 5–25; however, the confidence intervals are wide and overlapping.

In addition to type of antipsychotic, other risk factors for QTc prolongation include the following (Drew et al. 2010):

- Use of more than one QT-prolonging drug: Some of the other agents that contribute to the long QT syndrome include class III antiarrhythmics, methadone, macrolide antibiotics, quinolones, azole antifungals, antihistamines, some proton pump inhibitors, and some antiretroviral drugs.
- Rapid intravenous administration of a QT-prolonging agent
- Higher dosages of QT-prolonging agents
- Impaired elimination due to liver disease, kidney disease, or drug interactions
- Heart disease
- Advanced age
- Female sex
- Hypokalemia, hypomagnesemia, or hypocalcemia
- Diuretic use
- Impaired hepatic function
- Bradycardia
- Occult congenital long QT syndrome: This syndrome occurs in 5%–20% of cases of "drug-induced" TdP. Patients with congenital long QT syndrome will have a family history significant for syncope and sudden death as well as a personal history of symptomatic tachycardia and syncope.

Electrocardiographic Diagnosis

A prolonged corrected QT interval (QTc) is defined as greater than 0.450 seconds for men and greater than 0.470 seconds for women, and a QTc greater than 0.500 seconds confers an approximate two to three times greater risk of TdP among patients with congenital long QT (Drew et al. 2010). TdP occasionally occurs in patients with a normal QT interval. The 0.500-second cutoff is used by many as the threshold at which to discontinue, reduce dosage, or change therapy. If the QTc was prolonged before addition of a known QT-prolonging agent and did not increase after addition of the agent, then congenital long QT syndrome or another cause of acquired long QT should be investigated.

The QTc corrects estimates of appropriate QT length for different heart rates. Bazett's formula (QT interval/$\sqrt{RR}$ interval) is the most commonly used method to determine the QTc; however, it overestimates the correction for patients with a heart rate greater than 100 beats/minute.

Management

If the QTc interval is greater than 500 milliseconds or the current QTc interval is greater than 60 milliseconds more than the QTc interval prior to administration of the QT-prolonging agent, modifiable risk factors should be addressed first, as follows (Drew et al. 2010):

- Dosage reduction or cessation of the QT-prolonging agent
- Change of QT-prolonging medication to another psychotropic agent, particularly agents from the AZCERT website (www.CredibleMeds.org) "conditional risk of TdP" category or the "not yet classified" category, or agents not listed on the site.

TABLE 5–24. Risk of torsades de pointes (TdP) with psychotropic medications

Drug class	Drugs with known risk of TdP	Drugs with possible risk of TdP (prolong the QT interval but currently lack evidence for a risk of TdP when taken as directed)	Drugs with conditional risk of TdP (known risk only proven to occur with predisposing circumstances[a])	Drugs not yet classified as causing TdP	Drugs that need to be avoided in congenital long QT but do not prolong the QT interval
Antidepressants	Citalopram Escitalopram	Clomipramine Desipramine Imipramine Maprotiline Mirtazapine Nortriptyline Trimipramine Venlafaxine	Amitriptyline Doxepin Fluoxetine Fluvoxamine Paroxetine Sertraline Trazodone	Bupropion Duloxetine Nefazodone	
Antipsychotics	Chlorpromazine Haloperidol Pimozide Thioridazine	Aripiprazole Asenapine Clozapine Iloperidone Paliperidone Perphenazine Risperidone Pimavanserin	Olanzapine Quetiapine Ziprasidone	Brexpiprazole Fluphenazine Lurasidone	
Anxiolytics				Alprazolam Buspirone Clonazepam Diazepam Lorazepam Oxazepam Temazepam	

TABLE 5–24. Risk of torsades de pointes (TdP) with psychotropic medications *(continued)*

Drug class	Drugs with known risk of TdP	Drugs with possible risk of TdP (prolong the QT interval but currently lack evidence for a risk of TdP when taken as directed)	Drugs with conditional risk of TdP (known risk only proven to occur with predisposing circumstances[a])	Drugs not yet classified as causing TdP	Drugs that need to be avoided in congenital long QT but do not prolong the QT interval
Mood stabilizers		Lithium		Carbamazepine Valproic acid	
Other agents	Methadone Donepezil	Atomoxetine Buprenorphine Tetrabenazine Valbenazine			Amphetamines (isomers and salts) Methylphenidate Dexmethylphenidate

[a]Possible circumstances in which these agents may cause TdP include ingestion with other agents that confer risk of TdP, when there is a pharmacokinetic interaction with another agent, when taken in overdose, or in the setting of relevant electrolyte abnormalities.

Source. Data from Woosley et al. 2019.

TABLE 5–25.	QT-prolonging drugs and risk of sudden death
Drug	Odds ratio for sudden death (95% confidence interval)
Chlorpromazine	1.66 (0.83–3.29)
Clozapine	3.67 (1.94–6.94)
Fluphenazine	0.06 (0.00–6.00)
Haloperidol	2.97 (1.59–5.54)
Olanzapine	2.04 (1.52–2.74)
Quetiapine	1.72 (1.33–2.23)
Risperidone	3.04 (2.39–3.86)
Thioridazine	4.58 (2.09–10.05)

Source. Data from Salvo et al. 2016.

- Identification and cessation of other coprescribed QT-prolonging agents
- Treatment of hypokalemia, hypomagnesemia, and hypocalcemia
- Identification of drug interactions that impair clearance of the QT-prolonging agent

If the QT interval remains prolonged and the clinician is unable to reduce or discontinue the offending agent, the consulting internist or cardiologist should meet with the prescribing physician to carefully weigh the risks and benefits of continued treatment with this agent. This conversation should occur in the context of the patient's other risk factors for TdP, particularly a personal or family history of syncope or sudden death suggestive of occult congenital long QT syndrome.

Drug-Induced Orthostatic Hypotension

Antipsychotic drugs and TCAs antagonize α-adrenergic receptors and may cause orthostatic hypotension, in part through this mechanism. MAOIs can cause orthostatic hypotension, but the mechanism by which this occurs in unclear. Patients may be asymptomatic, and most do not experience dizziness; the latter symptom is neither sensitive nor specific for identifying orthostatic hypotension (Angelousi et al. 2014). Orthostatic hypotension causes falls, syncope, and associated trauma. Patients should have orthostatic blood pressure and pulse measured before initiating antipsychotics, TCAs, or MAOIs, and when steady state is reached after initiation or dosage adjustment. Inpatients should have their orthostatic vital signs measured on a daily basis (Angelousi et al. 2014).

Risk Factors

There are limited data ranking risk of orthostatic hypotension caused by psychotropic medications. Most estimates come from studies using imperfect surrogates such as orthostatic faintness or hypotension independent of positional change. Other than with chlorpromazine and haloperidol, there are few data on the relative orthostatic effects of other typical antipsychotics (Gugger 2011). Similarly, there has been only limited reporting about the relative hypotensive effects of newer agents such as iloperidone, aripiprazole, asenapine, and lurasidone (Freudenreich et al. 2016). The Clinical Antipsychotic Trials of Intervention Effectiveness (CATIE) trial (Stroup et al. 2009) investigated the discontinuation of antipsychotics due to different adverse effects (a summary of the rates of orthostatic intolerance during the trial is provided in Table 5–26). Given the available data, a reasonable ranking of some antipsychotics, from most to least effect on orthostatic blood pressure change, would divide antipsychotic agents into four risk categories, with Category 1 agents having the most risk and Category 4 agents having the least risk of orthostatic hypotension (Freudenreich et al. 2016; Gugger 2011):

- Category 1: Chlorpromazine and other low-potency first-generation agents
- Category 2: Clozapine, quetiapine, perphenazine, and iloperidone
- Category 3: Haloperidol, olanzapine, risperidone, and ziprasidone
- Category 4: Asenapine, lurasidone, and aripiprazole

Table 5–27 summarizes available data from systematic reviews on the relative risks of different antipsychotic agents compared with each other (as well as comparison of TCAs with placebo).

Evaluation and Management

The following approaches for evaluation and management of drug-induced orthostatic hypotension are recommended:

1. Assess for other reversible causes of orthostatic hypotension (e.g., nonpsychiatric medications, decreased oral intake, vomiting, diarrhea, bleeding).
2. Consider discontinuing or reducing dosage of the offending agent versus switching to an agent with less risk of orthostatic hypotension.
3. Encourage nonpharmacological measures to prevent complications.
   - Keep the head of the bed elevated more than 12 degrees.
   - Educate patients regarding countermeasures (leg crossing with isometric squeeze, arm tensing to reduce orthostatic hypotension and symptoms).
   - Eating six small meals instead of three large meals will reduce orthostatic symptoms (via reduced splanchnic pooling).
   - Drinking 500 mL of cold water 30 minutes before standing may reduce orthostatic symptoms (ingestion of free water increases plasma norepinephrine). This effect peaks 20–40 minutes after ingestion. Monitor serum sodium in these patients using this modality if they are prescribed an agent associated with SIADH (Jones et al. 2015).
   - Offer a tightly fitted abdominal binder to wear when standing and ankle-to-thigh compressive bandages to prevent mesenteric and lower-extremity venous pooling, respectively.
4. If nonpharmacological measures are inadequate and the patient has persistent symptomatic orthostasis on a low-risk psychotropic regimen, consider pharmacological therapy with midodrine or fludrocortisone with sodium chloride tablets (total NaCl intake/day of 10 g) (Ong et al. 2013). Patients prescribed lithium who are given fludrocortisone and/or sodium chloride tablets should be monitored for hypernatremia (Ong et al. 2013).

TABLE 5–26.   Rates of orthostatic intolerance for antipsychotics in the Clinical
               Antipsychotic Trials of Intervention Effectiveness (CATIE)

	Rate, %		Rate, %
Olanzapine	8	Risperidone	8
Perphenazine	11	Ziprasidone	9
Quetiapine	12	Clozapine	24

Source. Data from Essali et al. 2009; Hazell and Mirzaie 2013; Leucht et al. 2008; Srisurapanont et al. 2004; Stroup et al. 2009; Tuunainen et al. 2000.

TABLE 5–27.   Relative risk of hypotension in systematic reviews comparing
               antipsychotic agents

Drug comparison	Relative risk of orthostatic hypotension (95% confidence interval)
Haloperidol vs. chlorpromazine	0.31 (0.12–0.88)
Clozapine vs. haloperidol	1.29 (1.12–1.49)
Clozapine vs. chlorpromazine	0.33 (0.20–0.55)
Olanzapine vs. clozapine	0.13 (0.02–0.98)
Quetiapine vs. chlorpromazine	0.28 (0.11–0.71)
Quetiapine vs. haloperidol	2.12 (NA)
Quetiapine vs. risperidone	4.86 (1.69–13.97)
Tricyclic antidepressant vs. placebo	4.86 (1.69–13.97)

NA=not available.
Source. Data from Duggan et al. 2005; Essali et al. 2009; Gugger 2011; Hazell and Mirzaie 2013; Leucht et al. 2008; Tuunainen et al. 2000.

Conclusion

In this chapter we have provided an overview of drug, medication, and environmental exposures, as well as nutritional deficiencies, that may occur in patients with psychiatric illness. It is our hope that the data and recommendations presented here will equip physicians with the knowledge and confidence they need to successfully assess, diagnose, and treat patients presenting with these problems.

References

Abraham HD, Aldridge AM, Gogia P: The psychopharmacology of hallucinogens. Neuropsychopharmacology 14(4):285–298, 1996 8924196
Allen LH: Causes of vitamin B12 and folate deficiency. Food Nutr Bull 29(2 suppl):S20–S34; discussion S35–S37, 2008 18709879
American Association of Poison Control Centers: Synthetic Cannabinoids. Alexandria, VA, American Association of Poison Control Centers, 2017. Available at: https://aapcc.org/track/synthetic-cannabinoids. Accessed November 26, 2017.

Angelousi A, Girerd N, Benetos A, et al: Association between orthostatic hypotension and car-diovascular risk, cerebrovascular risk, cognitive decline and falls as well as overall mortal-ity: a systematic review and meta-analysis. J Hypertens 32(8):1562–1571, discussion 1571, 2014 24879490

Au JS, Pockros PJ: Drug-induced liver injury from antiepileptic drugs. Clin Liver Dis 17(4):687–697, x, 2013 24099025

Baumann MH, Partilla JS, Lehner KR, et al: Powerful cocaine-like actions of 3,4-methylenedi-oxypyrovalerone (MDPV), a principal constituent of psychoactive "bath salts" products. Neuropsychopharmacology 38(4):552–562, 2013 23072836

Baylen CA, Rosenberg H: A review of the acute subjective effects of MDMA/ecstasy. Addiction 101(7):933–947, 2006 16771886

Beers E, van Puijenbroek EP, Bartelink IH, et al: Syndrome of inappropriate antidiuretic hor-mone secretion (SIADH) or hyponatraemia associated with valproic acid: four case reports from the Netherlands and a case/non-case analysis of vigibase. Drug Saf 33(1):47–55, 2010 20000866

Berman BD: Neuroleptic malignant syndrome: a review for neurohospitalists. Neurohospitalist 1(1):41–47, 2011 23983836

Bey T, Patel A: Phencyclidine intoxication and adverse effects: a clinical and pharmacological review of an illicit drug. Cal J Emerg Med 8(1):9–14, 2007 20440387

Bjørklund G, Mutter J, Aaseth J: Metal chelators and neurotoxicity: lead, mercury, and arsenic. Arch Toxicol 91(12):3787–3797, 2017 29063135

Björnsson ES, Hoofnagle JH: Categorization of drugs implicated in causing liver injury: critical assessment based on published case reports. Hepatology 63(2):590–603, 2016 26517184

Bonnet U, Preuss UW: The cannabis withdrawal syndrome: current insights. Subst Abuse Re-habil 8:9–37, 2017 28490916

Bourre JM: Effects of nutrients (in food) on the structure and function of the nervous system: update on dietary requirements for brain, part 1: micronutrients. J Nutr Health Aging 10(5):377–385, 2006 17066209

Boyer EW, Shannon M: The serotonin syndrome. N Engl J Med 352(11):1112–1120, 2005 15784664

Bramness JG, Rognli EB: Psychosis induced by amphetamines. Curr Opin Psychiatry 29(4):236–241, 2016 27175554

Brown TM: Neuropsychiatric scurvy. Psychosomatics 56(1):12–20, 2015 25619670

Burns JM, Boyer EW: Antitussives and substance abuse. Subst Abuse Rehabil 4:75–82, 2013 24648790

Burns MJ, Linden CH, Graudins A, et al: A comparison of physostigmine and benzodiazepines for the treatment of anticholinergic poisoning. Ann Emerg Med 35(4):374–381, 2000 10736125

Cakic V, Potkonyak J, Marshall A: Dimethyltryptamine (DMT): subjective effects and patterns of use among Australian recreational users. Drug Alcohol Depend 111(1–2):30–37, 2010 20570058

Callaway JC, McKenna DJ, Grob CS, et al: Pharmacokinetics of hoasca alkaloids in healthy hu-mans. J Ethnopharmacol 65(3):243–256, 1999 10404423

Castaneto MS, Gorelick DA, Desrosiers NA, et al: Synthetic cannabinoids: epidemiology, phar-macodynamics, and clinical implications. Drug Alcohol Depend 144:12–41, 2014 25220897

Chopra A, Kolla BP, Mansukhani MP, et al: Valproate-induced hyperammonemic encephalop-athy: an update on risk factors, clinical correlates and management. Gen Hosp Psychiatry 34(3):290–298, 2012 22305367

Chouinard G: Issues in the clinical use of benzodiazepines: potency, withdrawal, and rebound. J Clin Psychiatry 65 (suppl 5):7–12, 2004 15078112

Coffey SF, Dansky BS, Carrigan MH, et al: Acute and protracted cocaine abstinence in an out-patient population: a prospective study of mood, sleep and withdrawal symptoms. Drug Alcohol Depend 59(3):277–286, 2000 10812287

Creeke PI, Dibari F, Cheung E, et al: Whole blood NAD and NADP concentrations are not de-pressed in subjects with clinical pellagra. J Nutr 137(9):2013–2017, 2007 17709435

Currier GW, Trenton AJ, Walsh PG: Innovations. Emergency psychiatry: relative accuracy of breath and serum alcohol readings in the psychiatric emergency service. Psychiatr Serv 57(1):34–36, 2006 16399960

Dawson AH, Buckley NA: Pharmacological management of anticholinergic delirium: theory, evidence and practice. Br J Clin Pharmacol 81(3):516–524, 2016 26589572

Dawson-Hughes B: Vitamin D and muscle function. J Steroid Biochem Mol Biol 173:313–316, 2017 28341251

De Picker L, Van Den Eede F, Dumont G, et al: Antidepressants and the risk of hyponatremia: a class-by-class review of literature. Psychosomatics 55(6):536–547, 2014 25262043

Delgado-Sanchez L, Godkar D, Niranjan S: Pellagra: rekindling of an old flame. Am J Ther 15(2):173–175, 2008 18356638

Devalia V, Hamilton MS, Molloy AM: Guidelines for the diagnosis and treatment of cobalamin and folate disorders. Br J Haematol 166(4):496–513, 2014 24942828

Drew BJ, Ackerman MJ, Funk M, et al: Prevention of torsade de pointes in hospital settings: a scientific statement from the American Heart Association and the American College of Cardiology Foundation. J Am Coll Cardiol 55(9):934–947, 2010 20185054

Duggan L, Fenton M, Rathbone J, et al: Olanzapine for schizophrenia. Cochrane Database Syst Rev (2):CD001359, 2005 15846619

Dunkley EJ, Isbister GK, Sibbritt D, et al: The Hunter serotonin toxicity criteria: simple and accurate diagnostic decision rules for serotonin toxicity. QJM 96(9):635–642, 2003 12925718

Durazo-Arvizu RA, Dawson-Hughes B, Sempos CT, et al: Three-phase model harmonizes estimates of the maximal suppression of parathyroid hormone by 25-hydroxyvitamin D in persons 65 years of age and older. J Nutr 140(3):595–599, 2010 20089790

Engelhard CP, Touquet G, Tansens A, et al: Alcohol-induced psychotic disorder: a systematic literature review. Tijdschr Psychiatr 57(3):192–201, 2015 25856742

Essali A, Al-Haj Haasan N, Li C, Rathbone J: Clozapine versus typical neuroleptic medication for schizophrenia. Cochrane Database Syst Rev (1):CD000059, 2009 19160174

Farrell CJ, Kirsch SH, Herrmann M: Red cell or serum folate: what to do in clinical practice? Clin Chem Lab Med 51(3):555–569, 2013 23449524

Forrester MB: Jimsonweed (Datura stramonium) exposures in Texas, 1998–2004. J Toxicol Environ Health A 69(19):1757–1762, 2006 16905506

Freudenreich O, Goff D, Henderson D: Antipsychotic drugs, in Massachusetts General Hospital Comprehensive Clinical Psychiatry, 6th Edition. Edited by Stern T, Fava M, Wilens T, et al. Boston, MA, Elsevier, 2016, pp 475–488

Friedrich ME, Akimova E, Huf W, et al: Drug-induced liver injury during antidepressant treatment: results of AMSP, a drug surveillance program. Int J Neuropsychopharmacol 19(4):pyv126, 2016 26721950

Gandhi S, Shariff SZ, Al-Jaishi A, et al: Second-generation antidepressants and hyponatremia risk: a population-based cohort study of older adults. Am J Kidney Dis 69(1):87–96, 2017 27773479

Gillman PK: The serotonin syndrome and its treatment. J Psychopharmacol 13(1):100–109, 1999 10221364

Gillman PK: A review of serotonin toxicity data: implications for the mechanisms of antidepressant drug action. Biol Psychiatry 59(11):1046–1051, 2006 16460699

Gillman PK: Triptans, serotonin agonists, and serotonin syndrome (serotonin toxicity): a review. Headache 50(2):264–272, 2010 19925619

Goldfrank LR, Hoffman RS, Lewin NA, et al: Goldfrank's Toxicologic Emergencies. New York, McGraw Hill Education, 2015

Gugger JJ: Antipsychotic pharmacotherapy and orthostatic hypotension: identification and management. CNS Drugs 25(8):659–671, 2011 21790209

Gurrera RJ, Caroff SN, Cohen A, et al: An international consensus study of neuroleptic malignant syndrome diagnostic criteria using the Delphi method. J Clin Psychiatry 72(9):1222–1228, 2011 21733489

Gurrera RJ, Mortillaro G, Velamoor V, et al: A validation study of the international consensus diagnostic criteria for neuroleptic malignant syndrome. J Clin Psychopharmacol 37(1):67–71, 2017 28027111

Halpern JH: Hallucinogens and dissociative agents naturally growing in the United States. Pharmacol Ther 102(2):131–138, 2004 15163594

Halpern JH, Pope HG Jr: Hallucinogen persisting perception disorder: what do we know after 50 years? Drug Alcohol Depend 69(2):109–119, 2003 12609692

Harris D, Batki SL: Stimulant psychosis: symptom profile and acute clinical course. Am J Addict 9(1):28–37, 2000 10914291

Hasnain M, Vieweg WV: QTc interval prolongation and torsade de pointes associated with second-generation antipsychotics and antidepressants: a comprehensive review. CNS Drugs 28(10):887–920, 2014 25168784

Hazell P, Mirzaie M: Tricyclic drugs for depression in children and adolescents. Cochrane Database Syst Rev (6):CD002317, 2013 23780719

Hegyi J, Schwartz RA, Hegyi V: Pellagra: dermatitis, dementia, and diarrhea. Int J Dermatol 43(1):1–5, 2004 14693013

Herbert V: The five possible causes of all nutrient deficiency: illustrated by deficiencies of vitamin B 12 and folic acid. Aust N Z J Med 2(1):69–77, 1972 4557822

Hess SY, Peerson JM, King JC, Brown KH: Use of serum zinc concentration as an indicator of population zinc status. Food Nutr Bull 28(3 suppl):S403–S429, 2007 17988005

Hild DH: Folate losses from the skin in exfoliative dermatitis. Arch Intern Med 123(1):51–57, 1969 4236056

Holick MF, Binkley NC, Bischoff-Ferrari HA, et al: Evaluation, treatment, and prevention of vitamin D deficiency: an Endocrine Society clinical practice guideline. J Clin Endocrinol Metab 96(7):1911–1930, 2011 21646368

Institute of Medicine (US) Committee to Review Dietary Reference Intakes for Vitamin D and Calcium: Dietary Reference Intakes for Calcium and Vitamin D. Edited by Ross AC, Taylor CL, Yaktine AL, et al. Washington, DC, National Academies Press, 2011. Available at: https://www.ncbi.nlm.nih.gov/pubmed/21796828. Accessed November 1, 2019.

Iqbal MM, Basil MJ, Kaplan J, et al: Overview of serotonin syndrome. Ann Clin Psychiatry 24(4):310–318, 2012 23145389

Isbister GK, Hackett LP, Dawson AH, et al: Moclobemide poisoning: toxicokinetics and occurrence of serotonin toxicity. Br J Clin Pharmacol 56(4):441–450, 2003 12968990

Isbister GK, Bowe SJ, Dawson A, Whyte IM: Relative toxicity of selective serotonin reuptake inhibitors (SSRIs) in overdose. J Toxicol Clin Toxicol 42(3):277–285, 2004 15362595

Johns A: Psychiatric effects of cannabis. Br J Psychiatry 178(2):116–122, 2001 11157424

Jones PK, Shaw BH, Raj SR: Orthostatic hypotension: managing a difficult problem. Expert Rev Cardiovasc Ther 13(11):1263–1276, 2015 26427904

Jung YC, Chanraud S, Sullivan EV: Neuroimaging of Wernicke's encephalopathy and Korsakoff's syndrome. Neuropsychol Rev 22(2):170–180, 2012 22577003

Kalant H: The pharmacology and toxicology of "ecstasy" (MDMA) and related drugs. CMAJ 165(7):917–928, 2001 11599334

Kanayama G, Brower KJ, Wood RI, et al: Treatment of anabolic-androgenic steroid dependence: emerging evidence and its implications. Drug Alcohol Depend 109(1–3):6–13, 2010 20188494

Katus LE, Frucht SJ: Management of serotonin syndrome and neuroleptic malignant syndrome. Curr Treat Options Neurol 18(9):39, 2016 27469512

Katz MM, Waskow IE, Olsson J: Characterizing the psychological state produced by LSD. J Abnorm Psychol 73(1):1–14, 1968 5639999

Kerr GW, McGuffie AC, Wilkie S: Tricyclic antidepressant overdose: a review. Emerg Med J 18(4):236–241, 2001 11435353

Lachner C, Steinle NI, Regenold WT: The neuropsychiatry of vitamin B12 deficiency in elderly patients. J Neuropsychiatry Clin Neurosci 24(1):5qP15, 2012 22450609

Lago JA, Kosten TR: Stimulant withdrawal. Addiction 89(11):1477–1481, 1994 7841859

Lai J, Moxey A, Nowak G, et al: The efficacy of zinc supplementation in depression: systematic review of randomised controlled trials. J Affect Disord 136(1–2):e31–e39, 2012 21798601

Lazarou C, Kapsou M: The role of folic acid in prevention and treatment of depression: an overview of existing evidence and implications for practice. Complement Ther Clin Pract 16(3):161–166, 2010 20621278

Lee JW: Serum iron in catatonia and neuroleptic malignant syndrome. Biol Psychiatry 44(6):499–507, 1998 9777183

Letmaier M, Painold A, Holl AK, et al: Hyponatraemia during psychopharmacological treatment: results of a drug surveillance programme. Int J Neuropsychopharmacol 15(6):739–748, 2012 21777511

Leucht C, Kitzmantel M, Chua L, et al: Haloperidol versus chlorpromazine for schizophrenia. Cochrane Database Syst Rev (1):CD004278, 2008 18254045

Levine M, Ruha AM: Overdose of atypical antipsychotics: clinical presentation, mechanisms of toxicity and management. CNS Drugs 26(7):601–611, 2012 22668123

Lewis C, Deshpande A, Tesar GE, et al: Valproate-induced hyperammonemic encephalopathy: a brief review. Curr Med Res Opin 28(6):1039–1042, 2012 22587482

Li Z, Li B, Song X, et al: Dietary zinc and iron intake and risk of depression: a meta-analysis. Psychiatry Res 251:41–47, 2017 28189077

Liechti ME, Quednow BB, Liakoni E, et al: Pharmacokinetics and pharmacodynamics of gamma-hydroxybutyrate in healthy subjects. Br J Clin Pharmacol 81(5):980–988, 2016 26659543

Lindenbaum J, Healton EB, Savage DG, et al: Neuropsychiatric disorders caused by cobalamin deficiency in the absence of anemia or macrocytosis. N Engl J Med 318(26):1720–1728, 1988 3374544

Liu BA, Mittmann N, Knowles SR, et al: Hyponatremia and the syndrome of inappropriate secretion of antidiuretic hormone associated with the use of selective serotonin reuptake inhibitors: a review of spontaneous reports. CMAJ 155(5):519–527, 1996 8804257

Livertox: Livertox: Clinical and Research Information on Drug-Induced Liver Injury (website). Bethesda, MD, U.S. National Library of Medicine, National Institute of Diabetes and Digestive and Kidney Diseases, 2017. Available at: http://livertox.nih.gov. Accessed November 24, 2017.

Long D, Long B, Koyfman A: The emergency medicine management of severe alcohol withdrawal. Am J Emerg Med 35(7):1005–1011, 2017 28188055

Lowe NM, Fekete K, Decsi T: Methods of assessment of zinc status in humans: a systematic review. Am J Clin Nutr 89(6):2040S–2051S, 2009 19420098

Mareck U, Geyer H, Opfermann G, et al: Factors influencing the steroid profile in doping control analysis. J Mass Spectrom 43(7):877–891, 2008 18570179

Marwick KF, Taylor M, Walker SW: Antipsychotics and abnormal liver function tests: systematic review. Clin Neuropharmacol 35(5):244–253, 2012 22986798

Mascarenhas R, Mobarhan S: Hypovitaminosis D–induced pain. Nutr Rev 62(9):354–349, 2004 15497769

Mason PE, Kerns WP 2nd: Gamma hydroxybutyric acid (GHB) intoxication. Acad Emerg Med 9(7):730–739, 2002 12093716

Meehan AD, Udumyan R, Kardell M, et al: Lithium-associated hypercalcemia: pathophysiology, prevalence, management. World J Surg 42(2):415–424, 2018 29260296

Meulendijks D, Mannesse CK, Jansen PA, et al: Antipsychotic-induced hyponatraemia: a systematic review of the published evidence. Drug Saf 33(2):101–114, 2010 20082537

Miech RA, Johnston LD, O'Malley PM, et al: Monitoring the Future national survey results on drug use, 1975–2018: Vol I, Secondary school students. Ann Arbor, MI, Institute for Social Research, The University of Michigan, June 2019. Available at http://monitoringthefuture.org/pubs.html#monographs. Accessed October 1, 2019.

Miotto K, Darakjian J, Basch J, et al: Gamma-hydroxybutyric acid: patterns of use, effects and withdrawal. Am J Addict 10(3):232–241, 2001 11579621

Mitchell MC Jr, Teigen EL, Ramchandani VA: Absorption and peak blood alcohol concentration after drinking beer, wine, or spirits. Alcohol Clin Exp Res 38(5):1200–1204, 2014 24655007

Modi S, Dharaiya D, Schultz L, et al: Neuroleptic malignant syndrome: complications, outcomes, and mortality. Neurocrit Care 24(1):97–103, 2016 26223336

Munns CF, Shaw N, Kiely M, et al: Global consensus recommendations on prevention and management of nutritional rickets. J Clin Endocrinol Metab 101(2):394–415, 2016 26745253

Murray RM, Quigley H, Quattrone D, et al: Traditional marijuana, high-potency cannabis and synthetic cannabinoids: increasing risk for psychosis. World Psychiatry 15(3):195–204, 2016 27717258

Ng BK, Cameron AJ: The role of methylene blue in serotonin syndrome: a systematic review. Psychosomatics 51(3):194–200, 2010 20484716

Nriagu JO: Zinc deficiency in human health, in Encyclopedia of Environmental Health. Edited by Nriagu JO. Amsterdam, Elsevier, 2011, pp 789–800

Núñez LA, Gurpegui M: Cannabis-induced psychosis: a cross-sectional comparison with acute schizophrenia. Acta Psychiatr Scand 105(3):173–178, 2002 11939970

O'Brien CP: Benzodiazepine use, abuse, and dependence. J Clin Psychiatry 66 (suppl 2):28–33, 2005 15762817

Ong AC, Myint PK, Shepstone L, et al: A systematic review of the pharmacological management of orthostatic hypotension. Int J Clin Pract 67(7):633–646, 2013 23758443

Pan Y, Liu Y, Guo H, et al: Associations between folate and vitamin B12 levels and inflammatory bowel disease: a meta-analysis. Nutrients 9(4):E382, 2017 28406440

Parfitt DN: An outbreak of atropine poisoning. J Neurol Neurosurg Psychiatry 10(2):85–88, 1947 20265614

Parker G, Brotchie H: "D" for depression: any role for vitamin D? "Food for Thought" II. Acta Psychiatr Scand 124(4):243–249, 2011 21480836

Parker GB, Brotchie H, Graham RK: Vitamin D and depression. J Affect Disord 208:56–61, 2017 27750060

Passie T, Seifert J, Schneider U, et al: The pharmacology of psilocybin. Addict Biol 7(4):357–364, 2002 14578010

Pétursson H: The benzodiazepine withdrawal syndrome. Addiction 89(11):1455–1459, 1994 7841856

Pitche PT: [Pellagra]. Sante 15(3):205–208, 2005 16207585

Popovich D, McAlhany A, Adewumi AO, et al: Scurvy: forgotten but definitely not gone. J Pediatr Health Care 23(6):405–415, 2009 19875028

Pragst F, Herre S, Bakdash A: Poisonings with diphenhydramine—a survey of 68 clinical and 55 death cases. Forensic Sci Int 161(2–3):189–197, 2006 16857332

Prasad AS: Discovery of human zinc deficiency: 50 years later. J Trace Elem Med Biol 26(2qP3):66–69, 2012 22664333

Prosser JM, Nelson LS: The toxicology of bath salts: a review of synthetic cathinones. J Med Toxicol 8(1):33–42, 2012 22108839

Ranjbar E, Shams J, Sabetkasaei M, et al: Effects of zinc supplementation on efficacy of antidepressant therapy, inflammatory cytokines, and brain-derived neurotrophic factor in patients with major depression. Nutr Neurosci 17(2):65–71, 2014 23602205

Raynaud-Simon A, Cohen-Bittan J, Gouronnec A, et al: Scurvy in hospitalized elderly patients. J Nutr Health Aging 14(6):407–410, 2010 20617280

Rehman K, Fatima F, Waheed I, et al: Prevalence of exposure of heavy metals and their impact on health consequences. J Cell Biochem 119(1):157–184, 2018 28643849

Ries RK, Fiellin DA, Miller SC (eds): The ASAM Principles of Addiction Medicine, 5th Edition. Philadelphia, PA, Wolters Kluwer Health, 2015

Roncero C, Ros-Cucurull E, Daigre C, et al: Prevalence and risk factors of psychotic symptoms in cocaine-dependent patients. Actas Esp Psiquiatr 40(4):187–197, 2012 22851479

Rosebush PI, Mazurek MF: Serum iron and neuroleptic malignant syndrome. Lancet 338(8760):149–151, 1991 1677067

Sachs J, McGlade E, Yurgelun-Todd D: Safety and toxicology of cannabinoids. Neurotherapeutics 12(4):735–746, 2015 26269228

Salahudeen MS, Duffull SB, Nishtala PS: Anticholinergic burden quantified by anticholinergic risk scales and adverse outcomes in older people: a systematic review. BMC Geriatr 15:31, 2015 25879993

Salvo F, Pariente A, Shakir S, et al: Sudden cardiac and sudden unexpected death related to antipsychotics: a meta-analysis of observational studies. Clin Pharmacol Ther 99(3):306–314, 2016 26272741

Santos C, Olmedo RE: Sedative-hypnotic drug withdrawal syndrome: recognition and treatment. Emerg Med Pract 19(3):1–20, 2017 28186869

Saper RB, Rash R: Zinc: an essential micronutrient. Am Fam Physician 79(9):768–772, 2009 20141096

Sauberlich HE: Human requirements and needs. Vitamin C status: methods and findings. Ann N Y Acad Sci 258:438–450, 1975 1060412

Schuckit MA: Recognition and management of withdrawal delirium (delirium tremens). N Engl J Med 371(22):2109–2113, 2014 25427113

Sechi G, Serra A: Wernicke's encephalopathy: new clinical settings and recent advances in diagnosis and management. Lancet Neurol 6(5):442–455, 2007 17434099

Singer HD: Mental and nervous disorders associated with pellagra. Arch Intern Med (Chic) 15(1):121–146, 1915. Available at: https://jamanetwork.com/journals/jamainternalmedicine/article-abstract/653858. Accessed June 5, 2019.

Solati Z, Jazayeri S, Tehrani-Doost M, et al: Zinc monotherapy increases serum brain-derived neurotrophic factor (BDNF) levels and decreases depressive symptoms in overweight or obese subjects: a double-blind, randomized, placebo-controlled trial. Nutr Neurosci 18(4):162–168, 2015 24621065

Srisurapanont M, Maneeton B, Maneeton N: Quetiapine for schizophrenia. Cochrane Database Syst Rev (2):CD000967, 2004 15106155

Sternbach H: The serotonin syndrome. Am J Psychiatry 148(6):705–713, 1991 2035713

Stroup TS, Lieberman JA, McEvoy JP, et al: Results of phase 3 of the CATIE schizophrenia trial. Schizophr Res 107(1):1–12, 2009 19027269

Substance Abuse and Mental Health Data Archive: National Household Survey on Drug Abuse (formerly called the National Household Survey), Part B (NHSDA-1994-DS0002). Rockville, MD, Office of Applied Studies, Substance Abuse and Mental Health Services Administration, June 1996. Available at: https://www.datafiles.samhsa.gov/study-data-set/part-b-nhsda-1994-ds0002-nid13785. Accessed October 1, 2019.

Substance Abuse and Mental Health Services Administration: Results From the 2016 National Survey on Drug Use and Health: Detailed Tables. Rockville, MD, Center for Behavioral Health Statistics and Quality, Substance Abuse and Mental Health Services Administration, 2017. Available at: https://www.samhsa.gov/data/sites/default/files/NSDUH-DetTabs-2016/NSDUH-DetTabs-2016.pdf. Accessed October 13, 2017.

Sun-Edelstein C, Tepper SJ, Shapiro RE: Drug-induced serotonin syndrome: a review. Expert Opin Drug Saf 7(5):587–596, 2008 18759711

Susman VL: Clinical management of neuroleptic malignant syndrome. Psychiatr Q 72(4):325–336, 2001 11525080

Swardfager W, Herrmann N, Mazereeuw G, et al: Zinc in depression: a meta-analysis. Biol Psychiatry 74(12):872–878, 2013 23806573

Taylor MJ, Carney SM, Goodwin GM, et al: Folate for depressive disorders: systematic review and meta-analysis of randomized controlled trials. J Psychopharmacol 18(2):251–256, 2004 15260915

Thomson AD, Cook CC, Touquet R, et al; Royal College of Physicians, London: The Royal College of Physicians report on alcohol: guidelines for managing Wernicke's encephalopathy in the accident and emergency department. Alcohol Alcohol 37(6):513–521, 2002 [Erratum in: Alcohol Alcohol 38(3):291, 2003] 12414541

Tse L, Barr AM, Scarapicchia V, et al: Neuroleptic malignant syndrome: a review from a clinically oriented perspective. Curr Neuropharmacol 13(3):395–406, 2015 26411967

Tuunainen A, Wahlbeck K, Gilbody SM: Newer atypical antipsychotic medication versus clozapine for schizophrenia. Cochrane Database Syst Rev (2):CD000966, 2000 10796559

Uddin MF, Alweis R, Shah SR, et al: Controversies in serotonin syndrome diagnosis and management: a review. J Clin Diagn Res 11(9):OE05–OE07, 2017 29207768

Vallersnes OM, Lund C, Duns AK, et al: Epidemic of poisoning caused by scopolamine disguised as Rohypnol tablets. Clin Toxicol (Phila) 47(9):889–893, 2009 19821638

Verrotti A, Trotta D, Morgese G, et al: Valproate-induced hyperammonemic encephalopathy. Metab Brain Dis 17(4):367–373, 2002 12602513

Verstraete AG: Detection times of drugs of abuse in blood, urine, and oral fluid. Ther Drug Monit 26(2):200–205, 2004 15228165

Voican CS, Corruble E, Naveau S, et al: Antidepressant-induced liver injury: a review for clinicians. Am J Psychiatry 171(4):404–415, 2014 24362450

Weller M, Kornhuber J: Serum iron levels in neuroleptic malignant syndrome. Biol Psychiatry 34(1–2):123–124, 1993 8373934

Whitfield KC, Bourassa MW, Adamolekun B, et al: Thiamine deficiency disorders: diagnosis, prevalence, and a roadmap for global control programs. Ann N Y Acad Sci 1430(1):3–43, 2018 30151974

Williamson S, Gossop M, Powis B, et al: Adverse effects of stimulant drugs in a community sample of drug users. Drug Alcohol Depend 44(2–3):87–94, 1997 9088780

Woodruff CW: Ascorbic acid—scurvy. Prog Food Nutr Sci 1(7–8):493–506, 1975 772754

Woosley R, Heise C, Gallo T, et al: QTdrugs Lists (www.CredibleMeds.org). Oro Valley, AZ, Arizona Center for Education and Research on Therapeutics (AZCERT), 2019. Available at: http://www.crediblemeds.org. Accessed on August 10, 2019.

Appendix

Laboratory Testing
for Toxicological Complications
and Conditions Associated With
Psychiatric Illness

The following table provides a listing of common laboratory and diagnostic tests for psychiatric patients.

Appendix: Laboratory Testing for Toxicological Complications and Conditions Associated With Psychiatric Illness

Test	Rationale/Indication	Comments
Cardiac testing		
EEG[a]	Monitor patients on QT-prolonging psychotropic medications	
	Screen for clozapine myocarditis/perimyocarditis	Check in all patients on clozapine with fever during the first 2 months of therapy or with chest pain or dyspnea.
	Rule out ischemic complications for sympathomimetic toxicities (i.e., stimulants, MDMA, hallucinogens with noradrenergic agonist properties)	
Troponin	Screen for clozapine myocarditis	Check in all patients on clozapine with fever during the first 2 months of therapy or with chest pain or dyspnea.
		Consider checking every 1–2 days for a week after any gastrointestinal or respiratory illness that occurs during the first 6 weeks of treatment. Viral-type gastrointestinal or respiratory symptoms often occur in the week preceding clozapine myocarditis.
	Rule out ischemic complications of sympathomimetic toxicities (i.e., stimulants, MDMA, hallucinogens with noradrenergic agonist properties)	
Drug testing		
Carbamazepine	Monitor for usual adult therapeutic levels: between 4 and 12 µg/L	Carbamazepine levels initially rise on medication initiation, then decrease slowly over 3–4 weeks due to auto-induction of its metabolism.
	Screen if concern about carbamazepine-induced hepatotoxicity, neurotoxicity	Carbamazepine has myriad drug-drug interactions, and all medications should be checked for possibility of interaction.
	Monitor levels if there are changes in dosing or changes in hepatic function, or if new medications are added	

Appendix: Laboratory Testing for Toxicological Complications and Conditions Associated With Psychiatric Illness (*continued*)

Test	Rationale/Indication	Comments
Drug testing (*continued*)		
Clozapine	Monitor for therapeutic levels: thought to be most effective at serum concentrations of ≥350 ng/mL	Cigarette smoking will reduce serum levels. Seizure risk is related to rapid dose escalation as well as high plasma concentrations (>700 ng/mL). Due to risk of agranulocytosis, patients on clozapine require weekly monitoring of ANC for the first 6 months, then every other week for 6 months, and then monthly for the duration of treatment. Discontinue clozapine if ANC <1,000 neutrophils/cm^3 (or <500 neutrophils/cm^3 with benign ethnic neutropenia). Consider hematology consult for all patients with ANC <1,000 neutrophils/cm^3.
Lithium	Monitor for therapeutic levels (normal range is 0.6–1.2 mEq/L) Workup for potential lithium-induced electrolyte changes, altered mental status due to toxicity, or other adverse effects Assess for effects of dosing changes, changes in renal function, and drug interactions	Check trough level 5–7 days after initial dose and each dose adjustment. Some patients may exhibit some toxicity above 0.8–1.0 mEq/L. Thiazide and loop diuretics, angiotensin-converting enzyme inhibitors, nonsteroidal anti-inflammatory drugs, metronidazole, and tetracycline may increase serum levels. Caffeine, urine-alkalinizing drugs, theophylline, and osmotic and potassium-sparing diuretics will decrease lithium.
Valproate	Monitor for therapeutic level or toxicity There is disagreement about the role for routine monitoring, but levels may be helpful in clarifying whether subtherapeutic level results in ineffectiveness, if nonadherence is a concern, or if toxicity may be occurring.	Normal range is 50–125 µg/mL. Higher concentrations may be needed initially to manage acute mania. Coadministration of carbamazepine with valproic acid will decrease levels of valproic acid; some SSRIs can increase levels of valproic acid.

Appendix: Laboratory Testing for Toxicological Complications and Conditions Associated With Psychiatric Illness *(continued)*

Test	Rationale/Indication	Comments
Drug testing (continued)		
Free valproate	Monitor for possible valproate toxicity in patients with critical illness or low albumin	Normal range is 5–17 µg/mL. In most patients, 90%–95% of valproate is bound to albumin. The free, unbound portion is the biologically active portion. Critical illness, uremia, hypoalbuminemia, and drug interactions may result in a higher active free fraction.
Lamotrigine	Monitor for drug interactions. There is not a recommendation for or against routine monitoring of levels, so doses should be titrated slowly to limit risk of serious cutaneous adverse effects that occur more frequently with toxic levels.	Therapeutic drug levels have not been established in bipolar disorder, but 2.5–15 mg/L is appropriate for epilepsy. Phenytoin, phenobarbital, carbamazepine, oxcarbazepine, and estrogenic agents may reduce levels, and valproate will increase levels.

TCAs	Occasionally used in monitoring for toxic level in overdose	Diagnosis and triage of TCA toxicity are usually determined based on patient report, ECG findings, and neurological and cardiovascular signs.
		
		Where available, TCA concentrations may be helpful. A concentration >450 mg/mL may be associated with delirium or agitation. Levels >1,000 ng/mL may be associated with major toxicity and death.
		
		Therapeutic levels are
		   nortriptyline: 50–150 ng/mL;
		   total imipramine: 175–350 ng/mL;
		   total amitriptyline: 93–140 ng/mL.

Standard toxicology studies:[a] opioids, methadone, benzodiazepines, barbiturates, amphetamines, cannabinoids, and phencyclidine	Diagnose substance use disorder, intoxication, and toxicity and assess risk of withdrawal	Routine opioid testing is insensitive for synthetic or semisynthetic opioids; it is sensitive for identifying heroin, morphine, and codeine. Routine benzodiazepine testing is insensitive for alprazolam, clonazepam, lorazepam, and midazolam.

Appendix: Laboratory Testing for Toxicological Complications and Conditions Associated With Psychiatric Illness *(continued)*

Test	Rationale/Indication	Comments
Electrolytes and renal function testing		
Serum sodium[a]	Assess for drug-induced hyponatremia, psychogenic polydipsia–induced hyponatremia, and lithium-induced hypernatremia (nephrogenic diabetes insipidus)	Hyponatremia/syndrome of inappropriate antidiuretic hormone secretion may be caused by SSRIs, TCAs, venlafaxine, carbamazepine, oxcarbazepine, and occasionally valproic acid and antipsychotic drugs. Psychogenic polydipsia is common in schizophrenia and intellectual disability.
Serum potassium and magnesium[a]	Reduce risk of arrhythmia in patients with psychotropic drug–induced long QT syndrome	Hypokalemia and hypomagnesemia increase QT prolongation and risk of torsades de pointes in patients on QT-prolonging drugs. Keep serum K+ and Mg++ concentrations closer to the upper range of normal in patients with a long QT interval.
Serum calcium[a]	Monitor for lithium-associated hyperparathyroidism Screen for hypercalcemia as cause of or contributor to depression, cognitive impairment, and occasionally psychosis.	Check serum calcium concentration at initiation of lithium, at 6 months, and then yearly.
Serum bicarbonate (total CO_2 in an electrolyte panel)[a]	Assess for respiratory acidosis in patients prescribed sedating psychotropic drugs or using other sedating agents	Almost all sedating drugs can cause hypoventilation. Patients with underlying respiratory disorders or taking combinations of sedating agents are at risk of respiratory acidosis. Within 3–5 days of onset of respiratory acidosis, serum bicarbonate will rise to a new steady state, reflecting compensatory metabolic acidosis. Blood gas assessment is necessary to capture an acute acid-base abnormality before that time window is complete.
Blood urea nitrogen and creatinine	Assess for acute kidney injury due to syndromes associated with drug toxicity, agitation, or prerenal failure due to decreased intake of water and solute. Assess for baseline renal function in lithium dosing Assess for lithium-induced nephrotoxicity	

Appendix: Laboratory Testing for Toxicological Complications and Conditions Associated With Psychiatric Illness *(continued)*

Test	Rationale/Indication	Comments
Electrolytes and renal function testing *(continued)*		
Urinalysis: specific gravity	Help in determining cause of hyponatremia	A urine specific gravity <1.008 suggests psychogenic polydipsia as the cause of hyponatremia. This point-of-care test is helpful while waiting for urine osmolality and sodium tests to be completed. In patients with glycosuria or albuminuria, specific gravity will overestimate urine osmolality.
	Assist in diagnosis of lithium-induced diabetes insipidus	A low specific gravity (<1.010 after a water deprivation test) in normonatremic or hypernatremic patients suggests lithium-induced nephrogenic diabetes insipidus.
Endocrine testing		
Hemoglobin A_{1c},[a] fasting glucose, and fasting lipid profile[a]	Assess risk of diabetes mellitus, metabolic syndrome, and cardiovascular disease in patients with anxiety disorder, bipolar disorder, depressive disorder, or schizophrenia.	Risk of metabolic syndrome is probably increased in all of the mental health diagnoses listed to the left, but the most robust evidence is for patients with schizophrenia. Atypical antipsychotics confer a higher risk of diabetes than typical agents. Hemoglobin A_{1c}, fasting glucose, and fasting lipid profile should be checked at baseline, at 6 and 12 weeks after initiation of therapy, and at least yearly thereafter.
TSH[a]	Screen for thyroid dysfunction as a cause of or contributor to specific psychiatric presentations	Usual range of normal for TSH (0.35–4.8 µIU/mL) expands to 0.2–20.0 µIU/mL in acute illness (including acute psychiatric illness). Thyroid dysfunction may be associated with neuropsychiatric findings: depressed mood, psychomotor retardation, anxiety, mania, psychosis, and cognitive impairment.
	Monitor for lithium-induced thyroid dysfunction	Different studies estimate a prevalence of hypothyroidism of approximately 5%–50% among patients prescribed lithium. Patients should have TSH and antithyroid peroxidase antibodies measured at baseline, at 6 and 12 months after initiation of therapy, and yearly thereafter if laboratory findings are normal. Most patients with TSH <10 and negative antibody studies will have subsequent normalization of thyroid function tests even if maintained on lithium.

Appendix: Laboratory Testing for Toxicological Complications and Conditions Associated With Psychiatric Illness (continued)

Test	Rationale/Indication	Comments
Endocrine testing (continued)		
TSH[a] (continued)	Monitor for lithium-induced thyroid dysfunction (continued)	The incidence of hyperthyroidism is also increased in patients prescribed lithium but is much less than hypothyroidism, at 0.25%.
Prolactin	Assess for antipsychotic-induced hyperprolactinemia	Guidelines disagree about whether to check baseline prolactin before initiating antipsychotic drugs, and/or timing and need for routine follow-up. For those patients who develop symptoms of galactorrhea and/or hypogonadism, a baseline prolactin level will help to distinguish antipsychotic-induced hyperprolactinemia from other causes. Because hyperprolactinemia increases risk of osteoporosis, some argue it may be prudent to check baseline and follow up in all patients.
		Risperidone and first-generation antipsychotics cause the most hyperprolactinemia.
Hematological testing: complete blood count		
WBC count/ANC[a]	Monitor for clozapine-induced neutropenia	Monitor hemogram every week for the first 6 months of clozapine therapy, less frequently but according to standard protocol thereafter. More information may be found at clozapinerems.com.
		Clozapine causes agranulocytosis in 1%–2% of patients when prescribed without appropriate monitoring.
	Monitor for rare but serious antiepileptic/mood stabilizer–induced agranulocytosis (e.g., treatment with carbamazepine, valproate, lamotrigine)	Obtain at baseline and periodically. Advise patients to seek prompt medical attention in case of fever, particularly if within the first few months of starting these agents.
Platelet count[a]	Monitor for valproate- or antipsychotic drug–associated thrombocytopenia	Obtain baseline platelet count and periodically thereafter. Severity of thrombocytopenia correlates with serum concentration of valproate. Thrombocytopenia occurs in 5% of patients with a level of 81–100 µg/mL and in 15% of patients with a level of 101–120 µg/mL.

Appendix: Laboratory Testing for Toxicological Complications and Conditions Associated With Psychiatric Illness *(continued)*

Test	Rationale/Indication	Comments
	Infectious disease screening	
Hepatitis serology	Screen for hepatitis B and C infections	Prevalence of hepatitis B and C infections is increased in patients with serious mental illness.
Syphilis serology[a]	Screen for neurosyphilis with psychiatric presentation	Neurosyphilis may manifest with delirium, dementia, depressed mood, personality changes, psychosis, and mania.
	Nutritional indices testing	
Vitamin B_{12} level[a]	Screen for B_{12} deficiency as cause of psychiatric presentation	Check fasting levels. Deficiency may manifest with depression, insomnia, hallucinations, delusions, and cognitive impairment.
Homocysteine and MMA	Assist in diagnosis of B_{12} deficiency when B_{12} levels are indeterminate (vitamin B_{12}=200–300 pg/mL)	Elevation of both homocysteine and MMA is predictive of neuropsychiatric complications of B_{12} deficiency.
Folate level[a]	Screen for a nutritional deficiency that may be associated with mental illness	Folate deficiency is associated with depressive disorders and may be associated with schizophrenia. Levels between 3 and 4.5 ng/mL are indeterminate. Although RBC folate levels may help clarify indeterminate results, empiric therapy with folic acid is probably more cost-effective.
	Other tests	
Creatine kinase	Assess for muscle injury/rhabdomyolysis in the agitated patient, the restrained patient, the catatonic patient, or the patient with drug-induced syndromes of hyperthermia and/or rigidity (neuroleptic malignant syndrome, serotonin toxicity, anticholinergic toxicity, and sympathomimetic toxicity).	

Appendix: Laboratory Testing for Toxicological Complications and Conditions Associated With Psychiatric Illness *(continued)*

Test	Rationale/Indication	Comments
Other tests *(continued)*		
Liver function tests[a]	Surveillance for psychotropic drug–induced liver injury: hepatocellular and cholestatic injury may occur.	There is increased risk of viral hepatitis in patients with serious mental illness.
	Transaminase elevation with aspartate transaminase>alanine transaminase may indicate occult alcohol use disorder and alcoholic liver disease or may indicate muscle injury.	

Note. ANC=absolute neutrophil count; EEG=electrocardiogram; MDMA=3,4-methylenedioxy-methamphetamine; MMA=methylmalonic acid; RBC=red blood cell; SSRIs=selective serotonin reuptake inhibitors; TCAs=tricyclic antidepressants; TSH=thyroid-stimulating hormone; WBC=white blood cell.
[a]Standard laboratory tests completed for inpatient psychiatric admission.

PART II

Psychiatric Considerations in
Medical Disorders

CHAPTER 6

Cardiovascular Disease

Peter A. Shapiro, M.D.

Heart disease (in particular, ischemic heart disease) and mental disorders (in particular, major depressive disorder [MDD]) are the leading causes of disability worldwide (Murray and Lopez 1997). Co-occurrence of psychiatric disorders with cardiovascular disease is extremely common. Diagnostic and management problems related to this comorbidity occur regularly in the course of everyday practice. Psychiatric disorders may mimic heart disease, predispose to its development, occur as a complication, or exacerbate its course and complications. Heart disease also can manifest with psychiatric symptoms. Patients with mental disorders often experience barriers to care—because of stigma, lack of resources, or difficulties in self-advocacy—as well as barriers to treatment adherence, all of which further exacerbate their risk of receiving inadequate diagnosis and treatment. The ideal of cardiac health maintenance is less likely to be achieved by individuals with depression, and patients with mental illnesses who are hospitalized for acute coronary syndromes are less likely than other patients to be offered revascularization procedures (De Hert et al. 2011; España-Romero et al. 2013; Young and Foster 2000).

In this chapter, I discuss the problem of overlapping symptoms (psychiatric problems presenting with somatic symptoms, and psychiatric symptoms due to cardiovascular disease and treatment); consider psychiatric disorders seen in adult patients with heart disease and their treatment; and review important drug interactions. I conclude with a brief note on extended cardiac life support with left ventricular assist devices (LVADs).

Overlapping Symptoms

Somatic Symptoms Due to Psychiatric Illness

Chest pain, shortness of breath, palpitations, and fatigue are common complaints whose differential diagnosis includes psychiatric disorders. When typical anginal pain with chest pressure occurs in a middle-aged or older patient with known coronary disease risk factors, it is easy to reach a presumptive diagnosis of coronary artery disease (CAD). However, many cases are atypical: the patient does not have traditional risk factors, the pain is atypical, or classically associated clinical features are absent. What is one to make of such cases?

It is important to consider both atypical presentations of heart disease and noncardiac causes of chest pain in addition to the possibility that cardiac-related symptoms are due to psychiatric illness. Of particular relevance is that, compared with men, women more frequently report atypical symptoms (especially upper abdominal pain and fatigue) as a presentation of myocardial ischemia, and they may be more likely to have nonspecific electrocardiogram (ECG) findings. Women are also more likely to have blood flow obstructions in smaller branches of the coronary arterial tree rather than in the major epicardial vessels, and this form of CAD may be associated with atypical symptoms. In addition to psychiatric disorders and coronary disease, many other illnesses can cause chest pain, including pericarditis, pleuritis, pulmonary embolism, gastroesophageal reflux, and esophagitis (Campbell et al. 2017).

Panic Disorder

Panic disorder tops the list of psychiatric disorders presenting with somatic symptoms suggesting cardiac disease (Table 6–1). Panic disorder is characterized by recurrent panic attacks (i.e., sudden episodes of intense fearfulness), with abrupt onset and a number of associated symptoms, such as palpitations; a sensation of heart racing; subjective sensations of shortness of breath, dyspnea, or choking; chest pain; nausea; paresthesias; dizziness or faintness; fear of dying, "going crazy," or losing control; and derealization or depersonalization (American Psychiatric Association 2013). Attacks usually tail off after several minutes. The ECG is normal or may show sinus tachycardia. Among emergency department visits for chest pain, 20%–40% can be attributed to panic disorder (Campbell et al. 2017). Features such as young age, atypical quality of chest pain, female sex, and absence of CAD risk factors or history increase the likelihood that panic disorder is the cause of the patient's symptoms (Campbell et al. 2017).

Somatic Symptom Disorder

Somatic symptom disorder is characterized by the persistence of one or more prominent somatic symptoms and excessive preoccupation and distress associated with them, regardless of whether the symptoms have a known cause. Its prevalence in the general population has been estimated at 5%–7% (American Psychiatric Association 2013). The prevalence of cardiac-related symptoms in somatic symptom disorder is not known. Syndromes such as chronic fatigue syndrome and fibromyalgia overlap with somatic symptom disorder because patients may experience what seems to physicians and others to be a high degree of preoccupation with symptoms.

Illness Anxiety Disorder

Illness anxiety disorder is characterized by the persistent fear of having an illness despite the absence of significant physical symptoms. This fear is at best only transiently relieved by testing and reassurance. Normal sensations such as momentary light-

TABLE 6–1.   **Psychiatric disorders that commonly present with cardiovascular symptoms**

Panic disorder	Generalized anxiety disorder
Somatic symptom disorder	Factitious disorder
Illness anxiety disorder	Malingering[a]
Major depressive disorder	

[a]Malingering is not a psychiatric disorder but is included here as part of differential diagnosis.

headedness on rising may become a focus of concern. Fear of having heart disease is a common form of illness anxiety. The 1-year prevalence of illness anxiety in the general population is estimated at 1%–10% (American Psychiatric Association 2013).

Major Depressive Disorder

Patients with MDD often present with nonspecific somatic complaints such as low energy, fatigue, and effort intolerance. MDD is characterized by a persistent change from one's normal state, with sadness or depressed mood, loss of interest or pleasure in usually engaging activities, or both, as well as disturbances in several domains (e.g., sleep, appetite, self-esteem, concentration), thoughts of death or suicide, and psychomotor activation or retardation. The signs and symptoms should not be due to a general medical disorder, substance (including medication) use or withdrawal, or another mental disorder (American Psychiatric Association 2013). These criteria may prove difficult when patients have heart disease, and psychiatrists generally choose to err in the direction of inclusion of symptoms toward a depression diagnosis. Over-inclusiveness and false-positive diagnoses also can occur; patients can register a high level of somatic depression symptoms on standardized rating scales such as the Beck Depression Inventory (Beck et al. 1961) and the Hamilton Rating Scale for Depression (Hamilton 1960) without endorsing either of the cardinal cognitive symptoms of depressed mood or loss of interest. Patients may be in such profound heart failure that symptoms are most plausibly attributable to a low output state. Thus, rating scale symptom scores are not specific or adequate as a basis for diagnosis.

Generalized Anxiety Disorder

Generalized anxiety disorder (GAD) is characterized by chronic overworrying, a subjective feeling of nervousness or fearfulness, and several associated symptoms, including restlessness or feeling "on edge," fatigue, difficulty concentrating, irritability, muscle tension, and sleep disturbance. None of these symptoms are attributable to other medical or mental illnesses or to the effects of substances or substance withdrawal. Cardiac awareness (i.e., a tendency toward awareness of one's heartbeat), palpitations, a subjective sense of heart racing, and dizziness can occur, although these symptoms are generally not as dramatic as they are in panic attacks. The 12-month prevalence of GAD in the general adult population in the United States is about 3%, and prevalence is higher in women than in men (American Psychiatric Association 2013).

Psychiatric Symptoms Due to Cardiovascular Disorders

The converse of the problem of somatic symptoms due to psychiatric disorders is psychiatric symptoms due to cardiovascular disorders (and their treatment) (Table 6–2).

Paroxysmal Supraventricular Tachycardia

Paroxysmal supraventricular tachycardia (PSVT) can occur in otherwise healthy young adults and is characterized by a regular rapid heart rate (150–200 beats per minute), with sudden onset and usually abrupt termination. Patients often present with intense anxiety and feelings of panic and also report palpitations, chest discomfort, dizziness, or tachycardia. The correct diagnosis should be evident from the ECG (Al-Zaiti and Magdic 2016; Lessmeier et al. 1997). Symptoms of PSVT respond well to treatment with vagal maneuvers or medication—or, if necessary, with cardioversion or catheter ablation of an ectopic atrial pacemaker or accessory conduction pathway.

Other Arrhythmias

Other arrhythmias, including bradyarrhythmias, intermittent heart block, ventricular premature beats, atrial fibrillation, and nonsustained ventricular tachycardia, may occur intermittently and may not be reflected in prominent physical symptoms but may cause subjective feelings of vague unease, unwellness, and anxiety. The patient does not know what is wrong, does not feel well, presents to ambulatory care with fearfulness, and may be misdiagnosed as having anxiety. Ambulatory ECG recording, electrophysiology studies, or stress testing may be necessary to identify arrhythmias.

Silent Myocardial Ischemia

Silent myocardial ischemia—that is, ischemia without typical chest pain or other typical anginal symptoms—is common in patients with CAD and also may generate vague uneasiness and a sense of unwellness that may be easily misdiagnosed as anxiety. To make matters more complicated, silent myocardial ischemia often occurs in response to mental stress, even in patents with no psychiatric disorder. About 20%–40% of CAD patients with exercise-induced ischemia also experience mental stress–induced myocardial ischemia that can be demonstrated with in-laboratory provocation of ST-segment depression, transient reduction in left ventricular ejection fraction, or regional ventricular wall motion abnormality (Strike and Steptoe 2003). In comparison with CAD patients without mental stress–induced myocardial ischemia, those with such ischemia have a higher likelihood of mortality (Jiang 2015; Sheps et al. 2002), a finding that underscores the importance of detecting and adequately treating ischemic disease. Treatment with the selective serotonin reuptake inhibitor (SSRI) escitalopram had been found to reduce mental stress–induced myocardial ischemia (Jiang et al. 2013), but distal effects on morbidity and mortality have yet to be shown.

Atrial Myxoma

Atrial myxoma is the most common cardiac tumor, with an estimated prevalence of 0.3% in the general population (Percell et al. 2003). Atrial myxoma can be asymptomatic or can cause embolic strokes or intermittent or persistent atrial outflow obstruction. Patients can have constitutional symptoms, including fever or weight loss. Physical findings may be absent, particularly in cases of intermittent outflow obstruction, leading to misattribution of transient somatic symptoms to anxiety or other psychiat-

TABLE 6–2.   **Cardiac conditions that may manifest with psychiatric symptoms**

Arrhythmias	Congestive heart failure
Silent myocardial ischemia	Cardiac medication–induced symptoms
Atrial myxoma	

ric symptoms. Psychoses have also been reported in atrial myxoma. Echocardiography has high sensitivity for diagnosis. Atrial myxoma can be recurrent and may occur as a familial syndrome.

Heart Failure

Heart failure patients may experience anxiety, sleep disturbance, cognitive impairment, low energy, cognitive dulling, and depressed or irritable mood. Although symptoms resemble those of a primary psychiatric disorder, they may in fact be due to orthopnea, paroxysmal nocturnal dyspnea, or diminished cardiac output and cardiac reserve. As noted previously (see earlier subsection "Major Depressive Disorder"), assessment of cognitive as opposed to somatic symptoms may be important in cases of diagnostic uncertainty.

Psychiatric Symptoms Due to Medications for Heart Disease

Psychiatric symptoms due to medications for heart disease include delirium as an effect of many antiarrhythmic agents; visual hallucinations, including change in color vision; confusion or other mental state changes due to digoxin; fatigue due to diuretic-induced hyponatremia; depression and cognitive impairment associated with hypothyroidism caused by amiodarone; fatigue and sexual dysfunction caused by β-adrenergic blockers; and mood elevation or depression associated with angiotensin-converting enzyme inhibitors and angiotensin receptor blockers (Shapiro 2017).

Psychiatric Disorders in Patients With Heart Disease

Stress, anger and hostility, anxiety, depression, schizophrenia and other psychotic disorders, posttraumatic stress disorder (PTSD), cognitive disorders, and sexual dysfunction are mental health problems of special significance with respect to heart disease. Personality disorders may affect adjustment to illness, the propensity for denial of illness, treatment adherence, and the doctor-patient relationship. Sleep apnea occupies a middle position between psychiatric and general medical disorders in that it can cause both psychiatric and cardiac effects.

Stress

Stress is an elusive concept but is generally understood as an increased demand (either objectively identifiable or subjectively perceived) on the organism that disrupts homeostasis (Shapiro 2013b). *Stressors* (i.e., circumstances or events external to the individual) can be distinguished from *stress* (i.e., the experience of the organism in response to stressors), but common usage often hides this verbal distinction. Nevertheless, interventions might be targeted at reducing stressor exposure, improving coping with stressors to reduce experienced stress, or both. Major life changes (even nominally positive and desired changes, such as marriage), minor irritations of everyday life, job strain, difficulties in intimate relationships, brief or momentary stressors such as arguments, cognitively challenging tasks, or the occurrence of catastrophic events (even when not directly endangering the individual) are examples of chronic and acute stressors that increase psychological stress. Stress experiences are associated with an increased incidence of acute coronary events, ventricular arrhythmias, atrial fibrillation, and sudden cardiac death (Dimsdale 2008). Stressors that appear suddenly, whether positive or negative (e.g., surprise parties, learning of the death of a loved one), are triggers for *Takotsubo cardiomyopathy,* an acute, transient, reversible illness characterized by chest pain, reduced left ventricular function, and apical ballooning (Wittstein 2007). The role of stress as a risk factor for cardiac events may be moderated by a personal propensity toward anger; cognitive-behavioral stress management with an emphasis on reducing anger has been shown to reduce recurrent cardiac events and mortality in patients who have had a myocardial infarction (Gulliksson et al. 2011).

Anger and Hostility

Hostility as a chronic personality trait increases the stressfulness of everyday life (every interaction with others is perceived as a potential battle), and momentary experiences of anger can provoke myocardial ischemia and infarction in vulnerable individuals. Many studies demonstrate a gradient or "dose" effect of hostility on coronary artery calcification and incident myocardial infarction. Acute anger has been estimated to be the trigger in about 5% of myocardial infarctions (Chida and Steptoe 2009; Jiang 2015).

Neither psychotherapy nor medication interventions to diminish anger and hostility have been found to be effective as primary prevention to reduce the incidence of coronary disease or acute coronary events, but cognitive-behavioral therapy (CBT) focused on diminishing anger has been found to reduce the risk of recurrent coronary events in post–myocardial infarction patients (Gulliksson et al. 2011).

Anxiety

Many, but not all, prospective studies of anxiety identify it as a risk factor for incident cardiovascular disease and sudden cardiac death. In a 2016 meta-analysis of 37 primary studies involving more than 1 million patients and follow-up periods ranging from 1 to 24 years, Batelaan et al. (2016) concluded that anxiety was associated with a 52% increased incidence of cardiovascular disease (hazard ratio=1.52; 95% confidence interval [CI]=1.36–1.71). In addition, anxiety is a common reaction to receiving a diagnosis of heart disease and being hospitalized for acute coronary events. Patients fear experiencing pain, suffering, and disability; being unable to provide for loved ones; becoming increasingly dependent on others; losing work, income, and social status; and dying. Procedures are risky, patients are surrounded by mysterious and disturbing alarms and monitor signals that might indicate danger, and ongoing symptoms seem threatening. Although a remarkable number of patients cope well, demonstrating a mixture of optimism, benign denial, and trust in their care providers, perhaps 5%–10% of patients have anxiety sufficient to cause subjective distress or interfere with their care. In-hospital anxiety is associated with increased short-term mortality (Moser and Dracup 1996; Moser et al. 2007). Education, benzodiazepines, supportive psychotherapy, and β-adrenergic blockers all may help reduce anxiety symptoms in the hospital. Stress management, meditation, supportive therapy, or CBT may reduce anxiety and anxiety-related distress after hospital discharge (Huffman et al. 2014). SSRIs are helpful for longer-term management of anxiety and are generally well tolerated in heart disease patients.

Depression

A major depressive episode is defined as a period of 2 weeks or longer in which symptoms of 1) sad or depressed mood or 2) loss of interest and pleasure in normally engaging activities, or both, are present, along with several associated symptoms, including insomnia or oversleeping; appetite disturbance; restlessness or psychomotor slowing; fatigue or low energy; loss of self-esteem or guilt; difficulty thinking, concentrating, and making decisions; and thoughts of death, wishes to be dead, or suicidal ideation (American Psychiatric Association 2013). The symptoms must be severe enough to cause subjective distress or impairment in daily functioning and must not be attributable to medical illness or to the effects of substance use or medications. Major depressive episodes occur in MDD and bipolar disorder, and phenomenologically similar symptom clusters can occur in other mental disorders. These symptoms may be secondary to medications, substance use, and medical illnesses, including heart disease. A history of depressive symptoms or MDD is clearly associated with an approximately doubled incidence of coronary disease and with more functional limitation, reduced quality of life, and a two- to fourfold increased risk of morbidity, recurrent cardiac events, and mortality in patients with established cardiac disease (Lichtman et al. 2008, 2014). Because depression is so common in the U.S. population, as evidenced by a 6%–10% current prevalence (Centers for Disease Control and Prevention 2010) and a 16% lifetime prevalence (Kessler et al. 2003), this relationship is of considerable epidemiological significance.

Pathways thought to mediate the relation of depression to coronary disease outcomes include altered hypothalamic-pituitary-adrenal axis function with elevated cortisol levels, increased inflammation, platelet activation, altered autonomic tone, and diminished adherence to healthful behaviors/lifestyle and medication use. No single pathway seems to account for all of the additional risk. In addition, depression might occur as an epiphenomenon of atherosclerotic disease affecting the brain as well as the coronary arteries (Kent and Shapiro 2009; Lichtman et al. 2014).

Depressive episodes occur in about 15%–20% of patients with coronary disease and at about the same rate in patients with heart failure (Shapiro 2009, 2015). The occurrence of significant depressive symptoms that do not meet the criteria for a diagnosis of major depressive episode is even more common. Because of the high prevalence of depression and the associated suffering, functional impairment, and morbidity, the American Heart Association has recommended that patients with heart disease receive routine screening for depression with validated screening tools (Lichtman et al. 2008). It should be noted, however, that screening is not likely to be helpful unless it is followed by appropriate intervention.

In randomized double-blind, placebo-controlled trials, the SSRIs sertraline, citalopram, fluoxetine, and escitalopram have been found to be effective and generally well-tolerated treatments for depression in the setting of coronary disease, including patients with recent acute coronary events. Evidence for the effectiveness of the tetracyclic antidepressant agent mirtazapine is equivocal at best. In medication trials in patients with heart failure, paroxetine was an effective antidepressant, but sertraline and escitalopram were not (Shapiro 2015). Despite their effectiveness, tricyclic antidepressants (TCAs) are no longer considered an appropriate first-line therapy for depression in the setting of cardiac disease because of their adverse effects, which include risk of arrhythmias. Problem-solving psychotherapy and CBT are at least modestly effective for depression in patients with coronary disease, and stepped-intensity collaborative care interventions that use combinations of psychotherapy with antidepressants have apparent benefit at relatively low cost. Clinical trials also indicate the efficacy of intensive exercise programs (35–45 minutes of aerobic activity, four or five sessions per week) to reduce depressive symptoms in patients with coronary disease or congestive heart failure (Shapiro 2015). Although recovery from depression is associated with reduced mortality in patients with heart disease over several years of longitudinal follow-up, it remains to be determined whether depression treatment reduces the recurrence of coronary disease events or mortality; more effective depression interventions, or interventions targeted at mediating mechanisms, may be necessary if improvements in long-term prognosis are to be achieved (Carney and Freedland 2009; Shapiro 2013a).

Schizophrenia and Other Psychotic Disorders

Patients with severe and persistent mental illness are at high risk of experiencing stigma, socioeconomic disadvantage, and poor access to medical care (De Hert et al. 2011; Young and Foster 2000). Patients with schizophrenia are likely to have many risk factors for coronary disease; for example, in comparison with the general population, individuals with schizophrenia are more likely to smoke cigarettes, and most second-generation antipsychotic drugs increase the risk of metabolic syndrome (Daumit et al. 2008; Mackin 2008; Newcomer and Hennekens 2007; Newcomer and Sernyak 2007). Antipsychotic drugs are associated with a number of adverse cardiac effects and also carry the potential for interaction with many medications used in the treatment of heart disease (Shapiro 2013b).

Acute Stress Disorder and Posttraumatic Stress Disorder

Preexisting PTSD is associated with an increased risk of CAD events and coronary mortality; furthermore, acute coronary syndromes, hospitalization, and treatment may themselves be traumatic events that set the stage for incident acute stress disorder and PTSD, creating a vicious cycle of pathology, morbidity, and mortality (Edmondson and von Känel 2017). Traumatic experiences include undergoing painful and invasive procedures, witnessing frightening events (e.g., emergency cardiopulmonary resuscitation of other patients) in the emergency department and cardiac care unit, and facing the prospect of one's own death. The estimated incidence of acute stress disorder progressing to PTSD in acute coronary syndrome hospitalizations is 5%–15%, and post–acute coronary syndrome PTSD is associated with a one and one-half– to twofold increase in risk for subsequent coronary events over 1–5 years of follow-up (Edmondson and von Känel 2017).

Cognitive Disorders

As a systemic disease, atherosclerosis affects not only the coronary and peripheral vasculature but also the cerebral circulation. Minor neurocognitive symptoms and even transient ischemic attacks may be unrecognized in the history of patients with heart failure and coronary disease but are indicators of cerebrovascular disease. The incidence of delirium after cardiac surgery is 10%–50% (Detroyer et al. 2008; Kazmierski et al. 2008; Koster et al. 2009; Rudolph et al. 2009), with greater risk in patients with preexisting cognitive dysfunction, and delirium is itself associated with an increased risk of persistent cognitive impairment (Crocker et al. 2016; Koster et al. 2009). Even in the absence of postoperative delirium, postsurgical neuropsychological impairment occurs in 5%–20% of cardiac patients, with older age being an important risk factor (Habib et al. 2014). "Off-pump" coronary artery bypass surgery has failed to demonstrate an advantage over conventional bypass surgery for preservation of cognitive function (Afilalo et al. 2012). Among patients with congestive heart failure, the adverse effects of low cardiac output on cognition are heightened in the elderly (Festa et al. 2011), reflecting loss of cerebral reserve associated with aging and preexisting cerebrovascular disease.

Sexual Dysfunction

Impaired sexual desire and arousal are common in patients with heart disease, and there are many potential contributing factors. Heart disease risk factors such as diabetes, hypertension, and dyslipidemia may damage neural and vascular systems necessary for sexual response. Medications may reduce desire and genital neurovascular inflow. Depression, fear, and fear on the part of the sexual partner of a patient with heart disease also contribute to impaired function. The American Heart Association has published extensive guidelines for cardiac patients and their partners with recommendations for counseling on safe sexual practices (Steinke et al. 2013). Patients may be reluctant to raise these issues with providers, and proactive inquiry into patients' sexual functioning and concerns may open the door for therapeutic intervention.

Sleep Apnea

Obstructive sleep apnea is a risk factor for both heart disease and a range of psychiatric symptoms. Breathing-related sleep disorders promote pulmonary hypertension and heart failure as well as depressed mood, fatigue, irritability, and cognitive dulling. Central sleep apnea, including Cheynes-Stokes respiratory pattern, is comparatively rare but may occur in patients with chronic heart disease and respiratory disease and may also contribute to psychiatric symptoms (Floras 2014).

Personality Styles and Disorders

Personality refers to an individual's enduring pattern of inner experience and behavior that is stable over time and situation—the person's characteristic mode of experiencing and responding to the vicissitudes of life (American Psychiatric Association

2013). Diagnosis of a personality disorder is based on the presence of inflexible, maladaptive responses; marked deviation from cultural norms and expectations; and distress or impaired functioning in daily life. Personality should be distinguished from the effects of acute or chronic medical or psychiatric illness on the patient's inner experience, interpersonal interactions, and coping; however, with chronic illness, these effects may be tantamount to an alteration of personality. Personality characteristics such as dependency, need for control, mistrust, interpersonal detachment, excessive emotionality, need for admiration, eccentricity of thinking and behavior, grandiosity and lack of empathy, propensity to worry, openness, agreeableness, and conscientiousness can affect a patient's experience of and response to illness. Most patients adapt quickly to the reality of acute illness and can normatively enter the patient role and a treatment relationship; however, the threat posed by illness can lead to intensification of customary coping mechanisms. Idiosyncratic understanding, distrust of providers, and the need to diminish intolerable affects can lead to denial, delay in seeking treatment, and poor acceptance of and adherence to treatment regimens. Therefore, providers must attempt to grasp the patient's experience of the meaning of the illness and characteristic response style and tailor communication and treatment accordingly (Groves and Muskin 2011).

Cardiovascular Effects of Treatments for Psychiatric Problems in Heart Disease Patients

Many psychotropic drugs have cardiovascular effects that may affect treatment for heart disease patients (Mackin 2008; Shapiro 2017).

Antidepressants

SSRIs may slow the heart rate, but usually not to a clinically significant degree. Modest QT interval prolongation occurs with most SSRIs; the effect is most significant for citalopram, resulting in a required black box warning about dosages higher than 40 mg/day (20 mg/day in the elderly), but large-scale epidemiological studies suggest that little to no excess risk of resulting ventricular tachyarrhythmia or death is present, even with high dosages of citalopram (Leonard et al. 2011; Weeke et al. 2012; Zivin et al. 2013). Serotonin-norepinephrine reuptake inhibitors have not been as extensively studied as SSRIs but have not been reported to cause significant QT interval prolongation. Hypertension has been reported as an adverse effect of the immediate-release formulation of venlafaxine. SSRIs impair platelet storage of serotonin and may thereby reduce platelet activation.

TCAs increase the risk of orthostatic hypotension and can cause first-, second-, or third-degree heart block at the level of the atrioventricular node–His bundle. In addition, TCAs have quinidine-like antiarrhythmic effects and proarrhythmic effects in overdose and in the setting of myocardial ischemia. Therefore, they are not suitable as first-line therapy for depression in patients with coronary disease.

Monoamine oxidase inhibitors (MAOIs) cause orthostatic hypotension and can cause hypertensive crisis after ingestion of tyramine-rich foods. Bupropion is generally well tolerated and has few cardiac effects. Within its therapeutic dosage range, bupropion does not cause QT interval prolongation. Bupropion carries a potential for many drug interactions. Nefazodone has no cardiovascular effects and was found to be well tolerated in an open trial in patients with depression and stable CAD (Lespérance et al. 2003). It is a strong inhibitor of cytochrome P450 (CYP) 3A4 and carries a potential for many drug interactions. Mirtazapine has no effect on heart rate, blood pressure, or cardiac conduction but was found to be the antidepressant most often associated with sudden cardiac death in a review of Swedish national registry data (Danielsson et al. 2016; Jasiak and Bostwick 2014).

Antipsychotics

Antipsychotic medications can cause QT interval prolongation, torsades de pointes, and metabolic syndrome. Cardiomyopathy is an adverse effect associated specifically with clozapine.

Torsades de pointes ("twisting of the points") is a polymorphic ventricular tachycardia that can degenerate into ventricular fibrillation and cardiac arrest. Prolonged ventricular repolarization, manifesting as prolongation of the T wave (and therefore of the QT interval) due to inhibition of potassium channels and the so-called potassium rectifier current, increases the risk of torsades de pointes. Female sex and presence of comorbid medical illness also increase the risk of this adverse effect. Genetic variation in the potassium channel can result in long QT syndrome, which may manifest with torsades de pointes either spontaneously or during treatment with medications that further prolong the QT interval. A personal or family history of unexplained syncope or seizure, sudden cardiac death, or cardiac arrest should raise suspicion for a genetic predisposition to torsades de pointes. Many antipsychotic agents affect the function of the potassium channel and prolong the QT interval, albeit to varying degrees. Among antipsychotic drugs marketed in the United States, aripiprazole and lurasidone have no or insignificant effects on the QT interval, whereas thioridazine, ziprasidone, and intravenous haloperidol commonly cause substantial QT interval prolongation; other antipsychotic agents have intermediate effects. The QT interval corrected to account for heart rate (QTc interval) is normally in the range of 380–450 ms, and the risk of torsades increases gradually and nonlinearly as QT interval prolongation increases, such that a QTc interval of 500 ms carries approximately double the risk associated with a QTc interval of 400 ms. However, even with a long QTc interval, the risk of torsades is low in the absence of other contributing risk factors such as bradycardia, hypokalemia, and hypomagnesemia (Beach et al. 2013; Hasnain and Vieweg 2014), and some antipsychotic drugs known to prolong the QT interval have not been associated with tachyarrhythmia.

Stimulants

Stimulants at low therapeutic dosages (e.g., methylphenidate 5–30 mg/day) can produce modest increases in heart rate and blood pressure. Although labeled as contraindicated in patients with structural heart disease, stimulants have been studied in several small depression treatment trials, including trials in the elderly and people with medical illness. While noting the limited data available, authors of a Cochrane review found no evidence of adverse cardiac effects from stimulant treatment for depression (Candy et al. 2008). Reviews of higher-dosage stimulant treatment of attention-deficit/hyperactivity disorder in young adults found very low rates of adverse cardiac events (Peyre et al. 2014). A high degree of caution, informed consent, and consultation with a cardiologist seem prudent before prescribing stimulants in patients with unstable coronary disease, arrhythmias, rapid heart rate, hypertension, or heart failure.

Lithium

Lithium affects sinoatrial node function and may cause sinus bradycardia or sick sinus syndrome. Isolated reports have linked lithium to cases of Brugada syndrome (Darbar et al. 2005; Mehta and Vannozzi 2017).

Important Drug Interactions

Pharmacodynamic and pharmacokinetic interactions between psychoactive and cardiac medications have the potential to reduce drug efficacy and increase risk of toxicity (Owen and Crouse 2017; Shapiro 2017). Direct effects of psychotropic agents on blood pressure, heart rate, and cardiac conduction effects will add to or counter the effects of certain cardiac medications. Antagonists of the renin-angiotensin system and thiazide diuretics reduce lithium clearance, whereas osmotic diuretics increase the drug's clearance. Hyponatremia, an effect of SSRIs, carbamazepine, and oxcarbazepine, can be exacerbated by concomitant use of diuretics. The anticholinergic effects of certain cardiac medications, such as procainamide and quinidine, digoxin, isosorbide dinitrate, and furosemide, can antagonize the effects of donepezil and rivastigmine. The vagomimetic effects of donepezil and rivastigmine may exacerbate β-blocker-induced bradycardia. The risk of bleeding associated with the antiplatelet effects of SSRIs is approximately doubled with concomitant use of warfarin and antiplatelet therapies. Severe hypotension can result from the interaction of phosphodiesterase-5 inhibitors with nitrates.

Many psychiatric and cardiac medications are substrates, strong inducers, or strong inhibitors of CYP isoenzymes, creating numerous potential pharmacokinetic interactions (Table 6–3). When a drug has only one predominant metabolic pathway and that pathway is inhibited, the likelihood of toxicity and adverse effects dramatically increases. Drugs metabolized through many pathways are less prone to be affected by pharmacokinetic interactions; however, a few drugs (e.g., amiodarone, barbiturates, carbamazepine) have effects on multiple CYP isoenzyme systems simultaneously.

Nefazodone, diltiazem, and amiodarone are especially notable inhibitors of CYP3A4, which is responsible for the metabolism of a host of psychoactive agents, including antipsychotics and methadone, thereby increasing the risk of QT interval prolongation. Bupropion and SSRIs inhibit CYP2D6, thereby increasing β-blocker effects.

TABLE 6–3.	Cytochrome P450 isoenzymes: some effects on cardiac and psychotropic agents		
Cytochrome	**Substrates**	**Inducers**	**Inhibitors**
1A2	Tricyclic antidepressants Many antipsychotics	Carbamazepine Modafinil Phenobarbital Phenytoin	Amiodarone Mexilitene Propafenone
2C9	Amiodarone Phenytoin	Carbamazepine Phenobarbital Phenytoin Valproate	Amiodarone Fluvoxamine Modafinil Many statins
2D6	β-Blockers Carvedilol Flecainide Mexilitene Propafenone Warfarin Many antipsychotics Many opiates	Carbamazepine Phenobarbital Phenytoin	Amiodarone Bupropion Clomipramine Desipramine Duloxetine Fluoxetine Haloperidol Moclobemide Paroxetine Propafenone Propranolol Quinidine
3A4	Amiodarone Bupropion Carbamazepine Cyclosporine Disopyramide Methadone Quinidine Rivaroxaban Sirolimus Tacrolimus Warfarin Many antipsychotics Many benzodiazepines Many calcium channel blockers Many opiates	Carbamazepine Phenytoin	Amiodarone Diltiazem Fluoxetine Nefazodone

Note. Not an exhaustive list. Drug labeling and online resources provide ready access to information.

Source. Flockhart DA: Drug Interactions: Cytochrome P450 Drug Interaction Table. Indianapolis, Indiana University School of Medicine, 2007. Available at: https://drug-interactions.medicine.iu.edu. Accessed August 28, 2019.

Left Ventricular Assist Devices

Heart transplantation is available to a very small portion of patients with end-stage heart failure (2,000–2,500 patients per year in the United States), whereas long-term cardiac life support with LVADs is not limited by donor supply and is becoming much more widely available (Kirklin et al. 2017). Common complications of LVAD therapy include infection, bleeding, and stroke, all of which contribute to a substantial risk of delirium, mood disorders, and neurocognitive dysfunction (Rosenberger et al. 2012). Attentive management of the LVAD power supply and controller, adherence to anticoagulant therapy, and prevention of drive-line infection require a high level of cognitive and executive function and can be extremely stressful for patients and their caregivers. Although LVADs reverse heart failure symptoms and improve quality of life, these gains may be impaired by device failure, stroke, and other complications; suicide and requests for hastened death via deactivation of the device are an increasingly recognized problem. Preimplantation counseling, clarification of patient and family understanding and expectations, psychiatric and palliative care, and ethics consultations are necessary components of care (Chamsi-Pasha et al. 2014).

Conclusion

Psychiatric problems can be both contributing causes and sequelae of heart disease, as well as coincidental comorbidities. In patients with preexisting psychiatric disorders, smoking, metabolic syndrome, limited access to medical care, and poor adherence to medical treatment all contribute to heart disease risk. Anxiety, cognitive problems, delirium, depression, posttraumatic stress, and sexual dysfunction are common in heart disease patients. Optimal management requires careful differential diagnosis and awareness of medication side effects and drug interactions. Promising treatments include exercise, stress management, and collaborative stepped-care interventions that incorporate brief evidence-based psychotherapy as well as medications. Because heart failure is a fatal illness, ethical and existential questions about meaning and value in living and the goals of care may ultimately become a focus of psychotherapy. Psychiatrists have much to offer to improve functional status, well-being, and survival of heart disease patients.

References

Afilalo J, Rasti M, Ohayon SM, et al: Off-pump vs. on-pump coronary artery bypass surgery: an updated meta-analysis and meta-regression of randomized trials. Eur Heart J 33(10):1257–1267, 2012 21987177

Al-Zaiti SS, Magdic KS: Paroxysmal supraventricular tachycardia: pathophysiology, diagnosis, and management. Crit Care Nurs Clin North Am 28(3):309–316, 2016 27484659

American Psychiatric Association: Diagnostic and Statistical Manual of Mental Disorders, 5th Edition. Arlington, VA, American Psychiatric Association, 2013

Batelaan NM, Seldenrijk A, Bot M, et al: Anxiety and new onset of cardiovascular disease: critical review and meta-analysis. Br J Psychiatry 208(3):223–231, 2016 26932485

Beach SR, Celano CM, Noseworthy PA, et al: QTc prolongation, torsades de pointes, and psychotropic medications. Psychosomatics 54(1):1–13, 2013 23295003

Beck A, Ward C, Mendelson M, et al: An inventory for measuring depression. Arch Gen Psychiatry 42:667–675, 1961 13688369

Campbell KA, Madva EN, Villegas AC, et al: Non-cardiac chest pain: a review for the consultation-liaison psychiatrist. Psychosomatics 58(3):252–265, 2017 28196622

Candy B, Jones L, Williams R, et al: Psychostimulants for depression. Cochrane Database Syst Rev (2):CD006722, 2008 18425966

Carney RM, Freedland KE: Treatment-resistant depression and mortality after acute coronary syndrome. Am J Psychiatry 166(4):410–417, 2009 19289455

Centers for Disease Control and Prevention: Current depression among adults—United States, 2006 and 2008. MMWR Morb Mortal Wkly Rep 59(38):1229–1235, 2010 20881934

Chamsi-Pasha H, Chamsi-Pasha MA, Albar MA: Ethical challenges of deactivation of cardiac devices in advanced heart failure. Curr Heart Fail Rep 11(2):119–125, 2014 24619521

Chida Y, Steptoe A: The association of anger and hostility with future coronary heart disease: a meta-analytic review of prospective evidence. J Am Coll Cardiol 53(11):936–946, 2009 19281923

Crocker E, Beggs T, Hassan A, et al: Long-term effects of postoperative delirium in patients undergoing cardiac operation: a systematic review. Ann Thorac Surg 102(4):1391–1399, 2016 27344279

Danielsson B, Collin J, Jonasdottir Bergman G, et al: Antidepressants and antipsychotics classified with torsades de pointes arrhythmia risk and mortality in older adults—a Swedish nationwide study. Br J Clin Pharmacol 81(4):773–783, 2016 26574175

Darbar D, Yang T, Churchwell K, et al: Unmasking of Brugada syndrome by lithium. Circulation 112(11):1527–1531, 2005 16144991

Daumit GL, Goff DC, Meyer JM, et al: Antipsychotic effects on estimated 10-year coronary heart disease risk in the CATIE schizophrenia study. Schizophr Res 105(1–3):175–187, 2008 18775645

De Hert M, Correll CU, Bobes J, et al: Physical illness in patients with severe mental disorders, I: prevalence, impact of medications and disparities in health care. World Psychiatry 10(1):52–77, 2011 21379357

Detroyer E, Dobbels F, Verfaillie E, et al: Is preoperative anxiety and depression associated with onset of delirium after cardiac surgery in older patients? A prospective cohort study. J Am Geriatr Soc 56(12):2278–2284, 2008 19112653

Dimsdale JE: Psychological stress and cardiovascular disease. J Am Coll Cardiol 51(13):1237–1246, 2008 18371552

Edmondson D, von Känel R: Post-traumatic stress disorder and cardiovascular disease. Lancet Psychiatry 4(4):320–329, 2017 28109646

España-Romero V, Artero EG, Lee DC, et al: A prospective study of ideal cardiovascular health and depressive symptoms. Psychosomatics 54(6):525–535, 2013 24012292

Festa JR, Jia X, Cheung K, et al: Association of low ejection fraction with impaired verbal memory in older patients with heart failure. Arch Neurol 68(8):1021–1026, 2011 21825237

Floras JS: Sleep apnea and cardiovascular risk. J Cardiol 63(1):3–8, 2014 24084492

Groves MR, Muskin PR: Psychological responses to illness, in Textbook of Psychosomatic Medicine, 2nd Edition. Edited by Levenson JL. Washington, DC, American Psychiatric Publishing, 2011, pp 45–67

Gulliksson M, Burell G, Vessby B, et al: Randomized controlled trial of cognitive behavioral therapy vs standard treatment to prevent recurrent cardiovascular events in patients with coronary heart disease: Secondary Prevention in Uppsala Primary Health Care project (SUPRIM). Arch Intern Med 171(2):134–140, 2011 21263103

Habib S, Khan Au, Afridi MI, et al: Frequency and predictors of cognitive decline in patients undergoing coronary artery bypass graft surgery. J Coll Physicians Surg Pak 24(8):543–548, 2014 25149830

Hamilton M: A rating scale for depression. J Neurol Neurosurg Psychiatry 23:56–62, 1960 14399272

Hasnain M, Vieweg WV: QTc interval prolongation and torsade de pointes associated with second-generation antipsychotics and antidepressants: a comprehensive review. CNS Drugs 28(10):887–920, 2014 25168784

Huffman JC, Mastromauro CA, Beach SR, et al: Collaborative care for depression and anxiety disorders in patients with recent cardiac events: the Management of Sadness and Anxiety in Cardiology (MOSAIC) randomized clinical trial. JAMA Intern Med 174(6):927–935, 2014 24733277

Jasiak NM, Bostwick JR: Risk of QT/QTc prolongation among newer non-SSRI antidepressants. Ann Pharmacother 48(12):1620–1628, 2014 25204465

Jiang W: Emotional triggering of cardiac dysfunction: the present and future. Curr Cardiol Rep 17(10):91, 2015 26298307

Jiang W, Velazquez EJ, Kuchibhatla M, et al: Effect of escitalopram on mental stress-induced myocardial ischemia: results of the REMIT trial. JAMA 309(20):2139–2149, 2013 23695483

Kazmierski J, Kowman M, Banach M, et al: Clinical utility and use of DSM-IV and ICD-10 Criteria and The Memorial Delirium Assessment Scale in establishing a diagnosis of delirium after cardiac surgery. Psychosomatics 49(1):73–76, 2008 18212180

Kent LK, Shapiro PA: Depression and related psychological factors in heart disease. Harv Rev Psychiatry 17(6):377–388, 2009 19968452

Kessler RC, Berglund P, Demler O, et al; National Comorbidity Survey Replication: The epidemiology of major depressive disorder: results from the National Comorbidity Survey Replication (NCS-R). JAMA 289(23):3095–3105, 2003 12813115

Kirklin JK, Pagani FD, Kormos RL, et al: Eighth annual INTERMACS report: special focus on framing the impact of adverse events. J Heart Lung Transplant 36(10):1080–1086, 2017 28942782

Koster S, Hensens AG, van der Palen J: The long-term cognitive and functional outcomes of postoperative delirium after cardiac surgery. Ann Thorac Surg 87(5):1469–1474, 2009 19379886

Leonard CE, Bilker WB, Newcomb C, et al: Antidepressants and the risk of sudden cardiac death and ventricular arrhythmia. Pharmacoepidemiol Drug Saf 20(9):903–913, 2011 21796718

Lespérance F, Frasure-Smith N, Laliberté MA, et al: An open-label study of nefazodone treatment of major depression in patients with congestive heart failure. Can J Psychiatry 48(10):695–701, 2003 14674053

Lessmeier TJ, Gamperling D, Johnson-Liddon V, et al: Unrecognized paroxysmal supraventricular tachycardia: potential for misdiagnosis as panic disorder. Arch Intern Med 157(5):537–543, 1997 9066458

Lichtman JH, Bigger JT Jr, Blumenthal JA, et al: Depression and coronary heart disease: recommendations for screening, referral, and treatment: a science advisory from the American Heart Association Prevention Committee of the Council on Cardiovascular Nursing, Council on Clinical Cardiology, Council on Epidemiology and Prevention, and Interdisciplinary Council on Quality of Care and Outcomes Research: endorsed by the American Psychiatric Association. Circulation 118(17):1768–1775, 2008 18824640

Lichtman JH, Froelicher ES, Blumenthal JA, et al: Depression as a risk factor for poor prognosis among patients with acute coronary syndrome: systematic review and recommendations: a scientific statement from the American Heart Association. Circulation 129(12):1350–1369, 2014 24566200

Mackin P: Cardiac side effects of psychiatric drugs. Hum Psychopharmacol 23 (suppl 1):3–14, 2008 18098218

Mehta N, Vannozzi R: Lithium-induced electrocardiographic changes: a complete review. Clin Cardiol 40(12):1363–1367, 2017 29247520

Moser DK, Dracup K: Is anxiety early after myocardial infarction associated with subsequent ischemic and arrhythmic events? Psychosom Med 58(5):395–401, 1996 8902890

Moser DK, Riegel B, McKinley S, et al: Impact of anxiety and perceived control on in-hospital complications after acute myocardial infarction. Psychosom Med 69(1):10–16, 2007 17244843

Murray CJ, Lopez AD: Alternative projections of mortality and disability by cause 1990–2020: Global Burden of Disease Study. Lancet 349(9064):1498–1504, 1997 9167458

Newcomer JW, Hennekens CH: Severe mental illness and risk of cardiovascular disease. JAMA 298(15):1794–1796, 2007 17940236

Newcomer JW, Sernyak MJ: Identifying metabolic risks with antipsychotics and monitoring and management strategies. J Clin Psychiatry 68(7):e17, 2007 17685728

Owen JA, Crouse EL: Pharmacokinetics, pharmacodynamics, and principles of drug-drug interactions, in Clinical Manual of Psychopharmacology in the Medically Ill, 2nd Edition. Edited by Levenson JL, Ferrando SJ. Arlington, VA, American Psychiatric Association Publishing, 2017, pp 3–44

Percell RLJ Jr, Henning RJ, Siddique Patel M: Atrial myxoma: case report and a review of the literature. Heart Dis 5(3):224–230, 2003 12783636

Peyre H, Hoertel N, Hatteea H, et al: Adulthood self-reported cardiovascular risk and ADHD medications: results from the 2004–2005 National Epidemiologic Survey on Alcohol and Related Conditions. J Clin Psychiatry 75(2):181–182, 2014 24602253

Rosenberger EM, Fox KR, DiMartini AF, Dew MA: Psychosocial factors and quality-of-life after heart transplantation and mechanical circulatory support. Curr Opin Organ Transplant 17(5):558–563, 2012 22890039

Rudolph JL, Jones RN, Levkoff SE, et al: Derivation and validation of a preoperative prediction rule for delirium after cardiac surgery. Circulation 119(2):229–236, 2009 19118253

Shapiro PA: Treatment of depression in patients with congestive heart failure. Heart Fail Rev 14(1):7–12, 2009 17955364

Shapiro PA: Depression treatment and coronary artery disease outcomes: time for reflection. J Psychosom Res 74(1):4–5, 2013a 23272981

Shapiro PA: Heart disease and stress, in Encyclopedia of Behavioral Medicine. Edited by Gellman M, Turner R. New York, Springer, 2013b, p 59

Shapiro PA: Management of depression after myocardial infarction. Curr Cardiol Rep 17(10):80, 2015 26277362

Shapiro PA: Cardiovascular disorders, in Clinical Manual of Psychopharmacology in the Medically Ill, 2nd Edition. Edited by Levenson JL, Ferrando SJ. Arlington, VA, American Psychiatric Association Publishing, 2017, pp 233–270

Sheps DS, McMahon RP, Becker L, et al: Mental stress-induced ischemia and all-cause mortality in patients with coronary artery disease: results from the Psychophysiological Investigations of Myocardial Ischemia study. Circulation 105(15):1780–1784, 2002 11956119

Steinke EE, Jaarsma T, Barnason SA, et al: Sexual counseling for individuals with cardiovascular disease and their partners: a consensus document from the American Heart Association and the ESC Council on Cardiovascular Nursing and Allied Professions (CCNAP). Circulation 128(18):2075–2096, 2013 23897867

Strike PC, Steptoe A: Systematic review of mental stress-induced myocardial ischaemia. Eur Heart J 24(8):690–703, 2003 12713764

Weeke P, Jensen A, Folke F, et al: Antidepressant use and risk of out-of-hospital cardiac arrest: a nationwide case-time-control study. Clin Pharmacol Ther 92(1):72–79, 2012 22588605

Wittstein IS: The broken heart syndrome. Cleve Clin J Med 74 (suppl 1):S17–S22, 2007 17455537

Young JK, Foster DA: Cardiovascular procedures in patients with mental disorders. JAMA 283(24):3198–3199, author reply 3198–3199, 2000 10866854

Zivin K, Pfeiffer PN, Bohnert AS, et al: Evaluation of the FDA warning against prescribing citalopram at doses exceeding 40 mg. Am J Psychiatry 170(6):642–650, 2013 23640689

CHAPTER 7

Endocrine Disorders and Their Psychiatric Manifestations

Jane P. Gagliardi, M.D., M.H.S., FACP, DFAPA

The group of disorders identified as endocrine disorders encompasses a wide array of syndromes and illnesses involving the hypothalamic-pituitary-adrenal (HPA) axis, autoimmune disorders, and other tumors or nodules directly affecting the target organs. The endocrine system encompasses a network of interconnected target organs including the pancreas, thyroid, adrenal glands, parathyroid glands, and reproductive organs. Dysfunction of the hypothalamus, pituitary, or target organ can result in impairment of the endocrine function and also can manifest with behavioral or psychiatric symptoms. Patients who present with symptoms consistent with mania, depression, anxiety, or even psychosis may have occult endocrine dysfunction. Many of the endocrinopathies are associated with cognitive changes, which may be subtle. For this reason, the presence of cognitive changes in association with behavioral symptoms should be considered a possible indicator of underlying medical or endocrine etiology, as should other unexplained general medical symptoms. Given the frequency with which endocrine disorders affect mental functioning, clinicians should maintain a high index of suspicion to ensure timely identification and management of endocrine disorders, treatment of which may also improve quality of life (QOL) and psychological well-being.

Diabetes Mellitus

Diabetes mellitus is a complex illness with a variety of manifestations involving impaired glucose metabolism and associated with increased risk of vascular disease. The direction of the association between diabetes mellitus and psychiatric disorders including mood disorders, anxiety, and schizophrenia is not clear; therefore, whether glycemic control will improve psychiatric outcomes or whether psychiatric treatment will improve outcomes in diabetes mellitus has been an area of investigation. Diabetes mellitus is increasing in prevalence, especially in low- and middle-income countries, and affects an estimated 11.4% of the North American population (Zaccardi et al. 2016).

Major Subtypes of Diabetes Mellitus

Initially classified as either "insulin-dependent" (implying immune-mediated loss of insulin-secreting pancreatic beta cells) or "non-insulin-dependent" (implying impaired peripheral effect of insulin, or insulin resistance), diabetes mellitus was reclassified as "type 1" (T1DM) or "type 2" (T2DM), respectively, in 1979; more recent developments include the recognition of components of both relative insufficiency of insulin production *and* insulin resistance in many patients (Zaccardi et al. 2016).

Etiological, Pathophysiological, and Genetic Factors in Diabetes Mellitus

The basic etiology of diabetes mellitus is impaired action of insulin on target cells; the disease can result from pancreatic beta-cell insufficiency, peripheral insulin resistance, or a combination (Zaccardi et al. 2016). T1DM is caused by autoimmune destruction of pancreatic beta cells; infections, nutritional exposures, and chemicals may precipitate autoimmunity in susceptible individuals. T2DM is associated with obesity and "continuous positive energy balance" (i.e., excess calories in combination with insufficient physical activity) leading to reduced insulin sensitivity (Zaccardi et al. 2016). The relatively recently identified autosomal dominant "maturity-onset diabetes of the young" (MODY) has been colloquially considered "T2DM with childhood onset." Latent autoimmune diabetes in adults (LADA) is diagnosed in adulthood and is associated with autoantibodies but is not insulin-requiring (Zaccardi et al. 2016). In addition to autoimmune and genetic causes, diabetes mellitus can be associated with genetic and chromosomal abnormalities that affect multiple organ systems. Diabetes mellitus is associated with an increased risk of coronary artery disease, stroke, and other vascular disease and also has been associated with increased risk of infection, liver disease, renal failure, central nervous system disorders, and psychological symptoms (Zaccardi et al. 2016).

Clinical Presentations of Diabetes Mellitus

The classic triad of polydipsia, polyuria, and weight loss is associated with some cases of diabetes mellitus; however, diabetes mellitus can present in a variety of ways, ranging from gradual onset of the classic symptoms to sudden presentation with abdominal pain, shortness of breath, nausea, and hyperglycemia associated with diabetic ketoacidosis (DKA). Patients with long-standing diabetes mellitus may have developed complications of the disease (including neuropathy, nephropathy, and retinopathy); patients also may develop associated cardiovascular disease, cerebrovascular disease, and hyperlipidemia. T2DM is associated with obesity and other features of the metabolic syndrome (i.e., hypertension, hyperlipidemia).

Diagnostic and Laboratory Findings in Diabetes Mellitus

The hallmark diagnostic sign of diabetes mellitus is hyperglycemia. Elevated random blood glucose levels (>200 mg/dL), elevated fasting blood glucose levels (>126 mg/dL), abnormal oral glucose tolerance test results (>200 mg/dL after 2 hours), and HbA_{1c} levels of 6.5% or greater are considered diagnostic of diabetes mellitus.

Treatment of Diabetes Mellitus

The goal of treatment in diabetes mellitus is to normalize blood glucose. Diet, exercise, oral agents, and injectable agents including insulin are prescribed in an effort to achieve a target hemoglobin A_{1c} (glycated hemoglobin; HbA_{1c}) level of 7% or lower (Owens et al. 2017).

Learning to accept chronic illness and the need for medical intervention is critical for patients diagnosed with diabetes mellitus. Patients with T1DM will require insulin therapy to avoid complications such as DKA. Some patients with mixed insulin deficiency and insulin resistance may need both oral and injectable agents. In all patients with diabetes mellitus, behavioral interventions are important (Owens et al. 2017). Patients will be asked to monitor their blood sugar through potentially noxious finger sticks and also may be required to self-administer insulin by injection. Dietary modification, with an emphasis on decreasing blood sugar spikes and avoiding high-carbohydrate foods, is advised for all patients with diabetes mellitus. In order to improve insulin sensitivity and body mass index (BMI), particularly among patients with diabetes mellitus associated with obesity, exercise and weight loss are recommended. Regardless of type or symptom burden, patients are advised to undergo regular (annual) foot examinations to assess for neuropathy and vasculopathy as well as annual ophthalmological examinations to assess for retinopathy.

Oral agents used in the treatment of diabetes mellitus include insulin-sensitizing agents and insulin secretagogues (i.e., substances that promote insulin secretion); metformin, an insulin-sensitizing agent with a low risk of inducing hypoglycemia, is frequently initially recommended for patients in whom diet and exercise do not result in adequate glycemic control (Owens et al. 2017). If after 3 months the HbA_{1c} level is not within goal, other medications may be tried, including sulfonylurea medications, thiazolidinediones, α-glucosidase inhibitors, dipeptidyl peptidase-4 inhibitors, glucagon-like peptide-1 receptor agonists, sodium-glucose cotransporter 2 inhibitors, or insulin (Owens et al. 2017). Many patients will require insulin therapy to achieve sufficient control of their diabetes mellitus, although there may be considerable delay in initiation of insulin due to a number of factors, including patient preference (including fear of needles), safety (concern for hypoglycemia), and side effects (insulin is associated with weight gain and increased hunger). Although evidence supports a role for tight glycemic control in prevention of some of the downstream complications of diabetes mellitus, patients with T1DM who take medications as prescribed and maintain HbA_{1c} levels at goal may still experience vascular complications, retinopathy, nephropathy, or neuropathy (Katsarou et al. 2017). Diabetes mellitus is a chronic disease that is complex to manage and places an ongoing burden on patients and their families. It requires ongoing support and attention to behavior in multiple domains, with real risks of other chronic disorders occurring over time.

Neuropsychiatric Presentations in Diabetes Mellitus

The impact of a diabetes mellitus diagnosis on behavioral and mental health can be significant, and comorbid psychiatric disorders can affect the management and course of the illness, especially with insulin-requiring varieties of diabetes mellitus (Ducat et al. 2015). When diabetes mellitus is diagnosed early in life, the illness and the procedures associated with it (e.g., glucose checks, insulin administration) can affect a child's relationships and worldview. Effects on body image and sense of mortality, fears of inexorable disease progression, and experiences of witnessing first-degree relatives with poor health outcomes related to diabetes mellitus all may contribute to psychological stress and problems in children and adolescents with diabetes mellitus. The biology of the disease also poses particular challenges: adolescent rebellion, challenging with healthy children, can become fatal if it involves skipping insulin doses or eating high-carbohydrate foods. Insulin administration (or lack thereof) can be a tool employed by individuals with eating disorders. Adolescent girls and adult women, in particular, may demonstrate abnormal eating behaviors, including binge eating and caloric restriction, which they may accomplish through insulin restriction (Ducat et al. 2015). Additionally, as a disease that affects micro- and macrovascular structures, diabetes mellitus can have a direct impact on brain structure and cognitive function. Depression, anxiety, eating disorders, and other serious mental illnesses have been associated with diabetes mellitus.

Depression

The full extent and direction of the relationship between depression and diabetes mellitus have not been entirely elucidated (Tabák et al. 2014), but 12%–18% of patients with diabetes mellitus will meet diagnostic criteria for major depressive disorder (MDD) (Katon 2008). Depression has been associated with abnormalities in the HPA axis, sympathetic nervous system, and inflammatory processes, and these mechanisms may themselves portend increased risk for development of diabetes as well as worse complications and outcomes in individuals with both diabetes and depression (Katon 2003). The presence of depression is a poor prognostic factor, with a 1.5-fold increase in all-cause mortality among patients with diabetes mellitus and depression compared with patients with diabetes mellitus without depression (Park et al. 2013). On average, patients who have diabetes mellitus and depression demonstrate more symptoms from diabetes, decreased adherence to diabetes treatment, increased health care utilization, and higher medical expenses than patients with diabetes mellitus who do not have depression (Park et al. 2013). There is some hope that effective treatment of depression could result in improved outcomes in diabetes mellitus, and vice versa.

Anxiety

Generalized anxiety disorder may be more prevalent among patients with diabetes mellitus than among those without, although the biology and causality of anxiety associated with diabetes mellitus are not well described (Smith et al. 2013). A specific fear of hypoglycemia, which can have a detrimental impact on disease control and long-term complications, can occur (Martyn-Nemeth et al. 2016). In addition, hypoglycemia caused by the adrenergic and related responses to low blood sugar can lead to tachycardia, sweating, and (in more severe cases) confusion. Fear of hypoglycemia may lead patients to overeat, avoid taking insulin, and maintain higher-than-recommended glucose levels. The associated glycemic fluctuations can result in more severe neurological and neuropsychiatric complications of diabetes mellitus itself (Ducat et al. 2015).

Eating Disorders

Adolescent girls with T1DM have an increased rate of developing eating disorders compared with adolescent girls without diabetes mellitus, and adult women with diabetes mellitus may restrict their use of insulin in an effort to avoid calorie consumption (Ducat et al. 2015). The presence of an eating disorder in the setting of diabetes mellitus is associated with higher rates of retinopathy, neuropathy, hospitalization, and early mortality (Ducat et al. 2015).

Psychosis and Severe Mental Illness

Prevalence rates of diabetes and obesity in individuals with schizophrenia and mood disorders are 1.5–2.0 times higher than those in the general population, although the etiology is uncertain. Likewise, the associations among antipsychotic treatment, metabolic syndrome, and diabetes mellitus make direct causal attributions between psychiatric illnesses and diabetes mellitus difficult (American Diabetes Association et al. 2004). An estimated 10%–12% of patients with psychotic disorders have diabetes (Holt and Mitchell 2015). Patients with diabetes mellitus and comorbid serious mental illness (SMI; defined by the CDC as "a mental illness or disorder with serious functional impairment that substantially interferes with or limits one or more major life activities") have higher rates of microvascular and macrovascular complications and mortality related to diabetes compared with diabetic persons without SMI. Many different factors, including genetics, environmental factors, pathophysiology of SMI itself, and the treatments provided for SMI, may be implicated (Holt and Mitchell 2015).

Treatment of Neuropsychiatric Symptoms in Diabetes Mellitus

Recommendations for the comprehensive treatment of diabetes mellitus include consideration of behavioral, psychological, psychiatric, and motivational aspects encompassing lifestyle modification as well as treatment of diagnosable psychiatric entities (Ducat et al. 2015).

Behavioral and psychiatric interventions to treat underlying or associated depression, anxiety, and eating disorders can improve medical outcomes and long-term complication rates in patients with diabetes mellitus (Ducat et al. 2015). Cognitive-behavioral therapy (CBT) for the treatment of depression is associated with improved mood and glycemic control (Li et al. 2017). Treating underlying depression and anxiety is likely to facilitate adherence to recommended treatments for diabetes mellitus as well as improve overall QOL (Ducat et al. 2015).

Neuropsychiatric Symptoms Associated With Treatments for Diabetes Mellitus

Patients with diabetes mellitus may develop fear of hypoglycemia, which can include tachycardia, confusion, and anxiety among its symptoms. Hypoglycemia can be associated with both oral agents and insulin (Ducat et al. 2015). Metformin, frequently used as a first-line treatment in patients with diabetes mellitus, has in rare cases been associated with anxiety, confusion, depression, and changes in sleep. Thiazolidine-diones have been associated with headaches, anxiety, confusion, and shakiness.

Significant Psychiatric Drug Interactions or Considerations in Diabetes Mellitus

There is a well-known association between antipsychotic medications, particularly the atypical antipsychotics, and the development of the metabolic syndrome and diabetes mellitus. The 2004 Consensus Development Conference on Antipsychotic Drugs and Obesity and Diabetes was convened to recommend monitoring parameters for patients taking antipsychotic medications (American Diabetes Association et al. 2004). Evidence still suggests, however, that a large number of patients are prescribed antipsychotic medications without proper monitoring of cardiometabolic risk factors (Mitchell and Hardy 2013). The recommended parameters for monitoring are as follows (American Diabetes Association et al. 2004):

- *Baseline:* Personal/family history, weight (BMI), waist circumference, blood pressure, fasting plasma glucose, fasting lipid profile
- *4 weeks:* Weight (BMI)
- *8 weeks:* Weight (BMI)
- *12 weeks:* Weight (BMI), blood pressure, fasting plasma glucose, fasting lipid profile
- *Quarterly:* Weight (BMI)
- *Annually:* Personal/family history, weight (BMI), waist circumference, blood pressure, fasting plasma glucose
- *Every 5 years:* Fasting lipid profile

Thyroid Disorders

The thyroid gland is involved in metabolic function and depends on hypothalamic (thyrotropin-releasing hormone [TRH]) and anterior pituitary (thyroid-stimulating hormone [TSH]) signals to secrete proper amounts of the two major thyroid hormones, thyroxine (T_4) (the precursor hormone) and triiodothyronine (T_3) (the biologically active hormone, 80% of which is converted from T_4 and 20% of which is secreted directly by the thyroid gland). Thyroid hormone concentrations vary over the course of the day in a diurnal or circadian pattern and are influenced by stimuli such as light and sleep patterns. TSH concentrations are lowest at midday and highest just before midnight. When making a diagnosis of hypothyroidism, it is important to consider the pulsatile and diurnal patterns of TSH release (Gorman and Chiasera 2013). The amount of thyroid hormone available intracellularly in the brain is influenced by a number of complex factors (Bauer et al. 2008).

As with other endocrine disorders, the subclinical manifestations of thyroid dysfunction can be subtle and difficult to detect. Three percent to 5% of adults have subclinical thyroid dysfunction, and an additional 0.5%–1% of adults have overt thyroid dysfunction. Disordered thyroid function can be underactive (hypothyroidism) or overactive (hyperthyroidism) (Rugge et al. 2014). The association between thyroid function and mental health has been recognized for more than a century, with thyroid dysfunction leading to prominent symptoms in affective, anxiety, and cognitive domains (Ritchie and Yeap 2015). Some studies, including a 2016 study by Delitala and colleagues, have found a "U-shaped" relationship between thyroid dysfunction and psychiatric symptomatology: depressive symptoms can result from either hyperthyroid or hypothyroid states, even though anxiety and mania are more commonly associated with hyperthyroidism, and depression and cognitive clouding are more commonly associated with hypothyroidism (Delitala et al. 2016). Similarly, psychotic symptoms are seen at both ends of the thyroid dysfunction spectrum (i.e., in both thyrotoxicosis and myxedema coma).

The most common treatment of hypothyroidism is supplementation of T_4 using levothyroxine. It takes 6–8 weeks for T_4 levels to equilibrate in the tissues. It is unclear whether a combination of T_4 and T_3 is more effective than T_4 alone for the general treatment of hypothyroidism (Samuels 2014). Thyroid hormone has been studied as an augmentation strategy for depression, with varying results (Feldman et al. 2013).

Major Subtypes of Thyroid Disorders

Thyroid disorders range from life threatening (on either the over- or underproduction spectrum) to subclinical. At the most severe hypothyroid end of the spectrum, *myxedema coma,* a life-threatening lack of thyroid hormone sufficient to maintain metabolic functions, can result in hypothermia, hypoventilation, seizures, and decreased consciousness. *Overt hypothyroidism* manifests as fatigue, cold intolerance, weight gain, hair loss, dry skin, constipation, and poor concentration. *Subclinical hypothyroidism* frequently has no specific physical symptomatology. *Subclinical hyperthyroidism* also tends to be physically asymptomatic. *Overt hyperthyroidism* can manifest as palpitations, emotional lability, anxiety, heat intolerance, sweating, weight loss, diarrhea, hyperactivity, and fatigue. Most patients with hyperthyroidism also have stare and lid lag (a condition in which the movement of the eyelids lags behind that of the eyes; in severe cases, the eyelids do not move at all) due to a hypersympathetic state. At the most severe hyperthyroid end of the spectrum, *thyroid storm* (i.e., thyrotoxicosis) is a potentially life-threatening overproduction of thyroid hormone and can manifest as fever, delirium, seizures, and coma (Ritchie and Yeap 2015; Rugge et al. 2014).

Etiological, Pathophysiological, and Genetic Factors in Thyroid Disorders

The most common cause of *hypothyroidism* is autoimmune thyroiditis, also known as Hashimoto's thyroiditis, diagnosed by the presence of thyroid peroxidase antibodies. Clinical manifestations can include slowing of thought and speech, decreased attentiveness, apathy, fatigue, and impaired concentration (Samuels 2014). Other causes include insufficient replacement treatment with levothyroxine, effects of external beam radiation to the head and neck, untreated adrenal insufficiency, and effects of medications (e.g., lithium or amiodarone). Risk factors for hypothyroidism include T1DM, family history, and Down syndrome.

The most common cause of *hyperthyroidism* is Graves' disease, which is thought to be related to autoantibodies to the thyrotropin receptor, although it can also be caused by drug exposure, including lithium. In addition to the typical symptoms of hyperthyroidism, Graves' disease is associated with diffuse goiter, Graves ophthalmopathy, and pretibial myxedema. Additionally, the initial phase of Hashimoto's thyroiditis can result in hyperthyroidism, also referred to as Hashithyrotoxicosis. In rare cases, Hashimoto's thyroiditis can be associated with a disorder known as Hashimoto's encephalopathy, which is of uncertain etiology but generally viewed as being immune mediated; this disorder can manifest as a slow onset of confusion and can progress to seizures, myoclonus, and altered consciousness. In other cases, there is an acute or subacute onset of focal deficits that can be associated with cognitive impairment. Other causes of hyperthyroidism include functional nodules and overtreatment with levothyroxine. Risk factors for hyperthyroidism include personal or family history and ingestion of iodine-containing drugs (or contrast media, such as iodinated contrast dye utilized for computed tomography [CT]).

In a systematic review and meta-analysis of 19 studies involving more than 36,000 participants, patients with autoimmune thyroiditis, Hashimoto's thyroiditis, or subclinical or overt hypothyroidism were found to have an increased hazard ratio for depressive disorders (3.56) or anxiety disorders (2.32) when compared with healthy control subjects (Siegmann et al. 2018).

Clinical Presentations of Thyroid Disorders

The range of subtle clinical presentations of thyroid disease as well as a lack of clear evidence of benefit from interventions targeting subclinical thyroid dysfunction prompted the U.S. Preventive Services Task Force to conclude that "the optimal screening interval for thyroid dysfunction (if one exists) is unknown" (p. 644) and that "current evidence is insufficient to assess the balance of benefits and harms of screening for thyroid dysfunction in nonpregnant, asymptomatic adults" (LeFevre and U.S. Preventive Services Task Force 2015, p. 649). By the same token, given the range of clinical presentations and the nonspecific nature of symptoms that can be associated with thyroid dysfunction, patients presenting with a variety of physical and mental health symptoms could be considered to fall outside of the category of "asymptomatic adults."

Symptoms of overproduction or overfunction of thyroid hormone (e.g., thyroid storm, overt hyperthyroidism, subclinical hyperthyroidism) are related to increased metabolic activity and can range from mild to severe. Subclinical hyperthyroidism may not have any symptoms at all, or patients may notice subtle cognitive changes. As severity increases, patients may develop symptoms of heat intolerance, sweating, diarrhea, fatigue, and anxiety; thyrotoxicosis can cause delirium, flushing, fevers, and even seizures or coma. Underproduction of thyroid hormone (e.g., myxedema coma, overt hypothyroidism, subclinical hypothyroidism) also results in a range of symptoms, with the mildest form involving mood symptoms or no symptoms. As patients develop subclinical and then overt hypothyroidism, they may experience fatigue, cold intolerance, hair loss, impaired concentration, dry skin, and constipation; myxedema coma is uncommon but potentially life threatening and can result in hypothermia, hypoventilation, altered consciousness, and seizures.

Diagnostic and Laboratory Findings in Thyroid Disorders

Table 7–1 depicts diagnostic and laboratory findings in various disorders of thyroid function.

Treatment of Thyroid Disorders

Treatment for overt hypothyroidism involves replacement of thyroid hormone (levothyroxine). Guidelines for treatment of subclinical hypothyroidism include watchful waiting or thyroid hormone replacement. Treatment of overt hyperthyroidism involves antithyroid medications (methimazole or propylthiouracil) or ablation therapy with radioactive iodine or surgery. Subclinical hyperthyroidism is managed with watchful waiting, because ablation of the gland can result in hypothyroidism, and the natural history of subclinical hyperthyroidism may be one of spontaneously resolving thyroiditis (Rugge et al. 2014).

Neuropsychiatric Presentations in Thyroid Disorders

MDD involves both affective and neurovegetative symptoms, and both hypothyroidism and apathetic hyperthyroidism can potentially manifest the neurovegetative and cognitive aspects of depressive illness (Bathla et al. 2016).

The etiology of neuropsychiatric changes in thyroid dysfunction is not clearly elucidated, but proposed mechanisms include a role for thyroid hormones as trophic or growth-promoting factors for the developing nervous system; nuclear receptor binding of the active form of thyroid hormone (T_3) with subsequent alteration in gene expression; and the proximity of thyroid receptors to many limbic structures. Additionally, some studies have demonstrated an association between thyroid hormone and norepinephrine or serotonin (Delitala et al. 2016).

In mild forms, hypothyroidism and hyperthyroidism can present with cognitive changes, depressed mood, or mild anxiety; alternatively, subclinical hypothyroidism can be asymptomatic. *Overt hypothyroidism* may be associated with poor concentration, slowed thought, fatigue, and depression, although some case series and case reports describe hypothyroid patients developing acute mania (Ritchie and Yeap 2015; Rugge et al. 2014). In rare cases, severely hypothyroid patients can present with T_4-reversible psychotic symptoms (Samuels 2014). Psychotic symptoms can include auditory and visual hallucinations, paranoid and other delusions, and even Capgras syndrome (Feldman et al. 2013). Melancholic depression—a subtype of major depressive disorder characterized by marked sadness and worse mood in the mornings, as well as neurovegetative symptoms such as weight loss and loss of appetite—also has been described. Patients with *myxedema coma* may have a decreased level of consciousness, although despite its name, they do not have to be comatose. Psychosis has historically been described, as in the report of the 1888 Committee of the Clinical Society in London, in which the description included "delusions and hallucinations. It takes the form of acute or chronic manias, dementia, or melancholia, with marked predominance of suspicion and self-accusation" (Ritchie and Yeap 2015, p. 267).

Subclinical hyperthyroidism may be asymptomatic or may be associated with some mood and cognitive symptoms (Ritchie and Yeap 2015). *Overt hyperthyroidism* is classically associated with emotional lability, anxiety, dysphoria, cognitive dysfunction,

TABLE 7–1.	Diagnostic and laboratory findings in various disorders of thyroid function
Disorder	**Findings**
Hyperthyroidism	
Subclinical hyperthyroidism	Low serum TSH, normal FT_4
Overt hyperthyroidism	Low serum TSH, normal or high FT_4
Thyroid storm	Low serum TSH, high FT_4
Hypothyroidism	
Subclinical hypothyroidism	High serum TSH, normal FT_4
Overt hypothyroidism	High TSH, normal or low FT_4
Myxedema coma	High TSH, low FT_4

Note. FT_4=free thyroxine (T_4); TSH=thyroid-stimulating hormone.

and manic symptoms. Manic symptoms are generally less severe than those seen in true manic episodes associated with bipolar disorder. True manic episodes can be precipitated by hyperthyroidism in patients with baseline bipolar disorder and have been described in patients with a strong family history of bipolar disorder (Samuels 2014). Depression also has been reported with hyperthyroidism (Ritchie and Yeap 2015). First described in the 1930s (Lahey 1931), *apathetic hyperthyroidism* is typically found in middle-aged and older individuals, who may present with weight loss, irritability, or amotivation—symptoms that can be indistinguishable from those of melancholic depression or dementia. These patients often have cardiovascular symptoms, including atrial fibrillation, high-output heart failure, or tachycardia (Wu et al. 2010). Apathetic hyperthyroidism may be found in up to 10%–15% of older individuals with thyrotoxicosis.

Patients with untreated hyperthyroidism demonstrate higher rates of anxiety and depression than the general population. In one case series (Brownlie et al. 2000) of 18 patients, thyrotoxicosis was associated with mania in seven patients, depression in seven, psychotic symptoms with an affective component in two, and psychotic symptoms with paranoia in one. The remaining patient demonstrated symptoms of delirium (Brownlie et al. 2000), which in severe cases can progress to coma.

Treatment of Neuropsychiatric Symptoms in Thyroid Disorders

In general, restoring a euthyroid state (through supplementation of thyroid hormone or ablation of the overproducing gland) is recommended to restore cognitive and affective functioning (Ritchie and Yeap 2015). With recognition that restoration of a euthyroid state is paramount, there may be a need for concomitant pharmacological treatment of depression, anxiety, or psychosis associated with hypo- or hyperthyroid states. Although no medications are specifically indicated for treatment of thyroid-associated neuropsychiatric syndromes, case series provide support for using medications targeting the specific neuropsychiatric symptoms. For instance, mood stabilizers or mood-stabilizing antipsychotic medications could be used for affective psychosis (i.e., schizoaffective disorder) or mood lability. Benzodiazepines and β-blockers could be helpful for the adrenergic overdrive and anxiety associated with hyperthyroidism. For the cognitive slowing associated with myxedema coma, stimulants should be avoided because of the concern for cardiovascular stress and arrhythmias, issues that can also occur with overly rapid repletion of thyroid hormone. In addition, sedatives including opioids can worsen severe hypothyroid states such as myxedema and should therefore be avoided.

Neuropsychiatric Symptoms Associated With Treatments for Thyroid Disorders

There are no neuropsychiatric symptoms specifically associated with treatment of thyroid disorder, although overshooting treatment of hyperthyroidism can result in hypothyroidism (and associated symptoms), and overshooting treatment of hypothyroidism can result in hyperthyroidism. In patients with eating disorders or a strong motivation to lose weight, overuse of levothyroxine can result in symptoms of hyperthyroidism (ranging from anxiety to mania).

Significant Psychiatric Drug Interactions or Considerations in Thyroid Disorders

Abnormal thyroid tests have been observed in a percentage of individuals with psychiatric disorders, including mood disorders. Depressed patients frequently lack the nocturnal surge of TSH that occurs in healthy individuals, possibly as a result of the disordered sleep associated with depression. As many as 25%–30% of patients with acute mood or psychotic symptoms exhibit a "blunted" TSH response to TRH administration, which normalizes with treatment of depression (Bauer et al. 2008). Another estimated 15% of depressed patients have an "enhanced" TSH response (Feldman et al. 2013). Both T_4 and T_3 preparations have been used in the primary treatment of depressive disorders, usually as augmentation strategies. When employing thyroid hormone augmentation, periodic assessment of thyroid function is essential.

Hyperthyroidism may be managed with propylthiouracil or methimazole as a temporizing measure before ablation or surgical resection. Methimazole may cause myelosuppression, which is a consideration in patients taking clozapine. Mirtazapine's product label includes a warning about the possibility of neutropenia. Although there are no published reports of neutropenia resulting from mirtazapine in combination with methimazole, it is worth keeping the possibility of this adverse effect in mind. Patients experiencing extreme anxiety or psychosis from hyperthyroidism may be hesitant to undergo radioactive iodine or surgical resection, and treatment with methimazole or propylthiouracil, careful monitoring, and input from proxy decision makers may be necessary.

Thyroid Function and Lithium

Although newer-generation antipsychotic and anticonvulsant medications may be used to treat bipolar disorder, lithium remains a highly effective option, including for many patients who achieve suboptimal response to the newer agents. For decades, lithium has been recognized as an agent that interferes with normal thyroid function. In the 1970s, authors reported that lithium-treated patients developed hypothyroidism and goiter (Barbesino 2010; McDermott et al. 1986). Later studies demonstrated lithium-induced inhibition of thyroid hormone synthesis (Barbesino 2010). In rare cases, lithium has been associated with hyperthyroidism (Barbesino 2010; McDermott et al. 1986). It is important to monitor thyroid function periodically in patients taking lithium and also to be aware of the possibility of thyroid derangements as causing or contributing to mood episodes (mania or depression).

Hyperparathyroidism

Primary hyperparathyroidism (PHPT) is a condition that results from oversecretion of parathyroid hormone (PTH) from the parathyroid glands, located in the neck, usually associated with parathyroid adenoma. Classically described as manifesting with bone pain, kidney stones, abdominal cramps, and psychological manifestations, PHPT has many manifestations. PHPT results in hypercalcemia, which has been demonstrated in a number of studies to be associated with cognitive slowing ranging from a foggy feeling to memory and cognitive impairment that is measurable with neurocognitive testing (Grant and Velusamy 2014). Guidelines for management of PHPT focus on physical manifestations of the illness, although treatment with parathyroidectomy has been demonstrated to result in improvements in QOL as well as in neurocognitive functioning (Grant and Velusamy 2014; Roman et al. 2011; Zanocco et al. 2015). Roman et al. (2011) demonstrated a correlation between degree of postparathyroidectomy PTH reduction and degree of anxiety improvement, with subsequent improvement in neurocognitive function.

Etiological, Pathophysiological, and Genetic Factors in Hyperparathyroidism

In addition to a long-recognized association between hypercalcemia and cognitive impairment (Grant and Velusamy 2014; Roman et al. 2011; Zanocco et al. 2015), some data suggest a direct impact of PTH in the brain. Roman et al. (2011) noted that there are PTH receptors in the brain and also cited studies identifying cerebral hypoperfusion in patients with PHPT; additionally, intact PTH is associated with peripheral vasoconstriction and increased stiffness of the vasculature, which could theoretically also occur in the central nervous system (Roman et al. 2011).

Clinical Presentations of Hyperparathyroidism

The classical presentation of PHPT has been characterized as involving "bones, stones, abdominal groans, and psychic moans" and can include osteoporosis and bone pain, kidney stones, pancreatitis, and cognitive impairment or psychiatric symptomatology. Physical symptoms can also include myalgia, headaches, abdominal pain, and proximal muscle weakness.

Diagnostic and Laboratory Findings in Hyperparathyroidism

The most common initial laboratory finding in PHPT is elevated serum calcium. Further testing reveals elevated PTH. If PTH is not elevated, secondary causes of hyperparathyroidism, including malignancy, should be considered.

Treatment of Hyperparathyroidism

Treatment of overtly symptomatic PHPT is parathyroidectomy. Guidelines continue to recommend parathyroidectomy for physical symptoms, although evidence is mounting that psychological and cognitive symptoms can be improved with it as well (Grant and Velusamy 2014; Roman et al. 2011).

Neuropsychiatric Presentations in Hyperparathyroidism

Hyperparathyroidism was noted in earlier literature to be associated with psychosis (paranoia, delusions, and visual hallucinations—symptoms that in more recent descriptions are attributed to delirium). Additional symptoms noted in recent overviews include, in addition to physical symptoms, fatigability, mood swings, feeling "blue" or depressed, weakness, irritability, and forgetfulness (Grant and Velusamy 2014). Determining whether cognitive symptoms (which occur mostly in older adults) are due to PHPT or are related to other factors can be challenging. PHPT is associated with elevated calcium levels, and cognitive slowing associated with hypercalcemia can range from a foggy-headed feeling to memory impairment, poor concentration, and grossly impaired recall. Vitamin D deficiency, which is present in a high proportion of aging adults, has been associated with impaired ability to shift tasks and slow processing speed (Grant and Velusamy 2014).

Treatment of Neuropsychiatric Symptoms in Hyperparathyroidism

When patients with PHPT present with cognitive fogging and serum calcium is elevated, interventions to normalize calcium—fluids, diuresis, and (in extreme cases) bisphosphonates—can be utilized. One recent study found that hydrochlorothiazide was a safe and effective treatment for PHPT-associated hypercalcemia (Tsvetov et al. 2017), although the theoretical risk of increasing serum calcium has limited this agent's use historically. The only definitive treatment for PHPT is parathyroidectomy (Zanocco et al. 2015). Current best evidence suggests that parathyroidectomy is underused and that this surgery may have beneficial effects on neurocognitive symptoms attributable to PHPT; use of parathyroidectomy for this indication is also recommended in the most recent guidelines for management of primary hyperparathyroidism from the American Association of Endocrine Surgeons, although the supporting evidence is of low quality (Wilhelm et al. 2016).

Neuropsychiatric Symptoms Associated With Treatment for Hyperparathyroidism

There are no specific neuropsychiatric syndromes reported with parathyroidectomy. Given the possibility of iatrogenic hypoparathyroidism as an effect of parathyroidectomy, clinicians should be aware that cases of major depressive symptoms associated with hypoparathyroidism have been reported in the literature (Montenegro et al. 2019; Rosa et al. 2014).

Polycystic Ovary Syndrome

Polycystic ovary syndrome (PCOS) refers to a condition first described by Stein and Leventhal in 1935 (therefore also known as Stein-Leventhal syndrome); it affects up to 7% of women of reproductive age and is the most common cause of infertility (Wang et al. 2017). The syndrome should be suspected in women who demonstrate ovarian dysfunction along with features of hyperandrogenism (acne, hirsutism) and polycystic ovaries (Andrade et al. 2016; Rotterdam ESHRE/ASRM-Sponsored PCOS Consensus Workshop Group 2004; Wang et al. 2017). PCOS is associated with irregular menses, increased rates of T2DM, and increased cardiovascular risk. Insulin resistance, hyperinsulinemia, dyslipidemia, and obesity are also associated with the disorder (Tsikouras et al. 2015).

Patients with PCOS may experience anovulatory infertility, spontaneous abortion, gestational diabetes, and pre-eclampsia, all of which are thought to be related to insulin resistance. The literature suggests a significant association between PCOS and depression and anxiety (Blay et al. 2016). Phenotypic features, the presence of infertility, and treatments targeting infertility may contribute to psychological distress.

Major Subtypes of Polycystic Ovary Syndrome

A somewhat heterogeneous cluster of symptoms, PCOS may manifest in various ways. Some patients will present with concerns about symptoms associated with androgen excess (e.g., acne, male-pattern hair growth), whereas others will experience infertility as the presenting concern (Tsikouras et al. 2015).

Etiological, Pathophysiological, and Genetic Factors in Polycystic Ovary Syndrome

Although causal factors remain unclear, PCOS is believed to result from interactions between genetic and environmental factors. With the rising prevalence of obesity among adolescent girls, authors predict higher rates of PCOS in the future (Tsikouras et al. 2015).

Clinical Presentations of Polycystic Ovary Syndrome

PCOS may go unrecognized and undiagnosed in many women, and its recognition may depend on cultural differences, age, and manifestations of the syndrome.

Younger women tend to present with symptoms of reproductive difficulties (oligo-ovulation or anovulation, with associated irregular menses or infertility) and also may exhibit obesity and insulin resistance (Boyle and Teede 2012). For other patients, the condition may be recognized when they seek medical treatment for acne or hirsutism. Still other patients may come to medical attention because of diabetes mellitus and other features of the metabolic syndrome (Chan et al. 2017). Some individuals may never be diagnosed, despite presenting with evidence of insulin resistance and inflammatory changes in the form of diabetes mellitus or coronary heart disease.

Diagnostic and Laboratory Findings in Polycystic Ovary Syndrome

Among the three separate sets of clinical criteria in use for diagnosing PCOS (the NIH criteria [1990], the Rotterdam criteria [2004], and the Androgen Excess and PCOS [AE-PCOS] Society criteria [2006]), the Rotterdam criteria (Rotterdam ESHRE/ ASRM-Sponsored PCOS Consensus Workshop Group 2004) are the most widely accepted. These criteria require two of the following three manifestations:

1. Oligo-ovulation or anovulation
2. Hyperandrogenism, as assessed clinically (hirsutism or [less commonly] male-pattern baldness) or biochemically (high free androgen index or free testosterone)
3. Polycystic ovaries on ultrasound

An NIH expert panel in 2012 discussed the merits and drawbacks of the three sets of PCOS criteria (i.e, the NIH criteria, the Rotterdam criteria, and the AE-PCOS Society criteria) and recommended specifying phenotype when diagnosing PCOS, as follows: 1) androgen excess and ovulatory dysfunction; 2) androgen excess and polycystic ovary morphology; 3) ovulatory dysfunction and polycystic ovary morphology; and 4) androgen excess, ovulatory dysfunction, and polycystic ovary morphology (Johnson et al. 2012). More recent recommendations advocate use of more rigorous study methodology to improve diagnostic and treatment options (Wang and Mol 2017).

Treatment of Polycystic Ovary Syndrome

The treatment of PCOS is directed at symptoms, because the underlying etiology has not been entirely elucidated. Table 7–2 summarizes the evidence on treatment options presented at the 2012 National Institutes of Health (NIH) expert panel (Johnson et al. 2012).

Neuropsychiatric Presentations in Polycystic Ovary Syndrome

PCOS is reported to be associated with anxiety, depression, disordered eating, and bipolar disorder (Blay et al. 2016). The strength and causality of these associations vary depending on the study. One group of authors (Scaruffi et al. 2014) who used structured psychological and psychiatric measures to evaluate 60 individuals with PCOS demonstrated significantly elevated rates of dysphoria, chronic emotional distress,

TABLE 7–2.   Treatment strategies for polycystic ovary syndrome

Treatment	Effect on manifestations			Comments
	Androgen excess	Anovulation/oligo-ovulation	Insulin sensitivity	
Lifestyle modification and weight loss	Decreases excess androgen	Increases ovulation/fertility	Improves insulin function	
Metformin	Decreases excess androgen	Modest (if any) effect on ovulation/fertility	No effect on insulin function	
Thiazolidinediones	No effect on excess androgen	No effect on ovulation/fertility	Increases insulin function	
Clomiphene, aromatase inhibitors	No effect on excess androgen	Stimulates ovulation and increases fertility	No effect on insulin function	Can lead to multiple gestation, bone loss, cardiovascular disease
Surgery	No effect on excess androgen	Can have short-term effect on ovarian function	No effect on insulin function	
Ovarian gonadotropin stimulation	No effect on excess androgen	Can improve ovarian function during the corresponding menstrual cycle	No effect on insulin function	Can lead to multiple gestation and potentially fatal overstimulation
Antiandrogen agents	Can mitigate hirsutism	No effect on ovarian function	No effect on insulin function	

Source.   Data from Johnson et al. 2012.

interpersonal difficulties, and even delusional disorder (Scaruffi et al. 2014). A systematic review and meta-analysis of high-quality studies using prospectively employed validated psychiatric diagnostic criteria found consistent evidence for higher rates of depression and anxiety among individuals with PCOS in comparison with individuals who do not have PCOS (Blay et al. 2016). The etiology of neuropsychiatric symptoms in PCOS could be multifactorial; biological factors (e.g., changes in the HPA axis, dysregulation of cortisol production, brain changes), psychological factors (e.g., self-esteem issues that could be related to physical manifestations of androgen excess and/or to problems with fertility), and social factors have been implicated (Blay et al. 2016).

Treatment of Neuropsychiatric Symptoms in Polycystic Ovary Syndrome

Neuropsychiatric symptoms of PCOS are treated symptomatically, such as with CBT or interpersonal therapy or selective serotonin reuptake inhibitors (SSRIs). Although experts agree that it is important to address potentially relevant psychosocial stressors (e.g., marital, family, social issues, QOL, sexual dysfunction, low self-esteem), evidence for improved outcomes from specific treatment modalities is lacking (Blay et al. 2016).

Neuropsychiatric Symptoms Associated With Treatments for Polycystic Ovary Syndrome

The various treatments employed for PCOS may have possible neuropsychiatric side effects, although the psychiatric and psychosocial impact of PCOS itself must be factored into the decision of when and how to treat. Metformin, used to help reduce insulin resistance and the risk of metabolic consequences, can occasionally be associated with anxiety, confusion, depression, or sleep changes. Thiazolidinediones, also used to target insulin function, commonly are associated with headache and in rare instances can induce anxiety, confusion, and shakiness. Clomiphene, used to promote fertility, may in rare cases be associated with depression, fatigue, restlessness, and insomnia. Aromatase inhibitors, used to enhance fertility, may be associated with cognitive changes.

Testosterone Deficiency

Testosterone is a hormone that is involved in the function of many organ systems and tissues and is involved in the regulation of lipid, carbohydrate, and protein metabolism as well as vascular physiology and action (Traish 2016). Testosterone is produced in the Leydig cells of the testes and is regulated by the hypothalamic-pituitary-gonadal (HPG) axis through luteinizing hormone (LH) production. Testosterone deficiency, or male hypogonadism, affects adult men and is diagnosed when serum testosterone levels are low in the presence of clinical signs and symptoms (Berkseth et al. 2016; Bhasin et al. 2010). Estimates of prevalence vary widely, as do thresholds for diagnosis and treatment in aging men (Millar et al. 2016). Testosterone deficiency can be associated with depressive and cognitive symptoms, but replacement therapy currently is recommended only for quantifiable symptoms such as sexual function, walking distance, and mood (Millar et al. 2016).

Major Subtypes of Testosterone Deficiency

Hypogonadism can be categorized as *primary* (related to testicular dysfunction) or *secondary* (related to pituitary or hypothalamic abnormalities). Older men may present with mixed forms of testosterone deficiency associated with mechanisms including decreased bioavailability, decreased production of testosterone, and blunted HPG axis diurnal variation (McBride et al. 2016).

Etiological, Pathophysiological, and Genetic Factors in Testosterone Deficiency

Primary hypogonadism can result from a number of factors, including prior treatment for testicular cancer, history of testicular infection, medications such as chemotherapeutic agents that are toxic to the gonads, other toxins such as environmental exposures, surgical removal, trauma, idiopathic atrophy, varicocele, or Klinefelter syndrome (McBride et al. 2016). Secondary hypogonadism, which results from insufficient LH production, can result from primary gonadotropin-releasing hormone deficiency; hypopituitarism from radiation, inflammation, infection, or trauma; or pituitary adenomas producing prolactin (McBride et al. 2016). As patients age, hypogonadism can be associated with metabolic syndrome and insulin resistance.

Although use of anabolic steroids was once thought to be a problem only among competitive athletes, current data estimate that 3%–4% of people worldwide (6.4% of males and 1.6% of females) have used anabolic steroids (Christou et al. 2017). Exogenous anabolic steroid use is associated with significant reductions in gonadotropin and testosterone levels; testosterone levels may remain low for months after discontinuation of anabolic steroids (Christou et al. 2017).

Chronic alcohol use and chronic disease, including HIV, can contribute to the development of testosterone deficiency (McBride et al. 2016; Morales et al. 2015). Medications including 5-α-reductase inhibitors (used to treat benign prostatic hypertrophy), alkylating agents, and glucocorticoids can contribute to testosterone deficiency, as can opioids, β-blockers, statins, and anabolic steroids (McBride et al. 2016).

Clinical Presentations of Testosterone Deficiency

Symptoms of testosterone deficiency can include incomplete or delayed sexual development; eunuchoidism; low libido; erectile dysfunction; gynecomastia; sparse axillary, facial, and pubic hair; small testes; infertility; pathological fractures or low bone mineral density; and hot flashes. Symptoms may be much less specific or may be attributed to other causes, in which case the deficiency may go unrecognized. Nonspecific signs and symptoms of testosterone deficiency include low energy, poor motivation, depressed mood, poor concentration, impaired memory, sleep disturbances, mild anemia, decreased muscle strength and mass, and poor physical performance (Bhasin et al. 2010; Millar et al. 2016). Deficiency of testosterone can also lead to anemia, increased body fat, decreased muscle mass, insulin resistance, osteopenia, metabolic syndrome, and other downstream negative consequences that could be attributed to myriad other causes (Traish 2016).

Diagnostic and Laboratory Findings in Testosterone Deficiency

Clinical practice guidelines for the evaluation and treatment of androgen deficiency syndromes recommend measuring morning total testosterone when the patient is not acutely ill and only after the patient has been ascertained to demonstrate specific or nonspecific signs and symptoms of testosterone deficiency (Bhasin et al. 2010; Morales et al. 2015). If the screening measurement is unequivocally low, the diagnosis of low testosterone can be made. If the screening measurement is on the borderline between the low and normal ranges, free (bioavailable) testosterone should be measured.

Once identified as exhibiting hypogonadism, the patient should undergo additional evaluation to determine primary versus secondary causes. Measurement of serum LH and follicle-stimulating hormone (FSH) can help determine whether pituitary hormone secretion is adequate. If LH and FSH are low (consistent with secondary hypogonadism), further evaluation to identify the cause is warranted, perhaps with measurement of serum prolactin and iron saturation, pituitary function testing, and magnetic resonance imaging using a pituitary-imaging protocol (Bhasin et al. 2010). If LH and FSH are normal or elevated (consistent with primary hypogonadism), additional evaluation, including assessment for chromosomal abnormalities (e.g., Klinefelter syndrome, 46XX), is warranted. For patients with pathological fractures or severe androgen deficiency, bone mineral density assessment is recommended (Bhasin et al. 2010).

Treatment of Testosterone Deficiency

Treatment of testosterone deficiency involves replacement of testosterone (intramuscularly, transdermally, or with a topical gel) with a goal of improving overall cardiovascular risk. The topic raises some controversy because although replacement therapy is most consistently recommended for men at risk of cardiovascular disease (Morales et al. 2015), some authorities advocate treatment of testosterone deficiency with a goal of improving overall well-being, energy, mood, and vitality (Traish 2016). Response to testosterone therapy (as assessed by testosterone levels) should be evaluated at 3 and 6 months and then regularly (with low-quality evidence suggesting annual measurement of testosterone levels), and patients should be monitored for improvement in symptoms and anemia and also for the development of prostatic hyperplasia or other adverse effects of testosterone replacement (Morales et al. 2015).

Neuropsychiatric Presentations in Testosterone Deficiency

Patients with hypogonadism and "nonspecific" presentations may report symptoms reminiscent of MDD, with low energy, low libido, impaired concentration, depressed mood, irritability, and sleep disturbances (Morales et al. 2015). Impaired cognitive function also has been reported (Giagulli et al. 2016).

Treatment of Neuropsychiatric Symptoms in Testosterone Deficiency

The use of testosterone to treat nonspecific neuropsychiatric symptoms is controversial and is not part of the recommendations outlined in comprehensive, evidence-based guidelines (Bhasin et al. 2010; Morales et al. 2015). Some authors recommend using testosterone to treat low energy, irritability, and depressive-like symptoms that can accompany low testosterone and criticize studies demonstrating a link between testosterone treatment and adverse cardiovascular outcomes (Traish 2016). Current best evidence is insufficient to support the safety and effectiveness of testosterone in the treatment of neuropsychiatric symptoms, although there is some evidence that testosterone replacement therapy is associated with increased energy, higher libido, and enhanced QOL (Parker et al. 2016).

Hyperprolactinemia

Hyperprolactinemia is associated with short-term effects ranging from galactorrhea to sexual dysfunction, as well as longer-term effects including infertility, osteoporosis, and increased cardiovascular risk. Treatment of hyperprolactinemia can include use of dopamine agonists or surgical resection of a pituitary adenoma. Psychotropic medications, including first-generation antipsychotic medications and some second-generation antipsychotic medications, can cause hyperprolactinemia, although the diagnosis may be missed, leaving patients at increased risk for osteoporosis, cancer, and cardiovascular mortality.

Major Subtypes of Hyperprolactinemia

Hyperprolactinemia occurs physiologically during pregnancy and lactation. Pathological hyperprolactinemia can arise from disinhibition of pituitary prolactin release (e.g., through dopamine antagonist treatment or disruption of dopamine-releasing neurons from the arcuate nucleus to the anterior pituitary) or from prolactin-secreting pituitary adenomas.

Etiological, Pathophysiological, and Genetic Factors in Hyperprolactinemia

Prolactin is produced in the anterior pituitary and has a very wide range of physiological actions, which can be considered essential for female reproductive function (transfer of energy to the offspring, nurturing) and are less clearly essential for male function, although prolactin may be involved in parenting behavior (Grattan 2015). The hypothalamic-pituitary regulation of prolactin secretion is unique in that dopamine released from the arcuate nucleus, acting through dopamine type 2 (D_2) and type 4 (D_4) receptors found in the pituitary gland, inhibits lactotroph function and thereby prolactin secretion (Grattan 2015). Normally under tight inhibitory control, prolactin levels undergo physiological elevation during pregnancy and lactation. Hyperprolactinemia may also be caused in association with hypothalamic or pituitary disease, drugs or medications (e.g., antipsychotics, opioids, others), or other organ dysfunction. Excess prolactin (i.e., levels greater than 50 ng/mL) can be associated with short-term effects, including amenorrhea, galactorrhea, gynecomastia, and sexual dysfunction, as well as long-term effects, such as osteoporosis, cardiovascular disease, tumorigenesis, and prolactinoma (Montejo et al. 2017).

Clinical Presentations of Hyperprolactinemia

Clinical presentations of hyperprolactinemia vary. In cases of severe elevation, patients may develop gynecomastia or galactorrhea. Irregular or anovulatory menstrual cycles may prompt a woman to seek medical attention, and assessment including laboratory testing for prolactin may reveal elevated levels. Elevated prolactin levels are associated with weight gain, and many patients with hyperprolactinemia will have gained weight, although prolactin's role may be unrecognized in many patients with weight gain. Decreased libido may be present in men and women with elevated prolactin levels, although this symptom may go unrecognized. Hypogonadism (resulting in vaginal dryness in women and erectile dysfunction in men) is associated with hyperprolactinemia. In cases of pituitary adenoma, some women and many men may remain asymptomatic until compression of the optic chiasm results in visual disturbances (classically known as bitemporal hemianopia) or increased pressure results in headaches.

Diagnostic and Laboratory Findings in Hyperprolactinemia

Prolactin elevation (>50 ng/mL) is diagnostic of hyperprolactinemia and warrants monitoring for long-term effects (e.g., osteoporosis, cardiovascular risk). In women presenting for evaluation of infertility or irregular menses, measurement of serum prolactin should be undertaken. Galactorrhea in a nonlactating woman or gynecomastia or galactorrhea in a male patient should prompt measurement of serum prolactin. Patients taking first-generation antipsychotic medications, risperidone, or paliperidone may be asymptomatic, but up to 30% of patients on these medications may experience severe hyperprolactinemia (level >100 ng/mL) (Montejo et al. 2017).

Treatment of Hyperprolactinemia

Hyperprolactinemia can be treated with medications (dopamine agonists such as cabergoline or bromocriptine) or surgery. In a retrospective cohort study comparing surgical and pharmacological treatments for hyperprolactinemia, about 80% of patients experienced improvement in their symptoms regardless of primary treatment strategy (Andereggen et al. 2017).

Medications that inhibit dopamine D_2 or D_4 receptors (an action common to many of the first-generation and some of the second-generation antipsychotics) release the dopamine-associated inhibition of prolactin secretion and cause hyperprolactinemia.

Treatment of antipsychotic-associated hyperprolactinemia with dopamine agonists can be problematic and associated with psychosis. The recommended approach involves decreasing the dosage, switching to an antipsychotic less likely to contribute to hyperprolactinemia, adding aripiprazole, adding a dopamine agonist (if tolerated), or considering other treatment (Montejo et al. 2017).

Neuropsychiatric Presentations in Hyperprolactinemia

Patients with hyperprolactinemia resulting in hypogonadism may experience loss of libido, low energy, erectile dysfunction, or other sexual dysfunction. Many instances of hyperprolactinemia may be symptomatically silent or subsyndromal, and the importance of recognizing and attempting to intervene to mitigate long-term sequelae of hyperprolactinemia has been emphasized in recent publications (Montejo et al. 2017).

Treatment of Neuropsychiatric Symptoms in Hyperprolactinemia

Treatment of neuropsychiatric symptoms with estrogen or estrogen/progesterone compounds or with testosterone can mitigate long-term effects and symptomatic hypogonadism resulting from hyperprolactinemia.

Neuropsychiatric Symptoms Associated With Treatment for Hyperprolactinemia

When patients experience hyperprolactinemia as the result of antipsychotic treatment, the decision to add dopamine agonist medications (e.g., cabergoline, bromocriptine) can be difficult, given the high risk of psychosis with these agents. When possible, experts recommend decreasing the antipsychotic dosage, switching the patient to an antipsychotic less likely to cause hyperprolactinemia, or adding aripiprazole to the existing antipsychotic regimen.

Pheochromocytoma

Pheochromocytoma, a rare tumor of the adrenal gland, arises in the medulla or chromaffin cells and secretes catecholamines (Kakoki et al. 2015; Lam 2017; Pillai et al. 2016). Pheochromocytoma may be associated with a wide variety of presentations and may go undetected for years. Cardinal features of pheochromocytoma include hypertension, headache, palpitations, sweating, anxiety, tremor, and other manifestations of catecholamine excess, although some patients who have familial pheochromocytoma may have less severe manifestations (Manger 2009).

Major Subtypes of Pheochromocytoma

Pheochromocytoma may be characterized as medullary or extra-adrenal paraganglionic (Lam 2017). Formerly characterized as malignant, pheochromocytoma is newly classified as metastatic and can be simple or composite (Lam 2017).

Etiological, Pathophysiological, and Genetic Factors in Pheochromocytoma

Pheochromocytoma is rare, estimated to be present in about 0.1%–0.6% of clinic patients with hypertension (Kakoki et al. 2015; Lenders et al. 2014). A significant proportion of pheochromocytomas are genetically mediated, and more than 20 sporadic or hereditary susceptibility genes have been identified (Lam 2017). The genetic abnormalities most commonly associated with pheochromocytoma include mutations in the von Hippel–Lindau gene, the rearranged during transfection (RET) proto-oncogene, and the neurofibromatosis type 1 gene. Multiple endocrine neoplasia (MEN) syndromes II and III and neurofibromatosis type 1 are associated with pheochromocytoma (Lam 2017). Pheochromocytoma typically presents in the fourth or fifth decade of life (Lam 2017). When associated with MEN II or neurofibromatosis type 1, pheochromocytoma typically produces epinephrine (Lam 2017). Pheochromocytoma associated with von Hippel–Lindau syndrome typically produces normetanephrines and norepinephrine; metastatic tumors are more likely to release dopamine (Lam 2017).

Clinical Presentations of Pheochromocytoma

The first presentation of a pheochromocytoma may be a variant of a panic attack, although these tumors have a wide range of manifestations and may go unrecognized and undiagnosed (Manger 2009). Sustained hypertension, headaches, palpitations, tachycardia, and sweating may be the presenting signs, although pheochromocytoma multisystem crisis (a potentially fatal condition characterized by multiple organ system failure, severe autonomic instability, high fever, and encephalopathy) may be the presenting syndrome and requires immediate management (Kakoki et al. 2015). Takotsubo cardiomyopathy (also known as "broken heart syndrome" or stress-related cardiomyopathy) has been associated with pheochromocytoma and should be included in the differential diagnosis in idiopathic systolic heart failure (Agarwal et al. 2011).

Diagnostic and Laboratory Findings in Pheochromocytoma

In a patient suspected of having a pheochromocytoma, initial testing of free plasma metanephrines (with blood drawn in the supine position) or of urinary fractionated metanephrines is recommended. If levels are elevated, the search for an explanation should be conducted using imaging. CT of the chest, abdomen, and pelvis is recommended to identify a tumor. If a metastatic or recurrent tumor is detected or suspected, ^{123}I-metaiodobenzylguanidine (MIBG) scanning is recommended. For known metastatic disease, positron emission tomography (PET) imaging is preferred (Lenders et al. 2014). Because of the genetic component and heritability of pheochromocytoma, guidelines recommend shared decision making with patients regarding further testing, with pre- and posttest counseling (Lenders et al. 2014).

Treatment of Pheochromocytoma

Surgical resection of the pheochromocytoma is recommended. Guidelines recommend minimally invasive (laparoscopic) adrenalectomy when feasible, although for large (>6 cm) or invasive masses, open resection is preferred in order to ensure complete resection without rupture (Lenders et al. 2014). Presurgery preparation should include preoperative α-adrenergic blockade, a high-sodium diet, and fluid intake designed to reverse catecholamine-mediated volume contraction and to normalize blood pressure and heart rate (Lenders et al. 2014). Once treated surgically, patients should undergo annual measurement of plasma free and urinary metanephrines to monitor for recurrence (Lenders et al. 2014).

Neuropsychiatric Presentations in Pheochromocytoma

For more than half a century, case reports have linked pheochromocytoma with neuropsychiatric symptoms presumed to be related to the excess catecholamine secretion and associated panic, anxiety, sweating, palpitations, and restlessness (Medvei and Cattell 1988).

Treatment of Neuropsychiatric Symptoms in Pheochromocytoma

Full resection of pheochromocytoma will result in resolution of elevated catecholamines and ultimately will lead to improvement in the associated hyperadrenergic symptomatology (Lenders et al. 2014). It is important to avoid precipitating adverse reactions in patients with pheochromocytoma, however, and many medications used to treat psychiatric conditions have the potential to cause adverse reactions or to precipitate a crisis in patients with suspected pheochromocytoma (Lenders et al. 2014).

Significant Psychiatric Drug Interactions or Considerations in Pheochromocytoma

A number of psychotropic medications have been implicated in adverse reactions in patients with pheochromocytoma and thus should not be prescribed in this population. Dopamine antagonists such as metoclopramide, chlorpromazine, and prochlorperazine should be avoided. Pheochromocytoma crisis has been reported with the use of antidepressants—including tricyclic agents (amitriptyline, imipramine), SSRIs (paroxetine, fluoxetine), and monoamine oxidase inhibitors (tranylcypromine, moclobemide, phenelzine)—and with sympathomimetics (pseudoephedrine, methylphenidate, dexamphetamine, fenfluramine, phentermine) (Lenders et al. 2014). Opioids, corticosteroids, peptides such as adrenocorticotropic hormone (ACTH) and glucagon, neuromuscular blocking agents, and β-blockers all have been associated with pheochromocytoma crisis and should also be avoided (Lenders et al. 2014).

Acromegaly

Acromegaly, a rare condition, usually results from pituitary adenoma with associated growth hormone excess and elevated insulin-like growth factor 1 (IGF-1) levels (Lavrentaki et al. 2017; Pivonello et al. 2017). The result of growth hormone excess is disproportionate skeletal, tissue, and organ growth (Melmed 2009). The onset of clinical manifestations can be insidious, and patients may present with associated metabolic or cardiovascular complications before they demonstrate the typical clinical phenotype of acral enlargement and coarsened facial features (Lavrentaki et al. 2017). Acromegaly is associated with increased mortality related to cardiomyopathy; patients may also experience respiratory and metabolic complications, including disordered glucose metabolism (Pivonello et al. 2017). Although therapy is appropriately targeted at removing the source of growth hormone excess and improving survival and overall health, the importance of QOL among patients with acromegaly both before and after treatment is increasingly recognized (Crespo et al. 2017).

Etiological, Pathophysiological, and Genetic Factors in Acromegaly

Acromegaly usually is diagnosed in the fifth decade of life, with an estimated annual incidence of 0.2–1.1 per 100,000 population and prevalence of 2.8–13.7 cases per 100,000 population (Lavrentaki et al. 2017). The presence of excess growth hormone (and IGF-1) can cause hypertrophy of multiple organ systems and structures and can have downstream effects on the cardiovascular system, with resulting cardiac hypertrophy, hypercontractility, and eventual diastolic dysfunction (which can lead to systolic dysfunction). Arrhythmias and valvular disease also may occur. Associated endothelial dysfunction can result in increased insulin resistance and accelerated arteriosclerosis (Pivonello et al. 2017). Long-term growth hormone and IGF-1 overexposure can result in pathological effects on bones, joints, heart, skin, pancreas, lung, kidney, reproductive organs, thyroid, muscle, fat, and abdominal organs (Melmed 2009) and can lead to dysfunction in any or all of these structures.

Mechanical effects of craniofacial hypertrophy and organ overgrowth can contribute to respiratory impairment, including obstructive sleep apnea, daytime sleepiness, and impaired breathing (Pivonello et al. 2017).

Clinical Presentations of Acromegaly

The development of the phenotype associated with acromegaly may be insidious; patients may present with facial coarsening, headaches, macroglossia, increased sweating, arthralgia, thickened skin, fatigue, and carpal tunnel syndrome—all associated with tissue and organ enlargement (Lavrentaki et al. 2017).

Diagnostic and Laboratory Findings in Acromegaly

Because acromegaly is associated with tonically increased growth hormone levels with suppressed secretory bursts, a low random growth hormone level ($<0.04\ \mu g/L$) would rule out the diagnosis (Melmed 2009). Impaired glucose suppression of growth hormone level is characteristic of acromegaly and signals impaired pituitary response to normally suppressive stimuli (Melmed 2009).

Treatment of Acromegaly

Treatment of acromegaly is intended to block the excess production or action of growth hormone, which can be accomplished with medication (somatostatin receptor ligands, such as octreotide or lanreotide, or growth hormone receptor antagonists), pituitary surgery, or sometimes radiation therapy (Crespo et al. 2017; Pivonello et al. 2017). Surgery can be challenging from an anatomical perspective but is curative in about 70% of cases (Melmed 2009). Radiation therapy is administered over the course of 6 weeks and can result in reduction in growth hormone levels (Melmed 2009).

Neuropsychiatric Presentations in Acromegaly

Patients with acromegaly experience a changed overall appearance, with detrimental effects on body image. Changes in appearance can persist even after resolution of excess growth hormone, and patients may develop a negative self-concept and impaired QOL (Crespo et al. 2017). Psychopathology has been reported among patients with acromegaly, including anxiety, depression, "maladaptive personality traits," and impaired cognitive performance. The cognitive impairment is thought to be more closely related to depression and anxiety and not clearly linked to the biochemical changes associated with acromegaly itself (Crespo et al. 2015, 2017).

Treatment of Neuropsychiatric Symptoms in Acromegaly

Anxiety and depression, which can accompany acromegaly, should be identified and treated with usual measures, including psychotherapy and consideration of medications such as SSRIs (Crespo et al. 2015).

Neuropsychiatric Symptoms Associated With Treatments for Acromegaly

Surgical resection or pharmacological suppression of growth hormone secretion in acromegaly is not correlated with improved QOL, anxiety, depression, or cognitive outcomes (Crespo et al. 2015, 2017). Surgical resection carries a small but defined risk (5%) of hypopituitarism, which can be associated with any or all of the deficiency syndromes outlined elsewhere in this chapter (e.g., hypogonadism, adrenal insufficiency, PCOS, hypothyroidism) as well as with impaired empathy related to lack of oxytocin (Higham et al. 2016).

Cushing's Syndrome

Endogenous hypercortisolism, also known as Cushing's syndrome, can be the result of a pituitary or hypothalamic neoplasm producing ACTH or an adrenal neoplasm producing cortisol. In other cases, metabolic effects of illnesses (including alcohol use disorder, chronic kidney disease, diabetes mellitus, anorexia) or physiological states such as pregnancy may contribute to excess cortisol. Initially recognized almost a century ago by Dr. Harvey Cushing (Doyle et al. 2017), Cushing's syndrome is now known to be only one of many contributors to obesity, and it must be suspected in order to be detected. Effects of Cushing's syndrome include central obesity, arterial hypertension, proximal muscle weakness, diabetes mellitus, hirsutism, oligomenorrhea, thin skin, and ecchymoses. In the current era of high prevalence of obesity, the presence of thin skin, ecchymosis, and osteoporosis are suggestive of Cushing's syndrome and warrant further evaluation. Cushing's syndrome has been associated with depression, mania, and other neuropsychiatric symptoms. Excess cortisol has been associated with alcohol use disorder and other states of chronic stress, including anorexia nervosa. Treatment through removal of the source of excess cortisol can be effective in halting the metabolic effects and in many cases can improve psychiatric symptoms.

Major Subtypes of Cushing's Syndrome

Cushing's syndrome can be classified as "corticotropin (ACTH) dependent" (usually pituitary or ectopic tumors that secrete ACTH) or "corticotropin independent" (e.g., an adrenal neoplasm secreting cortisol independently of ACTH action). Pituitary tumors that secrete ACTH cause a form of Cushing's syndrome known as Cushing's disease. Some neoplasms are malignant (usually secreting more than one hormone), whereas others are classified as benign. In some cases, chronic medical illness such as diabetes mellitus, anorexia nervosa, chronic kidney disease, or alcohol use disorder can be associated with elevated cortisol. Some patients will present with elevated cortisol related to glucocorticoid resistance and will exhibit evidence of hypokalemia and hypertension without the usual features of Cushing's syndrome (Findling and Raff 2017).

Etiological, Pathophysiological, and Genetic Factors in Cushing's Syndrome

In cases in which cortisol excess is not directly related to glucocorticoid administration (e.g., for therapeutic purposes), the HPA axis is implicated in Cushing's syndrome. Hypothalamic or pituitary tumors can secrete corticotropin and result in increased adrenal production of cortisol; alternatively, ACTH-independent tumors in the adrenal gland can autonomously overproduce cortisol.

Clinical Presentations of Cushing's Syndrome

The physical manifestations of Cushing's syndrome may be difficult to distinguish from other forms of obesity or from the metabolic syndrome, but patients classically present with central obesity, fat accumulations on the face, hypertension, proximal muscle weakness, hyperglycemia or diabetes mellitus, oligomenorrhea, hirsutism, thin skin, purple striae, ecchymoses, and supraclavicular fat pads (Loriaux 2017).

Diagnostic and Laboratory Findings in Cushing's Syndrome

Given the high prevalence of obesity and the metabolic syndrome in the general population, experts recommend maintaining a high index of suspicion for Cushing's disease, particularly because a percentage of cases can be caused by malignant cortisol- or ACTH-producing neoplasms (Loriaux 2017). Osteoporosis, thin skin (<2 mm on the nondominant index finger), and ecchymosis (three or more ecchymoses ≥1 cm in diameter, nontraumatic in etiology) are each associated with Cushing's syndrome; the presence of all three in a patient with obesity is highly suggestive (Loriaux 2017).

Historically (and still listed in guidelines), the dexamethasone suppression test has been used by some experts for its ability to rule out (rather than rule in) illness.

Treatment of Cushing's Syndrome

Treatment of Cushing's syndrome is aimed at removing the source of excess cortisol. In many cases, surgical resection of tumors and metastases is curative. Before proceeding with surgery, it is important for the surgeon to ascertain that the adenoma or mass is, in fact, contributing to hypercortisolism, because in one series, up to 40% of pituitary masses in patients with Cushing's disease turned out to be unrelated to the cortisol excess (Barker et al. 2003, cited by Loriaux 2017).

Neuropsychiatric Presentations in Cushing's Syndrome

Early characterizations of Cushing's syndrome described a relatively high incidence of psychosis and suicidality, with some evidence of manic behavior early on giving way to irritability, impaired concentration, and depressive symptomatology later in the course of the syndrome (Jeffcoate et al. 1979; Levenson 2006). The most common psychiatric presentations are irritability, emotional lability, depression, and anxiety. Hypomanic symptoms can be seen as well.

Treatment of Neuropsychiatric Symptoms in Cushing's Syndrome

Historically, normalization of cortisol levels in patients with Cushing's syndrome has been associated with improvement in severe depression and resolution of a significant proportion of mild to moderate depressive episodes associated with cortisol excess (Jeffcoate et al. 1979).

Primary Aldosteronism

Initially described in 1955 by the American endocrinologist Jerome Conn and therefore sometimes called Conn's syndrome, primary aldosteronism is recognized as an increasingly prevalent contributor to malignant and refractory hypertension (Gyamlani et al. 2016). Elevated aldosterone levels contribute to hypertension, hypokalemia, and increased cardiovascular risk. Historically, some authors reported an association between primary aldosteronism and depression or anxiety (Künzel 2012); fibrosis and inflammation are present in the syndrome. Treatment depends on the underlying cause; when a causative adrenal adenoma is identified, surgery can be curative (Gyamlani et al. 2016).

Major Subtypes of Primary Aldosteronism

Primary aldosteronism can result from aldosterone-producing adenomas, idiopathic hypertrophy of the adrenal cortical zona glomerulosa (where aldosterone is produced), unilateral adrenal hyperplasia, primary adrenal hyperplasia, familial ACTH-dependent activation of aldosterone synthase, and (in rare cases) carcinomas of the adrenal cortex or ectopic aldosterone-secreting tumors (Gyamlani et al. 2016).

Etiological, Pathophysiological, and Genetic Factors in Primary Aldosteronism

Primary aldosteronism may go unrecognized, and its etiology and genetic factors are still being elucidated (Gyamlani et al. 2016). A family history of hypertension—and, in particular, of refractory hypertension—should prompt an additional workup to identify possible primary hyperaldosteronism.

Clinical Presentations of Primary Aldosteronism

Primary aldosteronism is most commonly seen in patients 40–50 years of age and is a cause of refractory hypertension. The presence of inappropriately high levels of aldosterone can cause cardiovascular damage, sodium retention, potassium excretion, and end-organ damage, with fibrosis and inflammation of the myocardium (Gyamlani et al. 2016). Hypokalemia, sleep apnea, or a family history of early-onset hypertension or cardiovascular disease can be associated with primary aldosteronism. A causal relationship between hyperaldosteronism and neuropsychiatric symptoms such as depression and anxiety has not been established (Künzel 2012).

Diagnostic and Laboratory Findings in Primary Aldosteronism

Primary aldosteronism should be suspected in a patient with 3 separate days' blood pressure readings above 150/100 mmHg, hypertension resistant to treatment with three medications (including a diuretic), or the combination of hypertension plus hyperkalemia, adrenal incidentaloma, sleep apnea, or a family history of early-onset hypertension or heart disease (Gyamlani et al. 2016). Once suspected, the diagnosis can be supported with the measurement of plasma aldosterone concentration and plasma renin activity, with the subsequent production of a ratio. Optimally, the measurements would be undertaken with the patient off antihypertensive medications for 2 weeks; however, in the setting of uncontrolled hypertension, it usually is possible only to discontinue potassium-sparing diuretics and spironolactone and make sure potassium has been repleted. The presence of an elevated aldosterone level and elevated aldosterone-renin ratio is suggestive of primary hyperaldosteronism. The results then can be confirmed with an oral sodium load, saline infusion, fludrocortisone suppression test, or captopril challenge. Once the diagnosis is confirmed, imaging can be undertaken to localize an aldosterone-secreting tumor; selective adrenal vein sampling can be employed to determine whether the tumor is contributing to the syndrome and whether resection would be of benefit.

Treatment of Primary Aldosteronism

The goal of treatment for primary hyperaldosteronism is to normalize blood pressure, normalize potassium levels, and reverse the damage to the cardiovascular system. If the source of the elevated aldosterone can be identified and removed (surgically), associated symptoms and damage can resolve.

Neuropsychiatric Presentations in Primary Aldosteronism

Although a connection between aldosteronism and depression or anxiety was previously suspected, current data do not support an association between primary aldosteronism and psychiatric symptoms (Künzel 2012). Patients with untreated refractory hypertension are at risk for small-vessel ischemic changes, white matter changes, and lacunar infarcts, which in turn are associated with an increased risk for cognitive impairment (Rincon and Wright 2014). Over time, mild cognitive impairment or vascular dementia may manifest as stepwise decline with or without focal neurological signs.

Treatment of Neuropsychiatric Symptoms in Primary Aldosteronism

If present, depression and anxiety can be treated nonpharmacologically with CBT or pharmacologically with medications. It is best to avoid medications with the potential to increase blood pressure, such as serotonin-norepinephrine reuptake inhibitors. Medications to reduce blood pressure and strategies to optimize cognitive function may be employed.

Adrenal Insufficiency

Adrenal insufficiency is the insufficient production of cortisol. Symptoms of adrenal insufficiency include weight loss, weakness, fatigue, abdominal pain, depression, and anxiety. Symptoms can be sufficiently nonspecific to delay recognition and diagnosis until patients encounter adrenal crises, requiring urgent administration of corticosteroids (Bornstein et al. 2016).

Major Subtypes of Adrenal Insufficiency

Primary adrenal insufficiency (Addison's disease) results from the inability of the adrenal glands to secrete sufficient amounts of cortisol; it can be caused by autoimmune disease, infection (e.g., tuberculosis), adrenalectomy (e.g., Cushing's syndrome), neoplasia, or (more commonly in children) genetic abnormalities such as congenital adrenal hypoplasia (Bornstein et al. 2016). Secondary adrenal insufficiency results from the failure of the pituitary gland to secrete adequate amounts of corticotropin (ACTH) by the pituitary. A common contributor to adrenal insufficiency is the rapid withdrawal of corticosteroid medications.

Etiological, Pathophysiological, and Genetic Factors in Adrenal Insufficiency

Infections, infiltration (such as by amyloid), surgical removal, or drug-induced suppression of the adrenal glands can contribute to adrenal insufficiency. Primary adrenal insufficiency results in enhanced production of ACTH through activation of the proopiomelanocortin (POMC) gene, which can result in hyperpigmentation in palmar creases and other areas.

Clinical Presentations of Adrenal Insufficiency

The presentation of primary adrenal insufficiency can be nonspecific. Patients may present with weight loss, orthostatic changes, dehydration, and anemia. They may report low libido, low energy, and depressive symptoms. Patients with primary adrenal insufficiency can show hyperpigmentation secondary to the hypersecretion of ACTH. Nonspecific malaise or weakness is common, as is abdominal pain. In the absence of high clinical suspicion, the diagnosis of adrenal insufficiency may be missed in favor of MDD or anxiety disorder. Some patients may have an isolated glucocorticoid deficiency without significant hypotension. Adrenal insufficiency can manifest as a life-threatening adrenal crisis, including shock, fever, and confusion. Adrenal crisis is usually precipitated by some additional medical stress, such as illness, trauma, or surgery.

Diagnostic and Laboratory Findings in Adrenal Insufficiency

Once the diagnosis is suspected (based on orthostatic hypotension, listlessness, abdominal pain, and/or nausea), the morning cortisol level should be checked; if it is less than 5 μg/dL in the setting of an ACTH level that is at or above twice the upper limit of normal, the diagnosis is made.

Treatment of Adrenal Insufficiency

The goal of treatment in adrenal insufficiency is to normalize corticosteroid activity to maintain bodily functions; this goal is accomplished through exogenous administration of glucocorticoids. Guidelines recommend hydrocortisone (15–25 mg) or cortisone (20–35 mg) divided into two or three doses per day as the preferred approach; for patients who have a hard time taking multiple doses per day, prednisolone (3–5 mg) may be given in a single dose or divided into two doses each day. For a variety of reasons, dexamethasone is the least preferred glucocorticoid (Bornstein et al. 2016). If patients also exhibit evidence of aldosterone deficiency, fludrocortisone 50–100 μg daily is advised (decreasing the dosage if hypertension develops). When patients with primary adrenal insufficiency undergo physiological stress, they are prone to developing "adrenal crisis" and require administration of high-dose bolus corticosteroids (hydrocortisone 100 mg, followed by 200 mg/24 hours until the stressor is resolved). Pregnant women with primary adrenal insufficiency should be placed on high-dosage corticosteroids during labor and delivery in order to avoid adrenal crisis.

Neuropsychiatric Presentations in Adrenal Insufficiency

The presentation of adrenal insufficiency can closely mimic the neurovegetative symptoms of MDD, and patients may be diagnosed as depressed when, in fact, they instead or additionally have adrenal insufficiency. Anergia, malaise, low energy, and weight loss are common presentations.

Treatment of Neuropsychiatric Symptoms in Adrenal Insufficiency

Once glucocorticoids and mineralocorticoids are supplemented, women who continue to report low libido and depressive symptoms can be given a trial course of dehydro-epiandrosterone (DHEA) for 6 months to see whether symptoms improve. If patients have not improved by the end of 6 months, discontinuation of DHEA is recommended (Bornstein et al. 2016).

Neuropsychiatric Symptoms Associated With Corticosteroid Treatment for Adrenal Insufficiency

Exogenous corticosteroids can cause a wide range of neuropsychiatric symptoms, including depression and mania. In a review and meta-analysis of 13 uncontrolled studies (N=2,555) evaluating the efficacy of corticosteroids in various medical illnesses, severe psychiatric side effects—defined as those that were serious enough to require psychiatric treatment—were found in 5.7% of patients (Lewis and Smith 1983), with euphoria and hypomania being the most common early symptoms and depression developing with longer treatment (Warrington and Bostwick 2006). Psychiatric side effects tended to occur early in treatment (most often developing within 5 days of corticosteroid initiation [Ciriaco et al. 2013]), with higher corticosteroid dosage being the strongest risk factor for symptom development (Warrington and Bostwick 2006).

Conclusion

The HPA axis contributes to behavioral and mental wellness. Neuropsychiatric manifestations of endocrine disorders and neurovegetative manifestations of certain psychiatric disorders can be difficult to distinguish from each other. Some neuroendocrine disorders have an insidious onset. Although certain neuroendocrine disorders can be treated with medications, some of the disorders that initially manifest with vague and seemingly psychiatric symptomatology may be best treated with surgery. In order to detect treatable endocrine disorders and to improve patients' functioning and quality of life, it is important that clinicians maintain a high index of suspicion for disorders of the pancreas, thyroid, adrenal glands, gonads, and/or pituitary.

References

Agarwal V, Kant G, Hans N, et al: Takotsubo-like cardiomyopathy in pheochromocytoma. Int J Cardiol 153(3):241–248, 2011 21474192

American Diabetes Association, American Psychiatric Association, American Association of Clinical Endocrinologists, et al: Consensus development conference on antipsychotic drugs and obesity and diabetes. Diabetes Care 27(2):596–601, 2004 14747245

Andereggen L, Frey J, Andres RH, et al: 10-year follow-up study comparing primary medical vs. surgical therapy in women with prolactinomas. Endocrine 55(1):223–230, 2017 27688009

Andrade VH, Mata AM, Borges RS, et al: Current aspects of polycystic ovary syndrome: a literature review. Rev Assoc Med Bras (1992) 62(9):867–871, 2016 28001262

Barbesino G: Drugs affecting thyroid function. Thyroid 20(7):763–770, 2010 20578900

Barker FG 2nd, Klibanski A, Swearingen B: Transsphenoidal surgery for pituitary tumors in the United States, 1996–2000: mortality, morbidity, and the effects of hospital and surgeon volume. J Clin Endocrinol Metab 88(10):4709–4719, 2003 14557445

Bathla M, Singh M, Relan P: Prevalence of anxiety and depressive symptoms among patients with hypothyroidism. Indian J Endocrinol Metab 20(4):468–474, 2016 27366712

Bauer M, Goetz T, Glenn T, et al: The thyroid-brain interaction in thyroid disorders and mood disorders. J Neuroendocrinol 20(10):1101–1114, 2008 18673409

Berkseth KE, Thirumalai A, Amory JK: Pharmacologic therapy in men's health: hypogonadism, erectile dysfunction, and benign prostatic hyperplasia. Med Clin North Am 100(4):791–805, 2016 27235615

Bhasin S, Cunningham GR, Hayes FJ, et al: Testosterone therapy in men with androgen deficiency syndromes: an Endocrine Society clinical practice guideline. J Clin Endocrinol Metab 95(6):2536–2559, 2010 20525905

Blay SL, Aguiar JV, Passos IC: Polycystic ovary syndrome and mental disorders: a systematic review and exploratory meta-analysis. Neuropsychiatr Dis Treat 12:2895–2903, 2016 27877043

Bornstein SR, Allolio B, Arlt W, et al: Diagnosis and treatment of primary adrenal insufficiency: an Endocrine Society clinical practice guidelines. J Clin Endocrinol Metab 101(2):364–389, 2016 26760044

Boyle J, Teede HJ: Polycystic ovary syndrome: an update. Aust Fam Physician 41(10):752–756, 2012 23210095

Brownlie BEW, Rae AM, Walshe JWB, et al: Psychoses associated with thyrotoxicosis—"thyrotoxic psychosis." A report of 18 cases, with statistical analysis of incidence. Eur J Endocrinol 142(5):438–444, 2000 10802519

Chan JL, Kar S, Vanky E, et al: Racial and ethnic differences in the prevalence of metabolic syndrome and its components of metabolic syndrome in women with polycystic ovary syndrome: a regional cross-sectional study. Am J Obstet Gynecol 217(2):189.e1–189.e8, 2017 28400308

Christou MA, Christou PA, Markozannes G, et al: Effects of anabolic androgenic steroids on the reproductive system of athletes and recreational users: a systematic review and meta-analysis. Sports Med 47(9):1869–1883, 2017 28258581

Ciriaco M, Ventrice P, Russo G, et al: Corticosteroid-related central nervous system side effects. J Pharmacol Pharmacother 4 (suppl 1):S94–S98, 2013 24347992

Crespo I, Santos A, Valassi E, et al: Impaired decision making and delayed memory are related with anxiety and depressive symptoms in acromegaly. Endocrine 50(3):756–763, 2015 26018738

Crespo I, Valassi E, Webb SM: Update on quality of life in patients with acromegaly. Pituitary 20(1):185–188, 2017 27730455

Delitala AP, Terracciano A, Fiorillo E, et al: Depressive symptoms, thyroid hormone and autoimmunity in a population-based cohort from Sardinia. J Affect Disord 191:82–87, 2016 26655116

Doyle NM, Doyle JF, Walter EJ: The life and work of Harvey Cushing 1869–1939: a pioneer of neurosurgery. J Intensive Care Soc 18(2):157–158, 2017 28979564

Ducat L, Rubenstein A, Philipson LH, et al: A review of the mental health issues of diabetes conference. Diabetes Care 38(2):333–338, 2015 25614689

Feldman AZ, Shrestha RT, Hennessey JV: Neuropsychiatric manifestations of thyroid disease. Endocrinol Metab Clin North Am 42(3):453–476, 2013 24011880

Findling JW, Raff H: Diagnosis of endocrine disease: differentiation of pathologic/neoplastic hypercortisolism (Cushing's syndrome) from physiologic/non-neoplastic hypercortisolism (formerly known as pseudo-Cushing's syndrome). Eur J Endocrinol 176(5):R205–R216, 2017 28179447

Giagulli VA, Guastamacchia E, Licchelli B, et al: Serum testosterone and cognitive function in ageing male: updating the evidence. Recent Pat Endocr Metab Immune Drug Discov 10(1):22–30, 2016 27981914

Gorman LS, Chiasera JM: Endocrinology review—adrenal and thyroid disorders. Clin Lab Sci 26(2):107–111, 2013 23772478

Grant P, Velusamy A: What is the best way of assessing neurocognitive dysfunction in patients with primary hyperparathyroidism? J Clin Endocrinol Metab 99(1):49–55, 2014 24203059

Grattan DR: 60 years of neuroendocrinology: the hypothalamo-prolactin axis. J Endocrinol 226(2):T101–T122, 2015 26101377

Gyamlani G, Headley CM, Naseer A, et al: Primary aldosteronism: diagnosis and management. Am J Med Sci 352(4):391–398, 2016 27776721

Higham CE, Johannsson G, Shalet SM: Hypopituitarism. Lancet 388(10058):2403–2415, 2016 27041067

Holt RIG, Mitchell AJ: Diabetes mellitus and severe mental illness: mechanisms and clinical implications. Nat Rev Endocrinol 11(2):79–89, 2015 25445848

Jeffcoate WJ, Silverstone JT, Edwards CR, et al: Psychiatric manifestations of Cushing's syndrome: response to lowering of plasma cortisol. Q J Med 48(191):465–472, 1979 542586

Johnson TRB, Ouyang P, Kaplan LK, et al: National Institutes of Health Evidence-Based Methodology Workshop on Polycystic Ovary Syndrome, December 3–5, 2012: Executive Summary. Bethesda, MD, National Institutes of Health, 2012

Kakoki K, Miyata Y, Shida Y, et al: Pheochromocytoma multisystem crisis treated with emergency surgery: a case report and literature review. BMC Res Notes 8:758, 2015 26645353

Katon WJ: Clinical and health services relationships between major depression, depressive symptoms, and general medical illness. Biol Psychiatry 54(3):216–226, 2003 12893098

Katon WJ: The comorbidity of diabetes mellitus and depression. Am J Med 121 (11 suppl 2):S8–S15, 2008 18954592

Katsarou A, Gudbjörnsdottir S, Rawshani A, et al: Type 1 diabetes mellitus. Nat Rev Dis Primers 3:17016, 2017 28358037

Künzel HE: Psychopathological symptoms in patients with primary hyperaldosteronism—possible pathways. Horm Metab Res 44(3):202–207, 2012 22351473

Lahey FH: Apathetic thyroidism. Ann Surg 93(5):1026–1030, 1931 17866558

Lam AK: Update on adrenal tumours in 2017 World Health Organization (WHO) of endocrine tumours. Endocr Pathol 28(3):213–227, 2017 28477311

Lavrentaki A, Paluzzi A, Wass JA, et al: Epidemiology of acromegaly: review of population studies. Pituitary 20(1):4–9, 2017 27743174

LeFevre ML, U.S. Preventive Services Task Force: Screening for thyroid dysfunction: U.S. Preventive Services Task Force recommendation statement. Ann Intern Med 162(9):641–650, 2015 25798805

Lenders JW, Duh QY, Eisenhofer G, et al: Pheochromocytoma and paraganglioma: an endocrine society clinical practice guideline. J Clin Endocrinol Metab 99(6):1915–1942, 2014 24893135

Levenson JL: Psychiatric issues in endocrinology. Primary Psychiatry 13(4):27–30, 2006. Available at: http://primarypsychiatry.com/psychiatric-issues-in-endocrinology. Accessed March 27, 2019.

Lewis DA, Smith RE: Steroid-induced psychiatric syndromes. A report of 14 cases and a review of the literature. J Affect Disord 5(4):319–332, 1983 6319464

Li C, Xu D, Hu M, et al: A systematic review and meta-analysis of randomized controlled trials of cognitive behavior therapy for patients with diabetes and depression. J Psychosom Res 95:44–54, 2017 28314548

Loriaux DL: Diagnosis and differential diagnosis of Cushing's syndrome. N Engl J Med 376(15):1451–1459, 2017 28402781

Manger WM: The protean manifestations of pheochromocytoma. Horm Metab Res 41(9):658–663, 2009 19242899

Martyn-Nemeth P, Schwarz Farabi S, Mihailescu D, et al: Fear of hypoglycemia in adults with type 1 diabetes: impact of therapeutic advances and strategies for prevention—a review. J Diabetes Complications 30(1):167–177, 2016 26439754

McBride JA, Carson CC 3rd, Coward RM: Testosterone deficiency in the aging male. Ther Adv Urol 8(1):47–60, 2016 26834840

McDermott MT, Burman KD, Hofeldt FD, et al: Lithium-associated thyrotoxicosis. Am J Med 80(6):1245–1248, 1986 3755288

Medvei VC, Cattell WR: Mental symptoms presenting in phaeochromocytoma: a case report and review. J R Soc Med 81(9):550–551, 1988 3054110

Melmed S: Acromegaly pathogenesis and treatment. J Clin Invest 119(11):3189–3202, 2009 19884662

Millar AC, Lau AN, Tomlinson G, et al: Predicting low testosterone in aging men: a systematic review. CMAJ 188(13):E321–E330, 2016 27325129

Mitchell AJ, Hardy SA: Screening for metabolic risk among patients with severe mental illness and diabetes: a national comparison. Psychiatr Serv 64(10):1060–1063, 2013 24081407

Montejo AL, Arango C, Bernardo M, et al: Multidisciplinary consensus on the therapeutic recommendations for iatrogenic hyperprolactinemia secondary to antipsychotics. Front Neuroendocrinol 45:25–34, 2017 28235557

Montenegro FLM, Brescia MDG, Lourenço DM Jr, et al: Could the less-than subtotal parathyroidectomy be an option for treating young patients with multiple endocrine neoplasia type 1–related hyperparathyroidism? Front Endocrinol (Lausanne) 10:123, 2019 30899245

Morales A, Bebb RA, Manjoo P, et al: Diagnosis and management of testosterone deficiency syndrome in men: clinical practice guideline. CMAJ 187(18):1369–1377, 2015 26504097

Owens DR, Monnier L, Barnett AH: Future challenges and therapeutic opportunities in type 2 diabetes: changing the paradigm of current therapy. Diabetes Obes Metab 19(10):1339–1352, 2017 28432748

Park M, Katon WJ, Wolf FM: Depression and risk of mortality in individuals with diabetes: a meta-analysis and systematic review. Gen Hosp Psychiatry 35(3):217–225, 2013 23415577

Parker A, Bruha M, Akinola O, et al: A summary of the controversy surrounding off-label medications in men's health. Transl Androl Urol 5(2):201–206, 2016 27141447

Pillai S, Gopalan V, Smith RA, et al: Updates on the genetics and the clinical impacts on phaeochromocytoma and paraganglioma in the new era. Crit Rev Oncol Hematol 100:190–208, 2016 26839173

Pivonello R, Auriemma RS, Grasso LFS, et al: Complications of acromegaly: cardiovascular, respiratory and metabolic comorbidities. Pituitary 20(1):46–62, 2017 28224405

Rincon F, Wright CB: Current pathophysiological concepts in cerebral small vessel disease. Front Aging Neurosci 6:24, 2014 24715862

Ritchie M, Yeap BB: Thyroid hormone: influences on mood and cognition in adults. Maturitas 81(2):266–275, 2015 25896972

Roman SA, Sosa JA, Pietrzak RH, et al: The effects of serum calcium and parathyroid hormone changes on psychological and cognitive function in patients undergoing parathyroidectomy for primary hyperparathyroidism. Ann Surg 253(1):131–137, 2011 21233611

Rosa RG, Barros AJS, de Lima ARB, et al: Mood disorder as a manifestation of primary hypoparathyroidism: a case report. J Med Case Reports 8:326, 2014 25280468

Rotterdam ESHRE/ASRM-Sponsored PCOS Consensus Workshop Group: Revised 2003 consensus on diagnostic criteria and long-term health risks related to polycystic ovary syndrome (PCOS). Hum Reprod 19(1):41–47, 2004 14711538

Rugge JB, Bougatsos C, Chou R: Screening for and Treatment of Thyroid Dysfunction: An Evidence Review for the U.S. Preventive Services Task Force. Evidence Synthesis, No. 118. Rockville, MD, Agency for Healthcare Research and Quality, 2014

Samuels MH: Thyroid disease and cognition. Endocrinol Metab Clin North Am 43(2):529–543, 2014 24891176

Scaruffi E, Gambineri A, Cattaneo S, et al: Personality and psychiatric disorders in women affected by polycystic ovary syndrome. Front Endocrinol (Lausanne) 5:185, 2014 25429283

Siegmann EM, Müller HHO, Luecke C, et al: Association of depression and anxiety disorders with autoimmune thyroiditis: a systematic review and meta-analysis. JAMA Psychiatry 75(6):577–584, 2018 29800939

Smith KJ, Béland M, Clyde M, et al: Association of diabetes with anxiety: a systematic review and meta-analysis. J Psychosom Res 74(2):89–99, 2013 23332522

Tabák AG, Akbaraly TN, Batty GD, et al: Depression and type 2 diabetes: a causal association? Lancet Diabetes Endocrinol 2(3):236–245, 2014 24622754

Traish AM: Testosterone therapy in men with testosterone deficiency: are the benefits and cardiovascular risks real or imagined? Am J Physiol Regul Integr Comp Physiol 311(3):R566–R573, 2016 27488887

Tsikouras P, Spyros L, Manav B, et al: Features of polycystic ovary syndrome in adolescence. J Med Life 8(3):291–296, 2015 26351529

Tsvetov G, Hirsch D, Shimon I, et al: Thiazide treatment in primary hyperparathyroidism: a new indication for an old medication? J Clin Endocrinol Metab 102(4):1270–1276, 2017 28388724

Wang R, Mol BW: The Rotterdam criteria for polycystic ovary syndrome: evidence-based criteria? Hum Reprod 32(2):261–264, 2017 28119448

Wang R, Kim BV, van Wely M, et al: Treatment strategies for women with WHO group II anovulation: systematic review and network meta-analysis. BMJ 356:j138, 2017 28143834

Warrington TP, Bostwick JM: Psychiatric adverse effects of corticosteroids. Mayo Clin Proc 81(10):1361–1367, 2006 17036562

Wilhelm SM, Wang TS, Ruan DT, et al: The American Association of Endocrine Surgeons Guidelines for Definitive Management of Primary Hyperparathyroidism. JAMA Surg 151(10):959–968, 2016 27532368

Wu W, Sun Z, Yu J, et al: A clinical retrospective analysis of factors associated with apathetic hyperthyroidism. Pathobiology 77(1):46–51, 2010 20185967

Zaccardi F, Webb DR, Yates T, et al: Pathophysiology of type 1 and type 2 diabetes mellitus: a 90-year perspective. Postgrad Med J 92(1084):63–69, 2016 26621825

Zanocco K, Butt Z, Kaltman D, et al: Improvement in patient-reported physical and mental health after parathyroidectomy for primary hyperparathyroidism. Surgery 158(3):837–845, 2015 26032828

CHAPTER 8

Inflammatory Diseases and Their Psychiatric Manifestations

Rolando L. Gonzalez, M.D.

Charles B. Nemeroff, M.D., Ph.D.

Inflammation and the Immune System

The immune system plays a vital role in the maintenance of homeostasis. Through the adaptive and innate immune system, this balance has evolved to protect the body from internal and external insults, such as infections and toxins for the former and cancer development for the latter (Beurel 2015). The immune system in all its complexity provides stable equilibrium via recognition, regulation, and memory. The innate immune system, also referred to as native immunity, contains germline-encoded receptors that recognize and eliminate various pathogens and is often considered the first line of defense against infections. The principal components of the innate immune system are neutrophils, dendritic cells, natural killer cells, mast cells, cytokines, and macrophages, which play specific and overlapping roles. Infection and tissue injury are typically managed by the process of inflammation. Inflammation is characterized by the amassing of leukocytes (neutrophils) and plasma proteins in the circulation at the site of inflammation or infection. During this process, the induction of cytokines occurs. Cytokines are small molecules derived from various cells in the innate and adaptive immune system. Proinflammatory cytokines such as interleukin (IL)-6, IL-1, and tumor necrosis factor-α (TNF-α) further propagate the acute and systemic inflammatory response through enlistment of additional leukocytes, acute-phase proteins including C-reactive protein (CRP), and induction of fever through production of prostaglandin E2 and cyclooxygenase-2 (COX-2) (Abbas et al. 2015; Beurel 2015). The microglia (macrophages of the central nervous system [CNS]) play a central role in mediating proinflammatory cytokines in the CNS, accounting for nearly 20% of the CNS glial population. They also exert significant influence on neurodevelopment. The microglia and proinflammatory cytokines have been implicated in potential neurotoxic effects and can inhibit neurogenesis in states of excessive and chronic inflammation (Müller et al. 2015).

The adaptive immune system is often considered an evolutionary advance in the immune system due to the additional capacity of increased intensity and rapidity of immunological response to the subsequent interaction with a specific antigen. The adaptive immune system constitutes a more specialized mechanism of defense through the proliferation and specialization of lymphocytes into either B-lymphocytes or T-lymphocytes. Through the production of antibodies, B-lymphocytes direct the humoral immune response. Cell-mediated immunity is directed by T-lymphocytes through the production of cytokines, often initially IL-2, which by direction of helper T cells assists in further proliferation of lymphocytes (Abbas et al. 2015).

Unfortunately, when a breakdown in the innate and adaptive immune systems occurs, allergies and chronic inflammatory and autoimmune diseases may develop. *Autoimmunity* is the process of self-directed immune response present in healthy individuals with the development of autoimmune disease through failed regulation of self-reactivity and associated tissue damage (Abbas et al. 2015; Lawson et al. 1992).

Inflammation and Psychiatric Disorders

Increased inflammation has been linked to a variety of psychiatric disorders, including depression, schizophrenia, and bipolar disorder. Depression is frequently comorbid with diseases associated with pathological inflammatory mechanisms. Depressive illness occurs in 31%–45% of patients with coronary artery disease, 9%–26% of patients with diabetes, and 25% of patients with cancer (Anderson et al. 2001; Evans et al. 2005; Huffman et al. 2013; Raison and Miller 2003). Prior autoimmune disease has been shown to increase the risk for future mood disorder by 45% (Benros et al. 2013). Increased concentrations of inflammatory cytokines, chemokines, and other inflammatory markers have been repeatedly demonstrated in the peripheral blood and cerebrospinal fluid (CSF) of patients with depression when compared with control subjects (Miller et al. 2009). For example, in a meta-analysis, Dowlati et al. (2010) reported significantly higher levels of the proinflammatory cytokines TNF-α and IL-6 in depressed patients compared with healthy control subjects. These peripheral inflammatory cytokines have been shown to induce "sickness behavior" that is similar to the somatic and depressive symptoms characteristic of major depressive disorder (MDD) (Haroon et al. 2012).

Interferon-α, an immunomodulator that produces a robust inflammatory response that is used to treat hepatitis C and malignant melanoma, routinely induces depressive symptoms (Musselman et al. 2001; Raison et al. 2005). In contrast, the COX-2 inhibitor celecoxib, an anti-inflammatory agent, has been used as an adjunctive treatment with antidepressants for patients with depressive disorders (Köhler et al. 2014). A recent meta-analysis (Kappelmann et al. 2018) highlighted the evidence that the cytokine modulators adalimumab, etanercept, and infliximab can reduce depressive symptoms. One of the studies analyzed examined patients with treatment-resistant depression who were randomly assigned to receive either the monoclonal antibody infliximab or placebo; the TNF-α antagonist reduced depressive symptoms in patients with increased inflammation as delineated by CRP concentrations of 5 mg/L or higher (Raison et al. 2013). Depressed patients with elevated inflammatory markers are less likely to respond to standard antidepressant treatment (Yoshimura et al. 2009). Moreover, another meta-analysis (Strawbridge et al. 2015) found significant reductions of TNF α blood levels in patients whose depression responded to an antidepressant compared with those whose illness was treatment refractory. In a recent longitudinal study, depressed elderly patients with elevated CRP levels (>3 mg/L) had more persistent depressive symptoms over a longer period and a higher level of medical comorbidity (Gallagher et al. 2017).

Although most attention has been paid to the relationship between depression and inflammation, evidence of increased inflammation in other psychiatric disorders—including schizophrenia, bipolar disorder, and posttraumatic stress disorder (PTSD)—is mounting. The risk of developing schizophrenia and schizophrenia-related disorders is increased in individuals who have a history of both autoimmune disorders and severe infections (Benros et al. 2011).

In a meta-analysis (Miller et al. 2011), certain inflammatory cytokines were found to be altered in patients with schizophrenia even after treatment. Similarly, another meta-analysis (Modabbernia et al. 2013) found significant elevations in levels of both anti-inflammatory and proinflammatory biomarkers, including TNF-α, in bipolar manic, depressed, and euthymic states. Treatment of bipolar disorder with valproic acid or lithium has been shown to exert anti-inflammatory effects, such as reduction of IL-6 and TNF-α, with lithium providing an additional increase in the anti-inflammatory cytokine IL-10 (Leu et al. 2017).

Proposed pathophysiological relationships between inflammation and psychiatric disorders include stress-induced cytokine activation of the hypothalamic-pituitary-adrenal (HPA) axis as well as selective cytokine stimulation of indoleamine 2,3-dioxygenase (IDO). IDO stimulation can cause a depletion of tryptophan, a necessary precursor for serotonin, the neurotransmitter system most implicated in depression. Another aspect of this pathway is the increased production of kynurenine metabolites that can stimulate the *N*-methyl-D-aspartate receptor (NMDAR), which has been associated with glutamate alterations associated with psychosis in schizophrenia and anti-NMDAR encephalitis (Capuron and Castanon 2017).

With the plethora of studies indicating significant comorbidity and associations between psychiatric disorders and inflammatory disease, it comes as no surprise that there is substantial symptom overlap between certain psychiatric disorders and diseases of inflammation, which has often led to management difficulties. The goal of this chapter is to highlight the psychiatric manifestations of some of the more prevalent and severe inflammatory diseases: systemic lupus erythematosus (SLE), rheumatoid arthritis (RA), Sjogren's disease, scleroderma, Hashimoto's thyroiditis, Addison's disease, sarcoidosis, and anti-NMDAR encephalitis. A knowledge of these major illnesses will help the clinician to distinguish symptom causes more readily, make more accurate diagnoses, improve treatment efficacy, and, most importantly, reduce disease burden.

Systemic Lupus Erythematosus

SLE is a chronic, multisystem autoimmune disease that is highly variable in its clinical presentation, severity, prognosis, and treatment response. It is characterized by dysregulation in immune tolerance, autoantibodies targeted at self-antigens, deposition of immune complexes, and systemic and local inflammation (Jeltsch-David and Muller 2014). The disease primarily targets women of childbearing age, with the highest prevalence in African American women (Dall'Era 2013). SLE is notorious for the variety of its presentations and its waxing and waning course, which pose significant diagnostic challenges. Fever, joint pain, and rash represent the classic presenting triad of SLE, yet the manifestations of the disease are broad, including constitutional (fever, fatigue), mucocutaneous, musculoskeletal, renal, neuropsychiatric, cardiovascular, pulmonary, gastrointestinal, and hematological symptoms (Table 8–1).

Neuropsychiatric Manifestations of Systemic Lupus Erythematosus

The American College of Rheumatology (ACR) developed classification criteria for SLE that contain a total of 19 neuropsychiatric symptoms (Table 8–2) (American College of Rheumatology 1999). Five of the 11 CNS syndromes involve neuropsychiatric manifestations: acute confusional state, anxiety disorder, cognitive dysfunction, mood disorder, and psychosis. In establishing these syndromes, the ACR listed several possible etiologies. The ACR also utilized the *Diagnostic and Statistical Manual of Mental Disorders,* Fourth Edition (DSM-IV; American Psychiatric Association 1994), in developing its psychiatric terminology. In a meta-analysis of 10 prospective studies that included 2,039 patients, 56.3% of the patients had evidence of neuropsychiatric syndromes (Unterman et al. 2011). After headache, the two most frequent neuropsychiatric manifestations were mood disorders (20.7%) and cognitive dysfunction (19.7%) (Unterman et al. 2011). The reported prevalence of neuropsychiatric symptoms in SLE varies broadly, ranging from 21% to 95%, with 13%–38% of neuropsychiatric manifestations being directly attributable to SLE itself (Hanly 2011). There is a clear negative correlation between neuropsychiatric symptoms and patient quality of life, as well as a reported tenfold increase in mortality rate in patients with neuropsychiatric SLE compared with the general population (Magro-Checa et al. 2016).

Cognitive Dysfunction

Cognitive dysfunction has been found to be present in 20%–80% of individuals with SLE and is generally accepted as the most prevalent psychiatric manifestation of SLE (Denburg and Denburg 2003; Hanly 2011). Subclinical cognitive deficits have also been found in 11%–54% of patients, as identified in a review of 14 cross-sectional studies of cognitive dysfunction in SLE (Denburg and Denburg 2003). The most commonly identified cognitive symptoms have included impaired working memory, impaired executive function, decreased attention, and overall cognitive slowing (Hanly 2011). Autoimmune antiphospholipid antibodies, which are involved in the induction of a procoagulant state and the development of local ischemia, have also been associated with cognitive dysfunction in the absence of stroke (Hanly 2014). In a Tai-

TABLE 8–1.	Clinical features of systemic lupus erythematosus
Mucocutaneous	Malar rash, discoid rash, generalized erythema, alopecia, and oral ulcers
Musculoskeletal	Nonerosive arthritis, tenosynovitis, myositis, subcutaneous nodules, and avascular necrosis
Renal	Proteinuria and hematuria
Neuropsychiatric	Headache, cognitive dysfunction, psychosis, seizures, myelitis, mood disorder, anxiety disorder, polyneuropathy, cerebrovascular disease, and acute confusional state
Ophthalmic	Retinal ischemia, conjunctivitis, and uveitis (rare)
Cardiovascular	Pericarditis, premature atherosclerosis, and valvulitis
Pulmonary	Pleuritis, pleural effusions, and pulmonary hypertension
Hematological	Anemia, leukopenia, thrombocytopenia, vasculitis, and thrombosis
Gastrointestinal	Dyspepsia, abdominal pain, nausea, emesis, and hepatic disease

Source. Data from Bijlsma JWJ, da Silva JAP: "Systemic Lupus Erythematosus: Pathogenesis and Clinical Features," in *EULAR Textbook on Rheumatic Diseases.* Kilchberg, Switzerland, European League Against Rheumatism, 2012.

TABLE 8–2.	Neuropsychiatric syndromes observed in systemic lupus erythematosus

Central nervous system	
Aseptic meningitis	Seizure disorder
Cerebrovascular disease	Acute confusional state
Demyelinating syndrome	Anxiety disorder
Headache	Cognitive dysfunction
Movement disorder	Mood disorder
Myelopathy	Psychosis

Peripheral nervous system	
Guillain-Barré syndrome	Neuropathy
Autonomic disorder	Plexopathy
Mononeuropathy	Polyneuropathy
Myasthenia gravis	

Source. American College of Rheumatology 1999.

wanese cohort study, the incidence of dementia was found to be higher in SLE patients than in the general population (Lin et al. 2016). The study highlighted previously reported volumetric reductions in the hippocampus, amygdala, and cerebral cortex in neuropsychiatric SLE patients.

Mood Disorders

Depression is the second most common comorbid medical condition in SLE (Wolfe et al. 2010). A California cohort study of women with SLE ($n=326$) found a 49% lifetime prevalence of DSM-IV-diagnosed MDD in these patients, a rate twice that in the general population (Bachen et al. 2009). In an international cohort study involving 1,827 patients with SLE, the incidence of mood disorders was 12.7% (232) (Hanly et al. 2015). MDD (at 52.4%) was the most prevalent mood disorder diagnosis. The risk factors associated with depression included high-dosage prednisone (>20 mg daily), cutaneous activity, and myelitis (Huang et al. 2014). Autoantibodies against ribosomal-P and the NMDAR have been associated with depressive disorders in SLE, yet inconsistently (Kivity et al. 2015).

In the study by Bachen et al. (2009), the rate of bipolar I disorder in SLE was 6%, a rate six times that in the comparative general population without SLE. In an evaluation of 128 SLE patients, mood disorder with manic features was present in three (3%) of the cases (Brey et al. 2002).

Suicide risk.   Suicide risk in the SLE population has also been scrutinized. In a study of 367 Chinese SLE patients, 44 patients (12%) endorsed suicidal ideation in the prior month. Suicidal ideation was associated with higher SLE disease activity in the past year, more severe depressive and anxiety symptoms, unemployment, past psychiatric history, and history of suicide attempts, which was reported in 45 patients (12.4%), similar to previous studies (Mok et al. 2014). More recently, Hajduk et al. (2016) reported that among 53 patients with neuropsychiatric SLE, 14 (26%) reported suicidal ideation or hopelessness, which was associated with a notable increase in self-perceived cognitive dysfunction.

Anxiety Disorders

Anxiety is a prominent feature of SLE, with a 24% prevalence in one study (Brey et al. 2002). *Anxiety* is defined in DSM-5 (American Psychiatric Association 2013) as "the apprehensive anticipation of future danger or misfortune accompanied by a feeling of worry, distress, and/or somatic symptoms of tension" (p. 818). The symptom range of anxiety disorders includes excessive worry in regard to a variety of events (generalized anxiety disorder [GAD]), marked fear about a specific object (specific phobia) or social situation (social phobia), and abrupt surges of intense fear and somatic symptoms (panic disorder) (American Psychiatric Association 2013). In a study of 326 women with SLE, 65% of the patients received a diagnosis of an anxiety or mood disorder using the Composite International Diagnostic Interview (CIDI). Of those patients, 24% had specific phobia, 16% social phobia, 8% panic disorder, and 1% agoraphobia without panic symptoms (Bachen et al. 2009).

Obsessive-Compulsive Disorder

Obsessive-compulsive disorder (OCD) is characterized by recurrent, intrusive, unwanted thoughts, images, or urges that are often associated with repetitive acts or behaviors performed to reduce the anxiety associated with the obsessions (Slattery et al. 2004). The prevalence of OCD in SLE ranges from 9% to 16%, as assessed in two studies that utilized self-report questionnaires, the Yale-Brown Obsessive-Compulsive Scale and CIDI, as mentioned previously; these rates are significantly higher than those in the general population (2.3%) (Bachen et al. 2009; Kessler et al. 2012; Slattery et al. 2004).

Psychosis

Psychosis has been described as an impairment of reality testing that is often characterized by fixed false beliefs (delusions) and perceptual disturbances without external stimuli (hallucinations) (American Psychiatric Association 2013). The significance of psychosis in SLE is shown by its inclusion in the ACR classification criteria of SLE. The overall rate of psychosis in SLE has been estimated to be as high as 17% (Appenzeller et al. 2008). One of the major challenges of psychosis in the context of SLE is determining the cause, which may be attributed directly to SLE, corticosteroid treatment, or a primary psychiatric illness. In one study of 520 patients with SLE, acute psychosis was identified in 89 patients (17.1%). Of these, 19 patients had psychosis at disease onset, 40 patients developed psychosis during SLE, and 28 patients developed a corticosteroid-induced psychosis. The study found that psychosis considered due to SLE more frequently had other comorbid neuropsychiatric syndromes, greater SLE disease activity, and positive antiphospholipid antibodies (Appenzeller et al. 2008). In an evaluation of 485 patients, 11 (2.3%) had psychosis secondary to lupus. In 60% of patients, psychosis was the presenting symptom, and 80% of the patients experienced psychotic symptoms—including paranoia, visual hallucinations, and auditory hallucinations—within the first year of SLE diagnosis. The majority of these patients had cutaneous disease activity, and all had multisystem manifestations of lupus (Pego-Reigosa and Isenberg 2008). As with depression, anti-ribosomal P autoantibodies have been associated with lupus psychosis in some, but not all, studies (Kivity et al. 2015).

Acute Confusional State

According to the ACR nomenclature, *acute confusional state* is defined as "disturbance of consciousness or level of arousal with reduced ability to focus, maintain, or shift attention, accompanied by cognitive disturbance and/or changes in mood, behavior, or affect" (American College of Rheumatology 1999, p. 605). This description of acute confusional state in the ACR nomenclature is similar to the description of delirium in the DSM-5 criteria (American Psychiatric Association 2013). In a meta-analysis of 5,057 SLE patients, 155 (3.1%) had an acute confusional state (Unterman et al. 2011).

Other Neuropsychiatric Manifestations

One study of 45 patients with SLE compared with 60 control subjects found that the rate of personality disorders was 35.6% in SLE patients versus 11.7% in control subjects. The most prevalent personality disorder was obsessive-compulsive personality disorder, found in nine patients (20%) (Uguz et al. 2013). Self-report scores for symptoms of attention-deficit/hyperactivity disorder (ADHD) have been found to be elevated in patients with SLE compared with control subjects and were found to correlate with lupus disease activity in 49 patients (Garcia et al. 2013).

Corticosteroid-Induced Neuropsychiatric Symptoms

Corticosteroids are the mainstay of treatment for SLE flares and secondary manifestations and have been implicated in the production of euphoria, irritability, anxiety, depression, mania, cognitive deficits, and delirium (Dubovsky et al. 2012) (Figure 8–1). This association appears to be dose dependent, as initially established by the Boston Collaborative Drug Surveillance Program (1972). In a study of 674 patients, 18.3% showed severe neuropsychiatric symptoms at prednisolone dosages greater than 80 mg/day, whereas only 1.3% did so at dosages less than 40 mg/day (Boston Collaborative Drug Surveillance Program 1972). Kohen et al. (1993) highlighted the challenge of differentiating neuropsychiatric symptoms due to primary CNS lupus from those due to corticosteroids. Corticosteroid-induced neuropsychiatric side effects typically occur within 2 weeks of increasing the corticosteroid dosage, are rare at dosages less than 40 mg/day, and may manifest as mania, mixed mania/depression, depression with psychotic features, delirium, or psychosis. Other anti-inflammatory medications that can cause neuropsychiatric symptoms are reviewed in our discussion of rheumatoid arthritis later in this chapter (see section "Rheumatoid Arthritis").

Etiological Mechanisms of Neuropsychiatric Symptoms in Systemic Lupus Erythematosus

Potential mechanisms of neuropsychiatric symptoms in SLE include autoantibody production, microvascular damage, and proinflammatory cytokines. Some neuropsychiatric manifestations may also be an aspect of psychosocial stress related to disease severity or secondary manifestations of SLE treatment. In a review conducted by Hanly (2014), two pathogenic mechanisms were highlighted: 1) large- and small-vessel injury secondary to autoimmune antiphospholipid antibodies, immune complex, and leukocyte agglutination in cognitive dysfunction; and 2) an autoimmune-mediated inflammatory response with proinflammatory cytokine production, increased permeability of the blood-brain barrier, and intrathecal immune complex formation in psychosis and acute confusional state. The role of autoantibodies has been heavily investigated in neuropsychiatric syndromes. Most recently in a meta-analysis (Ho et al. 2016), there were positive associations of anticardiolipin antibodies with acute confusional state, antiphospholipid antibodies with cognitive dysfunction, and anti-ribosomal P with psychotic and mood manifestations.

Diagnosis and Management of Neuropsychiatric Symptoms in Systemic Lupus Erythematosus

The European League Against Rheumatism (EULAR) task force recommendations in 2014 indicated that investigations for new-onset neuropsychiatric symptoms in patients with SLE should be conducted in the same manner as for non-SLE patients with similar symptomatology (Bertsias et al. 2010). The initial goal should be to characterize the symptoms and rule out all possible causes, including infections, medications, and metabolic/endocrine abnormalities.

When evaluating these psychiatric manifestations, the clinician should obtain an extensive review of medications, complete metabolic panel, complete blood count, thyroid function tests, vitamin B_{12}, folate, and urine drug screen in addition to the clinical interview and an extensive neurological examination. In the case of delirium, a brain magnetic resonance imaging (MRI) scan and lumbar puncture are warranted to rule out malignancy, other neurological disease, and infection. In patients with cognitive dysfunction as well as a neurodegenerative disease, an MRI is warranted for similar exclusion, with the further requirement of neuropsychological testing to determine the severity and nature of the cognitive dysfunction. In patients with psychosis, an MRI may also be warranted. Recommended further studies in anxiety include urine screens for pheochromocytoma and carcinoid tumors (Magro-Checa et al. 2016). The sensitivity and specificity of serum anti-P antibodies for the diagnosis of

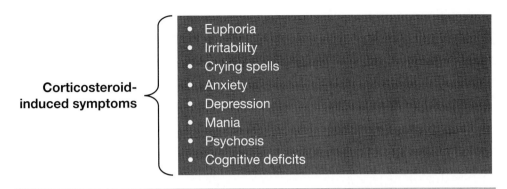

FIGURE 8–1. Corticosteroid-induced symptoms.

neuropsychiatric disorders in patients with SLE are 27% and 80%, respectively, indicating limited clinical utility (Zandman-Goddard et al. 2007). Due to a lack of specificity, measurement of CSF cytokines and autoantibodies is not recommended (Hanly 2014). One study found that 36%–72% of patients had not notified their health care provider of anxiety or mood symptoms yet had revealed such symptoms in self-reports in the form of standardized questionnaires, indicating the value of screening tools in this patient population (Bachen et al. 2009). Therefore, utilization of the Beck Depression Inventory (Beck et al. 1961) or the Hospital Anxiety and Depression Scale (Zigmond and Snaith 1983) may be helpful.

Treatment of Neuropsychiatric Symptoms in Systemic Lupus Erythematosus

Treatment should be focused on the underlying cause. In the case of an inflammatory or autoimmune cause, corticosteroids or immunosuppressive agents are indicated. An anticoagulant medication should be initiated if a hypercoagulable or vascular cause is discovered. In the case of severe psychosis or agitation associated with an acute confusional state, an antipsychotic (usually a second-generation agent) is indicated. The regimen should be continued until symptoms subside. In the case of medication-induced psychosis, tapering or withdrawal of the medication has been shown to be beneficial, specifically in patients on corticosteroids. Treatment of depression and anxiety follows the guidelines for these symptoms in non-SLE patients, and a trial of psychotherapy is recommended for mild to moderate cases. The benefit of cognitive-behavioral therapy (CBT) in reducing stress, depression, and anxiety in SLE patients was demonstrated in a small-scale study (Navarrete-Navarrete et al. 2010). Addition of a selective serotonin reuptake inhibitor (SSRI) would be indicated for patients with moderate to severe symptoms as well as for those who refuse or do not respond to CBT. Most importantly, the antidepressant needs to be prescribed at the optimal dosage and typically requires 6–8 weeks for full benefit, which should be explicitly explained to the patient at treatment onset. In a study of 127 patients with SLE, 53 of whom had moderate to severe depression (41.7%), only 26 patients (49%) were prescribed antidepressants, and only 8 were prescribed the maximum dosage of antidepressant (Karol et al. 2013). The same study also reported an association between severity of pain and lupus arthritis and depression severity scores.

Rheumatoid Arthritis

RA is a chronic inflammatory disease often associated with symmetrical synovitis of the peripheral joints that often progresses to systemic inflammation. The most commonly affected joints are the metacarpophalangeal and proximal interphalangeal joints. RA affects 0.5%–1% of the world population, with a female-to-male ratio of 2–3 to 1 (Shah and St. Clair 2015). The risk of developing RA is five times higher in individuals with a positive family history of RA than in those without such a history (Smolen et al. 2016). The pathogenesis of RA is multifactorial, with genetic, environmental, and inflammatory components. Diagnosis is often made clinically and augmented by serum antibodies, anti–cyclic citrullinated peptides (anti-CCPs), and rheumatoid factor as biomarkers. The goal of treatment is reduction of pain through use of nonsteroidal inflammatory drugs (NSAIDS) and reduction of inflammation, primarily through use of disease-modifying antirheumatic drugs (DMARDs). Corticosteroids also play a role in treatment, primarily for rapid symptomatic relief. The systemic inflammation in RA is evidenced by a high frequency of extra-articular involvement, reported in up to 40% of cases (Joaquim and Appenzeller 2015; Smolen et al. 2016). Extra-articular involvement in RA may include rheumatoid nodules, fatigue, weight loss, pulmonary involvement, vasculitis, or psychosocial manifestations.

Neuropsychiatric Manifestations of Rheumatoid Arthritis

Depression

Depression appears to be the most prevalent psychiatric manifestation in RA. In a study of 13,722 patients with RA, 15% reported depressive symptoms. Among the different comorbid conditions reported by patients, depression was most strongly associated with reduced quality of life (Wolfe et al. 2010). In a meta-analysis of 72 studies involving 13,189 patients, the prevalence of MDD was 16.8%. In addition, dysthymic disorder had a pooled prevalence of 18.7% (Matcham et al. 2013). Comorbid depression has been shown to reduce treatment adherence in RA, including increased likelihood of discontinuing DMARDs (Rathbun et al. 2013). Differentiation between symptoms of depression and RA is challenging because of the overlap of certain symptoms shared by both disorders. Examples of shared symptoms include disrupted sleep, fatigue, and reduced appetite (Matcham et al. 2013). Treatment of depressive symptoms has been associated with depressive symptom reduction as well as increased response to treatment of RA itself (Santiago et al. 2015). There is an increased risk of suicide in patients with RA and comorbid depression (Timonen et al. 2003). Given the interplay among pain, sleep disruption, and depression, each should be a target for overall improvement in patients with RA (Sturgeon et al. 2016).

Anxiety

Anxiety symptoms are highly prevalent in RA, with a prevalence of 21%–70% in one study (Uguz et al. 2009). In an Iranian cross-sectional study of 414 RA patients, 84.1% had moderate to severe anxiety, as assessed with a validated questionnaire (Jamshidi et al. 2016). The most common anxiety disorder in RA is GAD, as demonstrated in one clinical study of 200 Chinese patients, in which 5% were diagnosed with GAD, 4.5%

with specific phobia, and 4% with panic disorder (Lok et al. 2010). GAD was the most common anxiety disorder (16.9%) in a population of 82 patients with RA (Uguz et al. 2009). Anxiety symptoms correlate with poor quality of life and poorer treatment response in patients with RA (Matcham et al. 2016; Sturgeon et al. 2016).

Other Neuropsychiatric Manifestations

A variety of other neuropsychiatric illnesses and symptoms have been studied in RA. Cognitive dysfunction appears to be prevalent in the RA population. In a study involving 112 patients with RA (Shin et al. (2012), more than one-third ($n=41$) exhibited cognitive dysfunction, as assessed with a battery of standardized neuropsychological tests. Executive function, visuospatial learning/memory, and verbal learning/memory were the domains most prominently impaired (Shin et al. 2012). Additionally, risk factors for cardiovascular disease, current use of oral corticosteroids, low income, and low educational levels were all independent risk factors for worsening cognitive dysfunction in RA. In a population-based cohort study, RA was found to be a risk factor for subsequent development of bipolar disorder, with an incidence ratio of 2.13 (Hsu et al. 2014). Furthermore, being female and having comorbid alcohol use disorder, liver cirrhosis, or asthma with RA were found to be independent risk factors for bipolar disorder (Hsu et al. 2014).

Etiological Mechanisms of Neuropsychiatric Symptoms in Rheumatoid Arthritis

Disease-related causes of neuropsychiatric symptoms can include systemic inflammation, with direct CNS involvement. RA has also been associated with accelerated atherosclerosis, which may further contribute to the inflammatory damage (Joaquim and Appenzeller 2015). A variety of treatment options for RA have neuropsychiatric side effects, as summarized in Table 8–3. The effects of stress from disease-associated disability, pain, and sleep disruption have also been implicated. Inflammation itself has been implicated in the development of "sickness behaviors," which include social withdrawal, depression, fatigue, and abnormal sleep in both basic and experimental models (Irwin 2011). The severity of functional impairment in RA has been associated with rates and severity of anxiety as well as depression. Fatigue and sleep disturbance overlap with the symptoms of syndromal MDD and GAD. Additionally, patients with RA have been shown to exhibit HPA axis abnormalities, which may contribute to their chronic inflammatory state (Sturgeon et al. 2016).

Evaluation and Management of Neuropsychiatric Symptoms in Rheumatoid Arthritis

Differentiating psychiatric manifestations from nonpsychiatric etiology is of primary importance. A thorough history investigating the timeline, severity, and affiliating symptoms related to RA disease activity; medications; and any change in medical state will help guide treatment. Due to the lack of sensitive and specific diagnostic laboratory tests for psychiatric disorders, the evaluation will focus on ruling out nonpsychiatric causes, such as infection or metabolic changes, by use of a metabolic panel, complete blood count, and urinalysis. If acute changes in cognition or mental status

TABLE 8–3.   Psychiatric side effects of commonly used rheumatoid arthritis medications

Medication	Psychiatric manifestations
Nonsteroidal anti-inflammatory drugs (e.g., aspirin, ibuprofen)	Sleep disorders, anxiety, mood changes, psychosis, delirium (Browning 1996)
Corticosteroids	Insomnia, anxiety, depression, mania, cognitive impairment, delirium, psychosis (Dubovsky et al. 2012)
Cyclosporine A	Anxiety, depression, delirium, cognitive impairment, psychosis (Stevenson et al. 2016)
Sulfasalazine	Depression, insomnia, hallucinations (Stevenson et al. 2016)
Methotrexate	Delirium, irritability, personality changes (Turjanski and Lloyd 2005)
Interferon	Cognitive impairment, depression, delirium, sleep disturbance (Turjanski and Lloyd 2005)
Tacrolimus	Anxiety, depression, delirium, psychosis (Turjanski and Lloyd 2005)

are observed, a brain MRI to evaluate for focal CNS lesions possibly associated with the atherosclerotic risks of RA would be appropriate. Ongoing cognitive dysfunction requires a neuropsychological evaluation. Standardized self-report screening tools such as the Beck Depression Inventory were found to be useful in an evaluation of 258 patients with RA, showing a sensitivity of 87% and a specificity of 80% (Englbrecht et al. 2017). The Hospital Anxiety and Depression Scale has also been extensively used in research settings because of its lower reliance on overlapping somatic symptoms (Covic et al. 2012).

In the case of inflammation-induced psychiatric manifestations, the goal will be to amplify anti-inflammatory agents—either DMARDs alone or DMARDs in combination with short-term corticosteroids. Given the previously highlighted role of pain in mood disorder, pain management with NSAIDs—and possibly even a pain management consultation—may be beneficial. CBT, mindfulness-based stress reduction (MBSR), and Internet-based self-management approaches such as the Arthritis Self-Management Program have all been shown to provide benefit in the RA population, with direct reductions in anxiety or depressive symptoms and in pain and improvement in overall function with CBT; reductions in pain with MBSR; and improvement in self-efficacy and reduction in medical utilization with the self-management program (Knittle et al. 2010; Lorig et al. 2008; Zautra et al. 2008). The tricyclic antidepressant (TCA) amitriptyline was shown to have analgesic properties in a 32-week crossover trial in RA patients, yet in general this agent has an unfavorable side-effect profile (Frank et al. 1988). Despite these analgesic effects, amitriptyline did not reduce depressive or anxiety symptoms. In general, SSRIs are considered the first-line agents in treatment of anxiety and depression due to their favorable side-effect profile. In an open-label trial of 41 patients with MDD and RA, sertraline was found to be efficacious, with few side effects reported during a 15-month period (Slaughter et al. 2002). Although the evidence in RA remains scarce, the serotonin-norepinephrine reuptake inhibitors (SNRIs) venlafaxine, milnacipran, and duloxetine have been shown to be effective in the management of neuropathic pain, osteoarthritic pain, and fibromyalgia (Choy et al. 2011).

Sjogren's Syndrome

Sjogren's syndrome is predominantly an autoimmune disease that is chronic in nature, with a slow progression. It more commonly affects women, with a female-to-male ratio of 9:1 (Moutsopoulos and Tzioufas 2015). The disease can be primary or secondary to other autoimmune diseases such as RA or SLE. The prevalence of primary Sjogren's syndrome (pSS) is 0.5%–1% in the general population (Moutsopoulos and Tzioufas 2015). Histologically, there is lymphocytic infiltration of affected salivary and lacrimal glands. The nuclear and cytoplasmic antigens Ro/SS-A and La/SS-B have often been implicated and are considered strongly in the diagnosis, in combination with confirmation of oral and ocular involvement. Primary clinical manifestations include dryness of the mouth (xerostomia) and eyes (keratoconjuctivitis sicca). Extra-glandular manifestations of Sjogren's syndrome are present in nearly 30% of cases (Moutsopoulos and Tzioufas 2015). Extraglandular manifestations are often separated into the categories of nonvisceral (cutaneous, arthritis, myalgias) and visceral involvement that would include the pulmonary, cardiac, gastrointestinal, endocrine, and neurological systems (Fox 2005). Treatment is focused on symptomatic relief of xerostomia and sicca symptoms (i.e., use of ophthalmic preparations for sicca, or of procholinergic medications to induce saliva production in xerostomia). Treatment of systemic manifestations may require corticosteroids, NSAIDs, disease-modifying agents, or cytotoxic medications, depending on the severity and the organ system involved (Fox 2005; Moutsopoulos and Tzioufas 2015). CNS involvement, including neuropsychiatric manifestations, can be focal or nonfocal.

Neuropsychiatric Manifestations of Sjogren's Syndrome

Depression and Anxiety

Symptoms of depression and anxiety are highly prevalent in pSS. A meta-analysis conducted by Wan et al. (2016) evaluated the prevalence of anxiety and depression in patients with dry eye disease ($n=485,709$) compared with control subjects ($n=2,494,317$). Anxiety and depression had a threefold higher prevalence in patients with dry eye disease than in control subjects. Subgroup analysis of the 3,000 patients with pSS revealed a higher severity of anxiety and depression compared with control subjects. In a Taiwanese retrospective cohort study involving 2,686 patients with newly diagnosed pSS and 10,744 matched control patients without pSS, patients with pSS were shown to have a much higher risk of developing a depressive disorder (adjusted hazard ratio [HR], 1.829; 95% confidence interval [CI], 1.400–2.391) or an anxiety disorder (adjusted HR=1.856; 95% CI=1.384–2.489) in comparison with control patients (Shen et al. 2015). Symptoms of anxiety and depression have both been shown to negatively impact patient quality of life. In patients with pSS, anxiety has been more commonly associated with arthritis and fatigue, whereas depression has been more commonly associated with fatigue alone (Inal et al. 2010). Depression, anxiety, and neuroticism all independently impact Sjogren's syndrome–related fatigue, one of the most prominent symptoms of the disease, which negatively correlates with patient quality of life (Karageorgas et al. 2016).

Other Neuropsychiatric Manifestations

Cognitive deficits have been found in up to 50% of pSS cases (Morreale et al. 2014). The most commonly affected cognitive functions include impairments in memory, processing speed, verbal memory, executive dysfunction, and visuospatial perception, implicating subcortical dysfunction (Koçer et al. 2016; Morreale et al. 2014). Psychotic symptoms, dissociation, and somatization disorders have been observed in some case studies (Cox and Hales 1999).

Etiological Mechanisms of Neuropsychiatric Symptoms in Sjogren's Syndrome

The mechanisms of psychiatric manifestations remain unclear, yet direct CNS involvement and psychological distress related to pSS have been implicated (Figure 8–2). Ischemia-related damage due to CNS vasculitis may be one culprit (Alexander 1993). Anti-Ro/SSA antibodies have been associated with psychiatric disorders in Sjogren's syndrome, highlighting a potential inflammatory relationship that requires further investigation (Ampélas et al. 2001). The finding that corticosteroids produced improvement in some psychotic and affective symptoms in a few case studies also hints at a role for inflammation (Lin 2016). The psychological effects of this chronic disease that is fraught with discomfort, disability, and unpredictable systemic manifestations must also be considered as a chronic stressor. Reports of significant reductions in platelet serotonin levels due to functional serotonin transporter gene (*5-HTT*) polymorphisms in Sjogren's syndrome may provide another connection to mental disorders, specifically MDD and treatment-resistant depression (Markeljevic et al. 2015).

Evaluation and Management of Neuropsychiatric Symptoms in Sjogren's Syndrome

Consideration of the timing and severity of the psychiatric manifestations relative to Sjogren's syndrome activity and treatment may help clarify whether symptoms are secondary to or comorbid with Sjogren's syndrome. In one case study, psychiatric manifestations were present early in the illness and therefore may signal the presence of the disease itself (Pelizza et al. 2010). Self-rated assessment tools may also be useful in evaluating symptom severity and the need to treat. Evaluation and rule-out of other systemic manifestations of Sjogren's syndrome must also be performed, but there are no clear recommendations. Screening for autoantibodies (Anti-Ro/SS-A), erythrocyte sedimentation rate, CRP, and other markers of inflammation to determine symptom etiology is also useful. Although evidence is lacking, several case studies have reported beneficial effects from corticosteroids in combination with antidepressant and antipsychotic medications on the affective and psychotic manifestations of Sjogren's syndrome (Ampélas et al. 2001; Cox and Hales 1999; Lin 2016; Pelizza et al. 2010; Wong et al. 2014; Wyszynski and Wyszynski 1993). The benefit of psychiatric medications remains unclear. Medications with anticholinergic properties, such as TCAs, low-potency first-generation antipsychotics (e.g., chlorpromazine), and

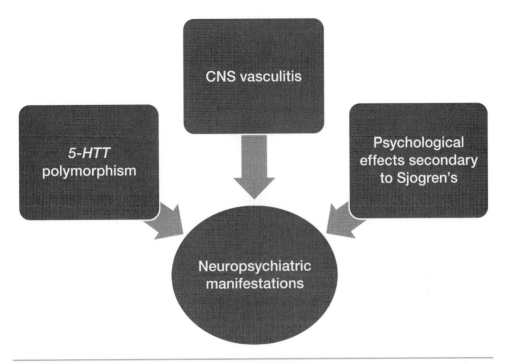

FIGURE 8–2. Etiological mechanisms of neuropsychiatric manifestations in primary Sjogren's syndrome.

5-HTT=serotonin transporter gene; CNS=central nervous system.

the second-generation antipsychotic clozapine, should be avoided. Neuropsychological testing is useful in the context of ongoing cognitive deficits. There are no available randomized controlled treatment trials in this patient population with either psychotherapy or psychiatric medications.

Scleroderma

Scleroderma is a rare disease of the connective tissue characterized by multisystem involvement associated with diffuse microangiopathy, immune dysregulation, and fibrosis of organ tissues. The reported incidence in the United States is 9–19 cases per million per year, with an estimated 100,000 cases in the United States currently (Varga 2015). There is a strong female predominance, mainly in the childbearing years. The illness is typically classified as either limited cutaneous scleroderma or diffuse cutaneous scleroderma. Clinical manifestations commonly include Raynaud's phenomenon, skin thickening, and visceral organ involvement including pulmonary, cardiac, kidney, and gastrointestinal systems (Khanna 2011). Diagnosis is clinically based on the presence of skin thickening, Raynaud's phenomenon, and visceral involvement, with laboratory investigations (antinuclear, anticentromere, and anti-topoisomerase-I antibodies) providing additional evidence (Khanna 2011). Treatment involves significant challenges due to differences in pathogenesis and disease presentation and the unpredictable course of the illness.

Neuropsychiatric Manifestations of Scleroderma

Clinically significant depression appears to be the most prominent psychiatric manifestation, with a prevalence of 36%–65% in one systematic review (Thombs et al. 2007). Anxiety symptoms are present in nearly one-third of scleroderma patients (Del Rosso et al. 2013). Baubet et al. (2011) interviewed 100 scleroderma patients and found a 35% prevalence rate of mood disorders, with 19% experiencing major depressive episode and 14% experiencing dysthymia. Remarkably, 49% of patients were diagnosed with an anxiety or related disorder, including 13% with GAD, 13% with social phobia, 9% with agoraphobia, 6% with panic disorder, 2% with OCD, and 2% with PTSD (Baubet et al. 2011). Some small-scale studies have observed cognitive impairment, delirium, and psychosis in patients with scleroderma (Cutolo et al. 2000; Hietaharju et al. 1993). In one study, somatization, interpersonal sensitivity, obsessive-compulsive symptoms, and paranoid ideation were more common in women with scleroderma compared with healthy women in a control group (Angelopoulos et al. 2001).

Etiological Mechanisms of Neuropsychiatric Symptoms in Scleroderma

Given the limited evidence implicating direct effects of inflammation, microangiopathy, and fibrosis on neuropsychiatric manifestations, the symptoms observed are likely secondary to the psychological impact of the illness (Del Rosso et al. 2013). Scleroderma is often associated with facial disfigurement and overall disability and is reliant on symptom control due to lack of a cure. Symptoms of depression and anxiety have shown direct correlations with overall disability, joint deformity, facial deformity, and skin deformity in a variety of studies (Del Rosso et al. 2013; Thombs et al. 2007).

Evaluation and Management of Neuropsychiatric Symptoms in Scleroderma

Patients with scleroderma benefit from an evaluation that considers the prevalent psychiatric comorbidity and investigates the severity of disability and perceived distress that this patient population encounters. Self-report rating scales that can highlight the presence of psychiatric symptoms are helpful. A collaborative approach between the psychiatrist and the primary treatment team, which may include a rheumatologist or dermatologist, is of primary importance. There is no clear evidence for treatment of patients currently, but improved psychoeducation, identification of social supports (e.g., family, support groups), psychotherapy, and psychiatric medications are options that appear to be useful in other patients with inflammatory-based neuropsychiatric manifestations, as previously discussed.

Hashimoto's Thyroiditis (Autoimmune Thyroiditis)

Hashimoto's thyroiditis (HT), the most common form of thyroiditis, is a chronic autoimmune disease characterized by inflammation of the thyroid gland. The key pathological finding is lymphocytic infiltration of the thyroid, similar to Graves' disease

(Caturegli et al. 2014). The prevalence is 8 cases per 1,000, with women having a greater risk than men (Caturegli et al. 2014; Jacobson et al. 1997). Diagnosis is primarily made by a combination of goiter development and serological findings. In the absence of goiter development, thyroid ultrasonography may be utilized. The presence of antithyroid antibodies, antithyroid peroxidase (abTPO; previously referred to as antimicrosomal antibodies), or antithyroglobulin (abTG) is utilized for diagnosis. Standard tests of thyroid function appear to be less useful (Amino et al. 2016). Clinical features of autoimmune thyroiditis include goiter development and systemic manifestations. Systemic manifestations include the classic findings of hypothyroidism, weakness, fatigue, weight gain, constipation, cold intolerance, and skin changes (dryness, thickening). Treatment is aimed at controlling symptoms through use of synthetic thyroid hormones or thyroid extract (Caturegli et al. 2014). HT can also be associated with a transient hyperthyroid phase known as Hashitoxicosis (Fatourechi et al. 1971). This phase is believed to be due to dysregulated release of thyroid hormone associated with chronic inflammatory damage to the thyroid gland (Nabhan et al. 2005). These signs and symptoms are similar to those in Graves' disease, which is discussed in the following section (Wasniewska et al. 2012).

Neuropsychiatric Manifestations of Hashimoto's Thyroiditis

Hypothyroidism can manifest with overlapping depressive-like symptoms, such as fatigue, impaired concentration, low appetite, and psychomotor retardation, that may cause either illness to be overlooked initially (Amino et al. 2016). At times, severe hypothyroidism may manifest similarly to melancholic depression (Schuff et al. 2013). Yet there has been evidence of psychiatric manifestations in the context of euthyroid HT. In one small-scale study, patients with abTPO-positive HT were shown to have a sixfold greater risk of developing depression compared with control subjects and nearly a fivefold greater risk of developing GAD compared with control subjects (Carta et al. 2005). In a study of 51 euthyroid HT patients compared with 68 control subjects, one-third of patients were diagnosed with a depressive disorder and 37.3% with an anxiety or related disorder, compared with 16% and 14.7% in the control group, respectively. The most common diagnoses were MDD, panic disorder, and OCD (Giynas Ayhan et al. 2014). Our group found a marked increase in autoimmune thyroid antibodies in depressed patients compared with control subjects (Nemeroff et al. 1985). In a study involving 226 outpatients with bipolar disorder, 3,190 psychiatric inpatients with any diagnosis, and 252 healthy population control subjects, Kupka et al. (2002) found a higher prevalence of antithyroid antibodies in the bipolar patients (28%) than in the individuals in the two control groups (3%–18%). In addition, children of bipolar patients exhibited an increased vulnerability to developing autoimmune thyroid disease (Hillegers et al. 2007). These findings were congruent with findings of elevated antithyroid antibodies more specifically in patients with bipolar disorder who experienced rapid cycling (Oomen et al. 1996). A meta-analysis of 19 case-control studies found that patients with autoimmune thyroiditis, HT, or overt or subclinical hypothyroidism had a higher risk of developing depression (odds ratio [OR]=3.56; 95% CI=2.14–5.94; I^2=92.1%) or anxiety (OR=2.32; 95% CI=1.40–3.85; I^2=89.8%) in comparison with healthy control subjects (Siegmann et al. 2018).

Cognitive Dysfunction

Cognitive dysfunction has been reported in hypothyroid and euthyroid patients with autoimmune thyroiditis. Patients with untreated hypothyroidism have difficulty in memory retrieval, more specifically in verbal information, without difficulties in attention or nonverbal tasks (Miller et al. 2007). Spatial, associative, and verbal memory were impaired in hypothyroid patients and were shown to partially improve with treatment (Correia et al. 2009). In comparison with control subjects, patients with euthyroid HT showed impairments in attention and response inhibition that correlated with abTPO titers (Leyhe et al. 2008).

Hashimoto's Encephalitis

First observed in 1966, Hashimoto's encephalitis (HE) is a clinically heterogeneous syndrome manifesting with a variety of symptoms that may include acute delirium, chronic dementia, depression, mania, seizures, focal neurological abnormalities, and acute psychosis with delusions or hallucinations. The syndrome is characterized by elevated antithyroid antibodies and an excellent response to corticosteroids, suggesting an inflammatory and autoimmune pathogenesis (Kirshner 2014). Olmez et al. (2013) showed the most common presentations as subacute deterioration of cognitive function (62%) and seizures (46%) in an evaluation of 13 patients with confirmed HE. The first-line treatment is corticosteroids, with clinical utilization and benefit of rituximab, methotrexate, intravenous immunoglobulin, and azathioprine (Chong et al. 2013; Olmez et al. 2013). Electroencephalography (EEG) findings have been characterized as diffuse slowing in 98% of the cases in one systematic review (Chong et al. 2003). Brain imaging findings are variable and nonspecific, as reviewed by Schiess and Pardo (2008).

Etiological Mechanisms of Neuropsychiatric Symptoms in Hashimoto's Thyroiditis

The relationship between mood alterations and thyroid dysfunction has been intensively studied, yet the relationship in the context of autoimmune thyroiditis remains unclear. Symptoms of anxiety and depression are more common in patients with positive abTPO than in control groups (Carta et al. 2004; Fountoulakis et al. 2004). Furthermore, as noted earlier, patients with depression have elevated rates of antithyroid antibodies, implicating inflammatory mechanisms (Musselman and Nemeroff 1996). There is a vast literature on the role of thyroid axis alterations, including subclinical hypothyroidism, in the pathogenesis of depression, which is outside the focus of the current review. Additionally, there is evidence of autoimmunity and CNS involvement, with findings of brain hypoperfusion in euthyroid autoimmune thyroiditis patients with elevated thyroid peroxidase antibodies (Piga et al. 2004).

Evaluation and Management of Neuropsychiatric Symptoms in Hashimoto's Thyroiditis

In addition to a thorough clinical interview, laboratory evaluation includes thyroid function tests (thyroid-stimulating hormone [TSH], free triiodothyronine [T_3], free thyroxine [T_4]), confirmation of autoimmune involvement (abTPO and abTG), and thyroid imaging. Although there are no laboratory examinations or imaging evaluations to confirm psychiatric involvement, EEG and MRI are useful, especially in patients with HE. The primary treatment goal is attaining euthyroid status by way of thyroid hormone replacement, which has been shown to reduce psychiatric manifestations, yet not completely in some instances (Davis and Tremont 2007; Saravanan et al. 2002). In a seminal study, Bunevicius et al. (1999) reported that the combination of T_3 and T_4 was superior to T_4 alone in improving mood and cognitive function in patients requiring thyroid hormone replacement. Corticosteroid management is typically indicated in cases of HE, as previously discussed.

Graves' Disease

Graves' disease is an autoimmune disorder of the thyroid gland that accounts for 80% of cases of hyperthyroidism (Jameson et al. 2015). The disease has a 2% prevalence in females and is one-tenth as common in males (Jameson et al. 2015). The disease is characterized by thyroid-stimulating antibodies that target the thyroid, thereby mimicking the function of TSH. Classic clinical manifestations include hyperthyroidism, goiter development, and ophthalmopathy (scleral irritation, dryness, proptosis), with ocular involvement occurring in 50% of cases (Bahn 2010; Menconi et al. 2014). Additional clinical manifestations include weight loss, decreased appetite, sinus tachycardia, palpitations, warm skin, heat intolerance, tremor, increased stool production, diarrhea, abnormalities in menstruation (in women), and erectile dysfunction (in men) (Jameson et al. 2015). Diagnosis is typically made by the presence of thyrotoxic symptoms, ophthalmic involvement, presence of thyrotropin receptor antibodies, or increased thyroid radioiodine uptake (Menconi et al. 2014). Management focuses on reduction of the hyperthyroid state by way of antithyroid medications, including propylthiouracil or methimazole. β-Adrenergic-blocking medications (e.g., propranolol) are useful in alleviating the acute sympathetic nervous system symptoms of thyrotoxicosis, such as tachycardia. Radioiodine, surgical reduction, or total removal of the thyroid are other reliable treatment options (Jameson et al. 2015).

Neuropsychiatric Manifestations of Graves' Disease

In general, symptoms of anxiety and depression appear to be more common in patients with hyperthyroidism than in the general population (Bunevicius and Prange 2006; Vogel et al. 2007). In one study of 137 patients with Graves' disease, the most common psychiatric symptoms were irritability (78.1%), anxious mood (72.3%), and somatic symptoms, most prominently insomnia (66.4%), fatigue (65.7%), and weight loss (62.8%) (Stern et al. 1996). These patients also reported significant concerns about cognitive function in regard to "slowed mental functioning" and memory impairment. Additional patient reports of difficulties with sustained attention and visuomotor performance have been described, yet cognitive test results have been inconclusive (Alvarez et al. 1983; Bunevicius and Prange 2006; Vogel et al. 2007). In regard to clinical diagnosis, Bunevicius et al. (2005) found social anxiety disorder, GAD, and MDD to be the most frequently diagnosed disorders in 30 women with Graves' disease.

Symptoms of mania have also been reported in one small-scale study and a case series of thyrotoxic patients with evident psychotic symptoms (Brownlie et al. 2000; Trzepacz et al. 1988b). Disease manifestations in elderly patients may differ from those in younger patients; one such presentation, described as "apathetic hyperthyroidism," is characterized by withdrawal, apathy, and depression (Mooradian 2008).

Etiological Mechanisms of Neuropsychiatric Symptoms in Graves' Disease

With the reported anecdotal improvement in depressive, anxious, manic, and cognitive symptoms after treatment with propranolol without associated alterations in thyroid hormone, a noradrenergic mechanism for Graves' disease has been posited (Bunevicius and Prange 2006; Trzepacz et al. 1988a). Although propranolol can cross the blood-brain barrier and exert direct effects on the CNS, its effects are likely focused on the peripheral nervous system. Propranolol is purported to have anxiolytic effects and is frequently used off-label in various anxiety disorders, which further supports the possibility of an adrenergic mechanism (Steenen et al. 2016). Other studies have found a reduction in anxiety and depression in association with antithyroid treatment, highlighting the seminal role of hyperthyroidism per se (Bunevicius and Prange 2006; Kathol et al. 1986). Finally, the presence of significant anxiety, depression, and cognitive dysfunction in euthyroid Graves' disease patients highlights the role of an autoimmune relationship (Bunevicius et al. 2005).

Evaluation and Management of Neuropsychiatric Symptoms in Graves' Disease

Because neuropsychiatric presentations are common in the disorder, the diagnosis of Graves' disease may initially be a challenge. In one study, 50% (n=47) of patients reported that it took 3–6 months (or longer) for them to receive a diagnosis of Graves' disease; this delay was likely attributable to the presence of neuropsychiatric symptoms, which apparently were perceived (by both patients and clinicians) as being primarily psychological in origin (Stern et al. 1996; Trzepacz et al. 1988b). Developing a clear timeline of symptom manifestations with differentiation of prominent somatic and psychological symptoms may be helpful. The goal for patients with psychiatric manifestations with confirmed thyrotoxicosis is attainment of euthyroid status. The evidence indicates that most neuropsychiatric manifestations and cognitive dysfunction are alleviated by use of antithyroid medications as well as propranolol (Bunevicius and Prange 2006; Bunevicius et al. 2005; Kathol et al. 1986; Trzepacz et al. 1988a). Psychotropic medications have been utilized in a variety of case studies, yet systematic evidence for benefits from psychotherapy or psychotropic medications is currently unavailable.

Sarcoidosis

Sarcoidosis is a multisystem inflammatory disease often associated with noncaseating granulomas of unknown origin that typically are associated with lung involvement. The disease prevalence ranges from 20 to 60 cases per 100,000 population, with higher rates being reported in African American and Nordic populations (Baughman and Lower 2015). Although the cause of sarcoidosis is unclear, noncaseating granuloma development with an exaggerated localized immune response is a hallmark finding of the illness. The disease manifestations are variable, ranging from asymptomatic cases to organ failure. The most commonly reported symptoms are respiratory—cough and shortness of breath. Symptoms may be nonspecific and may include fatigue, fever, night sweats, or weight loss. The cutaneous, ocular, and lymphatic systems are typically affected (Baughman and Lower 2015). CNS involvement occurs in up to 10% of cases; sarcoidosis with CNS involvement is termed *neurosarcoidosis*. There are a wide range of CNS symptoms, including headaches, ataxia, sensory disturbances, diplopia, confusion, depression, and psychosis (Nozaki and Judson 2012) (Figure 8–3).

Patients frequently show bilateral hilar lymphadenopathy or pulmonary involvement on chest radiograph, which—in combination with histological evidence of noncaseating granuloma—is required for diagnosis. Treatment is based on the disease manifestations and may require systemic corticosteroids, cytotoxic agents (e.g., methotrexate, cyclophosphamide), or cytokine modulators (e.g., thalidomide, infliximab), depending on symptom severity or the presence of cardiac, renal, or neurological involvement (Valeyre et al. 2014).

Neuropsychiatric Manifestations of Sarcoidosis

Depressive symptoms appear to be highly prevalent among individuals with sarcoidosis, with clinical depression—as assessed by a score of ≥9 on the Center for Epidemiologic Studies–Depression scale (Radloff 1977)—found in 60%–66% of patients (Chang et al. 2001; Cox et al. 2004). Chang et al. (2001) showed that depressive symptom severity increased with increasing organ system involvement; of the 154 sarcoidosis patients with involvement of three or more systems, 76% had clinically significant depressive symptoms. Nearly one-third of evaluated patients endorsed significant symptoms of anxiety, with severity of anxiety symptoms correlating with sarcoidosis disease severity (Holas et al. 2013; Ireland and Wilsher 2010). Patients with this disease have high rates of psychiatric comorbidity; in a study of 80 patients with sarcoidosis, the most common psychiatric diagnoses were MDD (25%), panic disorder (6.3%), bipolar disorder (6.3%), and GAD (5%) (Goracci et al. 2008). Altered sensorium, delusions, hallucinations, and cognitive dysfunction have also been identified in cases of sarcoidosis (Bourgeois et al. 2005; Shah et al. 2009; Westhout and Linskey 2008).

Etiological Mechanisms of Neuropsychiatric Symptoms in Sarcoidosis

A variety of mechanisms may magnify the prevalence of behavioral symptomatology in sarcoidosis, including direct CNS involvement and psychosocial factors. Direct granulomatous penetration of the CNS, leptomeningeal involvement, obstructing hydrocephalus, and white matter changes in the brain have all been associated with psychosis, delirium, or cognitive dysfunction, albeit not consistently (Nozaki and Judson 2012; Westhout and Linskey 2008). Fatigue, a common and disabling symptom of sar-

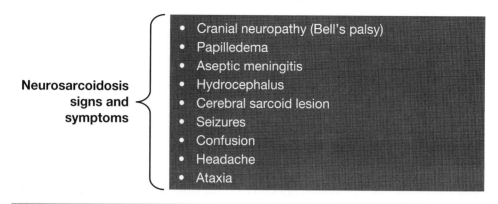

Neurosarcoidosis signs and symptoms

- Cranial neuropathy (Bell's palsy)
- Papilledema
- Aseptic meningitis
- Hydrocephalus
- Cerebral sarcoid lesion
- Seizures
- Confusion
- Headache
- Ataxia

FIGURE 8–3. Signs and symptoms of neurosarcoidosis.

coidosis, is also a necessary symptom for the diagnosis of both MDD and GAD, two prominent psychiatric diagnoses, and highlights a bidirectional relationship (de Kleijn et al. 2013). Corticosteroids, the first-line treatment for neurosarcoidosis, must also be considered as a potential culprit in the development of psychiatric sequelae.

Evaluation and Management of Neuropsychiatric Symptoms in Sarcoidosis

There is scant evidence available concerning treatment of psychiatric manifestations in sarcoidosis. An evaluation to rule out cranial nerve, brain, and meningeal manifestations is of primary importance. A thorough clinical and laboratory investigation of associated comorbid conditions that includes radiographic chest X rays, CSF, and MRI of the brain is necessary. Elevations in protein, lymphocytosis, and oligoclonal bands in CSF in neurosarcoidosis have been previously documented (Stern et al. 1985). A variety of brain MRI findings, including hydrocephalus, parenchymal lesions, and leptomeningeal involvement, have been previously associated with psychosis, cognitive deficits, and delirium (Nozaki and Judson 2012; Shah et al. 2009; Westhout and Linskey 2008). Self-report questionnaires (e.g., the Beck Depression Inventory) may be useful in screening for depression and anxiety, which may warrant a psychiatric consultation. Patients with confirmed neurosarcoidosis typically respond to corticosteroid, immune modulation, or cytotoxic agents (Nozaki and Judson 2012). Antidepressant or antipsychotic agents may be required to treat comorbid psychiatric diagnoses, but there are no randomized controlled trials to support the use of these agents in symptoms secondary to sarcoidosis.

Anti-NMDAR Encephalitis

Anti-NMDAR encephalitis is a severe antineuronal inflammatory brain disease, with antibodies targeted against the GluN1 subunit of the NMDAR (Dalmau et al. 2008). Anti-NMDAR encephalitis represents a specific form of limbic encephalitis that has garnered much attention in the past decade. Limbic encephalitis is classically associated with rapid progression of mood disturbance, delusions, hallucinations, memory loss, confusion, and seizures (Tüzün and Dalmau 2007). Identified forms of autoimmune encephalitis have been associated with cell surface receptors, intracellular antigens, ion channels, and antibodies against synaptic receptors (anti-NMDAR) (Graus et al. 2016). Although the incidence and prevalence of this disorder are currently unclear, a United Kingdom population-based study of 198 encephalitic patients showed that anti-NMDAR encephalitis was the second most common (4%) autoimmune cause of encephalitis (Granerod et al. 2010). Anti-NMDAR encephalitis was found in up to 40% (*n*=32) of patients evaluated in a California study (Gable et al. 2012). The disease typically develops in adolescent and young adult females (Dalmau et al. 2011). Disease manifestations include an early prodromal phase (involving flulike symptoms, with low-grade fever) and the appearance of neuropsychiatric symptoms (such as delusions, hallucinations, cognitive deficits, seizures, dyskinesias) and may progress to a hyporesponsive state (with autonomic instability and coma) (Maneta and Garcia 2014) (Figure 8–4). The disease was initially considered to be a paraneoplastic syndrome, yet nearly half of the cases evaluated did not involve a neoplasm (Maneta and Garcia 2014).

In an analysis of 464 cases of anti-NMDAR encephalitis that were individually described in the literature, the average age at illness onset was 27 years, and 79% of the patients were female (Al-Diwani et al. 2019). Thirty-two percent of the cases were attributed to ovarian teratoma. The most common psychiatric symptoms were agitation, aggression, depressed mood, mood instability, hallucinations, delusions, mutism, and irritability (Al-Diwani et al. 2019). Among the 464 patients with confirmed NMDAR-antibody encephalitis, behavioral disturbances were found in 68%, psychosis in 67%, mood symptoms in 47%, catatonia in 30%, and sleep disturbances in 21%. This mixed presentation and especially the overlap of mood and psychosis symptoms were distinctive findings of this analysis (Al-Diwani et al. 2019).

NMDA-associated psychiatric illness often develops rapidly, may have a viral prodrome (in up to 70% of cases), and is often accompanied by neurological symptoms, including movement abnormalities, short-term memory impairment, and confusion as the disease progresses (Warren et al. 2018). Agitation, aggression, and catatonia, particularly when fluctuating, were key findings in an analysis conducted by Warren et al. (2018). Among the 464 patients with anti-NMDAR encephalitis in the Al-Diwani et al. (2019) study, 257 (62%) had abnormal EEG scans and 135 (32%) had abnormal findings on brain MRI. Neurological abnormalities that developed over time were movement disorders, including choreoathetoid movements; seizures; and hyporesponsiveness. Early treatment with immunotherapy has been reported to be beneficial (Titulaer et al. 2013). Diagnosis is confirmed by the presence of positive serum or especially CSF antibodies to the NMDAR subunit (Al-Diwani et al. 2019; Dalmau et al. 2011; Warren et al. 2018).

First-line treatments for anti-NMDAR encephalitis include steroids, intravenous immunoglobulins, plasma exchange, plasmapheresis, and tumor removal. Approximately 75% of patients recover; the remainder experience either severe disability or death (Dalmau et al. 2011; Wang 2016).

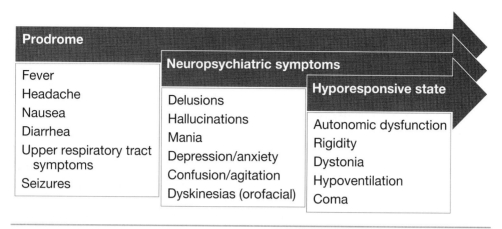

FIGURE 8–4. Symptom constellations of anti-NMDAR encephalitis.
NMDAR=N-methyl-D-aspartate receptor.

Neuropsychiatric Manifestations of Anti-NMDAR Encephalitis

Psychiatric manifestations are a prominent component of anti-NMDAR encephalitis presentations. Nearly 4% (n=23) of the cases evaluated by Kayser et al. (2013) had psychiatric symptoms as the sole manifestation of the disease, and 77% (n=77) of the 100 patients studied by Dalmau et al. (2008) were initially treated by a psychiatrist. Psychiatric symptoms are typically present at disease onset, with 72% of patients (n=164) presenting with anxiety, agitation, apathy, depression, delusions, bizarre behavior, cognitive deficits, or hallucinations (visual or auditory) (Zhang et al. 2017). Psychotic symptoms and agitation appear to dominate the presentation (Lejuste et al. 2016). Patients may develop catatonia, which manifests as purposeless motor activity, posturing, grimacing, mutism, echopraxia, echolalia, or extreme negativism (Consoli et al. 2011). Although adolescent patients may have presentations similar to those in adults, younger children seem to be more likely to manifest behavioral changes, temper tantrums, agitation, aggression, and impaired speech production, providing further challenges in identification (Florance et al. 2009). Individuals with anti-NMDAR encephalitis appear to be intolerant to antipsychotics; in one retrospective review, symptoms consistent with neuroleptic malignant syndrome were found in 21 (46.6%) of 45 patients initially hospitalized in a psychiatric unit (Lejuste et al. 2016). In two cases, patients developed hyperthermia, decreased alertness, muscle rigidity, rhabdomyolysis, and coma within days of initiating antipsychotics (Lejuste et al. 2016). Individuals with anti-NMDAR encephalitis may manifest rigidity and alterations in consciousness as part of disease development, resulting in diagnostic and treatment challenges. In a study of postrecovery cognitive performance in 9 patients with documented anti-NMDAR encephalitis (Finke et al. 2012), nearly 85% (n=8) showed persistent deficits (mean duration of 43 months). Deficits were most prominent in executive function, and included impulsivity, behavioral disinhibition, planning difficulty, and impairments in attention and working memory, indicating long-term challenges (Dalmau et al. 2011; Finke et al. 2012).

Etiological Mechanisms of Neuropsychiatric Symptoms in Anti-NMDAR Encephalitis

The disease is characterized by immune self-activation, possibly due to an immune response associated with tumor presence in more than half of cases, yet other immunological triggers are unclear (Dalmau et al. 2008). The autoimmune response leads to hypofunction of the NMDAR due to cross-linking and internalization of the GluN1 subunit of the receptor, resulting in a state of disinhibition and excitatory response associated with both glutamate and γ-aminobutyric acid (GABA) dysregulation. Dysregulation of GABA and glutamate may help explain the high prevalence of depressive symptoms, psychosis, cognitive dysfunction, and mania seen in anti-NMDAR encephalitis (Schwartz et al. 2012). Antibodies directed toward the NMDAR have also been found in patients with schizophrenia (Steiner et al. 2013). Further support for this mechanism is provided by the finding that psychosis and behavioral disturbance can be induced by drugs that antagonize the NMDAR (e.g., ketamine, phencyclidine) (Dowben et al. 2015).

Diagnosis and Management of Neuropsychiatric Symptoms in Anti-NMDAR Encephalitis

Diagnosis is confirmed by the presence of IgG antibodies toward the NR1 subunit of the NMDAR either by serum alone (sensitivity of 85.6%, specificity of 100%) or by CSF analysis (100% sensitivity and specificity), especially in cases of suspected anti-NMDAR encephalitis with a negative serum screen (Gresa-Arribas et al. 2014). Nonspecific pleocytosis and oligoclonal bands are also frequently seen (Zhang et al. 2017). EEG abnormalities, most commonly nonspecific disorganized slowing, have been identified in 90% ($n=21$) of cases (Schmitt et al. 2012). An extreme delta brush pattern has been identified in some patients, which typically is indicative of a worse prognosis (Dalmau et al. 2008; Schmitt et al. 2012; Titulaer et al. 2013). MRI abnormalities are evident in 40% of cases ($n=137$) in a variety of brain regions, including the hippocampus, cerebral cortex, corpus callosum, or insula (Zhang et al. 2017).

First-line treatments for anti-NMDAR encephalitis include steroids, intravenous immunoglobulins, plasma exchange, and plasmapheresis. The combination of corticosteroids and intravenous immunoglobulin appears to be most commonly used. Second-line options include rituximab, cyclophosphamide, methotrexate, mycophenolate mofetil, and azathioprine. In an observational cohort study of treatment outcomes in patients with anti-NMDAR encephalitis, 251 (53%) of the 472 patients who received first-line treatment with immunotherapy or tumor resection improved within 4 weeks (Titulaer et al. 2013). Among the 221 patients who did not respond to first-line treatment, 125 received second-line immunotherapy and experienced improvement. At the 24-month follow-up, 204 (81%) of the 252 patients evaluated were assessed as having good outcomes (Titulaer et al. 2013). In another study (a review of 83 studies [total $N=432$]) that examined treatments and outcomes in patients with anti-NMDAR encephalitis, 406 patients were treated with immunotherapy, of whom 301 received first-line immunotherapy alone and 104 received first-line immunotherapy combined with second-line immunotherapy (Zhang et al. 2017). Among the 301 patients treated with first-line immunotherapy, 128 (43%) experienced full recovery and 148 (49%) experienced substantial improvement. Findings for the 104 patients who received combined first-line and second-line immunotherapy were similar, with 50 (48%) experiencing full recovery and 43 (41%) experiencing substantial improvement (Zhang et al. 2017). Early identification and treatment are associated with better treatment outcomes in both children and adults (Byrne et al. 2015; Titulaer et al. 2013).

Psychiatric manifestations in anti-NMDAR encephalitis may require acute pharmacological management, particularly in cases of acute psychosis, mania, or delirium. First- and second-generation antipsychotics have similar efficacy in managing these symptoms. Because first-generation antipsychotics are associated with an increased risk of extrapyramidal symptoms—including acute dystonia, tremor, and akathisia—that may mimic the neurological manifestations of anti-NMDAR encephalitis, low-dosage second-generation antipsychotics should be used for treatment (Kuppuswamy et al. 2014).

Electroconvulsive therapy has been utilized in a few cases, with improvement in catatonic symptoms of anti-NMDAR encephalitis, and may be a viable option in treatment-resistant cases (Coffey and Cooper 2016). Current data are limited to case studies; therefore, an interdisciplinary approach, including neurology, immunology, and psychiatry, is recommended.

Conclusion

Neuropsychiatric presentations in the context of medical illnesses pose a significant challenge for any practitioner. Such symptoms often require prior experience or knowledge to thoroughly investigate and manage. As discussed in this chapter, there are strong associations between inflammatory disease and neuropsychiatric symptoms. Although the most common psychiatric comorbidities appear to be mood and anxiety disorders, it is clear that the neuropsychiatric manifestations of medical disease and its treatment can vary greatly and can negatively affect treatment outcomes. Patients require a thorough diagnostic evaluation to rule out other potential causes of symptoms. Mental health screening questionnaires such as the Beck Depression Inventory and the Hospital Anxiety and Depression Scale are efficient and useful tools for measuring the severity of mood and anxiety symptoms and can help to identify patients who may require further psychiatric management. Management should ideally be carried out by an interdisciplinary team with a focus on patient-specific care. Psychosocial and psychopharmacological management should follow the guidelines for noncomorbid psychiatric disorders.

References

Abbas AK, Lichtman AH, Pillai S: Properties and overview of immune responses, in Cellular and Molecular Immunology, 8th Edition. Edited by Abbas A, Lichtman A, Pillai S. Philadelphia, PA, Elsevier Saunders, 2015, pp 1–13

Al-Diwani A, Handel A, Townsend L, et al: The psychopathology of NMDAR-antibody encephalitis in adults: a systematic review and phenotypic analysis of individual patient data. Lancet Psychiatry 6(3):235–246, 2019. Available at: https://www.thelancet.com/journals/lanpsy/article/PIIS2215-0366(19)30001-X/fulltext. Accessed March 27, 2019.

Alexander EL: Neurologic disease in Sjögren's syndrome: mononuclear inflammatory vasculopathy affecting central/peripheral nervous system and muscle. A clinical review and update of immunopathogenesis. Rheum Dis Clin North Am 19(4):869–908, 1993 8265827

Alvarez MA, Gómez A, Alavez E, et al: Attention disturbance in Graves' disease. Psychoneuroendocrinology 8(4):451–454, 1983 6689536

American College of Rheumatology: The American College of Rheumatology nomenclature and case definitions for neuropsychiatric lupus syndromes. Arthritis Rheum 42(4):599–608, 1999 10211873

American Psychiatric Association: Diagnostic and Statistical Manual of Mental Disorders, 4th Edition. Washington, DC, American Psychiatric Association, 1994

American Psychiatric Association: Diagnostic and Statistical Manual of Mental Disorders, 5th Edition. Arlington, VA, American Psychiatric Association, 2013

Amino N, Lazarus J, De Groot L: Chronic (Hashimoto's) thyroiditis, in Endocrinology: Adult and Pediatric, 7th Edition. Edited by Jameson L, De Groot L, de Kretser D, et al. Philadelphia, PA, Elsevier Saunders, 2016, pp 1515–1527

Ampélas JF, Wattiaux MJ, Van Amerongen AP: [Psychiatric manifestations of lupus erythematosus systemic and Sjogren's syndrome]. Encephale 27(6):588–599, 2001 11865567

Angelopoulos NV, Drosos AA, Moutsopoulos HM: Psychiatric symptoms associated with scleroderma. Psychother Psychosom 70(3):145–150, 2001 11340416

Anderson RJ, Freedland KE, Clouse RE, et al: The prevalence of comorbid depression in adults with diabetes: a meta-analysis. Diabetes Care 24(6):1069–1078, 2001 11375373

Appenzeller S, Cendes F, Costallat LT: Acute psychosis in systemic lupus erythematosus. Rheumatol Int 28(3):237–243, 2008 17634902

Bachen EA, Chesney MA, Criswell LA: Prevalence of mood and anxiety disorders in women with systemic lupus erythematosus. Arthritis Rheum 61(6):822–829, 2009 19479699

Bahn RS: Graves' ophthalmopathy. N Engl J Med 362(8):726–738, 2010 20181974

Baubet T, Ranque B, Taïeb O, et al: Mood and anxiety disorders in systemic sclerosis patients. Presse Med 40(2):e111–e119, 2011 21055901

Baughman R, Lower E: Sarcoidosis, in Harrison's Principles of Internal Medicine, 19th Edition. Edited by Kasper D, Fauci A, Hauser S, et al. New York, McGraw-Hill, 2015

Beck AT, Ward CH, Mendelson M, et al: An inventory for measuring depression. Arch Gen Psychiatry 4(6):561–571, 1961 13688369

Benros ME, Nielsen PR, Nordentoft M, et al: Autoimmune diseases and severe infections as risk factors for schizophrenia: a 30-year population-based register study. Am J Psychiatry 168(12):1303–1310, 2011 22193673

Benros ME, Waltoft BL, Nordentoft M, et al: Autoimmune diseases and severe infections as risk factors for mood disorders: a nationwide study. JAMA Psychiatry 70(8):812–820, 2013 23760347

Bertsias GK, Ioannidis JP, Aringer M, et al: EULAR recommendations for the management of systemic lupus erythematosus with neuropsychiatric manifestations: report of a task force of the EULAR standing committee for clinical affairs. Ann Rheum Dis 69(12):2074–2082, 2010 20724309

Beurel E: A primer on inflammation for psychiatrists. Psychiatric Annals 45(5):226–231, 2015. Available at: https://www.healio.com/psychiatry/journals/psycann/2015-5-45-5/%7B40d227bd-b958-449e-8328-7641806ceb46%7D/a-primer-on-inflammation-for-psychiatrists. Accessed March 27, 2019.

Boston Collaborative Drug Surveillance Program: Acute adverse reactions to prednisone in relation to dosage. Clin Pharmacol Ther 13(5):694–698, 1972 5053810

Bourgeois JA, Maddock RJ, Rogers L, et al: Neurosarcoidosis and delirium. Psychosomatics 46(2):148–150, 2005 15774954

Brey RL, Holliday SL, Saklad AR, et al: Neuropsychiatric syndromes in lupus: prevalence using standardized definitions. Neurology 58(8):1214–1220, 2002 11971089

Browning CH: Nonsteroidal anti-inflammatory drugs and severe psychiatric side effects. Int J Psychiatry Med 26(1):25–34, 1996 8707453

Brownlie BE, Rae AM, Walshe JW, et al: Psychoses associated with thyrotoxicosis: "thyrotoxic psychosis." A report of 18 cases, with statistical analysis of incidence. Eur J Endocrinol 142(5):438–444, 2000 10802519

Bunevicius R, Prange AJ Jr: Psychiatric manifestations of Graves' hyperthyroidism: pathophysiology and treatment options. CNS Drugs 20(11):897–909, 2006 17044727

Bunevicius R, Kazanavicius G, Zalinkevicius R, et al: Effects of thyroxine as compared with thyroxine plus triiodothyronine in patients with hypothyroidism. N Engl J Med 340(6):424–429, 1999 9971866

Bunevicius R, Velickiene D, Prange AJ Jr: Mood and anxiety disorders in women with treated hyperthyroidism and ophthalmopathy caused by Graves' disease. Gen Hosp Psychiatry 27(2):133–139, 2005 15763125

Byrne S, Walsh C, Hacohen Y, et al: Earlier treatment of NMDAR antibody encephalitis in children results in a better outcome. Neurol Neuroimmunol Neuroinflamm 2(4):e130, 2015 26236759

Capuron L, Castanon N: Role of inflammation in the development of neuropsychiatric symptom domains: evidence and mechanisms. Curr Top Behav Neurosci 31:31–44, 2017 27221626

Carta MG, Loviselli A, Hardoy MC, et al: The link between thyroid autoimmunity (antithyroid peroxidase autoantibodies) with anxiety and mood disorders in the community: a field of interest for public health in the future. BMC Psychiatry 4:25, 2004 15317653

Carta MG, Hardoy MC, Carpiniello B, et al: A case control study on psychiatric disorders in Hashimoto disease and euthyroid goitre: not only depressive but also anxiety disorders are associated with thyroid autoimmunity. Clin Pract Epidemiol Ment Health 1:23, 2005 16285879

Caturegli P, De Remigis A, Rose NR: Hashimoto thyroiditis: clinical and diagnostic criteria. Autoimmun Rev 13(4–5):391–397, 2014 24434360

Chang B, Steimel J, Moller DR, et al: Depression in sarcoidosis. Am J Respir Crit Care Med 163(2):329–334, 2001 11179101

Chong JY, Rowland LP, Utiger RD: Hashimoto encephalopathy: syndrome or myth? Arch Neurol 60(2):164–171, 2003 12580699

Choy E, Marshall D, Gabriel ZL, et al: A systematic review and mixed treatment comparison of the efficacy of pharmacological treatments for fibromyalgia. Semin Arthritis Rheum 41(3):335–345, 2011 21868065

Coffey MJ, Cooper JJ: Electroconvulsive therapy in anti-N-methyl-D-aspartate receptor encephalitis: a case report and review of the literature. J ECT 32(4):225–229, 2016 27295461

Consoli A, Ronen K, An-Gourfinkel I, et al: Malignant catatonia due to anti-NMDA-receptor encephalitis in a 17-year-old girl: case report. Child Adolesc Psychiatry Ment Health 5(1):15, 2011 21569502

Correia N, Mullally S, Cooke G, et al: Evidence for a specific defect in hippocampal memory in overt and subclinical hypothyroidism. J Clin Endocrinol Metab 94(10):3789–3797, 2009 19584178

Covic T, Cumming SR, Pallant JF, et al: Depression and anxiety in patients with rheumatoid arthritis: prevalence rates based on a comparison of the Depression, Anxiety and Stress Scale (DASS) and the hospital, Anxiety and Depression Scale (HADS). BMC Psychiatry 12:6, 2012 22269280

Cox CE, Donohue JF, Brown CD, et al: Health-related quality of life of persons with sarcoidosis. Chest 125(3):997–1004, 2004 15006960

Cox PD, Hales RE: CNS Sjögren's syndrome: an underrecognized and underappreciated neuropsychiatric disorder. J Neuropsychiatry Clin Neurosci 11(2):241–247, 1999 10333995

Cutolo M, Nobili F, Sulli A, et al: Evidence of cerebral hypoperfusion in scleroderma patients. Rheumatology (Oxford) 39(12):1366–1373, 2000 11136880

Dall'Era M: Systemic lupus erythematosus, in Current Diagnosis and Treatment: Rheumatology, 3rd Edition. Edited by Imboden JB, Hellmann DB, Stone JH. New York, McGraw-Hill, 2013, pp 187–197

Dalmau J, Gleichman AJ, Hughes EG, et al: Anti-NMDA-receptor encephalitis: case series and analysis of the effects of antibodies. Lancet Neurol 7(12):1091–1098, 2008 18851928

Dalmau J, Lancaster E, Martinez-Hernandez E, et al: Clinical experience and laboratory investigations in patients with anti-NMDAR encephalitis. Lancet Neurol 10(1):63–74, 2011 21163445

Davis JD, Tremont G: Neuropsychiatric aspects of hypothyroidism and treatment reversibility. Minerva Endocrinol 32(1):49–65, 2007 17353866

de Kleijn WP, Drent M, De Vries J: Nature of fatigue moderates depressive symptoms and anxiety in sarcoidosis. Br J Health Psychol 18(2):439–452, 2013 22988824

Del Rosso A, Mikhaylova S, Baccini M, et al: In systemic sclerosis, anxiety and depression assessed by hospital anxiety depression scale are independently associated with disability and psychological factors. Biomed Res Int 2013:507493, 2013 23984376

Denburg SD, Denburg JA: Cognitive dysfunction and antiphospholipid antibodies in systemic lupus erythematosus. Lupus 12(12):883–890, 2003 14714906

Dowben JS, Kowalski PC, Keltner NL: Biological perspectives: anti-NMDA receptor encephalitis. Perspect Psychiatr Care 51(4):236–240, 2015 26220456

Dowlati Y, Herrmann N, Swardfager W, et al: A meta-analysis of cytokines in major depression. Biol Psychiatry 67(5):446–457, 2010 20015486

Dubovsky AN, Arvikar S, Stern TA, et al: The neuropsychiatric complications of glucocorticoid use: steroid psychosis revisited. Psychosomatics 53(2):103–115, 2012 22424158

Englbrecht M, Alten R, Aringer M, et al: Validation of standardized questionnaires evaluating symptoms of depression in rheumatoid arthritis patients: approaches to screening for a frequent yet underrated challenge. Arthritis Care Res 69(1):58–66, 2017 27482854

Evans DL, Charney DS, Lewis L, et al: Mood disorders in the medically ill: scientific review and recommendations. Biol Psychiatry 58(3):175–189, 2005 16084838

Fatourechi V, McConahey WM, Woolner LB: Hyperthyroidism associated with histologic Hashimoto's thyroiditis. Mayo Clin Proc 46(10):682–689, 1971 5171000

Finke C, Kopp UA, Prüss H, et al: Cognitive deficits following anti-NMDA receptor encephalitis. J Neurol Neurosurg Psychiatry 83(2):195–198, 2012 21933952

Florance NR, Davis RL, Lam C, et al: Anti-N-methyl-D-aspartate receptor (NMDAR) encephalitis in children and adolescents. Ann Neurol 66(1):11–18, 2009 19670433

Fountoulakis KN, Iacovides A, Grammaticos P, et al: Thyroid function in clinical subtypes of major depression: an exploratory study. BMC Psychiatry 4:6, 2004 15113438

Fox RI: Sjögren's syndrome. Lancet 366(9482):321–331, 2005 16039337

Frank RG, Kashani JH, Parker JC, et al: Antidepressant analgesia in rheumatoid arthritis. J Rheumatol 15(11):1632–1638, 1988 3236298

Gable MS, Sheriff H, Dalmau J, et al: The frequency of autoimmune N-methyl-D-aspartate receptor encephalitis surpasses that of individual viral etiologies in young individuals enrolled in the California Encephalitis Project. Clin Infect Dis 54(7):899–904, 2012 22281844

Gallagher D, Kiss A, Lanctot K, et al: Depression with inflammation: longitudinal analysis of a proposed depressive subtype in community dwelling older adults. Int J Geriatr Psychiatry 32(12):e18–e24, 2017 27911015

Garcia RJ, Francis L, Dawood M, et al: Attention deficit and hyperactivity disorder scores are elevated and respond to N-acetylcysteine treatment in patients with systemic lupus erythematosus. Arthritis Rheum 65(5):1313–1318, 2013 23400548

Giynas Ayhan M, Uguz F, Askin R, et al: The prevalence of depression and anxiety disorders in patients with euthyroid Hashimoto's thyroiditis: a comparative study. Gen Hosp Psychiatry 36(1):95–98, 2014 24211158

Goracci A, Fagiolini A, Martinucci M, et al: Quality of life, anxiety and depression in sarcoidosis. Gen Hosp Psychiatry 30(5):441–445, 2008 18774427

Granerod J, Ambrose HE, Davies NW, et al: Causes of encephalitis and differences in their clinical presentations in England: a multicentre, population-based prospective study. Lancet Infect Dis 10(12):835–844, 2010 20952256

Graus F, Titulaer MJ, Balu R, et al: A clinical approach to diagnosis of autoimmune encephalitis. Lancet Neurol 15(4):391–404, 2016 26906964

Gresa-Arribas N, Titulaer M, Torrents A, et al: Antibody titres at diagnosis and during follow-up of anti-NMDA receptor encephalitis: a retrospective study. Lancet Neurol 13(2):167–177, 2014 24360484

Hajduk A, Nowicka-Sauer K, Smoleńska Ż, et al: Prevalence and correlates of suicidal thoughts in patients with neuropsychiatric lupus. Lupus 25(2):185–192, 2016 26359173

Hanly J: The nervous system and lupus, in Systemic Lupus Erythematosus, 5th Edition. Edited by Lahita RG, Tsokos G, Buyon J, et al. San Diego, CA, Academic Press/Elsevier, 2011, pp 727–746

Hanly JG: Diagnosis and management of neuropsychiatric SLE. Nat Rev Rheumatol 10(6):338–347, 2014 24514913

Hanly JG, Su L, Urowitz MB, et al: Mood disorders in systemic lupus erythematosus: results from an international inception cohort study. Arthritis Rheumatol 67(7):1837–1847, 2015 25778456

Haroon E, Raison CL, Miller AH: Psychoneuroimmunology meets neuropsychopharmacology: translational implications of the impact of inflammation on behavior. Neuropsychopharmacology 37(1):137–162, 2012 21918508

Hietaharju A, Jääskeläinen S, Hietarinta M, et al: Central nervous system involvement and psychiatric manifestations in systemic sclerosis (scleroderma): clinical and neurophysiological evaluation. Acta Neurol Scand 87(5):382–387, 1993 8333243

Hillegers MH, Reichart CG, Wals M, et al: Signs of a higher prevalence of autoimmune thyroiditis in female offspring of bipolar parents. Eur Neuropsychopharmacol 17(6–7):394–399, 2007 17140771

Ho RC, Thiaghu C, Ong H, et al: A meta-analysis of serum and cerebrospinal fluid autoantibodies in neuropsychiatric systemic lupus erythematosus. Autoimmun Rev 15(2):124–138, 2016 26497108

Holas P, Krejtz I, Urbankowski T, et al: Anxiety, its relation to symptoms severity and anxiety sensitivity in sarcoidosis. Sarcoidosis Vasc Diffuse Lung Dis 30(4):282–288, 2013 24351619

Hsu CC, Chen SC, Liu CJ, et al: Rheumatoid arthritis and the risk of bipolar disorder: a nationwide population-based study. PLoS One 9(9):e107512, 2014 25229610

Huang X, Magder LS, Petri M: Predictors of incident depression in systemic lupus erythematosus. J Rheumatol 41(9):1823–1833, 2014 25128512

Huffman JC, Celano CM, Beach SR, et al: Depression and cardiac disease: epidemiology, mechanisms, and diagnosis. Cardiovasc Psychiatry Neurol 2013:695925, 2013 23653854

Inal V, Kitapcioglu G, Karabulut G, et al: Evaluation of quality of life in relation to anxiety and depression in primary Sjögren's syndrome. Mod Rheumatol 20(6):588–597, 2010 20585824

Ireland J, Wilsher M: Perceptions and beliefs in sarcoidosis. Sarcoidosis Vasc Diffuse Lung Dis 27(1):36–42, 2010 21086903

Irwin MR: Inflammation at the intersection of behavior and somatic symptoms. Psychiatr Clin North Am 34(3):605–620, 2011 21889682

Jacobson DL, Gange SJ, Rose NR, et al: Epidemiology and estimated population burden of selected autoimmune diseases in the United States. Clin Immunol Immunopathol 84(3):223–243, 1997 9281381

Jameson J, Mandel SJ, Weetman AP: Disorders of the thyroid gland, in Harrison's Principles of Internal Medicine, 19th Edition. Edited by Kasper D, Fauci A, Hauser S, et al. New York, McGraw-Hill, 2015, pp 2303–2305

Jamshidi AR, Banihashemi AT, Paragomi P, et al: Anxiety and depression in rheumatoid arthritis: an epidemiologic survey and investigation of clinical correlates in Iranian population. Rheumatol Int 36(8):1119–1125, 2016 27193469

Jeltsch-David H, Muller S: Neuropsychiatric systemic lupus erythematosus: pathogenesis and biomarkers. Nat Rev Neurol 10(10):579–596, 2014 25201240

Joaquim AF, Appenzeller S: Neuropsychiatric manifestations in rheumatoid arthritis. Autoimmun Rev 14(12):1116–1122, 2015 26238502

Kappelmann N, Lewis G, Dantzer R, et al: Antidepressant activity of anti-cytokine treatment: a systematic review and meta-analysis of clinical trials of chronic inflammatory conditions. Mol Psychiatry 23(2):335–343, 2018 27752078

Karageorgas T, Fragioudaki S, Nezos A, et al: Fatigue in primary Sjogren's syndrome: clinical, laboratory, psychometric, and biologic associations. Arthritis Care Res (Hoboken) 68(1):123–131, 2016 26315379

Karol DE, Criscione-Schreiber LG, Lin M, et al: Depressive symptoms and associated factors in systemic lupus erythematosus. Psychosomatics 54(5):443–450, 2013 23274009

Kathol RG, Turner R, Delahunt J: Depression and anxiety associated with hyperthyroidism: response to antithyroid therapy. Psychosomatics 27(7):501–505, 1986 3737839

Kayser MS, Titulaer MJ, Gresa-Arribas N, et al: Frequency and characteristics of isolated psychiatric episodes in anti–N-methyl-D-aspartate receptor encephalitis. JAMA Neurol 70(9):1133–1139, 2013 23877059

Kessler RC, Petukhova M, Sampson NA, et al: Twelve-month and lifetime prevalence and lifetime morbid risk of anxiety and mood disorders in the United States. Int J Methods Psychiatr Res 21(3):169–184, 2012 22865617

Khanna D: Diagnosis and treatment of systemic and localized scleroderma. Expert Rev Dermatol 6(3):287–302, 2011

Kirshner HS: Hashimoto's encephalopathy: a brief review. Curr Neurol Neurosci Rep 14(9):476, 2014 25027262

Kivity S, Agmon-Levin N, Zandman-Goddard G, et al: Neuropsychiatric lupus: a mosaic of clinical presentations. BMC Med 13:43, 2015 25858312

Knittle K, Maes S, de Gucht V: Psychological interventions for rheumatoid arthritis: examining the role of self-regulation with a systematic review and meta-analysis of randomized controlled trials. Arthritis Care Res (Hoboken) 62(10):1460–1472, 2010 20506175

Koçer B, Tezcan ME, Batur HZ, et al: Cognition, depression, fatigue, and quality of life in primary Sjögren's syndrome: correlations. Brain Behav 6(12):e00586, 2016 28032007

Kohen M, Asherson RA, Gharavi AE, et al: Lupus psychosis: differentiation from the steroid-induced state. Clin Exp Rheumatol 11(3):323–326, 1993 8353989

Köhler O, Benros ME, Nordentoft M, et al: Effect of anti-inflammatory treatment on depression, depressive symptoms, and adverse effects: a systematic review and meta-analysis of randomized clinical trials. JAMA Psychiatry 71(12):1381–1391, 2014 25322082

Kupka RW, Nolen WA, Post RM, et al: High rate of autoimmune thyroiditis in bipolar disorder: lack of association with lithium exposure. Biol Psychiatry 51(4):305–311, 2002 11958781

Kuppuswamy PS, Takala CR, Sola CL: Management of psychiatric symptoms in anti-NMDAR encephalitis: a case series, literature review and future directions. Gen Hosp Psychiatry 36(4):388–391, 2014 24731834

Lawson LJ, Perry VH, Gordon S: Turnover of resident microglia in the normal adult mouse brain. Neuroscience 48(2):405–415, 1992 1603325

Lejuste F, Thomas L, Picard G, et al: Neuroleptic intolerance in patients with anti-NMDAR encephalitis. Neurol Neuroimmunol Neuroinflamm 3(5):e280, 2016 27606355

Leu SJ, Yang YY, Liu HC, et al: Valproic acid and lithium mediate anti-inflammatory effects by differentially modulating dendritic cell differentiation and function. J Cell Physiol 232(5):1176–1186, 2017 27639185

Leyhe T, Müssig K, Weinert C, et al: Increased occurrence of weaknesses in attention testing in patients with Hashimoto's thyroiditis compared to patients with other thyroid illnesses. Psychoneuroendocrinology 33(10):1432–1436, 2008 18819753

Lin CE: One patient with Sjogren's syndrome presenting schizophrenia-like symptoms. Neuropsychiatr Dis Treat 12:661–663, 2016 27042076

Lin YR, Chou LC, Chen HC, et al: Increased risk of dementia in patients with systemic lupus erythematosus: a nationwide population-based cohort study. Arthritis Care Res (Hoboken) 68(12):1774–1779, 2016 27111329

Lok EY, Mok CC, Cheng CW, et al: Prevalence and determinants of psychiatric disorders in patients with rheumatoid arthritis. Psychosomatics 51(4):338, 2010 20587762

Lorig KR, Ritter PL, Laurent DD, et al: The Internet-based arthritis self-management program: a one-year randomized trial for patients with arthritis or fibromyalgia. Arthritis Rheum 59(7):1009–1017, 2008 18576310

Magro-Checa C, Zirkzee EJ, Huizinga TW, et al: Management of neuropsychiatric systemic lupus erythematosus: current approaches and future perspectives. Drugs 76(4):459–483, 2016 26809245

Maneta E, Garcia G: Psychiatric manifestations of anti-NMDA receptor encephalitis: neurobiological underpinnings and differential diagnostic implications. Psychosomatics 55(1):37–44, 2014 23932531

Markeljevic J, Sarac H, Bozina N, et al: Serotonin transporter gene polymorphisms: relation with platelet serotonin level in patients with primary Sjogren's syndrome. J Neuroimmunol 282:104–109, 2015 25903736

Matcham F, Rayner L, Steer S, et al: The prevalence of depression in rheumatoid arthritis: a systematic review and meta-analysis. Rheumatology (Oxford) 52(12):2136–2148, 2013 24003249

Matcham F, Norton S, Scott DL, et al: Symptoms of depression and anxiety predict treatment response and long-term physical health outcomes in rheumatoid arthritis: secondary analysis of a randomized controlled trial. Rheumatology (Oxford) 55(2):268–278, 2016 26350486

Menconi F, Marcocci C, Marinò M: Diagnosis and classification of Graves' disease. Autoimmun Rev 13(4–5):398–402, 2014 24424182

Miller AH, Maletic V, Raison CL: Inflammation and its discontents: the role of cytokines in the pathophysiology of major depression. Biol Psychiatry 65(9):732–741, 2009 19150053

Miller BJ, Buckley P, Seabolt W, et al: Meta-analysis of cytokine alterations in schizophrenia: clinical status and antipsychotic effects. Biol Psychiatry 70(7):663–671, 2011 21641581

Miller KJ, Parsons TD, Whybrow PC, et al: Verbal memory retrieval deficits associated with untreated hypothyroidism. J Neuropsychiatry Clin Neurosci 19(2):132–136, 2007 17431058

Modabbernia A, Taslimi S, Brietzke E, et al: Cytokine alterations in bipolar disorder: a meta-analysis of 30 studies. Biol Psychiatry 74(1):15–25, 2013 23419545

Mok CC, Chan KL, Cheung EF, et al: Suicidal ideation in patients with systemic lupus erythematosus: incidence and risk factors. Rheumatology (Oxford) 53(4):714–721, 2014 24361695

Mooradian AD: Asymptomatic hyperthyroidism in older adults: is it a distinct clinical and laboratory entity? Drugs Aging 25(5):371–380, 2008 18447402

Morreale M, Marchione P, Giacomini P, et al: Neurological involvement in primary Sjögren syndrome: a focus on central nervous system. PLoS One 9(1):e84605, 2014 24465419

Moutsopoulos HM, Tzioufas AG: Sjögren's syndrome, in Harrison's Principles of Internal Medicine, 19th Edition. Edited by Kasper D, Fauci A, Hauser S, et al. New York, McGraw-Hill, 2015, p 383

Müller N, Weidinger E, Leitner B, et al: The role of inflammation in schizophrenia. Front Neurosci 9(372):372, 2015 26539073

Musselman DL, Nemeroff CB: Depression and endocrine disorders: focus on the thyroid and adrenal system. Br J Psychiatry Suppl 30(30):123–128, 1996 8864158

Musselman DL, Lawson DH, Gumnick JF, et al: Paroxetine for the prevention of depression induced by high-dose interferon alfa. N Engl J Med 344(13):961–966, 2001 11274622

Nabhan ZM, Kreher NC, Eugster EA: Hashitoxicosis in children: clinical features and natural history. J Pediatr 146(4):533–536, 2005 15812459

Navarrete-Navarrete N, Peralta-Ramírez MI, Sabio-Sánchez JM, et al: Efficacy of cognitive behavioural therapy for the treatment of chronic stress in patients with lupus erythematosus: a randomized controlled trial. Psychother Psychosom 79(2):107–115, 2010 20090397

Nemeroff CB, Simon JS, Haggerty JJ Jr, et al: Antithyroid antibodies in depressed patients. Am J Psychiatry 142(7):840–843, 1985 4014506

Nozaki K, Judson MA: Neurosarcoidosis: clinical manifestations, diagnosis and treatment. Presse Med 41(6 Pt 2):e331–e348, 2012 22595777

Olmez I, Moses H, Sriram S, et al: Diagnostic and therapeutic aspects of Hashimoto's encephalopathy. J Neurol Sci 331(1–2):67–71, 2013 23759502

Oomen HA, Schipperijn AJ, Drexhage HA: The prevalence of affective disorder and in particular of a rapid cycling of bipolar disorder in patients with abnormal thyroid function tests. Clin Endocrinol (Oxf) 45(2):215–223, 1996 8881455

Pego-Reigosa JM, Isenberg DA: Psychosis due to systemic lupus erythematosus: characteristics and long-term outcome of this rare manifestation of the disease. Rheumatology (Oxford) 47(10):1498–1502, 2008 18658205

Pelizza L, Bonacini F, Ferrari A: Psychiatric disorder as clinical presentation of primary Sjögren's syndrome: two case reports. Ann Gen Psychiatry 9:12, 2010 20356417

Piga M, Serra A, Deiana L, et al: Brain perfusion abnormalities in patients with euthyroid auto-immune thyroiditis. Eur J Nucl Med Mol Imaging 31(12):1639–1644, 2004 15290119

Radloff LS: The CES-D scale: a self report depression scale for research in the general population. Applied Psychological Measurement 1(3):385 401, 1977. Available at: https://journals.sagepub.com/doi/10.1177/014662167700100306. Accessed August 28, 2019.

Raison CL, Miller AH: Depression in cancer: new developments regarding diagnosis and treatment. Biol Psychiatry 54(3):283–294, 2003 12893104

Raison CL, Borisov AS, Broadwell SD, et al: Depression during pegylated interferon-alpha plus ribavirin therapy: prevalence and prediction. J Clin Psychiatry 66(1):41–48, 2005 15669887

Raison CL, Rutherford RE, Woolwine BJ, et al: A randomized controlled trial of the tumor necrosis factor antagonist infliximab for treatment-resistant depression: the role of baseline inflammatory biomarkers. JAMA Psychiatry 70(1):31–41, 2013 22945416

Rathbun AM, Reed GW, Harrold LR: The temporal relationship between depression and rheumatoid arthritis disease activity, treatment persistence and response: a systematic review. Rheumatology (Oxf) 52(10):1785–1794, 2013 23236191

Santiago T, Geenen R, Jacobs JW, et al: Psychological factors associated with response to treatment in rheumatoid arthritis. Curr Pharm Des 21(2):257–269, 2015 25163734

Saravanan P, Chau WF, Roberts N, et al: Psychological well-being in patients on "adequate" doses of l-thyroxine: results of a large, controlled community-based questionnaire study. Clin Endocrinol (Oxf) 57(5):577–585, 2002 12390330

Schiess N, Pardo CA: Hashimoto's encephalopathy. Ann N Y Acad Sci 1142:254–265, 2008 18990131

Schmitt SE, Pargeon K, Frechette ES, et al: Extreme delta brush: a unique EEG pattern in adults with anti-NMDA receptor encephalitis. Neurology 79(11):1094–1100, 2012 22933737

Schuff K, Samuels M, Whybrow P, et al: Psychiatric and cognitive effects of hypothyroidism, in Werner and Ingbar's The Thyroid: A Fundamental and Clinical Text, 10th Edition. Edited by Braverman L, Cooper D. Philadelphia, PA, Lippincott Williams & Wilkins, 2013, pp 596–599

Schwartz TL, Sachdeva S, Stahl SM: Glutamate neurocircuitry: theoretical underpinnings in schizophrenia. Front Pharmacol 3(3):195, 2012 23189055

Shah A, St. Clair E: Rheumatoid arthritis, in Harrison's Principles of Internal Medicine, 19th Edition. Edited by Kasper D, Fauci A, Hauser S, et al. New York, McGraw-Hill, 2015, pp 2136–2149

Shah R, Roberson GH, Curé JK: Correlation of MR imaging findings and clinical manifestations in neurosarcoidosis. AJNR Am J Neuroradiol 30(5):953–961, 2009 19193748

Shen CC, Yang AC, Kuo BI, et al: Risk of psychiatric disorders following primary Sjögren syndrome: a nationwide population-based retrospective cohort study. J Rheumatol 42(7):1203–1208, 2015 25979721

Shin SY, Katz P, Wallhagen M, et al: Cognitive impairment in persons with rheumatoid arthritis. Arthritis Care Res (Hoboken) 64(8):1144–1150, 2012 22505279

Siegmann EM, Müller HHO, Luecke C, et al: Association of depression and anxiety disorders with autoimmune thyroiditis: a systematic review and meta-analysis. JAMA Psychiatry 75(6):577–584, 2018 29800939

Slattery MJ, Dubbert BK, Allen AJ, et al: Prevalence of obsessive-compulsive disorder in patients with systemic lupus erythematosus. J Clin Psychiatry 65(3):301–306, 2004 15096067

Slaughter JR, Parker JC, Martens MP, et al: Clinical outcomes following a trial of sertraline in rheumatoid arthritis. Psychosomatics 43(1):36–41, 2002 11927756

Smolen JS, Aletaha D, McInnes IB: Rheumatoid arthritis. Lancet 388(10055):2023–2038, 2016 27156434

Steenen SA, van Wijk AJ, van der Heijden GJ, et al: Propranolol for the treatment of anxiety disorders: systematic review and meta-analysis. J Psychopharmacol 30(2):128–139, 2016 26487439

Steiner J, Walter M, Glanz W, et al: Increased prevalence of diverse N-methyl-D-aspartate glutamate receptor antibodies in patients with an initial diagnosis of schizophrenia: specific relevance of IgG NR1a antibodies for distinction from N-methyl-D-aspartate glutamate receptor encephalitis. JAMA Psychiatry 70(3):271–278, 2013 23344076

Stern BJ, Krumholz A, Johns C, et al: Sarcoidosis and its neurological manifestations. Arch Neurol 42(9):909–917, 1985 3896208

Stern RA, Robinson B, Thorner AR, et al: A survey study of neuropsychiatric complaints in patients with Graves' disease. J Neuropsychiatry Clin Neurosci 8(2):181–185, 1996 9081554

Stevenson J, Dickens C, Irwin M: Rheumatology, in Clinical Manual of Psychopharmacology in the Medically Ill, 2nd Edition. Edited by Levenson J, Ferrand S. Washington, DC, American Psychiatric Association Publishing, 2016, pp 555–560

Strawbridge R, Arnone D, Danese A, et al: Inflammation and clinical response to treatment in depression: a meta-analysis. Eur Neuropsychopharmacol 25(10):1532–1543, 2015 26169573

Sturgeon JA, Finan PH, Zautra AJ: Affective disturbance in rheumatoid arthritis: psychological and disease-related pathways. Nat Rev Rheumatol 12(9):532–542, 2016 27411910

Thombs BD, Taillefer SS, Hudson M, et al: Depression in patients with systemic sclerosis: a systematic review of the evidence. Arthritis Rheum 57(6):1089–1097, 2007 17665491

Timonen M, Viilo K, Hakko H, et al: Suicides in persons suffering from rheumatoid arthritis. Rheumatology (Oxford) 42(2):287–291, 2003 12595624

Titulaer MJ, McCracken L, Gabilondo I, et al: Treatment and prognostic factors for long-term outcome in patients with anti-NMDA receptor encephalitis: an observational cohort study. Lancet Neurol 12(2):157–165, 2013 23290630

Turjanski N, Lloyd G: Psychiatric side-effects of medications: recent developments. Adv Psychiatr Treat 11(1):58–70, 2005

Tüzün E, Dalmau J: Limbic encephalitis and variants: classification, diagnosis and treatment. Neurologist 13(5):261–271, 2007 17848866

Trzepacz PT, McCue M, Klein I, et al: Psychiatric and neuropsychological response to propranolol in Graves' disease. Biol Psychiatry 23(7):678–688, 1988a 3370265

Trzepacz PT, McCue M, Klein I, et al: A psychiatric and neuropsychological study of patients with untreated Graves' disease. Gen Hosp Psychiatry 10(1):49–55, 1988b 3345907

Uguz F, Akman C, Kucuksarac S, et al: Anti-tumor necrosis factor-alpha therapy is associated with less frequent mood and anxiety disorders in patients with rheumatoid arthritis. Psychiatry Clin Neurosci 63(1):50–55, 2009 19154212

Uguz F, Kucuk A, Cicek E, et al: Mood, anxiety and personality disorders in patients with systemic lupus erythematosus. Compr Psychiatry 54(4):341–345, 2013 23246099

Unterman A, Nolte JE, Boaz M, et al: Neuropsychiatric syndromes in systemic lupus erythematosus: a meta-analysis. Semin Arthritis Rheum 41(1):1–11, 2011 20965549

Valeyre D, Prasse A, Nunes H, et al: Sarcoidosis. Lancet 383(9923):1155–1167, 2014 24090799

Varga J: Systemic sclerosis (scleroderma) and related disorders, in Harrison's Principles of Internal Medicine, 19th Edition. Edited by Kasper D, Fauci A, Hauser S, et al. New York, McGraw-Hill, 2015, pp 2154–2165

Vogel A, Elberling TV, Hørding M, et al: Affective symptoms and cognitive functions in the acute phase of Graves' thyrotoxicosis. Psychoneuroendocrinology 32(1):36–43, 2007 17097812

Wan KH, Chen LJ, Young AL: Depression and anxiety in dry eye disease: a systematic review and meta-analysis. Eye (Lond) 30(12):1558–1567, 2016 27518547

Wang H: Efficacies of treatments for anti-NMDA receptor encephalitis. Front Biosci 21:651–663, 2016 26709797

Warren N, Siskind D, O'Gorman C: Refining the psychiatric syndrome of anti-N-methyl-D-aspartate receptor encephalitis. Acta Psychiatr Scand 138(5):401–408, 2018 29992532

Wasniewska M, Corrias A, Salerno M, et al: Outcomes of children with hashitoxicosis. Horm Res Paediatr 77(1):36–40, 2012 22286076

Westhout FD, Linskey ME: Obstructive hydrocephalus and progressive psychosis: rare presentations of neurosarcoidosis. Surg Neurol 69(3):288–292, discussion 292, 2008 17976699

Wolfe F, Michaud K, Li T, et al: Chronic conditions and health problems in rheumatic diseases: comparisons with rheumatoid arthritis, noninflammatory rheumatic disorders, systemic lupus erythematosus, and fibromyalgia. J Rheumatol 37(2):305–315, 2010 20080915

Wong JK, Nortley R, Andrews T, et al: Psychiatric manifestations of primary Sjögren's syndrome: a case report and literature review. BMJ Case Rep 2014:bcr2012008038, 2014 24859541

Wyszynski AA, Wyszynski B: Treatment of depression with fluoxetine in corticosteroid-dependent central nervous system Sjögren's syndrome. Psychosomatics 34(2):173–177, 1993 8456162

Yoshimura R, Hori H, Ikenouchi-Sugita A, et al: Higher plasma interleukin-6 (IL-6) level is associated with SSRI- or SNRI-refractory depression. Prog Neuropsychopharmacol Biol Psychiatry 33(4):722–726, 2009 19332097

Zandman-Goddard G, Chapman J, Shoenfeld Y: Autoantibodies involved in neuropsychiatric SLE and antiphospholipid syndrome. Semin Arthritis Rheum 36(5):297–315, 2007 17258299

Zautra AJ, Davis MC, Reich JW, et al: Comparison of cognitive behavioral and mindfulness meditation interventions on adaptation to rheumatoid arthritis for patients with and without history of recurrent depression. J Consult Clin Psychol 76(3):408–421, 2008 18540734

Zhang L, Wu MQ, Hao ZL, et al: Clinical characteristics, treatments, and outcomes of patients with anti-N-methyl-D-aspartate receptor encephalitis: a systematic review of reported cases. Epilepsy Behav 68:57–65, 2017 28109991

Zigmond AS, Snaith RP: The hospital anxiety and depression scale. Acta Psychiatr Scand 67(6):361–370, 1983 29992532

Infectious Diseases and Their Psychiatric Manifestations

Oliver Freudenreich, M.D.
Kevin M. Donnelly-Boylen, M.D.
Rajesh T. Gandhi, M.D.

In this chapter, we review selected infectious agents relevant for psychiatrists practicing in the United States, with emphasis on neuropsychiatric presentations and aspects of psychiatric management. We highlight those infections that psychiatrists need to recognize because they are deadly if untreated (e.g., meningitis), they are common (e.g., pneumonia), or psychiatrists are routinely involved in their management due to significant psychiatric comorbidity (e.g., HIV, hepatitis C virus). Certain infections (e.g., Lyme disease) have neuropsychiatric sequelae that frequently lead to a psychiatric referral. For each infection, we delineate the roles psychiatrists can play in public health prevention efforts to control infections (e.g., risk reduction education and screening), we emphasize issues related to diagnostic referrals, and we outline approaches to optimizing medical treatment by addressing psychiatric obstacles to treatment of infectious diseases (e.g., nonadherence). Whereas in our global world any psychiatrist might encounter tropical infections and might even play a role in managing the psychological ramifications of an epidemic with an emerging agent, this chapter is neither a comprehensive listing of infections nor a guide for psychiatrists about diagnosing and treating infections that will usually fall under the purview of medicine. Excellent web-based resources are available for up-to-date information about infectious diseases (Table 9–1).

TABLE 9–1.   **Web-based resources for infectious diseases**

General information
   Centers for Disease Control and Prevention (CDC): www.cdc.gov
Viral hepatitis
   Veterans Administration viral hepatitis site: www.hepatitis.va.gov
HIV
   The Body Pro: www.thebodypro.com
   AIDSinfo: aidsinfo.nih.gov
   HIVInSite: hivinsite.ucsf.edu
   University of Liverpool HIV drug interactions site: www.hiv-druginteractions.org
Vaccinations
   Advisory Committee on Immunization Practices: www.cdc.gov/vaccines/acip
International travel
   Heading Home Healthy Program: www.headinghomehealthy.org
Practice guidelines
   Infectious Diseases of America (IDSA): www.idsociety.org

Infectious Disease Emergencies

Any psychiatrist, regardless of practice setting, might encounter a patient with seemingly psychiatric symptoms (e.g., depression, anxiety, fatigue) who instead has a potentially life-threatening infection. In typical cases, classic signs of infection (e.g., fever and malaise) will be clues to an infectious etiology of the patient's neuropsychiatric symptoms. In our global world, usual presentations in unusual places are easily missed (e.g., malaria manifesting with psychosis in an urban hospital in the United States).

A careful history (including a travel history and onset of illness), vital signs, a physical examination, and a cognitive examination focused on memory and attention followed by appropriate tests should lead to a diagnosis in most cases. However, a high index of suspicion is needed with patients in whom signs of infection might be obscured (e.g., patients on steroids, elderly patients with multiple comorbidities, patients referred by another physician who are believed to be medically stable) or from whom a history is difficult to obtain (e.g., because of language barriers, serious psychiatric symptoms such as psychosis or agitation, or limited symptom reporting due to negative symptoms).

Sepsis

Sepsis is a clinical syndrome of organ dysfunction that results from a dysregulated inflammatory response to an infection (Howell and Davis 2017). Although almost any type of infection can cause sepsis, respiratory and genitourinary infections are among the syndrome's major causes. The pathophysiology of sepsis includes the release of proinflammatory cytokines and blood-brain barrier disruption that can result in a delirium. The neuropsychiatric symptoms are thus not the result of a direct brain infection. Psychiatrists working in general hospitals are often involved in managing sepsis-associated delirium, which occurs in up to 70% of patients with severe systemic infection (Gofton and Young 2012).

Meningitis and Encephalitis

Bacterial meningitis is a serious infection that can be fatal if untreated. Delayed treatment can also lead to permanent neuropsychiatric sequelae (e.g., hearing loss, focal neurological deficits). Classic symptoms and signs of acute meningitis include headache, photophobia, nausea, vomiting, fever, and a stiff neck. Confusion is often present. Seizures are a late complication and an ominous prognostic sign. *Neisseria meningitidis* and *Streptococcus pneumoniae* are common causes of meningitis in adolescents and young adults; *N. meningitidis* can cause outbreaks in colleges and other institutional settings. Individuals who have been in close contact with a person with meningococcal meningitis may benefit from prophylactic antibiotics. In older adults, *Listeria monocytogenes* is an important, if at times cryptic, cause of bacterial meningitis. Listeriosis is a food-borne infection that usually manifests as a self-limited diarrheal illness with general malaise but can lead to meningitis in vulnerable individuals (e.g., immunocompromised or elderly hosts). Clouding of consciousness and neurological symptoms consistent with brain stem involvement (e.g., cranial nerve deficits) are typical; nuchal rigidity is less pronounced.

Encephalitis is usually caused by a viral infection that ranges in severity from asymptomatic to life threatening. Mild encephalitis may manifest as a flulike illness that lasts 2 or 3 weeks. Neuropsychiatric manifestations include headache, light sensitivity, unsteady gait, seizures, paralysis, delirium, and psychosis. Depending on the agent, severe encephalitis can leave the affected patient permanently neurologically damaged. Important causes of encephalitis include herpes simplex virus (HSV), varicella zoster virus, enteroviruses, arboviruses, and HIV. Season and geography play major roles in the risk for mosquito- or tick-borne causes of encephalitis.

Herpes simplex virus type 1 (HSV-1) is a common cause of encephalitis in adults. Infection occurs from a peripheral site by direct neural transmission. Following a prodrome of malaise, fever, and headache, patients may present with seizures or neuropsychiatric symptoms, including confusion, memory problems, and, at times, psychosis. Prompt treatment with intravenous acyclovir is effective in reducing mortality and neuropsychiatric sequelae. Untreated, herpes encephalitis has a mortality rate of 70% and in survivors often results in severe neurological deficits (Whitley et al. 1977). Treatment reduces mortality to 20% or 30%, but neurological sequelae may still occur. Because HSV-1 has a predilection for the temporal lobes, anterograde amnesia is a common complication.

In the United States, West Nile virus (WNV) is an important cause of mosquito-borne encephalitis. First described in the United States in 1999, WNV has since been seen in most states. The vast majority of infections are asymptomatic or mild and self-limited, but meningoencephalitis and an acute flaccid limb paralysis due to anterior poliomyelitis are possible complications of neuroinvasive disease (Kramer et al. 2007). The rare patient who develops encephalitis may fully recover, although permanent damage or death can occur. By contrast, Eastern equine encephalitis has a mortality rate of 30% or more, depending on the case series, and causes neurological damage in the majority of survivors (Silverman et al. 2013). Prevention of mosquito bites in endemic areas is critical.

Epidemics

Infectious agents with high case fatality rates have the potential to reach the United States. Even a few cases of such infections have a major impact on populations, not just because of actual deaths but because of their psychological effects. A case in point was the 2014 Ebola outbreak in West Africa that garnered extensive news coverage and stirred much anxiety and uncertainty in the United States, even though only four cases were diagnosed here (Centers for Disease Control and Prevention 2019a). Middle East respiratory syndrome (Arabi et al. 2017) and severe acute respiratory syndrome (Liang et al. 2004) are examples of lung infections with the potential to cause devastating epidemics, thus requiring substantial societal resources to prevent their spread and to manage the psychological ramifications in affected communities (Wu et al. 2009).

Some psychiatrists play a role in disaster preparedness to address the psychological aspects of managing large populations affected by an epidemic. Even if not directly affected by an epidemic and infection-control measures, many patients will ask about their personal risk, and psychiatrists can provide accurate information. Quarantine measures pose ethical and practical challenges that need to be collectively resolved (Folayan et al. 2016; Parmet 2007).

Pulmonary Infections

Lung infections are a major source of morbidity and mortality in the United States, accounting for 40% of deaths from infectious diseases (Hansen et al. 2016). In patients with schizophrenia, lung infections are the third leading cause of death after cardiovascular disease and cancer (Olfson et al. 2015), in part due to delayed treatment and exacerbation by high rates of tobacco use in patients with serious mental illness. Armed with an awareness of this risk, psychiatrists can ensure that such patients are referred for rapid assessment of possible pneumonia. In addition, psychiatrists can provide important education about the risks and benefits of vaccinations and assist primary care providers in vaccination campaigns, including those for the annual influenza vaccine. Misinformation, unfounded fears, complacency, and inconvenience all are factors that can lead to insufficient vaccination rates (Schmid et al. 2017).

Pneumonia

The most common etiologies of community-acquired pneumonia (CAP) are bacterial (e.g., *Streptococcus, Haemophilus, Moraxella*) and viral (e.g., rhinovirus, influenza) (Jain et al. 2015). Typical bacterial CAP manifests with fever, productive cough, dyspnea, and pleuritic chest pain. On examination, tachypnea is present, and rales can be heard over the affected lung segments. Atypical bacterial pneumonia may be caused by *Legionella spp., Mycoplasma pneumoniae,* or *Chlamydia pneumoniae.* In some cases, underlying illnesses can help determine likely pathogens. Patients with chronic obstructive pulmonary disease are at risk for *Streptococcus pneumoniae* and *Moraxella,* whereas patients with alcohol use disorder are at risk for *Klebsiella*. However, no constellation of symptoms and signs allows for a clinical diagnosis; a medical workup is required.

Aspiration pneumonia due to impaired swallowing is an often-missed cause of recurrent pneumonia. Many psychiatric patients have swallowing difficulties from a variety of causes. Patients on clozapine might be a particular risk group that is over-looked (Stoecker et al. 2017). Clozapine impairs deglutition and reduces the number of times a patient swallows, which causes a paradoxical (because clozapine is very anticholinergic) sialorrhea that is most pronounced at night. Unfortunately, treatment of clozapine-induced sialorrhea with dosage reduction or anticholinergic medications is often only partially effective; glycopyrrolate at night might be the best option (Man et al. 2017).

Unless delirium, sepsis, or meningitis is present, patients with uncomplicated pneumonia usually do not present neuropsychiatrically. However, systemic infections, including pneumonia, can induce cytokine-mediated adaptive sickness behaviors, including lethargy and withdrawal (Dantzer et al. 2008). Patients manifesting such behaviors can be misdiagnosed as depressed if the symptoms and signs of pneumonia are mild or overlooked.

Seasonal Influenza

Influenza viruses A and B usually cause outbreaks during the winter season. Influenza A is further subtyped based on two surface proteins, hemagglutinin (H) and neuraminidase (N). Influenza A in particular has the potential to cause pandemics with high morbidity and mortality. It has caused three pandemics since the early twentieth century: the 1918 H1N1 "Spanish flu" pandemic, the 1957 H2N2 pandemic, and the 1968 H3N2 pandemic. The Spanish flu pandemic caused 546,000 excess deaths in the United States and about 50 million deaths worldwide. In 2009, a new H1N1 strain caused the first pandemic in several decades (Cheng et al. 2012). The most common central nervous system (CNS) complication of influenza is febrile seizures in children; in rare cases, influenza causes acute encephalitis. Postencephalitic complications, including parkinsonism, have been linked to the Spanish flu.

A seasonal trivalent flu vaccine is updated annually and protects against circulating influenza A and B isolates. Since 2010, the U.S. Centers for Disease Control and Prevention (CDC) has recommended universal flu vaccination (Centers for Disease Control and Prevention 2019f). Vaccination should begin as early as October. The antiviral agents oseltamivir and zanamivir have some efficacy in treating influenza and in postexposure chemoprophylaxis.

Tuberculosis

With one-third of the world population infected, tuberculosis remains a major scourge of mankind. Globally, drug resistance has been increasing and is a substantial concern. In the United States, about 10,000 new tuberculosis cases are reported annually (Centers for Disease Control and Prevention 2019e), most of them in immigrants and in HIV-infected patients.

The clinical manifestations of tuberculosis can be understood as the immune system's attempt to eliminate or isolate mycobacteria. During latent tuberculosis infection (LTBI), a balance between interleukin-1 and type I interferons keeps the growth of mycobacteria in check (Friedland 2014). The fact that tuberculosis is merely contained by the immune system in LTBI explains tuberculosis reactivation in patients with an impaired immune system (e.g., due to chemotherapy for cancer, treatment with tumor necrosis factor-α [TNF-α]-blocking agents, or HIV infection). Patients with LTBI are asymptomatic, do not have pulmonary infiltrates on chest radiography, and are not infectious. Approximately 10% of infected patients will develop active tuberculosis over their lifetime; about half of those who develop active tuberculosis do so within the first 2 years after infection (LoBue and Mermin 2017). The decision of whether to treat LTBI is based on weighing the risks and benefits. The cardinal symptoms of active pulmonary tuberculosis are weight loss, fever, and cough. However, tuberculosis can disseminate into any organ, leading to extrapulmonary, organ-specific symptoms. A systemic illness, miliary tuberculosis, occurs because of a failure to contain the organism. CNS involvement includes tuberculous meningitis or tuberculomas in 1% of tuberculosis cases (Be et al. 2009) (Table 9–2). CNS tuberculosis should be considered if patients present with symptoms and signs of space-occupying lesions, increased intracranial pressure, mental status changes, or meningismus. In more severe cases, symptoms can include focal neurological deficits, cranial nerve abnormalities, or changes in level of consciousness.

Populations at clinically high risk for possible tuberculosis include patients with symptoms of tuberculosis, patients who have had exposure to tuberculosis (including certain immigrant populations), and patients with medical risk factors (e.g., HIV) or social risk factors (e.g., homelessness, poverty, alcoholism, drug use, incarceration). The Mantoux tuberculin skin test is used for screening, but increasingly patients are being tested for tuberculosis infection using interferon-γ release assays (IGRAs). IGRAs measure interferon-γ release after T-cell stimulation in response to tuberculosis-specific antigens. A positive screening test merely signifies the presence of tuberculosis infection, not necessarily active disease. Patients who screen positive require a physical examination and chest radiography to differentiate between latent and active pulmonary tuberculosis. Conversely, patients with active tuberculosis may have a negative tuberculin skin test or IGRA, so negative results of these tests should not be interpreted as excluding tuberculosis.

Treatment of tuberculosis is prolonged due to the sturdy nature of *Mycobacterium*, which divides slowly and is protected by a cell wall. Treatment relies on multidrug regimens that have to be taken over lengthy periods of time. Multidrug resistance (MDR)—defined as drug resistance to the standard agents isoniazid and rifampin—and extensive drug resistance (XDR)—MDR plus additional resistance to any fluoroquinolone and at least one of the three injectable second-line drugs (i.e., amikacin, kanamycin, or capreomycin)—are major concerns. Only two new drugs, bedaquiline and pretomanid, have been approved in recent years. The standard treatment for LTBI includes a 9-month course of isoniazid or a 4-month course of rifampin. A shorter-course regimen of isoniazid and rifapentine, sometimes given as directly observed therapy, is also effective (McClintock et al. 2017). Antimycobacterial drugs may cause psychiatric side effects and drug-drug interactions (Tables 9–3 and 9–4). Rifampin, in particular, is a potent pan-inducer of cytochrome P450 (CYP) enzymes (Doherty et al. 2013).

TABLE 9–2.	Central nervous system manifestations of tuberculosis

Intracranial

Tuberculous meningitis

Tuberculous encephalopathy

Tuberculous vasculopathy

Central nervous system tuberculoma (single or multiple)

Tuberculous brain abscess

Spinal

Pott's disease (vertebral osteomyelitis due to tuberculosis)

Non-osseous spinal tuberculoma

Source. Adapted from Cherian A, Thomas SV: "Central Nervous System Tuberculosis." *African Health Sciences* 11(1):116–127, 2011.

TABLE 9–3.	Selected drug-drug interactions between psychotropics and antibiotics/antivirals

Pharmacodynamic

Serotonin syndrome: linezolid added to SSRIs

Bone marrow suppression: trimethoprim/sulfamethoxazole added to clozapine

QTc prolongation: fluoroquinolones or macrolides added to ziprasidone

Pharmacokinetic

Erythromycin: increased clozapine levels from CYP3A4 inhibition

Rifampin: decreased psychotropic drug levels from CYP pan-induction

Antiretroviral drugs (ritonavir, other protease inhibitors, cobicistat): increased psychotropic drug levels from CYP3A4 inhibition

Note. CYP=cytochrome P450; SSRIs=selective serotonin reuptake inhibitors.

TABLE 9–4.	Severe psychiatric side effects of selected antibiotics/antivirals

Drug	Side effects
Tuberculosis drugs	
Cycloserine, isoniazid	Psychosis, mania
HIV drugs	
Efavirenz	Inner ear symptoms, suicidal ideation, agitation, depression
High-dose zidovudine	Mania
Hepatitis C virus drugs	
Interferon-α	Depression, anxiety, fatigue, irritability, mania, psychosis (rare), suicidal ideation, insomnia
Malaria prophylaxis	
Mefloquine	Nightmares, irritability, psychosis
Other	
Metronidazole	Disulfiram-like reactions

A major role for psychiatry lies in secondary prevention efforts. One case of active tuberculosis in a group home, for example, has the potential to infect many contacts, necessitating a major case-finding effort (Cavanaugh et al. 2012). Psychiatrists work with patients from crowded settings such as prisons, state hospitals, and homeless shelters, where person-to-person transmission is possible. For psychiatric patients who require treatment, psychiatrists can collaborate with internists and infectious disease specialists in determining and implementing the most appropriate treatment regimen (e.g., standard treatment or directly observed therapy) and in assessing a patient's capacity to refuse treatment. Tuberculosis is a reportable disease, and many states have mandated treatment mechanisms to ensure treatment for patients who cannot comply with voluntary outpatient treatment—issues that may be particularly important in more severely ill psychiatric patients who lack capacity or who may have difficulty adhering to mandated regimens.

HIV Infection

HIV, the virus that causes AIDS, continues to affect a great number of patients worldwide. As of 2018, 37.9 million individuals were infected worldwide, including 1.1 million in the United States (UNAIDS 2019). The CDC recommends screening of all individuals between the ages of 13 and 64 years at least once, as well as annual screening for those with specific risk factors (e.g., men who have sex with men, sexual activity with an HIV-positive partner, injection drug use, a diagnosis of hepatitis or tuberculosis) (Centers for Disease Control and Prevention 2019d; see Table 9–6, later in chapter). Testing should include an antibody/antigen combination immunoassay (detecting HIV-1 and HIV-2 antibodies and HIV-1 p24 antigen) to screen for both established (via antibodies) and early (via antigen) infection. If acute HIV infection is suspected, patients should also be tested for HIV RNA.

The relevance of HIV for psychiatry is threefold. First, patients with preexisting mental illness and substance use disorders are at significantly increased risk of developing HIV. Second, in addition to increasing the risk for infection, mental illness and substance abuse can negatively impact engagement in care and adherence to prescribed HIV treatment. Third, HIV infection itself and its medical complications due to immunosuppression can produce neuropsychiatric symptoms, particularly as the infection advances to AIDS. Psychiatrists are often asked to help differentiate between primary psychiatric illness and neuropsychiatric complications of HIV/AIDS (Table 9–5).

HIV Life Cycle and Treatment

HIV is spread by contact with body fluids—including blood, semen, vaginal and rectal fluids, and breast milk—from an HIV-infected individual. The most common methods of transmission are sexual contact and the sharing of equipment for drug injection. Almost all steps of the viral life cycle have been targeted by antiretroviral therapy (ART) (Gandhi and Gandhi 2014). Once in the blood, the virus binds to T cells expressing the CD4 (cluster of differentiation 4) glycoprotein and coreceptors (e.g., C-C chemokine receptor type 5 [CCR5]); CCR5 antagonists block this step. The next

TABLE 9–5. **Differential diagnosis of psychiatric and neurocognitive conditions in HIV/AIDS**

Delirium

HIV-associated neurocognitive disorder

    Asymptomatic neurocognitive impairment

    Mild neurocognitive disorder

    HIV-associated dementia

Affective conditions

    Demoralization

    Grief

    Secondary depression

    Secondary mania

Secondary psychosis

Substance intoxication or withdrawal

Acute HIV meningoencephalitis

Opportunistic infections

    Bacteria (*Mycobacterium avium-intracellulare* complex, tuberculosis, syphilis)

    Fungi (*Cryptococcus,* histoplasmosis, *Coccidioides, Pneumocystis*)

    Toxoplasmosis

    Viruses (herpes simplex, varicella zoster, cytomegalovirus)

    Progressive multifocal leukoencephalopathy

Neoplasms

    Primary central nervous system lymphoma

    Non-Hodgkin's lymphoma

Medication effects

Endocrinopathies and nutrient deficiencies

step in the viral life cycle is the fusion of the virus envelope to the CD4 cell membrane, followed by entry of the virus into the cell; fusion inhibitors block this step. Once in the cell, viral reverse transcriptase (an enzyme contained within the virus particle itself) helps create HIV DNA from HIV RNA; this step can be interrupted by nucleoside reverse transcriptase inhibitors and nonnucleoside reverse transcriptase inhibitors. HIV DNA then enters the CD4 cell nucleus and inserts itself into the cell's DNA with the assistance of integrase (another HIV enzyme); integrase inhibitors may be used to interrupt viral replication at this step. HIV proteins are then created by the hijacked cell itself, and new viral proteins and RNA move to the surface of the cell in a noninfectious form. Once at the cell membrane, the viral protease enzyme cleaves longer HIV proteins into smaller ones that combine to form mature HIV; this step may be interrupted by protease inhibitors.

    In all, seven medication classes currently exist that interrupt the virus's life cycle at multiple steps. Medications from two or more classes are combined to provide combination antiretroviral therapy (cART) that is highly effective and minimizes the risk of drug resistance. Current first-line treatments in the United States use a combination of two nucleoside/nucleotide reverse transcriptase inhibitors (abacavir/

lamivudine or tenofovir/emtricitabine) plus an integrase inhibitor (dolutegravir or raltegravir). A highly potent nonnucleoside reverse transcriptase inhibitor, efavirenz, used to be a first-line agent; in the United States, however, efavirenz has been relegated to a second-line medication because of its significant neuropsychiatric side effects (see Table 9–4). ART has the potential to cause drug-drug interactions due to interactions with the CYP enzyme system (see Table 9–3); for example, ritonavir, other protease inhibitors, and cobicistat inhibit CYP3A4. These interactions may affect psychiatric medications (e.g., alprazolam) that are metabolized by this system.

In the acute phase of infection, HIV multiplies rapidly and spreads widely. Some individuals develop flulike symptoms; others may develop an acute meningitis or meningoencephalitis. Chronic infection leads to slow damage to the immune system, primarily by reduction of CD4 T cells. AIDS develops once the immune system is severely compromised, usually after approximately 7–9 years of untreated HIV; AIDS is defined by a CD4 count lower than 200 cells/mm^3 or the occurrence of an AIDS-defining illness (e.g., *Pneumocystis* pneumonia, cryptococcosis, cytomegalovirus, Kaposi's sarcoma, progressive multifocal leukoencephalopathy, toxoplasmosis, *Mycobacterium avium-intracellulare* complex [MAC]). HIV enters the CNS within days of the initial infection, ultimately leading to injury to neurons and the significant neuropsychiatric symptom burden that may follow. Medication penetration into the CNS is variable and comes with its own risks; while intuitively one wants to target the virus in the CNS itself, medications that are able to do so may also be neurotoxic. Currently, the strategy for prophylaxis against and treatment of CNS complications focuses on peripheral viral suppression.

Opportunistic Infections

Opportunistic infections begin to appear at a higher rate when CD4 counts fall below 200 cells/mm^3. Therefore, new neuropsychiatric symptoms in severely immunocompromised patients should raise concern for an opportunistic infection. Common conditions affecting the CNS include toxoplasmosis, cytomegalovirus encephalitis, cryptococcal meningitis, and progressive multifocal leukoencephalopathy (PML).

In toxoplasmosis, *Toxoplasma gondii* is reactivated from a chronic, subclinical infection. The infection manifests as ring-enhancing lesions on computed tomography (CT) consistent with abscess formation. Further neuroimaging findings indicate multiple foci, usually in the basal ganglia. Patients are most often affected when the CD4 count drops below 100 cells/mm^3. Clinical features include change in mental status, headache, and focal neurological signs (Luft and Remington 1992). Antitoxoplasmosis therapy should be given until the patient improves clinically and shows evidence of viral suppression and CD4 cell reconstitution for a sustained period of time.

Cytomegalovirus encephalitis similarly involves the reactivation of dormant infection as the CD4 count falls below 100 cells/mm^3. Although cytomegalovirus more often causes chorioretinitis or radiculopathy in AIDS patients, a subacute encephalitis with personality changes, poor concentration, headaches, and somnolence can occur, as can a more acute encephalitis characterized by delirium, seizures, and fever.

Cryptococcosis may occur when *Cryptococcus neoformans*, a yeast present in the environment, is inhaled and, with impaired cell-mediated immunity, disseminates throughout the body. While pulmonary symptoms may occur, the CNS is the most common site of disseminated infection. Cryptococcal meningitis is most common among patients whose CD4 count is below 50 cells/mm^3. It is typically subacute, with headache, fever, and altered mental status; other features include papilledema, cerebellar dysfunction, and seizures. Treatment involves taking antifungal medications until the infection resolves and immune reconstitution is achieved.

PML occurs through reactivation of the John Cunningham polyomavirus and infection of oligodendrocytes, typically in patients with CD4 counts below 200 cells/mm^3 but also during immune reconstitution. PML produces multiple focal neurological signs, and CT or magnetic resonance imaging (MRI) shows nonenhancing subcortical lesions. Despite its name, PML is generally not progressive once cART is instituted. However, cART does not reverse brain damage, and the overall prognosis is less promising for PML than for some of the other opportunistic infections. One study found that after 5 years, only 33% of patients showed no significant disability, and 42% had moderate to severe disability (Lima et al. 2010).

HIV Prevention

As part of the National HIV/AIDS Strategy, the HIV Care Continuum initiative was established in 2013 (HIV.gov 2016). The Continuum initiative emphasized use of sequential steps to achieve optimal HIV control, including getting tested to learn one's HIV status, seeking medical attention and getting connected to HIV services, starting ART, and taking prescribed medications with sufficient adherence to achieve viral suppression. Remarkably, CDC findings from 2011 demonstrated that while 86% of HIV-positive patients in the United States were aware of their diagnosis, only 40% were engaged in care, only 37% were prescribed appropriate treatment, and a mere 30% had successfully achieved viral suppression (Bradley et al. 2014). HIV may be a manageable chronic illness only for the slim minority of people who are virally suppressed. Psychiatrists can play a role in helping monitor for and treat comorbid psychiatric and substance use disorders that interfere with HIV treatment engagement and cART adherence, thereby assisting more patients to achieve viral suppression.

In the absence of a cure for HIV, primary prevention remains an essential component in the control of HIV. Traditionally, prevention has included counseling patients about the dangers of sharing needles and the importance of safer-sex practices. Harm-reduction strategies have been shown to be effective in reducing the transmission of HIV, although strategies need to be adjusted for special populations (e.g., patients with serious mental illness). Needle exchange programs have been used for years to help reduce HIV among injection drug users. More recently, preexposure prophylaxis, a medication regimen provided to patient populations at increased risk of HIV exposure, provides an additional tool to reduce infection rates, in some populations by greater than 90% when adherence is complete (Grant et al. 2010). Early diagnosis of HIV is critical to prevent transmission to others (a strategy referred to as "treatment as prevention") and also to reduce the risk for complications. HIV treatment is now initiated at the earliest possible time and is no longer delayed (AIDSinfo 2018).

In addition to boosting primary and secondary prevention efforts, psychiatrists are often called on to assess patients with neuropsychiatric symptoms that may ultimately be conditions that result from the virus's effect on the brain itself. Earlier in the epidemic, more severe and acute psychiatric conditions (e.g., AIDS dementia) resulted from the progression of the illness to AIDS. Despite the availability of effective treatment, long-term cognitive impairment has emerged as a particular concern as patients with HIV are aging; even milder forms of HIV-associated neurocognitive disorder (HAND) can have functional consequences leading to disability.

Psychiatric Complications of HIV

People with HIV have higher rates of depression than the general population, and patients with depression are more likely to contract the virus. There is scant evidence that the virus itself causes a depressive disorder (in the absence of encephalopathy, dementia, other neuropsychiatric manifestations, or opportunistic infections). The effects of trauma and losses and psychosocial factors associated with having HIV should not be overlooked. Treatment of depression is similar to that in individuals without HIV; medication management (with consideration of potential medication interactions between ART and psychiatric medications), psychotherapy, and somatic treatments all are effective.

Mania can create diagnostic difficulties. A preexisting diagnosis of any mood disorder, including bipolar disorder, may predispose individuals to contracting the virus. However, effects of the virus itself, particularly when the CD4 count is low, may cause a primary encephalopathy with features of mania. While not pathognomonic, certain symptoms are more common in secondary mania than in bipolar disorder; these include irritability, aggressiveness, disruptive behavior, paranoia, and cognitive impairment (Nakimuli-Mpungu et al. 2006). Any patient with new-onset mania or psychosis should be tested for HIV.

HAND includes three categories: asymptomatic neurocognitive impairment, mild neurocognitive disorder, and HIV-associated dementia (Antinori et al. 2007). Each subsequent category has a progressively worse neuropsychological profile and level of functional impairment. Although a variety of screening tools are available, none is ideal and no standard exists; therefore, regular screening is not indicated in the absence of functional impairment. If clinical suspicion warrants further investigation, a patient should be referred for neurocognitive testing to delineate the cognitive domains most affected. Screening for other possible etiologies of cognitive impairment is essential. Assessment for thyroid dysfunction, vitamin B_{12} deficiency, neurosyphilis, stroke, substance use, and polypharmacy should be considered. No medications are approved by the U.S. Food and Drug Administration for HAND, and treatment relies on ART optimization. Simplification of medication regimens, coordination with other treaters to ensure cardiovascular health, and encouragement of patients to remain cognitively active all are critical.

Hepatitis B and Hepatitis C Virus Infections

Multiple viral hepatitides exist, including two major blood-borne forms: hepatitis B virus (HBV) and hepatitis C virus (HCV). Although these entities are clinically distinct and have different trajectories, prognoses, and treatments, both affect a large number of injection drug users and disproportionately affect individuals with mental disorders. Vaccination against HBV is available, but no vaccine exists for HCV. As of

2012, 850,000 individuals in the United States were living with chronic HBV (U.S. Department of Health & Human Services 2019). The long-term consequences of HBV infection differ greatly based on age; children usually develop chronic infection, while adults typically experience an acute hepatitis that clears (with only 2%–6% developing chronic HBV) (Centers for Disease Control and Prevention 2019b).

HCV, meanwhile, has a 70%–85% chronic infection rate (Centers for Disease Control and Prevention 2019c). Approximately 1% of the U.S. population, or 2.4 million people, are estimated to be infected with HCV (Centers for Disease Control and Prevention 2018a). Estimates indicate that a majority of those infected contracted the virus through injection drug use (Centers for Disease Control and Prevention 2019c). Individuals with severe mental illness are 10 to 20 times more likely than individuals in the general population to contract HCV. Many patients who are infected will go on to develop hepatic fibrosis, cirrhosis, and hepatocellular carcinoma. Screening is critical, because many patients are unaware of their HCV infection. For that reason, the CDC recommends both screening for high-risk patients and one-time cohort screening for the baby boom generation (Centers for Disease Control and Prevention 2019c). Screening is even more critical now that curative treatments have been developed (see Table 9–6, later in chapter).

Treatment for HCV began with interferon (IFN)-α monotherapy. However, this therapy failed to clear the virus in a majority of patients. Additionally, patients experienced multiple side effects, from pancytopenia and rash to neuropsychiatric symptoms including depression and fatigue. The treatment also required injections several times weekly. Some of these issues were mitigated by the creation of pegylated IFN, which is given only once weekly. When IFN is combined with the oral antiviral medication ribavirin, up to half of individuals achieve an undetectable viral load. Selective serotonin reuptake inhibitors have commonly been prescribed alongside IFN-based treatments to help prevent and treat depression. Improvements in side effects and efficacy have been achieved with the development of direct-acting antivirals, which lead to sustained viral remission (i.e., a cure) in almost all patients after a treatment course of 3 months in uncomplicated cases (American Association for the Study of Liver Diseases/Infectious Diseases Society of America 2018). As with cART, antiviral agents of different classes are combined for optimal efficacy, with several options available.

Although psychiatrists have traditionally played a role in helping to control the side effects of IFN treatment, the emphasis for psychiatrists has shifted to preventing new infections and improving adherence to curative treatment with newer antiviral agents among patients with HCV (Chasser et al. 2017). As with all communicable diseases, untreated mental illness and substance use increase the risk of new HCV infection. Adequate treatment of underlying psychiatric illness is essential for protecting patients from contracting the virus (including being reinfected) and for preventing secondary infections. Among the risk factors for contracting HCV, injection drug use is by far the most significant; there are, however, increasing numbers of cases of sexual transmission of HCV among men who have sex with men. Treating underlying substance use disorders, advocating for improved substance use services, and removing psychosocial treatment barriers can help turn the tide in the HCV epidemic. The cost of novel treatments remains very high; optimizing the chances of success by lowering adherence barriers is critical.

Syphilis and Other Sexually Transmitted Diseases

Syphilis

Syphilis is caused by *Treponema pallidum,* a spirochete bacterium. Whereas syphilis was once a common sexually transmitted disease (STD), successful treatment with penicillin has decreased its spread and morbidity significantly. However, with the advent of the AIDS epidemic in the early 1980s, neurosyphilis experienced a resurgence as a serious neuropsychiatric condition. Although syphilis typically takes 10–20 years to advance to the point of neurosyphilis, this progression occurs much more quickly in the setting of HIV coinfection. Moreover, primary and secondary syphilis are increasing in the United States, particularly among men who have sex with men (Centers for Disease Control and Prevention 2016).

The initial presentation of syphilis is as a primary infection, manifesting as a lesion on the genitalia or other sites of sexual exposure. Secondary syphilis follows, with a different set of symptoms (e.g., rash on the palms and soles) and lymphadenopathy, consistent with seeding of the spirochete. A lengthy period of latent, asymptomatic infection then ensues. Among some infected individuals, however, acute syphilitic meningitis (consisting of headache, fever, and meningismus) or meningovascular syphilis (symptoms appearing in a stroke-like manner) may occur. Eventually, demyelination of the dorsal columns of the spinal cord (tabes dorsalis) results in slowed gait (in which the feet "slap" the ground), paresthesias, diminished reflexes, and poor coordination. General paresis—infection of the cerebrum with *T. pallidum*—is the collection of symptoms most commonly described as neurosyphilis. Severe cognitive impairment, personality changes, hallucinations, and disorganized thinking are present. In addition to neuropsychiatric changes, signs including dysarthria, tremor, and the classic Argyll Robertson pupil (bilateral small pupils that constrict to accommodation but not to light) all indicate a diagnosis of neurosyphilis.

In many laboratories, screening for syphilis begins with treponemal antibody testing (see Table 9–6, later in chapter); if positive, rapid plasma reagin (RPR) testing is done to obtain a titer (Henao-Martinez and Johnson 2014). If there is a suspicion of neurosyphilis, a more aggressive approach to diagnosis is necessary. CDC recommendations for a diagnosis of neurosyphilis include serological testing as well as examination of cerebrospinal fluid (CSF) for Venereal Disease Research Laboratory (VDRL) testing, cell count, protein, and glucose. Although VDRL testing of CSF is highly specific, it is not sensitive; false-negatives occur in up to 40% of individuals with the infection (Henao-Martinez and Johnson 2014).

Penicillin remains the gold standard of treatment for syphilis. Treatment resistance has not been reported, but individuals who are allergic to penicillin require an alternative treatment (e.g., doxycycline). For patients who can tolerate penicillin, a diagnosis of primary or secondary syphilis warrants a single intramuscular injection of benzathine penicillin G (selection of the appropriate formulation is important to ensure effective treatment). Additionally, individuals known to have been exposed to the infection through sexual contact or blood transfusion should be treated prophylactically prior to test results. For patients found to have neurosyphilis, treatment requires parenteral penicillin for 10–14 days. Given the lack of sensitivity of CSF VDRL testing, a broad clinical review of symptoms, signs, laboratory results, and other factors (such as risk group and HIV status) should be undertaken before prematurely dismissing the diagnosis of neurosyphilis to ensure that all patients are treated appropriately. Patients previously treated for neurosyphilis should continue to be screened for reinfection.

Other Sexually Transmitted Diseases

Although STDs other than syphilis do not commonly affect the CNS, these infections remain burdensome. In 2017, 1.7 million cases of chlamydia and 556,000 cases of gonorrhea were reported in the United States (Centers for Disease Control and Prevention 2018b). As is the case with other infectious diseases, patients with mental illnesses and substance use disorders contract these STDs with higher frequency. Factors such as impulsivity and risk-taking behavior strongly influence the risk of contracting the illness, as does the presence of coinfection with other STDs. By addressing the underlying mental illnesses, psychiatrists can help reduce behaviors that place patients at risk. In addition, referral of high-risk patients for screening (Table 9–6) is an important part of the treatment cascade; mental health care providers are in a unique position to know details about people's lives and behaviors that may be overlooked by other medical professionals.

Tick-Borne Infections

Lyme disease is a tick-borne illness caused by the spirochete *Borrelia burgdorferi* that can lead to a host of symptoms in many organ systems (Gerstenblith and Stern 2014). In the early localized phase, the individual might notice erythema migrans—the typical bull's-eye skin rash—at the site of the tick bite. Once bacteria enter the bloodstream in the early disseminated phase, the individual might experience systemic symptoms and organ-specific manifestations, most commonly in the joints, the CNS (meningitis, radiculopathy, cranial neuropathies), and the heart (atrioventricular nodal block or myocarditis). In the late disseminated phase, months to years after tick exposure, an encephalomyelitis can mimic depression (Fallon and Nields 1994). The diagnosis of Lyme disease is based on exposure history and appropriate serological testing (Table 9–7). Neuroimaging yields nonspecific findings and is not helpful in making the diagnosis.

Standard treatment for early Lyme disease—a 14- to 21-day course of oral antibiotics—is very effective in eradicating the spirochete from the body, and almost all appropriately treated patients recover. CNS Lyme disease should be treated with parenteral ceftriaxone.

Other infections carried by the *Ixodes* tick, such as *Anaplasma phagocytophilum* (ehrlichiosis), human granulocytic anaplasmosis, and *Babesia microti* (babesiosis), should be considered (Sanchez et al. 2016). Powassen virus is also transmitted by ticks and can cause encephalitis. People with rickettsial diseases (e.g., Rocky Mountain spotted fever) present with fever, headache, and rash; early diagnosis and treatment are critical.

TABLE 9–6. **Screening for blood-borne infections and syphilis**

Infectious agent/ condition	Screening test	Comments
HIV	HIV antibody and antigen	Include HIV RNA if acute infection is suspected
HCV	HCV antibody	Include HCV RNA if acute infection is suspected or if HCV antibody test is positive
HBV	HBV surface antigen (HBsAg) HBV surface antibody HBV core antigen	Chronic HBV is defined as persistence of positive HBsAg for 6 months or longer
Syphilis	Treponemal antibody	If treponemal antibody test is positive, RPR titer should be obtained Screening for neurosyphilis requires CSF testing

Note. CSF=cerebrospinal fluid; HBV=hepatitis B virus; HCV=hepatitis C virus; RPR=rapid plasma reagin.

TABLE 9–7. **Diagnosis of Lyme disease**

Requirements

 History of possible exposure

 Presence of clinical features consistent with diagnosis

 Positive two-tier serological testing:
  First-tier enzyme immunoassay to detect potential antibodies
  Second-tier Western blot to confirm specific antibodies

Clinical comments

 Testing is not recommended if Lyme exposure is unlikely or if the clinical syndrome is not suggestive of Lyme (high false-positive rate in these scenarios).

 Serological testing in the acute phase has poor sensitivity; clinical diagnosis of Lyme should lead to treatment.

 If involvement of the central nervous system is suspected, lumbar puncture and examination of cerebrospinal fluid should be performed.

Source. Based on Lantos PM, Auwaerter PG, Nelson CA: "Lyme Disease Serology." *JAMA* 315(16):1780–1781, 2016.

Neuropsychiatric Presentations of Contested Illnesses

Contested illnesses sit uncomfortably between suffering patients who believe they know what ails them and physicians who feel that they have nothing to offer for symptoms that are not explained by accepted medical knowledge. Examples of contested infectious diseases include "chronic Lyme" as a postinfectious syndrome and delusional infestation. What is contested in this group of illnesses is the causal attribution of symptoms to specific triggers—often environmental toxins or infectious agents—as well as the optimal approach for managing symptoms. Psychiatric explanations are often specifically rejected by the patient. Although laboratory abnormalities suggestive of immune system dysregulation are frequently present in contested illnesses and are intriguing to patients, these abnormalities are nonspecific, and no single biomarker or biomarker profile has been identified that suggests a specific, targeted intervention. Contested illnesses make explicit that illness is negotiated and socially constructed; the Internet, for example, has empowered patients to challenge the monopoly on illness definition hitherto held by physicians (Dumit 2006). The general management principle in contested illnesses is to negotiate a safe and collaborative approach to patients that acknowledges the very real limits of knowledge and certainty in medicine without removing hope from or abandoning patients (Murphy et al. 2016). Doing no harm in the form of either over- or underdiagnosis is critical. Overdiagnosis results in poor and possibly dangerous treatments being offered (e.g., prolonged antibiotic treatment for Lyme disease); underdiagnosis may lead to delayed treatment (e.g., babesiosis coinfection in a patient with Lyme). Finally, regardless of the etiology or pathophysiology of the underlying disease, patients with contested illnesses often have comorbid psychological and psychiatric conditions that could benefit from treatment yet may not be noticed or diagnosed. Attention to these co-occurring conditions can substantially improve a patient's functioning and quality of life.

Postinfectious Syndromes

It has long been recognized that recovery from acute infection can lead to postinfectious syndromes (Bannister 1988). The classic example of this phenomenon is the persistent, profound postviral fatigue that follows infectious mononucleosis from Epstein-Barr virus (EBV) infection. In some patients with disabling fatigue, however, no clear link to EBV or other viruses can be established. A purely descriptive category of chronic fatigue syndrome (CFS) has been created to capture such patients. Nonspecific abnormalities in cytokines or stress hormones can often be found in CFS patients (Klimas et al. 2012). In 2015, the Institute of Medicine proposed that CFS be replaced with a new, less charged term—"systemic exertion intolerance disease"—to emphasize the core features of impaired recovery and nonresponse to rest after physical or mental effort (Clayton 2015). In a parallel-group randomized trial, patients who met the Oxford criteria for CFS were provided with medical care (including pharmacotherapy) by a specialist either alone or with the addition of adaptive pacing therapy (APT), graded exercise therapy (GET), or cognitive-behavioral therapy (CBT). At 1 year, patients receiving either GET or CBT showed decreased fatigue and increased physical function in comparison with patients receiving specialist care alone. No benefit was found for the APT group (White et al. 2011). Longer-term follow-up found improvement in the specialist care alone and APT groups equal to that in the GET and CBT groups (in which improvement was maintained) (Sharpe et al. 2015).

A small group of patients with well-documented Lyme disease experience ongoing fatigue, musculoskeletal pain, and cognitive difficulties despite treatment with antibiotics that successfully eradicated the *Borrelia burgdorferi* spirochete. In this group of patients with posttreatment Lyme disease syndrome, abnormalities in regional cerebral blood flow have been documented (Fallon et al. 2009). However, another group of patients believe themselves to be afflicted by the controversial entity of "chronic Lyme," with *persistent* infection as an explanation for a host of nonspecific pain, fatigue, and memory complaints, despite (in some cases) lack of good clinical and serological evidence of prior Lyme disease. What is contested in this group is the presence of persistent organisms and whether long-term antibiotic therapy is beneficial. Whereas the Infectious Disease Society of America does not recommend long-term use of antibiotics, the International Lyme and Associated Diseases Society, a more consumer-driven organization, does (Infectious Diseases Society of America 2019). Regardless of patient or clinician beliefs about the persistence of *Borrelia,* several randomized clinical trials have failed to substantiate clinical benefit from additional antimicrobial therapy beyond standard treatment for patients with persistent symptoms attributed to Lyme (Melia and Auwaerter 2016).

A prototype of a postinfectious autoimmune disease is Sydenham's chorea following rheumatic fever. In susceptible individuals, antibodies against group A streptococcus are misdirected due to cross-reactivity (molecular mimicry) against the basal ganglia, giving rise to involuntary movements. A similar pathogenic model—pediatric autoimmune neuropsychiatric disorders associated with streptococcal infections (PANDAS)—has been proposed for OCD symptoms that emerge in children after a streptococcal infection (Swedo et al. 1998). Although this pathophysiological model is becoming more accepted in principle, there is a risk of inappropriately extending the clinical phenotype to other psychiatric syndromes. Currently, the model is best established for very-acute-onset OCD with sleep difficulties and separation anxiety in a young child, but not for other neuropsychiatric syndromes (Swedo et al. 2015). The high prevalence of streptococcal infections in childhood can lead families and practitioners to mistakenly attribute behavioral symptoms to infections, leading to inappropriate antibiotic use.

Delusional Infestation

Patients who have delusional infestation attribute skin sensations such as pruritus to an infestation with an infectious parasite even if no parasite can be demonstrated (Freudenmann and Lepping 2009). Many patients dedicate their lives to a quest for "proof" and a cure. In a modern variant of delusional infestation, patients with self-diagnosed Morgellons disease attribute unexplained skin sensations to inanimate fibers that are excreted from the skin. An epidemiological study of 115 case patients by the CDC that used a case definition and skin biopsies for this unexplained dermopathy failed to demonstrate the presence of such fibers or other underlying pathologies (Pearson et al. 2012). Exclusion of actual infestations such as scabies, formication due to stimulant misuse, and dermatological conditions is important. Antipsychotic treatment can be at least partially effective (Huber et al. 2011) but is rarely accepted by patients. Among the 54 patients who agreed to see a psychiatrist, 40 (74%) had additional psychiatric conditions (Hylwa et al. 2011). Even if antipsychotics are rejected, treatment of comorbidities can enhance these patients' quality of life.

Epidemiological Linkage of Infections and Psychiatric Illness

A Danish registry analysis of more than 3.5 million persons born between 1945 and 1976 found that a hospital diagnosis of a mood disorder was increased in persons who had an earlier hospital contact for infectious or autoimmune disease (Benros et al. 2013). The incidence rate ratio (IRR) for autoimmune disorders was 1.45, and the IRR for infections was 1.62, with infections being far more common than autoimmune conditions.

The association between treated infections and subsequent risk of mental illness was investigated in a Danish population-based cohort study of individuals born between January 1, 1995, and June 30, 2012 (Köhler-Forsberg et al. 2019). Treated infections in the cohort were identified through records of hospitalization or prescriptions for anti-infective agents; mental disorders were similarly identified via records of hospitalization or redeemed psychotropic medication prescriptions. Hazard ratios for mental disorders were increased among individuals who had received hospital-based treatment of infections, and were lower but still increased among those who had received ambulatory treatment. There was a particularly strong association between antibiotic treatment and increased risk for mental illness. Risks for several psychiatric conditions, including obsessive-compulsive disorder (OCD) and tic disorders, were increased in children and adolescents with infectious disease histories (Köhler-Forsberg et al. 2019).

Treatment With Antibiotics

Antibiotics are among the most widely prescribed medications and are usually safe and well tolerated when combined with psychotropics. Systemic infections themselves can inhibit metabolizing enzymes such as CYP3A4, and this inhibition can lead to toxic levels of psychotropics metabolized by this enzyme. Although most psychotropics are well tolerated even if serum levels rise due to drug-drug interactions, there are exceptions. For example, higher drug levels of clozapine can lead to toxicity (sedation, orthostatic hypotension, seizures); QTc prolongation can become clinically relevant for psychotropics associated with dose-dependent QTc prolongation; and elevated alprazolam serum levels can lead to CNS suppression. Loss of psychotropic efficacy can occur if enzyme-inducing antibiotics (e.g., rifampin-containing tuberculosis regimens) are used. Pharmacodynamic drug interactions (e.g., added bone marrow suppression from trimethoprim/sulfamethoxazole) are frequently overlooked (see Table 9–3). Some medications used in infectious diseases can cause severe psychiatric side effects (see Table 9–4).

TABLE 9–8.	Roles for psychiatry in infectious diseases

Disease prevention

    Screen for infections (see Table 9–6)

    Educate patients about infectious diseases and risk reduction

    Collaborate with primary care physicians to ensure up-to-date vaccination

Disease diagnosis

    Exclude infectious diseases as the cause of psychiatric symptoms

    Diagnose psychiatric comorbidities in patients with infectious disease

Disease treatment

    Develop collaborative models to enhance psychiatric treatment in medical settings

    Address psychiatric obstacles to infectious disease treatment

    Address vaccination hesitancy

Disaster preparedness

    Manage psychological aspects of epidemics and bioterrorism

Conclusion: The Role of Psychiatry in Infectious Diseases

Psychiatrists are often at the forefront of caring for psychiatric patients who are at risk for infectious diseases due to their lower status in society and risk behaviors such as injection drug use. Table 9–8 summarizes possible tasks for psychiatrists in reducing the morbidity and mortality associated with infectious diseases. The underlying assumption of the mandate for shared responsibility and the need for collaboration between medicine and psychiatry in the care of patients with infectious diseases is that there is no medical health without mental health (*mens sana in corpore sano*). Providing effective psychiatric treatment to allow patients to participate in their own medical care is one obvious role for psychiatrists. Identifying new infections by screening to prevent not only disease progression but also secondary infections is a priority for the health care system (see Table 9–6). In addition, the provision of optimal addiction care (e.g., buprenorphine/naloxone [Suboxone] if indicated for an opioid use disorder) is a critical skill for physicians, given the link between substance use disorders and blood-borne infections. Where possible, close collaboration between infectious disease and psychiatric specialists is important in the care of patients with substance use or other psychiatric disorders who are at risk for acquiring an infection or who are being treated for an infection.

References

AIDSinfo: Guidelines for the Use of Antiretroviral Agents in Adults and Adolescents Living with HIV. Rockville, MD, U.S. Department of Health and Human Services, 2018. Available at: https://aidsinfo.nih.gov/guidelines/html/1/adult-and-adolescent-treatment-guidelines/0/. Accessed April 4, 2019.

American Association for the Study of Liver Diseases/Infectious Diseases Society of America: HCV Guidance: Recommendations for Testing, Managing, and Treating Hepatitis C. Alexandria and Arlington, VA, American Association for the Study of Liver Diseases/Infectious Diseases Society of America, May 24, 2018. Available at: https://www.hcvguidelines.org/. Accessed April 4, 2019.

Antinori A, Arendt G, Becker JT, et al: Updated research nosology for HIV-associated neurocognitive disorders. Neurology 69(18):1789–1799, 2007 17914061

Arabi YM, Balkhy HH, Hayden FG, et al: Middle East respiratory syndrome. N Engl J Med 376(6):584–594, 2017 28177862

Bannister BA: Post-infectious disease syndrome. Postgrad Med J 64(753):559–567, 1988 3074289

Be NA, Kim KS, Bishai WR, Jain SK: Pathogenesis of central nervous system tuberculosis. Curr Mol Med 9(2):94–99, 2009 19275620

Benros ME, Waltoft BL, Nordentoft M, et al: Autoimmune diseases and severe infections as risk factors for mood disorders: a nationwide study. JAMA Psychiatry 70(8):812–820, 2013 23760347

Bradley H, Hall HI, Wolitski RJ, et al: Vital Signs: HIV diagnosis, care, and treatment among persons living with HIV—United States, 2011. MMWR Morb Mortal Wkly Rep 63(47):1113–1117, 2014 25426654

Cavanaugh JS, Powell K, Renwick OJ, et al: An outbreak of tuberculosis among adults with mental illness. Am J Psychiatry 169(6):569–575, 2012 22684593

Centers for Disease Control and Prevention: Syphilis Statistics. Atlanta, GA, Division of STD Prevention, National Center for HIV/AIDS, Viral Hepatitis, STD, and TB Prevention, Centers for Disease Control and Prevention. Page last reviewed December 16, 2016. Available at: https://www.cdc.gov/std/syphilis/stats.htm. Accessed August 17, 2019.

Centers for Disease Control and Prevention: Hepatitis C Prevalence Estimates 2013–2016. Atlanta, GA, Division of Viral Hepatitis, National Center for HIV/AIDS, Viral Hepatitis, STD, and TB Prevention, Centers for Disease Control and Prevention. Page last reviewed November 6, 2018a. Available at: https://www.cdc.gov/nchhstp/newsroom/2018/hepatitis-c-prevalence-estimates.html. Accessed August 17, 2019.

Centers for Disease Control and Prevention: Sexually Transmitted Disease Surveillance 2017: National Profile. Atlanta, GA, Division of STD Prevention, National Center for HIV/AIDS, Viral Hepatitis, STD, and TB Prevention, Centers for Disease Control and Prevention. Page last reviewed July 24, 2018b. Available at: https://www.cdc.gov/std/stats17/natoverview.htm. Accessed August 17, 2019.

Centers for Disease Control and Prevention: 2014–2016 Ebola Outbreak in West Africa (web page). Atlanta, GA, National Center for Emerging and Zoonotic Infectious Diseases (NCEZID), Division of High-Consequence Pathogens and Pathology (DHCPP), Viral Special Pathogens Branch (VSPB), Centers for Disease Control and Prevention. Page last reviewed March 8, 2019a. Available at: https://www.cdc.gov/vhf/ebola/outbreaks/2014-west-africa/united-states-imported-case.html. Accessed April 4, 2019.

Centers for Disease Control and Prevention: Hepatitis B. Atlanta, GA, Division of Viral Hepatitis, National Center for HIV/AIDS, Viral Hepatitis, STD, and TB Prevention, Centers for Disease Control and Prevention. Page last reviewed June 13, 2019b. Available at: https://www.cdc.gov/hepatitis/hbv/index.htm. Accessed August 17, 2019.

Centers for Disease Control and Prevention: Hepatitis C. Atlanta, GA, Division of Viral Hepatitis, National Center for HIV/AIDS, Viral Hepatitis, STD, and TB Prevention, Centers for Disease Control and Prevention. Page last reviewed June 13, 2019c. Available at: https://www.cdc.gov/hepatitis/hcv/index.htm. Accessed August 17, 2019.

Centers for Disease Control and Prevention: Let's Stop HIV Together Campaign Resources. Atlanta, GA, Division of HIV/AIDS Prevention, National Center for HIV/AIDS, Viral Hepatitis, STD, and TB Prevention, Centers for Disease Control and Prevention. Page last reviewed September 3, 2019d. Available at: https://www.cdc.gov/actagainstaids/campaigns/hssc/. Accessed September 21, 2019.

Centers for Disease Control and Prevention: Tuberculosis—United States, 2018 (MMWR Media Summary). Atlanta, GA, National Center for HIV/AIDS, Viral Hepatitis, STD, and TB Prevention, Centers for Disease Control and Prevention. Page last reviewed March 21, 2019e.

Available at: https://www.cdc.gov/nchhstp/newsroom/2019/tb-united-states-2018-media-summary.html. Accessed August 17, 2019.

Centers for Disease Control and Prevention: Who Needs a Flu Vaccine and When. Atlanta, GA, National Center for Immunization and Respiratory Diseases (NCIRD), Centers for Disease Control and Prevention. Page last reviewed September 18, 2019f. Available at: https://www.cdc.gov/flu/prevent/vaccinations.htm. Accessed September 21, 2019.

Chasser Y, Kim AY, Freudenreich O: Hepatitis C treatment: clinical issues for psychiatrists in the post-interferon era. Psychosomatics 58(1):1–10, 2017 27871760

Cheng VC, To KK, Tse H, et al: Two years after pandemic influenza A/2009/H1N1: what have we learned? Clin Microbiol Rev 25(2):223–263, 2012 22491771

Clayton EW: Beyond myalgic encephalomyelitis/chronic fatigue syndrome: an IOM report on redefining an illness. JAMA 313(11):1101–1102, 2015 25668027

Dantzer R, O'Connor JC, Freund GG, et al: From inflammation to sickness and depression: when the immune system subjugates the brain. Nat Rev Neurosci 9(1):46–56, 2008 18073775

Doherty AM, Kelly J, McDonald C, et al: A review of the interplay between tuberculosis and mental health. Gen Hosp Psychiatry 35(4):398–406, 2013 23660587

Dumit J: Illnesses you have to fight to get: facts as forces in uncertain, emergent illnesses. Soc Sci Med 62(3):577–590, 2006 16085344

Fallon BA, Nields JA: Lyme disease: a neuropsychiatric illness. Am J Psychiatry 151(11):1571–1583, 1994 7943444

Fallon BA, Lipkin RB, Corbera KM, et al: Regional cerebral blood flow and metabolic rate in persistent Lyme encephalopathy. Arch Gen Psychiatry 66(5):554–563, 2009 19414715

Folayan MO, Haire BG, Brown B: Critical role of ethics in clinical management and public health response to the West Africa Ebola epidemic. Risk Manag Healthc Policy 9:55–65, 2016 27274326

Freudenmann RW, Lepping P: Delusional infestation. Clin Microbiol Rev 22(4):690–732, 2009 19822895

Friedland JS: Targeting the inflammatory response in tuberculosis. N Engl J Med 371(14):1354–1356, 2014 25271609

Gandhi M, Gandhi RT: Single-pill combination regimens for treatment of HIV-1 infection. N Engl J Med 371(3):248–259, 2014 25014689

Gerstenblith TA, Stern TA: Lyme disease: a review of its epidemiology, evaluation, and treatment. Psychosomatics 55(5):421–429, 2014 25016354

Gofton TE, Young GB: Sepsis-associated encephalopathy. Nat Rev Neurol 8(10):557–566, 2012 22986430

Grant RM, Lama JR, Anderson PL, et al: Preexposure chemoprophylaxis for HIV prevention in men who have sex with men. N Engl J Med 363(27):2587–2599, 2010 21091279

Hansen V, Oren E, Dennis LK, et al: Infectious disease mortality trends in the United States, 1980–2014. JAMA 316(20):2149–2151, 2016 27893119

Henao-Martinez AF, Johnson SC: Diagnostic tests for syphilis: new tests and new algorithms. Neurol Clin Pract 4(2):114–122, 2014 27606153

HIV.gov (an official U.S. Government website managed by the U.S. Department of Health & Human Services and supported by the Minority HIV/AIDS Fund): HIV Care Continuum. Page last updated December 30, 2016. Available at: https://www.hiv.gov/federal-response/policies-issues/hiv-aids-care-continuum. Accessed August 17, 2019.

Howell MD, Davis AM: Management of sepsis and septic shock. JAMA 317(8):847–848, 2017 28114603

Huber M, Lepping P, Pycha R, et al: Delusional infestation: treatment outcome with antipsychotics in 17 consecutive patients (using standardized reporting criteria). Gen Hosp Psychiatry 33(6):604–611, 2011 21762999

Hylwa SA, Bury JE, Davis MD, et al: Delusional infestation, including delusions of parasitosis: results of histologic examination of skin biopsy and patient-provided skin specimens. Arch Dermatol 147(9):1041–1045, 2011 21576554

Infectious Diseases Society of America: Lyme Disease. 2019. Available at: https://www.idsociety.org/public-health/lyme-disease/lyme-disease/. Accessed September 21, 2019.

Jain S, Self WH, Wunderink RG, et al: Community-acquired pneumonia requiring hospitalization among U.S. adults. N Engl J Med 373(5):415–427, 2015 26172429

Klimas NG, Broderick G, Fletcher MA: Biomarkers for chronic fatigue. Brain Behav Immun 26(8):1202–1210, 2012 22732129

Köhler-Forsberg O, Petersen L, Gasse C, et al: A nationwide study in Denmark of the association between treated infections and the subsequent risk of treated mental disorders in children and adolescents. JAMA Psychiatry 76(3):271–279, 2019 30516814

Kramer LD, Li J, Shi PY: West Nile virus. Lancet Neurol 6(2):171–181, 2007 17239804

Liang W, Zhu Z, Guo J, et al; Beijing Joint SARS Expert Group: Severe acute respiratory syndrome, Beijing, 2003. Emerg Infect Dis 10(1):25–31, 2004 15078593

Lima MA, Bernal-Cano F, Clifford DB, et al: Clinical outcome of long-term survivors of progressive multifocal leukoencephalopathy. J Neurol Neurosurg Psychiatry 81(11):1288–1291, 2010 20710013

LoBue PA, Mermin JH: Latent tuberculosis infection: the final frontier of tuberculosis elimination in the USA. Lancet Infect Dis 17(10):e327–e333, 2017 28495525

Luft BJ, Remington JS: Toxoplasmic encephalitis in AIDS. Clin Infect Dis 15(2):211–222, 1992 1520757

Man WH, Colen-de Koning JC, Schulte PF, et al: The effect of glycopyrrolate on nocturnal sialorrhea in patients using clozapine: a randomized, crossover, double-blind, placebo-controlled trial. J Clin Psychopharmacol 37(2):155–161, 2017 28129312

McClintock AH, Eastment M, McKinney CM, et al: Treatment completion for latent tuberculosis infection: a retrospective cohort study comparing 9 months of isoniazid, 4 months of rifampin and 3 months of isoniazid and rifapentine. BMC Infect Dis 17(1):146, 2017 28196479

Melia MT, Auwaerter PG: Time for a different approach to Lyme disease and long-term symptoms. N Engl J Med 374(13):1277–1278, 2016 27028918

Murphy M, Kontos N, Freudenreich O: Electronic support groups: an open line of communication in contested illness. Psychosomatics 57(6):547–555, 2016 27421707

Nakimuli-Mpungu E, Musisi S, Mpungu SK, et al: Primary mania versus HIV-related secondary mania in Uganda. Am J Psychiatry 163(8):1349–1354, quiz 1480, 2006 16877646

Olfson M, Gerhard T, Huang C, et al: Premature mortality among adults with schizophrenia in the United States. JAMA Psychiatry 72(12):1172–1181, 2015 26509694

Parmet WE: Legal power and legal rights—isolation and quarantine in the case of drug-resistant tuberculosis. N Engl J Med 357(5):433–435, 2007 17671251

Pearson ML, Selby JV, Katz KA, et al: Clinical, epidemiologic, histopathologic and molecular features of an unexplained dermopathy. PLoS One 7(1):e29908, 2012 22295070

Sanchez E, Vannier E, Wormser GP, et al: Diagnosis, treatment, and prevention of Lyme disease, human granulocytic anaplasmosis, and babesiosis: a review. JAMA 315(16):1767–1777, 2016 27115378

Schmid P, Rauber D, Betsch C, et al: Barriers of influenza vaccination intention and behavior—a systematic review of influenza vaccine hesitancy, 2005–2016. PLoS One 12(1):e0170550, 2017 28125629

Sharpe M, Goldsmith KA, Johnson AL, et al: Rehabilitative treatments for chronic fatigue syndrome: long-term follow-up from the PACE trial. Lancet Psychiatry 2(12):1067–1074, 2015 26521770

Silverman MA, Misasi J, Smole S, et al: Eastern equine encephalitis in children, Massachusetts and New Hampshire, USA, 1970–2010. Emerg Infect Dis 19(2):194–201; quiz 352, 2013 23343480

Stoecker ZR, George WT, O'Brien JB, et al: Clozapine usage increases the incidence of pneumonia compared with risperidone and the general population: a retrospective comparison of clozapine, risperidone, and the general population in a single hospital over 25 months. Int Clin Psychopharmacol 32(3):155–160, 2017 28059928

Swedo SE, Leonard HL, Garvey M, et al: Pediatric autoimmune neuropsychiatric disorders associated with streptococcal infections: clinical description of the first 50 cases. Am J Psychiatry 155(2):264–271, 1998 9464208

Swedo SE, Seidlitz J, Kovacevic M, et al: Clinical presentation of pediatric autoimmune neuropsychiatric disorders associated with streptococcal infections in research and community settings. J Child Adolesc Psychopharmacol 25(1):26–30, 2015 25695941

UNAIDS (Joint United Nations Programme on HIV/AIDS): Global HIV & AIDS statistics—2019 fact sheet. 2019. Available at: https://www.unaids.org/en/resources/fact-sheet. Accessed August 17, 2019.

U.S. Department of Health & Human Services: Hepatitis B Basic Information. Washington, DC, Office of Infectious Disease and HIV/AIDS Policy. Page last updated January 30, 2019. Available at: https://www.hhs.gov/hepatitis/learn-about-viral-hepatitis/hepatitis-b-basics/index.html. Accessed August 17, 2019.

White PD, Goldsmith KA, Johnson AL, et al: Comparison of adaptive pacing therapy, cognitive behaviour therapy, graded exercise therapy, and specialist medical care for chronic fatigue syndrome (PACE): a randomised trial. Lancet 377(9768):823–836, 2011 21334061

Whitley RJ, Soong SJ, Dolin R, et al: Adenine arabinoside therapy of biopsy-proved herpes simplex encephalitis. National Institute of Allergy and Infectious Diseases collaborative antiviral study. N Engl J Med 297(6):289–294, 1977 195208

Wu P, Fang Y, Guan Z, et al: The psychological impact of the SARS epidemic on hospital employees in China: exposure, risk perception, and altruistic acceptance of risk. Can J Psychiatry 54(5):302–311, 2009 19497162

CHAPTER 10

Gastroenterological Disease in Patients With Psychiatric Disorders

Ash Nadkarni, M.D.

David A. Silbersweig, M.D.

The relationship between the brain and the gut is a connection that humans have experienced for hundreds of years, giving rise to idioms such as "gut feeling." The gastrointestinal tract is a major visceral organ that processes food and digests waste. Historically, several categories of gastrointestinal disease, such as inflammatory bowel disease (IBD) and functional diseases, were conceptualized as purely psychosomatic diseases with a strong relationship between intestinal symptoms and psychological factors. In fact, the term *functional* is indicative of a lack of identified structural pathology.

In more recent decades, an explosion of research has established the complex pathways that underlie an organically mediated link between the gastrointestinal tract and psychiatric conditions. This research has clarified the role of the intestinal microbiome in protecting against pathogens, buoying the immune system, and affecting our physiological functioning. Impairment of the gut microbiome has also been implicated in the pathogenesis of autism spectrum disorder, major depressive disorder, and Parkinson's disease. Additionally, there has been a major growth in our knowledge of the brain-gut axis and the bidirectional interchange of neural, immune, and endocrine signals among the brain, gut, and intestinal microbiota. The significance of the brain-gut axis is further underscored by the fact that the enteric nervous system, which consists of 200–600 million neurons and governs gastrointestinal functioning, is the largest component of the peripheral nervous system (Furness et al. 2014). Finally, our understanding of the role of the hypothalamic-pituitary-adrenal (HPA) axis in explaining psychiatric illness, as well as tying together the link between depression and gut functioning, also has increased significantly.

In this chapter, we discuss the psychiatric issues occurring in gastrointestinal diseases commonly seen in a typical gastroenterology practice. We provide a basic overview of each disease topic, defining criteria, pathophysiological and genetic factors, clinical presentation, diagnostic and laboratory findings, and treatment recommendations.

Functional Gastrointestinal Disorders

Functional disorders are the most common gastrointestinal disorders and have been recognized for more than a century, beginning in 1862, when the American physician and scientist Jacob Mendes Da Costa first connected emotion to intestinal functioning (Da Costa 1871). *Functional gastrointestinal disorders* is a term that refers to a wide range of disorders attributable to the gastrointestinal tract that cannot be explained by structural or biochemical abnormalities (Drossman 2016). Since the time of Da Costa, our understanding of functional disorders has progressed considerably. In the twentieth century, the model of psychosomatic illness was used to understand functional gastroenterological disease. Current research has established the complex pathways that underlie an organically mediated link between the gastrointestinal tract and psychiatric conditions.

In this section we discuss in detail those categories of functional disorders that consultation-liaison psychiatrists most commonly encounter—esophageal, gastric, and intestinal functional disorders. The Rome IV criteria (Rome Foundation 2019; Schmulson and Drossman 2017) have drawn on scientific data to define criteria for the functional gastrointestinal disorders—now termed *disorders of gut-brain interaction*, including the esophageal disorders functional heartburn, functional dysphagia, and globus; the gastroduodenal disorder functional dyspepsia; and the functional intestinal disorder irritable bowel syndrome.

Subtypes and Defining Criteria

Functional esophageal disorders encompass five categories: functional chest pain, functional heartburn, reflux hypersensitivity, functional dysphagia, and globus. In these disorders, patients present with esophageal symptoms that are not explained by major motor disorders, gastroesophageal reflux disease (GERD), mechanical obstruction, or other structural or metabolic diseases (Aziz et al. 2016). These disorders have several exclusionary criteria in common. According to Rome IV criteria, *functional heartburn* is defined as typical heartburn symptoms in the presence of normal upper endoscopy findings (including normal biopsies), normal esophageal pH testing, and a negative association between symptoms and reflux events (Galmiche et al. 2006; Yamasaki et al. 2017). *Functional dysphagia* is the least prevalent of the functional esophageal disorders and, like functional heartburn, requires the exclusion of other gastrointestinal diseases, such as GERD or motility disorders. In *globus,* symptoms occur most commonly in the central neck but can also migrate laterally (Clouse et al. 1999).

Functional gastroduodenal disorders are divided into four categories: functional dyspepsia, belching disorders, chronic nausea and vomiting disorders, and rumination syndrome (Stanghellini et al. 2016). *Functional dyspepsia* has two subtypes: epigastric pain syndrome and postprandial distress syndrome (Talley and Ford 2015). Epigastric pain syndrome produces pain or burning in the epigastrium, occurring at least once per week. Postprandial distress syndrome involves either bothersome postprandial fullness occurring after normal-sized meals or early satiety that prevents the person from finishing a regular meal at least several times per week (Talley and Ford 2015). The most frequent co-occurring psychiatric disorders are depression, anxiety, and somatic symptom and related disorders (Aro et al. 2009; Gracie et al. 2015; Mak et al. 2012; Van Oudenhove et al. 2012; Zagari et al. 2010).

Functional bowel disorders include irritable bowel syndrome, functional bloating, functional constipation, functional diarrhea, and unspecified functional bowel disorder (Lacy et al. 2016). These disorders are characterized by predominant symptoms or signs of abdominal pain, bloating, distention, and/or bowel habit abnormalities (e.g., constipation, diarrhea, mixed constipation/diarrhea). These symptoms or signs are chronic (i.e., have been present for ≥6 months at the time of presentation); are currently active (i.e., have been present within the last 3 months); are experienced frequently (i.e., on average, at least 1 day per week); and cannot be attributed to any obvious anatomic or physiological abnormalities identified by routine diagnostic examinations, as deemed clinically appropriate (Lacy et al. 2016). In *irritable bowel syndrome* (IBS), the pattern of recurrent abdominal pain is associated with changes in bowel habit or defecation, symptoms of abdominal bloating or distension, and disordered bowel habits (e.g., constipation, diarrhea, mixed constipation/diarrhea). To qualify for a diagnosis of IBS, symptoms must have been present for 1 day a week for at least 6 months and must have been active during the last 3 months (Lacy et al. 2016). The three main subtypes of IBS are IBS-C (constipation predominant), IBS-D (diarrhea predominant), and IBS-M (mixed bowel symptoms). Subtypes are identified on the basis of the predominant stool type on days with at least one abnormal bowel movement; for example, in IBS-C, more than one-fourth (25%) of bowel movements will be hard or lumpy (Lacy et al. 2016). Given the anticholinergic side effects of many psychotropics, this differentiation can assist psychiatrists in choosing the optimal treatment. Other functional disorders such as fibromyalgia, chronic fatigue syndrome, and chronic pelvic pain often co-occur with IBS (Hausteiner-Wiehle and Henningsen 2014). The prevalence of psychiatric comorbidity in IBS is high, with up to 60% of patients having some sort of psychiatric diagnosis (Folks 2004). Associated with this comorbidity is the tendency to experience pain, worry, and hypervigilance focused on visceral and extraintestinal symptoms (Ballou and Keefer 2017).

Etiological, Pathophysiological, and Genetic Factors

The pathophysiological mechanisms implicated in functional disorders are intricately linked to the pathophysiological mechanisms implicated in psychiatric illnesses. These mechanisms include the HPA axis, the brain-gut axis, visceral hypersensitivity, and genetic etiologies.

The HPA axis represents the endocrine link between functional gastrointestinal disorders and diseases such as depression and anxiety (Folks 2004). While the HPA axis regulates autonomic and neuroendocrine function, it also has a role in the limbic system and influences emotional responses (Folks 2004). In both patients with IBS and patients with trauma, depression, or anxiety, there is a hyperresponse of the brain and gut to corticotropin-releasing hormone and alterations in adrenocorticotropic hormone, cortisol, and catecholamine levels (Woodman et al. 1998).

The brain-gut axis (i.e., the bidirectional interchange of neural, immune, and endocrine signals among the brain, gut, and intestinal microbiota) shares key pathways with depression (Fadgyas-Stanculete et al. 2014). The intestinal microbiome is connected to the brain and gut through both extrinsic and intrinsic neural pathways: the autonomic nervous system and the enteric nervous system, respectively (Fadgyas-Stanculete et al. 2014). In IBS, the occurrence of autonomic nervous system dysregulation, in which the locus coeruleus may be activated by painful gut stimuli, in turn incites fear- and arousal-mediating structures, such as the amygdala, periaqueductal gray, and medial hypothalamus (Folks 2004).

Visceral hypersensitivity, in which the threshold is lowered for low-intensity stimuli to be perceived as noxious, is strongly influenced by anxiety and depression (Folks 2004). For instance, anxiety has been demonstrated to cause hypervigilance and negative emotions and thoughts focused on visceral sensory input. Positron emission tomography studies have demonstrated that patients with functional disorders experience sustained activation of the locus coeruleus, which is also the case in patients with anxiety (Van Oudenhove et al. 2012). Also, during gastric distension, patients with functional disorders experience increased activation of the amygdala, a central node of emotional arousal circuitry involved in pain modulation (Jones et al. 2006; Vandenbergh et al. 2005; Van Oudenhove et al. 2012). Areas of the brain found to show changes in patients with functional disorders in comparison with healthy control subjects include the frontal cortex, somatosensory cortex, insula, anterior cingulate cortex, thalamus, hippocampus, and amygdala, which are also associated with visceral hypersensitivity, anxiety, and depression (Ly et al. 2015; Kano et al. 2018). Visceral hypersensitivity also plays a role in the pathogenesis of functional heartburn (Clouse et al. 1999). In the case of functional dysphagia, both abnormal motor events and abnormal perception of such events contribute to the pathophysiology (Clouse et al. 1999).

Finally, evidence also points to genetic etiologies. Functional gastrointestinal disorders cluster in families, with an increased concordance in monozygotic as compared with dizygotic twins (Saito 2011; Saito et al. 2010). Studies also indicate that polymorphisms in genes that encode proteins with immunomodulatory or neuromodulatory functioning, such as interleukin 4 (IL-4) and tumor necrosis factor (TNF), make a genetic contribution (Lee et al. 2016). Polymorphisms that affect many systems (e.g., serotonergic, adrenergic, and opioidergic) also may be involved (Adam et al. 2007; Woodman et al. 1998).

Clinical Presentation

Anxiety symptoms are quite common in globus. Patients report stressful life events over the year preceding symptom onset. Studies have shown alexithymia and low levels of extraversion (Galmiche et al. 2006). Rates of somatization and anxiety are higher in patients with functional heartburn than in those without the functional disorder (Clouse et al. 1999; Galmiche et al. 2006). In particular, patients with heartburn that is not correlated with reflux events on pH monitoring have been shown to have increased anxiety, poor social support, and emotional lability (Clouse et al. 1999). Although psychiatric disorders in functional dysphagia are poorly characterized, rates of anxiety and somatic symptom disorder are increased in this population (Clouse et al. 1999).

Women with functional dyspepsia are prone to generalized anxiety disorder (GAD) and depression (Mak et al. 2012). Onset of these psychiatric disorders tends to coincide with the time at which symptoms of functional disorders begin (Enck et al. 2016). Somatization is common and is predictive of epigastric pain (Van Oudenhove and Aziz 2013) as well as response to acid-lowering treatments such as ranitidine (Filipović et al. 2013). The inability to have normal food and drink intake strongly influences emotional distress (Van Oudenhove and Aziz 2013). Patients with refractory symptoms of functional dyspepsia display reduced physical activity, unhealthful eating, and unemployment and also complain frequently of insomnia (Holtmann et al. 2004).

The psychiatric disorders most commonly observed in IBS include depression, anxiety, and somatic symptom and related disorders (Folks 2004; Hausteiner-Wiehle and Henningsen 2014; Woodman et al. 1998). Rates of somatization in IBS are as high as 42% (Folks 2004). Other diagnoses, such as ICD-10 hypochondriasis, pain disorder, and conversion disorder, are observed frequently (Hausteiner-Wiehle and Henningsen 2014). The intensity of abdominal pain, diarrhea, and bloating is directly correlated to the severity of psychiatric symptoms (Folks 2004), including somatization, maladaptive coping, and catastrophizing (Hausteiner-Wiehle and Henningsen 2014).

Panic disorder (44% of IBS patients), GAD (32% of IBS patients), and posttraumatic stress disorder (PTSD) (36% of IBS patients) are the most frequently occurring anxiety- and stressor-related disorders (Folks 2004; Hausteiner-Wiehle and Henningsen 2014; Woodman et al. 1998). Panic attacks often amplify gastrointestinal symptoms such as nausea, diarrhea, and abdominal discomfort, which can be prominent in IBS patients' panic attacks (Woodman et al. 1998). Among anxiety symptoms, rumination about gastrointestinal symptoms (Hausteiner-Wiehle and Henningsen 2014) preoccupies patients and is escalated by visceral sensitivity (Woodman et al. 1998). The diagnosis of GAD also frequently co-occurs with depression (Woodman et al. 1998). Finally, a recent meta-analysis examining eight studies involving a total of 648,375 subjects found that PTSD was associated with an increased likelihood of IBS (Ng et al. 2019). Given that PTSD is a disorder in which hyperarousal and hypervigilance are prominent, the close link between PTSD and IBS is unsurprising but requires further investigation.

Psychological traits of illness behavior, low quality of life, stressful life events, and sexual or physical abuse history also are commonly observed in IBS patients (Folks 2004). Among depressive symptoms, exhaustion, insomnia, and reduced appetite are prominent (Hausteiner-Wiehle and Henningsen 2014).

Alcohol use disorder may be underdiagnosed in patients with IBS (Woodman et al. 1998). While bipolar disorder has not been shown to have an association with IBS, schizophrenia has been found to co-occur in 17%–19% of IBS patients (Woodman et al. 1998). Additionally, as many as two-thirds of patients with a current or former eating disorder also meet criteria for the diagnosis of IBS (Hausteiner-Wiehle and Henningsen 2014).

Diagnostic and Laboratory Findings

Given that functional disorders are defined as syndromes, the evaluation of a patient with a functional gastrointestinal disorder does not require extensive laboratory testing or imaging, but rather a clinical approach. However, a full medical workup to rule out organic causes of presenting symptomatology should always be undertaken prior to referring a patient for a psychiatric assessment. Symptoms inconsistent with the diagnosis of a functional illness include rectal bleeding, nocturnal or progressive abdominal pain, or weight loss; laboratory findings such as anemia, electrolyte disturbances, or inflammatory marker elevation would likewise point to a nonfunctional diagnosis. In these cases, further evaluation, imaging, or colonoscopy would be indicated (Jiang et al. 2015).

The psychiatric assessment should establish a therapeutic relationship and acknowledge the impact of illness attitudes on symptoms. Additionally, history of the onset, duration, and course of IBS symptoms and any pattern of symptoms in relation to psychiatric symptoms should be elicited.

Treatment Considerations

The goal of medication management is to achieve control of functional symptoms as well as psychiatric comorbidity. Pain, poor appetite, early satiety, bloating, disturbed motility, and nausea all are critical targets.

In functional esophageal disorders, low dosages of tricyclic antidepressants (TCAs) have been shown to alleviate symptoms due to their CNS antinociceptive properties that enable enhanced pain tolerance (Clouse et al. 1999; Galmiche et al. 2006). TCAs are also useful in functional dyspepsia (Talley et al. 2010, 2015), given that they reduce cortical excitability, affecting enteric nervous system function and descending pain pathways of the spinal cord. In the case of IBS, the number needed to treat with TCAs for the targets of pain reduction and IBS symptoms is four patients (Dekel et al. 2013). Amitriptyline, nortriptyline, and desipramine are the most commonly used TCAs, at daily dosages of 25–50 mg. The anticholinergic side effects of TCAs may make them particularly useful for patients with IBS-D.

Data from large, rigorously designed trials suggest that TCAs are superior to selective serotonin reuptake inhibitors (SSRIs) and serotonin-norepinephrine reuptake inhibitors (SNRIs) in the treatment of functional dyspepsia, although sufficient studies to support SSRIs are still lacking (Talley et al. 2015). In fact, SSRIs can cause dyspepsia (Talley et al. 2015).

For IBS, SSRIs can be useful for patients with IBS-C and high levels of anxiety, although SSRIs can also be associated with gastrointestinal side effects in some patients (Dekel et al. 2013). Citalopram has the greatest amount of evidence for the IBS targets of abdominal pain and bloating (Dekel et al. 2013). The SNRIs (duloxetine, venlafaxine, desvenlafaxine, and milnacipran) also have analgesic potential in IBS, particularly at higher dosages (150–225 mg/day) (Dekel et al. 2013); however, the use of SNRIs for treatment of functional dyspepsia requires further verification in prospective randomized, double-blind clinical trials with large sample sizes (Dekel et al. 2013).

Given its effects on sedation, appetite stimulation, weight gain, and nausea, the atypical antidepressant mirtazapine may be a useful adjunctive agent for functional dyspepsia (Tack et al. 2016). Additionally, buspirone, a nonbenzodiazepine anxiolytic, has been shown to reduce the severity of functional dyspepsia by improving gastric accommodation (Tack et al. 2012).

Evidence is accumulating for the use of atypical antipsychotics (e.g., olanzapine, quetiapine) in IBS patients with refractory and severe symptoms (Dekel et al. 2013). Quetiapine at low dosages (50–200 mg/day) has been shown to have efficacy in patients with functional disorder and pain (Dekel et al. 2013), and it has also been shown to improve sleep and reduce anxiety.

Clinicians should bear in mind that psychiatric illness in a patient with a functional gastrointestinal disorder may be primary rather than secondary to the functional disorder. For a patient with a functional gastrointestinal disorder who is also depressed or anxious, proceeding with the standard of care for the psychiatric disorder is the best approach.

Cognitive-behavioral therapy (CBT) has been demonstrated to have utility in patients with refractory functional dyspepsia (Talley et al. 2015). Additionally, hypnotherapy, which can produce a state of relaxation sufficient to assist the patient in regaining a sense of control over physiological sensations and symptoms, has been shown to be effective in small trials (Riehl and Keefer 2015).

For IBS, rigorous data support the use of CBT. CBT addresses IBS symptoms such as abdominal pain and diarrhea, as well as mood symptoms, and has been demonstrated to be most effective when combined with medication (Lackner et al. 2018, 2019; Laird et al. 2016; Windgassen et al. 2019). CBT helps the patient recognize the maladaptive thoughts and self-defeating patterns of behavior that increase functional symptomatology.

Finally, poor health behaviors are a key link between psychiatric disorders and gastrointestinal disease. The low-FODMAP (fermentable, oligo-, di-, and monosaccharides and polyols) diet is an important strategy for achieving symptom control in IBS. A study assessing the frequency of IBS symptoms in obese patients in a weight-loss program found that patients who consumed low-fat, high-fruit, and high-fiber diets and engaged in higher levels of physical activity experienced fewer symptoms (Levy et al. 2005). Thus, although the mechanism by which diet and exercise mediate the relationship between mood and gastrointestinal symptoms is unclear, the association between IBS symptom reduction and healthful lifestyle choices indicates the need to educate patients about pursuing such measures to achieve greater symptom control.

Gastrointestinal Pain Disorders: Centrally Mediated Abdominal Pain Syndrome and Narcotic Bowel Syndrome

Centrally mediated abdominal pain syndrome (CAPS), formerly called functional abdominal pain syndrome, is characterized by continuous or recurrent pain as a central complaint and is rarely related to gut function or a motility disturbance (Clouse et al. 2006; Keefer et al. 2016). To qualify for a CAPS diagnosis, symptoms must have been present for at least 6 months, must have met criteria for the last 3 months, and must cause limitations in some aspect of daily functioning (Keefer et al. 2016). The disorder is distinguishable from other functional complaints such as IBS by its lack of symptoms related to food intake or defecation (Keefer et al. 2016). CAPS has a close relationship with a variety of psychiatric disorders, including satisfying the pain criteria for DSM-IV somatization disorder (American Psychiatric Association 1994).

Subtypes and Defining Criteria

Narcotic bowel syndrome (NBS), also known as opioid-induced gastrointestinal hyperalgesia, produces a paradoxical increase in abdominal pain when opioid dosages are increased. NBS is called a centrally mediated pain disorder because it results from central nervous system (CNS) dysfunction (Drossman and Szigethy 2014; Grunkemeier et al. 2007). In NBS, pain escalates when opioid dosages are reduced and frequency, duration, and intensity of pain episodes progress. Additionally, a current gastrointestinal diagnosis must have been ruled out as the source of the pain. NBS must be distinguished from opioid tolerance (in which higher dosages of opioids are necessary to produce the same effect) and opioid withdrawal (in which a heightened sensitivity to pain is present, as are myalgias, restlessness, anxiety, lacrimation, yawning, and diaphoresis) (Drossman and Szigethy 2014). Demographic studies indicate that NBS tends to occur predominantly in educated Caucasian women (Drossman and Szigethy 2014).

Pain in CAPS is prolonged, widespread, and colicky. Burning also can be a common characteristic. CAPS most commonly occurs in women in their 40s and is associated with a high level of health care utilization (Keefer et al. 2016). In CAPS, anxiety, depression, and somatoform disorders are the most common psychiatric comorbidities (Clouse et al. 2006).

Along with CAPS, NBS is closely associated with other somatic syndromes (e.g., fibromyalgia) and psychological comorbidity (Drossman and Szigethy 2014; Grunkemeier et al. 2007). In one study of NBS patients ($N=39$), 28.2% were clinically depressed and 33.3% had clinically significant anxiety (Drossman and Szigethy 2014; Drossman et al. 2012; Grunkemeier et al. 2007).

Etiological, Pathophysiological, and Genetic Factors

Similar to other visceral pain disorders such as IBS, CAPS results from changes in CNS sensory processing of gastrointestinal pain (Keefer et al. 2016). Heightened sensitivity to stimuli results from modulation of descending pain pathways in the brain stem by cortical regions. Such regions include the midcingulate, insular, and somatosensory cortex and thalamus, which are involved in sensory functioning; the anterior cingulate cortex and amygdala, which are involved in emotional arousal; and the prefrontal cortical regions, which are involved in belief systems and coping styles (Clouse et al. 2006; Keefer et al. 2016), pointing to the role of emotional and cognitive input in influencing pain symptoms. However, given that CAPS symptoms do not have a relationship with food intake or defecation, input from visceral afferents in the gut is less likely to play a role (Keefer et al. 2016).

In NBS, hyperalgesia occurs as a result of CNS activation: chronic, escalating dosages of opioids activate glial cells (the immune cells of the CNS), which release cytokines and chemokines. These proinflammatory substances cause neuronal excitability, in turn enhancing pain perception (Drossman and Szigethy 2014). Additionally, long-term opioid administration causes glial activation and glutamate release in the ventral tegmental area, reinforcing reward effects. These dual mechanisms involving both inflammation and reward circuitry activation explain why individuals with NBS continue to seek drugs despite experiencing worsening pain (Drossman and Szigethy 2014).

Clinical Presentation

Patients with CAPS often experience pain intensity disproportionate to objective laboratory or diagnostic findings, deny that psychosocial issues contribute to their pain, continually seek health care services and diagnostic studies, request narcotic analgesics, and assume limited responsibility for self-management of symptoms (Keefer et al. 2016). Lack of social support, unresolved losses resulting in complex grief, and a history of sexual or physical abuse are common (Keefer et al. 2016). In NBS, poor coping skills and a tendency to catastrophize also characterize patients (Drossman and Szigethy 2014).

Diagnostic and Laboratory Findings

Observation of symptom-related behaviors, a psychosocial assessment, and a complete physical evaluation are essential to making the diagnosis of CAPS (Clouse et al. 2006; Keefer et al. 2016). Questions regarding trauma, psychiatric diagnoses, and the patient's illness attitude are useful (Clouse et al. 2006; Keefer et al. 2016). The clinical assessment will also require psychoeducation and a discussion of how increasing opioid doses paradoxically worsens pain, given that insight into this aspect of the disorder is key to recovery (Drossman and Szigethy 2014). Although abdominal X rays may show a partial intestinal obstruction due to a dynamic ileus or pseudo-obstruction, laboratory tests such as complete blood count, amylase, lipase, liver chemistries, and urinalysis are normal (Drossman and Szigethy 2014).

Treatment Considerations

Establishing an effective patient-physician relationship is essential to treatment of both CAPS and NBS (Keefer et al. 2016). Empathy, education, and validation of the illness all help to build rapport. TCAs such as amitriptyline and nortriptyline at low dosages provide some pain relief. SNRIs such as duloxetine and venlafaxine also are useful agents (Keefer et al. 2016). The antidepressant mirtazapine has been shown to be a useful antiemetic and appetite stimulant (Clouse et al. 2006). Although anticonvulsants such as carbamazepine, lamotrigine, gabapentin, and pregabalin have not been well evaluated, studies indicate that these agents may be useful for treatment of pain in CAPS (Keefer et al. 2016). Among nonpharmacological/behavioral interventions, CBT, interpersonal therapy, mindfulness-based acceptance therapy, and hypnotherapy hold the most promise in CAPS (Clouse et al. 2006; Keefer et al. 2016).

In NBS, physicians must weigh whether an outpatient or inpatient opioid withdrawal treatment protocol is suitable for the patient's needs (Drossman and Szigethy 2014). Antidepressants such as TCAs with fewer anticholinergic and antihistaminergic effects (e.g., desipramine, nortriptyline) at low dosages are helpful to target pain, although higher dosages are necessary if treatment of depression is a priority as well. The SNRIs duloxetine, venlafaxine, desvenlafaxine, and milnacipran all have been demonstrated to be effective treatments for both pain and mood (Drossman and

Szigethy 2014; Grunkemeier et al. 2007). Beginning antidepressant treatment before narcotic withdrawal further facilitates successful treatment (Clouse et al. 2006). Clonidine can reduce adrenergic symptoms in opioid withdrawal and functional symptoms such as diarrhea (Drossman and Szigethy 2014; Grunkemeier et al. 2007). Other promising agents include the atypical antipsychotic quetiapine, which has demonstrated efficacy in patients with functional disorder and pain, and the cognitive enhancing agent memantine, which has been shown to treat pain refractory to opioids (Drossman and Szigethy 2014). Additionally, behavioral treatments such as CBT and hypnotherapy have been found to be beneficial in reducing other causes of visceral pain (Drossman and Szigethy 2014; Grunkemeier et al. 2007).

Primary Gastrointestinal Diseases: Peptic Ulcer Disease and Gastroparesis

Peptic Ulcer Disease

Peptic ulcer disease (PUD) produces symptoms of pain, bloating, nausea, and epigastric fullness and is caused by breaks in the mucosa of the stomach or the first part of the small intestine (Malfertheiner et al. 2009). While nicotine and alcohol strongly influence the pathophysiology of PUD, an emerging role is now being defined for psychiatric disorders, illustrating the complex relationship between substance use disorders and PUD.

Subtypes and Defining Criteria

PUD consists of gastric and duodenal ulcers that measure 5 mm or greater, a criterion defined by clinical trials (Malfertheiner et al. 2009). For patients with gastric ulcers, meals produce immediate pain; for those with duodenal ulcers, pain occurs 2–3 hours after meals (Goodwin et al. 2009). Nicotine and alcohol use disorders are major risk factors (Goodwin et al. 2009), although bipolar disorder, schizophrenia, and dementia also have been shown to be associated with a higher incidence of PUD (Goodwin et al. 2009; Hsu et al. 2015b, 2016; Malfertheiner et al. 2009). While comorbid substance use disorders were thought to weaken the association between PUD and mood disorders (Goodwin et al. 2009), other data indicate that depression can independently increase the risk of PUD by as much as two times (Hsu et al. 2015a; Malfertheiner et al. 2009).

Etiological, Pathophysiological, and Genetic Factors

PUD is caused by defects in mucosal functioning and imbalances in gastric acid, both of which are exacerbated by nicotine and alcohol, which increase gastric acid production. Nicotine also reduces mucous production in the stomach and duodenum (Goodwin et al. 2009). The HPA axis plays a key role in the relationship between PUD and psychiatric disorders (Goodwin et al. 2009; Malfertheiner et al. 2009). Stress enhances the release of glucocorticoids, which can disrupt the healing of ulcers and increase the risk of recurrence (Malfertheiner et al. 2009). Bipolar disorder, psychotic illnesses, and neurodegenerative disorders also produce hypercortisolemia as a result of chronic neuroinflammation (Goodwin et al. 2009; Liao et al. 2014; Malfertheiner et al. 2009). Stress may also influence the inflammatory response to *Helicobacter pylori*, a bacterium that has been shown to cause ulcers (Goodwin et al. 2009; Hsu et al. 2015b). This influence of stress on *H. pylori* occurs because stress has an immunomodulatory effect and can change the inflammatory reaction to infections controlled by T helper type 1 (Th1) lymphocytes/cytokines such as *H. pylori* (Goodwin et al. 2009; Hsu et al. 2015b).

Clinical Presentation

The signs and symptoms of PUD are well established; however, further studies are needed to define the characteristics of psychiatric disorders that occur in PUD specifically as compared with other gastrointestinal illnesses. The hallmark symptom of PUD is epigastric pain. This pain is relieved by food and antacids for duodenal ulcers but not for gastric ulcers (Goodwin et al. 2009). Additional symptoms include belching, intolerance of fatty foods, bloating, and heartburn. If gastrointestinal bleeding occurs, hematemesis or melena can result (Goodwin et al. 2009).

Diagnostic and Laboratory Findings

There are no diagnostic or laboratory findings specific to psychiatric disorders comorbid with PUD. A standard medical assessment includes laboratory testing for *H. pylori* and endoscopy (Goodwin et al. 2009).

Treatment Considerations

A key issue in patients with comorbid PUD and psychiatric disorders is that psychotropic medications can have effects that either ameliorate or aggravate gastrointestinal symptoms. Patients with bleeding ulcers should be educated about the risk of upper gastrointestinal bleeding associated with SSRIs due to SSRIs' inhibition of platelet function; however, certain psychotropics can relieve poor appetite, nausea, and pain. For example, mirtazapine has been shown to improve nausea and poor appetite (Tack et al. 2016). A study in rats showed that mirtazapine had a gastroprotective effect on ulcers (Bilici et al. 2009). Additionally, TCAs are widely accepted as useful agents to improve visceral pain.

Gastroparesis

Gastroparesis is a syndrome in which gastric emptying is delayed, resulting from paresis of the stomach in the absence of mechanical obstruction (Bielefeldt 2012). Although gastroparesis occurs when the vagal nerve is damaged, keeping the muscles of the stomach and intestine from functioning properly, there are parallels between gastroparesis and functional gastrointestinal disorders: both occur predominantly in women, have an idiopathic nature, and co-occur with anxiety and depression (Camilleri et al. 2013).

Subtypes and Defining Criteria

Symptoms of gastroparesis include nausea, vomiting, bloating, early satiety, postprandial fullness, and upper abdominal pain (Bielefeldt 2012; Camilleri et al. 2013). The most common etiologies are diabetes, postsurgical complications, and idiopathic contributions (Bielefeldt 2012; Camilleri et al. 2013). Dyspeptic symptoms and a documented delay in gastric emptying without gastric outlet obstruction (as assessed by scintigraphy of a solid-phase meal over 4 hours) are required to make the diagnosis (Camilleri et al. 2013). In the case of idiopathic gastroparesis, symptoms often overlap with those of functional dyspepsia. Fatigue is also a prominent symptom (Cherian et al. 2012). An analysis of data from 146 gastroparesis patients seen over 6 years found that depression was associated with idiopathic gastroparesis in 23% of patients (Soykan et al. 1998). Additionally, 62% of women with idiopathic gastroparesis reported a history of physical or sexual abuse (Soykan et al. 1998). Depression and anxiety are two important contributors to perception of symptoms and pain.

Etiological, Pathophysiological, and Genetic Factors

While the etiology of gastroparesis has long been considered to involve disruption of gastrointestinal smooth muscle, the vagus nerve, the autonomic nervous system, and the enteric nervous system, further investigation has demonstrated a complex picture with a range of different mechanisms (Bielefeldt 2012). For instance, impairment of gastric accommodation, visceral hypersensitivity, and inflammatory infiltration of myenteric ganglia all can contribute to symptoms (Bielefeldt 2012). As with functional dyspepsia, mood disorders directly affect visceral hypersensitivity given that anxiety produces hypervigilance and negative emotions and thoughts focused on visceral sensory input (Bielefeldt 2012).

Clinical Presentation

Higher depression and anxiety scores on self-report symptom measures are associated with greater gastroparesis and pain intensity (Hasler et al. 2010). Depression is also a factor linked to treatment resistance (Hasler et al. 2013) and increases health care utilization (Pasricha et al. 2015). Additionally, fatigue, a common symptom in gastroparesis, has been noted to be strongly associated with depression (Cherian et al. 2012; Lacy et al. 2018).

Diagnostic and Laboratory Findings

As yet, no objective findings distinguish the patient with gastroparesis and comorbid psychiatric illness.

Treatment Considerations

Case studies support the rapid and effective improvement of nausea and vomiting in idiopathic gastroparesis with mirtazapine (Kundu et al. 2014). Mirtazapine improves gastric accommodation because receptive fundic relaxation is influenced by the stimulation of serotonin (5-hydroxytryptamine type 1A [5-HT$_{1A}$]) receptors (Kundu et al. 2014). Amitriptyline has also been shown to produce overall improvement of gastroparesis symptoms (Camilleri et al. 2013). Clonidine has been demonstrated to produce symptomatic relief in patients with diabetic gastroparesis (Rosa-e-Silva et al. 1995).

Inflammatory Disorders: Inflammatory Bowel Disease and Lymphocytic Colitis

Inflammatory Bowel Disease

IBD is defined as a chronic, inappropriate inflammatory response occurring anywhere in the gastrointestinal tract (Korzenik and Podolsky 2006). While IBD was historically viewed as a psychosomatic illness, the disorder is currently conceptualized as a primary inflammatory illness whose course may be influenced by psychiatric disorders (Sajadinejad et al. 2012).

Subtypes and Defining Criteria

IBD includes Crohn's disease and ulcerative colitis (Korzenik and Podolsky 2006). Symptoms include abdominal pain, diarrhea, fatigue, malnutrition, weight loss, anemia, joint pain, and skin lesions (Korzenik and Podolsky 2006). Depression, anxiety disorders, and substance use disorders are the psychiatric disorders that most commonly co-occur with IBD ((Sajadinejad et al. 2012; Walker et al. 2008). Psychiatric disorders lead to earlier and increased frequency of IBD relapse and interfere with response to biologics (i.e., powerful, selective anticytokine drugs used as a therapy for IBD; see Biancone et al. 2007) (Persoons et al. 2005).

Etiological, Pathophysiological, and Genetic Factors

Endocrine, neurological, and immunological mechanisms underlie the biological link between psychiatric illness and IBD.

Activation of the HPA axis results in release of corticotropin-releasing factor (CRF); signaling pathways triggered by CRF release have been shown to increase colonic permeability, transit, and secretion and to delay gastric emptying (Moss et al. 2007).

The brain-gut-microbiome axis, a set of complex and bidirectional interactions between the CNS and the enteric nervous system influenced by gut microbiota, is altered by emotional stress, which increases intestinal permeability (Moss et al. 2007; Petra et al. 2015). As a result, bacteria translocate across the epithelial barrier and catalyze the production of proinflammatory cytokines. The neurological link between psychiatric disorders and IBD is further evidenced by the finding of reduced volume in the anterior midcingulate cortex, which plays a role in the response to fear in Crohn's patients (Martin-Subero et al. 2016; Vogt 2013). In both depression and IBD, patients experience activation of peripheral Th1-like and Th17–like cells, increasing production of IL-2, interferon-gamma (IFN-γ), and IL-17 (Petra et al. 2015).

Clinical Presentation

Depression and anxiety are closely associated with the diagnosis of IBD (Mikocka-Walus et al. 2007), as illustrated by the high rates of depression and anxiety found among cohorts of IBD patients assessed for psychiatric disorders. In the Manitoba IBD cohort study, which investigated the rates of any anxiety or mood disorder (as diagnosed by DSM-IV [American Psychiatric Association 1994] criteria) in a large population-based cohort (N=351) of Canadian patients with IBD, the 12-month and lifetime prevalences were 22.2% and 45.3%, respectively (Walker et al. 2008). In an earlier study utilizing data from two large population-based surveys, the Canadian Community Health Survey 1.1 (CCHS; N=3,076 [2000–2001]) and the National Population Health Survey (NPHS; N=1,438 [1996–1997]), the prevalence rates of depression (as diagnosed by DSM-III [American Psychiatric Association 1980] criteria) among respondents with IBS were 16.3% in the CCHS and 14.7% in the NPHS (Fuller-Thomson and Sulman 2006). Depression rates have been noted to be higher in patients who are female, who have severe and active IBD, who are disabled or unemployed, or who are socioeconomically deprived (Fuller-Thomson and Sulman 2006; Nahon et al. 2012). In a study of 1,352 patients with IBD who were screened for depression at routine clinic visits, 71 patients expressed suicidal ideation; among these patients, low self-esteem, chronic pain, and narcotic use were common findings (Hashash et al. 2016). Depression heavily influences the presentation of comorbid IBS, as well as symptoms of visceral hypersensitivity, fatigue, cognitive dysfunction, and insomnia.

GAD, panic disorder, social anxiety disorder (social phobia), and PTSD also occur at higher rates in patients with IBD compared with individuals in the general population (Walker et al. 2008). Rumination about medical symptoms and worry about future disease underlie anxiety. Phobic objects/situations include fear of nausea, vomiting, fecal incontinence, and food and its impact on IBD symptoms. Fear of incontinence can precipitate agoraphobia. Food phobia, resulting in food restriction as a maladaptive response, can lead to eating disorders, and both anorexia and bulimia have been observed in patients with IBD (Ilzarbe et al. 2017).

PTSD is an important trauma- and stressor-related disorder associated with IBD. In a study examining PTSD among IBD patients in comparison with IBS patients (131 IBD, 57 IBS), 32% of IBD and 26% of IBS patients met criteria for PTSD (Taft et al. 2019). Crohn's disease patients with greater IBD symptom severity were more likely to experience PTSD, particularly those being hospitalized or undergoing ileostomy surgery (Taft et al. 2019).

The most frequent neurological disorders associated with IBD in the literature are cerebrovascular disease (with either arterial or venous events), demyelinating CNS disease such as multiple sclerosis, and peripheral neuropathy (either axonal or demyelinating). Although studies have noted that there is an association between epilepsy and IBD, the relationship has not been completely clarified. The question of whether psychiatric disorders are a manifestation of the direct effects of IBD on the brain remains unresolved (Morís 2014). Asymptomatic structural differences found in the brains of IBD patients compared with control subjects have included decreased gray matter volume in parts of the frontal gyrus and in the anterior midcingulate cortex (Dolapcioglu and Dolapcioglu 2015).

Cognitive dysfunction can occur in IBD and may include short-term memory and verbal IQ deficits, which have been attributed to white matter lesions (Vogt 2013).

Narcotic dependence is a major concern in patients with IBD. In a study that used the population-based Manitoba IBD Epidemiology Database, all IBD patient in Manitoba who were prescribed opioids before and after their diagnosis of IBD were identified (Targownik et al. 2014), and for each patient, the risk of becoming a heavy opioid user (defined as continuous use for 30 days at a dose exceeding 50 mg morphine/day or its equivalent) was calculated. Within 10 years of diagnosis, 5% of individuals with IBD had become heavy opioid users, with mortality rates nearly three times higher than those of individuals who were not heavy users (Targownik et al. 2014).

Diagnostic and Laboratory Findings

There are no current formal guidelines on diagnostic or laboratory findings that define patients with IBD and comorbid psychiatric disorders. C-reactive protein levels will often be normal, and inflammation can be absent on colonoscopy, indicating that these patients have no active inflammation.

Treatment Considerations

Evaluation of the patient with IBD should be the same as for any medically complex patient. The patient should be asked about the presence of IBD symptoms, whether mood influences the symptoms, and whether there is a history of treatment with biologics (i.e., anticytokine drugs) and, if so, their impact on mood. Screening for substance use (including tobacco) and eating disorders also is essential.

Antidepressants improve psychiatric symptoms and may reduce inflammation (as suggested in animal models and some small clinical studies) (Hall et al. 2018). Additionally, psychotropic medication can be useful in targeting symptoms such as poor appetite, nausea, frequent bowel movements, weight gain or loss, IBS overlay (i.e., IBS features superimposed on IBD), visceral hypersensitivity, fatigue, cognitive dysfunction, and insomnia. In animal models, the TCAs clomipramine and desipramine; the SSRIs citalopram, fluoxetine, and sertraline; the atypical antidepressant trazodone; and lithium have all been shown to have anti-inflammatory properties. In human studies, TCAs and SSRIs have been shown to reduce rates of IBD-specific medical therapy escalation (Hall et al. 2018; Mikocka-Walus et al. 2009). Bupropion has been shown to lower circulating levels of TNF-α (Kast 2003; Mikocka-Walus et al. 2009), while the SSRI paroxetine and the monoamine oxidase inhibitor phenelzine have also been demonstrated to improve IBD symptoms independently of their effect on patients' psychiatric symptoms (Goodhand et al. 2012). Further studies examining the influence of antidepressants on IBD outcomes are needed. CBT is the therapy that has garnered the most evidence for positive effects on IBD symptoms (McCombie et al. 2013).

Further guidelines on psychotropic choice in IBD are noted in Table 10–1.

Lymphocytic Colitis

Lymphocytic colitis, a subtype of microscopic colitis (in which inflammation of the large intestine causes sustained watery diarrhea), is an important consideration when patients are being treated with psychotropic medications. Patients with lymphocytic colitis have chronic nonbloody diarrhea with abdominal pain or weight loss, despite normal or near-normal findings on colonoscopy (Pascua et al. 2010). Histopathological features include an increase in intraepithelial lymphocytes and expansion of the lamina propria with acute and chronic inflammatory cells but preserved crypt architecture (Pascua et al. 2010). Lymphocytic colitis tends to occur predominantly in Caucasian women, with a peak incidence at approximately 60 years of age (Pascua et al. 2010).

The etiology of lymphocytic colitis is of relevance to psychiatrists. Case reports and descriptive data indicated that SSRI use may be a contributing factor (Pascua et al. 2010; Tong et al. 2015); however, a controlled study showed that among the SSRIs, only sertraline was more commonly used among individuals with lymphocytic colitis than among control subjects (Pascua et al. 2010). Although the exact mechanism of the relationship between sertraline and lymphocytic colitis remains unknown, it is also possible, given that a correlation but not a causal relationship has been established, that there is some other as-yet-unrecognized reason that the prevalence of microscopic colitis is increased among individuals who take sertraline (Pascua et al. 2010; Tong et al. 2015).

TABLE 10–1.   **Symptoms influencing psychotropic choice in inflammatory bowel disease with comorbid mood disorders**

Symptom	Preferred psychotropic
Visceral hypersensitivity	Duloxetine, venlafaxine, nortriptyline, amitriptyline, pregabalin, memantine
Insomnia	Mirtazapine
Nausea	Mirtazapine
Low appetite	Mirtazapine
Gastroparesis	Mirtazapine, buspirone
Fatigue	Bupropion, modafinil
Cognitive deficits	Bupropion, modafinil
Nicotine dependence	Bupropion
IBS overlay with diarrhea predominance	Citalopram, paroxetine, amitriptyline, nortriptyline

Note.   IBS overlay=irritable bowel syndrome features superimposed on inflammatory bowel disease.

Absorption Disorders: Celiac Disease

Celiac disease and gluten sensitivity are diseases caused by immune-mediated reactions to gluten, a protein found in wheat, barley, and rye. The classic symptom profile consists of steatorrhea, weight loss, and postprandial bloating (Jackson et al. 2012). However, for many years (Carta et al. 2002; Cascella et al. 2011), psychiatric manifestations have been observed as part of the presentation; in fact, up to one-third of patients with celiac disease present with psychiatric complications (Bushara 2005).

Subtypes and Defining Criteria

In celiac disease, present in approximately 1% of the population (Jackson et al. 2012), histological findings in the gut include villous atrophy, crypt hyperplasia, and increased intraepithelial lymphocytes. A diagnosis is made by testing for the presence of anti-endomysial antibodies, antitissue transglutaminase antibodies, and antigliadin antibodies (AGA) in the blood (Jackson et al. 2012). By contrast, gluten sensitivity occurs six times more frequently than celiac disease but results from a different immune reaction. Although individuals with gluten sensitivity do not show the villous atrophy or the laboratory evidence of anti-endomysial and antitissue transglutaminase antibodies seen in celiac disease, they do test positive for AGA (Jackson et al. 2012). Common psychiatric complications in celiac disease include schizophrenia, depression, anxiety disorders, attention-deficit/hyperactivity disorder (ADHD), and autism spectrum disorder.

Etiological, Pathophysiological, and Genetic Factors

Several mechanisms, including autoimmune, monoamine, and genetic pathways, may link gluten sensitivity to psychiatric disorders. First, wheat gluten, producing an immune-mediated response, could be a possible pathogenic factor for depression

(Carta et al. 2002), although gluten removal does not consistently relieve depression. In addition, given the increased prevalence of autoimmune thyroid disorder in patients with celiac disease, high levels of circulating thyroid antibodies may play a role (Carta et al. 2002). Malabsorption could also lead to both vitamin deficiency and decreased tryptophan availability, causing reductions in central serotonin. For example, reduced tryptophan levels have been found in patients with untreated celiac disease (Carta et al. 2002). The activation of T cells by gluten ingestion could additionally influence serotonin dysfunction (Porcelli et al. 2014). Although specific human leukocyte antigen (HLA) class II genes—*HLA-DQ2* and *HLA-DQ8*—are closely associated with celiac disease, studies in patients with schizophrenia have shown a different pathway for an immune response against gluten that is independent of transglutaminase and HLA-DQ2 and/or DQ8 molecules (Porcelli et al. 2014). Further studies are needed to elucidate the contribution of mechanisms such as an altered gut microbiome and changes in intestinal permeability, both of which influence infection risk, to the pathogenesis of psychiatric disorders (Porcelli et al. 2014).

Clinical Presentation

Social phobia, panic disorder, and GAD all have been linked to celiac disease (Jackson et al. 2012). In fact, a higher lifetime prevalence of panic disorder has been found in patients with celiac disease (Jackson et al. 2012). Depression is more common and more severe in patients with celiac disease than in healthy adults (Smith and Gerdes 2012), occurring in as many as one-third of patients (Bushara 2005). Irritability and apathy often characterize depressive episodes (Bushara 2005). Gluten intolerance also occurs at higher rates in individuals with autism spectrum disorder (Bushara 2005). These patients can benefit from gluten- and casein-free diets (Jackson et al. 2012). ADHD also may have an association with celiac disease (Jackson et al. 2012). Schizophrenia can co-occur with celiac disease, and a higher prevalence of celiac disease has been seen in patients with schizophrenia than in matched control subjects (Cascella et al. 2011).

Diagnostic and Laboratory Findings

The immunological markers for celiac disease and gluten sensitivity (anti-endomysial antibodies, antitissue transglutaminase antibodies, and AGA) have been assayed in patients with psychiatric disorders to identify implications for treatment. Results from a study in 1,401 schizophrenia patients and 900 control subjects indicated that 1 in 4.3 patients with schizophrenia had elevated levels of immunoglobulin A (IgA)-AGA, as compared with 1 in 32.1 control patients, indicating a specific immune response to gluten (Cascella et al. 2011).

Treatment Considerations

While elimination of gluten from the diet of schizophrenia patients has been shown to improve psychotic symptoms (Porcelli et al. 2014), the literature still lacks data regarding optimal treatment of psychiatric disorders co-occurring with celiac disease and gluten sensitivity. Given that celiac disease and gluten sensitivity manifest with weight loss and bloating, psychotropics that target comorbid psychiatric issues and that address gastrointestinal symptoms may be ideal choices. As an example, mirtaz-apine is a useful treatment for nausea, poor appetite, and weight loss. Additionally, duloxetine and venlafaxine are useful for their central antinociceptive properties, which facilitate improved pain tolerance.

Liver Diseases

Liver diseases cause a wide range of symptoms with manifestations throughout the body, often mimicking psychiatric and neurological disorders. While overt symptoms consist of ascites, palmar erythema, and spider angiomata, these can be preceded by fatigue, pruritus, personality and mood change, and memory loss (Crone et al. 2006). Thus, psychiatrists must learn to recognize and treat psychiatric manifestations in liver disease.

Liver diseases discussed in this section include viral hepatitis, alcoholic hepatitis, nonalcoholic fatty liver disease, hemochromatosis, and Wilson's disease, all of which can contribute to cirrhosis and liver failure.

Subtypes and Defining Criteria

While infection of the liver can occur with hepatitis A, B, C, D, and E viruses, it is infection with hepatitis C virus (HCV) that has become the most common cause of liver disease in the United States (Crone et al. 2006). Even with the rate of HCV dropping, the slowly progressive nature of the disease and the large pool of infected individuals contribute to rising prevalence (Crone et al. 2006). Symptoms of hepatitis include nausea, vomiting, jaundice, diarrhea, pruritus, fatigue, and pale bowel movements.

Transmission of HCV most commonly occurs through intravenous drug use. Following acute hepatitis, or inflammation of the liver, 85% of patients develop chronic infection, with 65%–80% progressing to chronic hepatitis (Crone et al. 2006). Another 7%–20% of patients develop cirrhosis (i.e., the formation of scar tissue within the liver), while 1%–5% develop hepatocellular cancer (Crone et al. 2006).

In alcoholic hepatitis, long-term heavy use of alcohol results in inflammatory liver injury. Regular alcohol use, even for just a few days per week, can result in a fatty liver (also called steatosis), in which liver cells fill with triglycerides (Lucey et al. 2009). However, steatosis can resolve with abstinence. In the case of alcoholic hepatitis, patients present with rapid onset of jaundice as well as fever, ascites, and a tender, enlarged liver. Cirrhosis of the liver develops in only a small proportion of heavy drinkers (Lucey et al. 2009).

Nonalcoholic steatohepatitis is marked by the buildup of extra fat in liver cells in the absence of alcohol use, resulting in inflammation (Stewart and Levenson 2012). This condition is closely linked to metabolic syndrome, with high levels of comorbidity in patients with heart disease and diabetes (Stewart and Levenson 2012).

In hereditary hemochromatosis, an autosomal recessive disorder prevalent among individuals of Northern European descent, iron deposits in organ tissue cause endocrine disorders (e.g., diabetes), cardiac problems (e.g., arrhythmias), liver disease (e.g., cirrhosis) and joint disease (e.g., destructive arthritis) (Cutler 1994; Pietrangelo 2004). Patients present with symptoms of these diseases as well as fatigue, right-upper-quadrant abdominal pain, arthralgias, impotence, decreased libido, and chondrocalcinosis (Cutler 1994).

Wilson's disease is an autosomal recessive illness that leads to copper accumulation in the brain, liver, and other tissues (Zimbrean and Schilsky 2014).

Liver failure can be complicated by hepatic encephalopathy, which produces disturbances in consciousness, mood, behavior, and cognition (Crone et al. 2006; Ferenci 2017). Minimal and covert hepatic encephalopathy may occur in up to 50% of patients with chronic liver disease (Ferenci 2017). Symptoms range from mild cognitive complaints to gross disorientation, agitation, and confusion (Crone et al. 2006). Fatigue and lethargy are also often present.

Etiological, Pathophysiological, and Genetic Factors

The causes of psychiatric manifestations of liver diseases vary according to the illness causing liver damage; however, a common pathway is the impact of liver damage on accumulation of toxic substances such as ammonia in the blood (Crone et al. 2006). Higher amounts of ammonia reach the brain because of both increased uptake and altered blood-brain barrier permeability (Crone et al. 2006). Manganese, a neurotoxic agent, also accumulates in the form of deposits in the basal ganglia in encephalopathy (Crone et al. 2006).

Although HCV infects the liver, there is accumulating evidence of its capacity for neuroinvasion (Adinolfi et al. 2015). HCV proteins have been hypothesized to produce neurotoxicity and to induce apoptosis in brain microvascular endothelial cells, resulting in changes in blood-brain barrier permeability, microglia activation, and diffusion of proinflammatory cytokines into the CNS (Adinolfi et al. 2015).

In alcoholic hepatitis, endotoxin is a key trigger of the inflammatory process in experimental models (Lucey et al. 2009). Endotoxin has biological activity associated with lipopolysaccharide, a component of the outer wall of gram-negative bacteria (Lucey et al. 2009). Lipopolysaccharide-endotoxin enters portal blood and triggers an inflammatory cascade. Additionally, alcohol ingestion causes oxidative stress and production of free radicals. TNF-α, produced by Kupffer cells, also appears to play a pivotal role in the genesis of alcoholic hepatitis (Lucey et al. 2009).

In Wilson's disease, copper accumulation occurs in the putamen, globus pallidus, thalami, and brain stem (Ranjan et al. 2015; Zimbrean and Schilsky 2014). Some authors have suggested that basal ganglia abnormalities can lead to psychiatric symptoms through dopamine dysregulation (Zimbrean and Schilsky 2014); however, studies have also considered the role of copper in schizophrenia and bipolar illness (Zimbrean and Schilsky 2014). In the case of hemochromatosis, iron overload has been shown to cause changes in gene expression and protein levels in the brain, leading to altered functioning (Milward et al. 2012).

Clinical Presentation

Cognitive impairment in HCV includes poor concentration and impaired working memory speed, diminished ability to sustain attention, and reduced psychomotor speed (Adinolfi et al. 2015). The most frequently reported psychiatric symptom is fatigue, often in association with depression and sleep disturbance (Adinolfi et al. 2015). Depression and anxiety have been found in up to one-third of patients with chronic HCV (Adinolfi et al. 2015); furthermore, one study found that brief, recurrent episodes of depression and anxiety occurred in 15% of 135 treatment-naive patients (Carta et al. 2012), suggesting that these episodes were not attributable to treatment effects. Neuropsychiatric effects of IFN-α and ribavirin therapy include cognitive impairment, depression, psychosis, mania, and delirium (Crone et al. 2006).

In Wilson's disease, a wide range of psychiatric disorders can occur, with great variability in prevalence—for example, rates of 4%–47% for major depressive disorder and of 1.4%–11.3% for psychosis (Zimbrean and Schilsky 2014). Psychiatric symptoms include psychosis, mania, schizophrenia-like syndromes, cognitive impairment, and depression and often precede other organ symptom presentations (Ranjan et al. 2015; Zimbrean and Schilsky 2014). Psychiatric symptoms can occur at any time during the course of the illness.

Reports reveal a high prevalence of anxiety and depressive disorders in adults with nonalcoholic steatohepatitis (Stewart and Levenson 2012). In addition to depression and anxiety, eating disorders (e.g., binge-eating disorder) commonly co-occur in patients with this disease.

Patients with psychiatric disorders are at risk for liver disease in multiple ways. For example, rates of drug abuse and of excessive alcohol consumption are higher in patients with chronic psychiatric disorders (e.g., schizophrenia, bipolar disorder) than in the general population. Long-term use of antipsychotics and other psychotropics can induce metabolic syndrome and associated steatohepatitis. Because of these risk factors, routine screening of psychiatric patients for liver diseases is essential (Carrier et al. 2016).

Psychiatric manifestations in hemochromatosis include depression, bipolar disorder, and cognitive impairment (Milward et al. 2012).

Hepatic encephalopathy, a common complication of cirrhosis, portends a poor prognosis. While hepatic encephalopathy can occur episodically, chronic encephalopathy also may develop. The West Haven criteria (Conn 1993; Table 10–2) provide a method of grading encephalopathy based on alterations in state of consciousness, intellectual function, and behavior, as well as on neuromuscular signs (Córdoba 2011). Sedating medications, including benzodiazepines, can worsen encephalopathic symptoms (Crone et al. 2006).

Diagnostic and Laboratory Findings

Liver disease is assessed by history taking, physical examination, and laboratory investigations for the particular disease. Diagnostic findings for psychiatric illnesses in patients with liver disease are the same as in any other medical condition. A comprehensive psychiatric interview, screening tools for assessment of mood disorders, and assessments of cognition all are essential elements of diagnosing patients, especially in the case of IFN-related mood disorders, in which a low threshold should be utilized for treatment. Screening for substance use disorders is likewise of great importance, because alcohol use is associated with diminished response to IFN-α treatment of HCV (Crone et al. 2006).

In hepatic encephalopathy, when cognitive disturbance is subtle, psychometric testing with the digit symbol test, the line-tracing test, and Trail Making parts A and B is useful (Crone et al. 2006). The electroencephalogram shows generalized slowing

TABLE 10–2.   **Stages of hepatic encephalopathy: West Haven criteria**

Stage	Clinical symptoms
0	No disturbances in mood, behavior, or personality; no neurological signs
1	Mild changes in mood, personality, and behavior and psychomotor slowing, attention deficits, sleep disturbance; asterixis
2	Obvious changes in mood and behavior with disinhibition; asterixis, drowsiness, lethargy, intermittent disorientation, and inappropriate behavior
3	Somnolence (but arousable), marked confusion, disorientation, perseveration, slurring of speech, pyramidal signs, muscle rigidity
4	Coma

Source.   Conn 1993; Córdoba 2011.

(Crone et al. 2006). Venous ammonia levels do not correlate with the severity of the encephalopathy but are relevant to the diagnosis. Magnetic resonance imaging scans in hepatic encephalopathy show bilateral, symmetrical hyperintensities of the globus pallidus on T1-weighted imaging, but these alterations are not specific to encephalopathy (Crone et al. 2006). The Child-Pugh score serves as a measure of liver functioning and can be used to help inform treatment decisions, such as determining whether a patient can safely take psychotropic medication (Crone et al. 2006).

Treatment Considerations

An initial consideration in the use of psychotropics in patients with liver disease is the effect of liver failure on basic aspects of pharmacokinetics. The Child-Pugh score (Child and Turcotte 1964; Pugh et al. 1973) enables clinicians to assess the severity of liver dysfunction and determine appropriate adjustments to dosing (Crone et al. 2006). For instance, patients with a Class A score can tolerate 75%–100% of a standard initial dosage, and those with a Class B score can tolerate 50%–75%. For patients with a Class C score, medication use should be monitored so as not to worsen hepatic encephalopathy. Drugs with high first-pass metabolism (Table 10–3) should be avoided (Telles-Correia et al. 2017), and drugs eliminated through glucuronidation (e.g., lorazepam, oxazepam) are preferable to those eliminated by oxidation (e.g., most SSRIs) (English et al. 2012).

The prevalence of psychotic, mood, personality, and substance use disorders is elevated in patients with HCV in comparison with the general population (Rifai et al. 2010). Although direct-acting antivirals and microRNA-targeting treatments have empirical support for the treatment of HCV (Janssen et al. 2013; Kardashian and Pockros 2017), current therapeutic regimens remain dependent on administration of pegylated interferon and ribavirin for 24–48 weeks. Unfortunately, subcutaneous IFN with oral ribavirin has numerous neuropsychiatric side effects, including significant depression (Crone et al. 2006). Therefore, in individuals with a history of depression, initiation of prophylactic antidepressant treatment may be necessary when IFN-α is warranted for HCV infection (Crone et al. 2006). The SSRIs paroxetine, sertraline, fluoxetine, and citalopram all have been demonstrated to be effective agents (Crone et al. 2006). Bupropion is useful for treatment of fatigue, cognitive impairment, and psy-

TABLE 10–3.	Drugs with high first-pass metabolism	
Antidepressants	TCAs:	amitriptyline, desipramine, doxepin, imipramine, nortriptyline
	SSRIs:	sertraline
	SNRIs:	venlafaxine
	Other:	bupropion
Antipsychotics	chlorpromazine, quetiapine, olanzapine	
Opiates	dextropropoxyphene, morphine	
Stimulants	methylphenidate	

Note. SSRIs=selective serotonin reuptake inhibitors; SNRIs=serotonin-norepinephrine reuptake inhibitors; TCAs=tricyclic antidepressants.
Source. Telles-Correia et al. 2017.

chomotor slowing in patients who receive IFN-α. In individuals without a history of substance use, psychostimulants and modafinil may serve a similar function. Mirtazapine can alleviate insomnia, anorexia, nausea, and pruritus caused by IFN-α (Crone et al. 2006), although monitoring for the rare outcome of agranulocytosis is advised.

For patients with mania in liver disease, valproate can be used, although liver functions tests require careful monitoring (Crone et al. 2006).

Delirium in hepatic encephalopathy is managed according to current standards, as in any other medical condition, through treatment of the underlying medical condition and use of medications that stabilize sleep and address issues with agitation.

In nonalcoholic steatohepatitis, the effect of psychotropics on weight gain is an important consideration. For this reason, mirtazapine, lithium, and antipsychotics may be less appealing choices for patients with this disease.

In Wilson's disease and hemochromatosis, treatment of the primary medical disorder alleviates most of the psychiatric symptoms (Zimbrean and Schilsky 2014); however, psychotropics have been shown to be useful in treating psychiatric symptoms. Lithium, the typical antipsychotic haloperidol, TCAs, benzodiazepines, and the atypical antipsychotics quetiapine, risperidone, and clozapine, as well as electroconvulsive therapy, all have been utilized for this purpose (Zimbrean and Schilsky 2014).

Pancreatic and Biliary Diseases

Pancreatic Cancer

The pancreas serves both essential digestive and endocrine roles and is the site of several important diseases that intersect with psychiatric illnesses.

Pancreatic cancer, among all other tumors of the digestive system, is associated with the highest incidence of depression (Mayr and Schmid 2010). Reports indicate that the prevalences of anxiety and of depression in patients with pancreatic cancer are nearly twice as high as those in the general population (Mayr and Schmid 2010). The bidirectional relationship between pancreatic cancer and depression can be traced to specific pathophysiological processes associated with pancreatic cancer and is not merely an effect of psychological adjustment to a fatal disease. For instance, almost 50% of individuals with pancreatic cancer show depressive symptoms before their tumor diagnosis is made (Mayr and Schmid 2010). Potential mechanisms for the link between depression and pancreatic cancer include possible paraneoplastic limbic encephalitis as well as a dysregulated immune response, in which increases in the levels of cytokines such as IL-6, IL-18, and TNF-α affect the HPA axis and corticotropin-releasing factor, producing depressive symptomatology (Mayr and Schmid 2010). Clinical trials have shown that antidepressant treatment, chosen on the basis of target symptoms and side effects, is an essential component of supportive care for pancreatic cancer patients. TCAs (e.g., amitriptyline) are commonly used for this purpose because of their effects on concomitant symptoms of neuropathic pain and insomnia. In some studies, mirtazapine had a more rapid onset of action and produced a higher rate of sustained remission in comparison with amitriptyline (Mayr and Schmid 2010).

Primary Sclerosing Cholangitis and Primary Biliary Cirrhosis

The biliary tract consists of the liver, gallbladder, and bile ducts, all of which work together to make, store, and secrete bile, which facilitates the absorption of dietary fats and oils. Primary sclerosing cholangitis and primary biliary cirrhosis are chronic cholestatic diseases that are associated with high rates of comorbid depression, with an estimated rate of 45% (as assessed by Beck Depression Inventory score > 10) in one study of 116 patients with primary biliary cirrhosis (Huet et al. 2000). In a cross-sectional study of 162 patients with primary sclerosing cholangitis, nearly 75% reported existential anxiety regarding disease progression and diminished life expectancy, with 25% reporting social isolation (Cheung et al. 2016). Given that fatigue is a common initial symptom of chronic cholestatic disease, depression must be ruled out as a contributor (Cheung et al. 2016; Huet et al. 2000).

Special Populations and Issues

Gastrointestinal Issues in Autism Spectrum Disorder

Autism spectrum disorder (ASD) is a neurodevelopmental disorder characterized by impaired communication and social interaction. Studies have revealed a high prevalence of gastrointestinal distress in children with ASD, with symptoms localized to the esophagus, stomach, small intestine, and colon (Hsiao 2014). Symptoms include gastroesophageal reflux, bloody stools, vomiting, and gaseousness as well as indications of gastrointestinal inflammation, such as lymphoid nodular hyperplasia, complement activation, elevated proinflammatory cytokines, and intestinal pathologies such as enterocolitis, gastritis, and esophagitis (Hsiao 2014). Non–gastrointestinal disease symptoms suggestive of gastroesophageal reflux and reflux esophagitis in children with ASD include sleep disturbance and sudden irritability or aggressive behavior. Evidence now suggests that impairment of the gut microbiota may play a role in the development or persistence of autism symptoms (Hsiao 2014; Mangiola et al. 2016). While conventional gastrointestinal treatments are effective in addressing symptoms, treatment of gastrointestinal issues often beneficially affects the behavioral components of ASD (Hsiao 2014).

Psychological Adjustment After Ostomy Surgery

An ostomy is a surgically created opening in the body that enables the stoma, or the ending of intestine or colon, to protrude through the abdominal wall so that intestinal waste can leave the body. Ostomies can be temporary or permanent; for instance, because the ostomy diverts stool away, it may allow for healing of the site of a surgery. Alternatively, permanent diversion may be necessary to treat a complicated gastrointestinal disease.

Literature has rigorously examined the psychological impact of ostomy creation. In one analysis of 545 patients who underwent permanent stoma creation after a rectal cancer diagnosis, 18% reported bodily limitations and mental suffering without a sense of acceptance nearly 3 years after the procedure (González et al. 2016). Findings from another study in which clinical interviews were conducted with patients who underwent ostomy revealed several dimensions of psychosocial symptomatology: patients struggled with psychological adjustment to physical problems with the ostomy (e.g., rash, leakage), financial demands of ostomy care, limitations on physical activity and travel, and problems with sexual functioning (Dabirian et al. 2010).

Conclusion

As we face a future in which the practice of collaborative care between medical specialties and psychiatry continues to rise in popularity, primary care physicians, psychiatrists, and other clinicians will require an understanding of the clinical issues most commonly faced by patients with gastroenterological disorders. Our hope is that this chapter not only broadens our readers' knowledge of key psychiatric issues in gastrointestinal diseases but also serves as a basis for clinicians to expand their research efforts and clinical collaborations in this exciting field.

References

Adam B, Liebregts T, Holtmann G: Mechanisms of disease: genetics of functional gastrointestinal disorders—searching the genes that matter. Nat Clin Gastroenterol Hepatol 4(2):102–110, 2007 17268545

Adinolfi LE, Nevola R, Lus G, et al: Chronic hepatitis C virus infection and neurological and psychiatric disorders: an overview. World J Gastroenterol 21(8):2269–2280, 2015 25741133

American Psychiatric Association: Diagnostic and Statistical Manual of Mental Disorders, 3rd Edition. Washington, DC, American Psychiatric Association, 1980

American Psychiatric Association: Diagnostic and Statistical Manual of Mental Disorders, 4th Edition. Washington, DC, American Psychiatric Association, 1994

American Psychiatric Association: Diagnostic and Statistical Manual of Mental Disorders, 4th Edition, Text Revision. Washington, DC, American Psychiatric Association, 2000

Aro P, Talley NJ, Ronkainen J, et al: Anxiety is associated with uninvestigated and functional dyspepsia (Rome III criteria) in a Swedish population-based study. Gastroenterology 137(1):94–100, 2009 19328797

Aziz Q, Fass R, Gyawali CP, et al: Functional esophageal disorders. Gastroenterology 150(6):1368–1379, 2016

Ballou S, Keefer L: Development of the Irritable Bowel Syndrome Cognitive Affective Scale: a brief self-report measure for clinical and research settings. Eur J Gastroenterol Hepatol 29(7):849–854, 2017 28338499

Biancone L, Calabrese E, Petruzziello C, Pallone F: Treatment with biologic therapies and the risk of cancer in patients with IBD. Nat Clin Pract Gastroenterol Hepatol 4(2):78–91, 2007 17268543

Bielefeldt K: Gastroparesis: concepts, controversies, and challenges. Scientifica (Cairo) 2012:424802, 2012 24278691

Bilici M, Ozturk C, Dursun H, et al: Protective effect of mirtazapine on indomethacin-induced ulcer in rats and its relationship with oxidant and antioxidant parameters. Dig Dis Sci 54(9):1868–1875, 2009 19034656

Bushara KO: Neurologic presentation of celiac disease. Gastroenterology 128 (4 suppl 1):S92–S97, 2005 15825133

Camilleri M, Parkman HP, Shafi MA, et al: Clinical guideline: management of gastroparesis. Am J Gastroenterol 108(1):18–37, quiz 38, 2013 23147521

Carrier P, Debette-Gratien M, Girard M, et al: Liver illness and psychiatric patients. Hepat Mon 16(12):e41564, 2016 28123443

Carta MG, Hardoy MC, Boi MF, et al: Association between panic disorder, major depressive disorder and celiac disease: a possible role of thyroid autoimmunity. J Psychosom Res 53(3):789–793, 2002 12217453

Carta MG, Angst J, Moro MF, et al: Association of chronic hepatitis C with recurrent brief depression. J Affect Disord 141(2–3):361–366, 2012 22609196

Cascella NG, Kryszak D, Bhatti B, et al: Prevalence of celiac disease and gluten sensitivity in the United States clinical antipsychotic trials of intervention effectiveness study population. Schizophr Bull 37(1):94–100, 2011 19494248

Cherian D, Paladugu S, Pathikonda M, et al: Fatigue: a prevalent symptom in gastroparesis. Dig Dis Sci 57(8):2088–2095, 2012 22669206

Cheung AC, Patel H, Meza-Cardona J, et al: Factors that influence health-related quality of life in patients with primary sclerosing cholangitis. Dig Dis Sci 61(6):1692–1699, 2016 26743764

Child CG, Turcotte JG: Surgery and portal hypertension. Major Probl Clin Surg 1:1–85, 1964 4950264

Clouse RE, Richter JE, Heading RC, et al: Functional esophageal disorders. Gut 45 (suppl 2):II31–II36, 1999 10457042

Clouse RE, Mayer EA, Aziz Q, et al: Functional abdominal pain syndrome. Gastroenterology 130(5):1492–1497, 2006 16678562

Conn HO: Hepatic encephalopathy, in Diseases of the Liver, 7th Edition. Edited by Schiff L, Schiff ER. Philadelphia, PA, Lippincott, 1993, pp 1036–1060

Córdoba J: New assessment of hepatic encephalopathy. J Hepatol 54(5):1030–1040, 2011 21145874

Crone CC, Gabriel GM, DiMartini A: An overview of psychiatric issues in liver disease for the consultation-liaison psychiatrist. Psychosomatics 47(3):188–205, 2006 16684936

Cutler P: Iron overload and psychiatric illness. Can J Psychiatry 39(1):8–11, 1994 8194001

Dabirian A, Yaghmaei F, Rassouli M, et al: Quality of life in ostomy patients: a qualitative study. Patient Prefer Adherence 5:1–5, 2010 21311696

Da Costa JM: Mucous enteritis. American Journal of Medical Sciences 89:321–335, 1871

Dekel R, Drossman DA, Sperber AD: The use of psychotropic drugs in irritable bowel syndrome. Expert Opin Investig Drugs 22(3):329–339, 2013 23316916

Dolapcioglu C, Dolapcioglu H: Structural brain lesions in inflammatory bowel disease. World J Gastrointest Pathophysiol 6(4):124–130, 2015 26600970

Drossman D: Functional gastrointestinal disorders: history, pathophysiology, clinical features, and Rome IV. Gastroenterology 150(6):1262–1279, 2016 27144617

Drossman D, Szigethy E: The narcotic bowel syndrome: a recent update. Am J Gastroenterol Suppl 2(1):22–30, 2014 25207609

Drossman D, Morris CB, Edwards H, et al: Diagnosis, characterization, and 3-month outcome after detoxification of 39 patients with narcotic bowel syndrome. Am J Gastroenterol 107(9):1426–1440, 2012 22710577

Enck P, Aziz Q, Barbara G, et al: Irritable bowel syndrome. Nat Rev Dis Primers 2:16014, 2016
    27159638

English BA, Dortch M, Ereshefsky L, Jhee S: Clinically significant psychotropic drug-drug in-
    teractions in the primary care setting. Curr Psychiatry Rep 14(4):376–390, 2012 22707017

Fadgyas-Stanculete M, Buga AM, Popa-Wagner A, et al: The relationship between irritable bowel
    syndrome and psychiatric disorders: from molecular changes to clinical manifestations. J Mol
    Psychiatry 2(1):4, 2014 25408914

Ferenci P: Hepatic encephalopathy. Gastroenterol Rep (Oxf) 5(2):138–147, 2017 28533911

Filipović BF, Randjelovic T, Ille T, et al: Anxiety, personality traits and quality of life in func-
    tional dyspepsia-suffering patients. Eur J Intern Med 24(1):83–86, 2013 22857883

Folks DG: The interface of psychiatry and irritable bowel syndrome. Curr Psychiatry Rep 6(3):210–
    215, 2004 15142474

Ford AC, Talley NJ, Schoenfeld PS, et al: Efficacy of antidepressants and psychological therapies
    in irritable bowel syndrome: systematic review and meta-analysis. Gut 58(3):367–378, 2009
    19001059

Fuller-Thomson E, Sulman J: Depression and inflammatory bowel disease: findings from two na-
    tionally representative Canadian surveys. Inflamm Bowel Dis 12(8):697–707, 2006 16917224

Furness JB, Callaghan BP, Rivera LR, Cho HJ: The enteric nervous system and gastrointestinal in-
    nervation: integrated local and central control, in Microbial Endocrinology: The Microbiota-
    Gut-Brain Axis in Health and Disease. Edited by Lyte M, Cryan JF. New York, Springer, 2014,
    pp 39–71

Galmiche JP, Clouse RE, Bálint A, et al: Functional esophageal disorders. Gastroenterology
    130(5):1459–1465, 2006 16678559

González E, Holm K, Wennström B, et al: Self-reported wellbeing and body image after abdom-
    inoperineal excision for rectal cancer. Int J Colorectal Dis 31(10):1711–1717, 2016 27506432

Goodhand JR, Greig FI, Koodun Y, et al: Do antidepressants influence the disease course in in-
    flammatory bowel disease? A retrospective case-matched observational study. Inflamm
    Bowel Dis 18(7):1232–1239, 2012 22234954

Goodwin RD, Keyes KM, Stein MB, et al: Peptic ulcer and mental disorders among adults in the
    community: the role of nicotine and alcohol use disorders. Psychosom Med 71(4):463–468,
    2009 19443694

Gracie DJ, Bercik P, Morgan DG, et al: No increase in prevalence of somatization in functional vs
    organic dyspepsia: a cross-sectional survey. Neurogastroenterol Motil 27(7):1024–1031, 2015
    25931163

Grunkemeier DM, Cassara JE, Dalton CB, et al: The narcotic bowel syndrome: clinical features,
    pathophysiology, and management. Clin Gastroenterol Hepatol 5(10):1126–1139, quiz
    1121–1122, 2007 17916540

Hall BJ, Hamlin PJ, Gracie DJ, Ford AC: The effect of antidepressants on the course of inflam-
    matory bowel disease. Can J Gastroenterol Hepatol 2018:2047242, 2018 30271765

Hashash J, Vachon A, Altman L, et al: P-028 predictors of suicidal severity amongst suicidal IBD
    patients. Inflammatory Bowel Diseases 22 (suppl 1):S18, 2016

Hasler WL, Parkman HP, Wilson LA, et al: Psychological dysfunction is associated with symp-
    tom severity but not disease etiology or degree of gastric retention in patients with gast-
    roparesis. Am J Gastroenterol 105(11):2357–2367, 2010 20588262

Hasler WL, Wilson LA, Parkman HP, et al: Factors related to abdominal pain in gastroparesis:
    contrast to patients with predominant nausea and vomiting. Neurogastroenterol Motil
    25(5):427–438, 2013 23414452

Hausteiner-Wiehle C, Henningsen P: Irritable bowel syndrome: relations with functional, men-
    tal, and somatoform disorders. World J Gastroenterol 20(20):6024–6030, 2014 24876725

Holtmann G, Kutscher SU, Haag S, et al: Clinical presentation and personality factors are pre-
    dictors of the response to treatment in patients with functional dyspepsia; a randomized,
    double-blind placebo-controlled crossover study. Dig Dis Sci 49(4):672–679, 2004 15185877

Hsiao EY: Gastrointestinal issues in autism spectrum disorder. Harv Rev Psychiatry 22(2):104–
    111, 2014 24614765

Hsu CC, Hsu YC, Chang KH, et al: Depression and the risk of peptic ulcer disease: a nationwide population-based study. Medicine 94(51):e2333, 2015a 26705225

Hsu YC, Hsu CC, Chang KH, et al: Increased subsequent risk of peptic ulcer diseases in patients with bipolar disorders. Medicine 94(29):e1203, 2015b 26200637

Hsu CC, Hsu YC, Chang KH, et al: Association of dementia and peptic ulcer disease: a nationwide population-based study. Am J Alzheimers Dis Other Demen 31(5):389–394, 2016 26802077

Huet PM, Deslauriers J, Tran A, et al: Impact of fatigue on the quality of life of patients with primary biliary cirrhosis. Am J Gastroenterol 95(3):760–767, 2000 10710071

Ilzarbe L, Fàbrega M, Quintero R, et al: Inflammatory bowel disease and eating disorders: a systematized review of comorbidity. J Psychosom Res 102:47–53, 2017 28992897

Jackson JR, Eaton WW, Cascella NG, et al: Neurologic and psychiatric manifestations of celiac disease and gluten sensitivity. Psychiatr Q 83(1):91–102, 2012 21877216

Janssen HL, Reesink HW, Lawitz EJ, et al: Treatment of HCV infection by targeting microRNA. N Engl J Med 368(18):1685–1694, 2013 23534542

Jiang SM, Jia L, Lei XG, et al: Incidence and psychological-behavioral characteristics of refractory functional dyspepsia: a large, multi-center, prospective investigation from China. World J Gastroenterol 21(6):1932–1937, 2015 25684962

Jones MP, Dilley JB, Drossman D, et al: Brain-gut connections in functional GI disorders: anatomic and physiologic relationships. Neurogastroenterol Motil 18(2):91–103, 2006 16420287

Kano M, Dupont P, Aziz Q, Fukudo S: Understanding neurogastroenterology from neuroimaging perspective: a comprehensive review of functional and structural brain imaging in functional gastrointestinal disorders. J Neurogastroenterol Motil 24(4):512–527, 2018 30041284

Kardashian AA, Pockros PJ: Novel emerging treatments for hepatitis C infection: a fast-moving pipeline. Therap Adv Gastroenterol 10(2):277–282, 2017 28203284

Kast RE: Anti- and pro-inflammatory considerations in antidepressant use during medical illness: bupropion lowers and mirtazapine increases circulating tumor necrosis factor-alpha levels. Gen Hosp Psychiatry 25(6):495–496, 2003 14706417

Keefer L, Drossman DA, Guthrie E, et al: Centrally mediated disorders of gastrointestinal pain. Gastroenterology 150(6):1408–1419, 2016 27144628

Korzenik JR, Podolsky DK: Evolving knowledge and therapy of inflammatory bowel disease. Nat Rev Drug Discov 5(3):197–209, 2006 16518373

Kundu S, Rogal S, Alam A, et al: Rapid improvement in post-infectious gastroparesis symptoms with mirtazapine. World J Gastroenterol 20(21):6671–6674, 2014 24914393

Lackner JM, Jaccard J, Keefer L, et al: Improvement in gastrointestinal symptoms after cognitive behavior therapy for refractory irritable bowel syndrome. Gastroenterology 155(1):47–57, 2018 [Erratum in: Gastroenterology 155(4):1281, 2018] 29702118

Lackner JM, Jaccard J; IBS Outcome Study Research Group: Factors associated with efficacy of cognitive behavior therapy vs education for patients with irritable bowel syndrome. Clin Gastroenterol Hepatol 17(8):1500–1508.e3, 2019 30613000

Lacy BE, Mearin F, Chang L, et al: Bowel disorders. Gastroenterology 150(6):1393–1407.e5, 2016

Lacy BE, Crowell MD, Mathis C, et al: Gastroparesis: quality of life and health care utilization. J Clin Gastroenterol 52(1):20–24, 2018 27775961

Laird KT, Tanner-Smith EE, Russell AC, et al: Short-term and long-term efficacy of psychological therapies for irritable bowel syndrome: a systematic review and meta-analysis. Clin Gastroenterol Hepatol 14(7):937–947.e4, 2016 26721342

Lee IS, Wang H, Chae Y, et al: Functional neuroimaging studies in functional dyspepsia patients: a systematic review. Neurogastroenterol Motil 28(6):793–805, 2016 26940430

Levy RL, Linde JA, Feld KA, et al: The association of gastrointestinal symptoms with weight, diet, and exercise in weight-loss program participants. Clin Gastroenterol Hepatol 3(10):992–996, 2005 16234045

Liao CH, Chang CS, Chang SN, et al: The association of peptic ulcer and schizophrenia: a population-based study. J Psychosom Res 77(6):541–546, 2014 25199406

Lucey MR, Mathurin P, Morgan TR: Alcoholic hepatitis. N Engl J Med 360(26):2758–2769, 2009 19553649

Ly HG, Weltens N, Tack J, et al: Acute anxiety and anxiety disorders are associated with im-
    paired gastric accommodation in patients with functional dyspepsia. Clin Gastroenterol
    Hepatol 13(9):1584–91.e3, 2015 25869636

Mak ADP, Wu JCY, Chan Y, et al: Dyspepsia is strongly associated with major depression and
    generalised anxiety disorder—a community study. Aliment Pharmacol Ther 36(8):800–
    810, 2012 22957985

Malfertheiner P, Chan FKL, McColl KEL: Peptic ulcer disease. Lancet 374(9699):1449–1461, 2009
    19683340

Mangiola F, Ianiro G, Franceschi F, et al: Gut microbiota in autism and mood disorders. World
    J Gastroenterol 22(1):361–368, 2016 26755882

Martin-Subero M, Anderson G, Kanchanatawan B, et al: Comorbidity between depression and
    inflammatory bowel disease explained by immune-inflammatory, oxidative, and nitrosa-
    tive stress; tryptophan catabolite; and gut-brain pathways. CNS Spectr 21(2):184–198, 2016
    26307347

Mayr M, Schmid RM: Pancreatic cancer and depression: myth and truth. BMC Cancer 10:569,
    2010 20961421

McCombie AM, Mulder RT, Gearry RB: Psychotherapy for inflammatory bowel disease: a re-
    view and update. J Crohn's Colitis 7(12):935–949, 2013 23466412

Mikocka-Walus AA, Turnbull DA, Moulding NT, et al: Controversies surrounding the comor-
    bidity of depression and anxiety in inflammatory bowel disease patients: a literature re-
    view. Inflamm Bowel Dis 13(2):225–234, 2007 17206706

Mikocka-Walus A, Clarke D, Gibson P: Can antidepressants influence the course of inflammatory
    bowel disease? The current state of research. European Gastroenterology and Hepatology Re-
    view 5(1):48–53, 2009

Milward E, Acikyol B, Bassett B, et al: Brain changes in iron loading disorders, in Metal Ions in
    Neurological Systems. Edited by Linert W, Kozlowski H. Berlin, Germany, Springer, 2012,
    pp 17–29

Morís G: Inflammatory bowel disease: an increased risk factor for neurologic complications.
    World J Gastroenterol 20(5):1228–1237, 2014 24574797

Moss AC, Anton P, Savidge T, et al: Urocortin II mediates pro-inflammatory effects in human
    colonocytes via corticotropin-releasing hormone receptor 2alpha. Gut 56(9):1210–1217,
    2007 17412781

Nahon S, Lahmek P, Durance C, et al: Risk factors of anxiety and depression in inflammatory
    bowel disease. Inflamm Bowel Dis 18(11):2086–2091, 2012 22294486

Ng QX, Soh AYS, Loke W, et al: Systematic review with meta-analysis: the association between
    post-traumatic stress disorder and irritable bowel syndrome. J Gastroenterol Hepatol
    34(1):68–73, 2019 30144372

O'Connor OJ, McSweeney SE, McWilliams S, et al: Role of radiologic imaging in irritable bowel
    syndrome: evidence-based review. Radiology 262(2):485–494, 2012 22156992

Pascua MF, Kedia P, Weiner MG, et al: Microscopic colitis and medication use. Clin Med In-
    sights Gastroenterol 2010(3):11–19, 2010 20640056

Pasricha PJ, Yates KP, Nguyen L, et al: Outcomes and factors associated with reduced symp-
    toms in patients with gastroparesis. Gastroenterology 149(7):1762–1774, 2015 26299414

Persoons P, Vermeire S, Demyttenaere K, et al: The impact of major depressive disorder on the
    short- and long-term outcome of Crohn's disease treatment with infliximab. Aliment Phar-
    macol Ther 22(2):101–110, 2005 16011668

Petra AI, Panagiotidou S, Hatziagelaki E, et al: Gut-microbiota-brain axis and its effect on neuro-
    psychiatric disorders with suspected immune dysregulation. Clin Ther 37(5):984–995, 2015
    26046241

Pietrangelo A: Hereditary hemochromatosis--a new look at an old disease. N Engl J Med
    350(23):2383–2397, 2004 15175440

Porcelli B, Verdino V, Bossini L, et al: Celiac and non-celiac gluten sensitivity: a review on the
    association with schizophrenia and mood disorders. Auto Immun Highlights 5(2):55–61,
    2014 26000156

Pugh RN, Murray-Lyon IM, Dawson JL, et al: Transection of the oesophagus for bleeding oesophageal varices. Br J Surg 60(8):646–649, 1973 4541913

Ranjan A, Kalita J, Kumar S, et al: A study of MRI changes in Wilson disease and its correlation with clinical features and outcome. Clin Neurol Neurosurg 138:31–36, 2015 26278999

Riehl ME, Keefer L: Hypnotherapy for esophageal disorders. Am J Clin Hypn 58(1):22–33, 2015 26046715

Rifai MA, Gleason OC, Sabouni D: Psychiatric care of the patient with hepatitis C: a review of the literature. Prim Care Companion J Clin Psychiatry 12(6):6, 2010 21494349

Rome Foundation: What's New for Rome IV (web page). Raleigh, NC, The Rome Foundation, 2019. Available at: https://theromefoundation.org/rome-iv/whats-new-for-rome-iv/. Accessed August 3, 2019.

Rosa-e-Silva L, Troncon LE, Oliveira RB, et al: Treatment of diabetic gastroparesis with oral clonidine. Aliment Pharmacol Ther 9(2):179–183, 1995 7605859

Saito YA: The role of genetics in IBS. Gastroenterol Clin North Am 40(1):45–67, 2011 21333900

Saito YA, Mitra N, Mayer EA: Genetic approaches to functional gastrointestinal disorders. Gastroenterology 138(4):1276–1285, 2010 [Erratum in: Gastroenterology 139(1):360, 2010] 20176021

Sajadinejad MS, Asgari K, Molavi H, et al: Psychological issues in inflammatory bowel disease: an overview. Gastroenterol Res Pract 2012:106502, 2012 22778720

Schmulson MJ, Drossman DA: What is new in Rome IV. J Neurogastroenterol Motil 23(2):151–163, 2017 28274109

Smith DF, Gerdes LU: Meta-analysis on anxiety and depression in adult celiac disease. Acta Psychiatr Scand 125(3):189–193, 2012 22128768

Soykan I, Sivri B, Sarosiek I, et al: Demography, clinical characteristics, psychological and abuse profiles, treatment, and long-term follow-up of patients with gastroparesis. Dig Dis Sci 43(11):2398–2404, 1998 9824125

Stanghellini V, Chan FK, Hasler WL, et al: Gastroduodenal disorders. Gastroenterology 150(6):1380–1392, 2016 27147122

Stewart KE, Levenson JL: Psychological and psychiatric aspects of treatment of obesity and nonalcoholic fatty liver disease. Clin Liver Dis 16(3):615–629, 2012 22824484

Tack J, Janssen P, Masaoka T, et al: Efficacy of buspirone, a fundus-relaxing drug, in patients with functional dyspepsia. Clin Gastroenterol Hepatol 10(11):1239–1245, 2012 22813445

Tack J, Ly HG, Carbone F, et al: Efficacy of mirtazapine in patients with functional dyspepsia and weight loss. Clin Gastroenterol Hepatol 14(3):385–392.e4, 2016 26538208

Taft TH, Bedell A, Craven MR, et al: Initial assessment of post-traumatic stress in a US cohort of inflammatory bowel disease patients. Inflamm Bowel Dis 25(9):1577–1585, 2019 30840762

Talley NJ, Ford AC: Functional dyspepsia. N Engl J Med 373(19):1853–1863, 2015 26535514

Talley NJ, Herrick L, Locke GR: Antidepressants in functional dyspepsia. Expert Rev Gastroenterol Hepatol 4(1):5–8, 2010 20136584

Talley NJ, Holtmann G, Walker MM: Therapeutic strategies for functional dyspepsia and irritable bowel syndrome based on pathophysiology. J Gastroenterol 50(6):601–613, 2015 25917563

Targownik LE, Nugent Z, Singh H, et al: The prevalence and predictors of opioid use in inflammatory bowel disease: a population-based analysis. Am J Gastroenterol 109(10):1613–1620, 2014 25178702

Telles-Correia D, Barbosa A, Cortez-Pinto H, et al: Psychotropic drugs and liver disease: a critical review of pharmacokinetics and liver toxicity. World J Gastrointest Pharmacol Ther 8(1):26–38, 2017 28217372

Tong J, Zheng Q, Zhang C, et al: Incidence, prevalence, and temporal trends of microscopic colitis: a systematic review and meta-analysis. Am J Gastroenterol 110(2):265–277, 2015 25623658

Vandenbergh J, Dupont P, Fischler B, et al: Regional brain activation during proximal stomach distention in humans: a positron emission tomography study. Gastroenterology 128(3):564–573, 2005 15765391

Van Oudenhove L, Aziz Q: The role of psychosocial factors and psychiatric disorders in functional dyspepsia. Nat Rev Gastroenterol Hepatol 10(3):158–167, 2013 23358396

Van Oudenhove L, Talley NJ, Jones MP, et al: 32 psychological factors and somatization at baseline predict gastrointestinal symptom severity and consulting behavior at 18 months follow-up. Gastroenterology 142 (5 suppl):S-9, 2012

Vogt BA: Inflammatory bowel disease: perspectives from cingulate cortex in the first brain. Neurogastroenterol Motil 25(2):93–98, 2013 23336589

Walker JR, Ediger JP, Graff LA, et al: The Manitoba IBD cohort study: a population-based study of the prevalence of lifetime and 12-month anxiety and mood disorders. Am J Gastroenterol 103(8):1989–1997, 2008 18796096

Wilkins T, Pepitone C, Alex B, Schade RR: Diagnosis and management of IBS in adults. Am Fam Physician 86(5):419–426, 2012 22963061

Windgassen S, Moss-Morris R, Goldsmith K, Chalder T: Key mechanisms of cognitive behavioural therapy in irritable bowel syndrome: the importance of gastrointestinal related cognitions, behaviours and general anxiety. J Psychosom Res 118:73–82, 2019 30522750

Woodman CL, Breen K, Noyes R Jr, et al: The relationship between irritable bowel syndrome and psychiatric illness. A family study. Psychosomatics 39(1):45–54, 1998 9538675

Yamasaki T, O'Neil J, Fass R: Update on functional heartburn. Gastroenterol Hepatol (N Y) 13(12):725–734, 2017 29339948

Zagari RM, Law GR, Fuccio L, et al: Epidemiology of functional dyspepsia and subgroups in the Italian general population: an endoscopic study. Gastroenterology 138(4):1302–1311, 2010 20074574

Zimbrean PC, Schilsky ML: Psychiatric aspects of Wilson disease: a review. Gen Hosp Psychiatry 36(1):53–62, 2014 24120023

CHAPTER 11

Renal Disease in Patients With Psychiatric Illness

Lily Chan, M.D.

J. Michael Bostwick, M.D.

Psychiatric illness is common in patients with chronic disease; chronic kidney disease (CKD) and end-stage renal disease (ESRD) are no exception. The stages of CKD, with the fifth and final stage referred to as end-stage renal disease, are defined by the estimated glomerular filtration rate (GFR), which is calculated by a serum creatinine that has been adjusted for sex, age, and race. The risk of hospitalization with a psychiatric diagnosis is 1.5–3 times higher in patients with renal failure in comparison with patients with other chronic conditions, including diabetes, heart disease, and cerebrovascular disease (Kimmel et al. 1998). Male, African American, and younger (ages 18–44 years) ESRD patients have been found to be more likely than female, white, and older patients to be hospitalized for a psychiatric condition (Kimmel et al. 1998).

In 2016, the number of ESRD patients in the United States was estimated to be greater than 726,000 (United States Renal Data System 2018). This number has been steadily increasing due to increasing prevalence of underlying causes of ESRD, most notably diabetes mellitus and hypertension. Additional causes of renal disease include hereditary conditions (e.g., polycystic kidney disease), connective tissue disorders, medication toxicity (particularly acyclovir and long-term lithium use), and rheumatological diseases (e.g., systemic lupus erythematosus). African Americans and, to a lesser extent, other racial and ethnic minorities have disproportionately higher incidence rates of ESRD in comparison with white Americans, and African Americans and Hispanics tend to experience a more rapid disease progression (United States Renal Data System 2018).

Underlying renal disease may initially manifest as alterations in mood, energy, sleep, appetite, sexual function, and mental status. These symptoms are secondary to a number of related pathophysiological mechanisms, including anemia and metabolic disturbances (e.g., hyperparathyroidism, which has been associated with psychiatric syndromes including mood and anxiety disorders). Other common metabolic abnormalities include hyperuricemia, hypogonadism, and alterations in the renin-angiotensin-aldosterone system leading to electrolyte abnormalities and changes in sympathetic activity, as well as compromised drug clearance and medication side effects. Uremia is a clinical syndrome that results from fluid, electrolyte, hormone, and metabolic changes in the setting of decreased renal function; it manifests with anorexia, nausea and vomiting, pruritus, muscle cramps, and central nervous system abnormalities ranging from lethargy to seizures, coma, and death. While no single uremic toxin has been identified, substances suspected to contribute to the constellation of uremic symptoms include parathyroid hormone (PTH), beta-2 microglobulin, and polyamines.

In the setting of known CKD and ESRD, psychosocial stressors may arise from the process of transplantation, including the wait for a suitable donor, concerns about impending transplant rejection and functional loss, social and financial burdens, dietary and fluid restrictions that may impede social functioning, and persistent physical discomfort such as chronic pain and pruritus associated with buildup of uremic toxins. Renal disease is distinct from other diseases of organ failure in that dialysis often extends life, sometimes for decades. Kidney transplants, while still in short supply, are relatively more common in comparison with other types of organ transplants and in some cases may cure the renal disease; however, studies have found that nearly half of renal transplant and hemodialysis patients experience psychiatric comorbidities (Kalman et al. 1983). The road to kidney transplantation involves significant immunological, endocrine, and metabolic stress. Patients may also experience high levels of psychosocial stress, particularly if the donated kidney comes from a family member. Depression and pain are symptoms that commonly affect patients on chronic dialysis, and both are strongly associated with decreased quality of life (Kimmel et al. 1998; Weisbord 2016).

For patients with premorbid psychiatric conditions, early mobilization of social and family support, involvement of psychiatrists and other mental health care providers, review of current psychiatric medications for suitability in renal compromise, and routine screening for new or worsening symptoms are advisable. Patients who develop renal disease commonly have a history of challenging life circumstances and difficulty with treatment adherence (e.g., a patient with poorly managed or complex diabetes who eventually develops renal nephropathy, or a patient with substance use disorder who develops drug-induced nephropathy). Retrospective studies have found that depressive episodes precede the onset of renal disease in 17%–30% of patients (Rubin et al. 2004). Regardless of which comorbidity precedes the other, depressive disorders have been found to be associated with multiple adverse consequences in CKD, including increased mortality and hospitalization rates (Kimmel et al. 1993). Depressive disorders in CKD may be viewed as a modifiable risk factor for the development of ESRD (Silva Junior et al. 2014).

Individuals with chronic renal disease face a number of unique challenges related to general functionality, employment, alterations in family and gender roles, and bodily control. An understanding of the physical and psychosocial challenges of coping with chronic renal disease may assist the clinician in selecting treatments that are tailored to patients' personalities and their most prominent concerns—for example, considering peritoneal dialysis as opposed to hemodialysis in a patient with a more independent personality, or scheduling counseling during a patient's hemodialysis sessions (Morton et al. 2010). The longitudinal nature of the patient-physician relationship in the primary care setting provides opportunities to attend to the patient's emotional and mental well-being. The patient may respond to this attention with improved adherence to dialysis and other medical treatments.

Renal Dosing of Psychiatric Medications

Physicians should be aware of possible interactions psychiatric medications may have with other medications, as well as the potential need for serum level monitoring and adjusted dosing in the renally compromised patient. Drugs are typically cleared via renal or hepatic routes or a combination of both. If renal clearance of the drug constitutes less than 30% of total clearance, the renal compromise does not usually significantly affect pharmacokinetics, and thus no dosage adjustment is required. Examples of antidepressants that do not require dosage adjustments in renal failure include fluoxetine, sertraline, and citalopram. Venlafaxine, paroxetine, and bupropion require dosage adjustments in renal failure (Cohen et al. 2004; Nagler et al. 2012). Other drugs, such as certain tricyclic antidepressants (TCAs; e.g., imipramine, clomipramine), are converted in the liver to active metabolites, which are then renally cleared, thus necessitating dosage adjustment (Nagler et al. 2012).

Two major factors affect free drug concentrations in the body: protein binding and volume of distribution (V_D). Proteinuria and hypoalbuminemia, common in renal failure, lead to fewer binding sites and thus elevated serum drug levels. The accumulation of organic acids, which act as protein-binding inhibitors, also contributes to increased free drug concentration. Cachectic ESRD patients, with their reduced fluid and body mass, have decreased V_D. Thus, standard medication dosages will reach higher concentrations in these patients than in those with normal V_D. The V_D of most psychotherapeutic agents is large, and the drugs have extensive protein binding, making it unlikely that significant quantities will be removed by dialysis. Strategies for addressing the resultant drug accumulation include dosage reduction, dosing interval increase, and replacement with a drug unaffected by renal clearance.

Dialysis Regimens

Adjustment of a dialysis regimen can ameliorate social stressors, sleep disorders, and sexual dysfunction in CKD and ESRD patients. A brief discussion of different dialysis modalities follows.

There are two general modalities of dialysis: peritoneal dialysis and hemodialysis. In peritoneal dialysis, patients are able to go about their regular activities while the dialysate fluid remains in their peritoneum. After approximately 4–6 hours, or overnight, the dialysate fluid is then removed. Each exchange takes approximately 30 minutes. The peritoneum serves as a semipermeable membrane, and wastes are removed with the dialysate. Peritoneal dialysis may be performed manually at home four to six times per day (known as continuous ambulatory peritoneal dialysis). Alternatively, a home machine may perform peritoneal dialysis at night, a method referred to as continuous cycler peritoneal dialysis or automated peritoneal dialysis. In continuous cycler peritoneal dialysis, a cycler fills and empties the peritoneal cavity three to five times overnight while the patient sleeps, and an additional exchange may be performed during the day. Depending on the patient's needs and preferences, a combination of continuous ambulatory peritoneal dialysis and automated peritoneal dialysis also may be used (e.g., a cycler at night and one exchange during the day).

The more common dialysis modality, hemodialysis, is typically conducted at an outpatient dialysis unit, usually three times weekly for 3–4 hours per session. Hemodialysis may also be performed at home, affording the patient more flexibility in scheduling and offering a way to avoid difficult travel to and from an outpatient unit. Home dialysis requires assistance from another person as well as 3–8 weeks of patient education and training. Hemodialysis requires strict limitations on fluid intake, potassium, sodium, and phosphorus. Other common issues include problems with vascular access, muscle cramps, and hypotension associated with rapid shifts in electrolyte balance.

Although randomized controlled trials of different dialysis modalities have not been performed, patients receiving peritoneal dialysis appear to rate their care more favorably than do patients receiving other dialysis modalities (Rubin et al. 2004). Patients on peritoneal dialysis have also been found to have lower rates of hospitalization for mental illness in comparison with patients on hemodialysis (Kimmel et al. 1998). These findings should be interpreted with caution, because patients who are offered the option of peritoneal dialysis may have different baseline characteristics from those who undergo hemodialysis.

Mood and Affective Disorders

Depressive Disorders

Major depressive disorder (MDD) may disproportionately increase morbidity and mortality in patients with renal disease, independent of renal disease severity (Hedayati et al. 2012; Kimmel et al. 1993). Meta-analyses and studies of dialysis patients have estimated the prevalence of MDD in this population as 23%–37%, in comparison with a general population prevalence of 6.7% (Palmer et al. 2013). Psychosocial stressors such as job loss, alterations in the hypothalamic-pituitary-adrenal (HPA) axis, and increased inflammation may contribute to depressive symptoms in CKD patients. Among chronic hemodialysis patients, diabetic, unemployed, and elderly patients are particularly vulnerable to depressive disorders (Chen et al. 2003).

MDD typically manifests with anhedonia, guilt, and nonspecific alterations in mood, energy, appetite, or sleep. Metabolic derangements common in renal disease—including anemia, electrolyte abnormalities (hyperkalemia and uremia), hypothyroidism, and nutritional deficiencies—may manifest with symptoms similar to those of MDD. Blood pressure or blood glucose fluctuations, primary sleep disorders, and nausea also may manifest with mood symptoms.

Demoralization is distinct from depression but at times is similar in presentation. The symptoms of demoralization do not rise to the level of MDD but manifest as a loss of efficacy in coping with stressors. The key differentiating factor between demoralization and MDD is that demoralized patients have a reactive mood and are able to enjoy some activities. The intensity of demoralization may wax and wane without ever reaching the level of MDD (Mangelli et al. 2005). Other psychiatric diagnoses that may be considered in a patient who presents with mood changes include anxiety disorders and adjustment disorders.

Given the prevalence of depression in CKD patients, routine screening is recommended (Hedayati et al. 2009a). Patients who have reached the point at which they need dialysis should also be screened at the time of dialysis initiation, after 6 months of dialysis, and then annually (Hedayati et al. 2012). Rapid screening may be performed by asking the patient the first two questions of the 9-item Patient Health Questionnaire (PHQ-9) (Kroenke et al. 2001), also known as the PHQ-2: "In the past 2 weeks, have you felt down, depressed, or hopeless?" and "In the past 2 weeks, have you had little pleasure or interest in doing things?" If a patient answers "Yes" to either of these questions, formal screening may be conducted. The Beck Depression Inventory (BDI; Beck et al. 1961), the Hamilton Rating Scale for Depression (Hamilton 1960), the Quick Inventory of Depressive Symptomatology—Self Report (Rush et al. 2003), and the PHQ-2 all are possible screening tools available in the primary care setting. Of these, the BDI has received the most study in renal disease. Modification of cutoff scores may improve diagnostic accuracy for depressive disorders in patients with ESRD (given this population's higher incidence of somatic symptoms that overlap with depression), but standard cutoff values should be sufficiently accurate for diagnosis of depression in predialysis patients with stages 2–5 CKD (Hedayati et al. 2009b). If depression is detected on a screening test, a more complete clinical interview should be conducted to assess safety, including the presence of suicidal ideation, and to determine subsequent management, which may involve referral of the patient to a psychiatrist.

Patients with uremia may present with somatic symptoms that mimic depression, including fatigue; however, affective symptoms such as sadness, feelings of guilt or worthlessness, or anhedonia must be present alongside somatic symptoms to make the diagnosis of MDD in CKD and ESRD patients; in the absence of these hallmark symptoms of depressive illness, alternative diagnoses should be considered. Uremia alone never causes suicidal ideation, and the presence of any suicidal ideation must be addressed by obtaining more information about the nature of the patient's suicidal thoughts, determining whether the patient has a plan or the means to attempt suicide, and ascertaining whether there is a history of suicidal behaviors in the patient and/ or the patient's family (Hedayati et al. 2012).

Management of depression in the setting of renal disease initially prioritizes non-pharmacological approaches, including lifestyle changes (e.g., improving sleep hygiene, encouraging social contact) if applicable, as well as psychosocial support in the form of counseling or psychotherapy. Studies have underscored the importance of social support in CKD and have suggested that higher levels of perceived social support are associated with higher levels of treatment adherence and reduced mortality (Kimmel 2001). Although studies suggest that antidepressant medications including citalopram and fluoxetine alleviate symptoms in CKD patients (Blumenfeld et al.

1997; Kalender et al. 2007), a more recent Cochrane review has suggested that antidepressant medications have mixed efficacy in the dialysis patient (Palmer et al. 2016). This review concluded that the body of research on antidepressant treatment in ESRD was sparse and incomplete—for instance, no data had been collected regarding antidepressant treatment effects on quality of life. The review also noted that although the evidence for antidepressant-associated side effects was limited and inconsistent, side effects potentially included hypotension, sexual dysfunction, headache, and nausea (Palmer et al. 2016). Nonetheless, it is reasonable to initiate a trial of antidepressant pharmacotherapy in CKD patients whose depressive symptoms are affecting their quality of life or their adherence to other aspects of their health care. In general, antidepressants should be initiated at a low dosage and gradually increased, with regular monitoring for side effects. Selective serotonin reuptake inhibitors (SSRIs) are the best-studied antidepressants and when renally dosed are tolerated as well in ESRD patients as they are in the general population. A full trial of an antidepressant in the CKD patient should last approximately 8–12 weeks, as opposed to a shorter trial period of up to 8 weeks in the general population, because studies have indicated a longer lag time to symptom improvement in the CKD population (Nagler et al. 2012). Possible explanations for this difference, which have not yet been fully studied, include inadequate dosing, increased nonadherence, and variations in drug availability or receptor-drug processing in the CKD population.

TCAs at dosages sufficient to treat depression should generally be avoided in the CKD population due to their anticholinergic side effects, narrow therapeutic range, potential for causing cardiac arrhythmias in vulnerable patients, and propensity to cause orthostatic hypotension, leading to increased risk of falls. Cardiotoxic TCA metabolites have been demonstrated to accumulate in CKD patients (Lieberman et al. 1985); however, doxepin has been successfully used to treat uremic pruritus and neuropathic pain in the ESRD population and may be used without dosage adjustment, because it is hepatically metabolized (Berger and Steinhoff 2011).

Mirtazapine is an α_2 and a serotonin (5-hydroxytryptamine type 2 [5-HT$_2$]) receptor antagonist. It is used for its antidepressant, anxiolytic, sedating, and appetite-stimulating effects, the latter of which may be beneficial in a CKD patient who, in addition to depressive symptoms, has a poor nutritional status. Mirtazapine has been used successfully to treat uremic pruritus in the ESRD population. Pharmacokinetic studies demonstrate the need for renal dosing, because mirtazapine is 85% protein bound and thus is not substantially removed by hemodialysis in the setting of hypoproteinemia (Eyler et al. 2015).

In the general medical setting, making support groups and brief supportive counseling available to patients can help manage anxiety and depressive symptoms as well as improve quality of life in patients with ESRD on hemodialysis (Lerma et al. 2017). Cognitive-behavioral therapy (CBT) also has been demonstrated to reduce depressive symptoms in hemodialysis patients (Lerma et al. 2017).

Anxiety Disorders and Adjustment Disorders

In patients with severe or chronic illness, including CKD, anxiety disorders are often perceived as symptoms of depression rather than a separate condition. Anxiety and depressive symptoms frequently co-occur, and the presence of comorbid anxiety and depressive symptoms correlates with a more persistent course of psychiatric illness in comparison with the presence of solely depressive or anxiety symptoms (Cukor et al. 2008b). Treatment targeted to anxiety may alleviate depressive symptoms (Lerma et al. 2017). The prevalence of anxiety disorders in patients undergoing chronic hemo-dialysis has been estimated at 12%–52% (Murtagh et al. 2007a).

An anxiety disorder can manifest in a variety of ways, including treatment nonad-herence, irritability, decreased sleep (notably early insomnia), poor concentration, physical tension, fatigue, or a sense of restlessness. Persistent anxiety may arise when renal transplant patients are anticipating eventual or inevitable organ rejection; this fear is known as the Damocles syndrome (Reinhart and Kemph 1988). As is the case in depression, it is important to rule out other causes of anxiety symptoms, most no-tably uremia. Routine screening tests for organic causes of new-onset anxiety may in-clude serum chemistries, liver function tests, renal function tests, serum glucose, and thyroid-stimulating hormone; an electrocardiogram, Holter monitoring, stress test, and echocardiogram should also be considered.

Anxiety disorders in ESRD patients have been relatively less well studied than have depressive disorders. The Hospital Anxiety and Depression Scale (HADS; Zig-mond and Snaith 1983) has been used for screening, although it has been found to have poor predictive value for anxiety in ESRD patients and does not reliably differ-entiate between anxiety and depression (Cukor et al. 2008a). Other appropriate screening tools for anxiety disorders include the Beck Anxiety Inventory (Beck et al. 1988) and the Hamilton Anxiety Scale (Hamilton 1959).

In the renally compromised patient, reasonable first-line choices for treatment of anxiety disorders include benzodiazepines such as clonazepam and lorazepam. Care must be taken, however, because benzodiazepines can cause sedation at higher dos-ages and agitation in the setting of delirium. Lorazepam is first hepatically trans-formed into an inactive, nontoxic metabolite and then eliminated by the kidneys. Because renal disease does not affect clearance, no renal dosage adjustment is neces-sary (Morrison et al. 1984). In general, benzodiazepines do not require dosage adjust-ments in renal failure; rather, limitations to their use stem from the risk of dependence and abuse, especially in patients with past histories of substance use disorders. Because of this risk, benzodiazepines are best used as short-term pharmacological manage-ment, with only limited amounts prescribed. The patient's need for benzodiazepines should be reassessed at regular intervals to avoid overtreatment. Buspirone, a $5-HT_{1A}$ receptor partial agonist, may be used in ESRD and may have a more benign side-effect profile compared with benzodiazepines (Caccia et al. 1988); however, clinical effects may take several weeks to appear. Short-term use of zolpidem or zaleplon may be ap-propriate for patients who experience insomnia in addition to or as a consequence of an anxiety disorder.

Adjustment disorders are defined as response to a recent (within the past 3 months) identifiable stressor that includes 1) marked distress out of proportion to the severity or intensity of the stressor, after context and cultural factors that might influence symptom severity are taken into account, or 2) significant impairment in social, occu-pational, or other areas of functioning (American Psychiatric Association 2013). Ad-justment disorders are now conceptualized as being on the spectrum of trauma- and stressor-related disorders. This diagnosis may apply when patients do not meet criteria for posttraumatic stress disorder (PTSD) or generalized anxiety disorder (GAD) due to the narrow scope and shorter duration of symptomatology (Carta et al. 2009). For example, a patient who has been newly diagnosed with CKD or started on dialysis within the past 3 months may acutely experience symptoms of depressed mood that interfere with daily activities, but such symptoms have not persisted for more than 2 weeks or risen to the level of GAD or PTSD. Management should focus on psychosocial support and emotional coping strategies rather than pharmacotherapy.

An additional period during which adjustment disorder may become particularly relevant is the peritransplant period (Stukas et al. 1999). Receiving an organ may evoke strong emotions ranging from anguish and guilt to hope and revival. The process of transplantation causes significant changes in both patients' and caregivers' routines and requires strict adherence to medication, medical follow-up, and dietary restrictions. After the transplant, the patient may confront anxiety surrounding organ rejection and both physical and neuropsychiatric side effects of newly started immunosuppressant medications. Psychotherapy, particularly individual psychotherapy, serves an important role in helping patients cope with the transplantation process. Studies have demonstrated that psychotherapy improved BDI scores and adherence to immunosuppressive medication in patients during the posttransplant period (Baines et al. 2004; De Geest et al. 2006).

Panic disorder has a more acute onset and a shorter duration compared with GAD. Symptoms include some combination of sudden breathlessness, palpitations, chest pain, diaphoresis, fear of dying, and other abnormal somatic sensations and generally peak within 10 minutes of panic attack onset and last around 30 minutes or less. In the renal disease patient, panic episodes may be related to hypervigilance to bodily sensations, or they can be associated with fluid overload and associated shortness of breath. While triggers of the episodes may or may not be clearly identifiable, patients may respond to these unpleasant episodes with conscious or unconscious avoidance of situations they perceive as triggers. It is important to recognize and manage panic disorder in the renal disease patient because, in addition to contributing to decreased quality of life, the subsequent avoidance of perceived triggers may contribute to treatment nonadherence. For example, a patient who feels that needles are a trigger for his or her panic attacks or who associates the attacks with the dialysis center may skip dialysis sessions (Cohen et al. 2016). Symptoms may be characterized with the Severity Measure for Panic Disorder (Craske et al. 2013), a free screening tool. After symptoms have been clarified and possible triggers have been explored, the patient can be offered CBT, with or without additional pharmacotherapy.

Sleep Disorders

Approximately 80% of ESRD patients have some sort of sleep-related complaint, most commonly excessive daytime sleepiness (Murtagh et al. 2007a). Other sleep disruptions include insomnia, restless legs syndrome (RLS), periodic limb movement disorder (PLMD), and obstructive sleep apnea (OSA). The underlying pathophysiology of sleep disorders in the setting of ESRD is thought to be related to interactions of increased sympathetic activation, decreased melatonin levels, increased orexin production, subclinical uremic encephalopathy, deficiency of tyrosine (a dopamine precursor), sleep-inducing cytokine release during hemodialysis, persistence of melatonin in daytime, and alterations in body temperature. A study comparing 30 ESRD patients undergoing hemodialysis and 20 healthy participants demonstrated significantly lower nocturnal melatonin in ESRD patients (Maung et al. 2016). Disrupted sleep may also stem from an anxiety disorder or a depressive disorder.

Insomnia

Excessive daytime sleepiness is most commonly caused by inefficient or nonrestorative nocturnal sleep. In ESRD, stage 1 and stage 2 non–rapid eye movement sleep are increased, whereas slow-wave sleep and rapid eye movement sleep are reduced due to autonomic dysregulation that increases sympathetic tone and decreases vagal tone (Roumelioti et al. 2010). The initial assessment of insomnia in renal patients does not differ from that in other patients. This assessment includes a thorough history and physical examination to exclude, or to prompt further investigation of, underlying conditions (e.g., sleep apnea, RLS) that can be exacerbated by anemia, which is not uncommon in CKD and ESRD patients. A sleep log may help identify factors that contribute to poor sleep quality, such as medications or the demands of waking up early to travel to a dialysis center.

An important approach to treating insomnia in the renal patient is adjustment of the patient's dialysis regimen. One study demonstrated reduced daytime sleepiness after ESRD patients were switched from conventional to nocturnal hemodialysis; however, this treatment approach may not work for all patients, because nocturnal hemodialysis may potentially cause sleep disruption due to technical difficulties associated with home dialysis as well as anxiety about receiving nighttime dialysis (Hanly et al. 2003).

Behavioral modifications include sleep hygiene improvement and CBT for insomnia. Patients may tend to nap during dialysis, but this may worsen insomnia and should be discouraged (Shibata et al. 2014).

Studies have shown that 3 mg of melatonin given several hours before bedtime is typically well tolerated and can help regulate the sleep-wake cycle in ESRD patients with insomnia (Russcher et al. 2012). With the exception of melatonin, chronic pharmacological treatment of insomnia is less favored due to the metabolic derangements and polypharmacy in many CKD patients. For transient insomnia, benzodiazepines and nonbenzodiazepine hypnotics such as zolpidem and zaleplon, which do not require any dosage adjustment in renal compromise, may be helpful (Drover 2004). Side effects and risks include further disruption of sleep architecture and development of tolerance, dependence, and withdrawal, although the abuse potential of nonbenzodiazepine hypnotics is lower than that of benzodiazepines.

Obstructive Sleep Apnea

OSA is a sleep disorder characterized by transient and repetitive obstruction of the airway during sleep. Evidence suggests that OSA is more prevalent in patients with renal disease than in the general population. A cross-sectional study of CKD patients demonstrated that the majority had OSA (Sim et al. 2009). It is estimated that OSA affects approximately 50% of CKD patients (Unruh 2007). Sleep apnea is especially problematic in the renally compromised patient population because it causes nocturnal hypoxemia and sleep fragmentation. Hypoxemia activates the sympathetic nervous system and the renin-angiotensin-aldosterone system, thereby further aggravating renal pathology through increased inflammation and free radical generation.

Independent of obesity, OSA is associated with glomerular hyperfiltration, a risk factor for CKD progression (Adeseun and Rosas 2010).

It is important to maintain a high index of suspicion for OSA because of its nonspecific presentation and the fact that patients may not recognize that they experience apneic episodes during sleep. OSA commonly manifests with snoring and daytime sleepiness. Nocturnal choking and gasping is highly suggestive of the diagnosis (Myers et al. 2013). OSA may also cause symptoms suggestive of depression or other mood disorders. Assessment of OSA in the renal disease patient is not significantly different from that in the average patient. First-line evaluation is pulse oximetry to establish the presence of repetitive hypoxic episodes during sleep, followed by overnight polysomnography. The diagnosis is made when five or more obstructive respiratory events per hour are noted during sleep in a patient exhibiting OSA symptoms. Weight loss and continuous positive airway pressure constitute the mainstays of OSA therapy.

Restless Legs Syndrome and Periodic Limb Movement Disorder

RLS is characterized by an unpleasant sensation in the lower extremities that worsens with rest and is transiently relieved by movement. Approximately 20%–30% of hemodialysis patients experience RLS, in comparison with approximately 10% of the general population (Murtagh et al. 2007a). Although RLS typically occurs during the evening hours, it may be bothersome during the daytime, while also potentially interfering with initiation and maintenance of sleep. Two studies have reported findings indicating that 200–300 mg of gabapentin after each dialysis session may be an effective treatment for RLS in hemodialysis patients (Micozkadioglu et al. 2004; Thorp et al. 2001). Other studies have shown exercise to have some promise in managing RLS in CKD patients (Giannaki et al. 2010; Sakkas et al. 2008). Whether traditional RLS treatments such as ropinirole and pramipexole are effective is unclear. A study of pramipexole found reductions in periodic leg movements during sleep but no change in sleep latency, total hours of sleep, number of awakenings, or sleep efficiency after 1 month of therapy (Miranda et al. 2004).

PLMD refers to involuntary jerking movement of the legs (and occasionally the arms) during sleep. RLS is almost always associated with PLMD, but PLMD can occur in the absence of RLS. Diagnosis is by polysomnography. Few independent studies have examined the efficacy of treatments specifically for PLMD; therefore, treatment of PLMD is based on treatment used in clinical practice for RLS (Aurora et al. 2012).

Sexual and Reproductive Function

Although frequently overlooked in the setting of numerous medical comorbidities, sexual function can be a major indicator of quality of life. CKD is associated with multiple endocrine disturbances that can contribute to sexual dysfunction, including loss of libido and infertility in both sexes. The psychological stress of coping with CKD and ESRD can further exacerbate sexual dysfunction; in depressed CKD patients, as with all patients, sexual dysfunction may be a side effect of antidepressant medications as well as of the depressive disorder itself. CKD and its associated derangements in the hypothalamic-pituitary-gonadal (HPG) axis can lead to menstrual disturbances and anovulation in women and to erectile dysfunction in men (Anantharaman and Schmidt 2007). An estimated 65% of hemodialysis patients report sexual dysfunction, and only 60% report having regular intercourse (Milde et al. 1996). Screening questions include the following: "Have there been any changes in your sex life?" "Are you satisfied with your current sex life?" and "How has your kidney disease affected your sex life?" Direct inquiry about menstrual cycle regularity in women and erectile dysfunction in men is appropriate (Anantharaman and Schmidt 2007). A physical examination may be performed to evaluate for physical signs of hypogonadism.

The primary endocrine alteration in males is hypogonadism due to altered pulsatile secretion of gonadotropin-releasing hormone, which in turn causes low testosterone. Low testosterone levels have been shown to increase mortality risk in men with ESRD (Carrero et al. 2009). Treatment of hypogonadism in CKD patients, as in the general population, involves testosterone supplementation. Testosterone should be increased only up to the lower end of the normal range, because further increments do not appear to yield greater beneficial effects on sexual function (Johansen 2004). Side effects include deleterious effects on lipid levels, while potentially beneficial effects include an anabolic effect and a slight increase in hematocrit (Anantharaman and Schmidt 2007).

Psychological factors also may play a role in the pathophysiology of erectile dysfunction, as may neurovascular damage or endocrinological derangements. If a patient has normal nocturnal erections during sleep, psychological factors are more likely to be a contributing factor. Erectile dysfunction may be treated empirically with phosphodiesterase-5 (PDE-5) inhibitors (Vecchio et al. 2010). No dosage adjustment is needed for renal patients, although starting at half-dosage (25 mg of sildenafil) and slowly titrating up to a maximum dosage of 100 mg is recommended, because the maximum dosage may not be necessary to achieve a response (Ghafari et al. 2010; Lasaponara et al. 2013).

A general treatment approach to sexual dysfunction includes optimizing the patient's dialysis regimen—for example, changing dialysis to six times weekly for shorter durations; however, one study demonstrated that hemodialysis adequacy did not necessarily impact sexual dysfunction in women (Carrero et al. 2009). Although HPA and HPG axis dysfunction initially worsens when hemodialysis is commenced, the symptomatic manifestations may improve but rarely normalize during the maintenance phase of dialysis. Successful kidney transplantation may improve sexual function and fertility, especially in younger patients, albeit not necessarily to the degree of function prior to renal failure.

Delirium

Delirium is characterized by acute onset (hours to days) and fluctuating disturbances in attention and cognition (memory deficits, disorientation, or impairments in language, visuospatial ability, or perception) that are not better explained by another preexisting neurocognitive disorder. Delirium is, by definition, caused by a medical condition. Therefore, aside from symptomatic management, it is imperative to identify and treat the underlying cause. In CKD, this might involve obtaining serum electrolytes, assessing the patient's hydration status, reviewing medications, and (if the patient is on dialysis), reviewing the regimen and making adjustments as necessary. A blood urea nitrogen to creatinine ratio above 18 is a common cause of encephalopathy in kidney disease, although delirium is a clinical syndrome and is not diagnosed on the basis of laboratory findings alone (Inouye et al. 1993; Meyer and Hostetter 2007).

Part of the challenge in diagnosing delirium is the broad spectrum of symptoms manifested in altered mental states. Patients may appear agitated, lethargic, or somnolent. They can also seem wide awake while demonstrating deficits in memory, thought process, and orientation. Speech may be incoherent, tangential, or disorganized. Asking nursing staff and family whether the patient's level of alertness and confusion has waxed and waned in recent hours or days can aid in diagnosis.

The Confusion Assessment Method is a highly sensitive and specific tool used to rapidly evaluate a patient for delirium (Inouye et al. 1990). Developed by an internist for use by non–psychiatrically trained clinicians, the four-item inventory reviews whether 1) the patient's apparent altered state is acute in onset with a fluctuating course; 2) the patient shows inattention; 3) the patient manifests disorganized thinking; or 4) the patient has an altered level of consciousness. For delirium to be diagnosed, both of the first two features must be present in addition to either the third or fourth feature.

The fluctuating course usually differentiates delirium from depression and dementia. Further evaluation in this regard may include serial administrations of the Mini-Mental Status Examination. Delirium should be distinguished from "sundowning," a common phenomenon in patients with dementia in which behavior deteriorates in the late afternoon or evening hours. Sundowning is associated with impaired circadian rhythmicity secondary to degeneration of the suprachiasmatic nucleus, leading to confusion as daylight yields to darkness. Sundowning should be distinguished from dialysis disequilibrium syndrome, a neurological syndrome occurring in patients newly started on dialysis and thought to stem from cerebral edema.

Once delirium is suspected, the general approach includes a review of the patient's history and medication list. Physical examination may include assessment of vital signs, hydration status, and potential sources of infection. Laboratory studies may include electrolytes, ammonia, and medication levels. Less commonly, brain imaging or a lumbar puncture may be diagnostically useful.

Contributions to delirium in the setting of renal disease include dehydration, uremia, anemia, hyperparathyroidism, and drug toxicity. The drugs that most commonly precipitate delirium in renal failure include anticholinergics, corticosteroids, H_2 blockers, opioid analgesics, and benzodiazepines. In transplant patients, supratherapeutic levels of immunosuppressant drugs—including cyclosporine, tacrolimus, sirolimus, and mycophenolate mofetil—pose a significant delirium risk (Mohammadpour et al. 2011).

Management includes both behavioral and medical approaches. Nonpharmacological approaches, such as treatment of precipitating factors, are strongly preferred as first-line treatments. Measures for prevention of delirium in hospitalized patients may include repeated reorientation to time and place, promotion of sleep hygiene, patient mobilization, adequate hydration, ensuring that sensory aids (e.g., hearing aids, glasses) are in place, and minimization of unnecessary noise and other stimuli. Pharmacological management includes antipsychotics such as haloperidol, although use of antipsychotics should be reserved for agitated patients who are in danger of harming themselves or others. No dosage adjustments for antipsychotics are necessary in the renal patient. The benzodiazepine lorazepam may be used cautiously but can cause paradoxical agitation in elderly patients, especially those with renal compromise.

Pain Management

Approximately half of ESRD patients experience pain (Murtagh et al. 2007a). Causes are multifactorial and may include calciphylaxis (a syndrome that involves vascular calcification and skin necrosis), bone disease, the placement of large-bore needles for dialysis, cramps from osmolar shifts, vascular steal secondary to an arteriovenous fistula or graft, diffuse pain associated with polycystic kidney disease, and neuropathic pain associated with diabetes (Olivo et al. 2015). Much like depression, pain is linked with adverse outcomes, including impaired sleep and mood, decreased quality of life, and increased contemplation of dialysis withdrawal (Weisbord 2016). Recognizing and treating psychological factors that may be aggravating the patient's perception of pain can improve the effectiveness of pain management. Counseling patients to establish clear and realistic expectations regarding pain relief may also help improve management.

Because many analgesics, particularly opioids, are renally cleared, serum levels will be unpredictable. Nonsteroidal anti-inflammatory drugs (NSAIDs), which cause renal vasoconstriction by inhibition of prostaglandins, are well known to have direct nephrotoxic effects, and may induce interstitial nephritis, with or without nephrotic syndrome; fluid and electrolyte abnormalities including hyponatremia and hyperkalemia; renal tubular acidosis; edema; hypertension; and acute or chronic renal papillary necrosis. Therefore, NSAIDs should be used with caution in renally compromised patients.

Challenges to managing chronic pain in CKD patients include the lack of dosing guidelines and the risk of opioid misuse or dependence. Long-term opioid use in the hemodialysis population was found to range from 5% to 36% in one systematic review (Wyne et al. 2011), and use of opioids and benzodiazepines tended to increase with duration of dialysis (Butler et al. 2014; Wyne et al. 2011). Guidelines for optimal management include regular reassessment of pain and analgesic side effects, thorough documentation of sources of all prescribed pain medications, patient education, and maintenance of a pain contract setting realistic expectations of pain management with the goals of preventing polypharmacy and encouraging adherence.

Depending on the type of pain, first-line management starts with conservative topical therapy, including ice and heat. Lidocaine patches can be safely used as adjunctive therapy in both renally impaired and dialysis patients. In 1986, the World Health Organization delineated a three-step approach to pharmacological management of pain that was subsequently adapted for use in pain associated with other illnesses, including CKD (Pham et al. 2009). The first step involves deployment of NSAIDs and nonopioid analgesics. Aspirin would be a reasonable first choice, given that it has the fewest adverse effects on GFR among the NSAIDs (Pham et al. 2009). If pain persists, the next step involves addition of low-potency opioids. Tramadol is a norepinephrine and serotonin reuptake inhibitor and μ opioid receptor agonist. Although its metabolites are both hepatically and renally excreted, tramadol is not known to be nephro-toxic and may be considered for CKD patients with appropriate adjustments (dosage reductions and increased dosing intervals). The third step involves addition of higher-potency opioids. Oral hydrocodone, methadone, and hydromorphone are considered the safest choices for renally impaired and dialysis patients with acute, unstable pain. Transdermal fentanyl may be used for chronic, stable pain (Murtagh et al. 2007b). Be-cause metabolites of morphine are toxic and renally cleared, morphine is not recom-mended in CKD patients. Side effects of metabolite accumulation include nausea, vomiting, myoclonus, seizures, and sedation. Opioids should be taken on a regular schedule, with as-needed medication available for "breakthrough" pain.

Treatment Nonadherence and Suicide in End-Stage Renal Disease

Patients may not follow their health care provider's instructions for a multitude of reasons: lack of comprehension due to limited health literacy, inadequate social or lo-gistical support, dementia or reduced cognitive capacity, depressive symptoms in-cluding feelings of hopelessness, intolerance of certain side effects that compromise quality of life, concern about possible side effects, or a conscious wish to stop treat-ment (Kimmel 2001). Other risk factors associated with nonadherence in CKD patients include being of lower socioeconomic status, using tobacco, and being male, particu-larly if young. Depression is independently associated with treatment nonadherence, and psychosocial support has been shown to improve adherence (DiMatteo et al. 2000; Unruh et al. 2005). A general practitioner can help identify obstacles driving nonad-herence and suggest solutions whenever possible. Care includes screening for, diag-nosing, and treating psychiatric comorbidities and referring patients whose emotional concerns might respond to psychotherapy or whose psychiatric complexity warrants specialist intervention. The general practitioner may also engage the patient in end-of-life discussions centered on decisions regarding whether and when to stop dialysis.

The most ethically or perhaps philosophically challenging aspect of managing dialysis-dependent patients is that withdrawal of dialysis almost always precipitates death. Although individual circumstances and personal beliefs determine whether withdrawal constitutes suicide, regardless of its ultimate designation, the rates of dial-ysis withdrawal and nonadherence—both intentional and unintentional—make it necessary to assess and differentiate among end-of-life planning, suicidality, and ob-stacles to treatment adherence.

Suicide rates in patients with ESRD are modestly elevated in comparison with rates in the general population. Independent predictors of suicide include age greater than 75 years, male sex, Caucasian or Asian race, alcohol or drug dependence, and re-cent hospitalization with mental illness (Kurella et al. 2005). In ESRD patients, the risk is greatest within the first 3 months of dialysis initiation (Kurella et al. 2005; Raue et al. 2014).

Withdrawal from dialysis prior to death occurs approximately 100 times more fre-quently than suicide does in the ESRD population (Kurella et al. 2005). The U.S. Renal Data System survey has demonstrated that 19%–25% of hemodialysis and peritoneal dialysis patients withdrew from dialysis prior to death (United States Renal Data System 2018). Rates of dialysis withdrawal and suicide are difficult to estimate accurately, because decisions to withdraw from dialysis can sometimes be a proxy for other impending causes of death or, in fact, good management. The constellation of risk factors for dialysis withdrawal are distinct from predictors of suicide—that is, female sex, older age, and recent hospitalization are stronger risks for dialysis withdrawal than for suicide (Kurella et al. 2005).

While no definitive evidence has determined that routine screening for suicidal ideation in outpatient settings reduces mortality, it is still reasonable to screen for suicidal ideation. Screening is particularly important at times of treatment initiation, hospitalization, and events possibly perceived as stressors or setbacks. The act of simply asking patients if they have experienced thoughts of ending their life does not increase the risk of suicide. If the patient answers affirmatively, further assessment should establish the seriousness of the suicidal ideation, including the intent and plan. If questions remain about acute risk, need for hospitalization, or medication changes, referrals should be made as needed to psychiatric, palliative care, or other specialists.

Conclusion

Chronic kidney disease may lead to physical, emotional, spiritual, or social challenges that can affect many aspects of a patient's daily life. In common with other chronic illnesses, CKD has the potential to cause or exacerbate depression, anxiety, and demoralization. In addition, patients with CKD may experience sleep disturbances, sexual dysfunction, pain, and the challenge of coping with dietary and fluid restrictions. Long-term dependency on the life-prolonging treatment of dialysis creates existentially complex circumstances, particularly when the patient is not eligible for a curative organ transplant or faces treatment withdrawal at the end of life. Clinicians' attention to patients' mental and emotional aspects of well-being, particularly at major treatment decision points such as dialysis initiation or withdrawal, may improve not only treatment adherence but also quality of life.

References

Adeseun GA, Rosas SE: The impact of obstructive sleep apnea on chronic kidney disease. Curr Hypertens Rep 12(5):378–383, 2010 20676805

American Psychiatric Association: Diagnostic and Statistical Manual of Mental Disorders, 5th Edition. Arlington, VA, American Psychiatric Association, 2013

Anantharaman P, Schmidt RJ: Sexual function in chronic kidney disease. Adv Chronic Kidney Dis 14(2):119–125, 2007 17395114

Aurora RN, Kristo DA, Bista SR, et al: The treatment of restless legs syndrome and periodic limb movement disorder in adults—an update for 2012: practice parameters with an evidence-based systematic review and meta-analyses. Sleep 35(8):1039–1062, 2012 22851801

Baines LS, Joseph JT, Jindal RM: Prospective randomized study of individual and group psychotherapy versus controls in recipients of renal transplants. Kidney Int 65(5):1937–1942, 2004 15086937

Beck A, Ward C, Mendelson M, et al: An inventory for measuring depression. Arch Gen Psychiatry 42:667–675, 1961 13688369

Beck AT, Epstein N, Brown G, et al: An inventory for measuring clinical anxiety: psychometric properties. J Consult Clin Psychol 56(6):893–897, 1988 3204199

Berger TG, Steinhoff M: Pruritus and renal failure. Semin Cutan Med Surg 30(2):99–100, 2011 21767770

Blumenfield M, Levy NB, Spinowitz B, et al: Fluoxetine in depressed patients on dialysis. Int J Psychiatry Med 27(1):71–80, 1997 9565715

Butler AM, Kshirsagar AV, Brookhart MA: Opioid use in the US hemodialysis population. Am J Kidney Dis 63(1):171–173, 2014 24145020

Caccia S, Vigano GL, Mingardi G, et al: Clinical pharmacokinetics of oral buspirone in patients with impaired renal function. Clin Pharmacokinet 14(3):171–177, 1988 3370902

Carrero JJ, Qureshi AR, Parini P, et al: Low serum testosterone increases mortality risk among male dialysis patients. J Am Soc Nephrol 20(3):613–620, 2009 19144759

Carta MG, Balestrieri M, Murru A, et al: Adjustment disorder: epidemiology, diagnosis and treatment. Clin Pract Epidemiol Ment Health 5(1):15, 2009 19558652

Chen YS, Wu SC, Wang SY, et al: Depression in chronic haemodialysed patients. Nephrology (Carlton) 8(3):121–126, 2003 15012727

Cohen LM, Tessier EG, Germain MJ, et al: Update on psychotropic medication use in renal disease. Psychosomatics 45(1):34–48, 2004 14709759

Cohen SD, Cukor D, Kimmel PL: Anxiety in patients treated with hemodialysis. Clin J Am Soc Nephrol 11(12):2250–2255, 2016 27660303

Craske M, Wittchen U, Bogels S, et al: Severity Measure for Panic Disorder—Adult. Washington, DC, American Psychiatric Association, 2013. Available at: https://www.psychiatry.org/File%20Library/Psychiatrists/Practice/DSM/APA_DSM5_Severity-Measure-For-Panic-Disorder-Adult.pdf. Accessed September 9, 2019.

Cukor D, Coplan J, Brown C, et al: Anxiety disorders in adults treated by hemodialysis: a single-center study. Am J Kidney Dis 52(1):128–136, 2008a 18440682

Cukor D, Coplan J, Brown C, et al: Course of depression and anxiety diagnosis in patients treated with hemodialysis: a 16-month follow-up. Clin J Am Soc Nephrol 3(6):1752–1758, 2008b 18684897

De Geest S, Schäfer-Keller P, Denhaerynck K, et al: Supporting medication adherence in renal transplantation (SMART): a pilot RCT to improve adherence to immunosuppressive regimens. Clin Transplant 20(3):359–368, 2006 16824155

DiMatteo MR, Lepper HS, Croghan TW: Depression is a risk factor for noncompliance with medical treatment: meta-analysis of the effects of anxiety and depression on patient adherence. Arch Intern Med 160(14):2101–2107, 2000 10904452

Drover DR: Comparative pharmacokinetics and pharmacodynamics of short-acting hypnosedatives: zaleplon, zolpidem and zopiclone. Clin Pharmacokinet 43(4):227–238, 2004 15005637

Eyler RF, Unruh ML, Quinn DK, et al: Psychotherapeutic agents in end-stage renal disease. Semin Dial 28(4):417–426, 2015 25857865

Ghafari A, Farshid B, Afshari AT, et al: Sildenafil citrate can improve erectile dysfunction among chronic hemodialysis patients. Indian J Nephrol 20(3):142–145, 2010 21072154

Giannaki, Sakkas GK, Hadjigeorgiou GM, et al: Non-pharmacological management of periodic limb movements during hemodialysis session in patients with uremic restless legs syndrome. ASAIO J 56(6):538–542, 2010 21245801

Hamilton M: The assessment of anxiety states by rating. Br J Med Psychol 32(1):50–55, 1959 13638508

Hamilton M: A rating scale for depression. J Neurol Neurosurg Psychiatry 23:56–62, 1960 14399272

Hanly PJ, Gabor JY, Chan C, et al: Daytime sleepiness in patients with CRF: impact of nocturnal hemodialysis. Am J Kidney Dis 41(2):403–410, 2003 12552503

Hedayati SS, Minhajuddin AT, Toto RD, et al: Prevalence of major depressive episode in CKD. Am J Kidney Dis 54(3):424–432, 2009a 19493599

Hedayati SS, Minhajuddin AT, Toto RD, et al: Validation of depression screening scales in patients with CKD. Am J Kidney Dis 54(3):433–439, 2009b 19493600

Hedayati SS, Yalamanchili V, Finkelstein FO: A practical approach to the treatment of depression in patients with chronic kidney disease and end-stage renal disease. Kidney Int 81(3):247–255, 2012 22012131

Inouye SK, van Dyck CH, Alessi CA, et al: Clarifying confusion: the confusion assessment method. A new method for detection of delirium. Ann Intern Med 113(12):941–948, 1990 2240918

Inouye SK, Viscoli CM, Horwitz RI, et al: A predictive model for delirium in hospitalized elderly medical patients based on admission characteristics. Ann Intern Med 119(6):474–481, 1993 8357112

Johansen KL: Treatment of hypogonadism in men with chronic kidney disease. Adv Chronic Kidney Dis 11(4):348–356, 2004 15492971

Kalender B, Ozdemir AC, Yalug I, et al: Antidepressant treatment increases quality of life in patients with chronic renal failure. Ren Fail 29(7):817–822, 2007 17994449

Kalman TP, Wilson PG, Kalman CM: Psychiatric morbidity in long-term renal transplant recipients and patients undergoing hemodialysis. A comparative study. JAMA 250(1):55–58, 1983 6343654

Kimmel PL: Psychosocial factors in dialysis patients. Kidney Int 59(4):1599–1613, 2001 11260433

Kimmel PL, Weihs K, Peterson RA: Survival in hemodialysis patients: the role of depression. J Am Soc Nephrol 4(1):12–27, 1993 8400064

Kimmel PL, Thamer M, Richard CM, et al: Psychiatric illness in patients with end-stage renal disease. Am J Med 105(3):214–221, 1998 9753024

Kroenke K, Spitzer RL, Williams JB: The PHQ-9: validity of a brief depression severity measure. J Gen Intern Med 16(9):606–613, 2001 11556941

Kurella M, Kimmel PL, Young BS, et al: Suicide in the United States end-stage renal disease program. J Am Soc Nephrol 16(3):774–781, 2005 15659561

Lasaponara F, Sedigh O, Pasquale G, et al: Phosphodiesterase type 5 inhibitor treatment for erectile dysfunction in patients with end-stage renal disease receiving dialysis or after renal transplantation. J Sex Med 10(11):2798–2814, 2013 23346948

Lerma A, Perez-Grovas H, Bermudez L, et al: Brief cognitive behavioural intervention for depression and anxiety symptoms improves quality of life in chronic haemodialysis patients. Psychol Psychother 90(1):105–123, 2017 27435635

Lieberman JA, Cooper TB, Suckow RF, et al: Tricyclic antidepressant and metabolite levels in chronic renal failure. Clin Pharmacol Ther 37(3):301–307, 1985 3971655

Mangelli L, Fava GA, Grandi S, et al: Assessing demoralization and depression in the setting of medical disease. J Clin Psychiatry 66(3):391–394, 2005 15766307

Maung SC, El Sara A, Chapman C, et al: Sleep disorders and chronic kidney disease. World J Nephrol 5(3):224–232, 2016 27152260

Meyer TW, Hostetter TH: Uremia. N Engl J Med 357(13):1316–1325, 2007 17898101

Micozkadioglu H, Ozdemir FN, Kut A, et al: Gabapentin versus levodopa for the treatment of restless legs syndrome in hemodialysis patients: an open-label study. Ren Fail 26(4):393–397, 2004 15462107

Milde FK, Hart LK, Fearing MO: Sexuality and fertility concerns of dialysis patients. ANNA J 23(3):307–313, 315; discussion 314–315, 1996 8716990

Miranda M, Kagi M, Fabres L, et al: Pramipexole for the treatment of uremic restless legs in patients undergoing hemodialysis. Neurology 62(5):831–832, 2004 15007148

Mohammadpour N, Elyasi S, Vahdati N, et al: A review on therapeutic drug monitoring of immunosuppressant drugs. Iran J Basic Med Sci 14(6):485–498, 2011 23493821

Morrison G, Chiang ST, Koepke HH, Walker BR: Effect of renal impairment and hemodialysis on lorazepam kinetics. Clin Pharmacol Ther 35(5):646–652, 1984 6713774

Morton RL, Tong A, Howard K, et al: The views of patients and carers in treatment decision making for chronic kidney disease: systematic review and thematic synthesis of qualitative studies. BMJ 340(January):c112, 2010 20085970

Murtagh FE, Addington-Hall J, Higginson IJ: The prevalence of symptoms in end-stage renal disease: a systematic review. Adv Chron Kidney Dis 14(1):82–99, 2007a 17200048

Murtagh FE, Chai MO, Donohoe P, et al: The use of opioid analgesia in end-stage renal disease patients managed without dialysis: recommendations for practice. J Pain Palliat Care Pharmacother 21(2):5–16, 2007b 17844723

Myers KA, Mrkobrada M, Simel DL: Does this patient have obstructive sleep apnea? The Rational Clinical Examination systematic review. JAMA 310(7):731–741, 2013 23989984

Nagler EV, Webster AC, Vanholder R, et al: Antidepressants for depression in stage 3–5 chronic kidney disease: a systematic review of pharmacokinetics, efficacy and safety with recommendations by European Renal Best Practice (ERBP). Nephrol Dial Transplant 27(10):3736–3745, 2012 22859791

Olivo RE, Hensley RL, Lewis JB, Saha S: Opioid use in hemodialysis patients. Am J Kidney Dis 66(6):1103–1105, 2015 26421755

Palmer S, Vecchio M, Craig JC, et al: Prevalence of depression in chronic kidney disease: systematic review and meta-analysis of observational studies. Kidney Int 84(1):179–191, 2013 23486521

Palmer SC, Natale P, Ruospo M, et al: Antidepressants for treating depression in adults with end-stage kidney disease treated with dialysis. Cochrane Database Syst Rev (5):CD004541, 2016 27210414

Pham PC, Toscano E, Pham PM, et al: Pain management in patients with chronic kidney disease. NDT Plus 2(2):111–118, 2009 25949305

Raue PJ, Ghesquiere AR, Bruce ML: Suicide risk in primary care: identification and management in older adults. Curr Psychiatry Rep 16(9):466, 2014 25030971

Reinhart JB, Kemph JP: Renal transplantation for children: another view. JAMA 260(22):3327–3328, 1988 3054195

Roumelioti ME, Ranpuria R, Hall M, et al: Abnormal nocturnal heart rate variability response among chronic kidney disease and dialysis patients during wakefulness and sleep. Nephrol Dial Transplant 25(11):3733–3741, 2010 20466675

Rubin HR, Fink NE, Plantinga LC, et al: Patient ratings of dialysis care with peritoneal dialysis vs hemodialysis. JAMA 291(6):697–703, 2004 14871912

Rush AJ, Trivedi MH, Ibrahim HM, et al: The 16-Item Quick Inventory of Depressive Symptomatology (QIDS), clinician rating (QIDS-C), and self-report (QIDS-SR): a psychometric evaluation in patients with chronic major depression. Biol Psychiatry 54(5):573–583, 2003 [Erratum in: Biol Psychiatry 54(5):585, 2003] 12946886

Russcher M, Koch B, Nagtegaal E, et al: The role of melatonin treatment in chronic kidney disease. Front Biosci 17:2644–2656, 2012 22652802

Sakkas GK, Hadjigeorgiou GM, Karatzaferi C, et al: Intradialytic aerobic exercise training ameliorates symptoms of restless legs syndrome and improves functional capacity in patients on hemodialysis: a pilot study. ASAIO J 54(2):185–190, 2008 18356653

Shibata S, Tsutou A, Shiotani H: Relation between sleep quality and daily physical activity in hemodialysis outpatients. Kobe J Med Sci 59(5):E161–E166, 2014 24854994

Silva Junior GB, Daher EF, Buosi AP, et al: Depression among patients with end-stage renal disease in hemodialysis. Psychol Health Med 19(5):547–551, 2014 24160459

Sim JJ, Rasgon SA, Kujubu DA, et al: Sleep apnea in early and advanced chronic kidney disease: Kaiser Permanente Southern California cohort. Chest 135(3):710–716, 2009 19029435

Stukas AA Jr, Dew MA, Switzer GE, et al: PTSD in heart transplant recipients and their primary family caregivers. Psychosomatics 40(3):212–221, 1999 10341533

Thorp ML, Morris CD, Bagby SP: A crossover study of gabapentin in treatment of restless legs syndrome among hemodialysis patients. Am J Kidney Dis 38(1):104–108, 2001 11431189

United States Renal Data System: 2018 USRDS Annual Data Report: Epidemiology of Kidney Disease in the United States. Bethesda, MD, National Institutes of Health, National Institute of Diabetes and Digestive and Kidney Diseases, November 2018. Available at: https://www.usrds.org/2018/view/Default.aspx. Accessed September 9, 2019.

Unruh ML: Sleep apnea and dialysis therapies: things that go bump in the night? Hemodial Int 11(4):369–378, 2007 17922730

Unruh ML, Evans IV, Fink NE, et al: Skipped treatments, markers of nutritional nonadherence, and survival among incident hemodialysis patients. Am J Kidney Dis 46(6):1107–1116, 2005 16310577

Vecchio M, Navaneethan SD, Johnson DW, et al: Treatment options for sexual dysfunction in patients with chronic kidney disease: a systematic review of randomized controlled trials. Clin J Am Soc Nephrol 5(6):985–995, 2010 20498250

Weisbord SD: Patient-centered dialysis care: depression, pain, and quality of life. Semin Dial 29(2):158–164, 2016 26748494

Wyne A, Rai R, Cuerden M, et al: Opioid and benzodiazepine use in end-stage renal disease: a systematic review. Clin J Am Soc Nephrol 6(2):326–333, 2011 21071517

Zigmond AS, Snaith RP: The hospital anxiety and depression scale. Acta Psychiatr Scand 67(6):361–370, 1983 6880820

CHAPTER 12

Neurological Conditions and Their Psychiatric Manifestations

Barry S. Fogel, M.D.

Gaston C. Baslet, M.D.

Laura T. Safar, M.D.

Geoffrey S. Raynor, M.D.

David A. Silbersweig, M.D.

Neurology and psychiatry are medical specialties with intersecting concerns. Both diagnose and treat diseases, syndromes, and symptoms that are produced by dysfunction of the hardware or software of the brain and that are influenced by a patient's developmental history and physical and social environment. In the history of medicine, conditions have moved from psychiatry to neurology when consistent abnormalities of brain anatomy or physiology have been identified, and a psychiatric perspective has been added to neurology in conditions where successful treatment of a brain disease has evidently required addressing its cognitive, emotional, and behavioral dimensions. Epilepsy moved decisively from psychiatry to neurology after the introduction of electroencephalography (EEG), and psychiatry gained a greater role in chronic pain management when the benefits of cognitive and behavioral interventions in relieving distress and dysfunction were definitively established. For the purposes of this chapter, psychiatric symptoms, syndromes, diseases, disorders, and illnesses are changes in mood, cognition, or behavior that cause distress or impair function; neurological symptoms are those related to characteristic changes in the function of the brain, spinal cord, peripheral nerves, or muscles, including functional changes associated with anatomical changes at the gross or microscopic level.

Neurological diseases often produce psychiatric symptoms. Neurologists and neurosurgeons ask psychiatrists' assistance with these symptoms when 1) the patient has psychiatric symptoms not fully explained by the known neurological condition; 2) the patient has psychiatric symptoms—either due to the known brain disease or due to a known primary mental disorder—that require specialized treatment or management beyond the scope of the neurologist's or neurosurgeon's practice; 3) the patient has a chronic neurological disease for which optimal long-term management requires an enduring change in the patient's beliefs or behavior; or 4) the patient has neurological symptoms with presence or severity not accounted for by any neurological disease the patient is thought to have, raising the possibility that the neurological syndrome or the severity of its symptoms is an expression of a primary psychiatric disorder.

In some settings, including those of emergency medicine and trauma care, psychiatrists are called upon to opine whether a patient's psychiatric symptoms might be secondary to a neurological or general medical condition that should be the top priority for treatment—that is, to assist in assessing a neurological disorder as the primary cause for the patient's condition. The presenting syndromes most requiring specialized clinical psychiatric skills are those that do not include acute impairment of cognition (including memory) or where the patient's abnormality of behavior, mood, or perception is disproportionate to impairment of cognition. In such cases, the psychiatrist must determine that the presenting symptoms, the mental status examination, and the context of the illness (e.g., environmental exposures, known preexisting medical conditions, recent travel, brain trauma) taken together imply a significant probability that the psychiatric symptoms are secondary. The psychiatrist then suggests additional history to be gathered, observations to be made, laboratory and imaging tests to be done, or other specialties to be consulted. More problematic is the situation where the psychiatrist is told that a patient has been thought to be free of causative medical disorders when there are open questions about neurological and general medical factors contributing to the patient's mental state. In these cases, the psychiatrist should identify the open questions and establish who will be responsible for following up on them. It is not unusual for a patient to be referred for emergency psychiatric treatment when important diagnostic issues remain unresolved.

Psychiatrists sometimes diagnose neurological diseases unexpected by other physicians. Characteristic examples are cases of encephalitis that manifest as acute psychosis and cases of subdural hematoma or normal-pressure hydrocephalus with an initial subacute presentation of disinhibited behavior or apathy. In another scenario, a psychiatrist follows a patient long term for a chronic psychiatric illness such as bipolar disorder or schizophrenia, and the patient develops a comorbid neurological disorder such as cerebrovascular disease, multiple sclerosis (MS), or Parkinson's disease that the psychiatrist is the first physician to notice. Many patients with chronic mental illness get infrequent or perfunctory general medical care, and the psychiatrist is in the best position to identify new neurological disorders in need of treatment.

Because of the historical splitting of psychiatry and mental health conditions from the remainder of medical care, which regrettably continues today in many systems for the delivery and financing of health care, psychiatrists and neurologists often are asked to categorize patients as either "neurological" or "psychiatric." However, some neurological conditions so frequently have functionally significant psychiatric symptoms that their characterization as neurological or psychiatric is not in the patients' best interest. Complex partial epilepsy, MS, migraine, Parkinson's disease, and sequelae of traumatic brain injury (TBI) are five examples of such conditions.

Psychiatric symptoms that accompany a neurological disease can be a symptomatic expression of the patient's reaction to the physical discomfort, functional impairment, practical consequences, stigma associated with the disease, or prognosis of the condition. The latter is a common concern in cases of progressive neurological diseases such as amyotrophic lateral sclerosis (ALS), Huntington's disease, late-stage Parkinson's disease, or chronic progressive MS, as well as progressive dementias such as Alzheimer's disease and frontotemporal dementia, which are discussed elsewhere in this volume (see Chapter 22, "Neurocognitive Disorders"). The stigma of neurological disease is greatest when the patient is distressed and functionally impaired but has no obvious, visible sign of physical illness. Epilepsy, an invisible disability of this kind, has been stigmatized and feared for millennia, and still is in many places. In diseases of the frontal and temporal lobes, personality changes can precede other neurological signs and any neurological diagnosis.

Neurological and psychiatric symptoms can arise from a common underlying general medical condition, such as a nutritional deficiency, a systemic or central nervous system (CNS) infection, an endocrine disorder, an autoimmune disease, or toxic effects of medications or environmental exposures. The condition can manifest with either a neurological or a psychiatric face; in the latter case, it may fall to the psychiatrist to recognize the scope of the problem and to assist in timely identification of the cause. Biological treatments for psychiatric disorders can have neurological adverse effects, treatments for neurological diseases can have psychiatric adverse effects, and treatments for neurological and psychiatric illness can interact in a way that requires modification of one or more treatments to optimize clinical outcomes. There are so many potential interactions between drugs with primary psychiatric indications and primary neurological indications that it is beyond the scope of this chapter to list all of them. In all cases where a patient receives both categories of medications, an automated search for relevant interactions should be done. Biological treatments for neurological and psychiatric conditions are not limited to medications; deep brain stimulation, transcranial magnetic stimulation (TMS), and vagus nerve stimulation are being used more often than a decade ago and for a wider range of indications. All are used for both primary neurological and primary psychiatric conditions, and in either case they can have off-target effects with which a psychiatric consultant to a neurological service and other clinicians should be familiar.

In chronic neurological conditions such as MS, Parkinson's disease, epilepsy, and migraine, psychiatrists can assist neurologists and their patients in choosing among treatments when there are several viable options. In addition to estimating patients' vulnerability to potential drug interactions and psychiatric adverse effects, they can consider cognitive and behavioral barriers to consistent treatment adherence and can evaluate the impact of prior treatments on mental status, social competence, instrumental activities of daily living (IADLs), and overall well-being.

Many of the psychiatric reactions that patients have to neurological diseases are general responses to major illness, with depression and anxiety especially common. Many brain diseases are associated with a prevalence of comorbid clinical depression (i.e., major depressive disorder, bipolar depression, mood disorders with mixed symptoms, and subsyndromal depression with functional impairment, significant distress, suicidal ideation, or self-harm) that is greater than the prevalence of depression in general medical conditions that cause similar pain, discomfort, and functional impairment but do not directly involve the CNS. Among these general medical conditions is a subset in which the prevalence of comorbid bipolar disorder is greater than would be expected, even taking the increased prevalence of depression into account. Secondary bipolar disorder is remarkable because nonpsychiatrists rarely are surprised when a chronically ill person becomes depressed but often are unaware that medical disorders can cause euphoria, grandiosity, or frenetic activity. Furthermore, the usual screening tests for depression used in primary care, such as the 9-item Patient Health Questionnaire (PHQ-9) for depression (Kroenke et al. 2001), do not screen for a history of hypomania.

Mania secondary to brain lesions occurs most commonly with lesions affecting frontal, temporal, and subcortical limbic brain areas. Right-sided lesions causing decreased local brain function or disconnection and left-sided excitatory lesions (epileptic foci) are implicated most frequently. Such lesions may be caused by strokes, tumors, or MS plaques (Satzer and Bond 2016). In addition, bipolar disorder is associated with migraine, perhaps reflecting a shared genetic factor or underlying neurophysiological disturbance; in a review of reports of migraine–bipolar disorder comorbidity, 30.7% of patients with bipolar disorder had comorbid migraine, and 5.9% of the population with migraine had bipolar disorder (Leo and Singh 2016). It is especially important to recognize depression associated with disorders in the bipolar spectrum, including depression with mixed symptoms and depression with a history of prior hypomanic symptoms. These conditions carry a higher suicide risk than does ordinary unipolar depression, and treating these conditions with antidepressants sometimes precipitates hypomania, rapid cycling, or an agitated dysphoric state. Antidepressant treatment is not necessarily contraindicated, but the plan for monitoring antidepressant treatment should consider the increased risk of hypomania. A mood-stabilizing antiepileptic drug and/or an atypical antipsychotic drug might be a more appropriate initial treatment than single-drug treatment with an antidepressant. There are several chronic neurological diseases—including recurrent strokes, MS, epilepsy, and migraine—for which the best long-term outcome requires that a patient adhere to a treatment that is taken when the patient is asymptomatic. A patient's consistent adherence to such a treatment might only be possible if psychiatric treatment addresses a behavioral impediment such as apathy, a passive-dependent personality, self-destructiveness, denial or minimization of illness, or the hopelessness of depression.

Patients with gross brain disease may be less able to describe their psychiatric symptoms than those who are neurologically intact. When patients cannot give an accurate and complete history, collateral information from observers—usually caregivers—is invaluable. Such history should be sought, but with the recognition that it also can be incomplete, unreliable, or biased. Patients with significant psychiatric comorbidity sometimes exaggerate, minimize, or deny their neurological symptoms and deficits. Nonetheless, it should not be assumed that patients with clinical depression and severe neurological symptoms are amplifying their neurological symptoms; highly disruptive or distressing neurological symptoms can precipitate a severe emotional reaction. The temporal sequence of the neurological and psychiatric symptoms can help in deciding whether a hypothesis of symptom amplification deserves consideration.

The assessment of psychiatric symptoms in neurological patients, including screening for and measurement of syndromes that accompany specific neurological diseases, is aided by using validated, standardized rating scales that are tailored to the neurological context. Many such scales are available in multiple forms specifically adapted for patients, informants, or clinicians. Scales that target specific neuropsychiatric syndromes are more useful than generic rating scales for depression, anxiety, or mental distress or wide-ranging symptom inventories. Several such scales are covered later in this chapter. Increasingly, diagnosing and tracking psychiatric syndromes in neurological patients may make use of mobile, wearable, or home-based devices. Such devices may circumvent issues with reporting errors and inconsistencies, because they do not require long-term recall or record keeping by patients or caregivers.

When assessing patients who have both a neurological disease and a psychiatric disorder such as major depressive disorder (MDD) or generalized anxiety disorder (GAD), the following contextual features should be considered:

1. Does the patient's neurological disorder affect his or her ability to accurately perceive, recall, or relate the details of neurological or psychiatric symptoms—for example, does it influence awareness of deficits, recall of experiences, or language abilities? If so, is there a reliable alternative source of data on the patient's psychiatric symptoms apart from self-report?
2. Are there cultural reasons that a patient or informant (usually a family member) would emphasize symptoms typically associated with general medical illnesses or brain diseases and understate symptoms typically regarded as psychiatric?
3. Are there aspects of the patient's physical or social environment that could be contributing to either the neurological or the psychiatric symptoms—for example, noise, chemical exposures, or violence in the family or the neighborhood?
4. Is the patient ingesting a potentially neurotoxic substance, such as a prescribed medication, an over-the-counter medication with potential CNS side effects, or a recreational drug?

The impact of inadequate sleep or poor nutrition on physical and mental functioning is greater in individuals whose brains are not structurally normal, particularly when diffuse or multifocal brain disease is present that makes it difficult and effortful to perform cognitive or physical tasks. For such patients, adequate sleep and nutrition may be necessary conditions for success that are not required by people with totally intact brains. Neurological patients with impaired function should be screened for sleep quality, excessive daytime sleepiness, and adequacy of nutrition. If the patient is obese or snores, consideration of obstructive sleep apnea would be part of the process. Endocrine dysfunction such as mild hypothyroidism or hypoadrenalism can have greater functional impact in patients with abnormal brains at baseline. Reviewing the patient's clinical history, physical and neurological examination findings, and recent laboratory studies (or lack thereof) and ordering additional laboratory tests, such as thyroid-stimulating hormone (TSH), morning cortisol level, serum calcium and magnesium levels, and levels of 25-hydroxy (OH) vitamin D, vitamin B_{12}, and red blood cell folate, might be appropriate to screen for the most common nutritional and endocrine conditions that can exacerbate the functional and psychiatric impact of brain lesions.

The remainder of this chapter presents methodology for psychiatric assessment and treatment of patients with known or suspected neurological diseases. Several common neurological conditions are discussed specifically. Many less common but clinically important diseases such as ALS, progressive supranuclear palsy, and genetic diseases with prominent neurological features such as fragile X syndrome and Down syndrome are not included. However, many aspects of the approach to assessment and treatment described for the more common conditions often are applicable to these rarer conditions.

Two Critical Concepts: Executive Function and Metacognition

Executive function, supported by the frontal lobes anterior to the motor strip and by their connections to the basal ganglia and cerebellum, comprises organization, planning, persistence in goal-directed behavior, resistance to distraction, accurate perception of social and environmental context, and impulse control. Executive functioning is the critical higher cognitive component of brain function required for translating a goal into an action that is performed effectively and efficiently, at an appropriate place and time, and with consideration of environmental contingencies. Impairments in executive function are associated with impairments in IADLs (e.g., shopping, driving, working at a job). The association of impaired executive function with impaired IADLs is consistent across a wide range of neurological/psychiatric diagnoses, from Alzheimer's disease to schizophrenia, as well as in medical diagnoses that can affect brain function on a metabolic basis (e.g., liver failure, advanced heart failure, end-stage renal disease) (Royall et al. 2007). Impairments in executive function fall on a spectrum from inability to carry out simple IADLs to being able to deal normally with everyday life but not with the demands of a cognitively intense job, or not being able to maintain functional performance in a distracting or emotionally stressful environment. Driving, adhering to a complex medication regimen, and managing finances are three examples of consequential instrumental activities that are dependent on executive functioning and capable of failing at a time when a casual assessment of physical and social functioning is normal. Executive functioning also is diminished when a patient is fatigued, sleep deprived, intoxicated, or depressed.

Two useful bedside screening tests for executive dysfunction are the Executive Interview Test (Royall et al. 1992) and the Clock Drawing Test (Terwindt et al. 2016). Both are brief but sensitive to executive impairment of disabling proportions caused by gross brain disease. Findings from generic bedside cognitive tests—such as the Mini-Mental State Examination (MMSE; Folstein et al. 1975) and the Montreal Cognitive Assessments (MoCA; Nasreddine et al. 2005)—may be normal in patients with functionally significant executive impairment. The patient's score on the test might not be perfect, but if the problem is executive functioning alone, the score will be above the test's cutoff score for abnormality.

Metacognition is defined as an accurate awareness of one's own cognitive function and its limitations and deficits coupled with an ability to consider one's cognitive capacities in decision making. Impaired metacognition is to cognition what denial of deficits is to paralysis or sensory loss. A person with cognitive impairment and intact metacognition will experience far fewer adverse consequences than one who is either unaware of cognitive deficits or unable to translate awareness of deficits into necessary changes in behavior. Impairment in metacognition falls on a spectrum. Patients with severely impaired metacognition do not acknowledge cognitive deficits, even when they are directly and repeatedly confronted with evidence of them. Patients with mildly impaired metacognition can describe their cognitive problems and what they ought to do to compensate for them, but these patients do not in fact make the changes in their daily activities that they have recognized as being necessary.

Cognitively impaired patients can be screened for moderate to severe impairment of metacognition by asking them how they thought they did after they complete a cognitive test on which they had difficulty. Patients who do not recognize that they have done poorly can be shown their errors and asked again.

Fatigue

Fatigue and fatigability are common accompaniments of brain disease. Between normal ability to carry out a physical or cognitive task and complete inability to complete the task lies a state in which the task can be done with more-than-usual effort. When neurological disease makes people's daily activities more effortful, they will develop fatigue under circumstances that would not have fatigued them before their neurological illness began. People with severe fatigue may be unable to complete energy-intensive tasks. Sometimes relief of fatigue with stimulants (subject to a careful review of risks) or with a timely nap (no longer than 20 minutes to prevent insomnia) will improve the patient's functional performance.

Fatigue is a major contributor to disability in neurological disease. It has a bidirectional relationship with depression, but, like apathy, it can be distinguished from depression. A useful fatigue screening test/rating scale is the Fatigue Severity Scale (Krupp et al. 1989), a questionnaire that asks patients to rate each of nine aspects of fatigue on a seven-point Likert scale (from 1 [strongly disagree] to 7 [strongly agree], with higher mean scores denoting greater fatigue severity). The nine aspects relate to decreased motivation; fatigability with exercise; easy fatigability; interference with physical function; frequent fatigue-related problems; inability to sustain physical function; interference with duties and responsibilities; interference with work, family, or social life; and the patient's regarding fatigue as one of the most disabling symptoms of his or her illness. An average score of 4 or higher is diagnostic of clinically significant fatigue. Originally developed for use in patients with MS and systemic lupus erythematosus, the Fatigue Severity Scale has demonstrated its usefulness across a range of chronic diseases associated with fatigue, including stroke and HIV/AIDS (Johansson et al. 2014).

Apathy

Apathy can be a feature of depression, but in several neurological diseases it occurs as a prominent behavioral symptom in the absence of depressed mood or negative thoughts and memories. Apathy comprises cognitive, affective, and behavioral/motivational dimensions. Conditions that reduce dopaminergic input to the frontal lobes and those that impair functional connectivity in the medial frontal region can cause reduced motivation, decreased emotional reactivity, and diminished spontaneous thought. Apathy is distinguishable from depression, and when patients have both apathy and depression, the two symptoms types are not necessarily of similar severity. Patients with mild depression alone have at most mild apathy; in more severe depression, there might be a significant loss of motivation, but this loss would be accompanied by negative thoughts or feelings and potentially by suicidal ideation or intent. It is not uncommon, however, to have the withdrawal associated with neurological disorders misconstrued as MDD or another primary psychiatric condition.

A useful screening test and rating scale for apathy is the Apathy Evaluation Scale (AES; Clarke et al. 2011; Marin et al. 1991). The scale, an instrument with clinician, subject, and informant versions, rates the three dimensions of apathy using 18 items, each rated on a scale of 1–4. Psychometric properties of the scale are favorable (Mohammad et al. 2018; Radakovic et al. 2015; Raimo et al. 2014; Stankevich et al. 2018). The AES can distinguish between apathy and depression; patients with Parkinson's disease who are apathetic but not depressed will score high on the AES but not on a standard depression rating scale.

Pseudobulbar Affect

Pseudobulbar affect is a syndrome of episodes of exaggerated laughing and crying lasting seconds to minutes that can be triggered by minor stimuli and are inconsistent or exaggerated with respect to felt emotion. The patient's mood and affect, which may otherwise be normal, return to their baselines between episodes. Pseudobulbar affect is seen in a clinically significant minority of patients with stroke, MS, moderate to severe TBI, Parkinson's disease, and degenerative dementias (Miller et al. 2011). Patients with pseudobulbar affect typically feel embarrassed by their symptoms and may avoid social encounters; the condition interferes with work in patients whose occupations require social interaction. Patients with pseudobulbar affect and patients with MDD both cry, and both may feel distressed about their condition, but those with pseudobulbar affect suddenly cry when they are not sad or laugh when they are not amused, and the range and intensity of their responses are often greater than those in individuals without the condition. Pseudobulbar affect usually responds to treatment with a dextromethorphan/quinidine combination—a treatment approved by the U.S. Food and Drug Administration (FDA) for the specific indication. Treatments sometimes helpful for pseudobulbar affect but not specifically approved for it include tricyclic antidepressants (TCAs) and selective serotonin reuptake inhibitors (SSRIs) (Pioro 2011).

The Center for Neurologic Study–Lability Scale (Moore et al. 1997) screens for and measures the severity of pseudobulbar affect. It is a seven-item questionnaire that asks patients to rate—on a five-point scale ranging from never (1) to most of the time (5)—how often they have experienced symptoms of pseudobulbar affect during the past week. Four items concern pathological laughing and three concern pathological crying. A score of 13 or higher suggests the diagnosis. Because of the design of the scale, it is unlikely that a patient with depression alone would screen positive for pseudobulbar affect.

Impulsive-Compulsive Syndrome of Parkinson's Disease

Patients with Parkinson's disease, mainly those treated with direct dopamine agonists such as pramipexole or ropinirole, can develop a distinctive syndrome of an impulse-control disorder with compulsive features—an "impulsive-compulsive disorder." Variations include compulsive gambling, hypersexuality, compulsive shopping, "hobbyism" (excessive engagement in an avocation), and "punding" (repetitive pointless but organized activity, such as lining up pebbles in a row or reorganizing the contents of a drawer). Affected patients may become irritable or angry if someone tries to interfere with their compulsive activity. Unlike hypomania, the behavior is not associated with euphoria or speeding up of thought or action. Impulsive-compulsive behavior is exhibited by approximately 30% of patients with Parkinson's disease at some point in the disease course, with a higher prevalence reported in patients from Denmark and Norway and a lower prevalence in patients from China and Japan (Callesen et al. 2014; Erga et al. 2017; Tanaka et al. 2013; Zhang et al. 2014). It is more common in male patients, in those with early-onset Parkinson's, in those treated with direct dopamine agonists, and in those with dyskinesia. Reduction in the dosage of a direct dopamine agonist drug may, but does not always, relieve symptoms. Dopamine antagonists will reduce impulsive-compulsive symptoms but will exacerbate the motor symptoms of Parkinson's disease.

The Questionnaire for Impulsive-Compulsive Disorders in Parkinson's Disease (QUIP) rating scale (Weintraub et al. 2012) assesses four types of impulsive-compulsive behaviors—gambling, sex, shopping, and eating—and three types of abnormal goal-directed behavior—hobbyism, punding, and medication misuse. Each is rated on a scale of 0–4 for frequency in the preceding 4 weeks with respect to thoughts, urges, difficulty in resisting urges, and behavior; thus, there are four responses and from 0 to 16 points for each of seven expressions of impulsive-compulsive behavior. Ratings can be completed by a patient, a caregiver, or both. The summary score is between 0 and 112, averaging 8.51 for Parkinson's patients with no impulsive-compulsive–related behaviors and 29.13 for Parkinson's disease patients with one or more such behaviors.

Interictal Personality of Temporal Lobe Epilepsy (Geschwind Syndrome)

People with temporal lobe epilepsy (TLE) due to an anterior medial focus often (but by no means always) exhibit a constellation of personality traits that would be unusual in a person without a primary neurological disease. The syndrome, which is associated with the name of the pioneering American behavioral neurologist Norman Geschwind, comprises hypergraphia, increased religious or philosophical preoccupations, decreased or altered sexuality, "stickiness" or "viscosity" (e.g., difficulty leaving the physician's office at the end of an appointment), obsessions, humorlessness, and intermittent irritability and anger (Geschwind 2009; Waxman and Geschwind 1975). As described by Geschwind, people with personality changes related to right-temporal epileptic foci tend to minimize their negative behavior and emphasize their strong points, while those with left-sided foci have lower self-esteem and are more self-critical (Perini 1986; Wuerfel et al. 2004). The behavioral features of TLE and the associated self-assessments are independent of any mood disorder or psychosis, although of course people with epilepsy can develop depression, hypomania, or a thought disorder.

The Bear-Fedio questionnaire (Bear 1979; Bear and Fedio 1977) is a systematic inventory of symptoms of the interictal personality syndrome of TLE. It is more sensitive to the syndrome's distinctive combination of traits than are generic personality tests. The Geschwind syndrome also can be seen in patients with epilepsy with nontemporal foci, as well as in patients without epilepsy. When patients with TLE were compared with healthy control subjects on the NEO Five-Factor Inventory (McCrae and Costa 2010), they differed only in having greater neuroticism (Rivera Bonet et al. 2019). The unique characteristics of the Geschwind syndrome are not captured by a generic personality test, and must be assessed specifically.

Among other specialized rating scales useful for identifying and quantifying psychiatric symptoms of neurological disease, three instruments with broad utility are the Neuropsychiatric Inventory (NPI), the Aggression Questionnaire (AQ), and the Neurological Disorders Depression Inventory for Epilepsy (NDDI-E).

The NPI (Cummings et al. 1994), initially developed for use in the assessment of dementia patients, is also useful in a broader range of individuals with brain diseases and psychiatric symptoms. It is a structured interview aimed at caregivers of patients and designed to be administered by a clinician, who questions the caregiver about 10 symptom domains, following up with questions about frequency and severity if symptoms are present. The 10 domains are delusions, hallucinations, dysphoria, anxiety, agitation/aggression, euphoria, disinhibition, irritability/lability, apathy, and aberrant motor activity. A briefer version, the NPI-Q, can be completed by a caregiver without clinician involvement and reviewed at a clinical encounter (Kaufer et al. 2000); this version includes questions about nighttime patient behavioral disturbances, patient appetite/eating changes, and caregiver distress.

The AQ (Buss and Perry 1992) is a 29-item self-rating questionnaire comprising five-point Likert-scale items that measure self-assessed aspects of anger, hostility, physical aggression, and verbal aggression. A short form of the instrument, the Brief Aggression Questionnaire (BAQ), accomplishes a result similar to that of the AQ with 12 items (Webster et al. 2014). The clinical impact of a neurological disorder that increases arousal, increases negative affect, decreases behavioral inhibition, or causes misperceptions of others' emotions and intentions will be more significant in patients with a propensity to engage in aggressive thinking and behavior. Because concern about aggressive behavior is a common reason for a request for psychiatric consultation, the AQ is a useful tool for the consultant. However, a valid score is dependent on a sufficient level of self-awareness by the patient. An informant might be asked to complete the scale on the patient's behalf.

The NDDI-E is a short questionnaire that asks patients to rate, on a four-point scale (from 1 [never] to 4 [always/often]), how often in the past 2 weeks they have experienced six specific feelings or thoughts: feeling that everything they do is a struggle, feeling that nothing they do is right, feeling guilty, thinking that they would be better off dead, feeling frustrated, and having difficulty finding pleasure. Scores of 15 or higher were 81% sensitive and 90% specific for a clinical diagnosis of MDD based on a structured interview with a sample of 192 patients drawn from an epilepsy clinic in a large public hospital (Friedman et al. 2009). Systematic screening identified clinical depression in more than 25% of patients screened, whereas only 2.9% of patients in a nonscreened sample were identified by their clinicians as depressed (Friedman et al. 2009). A systematic review of depression tools for people with epilepsy reported on 26 validation studies of the NDDI-E with the criterion of predicting a diagnosis of major depressive disorder on a structured diagnostic interview. The studies included evaluation of translations of the questionnaire into Arabic, Chinese, French, German, Greek, Portuguese, and Serbian. Twelve studies evaluated a cut point of 15/16; for these studies, the median sensitivity was 80.5%, the median specificity was 86.2%, the median positive predictive value was 59.3%, and the median negative predictive value was 96.0% (Gill et al. 2017).

Given the simplicity and minimal cost of a six-item screening test and the impact of depression on health-related quality of life, occupational function, and suicide risk, the NDDI-E has obvious value in routine clinical practice, particularly in a high-volume clinic with relatively brief time allotments for patient visits. It is noteworthy that the NDDI-E intentionally excludes items that might be explained by the epilepsy or its pharmacological treatment rather than by depression, such as cognitive symptoms, sleep disturbance, and psychomotor slowing. The NDDI-E was compared with the more generic Hospital Anxiety and Depression Scale (Zigmond and Snaith 1983) and was found to be more sensitive (Gandy et al. 2012).

Pain in Neurological Patients

Patients with primary neurological diseases may present with pain syndromes due to disruption of central pain processing pathways or due to physical problems such as spasticity that are consequences of their neurological illness. Their pain can come to psychiatric attention because it often is undertreated or ineffectively treated, causing or worsening depression and suicidal risk or leading to misuse of opioids or other analgesics. For example, approximately one-half of stroke patients experience pain (Harrison and Field 2015), but pain is seldom the leading item physicians—and caregivers—have in mind when they think about stroke. Pain syndromes include central pain syndromes, pain due to spasticity or contractures, and poststroke headaches. Psychiatrists consulting on patients with neurological diseases should inquire about pain; psychiatrists may have a useful role in bringing the problem of pain to the foreground and in assisting the medical team in addressing pain while minimizing the risks of medication misuse.

General Effects of Depression on Neurological Diseases

Mood disorders, particularly depression, are a frequent accompaniment of all chronic neurological diseases, both because these disorders are highly prevalent and because mood symptoms are a common reaction to the losses, disruptions, and distress associated with major illness. Depression makes some specific neurological symptoms worse—for example, the apathy and bradykinesia of Parkinson's disease; the fatigue associated with cerebral diseases including MS, stroke, and major TBI; and the fatigue, headaches, impaired concentration, and memory deficits of the postconcussion syndrome. Depression can bring out focal cognitive deficits, including those related to executive function, verbal fluency, and constructional praxis, and it can make symptoms and impairments less tolerable, as it often does with neuropathic pain. If depression is associated with significant insomnia, it will exacerbate fatigue, diminish attention and concentration, and increase the risk of seizures in disorders associated with them. The state of systemic inflammation often associated with MDD can increase the risk of progression of neurological diseases with inflammatory pathophysiology. Finally, depression can alter the way in which patients describe the symptoms of their neurological diseases, because it often increases patients' recall of negative experiences and the distress associated with specific symptoms.

Neurological Disease and Suicide Risk

Chronic diseases associated with pain or loss of function are risk factors for suicide. Beyond an association with depression, specific attributes of a neurological disease that can increase suicide risk include 1) functional deficits that interfere with the activities that give meaning and purpose to the patient's life; 2) decreased impulse control; 3) affective instability; and 4) loss of executive function with the consequence of impaired problem solving. The risk of suicide in depressed patients with neurological disorders is disproportionate to the risk associated with depression and patient demographic risk factors. When a profile of neuropsychiatric symptoms and signs associated with increased suicide risk is recognized, the psychiatrist should consider whether the patient has easy access to highly lethal means of impulsive self-harm such as firearms and potent poisons. When patients have intermittent and transient suicidal impulses combined with cognitive or physical impairments that would make it difficult to form and execute a complex suicidal plan, restriction of access to lethal means will reduce suicidal risk. If simple and highly lethal means of suicide are unavailable, suicidal thoughts are more likely to weaken or subside before patients can act on them.

A recent case-control study of 8,974 suicide attempts using a Danish case registry, matching each case with 10 control subjects, revealed an association of suicide attempts with nine different neurological diseases (Eliasen et al. 2018). They were (with the estimated odds ratios relative to the general population given in parentheses): stroke (3.1), Huntington's disease (8.8), ALS (5.0), Parkinson's disease (2.9), MS (1.5), epilepsy (4.5), neuropathy (2.2), myasthenia gravis (4.3), and degenerative dementias including Alzheimer's disease (4.8) (Eliasen et al. 2018). Estimates for odds ratios for death by suicide vary among publications because of differences in the population sampled, but findings are consistent with the data on suicide attempts.

Bidirectional Relationship Between Neurological and Psychiatric Disorders

Neurological diseases can produce psychiatric disorders by psychological-behavioral pathways or by direct physiological pathways, or a neurological disorder and a psychiatric disorder can share a common underlying cause, such as systemic inflammation or a genetic abnormality. A fourth pathway of relationship is the influence of neurological disease on the ability of a patient with a psychiatric illness to adhere to and benefit from treatment that would ordinarily be effective in a patient with the same illness and a grossly intact brain. For example, a neurological patient with apathy and executive cognitive dysfunction might have difficulty independently adhering to a regular regimen of antidepressant medication. Depression is associated with endocrine dysfunction, sleep disturbance, and systemic inflammation that can worsen neurological conditions, including epilepsy and migraine, and depressive symptoms, chronic stress, and hostility have been associated with an increased risk of incident transient ischemic attack and stroke (Everson-Rose et al. 2014). In addition, many psychiatric disorders have the potential to interfere with adherence to outpatient treatment of neurological disease.

Specific Neurological Diseases

Stroke

By producing focal anatomical lesions in the brain and by disrupting connections, strokes cause a loss of sensory, motor, perceptual, or cognitive function, usually leading to impairment in physical, instrumental, or social functioning. Strokes can cause characteristic and stereotypic symptoms and syndromes, including those just described, that occur with gross brain disease and rarely occur as *isolated* phenomena in primary psychiatric illness. The loss of function, ongoing symptoms, and social or financial consequences associated with strokes predictably cause emotional reactions, including anxiety and depression, but the incidence and prevalence rates of depressive and anxiety disorders exceed those seen with non-CNS diseases that cause equivalent levels of impairment and physical discomfort.

Depression following stroke is commonplace; the reported prevalence is no less than one-third of patients within 6 months of the stroke, and in many reports, the prevalence is considerably higher (Villa et al. 2018). Less obviously, the prevalence of depression in stroke patients immediately *preceding* their strokes is higher than the prevalence of depression in the general population. A meta-analysis of 29 studies comprising 164,993 stroke patients found that prestroke depression had a pooled prevalence of 11.6% (Taylor-Rowan et al. 2019). In a Danish stroke registry study of 5,070 first-ever ischemic stroke patients treated in a single county between 2003 and 2010, 35.2% of the patients received an antidepressant drug prescription during the first 6 months poststroke; of these patients, nearly half (48.1%) were started on anti-depressant treatment within the first 2 weeks poststroke (Mortensen et al. 2018).

Poststroke depression (PSD) is associated with poorer functional recovery and with a higher risk of recurrent stroke. PSD has a higher incidence in patients with a prestroke history of depression and in patients with low education. Strokes in the anterior circulation, left-hemisphere strokes, and strokes causing aphasia are more likely to cause PSD (Mitchell et al. 2017). The incidence of PSD is higher in patients with large-vessel strokes than in those with lacunar (small-vessel) infarctions (Tu et al. 2018). Underlying mechanisms of PSD include disruption of frontal-subcortical pathways involved in regulation of mood; impairment of connections between the cortex and the brain stem, resulting in a decrease in monoaminergic transmission; increased inflammation, both systemically and in the brain; reduced production of neurotrophic factors such as brain-derived neurotrophic factor (BDNF); and dysregulation of the hypothalamic-pituitary-adrenal axis.

In patients with mild strokes, PSD is associated with lower rates of return to prestroke activities, even those that remain feasible despite recently acquired neurological deficits (Tse et al. 2017). Among patients who are treated for PSD with antidepressant medications, the risk of stroke recurrence is significantly higher for those who are poorly adherent or nonadherent to poststroke antidepressant therapy (Krivoy et al. 2017).

Fatigue following stroke is even more common than PSD, affecting approximately 50% of stroke patients (Bivard et al. 2017). The relationship between poststroke fatigue and PSD is circular; fatigue can precipitate or exacerbate depression, and depression can worsen fatigue. Clinical experience and case series findings suggest that treatment of fatigue with modafinil or a stimulant (if not medically contraindicated) can relieve fatigue and reduce symptoms of depression as well (Bivard et al. 2017; Sinita and Coghill 2014).

Poststroke pain syndromes affect more than 40% of stroke patients at some point during their recovery. These syndromes contribute significantly to stroke patients' distress and disability and have a circular relationship with depression. Furthermore, stroke patients with poststroke pain were found to have a higher suicide risk after adjustment for the presence of depression and demographic risk factors (Eriksson et al. 2015). Poststroke pain comprises pain due to spasticity, shoulder pain, complex regional pain syndromes, poststroke headache, and central pain syndromes. Central poststroke pain develops gradually, typically between 3 and 6 months following the stroke. It can be severe and can be difficult to treat. Brain stimulation including TMS has been used successfully, as have a range of antiepileptic drugs (AEDs) and psychotropic drugs in small case series, but there is not an established standard of practice (Harrison and Field 2015).

PSD can be treated with the usual antidepressant therapies, which include medications, electroconvulsive therapy (ECT), TMS, and psychotherapy (assuming that the latter is feasible in the context of any impairment in cognition, communication, and mobility the patient might have). Randomized controlled trials have shown several specific antidepressants to be superior to placebo for PSD, including nortriptyline, paroxetine, and duloxetine (Paolucci 2017; Sun et al. 2017). Because head-to-head comparisons of alternative drug therapies for PSD have not been conducted, it is not known whether any specific antidepressant class is preferable to another. Antidepressant treatment of PSD should be selected for tolerability and acceptability to the patient, and the chosen medication should be given at an adequate dosage and duration according to conventional guidelines. If there is little or no improvement, a different antidepressant should be tried, preferably one with a different pharmacology. If there is partial improvement, the treatment should be augmented, with the choice of augmentation dependent on the specific persistent symptoms and influenced by consideration of the rest of the patient's medical diagnoses and treatments. ECT deserves consideration without first requiring two unsuccessful drug trials if one or more of the following conditions apply: 1) the patient is psychotic; 2) there are prominent melancholic features (i.e., severe anhedonia, lack of reactivity to positive stimuli, significant weight loss, excessive or inappropriate guilt, early-morning awakening, and diurnal variation with worse symptoms in the morning), 3) there is a high suicide risk; 4) the patient's depression is preventing effective poststroke rehabilitation; 5) the patient's general medical status is deteriorating as a consequence of depression-related behavior or physiological changes; or 6) there is a history of depression that remitted rapidly with ECT. If the patient has a prestroke history of depression that *remitted* with a specific treatment such as TMS or a second-line drug combination (e.g., TCA plus low-dose lithium), the prior treatment should be instituted promptly if there is no new medical contraindication. PSD can be so disruptive to recovery that a prompt remission can have a large positive impact on the overall clinical outcome. In a case of severe PSD, a consulting psychiatrist might be much better able to identify the optimal first treatment and sequence of follow-up treatments than the neurologist or internist who has primary responsibility for the patient's care. When PSD requires aggressive treatment because of its severity or functional impact, ongoing concurrent or collaborative care is more likely to achieve a remission than a one-time consultation and follow-up by the internist or neurologist.

A variety of nonpharmacological treatments—such as psychotherapies (including cognitive-behavioral therapy and motivational interviewing), light therapy, TMS, and exercise—have shown promise in small-scale trials for PSD (Hadidi et al. 2017; Wang et al. 2018).

Administration of antidepressants beginning in the first week after a stroke to *prevent* PSD is rational, and this strategy has been tried with success (Villa et al. 2018) but is not established as a routine practice. Prophylactic antidepressant treatment should be considered in patients with a prestroke history of one or more episodes of clinical depression or with an anterior large-vessel stroke—both conditions that raise the probability of PSD above 50% (Villa et al. 2018).

Epilepsy

Psychiatric issues in patients with seizure disorders can be subdivided into psychiatric *manifestations* of epilepsy, psychiatric *comorbidities* of epilepsy, and psychogenic nonepileptic seizures, a DSM-5 conversion disorder with phenomenology overlapping that of epilepsy. Psychogenic nonepileptic seizures are discussed elsewhere in this volume (see Chapter 25, "Somatic Symptom and Related Disorders"). Psychiatric manifestations in epilepsy are described, when possible, based on the temporal relationship between the seizures and the psychiatric symptoms: preictal, ictal, postictal, and interictal.

The diagnosis of epilepsy is associated with an increased prevalence of several major psychiatric comorbidities; the increase is greater than that seen in chronic diseases, such as asthma, that are not based on continual dysfunction of the brain. Approximately one-third of people with epilepsy have an anxiety disorder or a depressive disorder, with disproportionately high rates of social anxiety disorder and agoraphobia among those who have anxiety disorders (Rai et al. 2012). The prevalence of autism spectrum disorder among people with epilepsy is more than seven times higher than that in the general population (Rai et al. 2012).

The incidence of depression, anxiety, and psychosis is increased in the 3 years before the diagnosis of epilepsy and in the 3 years following the diagnosis of epilepsy (Hesdorffer et al. 2012), suggesting common underlying risk factors for epilepsy and the other diagnoses as well as overlap in mechanisms related to the symptomatic expression of the illnesses. Patients with well-controlled seizures are less likely than those with uncontrolled seizures to have psychiatric comorbidity. In both well-controlled and treatment-refractory epilepsy, depression may be the single most important predictor of patient quality of life (Boylan et al. 2004).

Patients with epilepsy and psychiatric comorbidity may have typical presentations of their psychiatric disorders or may have epilepsy-specific presentations. Table 12–1 shows the features of several psychiatric syndromes that are relatively specific to patients with epilepsy.

Psychiatric symptoms ranging from panic attacks to stereotyped hallucinations can in themselves be expressions of epileptic seizures—that is, ictal psychiatric symptoms. Ictal psychiatric symptoms are easily identified when they are linked to recurrent epileptiform discharges on scalp EEG; however, such linkage is not always possible. If the symptoms are generated by an epileptic focus in the orbital frontal region or medial temporal region, the electrical disturbance may not be detectable by electrodes on the scalp, relatively far from the focus. If seizures are infrequent, prolonged monitoring may be needed to capture a psychiatric symptom with its associated electrical discharge. Distinguishing features that favor episodic psychiatric symptoms being ictal include a paroxysmal character (sudden onset and offset), brief duration (seconds to minutes), and stereotyped characteristics that do not vary between episodes. Progression to a generalized seizure or to a distinctive postictal period of reduced function would also suggest ictal psychiatric symptoms. Table 12–2 lists potential ictal psychiatric symptoms and the primary psychiatric symptoms that they resemble.

When selecting and managing the treatment of epileptic patients with current or past psychiatric comorbidity, clinicians should consider the potential of AEDs to cause adverse psychiatric effects. Such potential is rarely an absolute contraindication to the use of an AED, but it should be a factor in the decision process, in conjunction with factors such as efficacy, other potential adverse effects, drug interactions, and cost. An increase in depressive symptoms can be seen with barbiturates, levetiracetam, zonisamide, topiramate, and tiagabine. Carbamazepine and oxcarbazepine, with some actions overlapping with those of the TCAs, occasionally induce hypomania or mania in patients with bipolar vulnerabilities. Psychosis is a rare adverse effect of phenytoin, vigabatrin, tiagabine, and zonisamide. Irritability and aggression are frequently reported adverse effects of levetiracetam, tiagabine, and perampanel (Chen et al. 2017; Schmitz 2011).

TABLE 12–1.	Distinctive psychiatric syndromes in people with epilepsy

Depressive syndromes

Interictal dysphoric disorder (Blumer et al. 2004)
Three symptom clusters:
Labile depressive symptoms (anergia, depressed mood, insomnia, pain)
Labile affective symptoms (fear, anxiety)
Specific symptoms (euphoric moods, paroxysmal irritability)
Symptoms last hours to days and are separated by symptom-free periods

Dysthymic disorder of epilepsy (Kanner 2003)
Chronic dysthymia
Frequently interrupted by periods of normal mood
Irritability, anhedonia, fatigue, anxiety, low frustration tolerance, mood lability with bouts of crying

Postictal depression (Kanner et al. 2010)
Begins after the seizure and lasts up to a week
More common in patients with history of interictal depression and anxiety
Median duration 24 hours

Preictal dysphoria (Blanchet and Frommer 1986)
Depressed mood as a prodromal aspect of a seizure

Psychotic syndromes

Postictal psychosis (Devinsky et al. 1995)
Onset after a lucid period of at least 24 hours postseizure
Lasts from 16 hours to 18 days
Paranoid, religious, or grandiose delusions
Change in mood
Violent behaviors
Auditory, visual, or somatic hallucinations

Schizophrenia-like psychosis of epilepsy (Mendez et al. 1993)
Usually develops after 10–15 years of epilepsy
Presentation similar to that of schizophrenia
Absence of premorbid personality abnormalities seen in schizophrenia
Loss of affective response and catatonia less common than in schizophrenia

"Forced normalization" or "alternative psychosis" (Krishnamoorthy and Trimble 1999)
May be seen after epilepsy surgery
Seizures remit and electroencephalographic abnormalities resolve as psychotic symptoms emerge

At therapeutic dosages (but not in overdose), antidepressants reduce seizure frequency or have no adverse effect, excepting clomipramine and immediate-release bupropion. TCAs can cause seizures in overdose, as can citalopram and venlafaxine (Judge and Rentmeester 2011). Antipsychotic drugs are associated with an increased risk of seizures, with the greatest effect seen with clozapine (Druschky et al. 2018). Most cases of antipsychotic-induced seizures in patients without epilepsy occur in the context of polypharmacy or the use of clozapine. Population-level data on patients with epilepsy who are taking both AEDs and antipsychotics are limited, and in many cases of epilepsy with psychosis, drug interactions or treatment nonadherence may be of greater concern than the seizure-inducing effects of antipsychotic drugs. Relevant to the diagnosis of episodic symptoms in patients treated for psychosis,

TABLE 12–2.   Ictal manifestations resembling symptoms of primary psychiatric illness

Ictal psychiatric symptom	Location of seizure focus	Primary psychiatric syndrome with similar symptoms
Hallucinations (stereotyped and usually simple) Visual Auditory Somatosensory Olfactory	Occipital lobe Auditory cortex Parietal lobe Medial or basal temporal lobe	Psychotic disorders
Fear (most common ictal emotion) Stereotyped symptoms and signs Short duration (1–2 min) Postictal confusion may also be present. Fear maximal at onset	Limbic system	Panic attacks
Forced thinking Recurring intrusive or irresistible thoughts, ideas, or crowding of thoughts Can occur as an aura preceding frontal or temporal lobe seizures Symptoms are stereotyped Occurs less frequently than the obsessions of obsessive-compulsive disorder, and involves less anxiety Intrusive thoughts may be expressed in behavior.	Frontal or temporal lobe	Obsessive-compulsive disorder Psychotic disorders with thought insertion
Automatisms Stereotyped repetitive movements Complex; may be fragments of purposeful behavior Spontaneous or in reaction to external stimuli	Frontal or temporal lobe	Psychotic disorders Delirium Autism spectrum disorder
Misperceptions Perception of formed body distortions Patients may be aware that their perceptions are abnormal.	Parietal association cortex	Psychotic disorders
Depersonalization/derealization	Mesial temporal cortex	Dissociative disorders Posttraumatic stress disorder Severe anxiety

more than half of patients with normal pretreatment EEGs may develop nonspecific EEG abnormalities when treated with second-generation antipsychotics (Dias Alves et al. 2018).

There are numerous potential drug interactions between AEDs and common psychiatric medications, many of which are based on induction or inhibition of cytochrome P450 (CYP) enzymes involved in the hepatic metabolism of the two interacting drugs. Some common significant interactions between AEDs and psychiatric drugs are shown in Table 12–3.

Surgical treatment by removal of a single seizure focus—when feasible given its location in the brain and the expected consequences of removing it—has become a standard option for treatment of epilepsy not controlled despite multiple AED regimens. Surgical treatment can provide full seizure control or a significant reduction in seizure frequency in individuals with medically intractable epilepsy. While functional outcomes can be favorable after surgery, psychiatric complications can appear for the first time after epilepsy surgery, or a preexisting psychiatric comorbidity can worsen. Transient depression or labile mood in the 3 months following epilepsy surgery is common. More prolonged depression can develop postoperatively; preoperative depression, poor postoperative seizure control, and being an older male are risk factors. Persistent anxiety postoperatively is most often seen in patients with preoperative anxiety or depression. While successful surgical treatment of medically refractory epilepsy often resolves interictal psychotic disorders, de novo postoperative psychosis occurs infrequently, affecting fewer than 5% of patients (Buranee et al. 2016).

People with epilepsy have an increased risk of death by suicide compared with the general population. This issue was studied quantitatively in a Danish population study that compared death registry data for 21,169 individuals who committed suicide with data for 423,218 population control subjects. It was found that 492 (2.32%) of the persons who died by suicide had epilepsy, compared with 3,140 (0.74%) of the control subjects (Christensen et al. 2007). The raw risk ratio for suicide associated with epilepsy was 3.17. When people with a history of psychiatric illness were excluded from the analysis and adjustment was made for demographics and socioeconomic status, the risk ratio was 1.99. People with both epilepsy and a formal psychiatric diagnosis had a risk ratio of 13.7 compared with people with neither condition. The risk of suicide in people with epilepsy was highest in the 6 months immediately following their epilepsy diagnosis (Christensen et al. 2007). Aspects of epilepsy associated with increased suicide risk include newly diagnosed epilepsy, treatment at a tertiary-care epilepsy center, epilepsy with a temporal lobe focus, and a history of epilepsy surgery. In a British longitudinal cohort study of patient records from a general practice database, 14,059 patients newly diagnosed with epilepsy were compared with control patients matched for age and sex. Investigators found that the risk of a first suicide attempt prior to the day of diagnosis was 2.9 times greater in the patients with epilepsy, suggesting that a common factor might increase vulnerability to epilepsy and to suicidal behavior (Hesdorffer et al. 2012). The association of epilepsy with suicide attempts and death by suicide should be considered when estimating the suicide risk of a patient with epilepsy who expresses death wishes, hopelessness, or suicidal ideation.

ECT has been demonstrated to be a safe and effective treatment for severe depression in patients with epilepsy, with induced seizure lengths being similar to those in

TABLE 12–3.	Psychotropic-antiepileptic drug interactions based on hepatic metabolism		
Isoenzyme	Substrate	Inhibitor	Inducer
CYP1A2	Asenapine Clozapine Duloxetine Fluvoxamine Olanzapine	Fluvoxamine	Carbamazepine Phenobarbital Phenytoin Primidone
CYP2C9	Phenobarbital Primidone	Valproic acid Fluoxetine Fluvoxamine	Carbamazepine Phenobarbital Phenytoin Primidone
CYP2C19	Citalopram Escitalopram Lacosamide	Felbamate Fluoxetine Fluvoxamine	Carbamazepine Phenytoin Phenobarbital Primidone
CYP2D6	Aripiprazole Brexpiprazole Fluoxetine Fluvoxamine Iloperidone Mirtazapine Paroxetine Risperidone Venlafaxine Vortioxetine	Fluoxetine Paroxetine Sertraline Duloxetine Bupropion	
CYP3A4	Aripiprazole Brexpiprazole Carbamazepine Clobazam Ethosuximide Felbamate Lurasidone Mirtazapine Perampanel Quetiapine Risperidone Reboxetine Tiagabine Trazodone Vilazodone Zonisamide	Fluoxetine Fluvoxamine	Carbamazepine Phenobarbital Phenytoin Primidone
CYP2B6	Bupropion Sertraline		Carbamazepine Phenobarbital Phenytoin Primidone

Note.   CYP=cytochrome P450.
Source.   Adapted from Spina et al. 2016.

nonepilepsy populations. Potential challenges of using ECT in epilepsy patients include risk of inducing spontaneous seizure activity, especially if AED dosages are lowered to allow planned seizure induction, and difficulty inducing seizures of adequate length for antidepressant effect. However, even in patients with well-controlled epilepsy, it is usually not necessary to discontinue AEDs. The patient's AED dose can be omitted on the morning of each treatment and the intensity of electrical stimulation increased if necessary (Ducharme et al. 2015; Lunde et al. 2006).

TMS is efficacious for treating MDD; with appropriate parameters, it can simultaneously reduce seizure frequency in patients with incompletely controlled epilepsy (Fregni et al. 2005). Transcranial direct current stimulation (tDCS) may be efficacious for some cases of depression in patients with epilepsy, and the limited evidence available to date suggests that low-current tDCS does not provoke seizures, increase the activity of seizure foci, or otherwise injure the brain (Bikson et al. 2016). Like TMS, tDCS can in some cases decrease seizure frequency in patients with medically uncontrolled seizures. Far more research is needed before TMS and tDCS become first-line treatments for patients with comorbid epilepsy and depression, but both modalities are reasonable to consider in such patients for whom current first-line treatments are ineffective, not tolerated, not feasible, or unacceptable to the patient.

Multiple Sclerosis

MS is an autoimmune disease of the CNS characterized by multiple inflammatory demyelinating white matter lesions disseminated in space and in time—that is, with at least two discrete sites of demyelination and two times at which new lesions occurred or old ones progressed. A clinically isolated syndrome (CIS) is a single-episode attack of inflammatory demyelinating disease; within 20 years, 85% of patients with a CIS will develop MS (Hou et al. 2018). MS typically begins between the ages of 20 and 50 years. Its lifetime prevalence is more than twice as great in women as it is in men. Disease with later onset tends to progress more rapidly. MS has three forms: relapsing-remitting (RRMS), primary progressive (PPMS), and secondary progressive (SPMS). PPMS accounts for about 10% of MS cases (Laakso et al. 2019; Salter et al. 2018). In RRMS, there are discrete attacks during which new neurological symptoms and signs occur; between attacks, there is complete or partial improvement in symptoms and signs. In both forms, there is an accumulation of brain lesions and associated deficits. Historically, more than 80% of patients initially diagnosed with RRMS have developed SPMS within 25 years of their diagnosis, with a median time to progression ranging from approximately 15 to 21 years after disease onset. Looking forward, the rate and speed of conversion to SPMS might be reduced by disease-modifying therapy during the relapsing-remitting phase (Kappos et al. 2015). Progressive neurological deficits related to the accumulating lesions cause impairment in physical and instrumental functioning, the latter including the ability to work.

Treatment of MS comprises three categories. *Treatment of relapses* involves the suppression of autoimmune inflammation through use of high-dose corticosteroids, adrenocorticotropic hormone (ACTH), plasmapheresis, or intravenous immunoglobulin (Berkovich 2016). *Disease-modifying therapies* modulate the function of the immune system to prevent autoimmune attack on white matter or to attenuate its severity if it occurs. In the case of progressive MS, the aim of disease-modifying therapy is to halt or slow disease progression. *Symptomatic treatments* of MS address distressing symptoms of the disease, such as fatigue, weakness, spasticity, incontinence, and sexual dysfunction (Grand'Maison et al. 2018).

Psychiatric disorders are more prevalent in people with MS than in the general population matched for age and gender (Marrie et al. 2015); conditions with increased prevalence include depression, anxiety, mania/hypomania, and suicidal behavior. Estimates of the lifetime prevalence of depression in MS patients range from 37% to 54%, and estimates for anxiety range from 25% to 36% (Marrie et al. 2015). The increased risk of depression and anxiety in MS patients is also found in the 2-year period before MS diagnosis (Hoang et al. 2016). The lifetime prevalence of bipolar disorder in individuals with MS is estimated to be 5.8%. Lifetime prevalence estimates for psychosis and for alcohol use disorder vary so widely that it is not clear whether the conditions are more prevalent in MS patients than in the general population (Rocca et al. 2015).

While most patients with MS seen by psychiatrists have been referred to them after MS has developed and the treating neurologist has identified comorbid psychiatric symptoms, MS can initially manifest as a psychiatric disorder in two distinct scenarios. In the first, a patient presents with depression, anxiety, manic or hypomanic, or psychotic symptoms (Lo Fermo et al. 2010). Subsequently, within the next 3 years, the patient develops neurological symptoms such as altered sensory or motor function that lead to a diagnosis of MS. In the second scenario, a patient presents with neurological symptoms that suggest a somatic symptom disorder, either because symptoms are more severe than physical signs on examination or because symptoms are vague, transient, or fluctuating. A prompt diagnosis of MS can make a difference in the second scenario, because it can lead to the institution of disease-modifying therapy prior to the occurrence of additional relapses that could significantly add to the patient's disability.

Any patient with a new diagnosis of a major psychiatric disorder should be questioned carefully about neurological symptoms, not only current ones but also ones that occurred in the past and resolved. Clinicians must be careful to ask about neurological symptoms such as nonpainful numbness or paresthesia, or minor problems with coordination, that a patient might not seek treatment for and might misattribute to other causes. In an adult less than 50 years old, discrete periods of neurological symptoms lasting days to weeks and then resolving suggest episodes of RRMS. The diagnosis of RRMS should likewise be considered in an adult under 50 who presents with episodic, unexplained neurological symptoms accompanied by fatigue disproportionate to any known general medical condition. The presence of unexpected and otherwise unexplained cognitive impairment would add to the likelihood of MS. Knowing the population prevalence of MS for those of the same ethnicity and gender in the area in which the patient lives can be helpful in the differential diagnosis in cases where the neurological workup is suggestive but not decisive (Leray et al. 2016). Geographically, the prevalence of MS is highest (170–350 cases per 100,000 population) in Canada, Scotland, and parts of Sweden, Finland, and Ireland. The prevalence is high (70–170 per 100,000) in the United States except for the South, and in Denmark, Norway, and Iceland. Some countries on the European continent, including Germany, Austria, and Switzerland, have rates exceeding 70 cases per 100,000 population. Russia, Spain, and Greece have rates between 38 and 70 per 100,000. The prevalence of MS is very low (13 or fewer cases per 100,000 population) in Mexico, in the major nations of East Asia, and in South America (except for Argentina). When people immigrate as adults, their risk of MS is determined by their native country; for those who immigrate as children, their risk is determined by their new homeland (Kingwell et al. 2013; Wade 2014). Within a given country, MS can cluster in specific regions; for example, its prevalence in Tuscany is higher than its prevalence in Italy overall (Bezzini et al. 2017).

When MS is suspected in a patient who presents psychiatrically, a careful neurological examination and magnetic resonance imaging (MRI) of the brain usually are sufficient to establish the diagnosis. The diagnosis requires establishing 1) that at least two separate episodes of disease activity occurred and 2) that two discrete anatomic areas were involved. A single MRI can establish that both conditions are met if, for example, it shows two discrete lesions of different ages, one showing signs of acute inflammation and the other showing demyelination without acute inflammation (Igra et al. 2017). If the MRI strongly suggests the diagnosis but is not conclusive, it can be supplemented by either a cerebrospinal fluid (CSF) examination or evoked potential studies. Multiple oligoclonal immunoglobulin G bands found in the CSF but not in the serum—that is, "isolated oligoclonal bands"—can distinguish MS from other autoimmune CNS diseases such as CNS lupus and CNS sarcoidosis. In one study, having four or more isolated oligoclonal bands was 98% sensitive and 87% specific for MS (Bernitsas et al. 2017). Visual, somatosensory, and auditory evoked potentials can demonstrate slowed conduction of sensory signals, implying demyelination of the involved pathways; this can establish a second site of disease when only one is seen on the MRI (Lascano et al. 2017). Evoked potentials are especially useful when a patient has a sensory complaint that could reflect either demyelinating disease or a somatic symptom–related disorder. Sensory changes due to MS that are sufficiently severe to be distressing and functionally significant are reliably associated with abnormalities in the corresponding evoked potentials (Leocani and Comi 2014).

Almost all patients in MS clinics have one or more neuropsychiatric symptoms. For example, 95% of 44 patients in a tertiary care MS clinic in Mexico City endorsed at least one symptom on the NPI, compared with 16% of 25 healthy control subjects similar in age, education, gender, and MMSE scores (Diaz-Olavarrieta et al. 1999). Some patients will have syndromes of primary psychiatric disorders; others will have symptoms more often seen secondary to neurological or general medical conditions, such as apathy or visual hallucinations. When patients with MS have primary psychiatric disorders, the pattern of symptoms is influenced by the underlying brain pathology. Patients with MS and depression are especially likely to display apathy, fatigue, psychomotor retardation, or cognitive impairment; these are common symptoms of MS without depression that can be made worse or reach a clinical level of severity because of comorbid depression (Murphy et al. 2017). Similarly, comorbid anxiety in a patient with MS may be associated with more cognitive disorganization or tremulousness than might be seen in an anxious patient without MS. Anxiety tends to worsen shortly after MS diagnosis and MS relapses, and the unpredictable prognosis of MS tends to be a contributing factor. Characteristics of anxiety disorders specific to MS may include the development of "self-injection anxiety" in patients who use self-injected disease-modifying therapies and a high level of health anxiety, with misattribution of common bodily symptoms to MS (Hayter et al. 2016).

Most patients with early MS have mild cognitive deficits detectable on neuropsychological examination but not necessarily symptomatic or recognizable on routine psychiatric or neurological examination without special attention to cognitive function. The brain's capacity to reorganize and to form new synapses during periods of remission underlies the improvement in cognition often seen in remissions early in the disease course. As the disease progresses and lesions accumulate (reflected by an increasing volume of cerebral and cerebellar lesions on T1- and T2-weighted MRIs), cognitive deficits develop that are symptomatic and/or evident on routine mental status testing.

Bipolar disorder is more common among patients with MS than in the general population. Bipolar patients with MS may present with isolated euphoria or with predominant irritability. Hypomania can occur with little or no insight; patients with MS lesions that affect metacognition and self-awareness will manifest denial of illness that would not ordinarily be seen with primary hypomania of the same severity. Cyclothymia and subsyndromal hypomania are considerations when a patient with MS presents with euphoria or irritability but does not fully meet criteria for a hypomanic episode.

Psychotic disorders are less common than other psychiatric comorbidities of MS. However, in rare cases, MS can initially manifest as psychosis. If no obvious motor or sensory impairments are present, the diagnosis of MS can be delayed for years. Features of new-onset psychosis that suggest a primary neurological cause (of which demyelinating disease is one and subacute encephalitis is another) include visual hallucinations, rapid onset, cognitive deficits, and absence of any negative or prodromal symptoms of schizophrenia (Camara-Lemarroy et al. 2017). Patients with new-onset psychosis due to MS typically have normal social and occupational function before the onset of their illness.

In patients with MS, bilateral involvement of pathways from the cerebrum to the facial motor nuclei can lead to pseudobulbar affect, a distressing condition clearly distinguishable from depression and hypomania and responsive to different treatments. About 10% of MS patients experience pseudobulbar affect, usually at a later stage in their illness (Schiffer and Pope 2005).

Psychiatric Aspects of Multiple Sclerosis Treatments

The primary treatment for acute MS relapses is high-dose corticosteroids. The most common dosing is 3–5 days of intravenous methylprednisolone, which may be followed with an oral prednisone taper. ACTH injections are a more expensive alternative that may be more efficacious in some patients because of other effects of ACTH on the CNS that are not mediated by increased corticosteroid level effects on the CNS (Philbin et al. 2017). Either of these treatments—corticosteroids or ACTH—carries the usual psychiatric risk of precipitating hypomania, depression, or psychotic symptoms. Corticosteroids usually are not continued long enough to produce adrenal suppression. The second-line treatment options for acute relapses of MS—either plasmapheresis or intravenous immune globulin—are not associated with specific psychiatric risks (Berkovich 2016).

The principal focus of MS treatment is prevention of relapses—new episodes of illness with new demyelinating brain lesions—in patients with RRMS. Drugs used to prevent such relapses are known as disease-modifying therapies (DMTs). DMTs can also be used to prevent the development of MS after a single episode of autoimmune demyelinating disease (i.e., a CIS) and to halt progression of disease in PPMS or

SPMS. In the United States, nine drugs are approved for the treatment of RRMS; only one of these, ocrelizumab, is also approved for PPMS, and none are approved for SPMS. Ocrelizumab and rituximab are used off-label for SPMS. Several other drugs are in clinical trials for SPMS (Baldassari and Fox 2018; Ciotti and Cross 2018; Gholamzad et al. 2019). One of these drugs, siponimod, a sphingosine-1-phosphate receptor antagonist, is under consideration for FDA approval. Two other options in clinical trials involve repurposing of nontoxic and inexpensive agents—i.e., high-dose simvastatin and the antioxidant alpha-lipoic acid. If the efficacy of either of these agents in MS is confirmed, its adoption will likely be rapid. Effective treatment of MS with DMTs can improve psychiatric comorbidities, including emotional and cognitive symptoms, by treating an element of their MS-related pathogenesis (Chan et al. 2017; Grand'Maison et al. 2018; Miller et al. 2017; Montalban et al. 2011).

With so many options for DMT following the initial diagnosis of a CIS or RRMS, the selection of an initial DMT—and a follow-on DMT if the initial agent does not prevent a relapse—is a complex issue in which a consulting psychiatrist can at times play a useful role. Specifically, the DMTs have different risks, and a patient's concerns about various risks can be explored by the psychiatrist and conveyed to the neurologist. Some DMTs require frequent injections, and if a patient is afraid of injections, behavioral interventions might make them more tolerable. DMTs have been associated with depression as an adverse effect, but a systematic review of the issue does not establish causality or a consistent and significant difference among them (Gasim et al. 2018). Clinical experience suggests that individual patients might develop depression as an expression of their intolerance of a specific DMT. If the depression is severe or accompanied by suicidal ideation or increased disability, switching to an alternative DMT should be considered. The immunomodulator glatiramer can be associated with anxiety, especially in the short term after the subcutaneous injection and in combination with flushing and other physical symptoms (La Mantia et al. 2010). Even when a DMT has a propensity to cause depression, there may be good reasons for choosing it and then managing the depression if and when it occurs; for example, a patient might have had an excellent past response to that DMT without major medical adverse effects. As previously noted, patients receiving DMT by subcutaneous injection can develop injection anxiety, which if not treated can interfere with their adherence to treatment. The monoclonal antibody alemtuzumab is given by infusion over 5 consecutive days, with 3 more days of infusion 1 year later and no need for regular oral or injected medication in the interim. If a psychiatrist determines that a patient has a very high risk of nonadherence to oral and injectable medications and the risk of relapse is high, a recommendation could be made to the neurologist in support of this costly treatment option.

The immunosuppressive drug fingolimod may cause atrioventricular block and bradyarrhythmia. Its use is contraindicated in patients with a baseline QTc interval greater than 500 msec. In MS patients with depression or anxiety who are taking fingolimod, it is preferable to avoid concurrent use of psychotropics that can lengthen the QTc interval—such as citalopram, escitalopram, TCAs, quetiapine, and ziprasidone—in favor of other agents for the same indication that are not associated with QT prolongation.

Several DMTs can increase the risk of autoimmune diseases or opportunistic infections that can initially manifest as mental status changes. If an MS patient is seeing a psychiatrist much more frequently than the treating neurologist, the psychiatrist may be the first to recognize a change in the patient's cognition or behavior that potentially may be caused by an infection or a new autoimmune disease. A change in a patient's psychiatric status developing over several days should prompt a comprehensive review of systems, communication with the treating neurologist, and appropriate screening laboratory tests.

Psychiatrists involved in the long-term management of the psychiatric comorbidities of MS can also contribute significantly to the management of the MS itself through their continual observation of their patients and the time spent during outpatient visits. Neurologists sometimes miss the earliest signs of MS relapses, especially when such signs are primarily cognitive or behavioral. Psychiatrists seeing patients frequently may notice evidence of cognitive or behavioral symptoms or hear about changes in patients' everyday activities that suggest new disease activity. They can follow up with additional history taking and examination and communication with the treating neurologist. Earlier intervention can shorten relapses and make them less severe. Identifying sooner that a DMT has not prevented relapses can accelerate the switch to a more effective agent. Precipitating stressors or nonadherence to DMT can also be addressed.

Chronic or frequent nontraumatic stress, such as that associated with family conflicts and financial problems, increases the risk of MS relapses. The adverse effects of stress are greater than the therapeutic benefits of some approved DMTs (Artemiadis et al. 2011; Kalincik 2015). The significant potential for stress to trigger MS relapses suggests that teaching patients how to better manage stress through mindfulness meditation, progressive relaxation, breathing exercises, biofeedback, or physical exercise can potentially alter the course of the illness. Although no specific stress management method has been shown to reduce MS relapses, the argument from the mechanism of disease is worthy of consideration. In addition, stress management techniques are helpful in managing anxiety and reducing the risk of clinical depression. Comorbid posttraumatic stress disorder (PTSD), if present, should be treated.

Symptomatic treatment of MS targets symptoms such as spasticity, weakness, fatigue, incontinence, and sexual dysfunction, which can have major effects on patients' health-related quality of life and on their levels of depression and anxiety. In some cases, specific distressing symptoms can increase suicide risk because they are especially intolerable or because they interfere with activities that make the patient's life worth living. For example, MS patients with severe fatigue are more likely than those without this burden to be suicidal. It has been noted that men with MS are particularly strongly affected by symptoms that impair their ability to work or their ability to perform sexually. Although such symptoms are also distressing to women with MS, they are not as closely linked with clinical depression and with suicidal ideation in women as they are in men.

Specific symptomatic treatments are available for these symptoms. Fatigue can be treated with modafinil or stimulants; weakness can be treated with dalfampridine; and spasticity can be treated with dantrolene, tizanidine, or botulinum toxin injections (Nicholas and Rashid 2012). The psychiatrist can identify when a specific physical symptom of MS may be implicated in the patient's emotional distress or suicidal thinking and bring that symptom to the attention of the neurologist managing the patient's MS treatment.

Migraine

While not perceived by some generalist physicians or psychiatrists as a major neuro-logical disease, migraine is significant as a highly prevalent cause of neurological symptoms, disability, and psychiatric comorbidity. Migraine—throbbing headache, usually unilateral but sometimes bilateral, often associated with nausea and vomiting or photophobia or phonophobia—affects 12%–16% of the U.S. population (Smither-man et al. 2013). Women are affected about twice as often as men. Migraine can occur with or without *aura*—a preceding period of neurological symptoms such as visual or other sensory disturbances (e.g., scintillating scotomata) or changes in mental state that are followed by the headache. Auras typically last 20–30 minutes, but a minority of patients may occasionally have prolonged auras lasting 2 hours or longer. Head-aches typically last several hours, often ending with the patient going to sleep. Mi-graine is a leading cause of disability in young adults, and severe headache, including migraine, is a common cause of emergency department (ED) visits. Migraine is clas-sified as episodic or chronic; the criteria for chronic migraine require the presence of 15 or more headache days per month for a minimum of 3 months, with at least 8 of the headache days each month being migraine days (a patient with chronic migraine may have headaches of other types, such as tension headaches) (Ruscheweyh et al. 2014). A diagnosis of medication overuse headaches rules out a diagnosis of chronic migraine; the latter diagnosis can only be made if the patient's headaches meet chronic migraine criteria after he or she is fully withdrawn from daily medication (typically daily analgesics) (Negro and Martelletti 2011). Chronic migraine has a prevalence of almost 1% in the general population; the prevalence is higher in women, in middle-aged people, and in those with lower incomes (Buse et al. 2012).

Episodes of migraine may respond to a range of drugs, among which the triptans—serotonin (5-hydroxytryptamine type 1B and type 1D [$5\text{-HT}_{1B/1D}$]) receptor agonists—are the most consistently effective. Triptans are available in various formulations, in-cluding ones that can be given intranasally or by injection if the patient is too nause-ated to take an oral medication. The nausea and vomiting that accompany migraine have traditionally been treated with dopamine antagonists such as metoclopramide or prochlorperazine. However, these drugs can cause extrapyramidal side effects. Nau-sea and vomiting can be treated with 5-HT_3 receptor antagonists such as ondansetron, although controlled studies of these agents' use specifically in migraine are lacking. Triptans have been linked to the serotonin syndrome in patients also taking SSRIs or serotonin-norepinephrine reuptake inhibitors (SNRIs), although a recent analysis sug-gested that the risk may be lower than initially reported (Orlova et al. 2018).

Triptans can be combined with nonsteroidal anti-inflammatory drugs (NSAIDs) when a triptan alone is insufficient. Opiates are less efficacious for migraines than are triptans and NSAIDs. In a patient presenting emergently with a severe headache, the clinician, after ruling out a neurological emergency such as subarachnoid hemor-rhage, should diagnose migraine if it is present and begin specific treatment immedi-ately. Timely diagnosis and treatment of migraine can prevent unnecessary use of opiates, with their potential for misuse.

Episodic migraines that occur frequently enough to disrupt life and work or to cause major distress should be treated preventively. Drug treatments that have shown efficacy and that have traditionally been used for migraine prevention include propranolol, timolol, topiramate, and valproate, which are FDA approved for migraine prevention, as well as the off-label options of amitriptyline, candesartan, and lisinopril (Loder and Rizzoli 2018). Propranolol or timolol can cause fatigue and psychomotor slowing without clinical depression. Amitriptyline, sometimes used as a preventive for chronic headache, can precipitate secondary hypomania or rapid cycling in a patient with bipolar disorder. This possibility is especially relevant for patients with migraine, because the prevalence of comorbid bipolar disorder in patients with migraine has averaged 9% in clinic-based studies and 5.9% in epidemiological studies. Furthermore, the weighted average prevalence of migraine among patients with bipolar disorder in published studies through 2015 was 30.7% (Leo and Singh 2016). Topiramate can cause cognitive symptoms. Among the approved agents for migraine prevention, valproate would be an attractive choice for a patient with comorbid bipolar disorder because of its efficacy as a mood stabilizer.

Standard migraine preventive treatments are not effective for many patients, especially those with chronic migraine. New pharmacological treatments have emerged for chronic migraine that are significantly more effective than TCAs and β-blockers. The two main options are botulinum toxin (injected at multiple sites around the face and skull) and monoclonal antibodies against calcitonin gene-related peptide (CGRP) or its receptor (CLR+RAMP1). Three CGRP antagonists have been approved to date: erenumab, fremanezumab, and galcanezumab. CGRP antagonists are given by monthly subcutaneous injection. Botulinum toxin injections for chronic migraine are given on a quarterly schedule. Both botulinum toxin and CGRP antagonists are much more efficacious than other preventive therapies, and neither has a significant incidence of psychiatric side effects. When they are effective, the CGRP antagonists can eliminate the patient's migraines, not merely reduce their frequency and intensity (Rosen et al. 2018). However, these agents are expensive. Lack of access to them for reasons of cost can be a major emotional issue for patients whose migraines have interfered with their work or education or have affected the quality of important relationships. When a patient with chronic migraine has health insurance but the insurance company has not authorized payment for medically necessary migraine-preventive therapy, a psychiatric consultant sometimes can help by documenting the range of adverse effects of the patient's migraines on mood, behavior, and occupational function, and the risk of ED visits or hospitalizations.

Prophylactic treatment can reduce the frequency and severity of episodic migraines, prevent episodic migraines from becoming chronic, and treat chronic migraine if it does develop. However, successful long-term treatment of patients with migraine often requires adjunctive treatment of patients' psychiatric comorbidity. Most patients with migraine have at least one psychiatric diagnosis, and many patients have more than one (Minen et al. 2016).

Migraine is associated with several psychiatric disorders, all of which are more prevalent in patients with chronic migraine than in those with episodic migraine. While the rates of depression in people with migraine as determined by surveys vary greatly according to study methodology, the prevalence of MDD in patients with episodic migraine may be as high as 25%, and the prevalence of MDD in those with chronic migraine may exceed 40% (Buse et al. 2013). The risk of conversion of episodic migraine to chronic migraine is higher in the presence of comorbid depression. Successful treatment of chronic migraine is associated with a reduction in depression severity.

More than half of patients with migraine will meet criteria for a DSM anxiety disorder (e.g., GAD, panic disorder) or a related disorder (e.g., obsessive-compulsive disorder, PTSD) at some point in their lives. Anxiety and related disorders are more common in patients with chronic migraine than in those with acute migraine. The bidirectional relationship of these disorders and migraine might be partially explained by common genetic and epigenetic factors. For example, anxiety disorders and migraine both are associated with the *s* allele of the 5HTTLPR polymorphism of the serotonin transporter gene, and both have an increased lifetime prevalence in patients with adverse childhood experiences known to be associated with epigenetic alterations (Minen et al. 2016). The prevalence of anxiety disorders is higher in patients with chronic migraine, and the presence of a comorbid anxiety or related disorder increases the risk that episodic migraines will become chronic. Finally, migraine is associated with PTSD. In a study of 593 patients with episodic or chronic migraine from six headache centers, PTSD was found in 30.3% of patients with chronic migraine and 22.4% of those with episodic migraine (Peterlin et al. 2009). In the National Comorbidity Survey of 2001–2003, a study of psychiatric and general medical illness prevalence in the general population, 22.4% of 304 respondents with migraine had PTSD, and 21.8% of 312 respondents with PTSD experienced migraine (Rao et al. 2015).

The association of migraine with bipolar disorder is strong and bidirectional. More than half of patients with bipolar II disorder have comorbid migraine, and approximately one-third of patients with bipolar I disorder have comorbid migraine (Sinha et al. 2018). In comparison with bipolar patients without migraine, those with migraine tend to have more frequent and prolonged episodes of depression and are more likely to have rapid cycling or mixed episodes (Sinha et al. 2018). A representative estimate of the prevalence of bipolar disorder in migraine patients in a headache clinic is 4.9% for bipolar I and 7.8% for bipolar II (Ortiz et al. 2010). Leo and Singh (2016) conducted a comprehensive literature review and derived a rate of 9% for bipolar disorder comorbidity in clinic samples. Kivilcim et al. (2017) found a prevalence of 19.2% in a migraine clinic at a tertiary care hospital. In the latter study, the investigators screened all patients with the Hypomania Checklist–32–Revised (Angst et al. 2005) and the Mood Disorder Questionnaire (Hirschfeld et al. 2000) and followed up with the Structured Clinical Interview for DSM-IV Axis I Disorders (First et al. 1997). The differences between the findings of Kivilcim and colleagues and the findings of other studies that reported a lower prevalence of bipolar comorbidity in migraine patients might be due to the patient mix at a tertiary care center, but it is likely that the thoroughness of their screening methodology played a role. Taken together, the evidence supports systematic, structured screening for bipolar disorder in patients with chronic migraine, high health care utilization, or headache-related disability.

The presence of a comorbid mood disorder makes effective management of the migraine—ideally with preventive treatment—especially important because of the patient's greater impairment of function and health-related quality of life and greater potential for suicide. Regarding choice of preventive agents, β-blockers can worsen depression and TCAs can cause secondary hypomania and are dangerous in overdose. Comorbid psychiatric illness can be advanced as an argument to payers for authorization of more expensive preventive treatments that may be more effective, do not carry the risks of making mood disorders worse, and cannot be abused or used in an overdose.

In some patients with migraine, the aura may occasionally be prolonged and be more clinically significant than the headache that follows it. Auras can be "complicated," involving behavioral disturbances or changes in cognition or memory. Infrequently, the phenomenology of complex migraine auras can suggest the presence of a dissociative or somatic symptom–related disorder. The headache history usually permits the diagnosis, and treatment that prevents the headaches will prevent the auras. Complex partial epilepsy with ictal or postictal headache should be considered in the differential diagnosis; the potential for comorbid anxiety or depression is similarly increased. Epilepsy has a much greater impact on suicide risk than does migraine.

In cases of complicated migraine and migraine with psychiatric comorbidity, psychiatrists may be consulted to help determine whether the symptoms of the aura are psychiatric problems or are expressions of the migraine or whether to treat the depression, anxiety, or bipolar symptoms displayed by the patient. In these situations, the headache should not be neglected. If the patient has frequent, severe episodic migraines or has chronic migraines, efforts to prevent the migraine should be concurrent with treatment of the psychiatric condition. It is more likely a patient will have a complete remission of a psychiatric disorder if the patient does not have frequent headaches that interfere with work and other purposeful life activities. If the psychiatric symptoms cause much more distress or dysfunction than the headaches, they can be treated first; if so, the frequency and severity of headaches, whether the headaches are migraines, and the nature and severity of the aura should be monitored. The issue of the need for migraine prevention should be revisited if necessary, because the headaches may emerge as a bigger problem as the patient's depression, anxiety, or bipolar disorder improves.

Conditions Commonly Treated by Neurosurgeons

Brain conditions commonly treated by neurosurgeons include brain tumors (malignant and benign), subdural hematoma, hydrocephalus, cerebral hemorrhage from aneurysm or arteriovenous malformation, and brain abscess. Neurosurgeons also deal with pituitary adenomas—extracerebral tumors that can anatomically impinge on the brain as well as affect brain function through their endocrine effects. In addition to consulting psychiatrists for the same reasons as neurologists do, neurosurgeons have two other notable reasons for consulting psychiatrists. The first is determining whether a patient has the capacity to consent to a neurosurgical procedure with nontrivial risks and uncertain outcome. The issue usually comes up when a patient who has a strong clinical indication for neurosurgery is reluctant to undergo the proposed procedure. The cognitive effects of the brain disease to be treated, any concurrent primary psychiatric disorder, and the patient's emotional reaction to the illness interact to influence the patient's decision-making processes. Beyond a role in assessment, the psychiatrist can play a useful role in facilitating understanding and communication between the neurosurgeon and the patient. The psychiatrist can help the neurosurgeon to understand the patient's reluctance to have surgery by deconstructing and explaining the patient's view of the proposed procedure in relation to any cognitive deficits, psychiatric issues, and personal concerns that may be present. Implementing an intervention to reduce patient anxiety, explaining the procedure differently (e.g., with a teaching video or with the assistance of a trusted family member), or simply delaying a procedure by a day sometimes enables a reluctant patient to accept needed surgery, thus avoiding legal and administrative problems. Psychiatrists may also be called to consult on patients in whom new-onset psychiatric or cognitive symptoms may not yet have been recognized as secondary to their neurological illness. Careful attention to the age of the patient and the pattern of symptom onset, especially when psychiatric symptoms appear over days to weeks in later life, should alert the psychiatrist to a possible primary neurological cause. A careful history (including family history and perspectives on the illness), a meticulous review of medical and laboratory records, and a full cognitive mental status examination and detailed neurological examination are essential to ensure that any new neurological etiologies are not missed.

Another special reason that neurosurgeons seek a psychiatric consultation for a patient is for assistance in deciding whether to treat a chronic brain disease, such as normal-pressure hydrocephalus or a small meningioma, when the mildness of the major neurological symptoms or the size of the lesion suggests that treatment is not urgent. In this situation, the psychiatrist is asked to help determine whether the patient has cognitive or behavioral issues likely to be due to the known brain disease and likely to improve if it is treated. For example, consider the case of an 80-year-old patient with mild normal-pressure hydrocephalus, subtle gait disturbance without a history of falls, and rare episodes of urinary incontinence. In this situation, there might be concern that surgery would not improve the patient's quality of life enough to warrant the operation. If the psychiatrist's history and mental status examination established a new onset of apathy and impaired judgment that paralleled the onset of the gait changes and incontinence and demonstrated that cognition was intact apart from high-level executive functioning, these facts would favor surgery to correct the normal-pressure hydrocephalus. If the psychiatrist found mild dementia and no suggestion of a change in cognitive function, mood, motivation, or social behavior coincident with the changes in gait and continence, the recommendation might be for additional testing of CSF dynamics before deciding upon surgery.

In a patient with a known focal lesion of the brain, such as a tumor, brain abscess, or lobar cerebral hemorrhage, any psychiatric problems would follow from the location of the lesion and from the context and prognosis of the disease that produced it. A patient with a benign tumor or a brain abscess that can be cured by excision would face the challenges of recovering from brain damage and perhaps of adapting to some permanent deficits, but this patient would not face the additional threat of progressive disease that would be faced by a patient with a glioblastoma or a cerebral metastasis from a cancer elsewhere in the body. Psychiatrists may be asked to help with the specific problem of denial or minimization of neurological deficits following brain surgery—an occurrence most likely in patients with lesions involving the right parietal lobe or the frontal lobes—or the denial or minimization of new behavioral symptoms. Neurological physical therapists and occupational therapists will address the rehabilitative aspects of anosognosia and impaired metacognition, but the psychiatrist may need to help the patient's family deal with the strangeness of the situation, offer advice on making the patient's environment safer, and treat symptoms such as depressed mood, apathy, and pseudobulbar affect, which can further impede recovery.

Psychiatric Sequelae of Brain Cancer Treatment

Malignant tumors of the brain, whether primary or metastatic, are treated with some combination of biopsy or resection, radiation therapy, and chemotherapy. Following treatment, patients have primary neurological deficits accompanied by cognitive, emotional, and behavioral changes associated with the foci of their lesions. Depression is a common sequel of brain cancer treatment; the emotional impact of the diagnosis, functional impairments, and prognosis of the cancer combine with the direct effects of the brain lesion on brain circuits and neurotransmitters related to mood regulation, which are similar to those seen with strokes.

Subarachnoid Hemorrhage and Cerebral Aneurysm

Subarachnoid hemorrhage from a ruptured (or leaky) aneurysm is a life-threatening condition. If a patient survives an initial hemorrhage, he or she will need to undergo neurosurgery to prevent a potentially fatal recurrence. Depending on the location of the aneurysm, the surgery can be risky, and the patient's decision of whether to have surgery—and where to have it—can be difficult. The most common location for an aneurysmal bleed is the anterior communicating artery. Bleeding in this area, especially if followed by vasospasm and local ischemia, can cause severe apathy, and sometimes even akinetic mutism. The psychiatrist can diagnose apathy, distinguish it from depression, and—if it is persistent—suggest (or implement) treatment with a stimulant or dopamine agonist.

When a psychiatrist provides frequent ongoing outpatient follow-up for a patient after a subarachnoid hemorrhage and notices a slow decline in mental state, a combination of apathy, disinhibition, and impaired executive functioning would suggest a frontal lobe syndrome possibly due to hydrocephalus. The psychiatrist can assess this finding with office-based testing and, if concern is warranted, could bring it to the attention of the neurologist or neurosurgeon responsible for the patient's neurological follow-up.

Subdural Hematoma

A slowly progressive change in behavior—often a dysexecutive syndrome—accompanied by headache is a typical presentation of a chronic frontal subdural hematoma. The patient is typically a middle-aged or older person with a vague history of a fall or a blow to the head, whose headache may be so mild that it is not complained of spontaneously. Such a patient can present to a psychiatrist because of a depressed mood or a family member's concern about a change in behavior. The story should initiate a neurological examination (either by the psychiatrist or by a colleague) and imaging of the brain. The diagnosis is made on the basis of findings on brain imaging.

Patients with chronic frontal subdural hematomas will not necessarily perform poorly on generic bedside cognitive screening tests such as the MMSE or MoCA. In behaviorally significant cases, deficits will be clearer if the clinician uses bedside tests that are more focused on executive functioning, such as the Clock Drawing Test (Terwindt et al. 2016) or the Executive Interview Test (Royall et al. 1992). The neurological examination should specifically include testing for frontal release signs, careful assessment of the plantar reflexes, and stress testing of gait and balance. It is not uncommon for these tests to be omitted in the so-called medical clearance of a patient initially thought to have a primary psychiatric disorder. If such omissions are found in the record of a patient's neurological examination, a psychiatrist can easily rectify them by performing these tests during the mental status examination.

Meningioma

Meningiomas are the most common benign tumors affecting the cerebral cortex and potentially manifesting as changes in mood, behavior, or cognition. Because typical meningiomas do not invade the brain, they usually do not produce symptoms when they are small. When meningiomas reach a size sufficient to displace brain structures, they become symptomatic. At that point, patients may present with seizures or with focal neurological symptoms and signs. Psychiatrists get involved with meningiomas when a patient has psychiatric symptoms potentially secondary to brain disease and a meningioma is found on brain imaging. The two usual questions are whether the meningioma is related to the psychiatric syndrome and whether there are psychiatric reasons in favor of or against treatment of the meningioma by surgery or radiation therapy.

For a psychiatrist, answering the first question usually begins with characterizing the neuropsychiatric syndrome one symptom at a time, even though the psychiatrist might also assemble a combination of symptoms that support a diagnosis of MDD. A patient might exhibit apathy, pseudobulbar affect, socially inappropriate behavior ("frontal lobe syndrome"), or behavioral dyscontrol in addition to a depressive syndrome. Meningiomas in the medial and basal frontal regions often manifest with apathy. Orbital groove meningiomas can present with behavioral dyscontrol or socially inappropriate behavior. Anterior frontal lesions can manifest with antisocial behavior. Dorsolateral frontal meningiomas can manifest with impaired executive function and working memory. Temporal lobe meningiomas can manifest with modality-specific memory loss. When the qualitative features of slowly progressive changes in cognition and behavior match the location of the meningioma visualized on imaging, it is likely that the tumor is the primary cause of the neuropsychiatric symptoms as well as of the depression that usually accompanies the more specific neurobehavioral symptoms.

The psychiatrist's contribution to the therapeutic decision making of the neurosurgeon and the patient consists of attempting to estimate how much of the patient's current neuropsychiatric symptoms are due to the meningioma, how much distress and dysfunction the symptoms are causing, and how vulnerable the patient might be to potential adverse outcomes of the surgery or radiotherapy. These opinions can be useful in informed consent as well as shared decision making. When a frontal meningioma has caused significant impairment of the patient's judgment, it is likely that treatment is needed, but the patient might refuse it. In this situation, the psychiatrist should assess the patient's decision-making capacity with a special focus on the element of *appreciation*. It is likely that the patient will be able to understand the diagnosis and treatment, communicate a preference, and offer a reason for the choice. The element that may be missing is realistic appreciation of the consequences of not dealing with the tumor.

Cognitive Changes After Cancer Chemotherapy

Patients who have undergone treatment for cancer with systemic chemotherapy often experience significant impairment of cognitive function, including executive impairment, apathy or mental fatigability, and problems with attention, concentration, and memory. These symptoms—known as chemotherapy-associated cognitive impairment (CACI) or cancer-related cognitive impairment (CRCI), and also known colloquially as "brain fog" or "chemo brain"—occur independently of whether the chemotherapy or radiation was effective in treating the cancer. CACI symptoms may appear immediately after treatment or after a delay of several weeks. The symptoms usually remit after several months but can be permanent. Although CACI symptoms may co-occur with depression or anxiety, they are not secondary to the depression or anxiety, and they will persist after the depression or anxiety is successfully treated. First-level screening for CRCI/CACI involves screening for cognitive symptoms and cognition-related functional impairment. The MoCA and the Clock Drawing Test are currently the preferred instruments for brief screening. When interpreting them, the psychiatrist should consider results in relation to the patient's known or probable baseline function and in relation to the cognitive demands of the patient's work and life. The Functional Assessment of Cancer Therapy—Cognitive Function (available from www.facit.org) provides a practical, structured look at the impact of cognitive symptoms on the patient's life (Isenberg-Grzeda et al. 2017). It is a self-rated questionnaire that rates items for frequency or severity on a 0–4 scale comprising domains of perceived cognitive impairments, cognitive abilities, impact on quality of life, and comments by others about the patient's memory, cognition, and communication. Using this instrument in conjunction with a psychiatric interview allows time-efficient identification of mild CACI when cognitive complaints are not the presenting problem. Ruling out CACI is important because a cancer patient's presenting symptoms of depression or anxiety might be partly or entirely due to his or her experience of impaired cognition or cognition-related functions.

The mechanisms that underlie CACI include inflammation, a decrease in nerve growth factors, oxidative stress, and accelerated aging processes, among others. White matter damage often can be demonstrated on MRI using diffusion-weighted imaging and diffusion tensor imaging in the weeks following completion of the cancer treatment. While evidence from controlled trials is lacking, the usual steps to optimize brain health should be maintained during the weeks after radiation or chemotherapy. Depression, if present, should be treated promptly because of its association with elevated inflammatory markers and decreased levels of the neurotrophic factors (e.g., BDNF) needed to restore normal function of the brain after the insult of chemotherapy or radiation. Patients should be encouraged to engage in regular moderate to vigorous physical exercise, because this is known to stimulate dendritic growth and synaptic development and was directly shown to improve CRCI in breast cancer survivors (Ehlers et al. 2018). Cognitive rehabilitation, either in person or via mobile apps, may be considered; it will become evident after several sessions whether the patient will benefit from it. Anti-inflammatory and antioxidant treatments show benefit in some animal models of CACI, but none has yet become the standard of practice (Matsos et al. 2017).

In patients with CACI, pharmacological treatment of apathy and mental fatigue should be considered if these symptoms are functionally significant and persist despite efforts to ensure adequate sleep and nutrition and to discontinue medications with adverse CNS side effects. A cholinergic agonist such as donepezil could be considered. As with any off-label use of a drug in a neuropsychiatric context, the patient should be informed that the drug is not approved for that specific indication, the rationale should be explained, and a quantitative measure of target symptoms should be selected and followed to assess treatment response.

Late Effects of Traumatic Brain Injury

TBI is defined by the Centers for Disease Control and Prevention (2019) as "a disruption in the normal function of the brain that can be caused by a bump, blow, or jolt to the head, or penetrating head injury." TBI is epidemic in the United States. In 2010, TBIs were the cause of more than 2.5 million civilian ED visits. Of TBI patients seen in EDs, 87% were treated and released, 11% were hospitalized and eventually discharged, and 2% died (Centers for Disease Control and Prevention 2015). Additional cases of TBI are seen in military and veterans' hospitals, and in both civilian and military settings, many individuals with mild TBI do not immediately seek medical treatment. The most common causes of TBI are falls, motor vehicle crashes, and blows to the head. People who engage in contact sports or military combat may sustain multiple TBIs; these injuries are particularly damaging when a second TBI occurs before a person has recovered from the first one. Combat-acquired TBI can involve blast injuries from explosions, where shock waves cause diffuse brain damage. Accurate and current estimates of the prevalence of TBI-related disability in the United States are not available—a gap that the CDC has recommended addressing. However, estimates of the U.S. prevalence of TBI-related disability based on extrapolations of data from state-level studies have been reported, and they indicate that in 2008, between 3.2 million and 5.3 million people were living with a TBI-related disability (Centers for Disease Control and Prevention 2015, p.19).

In several contexts, including combat-related TBI, TBI due to intimate partner violence, or TBI sustained during a criminal assault, the neuropsychiatric sequelae of TBI are accompanied by PTSD. When PTSD is present as a comorbidity, it should be treated, because comorbid PTSD contributes to the patient's overall distress and impairment and can markedly increase suicide risk.

The neuropsychiatry of TBI is a vast topic that this chapter cannot survey comprehensively. We concentrate on the sequelae of mild TBI, the type with the highest incidence and the type most often leading to consultations with general psychiatrists. Mild TBI, also referred to as "concussion," is defined as a loss of consciousness lasting less than 30 minutes, posttraumatic amnesia lasting less than 24 hours, and a Glasgow Coma Scale score of 13–15 (Teasdale and Jennett 1974). Thus, mild TBI covers a wide spectrum of injury severity, a fact that helps explain the marked variation in its outcomes (Katz et al. 2015). When conducting a psychiatric assessment of a patient with mild TBI, it is very helpful to know where on the continuum of "mildness" the patient's injury falls.

A computed tomography (CT) scan of the head immediately following mild TBI usually shows a normal brain. The outcome is highly variable; patients with more severe or persistent symptoms following mild TBI are referred to psychiatrists because of concern about comorbidities such as clinical depression, anxiety disorders, PTSD, or a substance use disorder or because of concern that the patient has symptoms suggestive of a somatic symptom disorder or malingering. Symptoms in the first 2 weeks (1 month in children) following mild TBI are typical; however, a sizable minority of patients with mild TBI—probably more than 15%—have postconcussion symptoms 1 year later (Barker-Collo et al. 2015). In a Norwegian study of patients admitted to the hospital for treatment after a TBI, 40 patients had mild injuries with an average of 3.5 hours of posttraumatic amnesia. Of these patients with mild TBI, 40% reported postconcussion symptoms 3 months later (Sigurdardottir et al. 2009). Postconcussion symptoms are of four types: vestibular (e.g., imbalance or dizziness), sensory (e.g., photophobia, phonophobia, tinnitus), cognitive (e.g., difficulties with concentration and memory), and "psychiatric" (e.g., irritability, depressed mood, insomnia, fatigue). Standardized questionnaires both screen for and measure postconcussion symptoms; two widely used instruments are the Rivermead Post-Concussion Symptoms Questionnaire (King et al. 1995) and the Post-Concussion Symptom Scale (Lovell and Collins 1998). When symptoms are identified, specific scales such as the PHQ-9 for depression (Kroenke et al. 2001), the Fatigue Severity Scale (Krupp et al. 1989), the Pittsburgh Sleep Quality Index (Buysse et al. 1989), and tinnitus scales such as the Tinnitus Handicap Inventory (Newman et al. 1996) can be used to further delineate the nature and severity of the symptoms.

DSM-5 (American Psychiatric Association 2013) does not recognize a postconcussion syndrome as such; instead, psychiatrists are encouraged to diagnose a neurocognitive disorder if cognitive symptoms are present and supported by examination. However, patients with distressing symptoms following mild TBI may not have cognitive complaints, or such complaints may not be accompanied by definite abnormalities on cognitive testing, particularly if the patient had high baseline functioning. Psychiatrists are left to diagnose comorbid psychiatric disorders such as depression or PTSD and one or more medical conditions. ICD-10 (World Health Organization 1992) does recognize a postconcussion syndrome; diagnosing it requires a history of concussion within 4 weeks preceding the onset of symptoms and at least three out of six symptoms: complaints of unpleasant sensations and pains; emotional changes; subjective cognitive complaints without objective evidence of marked cognitive impairment; insomnia; reduced alcohol tolerance; and preoccupation with symptoms and fear of permanent brain damage, including adoption of the sick role (Quinn et al. 2018).

People with symptoms following mild TBI have the usual vulnerabilities of people with general medical illness to clinical depression and anxiety, with increased risk of these comorbidities because there has been physical injury to the brain. Moreover, they often must contend with others' doubts about the validity of their symptoms, especially if loss of consciousness was brief and the patient did not initially seek medical care. Preinjury risk factors associated with more severe or prolonged postconcussion symptoms include the following, in decreasing order of effect size: three or more prior mild TBIs, attention-deficit/hyperactivity disorder, substance use, less than a high school education, unemployment, history of a psychiatric diagnosis, one or more prior mild TBIs, age younger than 18 years or older than 65 years, female gender, and any chronic medical condition. Risk is higher if the TBI was acquired in connection with combat or a criminal assault. While CT scans in mild TBI typically are normal, MRI scans may show evidence of contusions or axonal injury; such MRI abnormalities also predict greater severity and longer duration of symptoms (Quinn et al. 2018). Psychiatric comorbidities such as depression, anxiety, and PTSD have a circular relationship with postconcussion symptoms. Specific sleep disorders and migraine also have a circular relationship with postconcussion symptoms.

A general strategy for assessing and treating postconcussion symptoms begins with eliciting or collecting a full preinjury psychiatric and general medical history. A physical and neurological examination should be done with special attention to domains most likely to be affected by mild TBI and not necessarily examined fully on routine neurological examination. These areas include olfaction, oculomotor/vestibular function, gait, and balance, as well as the cervical spine and motor and sensory function and reflexes in the upper extremities that might indicate involvement of cervical nerve roots. Orthostatic vital signs should be checked. If there is doubt about the severity of the traumatic injury and no MRI was performed at the time, an MRI should be done. The neuroradiologist should be informed of the history and questions and should apply imaging methodology sensitive to white matter injuries. If the patient has paroxysmal stereotyped symptoms suggesting seizures, an EEG should be performed, with the diagnostic question discussed in advance with the neurologist involved to ensure that the correct EEG procedure is done (e.g., with sleep deprivation; anterior temporal or nasopharyngeal leads). Neuropsychological testing is not always needed but should be considered if cognitive complaints are prominent.

Treatment involves three components. First, the patient—and, if applicable, family members—should be informed of the findings of the psychiatrist's evaluation. Second, comorbid psychiatric disorders such as depression, PTSD, and substance use disorders should be treated, and comorbid medical conditions such as migraine should be addressed. Finally, symptoms such as fatigue, apathy, insomnia, tinnitus, and pain from cervical injury should be treated specifically with medications, physical therapy, or cognitive-behavioral therapy, as appropriate. An important goal is to help the patient return to preinjury physical, social, and occupational activity as soon as possible, because longer periods of inactivity worsen the patient's prognosis for full and timely recovery.

Chronic Traumatic Encephalopathy: A Real Syndrome With a Complex History

Psychiatrists may be asked to consult on patients who have experienced repetitive mild concussions, typically from contact sports or from military service in which they were exposed to explosive blasts. The patient will have some combination of depressed mood, suicidal ideation, apathy, irritability, and excessive anger, often accompanied by somatic symptoms including headache, body pain, and insomnia. The somatic, mood, and behavioral symptoms are accompanied by problems with executive functioning, attention, concentration, or memory, although these might be mild and evident only on neuropsychological testing or high-sensitivity cognitive screening. Focusing only on the patient's mood and behavior, several diagnoses would be considerations. However, if typical affective and behavioral symptoms are associated with history of repeated brain trauma, cognitive symptoms and signs, and somatic complaints such as headache or insomnia, the patient may have chronic traumatic encephalopathy (CTE). CTE, originally reported in professional boxers, has received much attention since it was identified in professional football players (Korngold et al. 2013; Solomon 2018; Yi et al. 2013).

CTE is a neuropathological diagnosis that at this time can be made definitively only at autopsy, although there has been considerable progress in developing in vivo biomarkers, including positron emission tomography (PET) imaging of tau protein with flortaucipir and detection of white matter tract disruption with diffusion tensor imaging (DTI) (Dallmeier et al. 2019). CTE is a "tauopathy"—a degenerative condition involving abnormal deposits of hyperphosphorylated tau in the neurons of the cerebral cortex. Tau protein is a normal part of the microtubules inside neurons. In several neurodegenerative conditions, excessive phosphorylation of tau protein causes the protein to dissociate from microtubules and form insoluble aggregates called *neurofibrillary tangles.* The presence of tangles and the disruption of normal microtubular architecture alter neuronal function. Abnormal accumulations of phosphorylated tau occur in frontotemporal degeneration, corticobasal degeneration, progressive supranuclear palsy, and Alzheimer's disease, as well as in CTE, but in each of these other conditions, the abnormal tau aggregates result in distinctive neuropathology and imaging findings. In CTE, aggregates of hyperphosphorylated tau accumulate in neurons, astrocytes, and cell processes around small vessels in an irregular pattern at the depths of cortical sulci—a pattern pathognomonic of the condition (Dallmeier et al. 2019).

Autopsies of former athletes who played contact sports and had histories of repetitive mild TBI showed the characteristic findings of CTE in fewer than half of all cases; these findings are not seen at all in the brains of people with no TBI history or a history of a single TBI, so the pathology is strongly linked to repeated brain trauma (Bieniek et al. 2015). While there is general agreement on a *neuropathological* syndrome occurring in former athletes with multiple mild TBIs, the clinical-neuropathological correlation is less settled. Some athletes who died and showed CTE postmortem had no neurological or psychiatric symptoms in life, and others who had neuropsychiatric symptoms did not have CTE at autopsy (Zuckerman et al. 2018). It is not known whether the changes of CTE are progressive in the absence of additional insults to the brain, nor is it known whether CTE results from repetitive TBI *alone* or requires a second factor—such as alcohol use, a comorbid neurodegenerative condition, or genetic risk factors—for its occurrence (Zuckerman et al. 2018). It is currently not possible either to make a confident diagnosis of CTE in life or to predict whether a patient will have a progressive disorder.

Brain-imaging studies of former NFL players compared with control subjects have shown reduced volumes bilaterally in the amygdala, hippocampus, and cingulate gyrus. Volume reductions in the cingulate gyri were associated with worse psychomotor speed and worse executive functioning, and volume reduction in the right hippocampus was associated with worse visual memory. Overall, the former players had more mood and behavioral symptoms than a control group and worse verbal memory (McKee et al. 2016). These findings suggest that players with lesser cognitive reserves who have had greater-than-average trauma exposure might end their football careers with diagnosable neuropsychiatric syndromes with imaging accompaniments or might develop them decades later as their subclinical deficits interact with the effects of normal or pathological brain aging.

When a psychiatrist encounters a patient who has a chronic neuropsychiatric condition with mixed cognitive, mood, and behavioral symptoms atypical for MDD alone and a history of repetitive mild TBI, the diagnostic agenda should include a careful neurological examination; an MRI with special attention to the frontal and temporal regions, if possible looking at white matter integrity with diffusion tensor imaging; an EEG; and neuropsychological testing (or detailed neurocognitive assessment if the former is feasible). Screening for alcohol and other substance use disorders is important, because they can both cause symptoms similar to those of symptomatic CTE and be symptoms of impaired judgment and impulse control due to symptomatic CTE.

In people with CTE, the MRI may show focal atrophy in the frontal or temporal regions or disruption of white matter tracts in those areas; the EEG may show focal changes that usually are nonspecific. If the MRI shows frontal or temporal lobe damage and there are demonstrable changes in memory or executive functioning associable with the areas of structural damage, it may be appropriate to diagnose a secondary neuropsychiatric syndrome due to multifocal brain injury from multiple TBIs. Repeating the neuropsychological examination or cognitive testing in a year will help establish whether the condition is progressive or static.

Treatment is focused on addressing specific neuropsychiatric symptoms and optimizing brain health, beginning with treating any mood disorder or substance use disorder that is present. If there is apathy, impaired attention, pathological anger, or pseudobulbar affect after mood and substance use problems are addressed, these can be treated specifically using problem-specific rating scales to track the response to treatment. Optimizing brain health includes ensuring adequate nutrition and sufficient high-quality sleep, avoiding alcohol, and avoiding additional TBI. In football players, who often have a high body mass index, screening for sleep apnea is especially relevant. In older patients with possible CTE, the potential for a comorbid degenerative condition such as Alzheimer's disease should be considered, and an additional workup—for example, a CSF examination—might be done if the patient's symptoms progress.

Acute and Subacute Encephalitis, Meningoencephalitis, and Autoimmune Encephalopathy With Prominent Psychiatric Symptoms

Infectious encephalitis, meningoencephalitis, or autoimmune encephalopathy typically manifests with a combination of cognitive or memory impairment and altered behavior, including symptoms of psychosis or new-onset anxiety or mood symptoms, often preceded by or accompanied by headache or signs of a general medical illness, such as fever or abnormal laboratory tests. If the disease attacks the limbic system selectively, memory impairment and emotional and/or behavioral symptoms may be present in the absence of disorientation, confusion, or altered consciousness. Depending on the setting of care and the severity of the psychiatric symptoms relative to the cognitive and systemic ones, the patient will present either to a psychiatrist or to a nonpsychiatric physician. The patient comes to the psychiatrist either with or without a diagnosis of encephalitis (or encephalopathy). In the former case, the reason for the consultation is management of behavior or treatment of psychiatric symptoms and syndromes, such as psychosis, agitation, depression, anxiety, apathy, or pseudobulbar affect. In the latter case, the patient is suspected of having a primary psychiatric disorder, and the challenge for the psychiatrist is to initiate a timely and adequate workup for the underlying neurological condition. The prognosis for treatable CNS infections and for autoimmune encephalopathies is much better if treatment is instituted early. A consulting psychiatrist who has seen hundreds of cases of new-onset primary psychosis may be more able than a neurologist or internist to determine whether a patient's presentation is atypical for—or even inconsistent with—

primary psychiatric illness. Careful attention to pre-illness history, unexplained symptoms, and subtle neurological findings is important.

Acute infectious encephalitis usually manifests with some signs of general medical illness—fever and/or headache—in addition to mental status changes. Herpes simplex encephalitis, Western and Eastern equine encephalitis, and Zika virus encephalitis virtually always present in this way. Patients with subacute or chronic CNS infections such as fungal meningitis or cysticercosis can present without fever; the main presenting symptoms may be neuropsychiatric, and headache, if present, may be minor or may blend in with a lifetime headache history. Given that nearly half of the global adult population experiences some form of headache disorder (Stovner et al. 2007), a headache due to a new infection might not be differentiated by the patient. Therefore, the psychiatrist should ask the patient about headaches and, if they are present, should attempt to determine if they are different in any way from the patient's usual headaches. As with all neuropsychiatric symptoms that might be due to focal or multifocal lesions, the history should include questions about paroxysmal stereotyped symptoms that might be seizures. In the typical case, seizures have not been diagnosed at the time of the first psychiatric consultation, but they might be present. If the history is of frequent paroxysmal symptoms, long-term EEG monitoring may find diagnostic abnormalities that would not be seen on a routine EEG.

Because fungal meningitis, tuberculous meningitis, secondary syphilis, herpes simplex encephalitis (HSE), and cysticercosis all have efficacious specific treatments, it is important to look for them in a timely way if one or more of them are suspected. MRI followed by CSF examination with appropriate special testing (cultures, immunology, polymerase chain reaction testing) is the next step in the neurological workup. The psychiatrist should advocate for such testing if the pace and symptomatology of the patient's neuropsychiatric illness are atypical for primary psychiatric illness, if the patient has been systemically ill from an infectious agent that potentially involves the CNS, if the patient is immunosuppressed, or if the patient has been exposed to infectious agents that can attack people with normal immune systems and that are either epidemic or endemic in a place the patient has been. For example, if a patient has been to the American Southwest, coccidioidomycosis would be considered; if the patient has recently been to tropical areas, Zika virus would be more likely. Exposure to parasites that can invade the brain can occur in immigrants as well as travelers. Cysticercosis, the most common CNS parasitosis in developed countries, is most often seen in patients who have emigrated from countries or who are visiting from countries in which contaminated pork might be consumed. Concise guidelines for how to question returning travelers regarding exposure to CNS infectious agents were recently provided by Bharucha and Manji (2018).

Consulting psychiatrists usually work with a consistent population for whom the most common causes of CNS infection can be defined and thus focused on in history taking and in the diagnostic workup. In hospitals with a highly diverse patient population, the psychiatric consultant can keep lists of suspected agents that match with specific locales and subcultures. Narrowing the differential diagnosis from CNS infections in general to specific infections can facilitate the consultation process with neurologists and internists by focusing the workup and establishing the psychiatrist's value as a member of the medical team. By proposing specific and realistic possibilities for infectious agents and providing cogent symptomatic and contextual reasons for suspecting these agents, the psychiatrist can help ensure that the consulting physician is well equipped to conduct a timely and targeted workup.

Autoimmune encephalopathies can have purely psychiatric presentations, with no general medical symptoms or signs initially evident. For example, autoimmune encephalitis due to AMPA (α-amino-3-hydroxy-5-methyl-4-isoxazolepropionic acid) receptor antibodies can manifest with "Ophelia syndrome," in which the patient shows profound memory loss and may no longer recognize familiar people (Hermetter et al. 2018). Autoimmune encephalopathies are postinfectious and are associated with other autoimmune disease, paraneoplastic, or idiopathic. Finding autoantibodies to neurotransmitter receptors or to intraneuronal proteins in the CSF at levels disproportionate to any levels in the serum is diagnostic. However, they are found in only about half of cases, and when they are present in a patient's CSF, the results of testing might not be available for weeks following the lumbar puncture, thus arriving too late to inform crucial decisions about treatment. When a patient has a cancer known to cause paraneoplastic encephalopathy or has Hashimoto's thyroiditis, the serum would be tested for the characteristic antibodies—for example, γ-aminobutyric acid $(GABA)_B$-RI and anti-Hu in lung cancer (Shen et al. 2018); anti-Yo, anti-Ri, anti-amphiphysin, and anti-N-methyl-D-aspartate receptor (NMDAR) in ovarian cancer (Zaborowski et al. 2015); and antithyroid microsomal antibodies in Hashimoto's disease. If the antibodies were present in the serum and the patient had a characteristic syndrome for autoimmune encephalopathy, the latter would be treated along with treatment of the initiating medical condition. Another instance of secondary autoimmune encephalopathy is that associated with HSE: a patient develops HSE and is treated with antiviral agents, recovers well, and then has a relapse of encephalopathic symptoms. The likely cause is a postviral autoimmune condition, often associated with anti-NMDAR antibodies and treatable with corticosteroids or immune modulators. Psychiatrists get involved in this situation because a patient is thought to have recovered from HSE, and the recurrence of symptoms is attributed to late-occurring psychiatric effects of brain injury or a reaction triggered by the experience and consequences of having an acute, life-threatening illness. The subacute onset, progressiveness, cognitive dimension, possible seizure-like episodes by history or on EEG, and evidence on imaging of an active inflammatory process suggest the diagnosis. The psychiatrist should either initiate the imaging or EEG or refer the patient back to the neurologist with a recommendation, depending on the psychiatrist's personal expertise and the customs of the clinical setting (Hermetter et al. 2018).

If a patient with acute psychosis is admitted to a psychiatric service, the occurrence of a seizure, a new movement disorder, or a change in vital signs not associated with a medication side effect should prompt reconsideration of the diagnosis of an acute or subacute encephalopathy.

In an analysis of 464 cases of anti-NMDAR encephalitis that were individually described in the literature, the average age at illness onset was 27 years, and 79% of patients were female (Al-Diwani et al. 2019). Thirty-two percent of cases were attributed to ovarian teratoma. The most common psychiatric symptoms were agitation, aggression, depressed mood, mood instability, hallucinations, delusions, mutism, and irritability (Al-Diwani et al. 2019). When these symptoms were grouped into higher-level categories, five categories accounted for the greatest proportion of patient symptoms: behavioral disturbances (present in 68% of cases), psychosis (67%), mood symptoms

(47%), catatonia (30%), and sleep disturbances (21%). This mixed presentation and especially the overlap of mood and psychosis symptoms were distinctive findings of this analysis (Al-Diwani et al. 2019).

NMDA-associated psychiatric illness often develops rapidly, may have a viral prodrome (in up to 70% of cases), and is often accompanied by neurological symptoms, including movement abnormalities, short-term memory impairment, and confusion as the disease progresses (Warren et al. 2018). Agitation, aggression, and catatonia, particularly when fluctuating, were key findings in an analysis by Warren et al. (2018). Among the 464 patients with anti-NMDAR encephalitis in the Al-Diwani et al. (2019) study, 257 (62%) had abnormal EEG scans and 135 (32%) had abnormal findings on brain MRI. Neurological abnormalities that developed over time were movement disorders, including choreoathetoid movements; seizures; and hyporesponsiveness. Early treatment with immunotherapy has been reported to be beneficial (Titulaer et al. 2013). Diagnosis is confirmed by the presence of positive serum or especially CSF antibodies to the NMDAR subunit (Al-Diwani et al. 2019; Dalmau et al. 2011; Warren et al. 2018).

Encephalitis due to viruses or to tick-borne bacteria is considered when a patient's residence, recent travel, or lifestyle makes exposure to the pathogen a realistic possibility. Paraneoplastic autoimmune encephalopathy can be the initial presentation of a cancer, and a steroid-responsive encephalopathy can be the first presentation of Hashimoto's thyroiditis, also known as Hashimoto's encephalopathy, which is discussed elsewhere in this volume (see Chapter 7, "Endocrine Disorders and Their Psychiatric Manifestations").

When a previously high-functioning person develops symptoms of psychosis or markedly abnormal, unusual behavior over a period of several days, an underlying medical cause should be suspected. Nonetheless, sometimes such people seek emergency care and are summarily thought to be without medical illness or are not carefully investigated for the same, and are referred to a consulting psychiatrist. In addition to noting that a patient's history is atypical for primary psychiatric illness, the psychiatrist should assemble additional data to help with a correct diagnosis and should request neurological consultation. The consultation is more likely to produce a correct diagnosis if the stage has been set. In gathering the data, it is usually necessary to rely on one or more informants as well as the patient, because the patient often has impaired memory, may be fearful or delusional, or may be unable to cooperate with an interview.

A history of the patient's recent activities, residence, and travel should be obtained to identify potential exposures to infectious agents. Relevant infections can be either epidemic or endemic in places the patient has recently been. Sleep should be reviewed, focusing on any new insomnia, hypersomnia, parasomnia, nocturnal confusion, or unusual nighttime behavior. The patient or informant should be asked about symptoms suggestive of viral infection, such as fever, headache, muscle aches, or fatigue, over the preceding few weeks, including symptoms that appeared to resolve. A review of the patient's medical history, including electronic medical records if available, should include a search for diagnosed cancer, rheumatological disease, or endocrine disease as well as for nonspecific, not-yet-explained laboratory abnormalities.

If the patient will not see a neurologist promptly, the psychiatrist should conduct a neurological examination, focusing on areas that might have been omitted during the patient's prior medical evaluation. Parts of the neurological examination often omitted by non-neurologists in urgent care settings include testing of olfactory sensation (relevant to temporal lobe disease or dysfunction), examination of visual fields, evaluation of dysmetria of the eyes and limbs, sensitive testing of gait and balance, testing of lower-extremity sensation, and checking for frontal release signs such as grasp reflexes. It is common for a physician examining an acutely psychotic patients to note in some way that the patient's behavior made it hard to determine the plantar reflex with certainty (e.g.,"the Babinski sign was equivocal" or "the patient withdrew"). However, the presence of an extensor plantar reflex in a patient with no history of CNS disease can immediately reclassify the cause of the patient's disturbance as potentially neurological, making a big difference to subsequent care and potentially to the clinical outcome. For this reason, it is worth the effort to elicit a valid plantar reflex, even though it can be difficult in an agitated, confused, or uncooperative patient. If the patient's withdrawal prevents ascertainment of a plantar response by stimulating the sole of the foot, the examiner can use an alternative mode of stimulation, such as stroking the lateral dorsum of the foot distally from the ankle (an extensor plantar reflex obtained with this stimulus is known as Chaddock's sign (Singerman and Lee 2008).

When working in a setting where neurological consultation is not easily obtained but EEG and MRI are available, getting these tests is useful, because limbic encephalitis is associated with characteristic abnormalities on these tests. If an abnormality typical of encephalitis is found by either modality, it will motivate and focus further diagnostic testing, including targeted examination of the CSF. In autoimmune encephalitis due to anti-NMDAR antibodies (the most common type of autoimmune encephalitis, also discussed elsewhere in this volume [see Chapter 8, "Inflammatory Diseases and Their Psychiatric Manifestations"]), the EEG shows a "brush" pattern of high-frequency activity superimposed on high-voltage delta waves. Any EEG abnormality, even a nonspecific one, will support reconsideration of the general medical/neurological dimension of the patient's illness. (See also Chapter 4, "Neuroimaging, Electroencephalography, and Lumbar Puncture in Medical Psychiatry.")

It has been increasingly noted that half or more of cases of encephalitis in high-income countries are autoimmune rather than infectious (Dubey et al. 2018a, 2018b). Autoimmune encephalitis does not necessarily entail fever or alteration in consciousness. However, because it typically affects the temporal lobes and the limbic system, autoimmune encephalitis consistently involves alterations in memory, with loss of working memory a consistent finding and loss of long-term memory seen in many cases. If the loss of working memory is of subacute onset (i.e., developing over a period less than 3 months) and is accompanied by one or more of the following—new focal neurological signs, seizures, an MRI suggestive of encephalitis, or CSF pleocytosis—and if alternative causes have been reasonably excluded, the diagnosis would be possible autoimmune encephalitis (Graus et al. 2016). If an MRI shows T2 lesions restricted to the medial temporal regions or an EEG shows temporal lobe slow-wave or epileptiform activity, the diagnosis would be probable autoimmune limbic encephalitis. Confirming the presence of specific antibodies in the CSF or the serum to identify the cause is not required for the diagnosis, because in many cases no such antibodies can be identified (Graus et al. 2016).

Brain Dysfunction and Psychiatric Symptoms in Treated HIV Infections

Before effective antiviral therapy for HIV was available, and HIV inevitably culminated in death from AIDS, it was common to see a progressive dementia due to HIV infection. The condition was called AIDS dementia complex or HIV encephalopathy. In the current era, HIV infection is treated with combined antiretroviral therapy (cART), HIV titers are suppressed, CD4 counts are maintained, and HIV-associated dementia affects less than 5% of patients treated for HIV. However, even when HIV cannot be detected in peripheral blood, up to 50% of patients experience brain dysfunction related to the persistence of the HIV in the brain and its downstream effects on the immune system—termed HIV-associated neurocognitive disorder (HAND) (Chan and Brew 2014; Eggers et al. 2017). HAND impacts the health-related quality of life of HIV patients, and it can affect adherence to cART and consequently its effectiveness. The disorder has three forms: 1) asymptomatic, with measurable impairment in two neuropsychological domains but no impairment in social or instrumental functioning; 2) mild, with measurable impairment in two domains accompanied by mild impairment in social or instrumental functioning; and 3) HIV-associated dementia, with cognitive performance at least two standard deviations below the mean on standardized testing and marked interference with day-to-day functioning.

The typical early symptoms of HAND are impaired memory, concentration, and executive function. Onset is insidious, and progression is gradual. Eventually patients develop changes in mood and behavior, such as depression and irritability. Seizures develop in about 5%–10% of patients as the disease progresses (Eggers et al. 2017). Patients with HAND have impaired metacognition. Early in the disease course, patients tend to minimize cognitive deficits or their functional impact; if they become depressed, they may catastrophize them.

HAND is more likely to occur in patients whose CD4 counts were already low at cART initiation. Other risk factors are lower education, older age, and higher plasma levels of tumor necrosis factor-α and monocyte chemoattractant protein-1 (Eggers et al. 2017). HAND can progress when there is no detectable virus in the CSF. It is hypothesized that HIV infection persists in CNS monocytes and macrophages, causing them to release markers of inflammation and creating a persistent inflammatory state (Clifford 2017). Prompt initiation of cART may prevent or delay the development of HAND, but numerous patients develop HAND despite prompt institution of cART. It is possible but not confirmed that cART agents with better brain penetration will be more efficacious in preventing, arresting, or reversing HAND. In any case, progression of the symptoms and signs of HAND should prompt reconsideration of the patient's cART.

When a psychiatrist consults on the care of a patient with HIV, the possibility of HAND should always be considered. Bearing in mind that patients with early HAND may deny or minimize their deficits, or simply be unaware of them, an evaluation should include sensitive testing of cognition and, if possible, information from a collateral source about the patient's functional performance. If new cognitive impairment is found, the response differs according to how rapidly it developed. If the impairment is subacute (i.e., developing over less than a month), the patient needs a full neurological workup for a secondary cause of the cognitive changes, including the possibility of an opportunistic infection of the CNS. If the impairment developed more slowly, the more important clinical question is whether the patient's cART is adequate. Treatment adherence and potential barriers to it should be assessed by the psychiatrist. If the patient appears to be taking medication as prescribed, the consulting psychiatrist should inform the principal physician treating the HIV infection that the patient's neurological impairment has progressed despite the currently prescribed antiviral therapy. The treating physician's expected response is to assess the patient's current viral load in the serum and CSF, and to switch to a different cART if the current antiretroviral regimen has not adequately suppressed HIV titers.

Because patients with HAND usually have impaired metacognition, the psychiatrist should consider the question of whether the patient's current activities and responsibilities are appropriate given his or her current cognitive state. In this respect, considerations regarding work, driving, and financial management are similar to those that arise with a patient in the early stages of a dementing illness.

Treatments for depression, apathy, cognitive fatigue, or impaired concentration in patients with HAND are managed with a focus on alleviating symptoms while minimizing side effects. In most cases of symptomatic neuropsychiatric treatment, medications will be used off-label, making it especially important to obtain informed consent and to regularly and systematically measure the symptom or syndrome being treated. Cholinesterase inhibitors, memantine, and stimulants have not proved efficacious for treating the cognitive dysfunction of HAND. Notwithstanding, it would be rational to consider using a stimulant to treat a patient with HAND and severe mental and physical fatigue or to consider using donepezil in an HIV patient older than 70 years who might well have concomitant Alzheimer's disease pathology.

Movement Disorders: Parkinson's Disease and Essential Tremor

The two most prevalent movement disorders in adults are Parkinson's disease and essential tremor. The primary signs of Parkinson's disease are resting tremor, rigidity, and bradykinesia. The frequency of the resting tremor is approximately 3 Hz. A diagnosis of "clinically established" Parkinson's disease requires at least two supportive criteria and no exclusionary criteria (Postuma et al. 2015). Supportive criteria include asymmetry of the resting tremor, olfactory loss, evidence of cardiac sympathetic denervation, and a positive response to treatment with levodopa or a dopamine agonist. Exclusionary criteria include current treatment with a dopamine antagonist drug, cerebellar abnormalities, signs of frontotemporal dementia, supranuclear gaze palsy, and lack of a response to a dopamine agonist or levodopa. When the diagnosis of Parkinson's disease is likely but not firmly established, a single-photon emission computed tomography (SPECT) scan to image the dopamine transmitter ("DaT scan") can help settle the issue by demonstrating a loss of dopaminergic neurons in the midbrain. The prevalence of Parkinson's disease is 1–2 per 1,000 in the general population (Tysnes and Storstein 2017). The prevalence is approximately 1% among people older than 60 years and approximately 4% in the oldest patients. Parkinson's disease is unusual in people younger than 50 years (Tysnes and Storstein 2017).

Essential tremor is a persistent visible bilateral, largely symmetric kinetic tremor of gradual onset involving the hands and forearms; the frequency ranges from 4 to 12 Hz, with higher frequencies in younger people. It is sometimes accompanied by postural tremor or tremor of the head. The prevalence of essential tremor in the United States is estimated to be seven million, or about 2.2% of the population (Louis and Ottman 2014). The prevalence increases with age; more than 4% of people older than 40 years have the condition (Louis 2011). Thus, essential tremor is many times more prevalent than Parkinson's disease and affects many more people of working age.

Parkinson's disease is associated with an increased prevalence of depression, anxiety, apathy, and cognitive impairment. A systematic review of prevalence studies of depressive disorders in patients with Parkinson's disease found a prevalence of 17% for MDD, 22% for minor depression, and 13% for dysthymia (Reijnders et al. 2008). Estimates of the prevalence of clinical anxiety—GAD, panic disorder, or phobia—in Parkinson's disease range from 25% to 40% (Pfeiffer 2016). Apathy affects 40% of patients with Parkinson's disease (Pfeiffer 2016). Parkinson's disease is accompanied by progressive cognitive impairment, although cognition can be normal for several years while the patient has significant motor symptoms. Early in the illness, approximately 25% of patients have mild cognitive impairment; among those who survive 20 years with Parkinson's disease, the prevalence of dementia is 80% (Pfeiffer 2016). Sexual dysfunction is experienced by most patients with Parkinson's disease; men have erectile dysfunction, difficulty reaching orgasm, or premature ejaculation, and women have reduced desire or difficulties with arousal and orgasm. Sexual dysfunction in Parkinson's disease can adversely affect self-esteem and marital relationships. The rate of death by suicide in Parkinson's disease was estimated at twice the rate of the general population in a South Korean study (Lee et al. 2016). The increase in suicide rate observed is compatible with the increased rate of suicide attempts in Parkinson's disease patients found in the Danish study cited earlier (Eliasen et al. 2018).

The syndromes of depression, anxiety, and apathy are treated in patients with Parkinson's disease much as they would be in patients without Parkinson's disease, with two important exceptions. Antipsychotic drugs are avoided to the greatest feasible extent because they predictably exacerbate the symptoms of Parkinson's disease. Thus, for example, the preferred treatment for melancholia with delusions in a patient with Parkinson's disease would be ECT rather than drug treatment with an antidepressant-antipsychotic combination. ECT can *improve* motor function in this situation (Grover et al. 2018), whereas even a second-generation antipsychotic drug will make it worse. When antidepressants are prescribed, bupropion, SNRIs, or TCAs may be more efficacious than SSRIs (Peña et al. 2018), although head-to-head comparison trials have not been done. When treating anxiety, benzodiazepines will not worsen the principal symptoms of Parkinson's disease and can help kinetic tremors (as opposed to resting tremor of Parkinson's disease), but they can exacerbate cognitive dysfunction and can increase fall risk. Because of their greater susceptibility to psychotropic drug side effects, patients with Parkinson's disease should receive frequent follow-up contacts—via either in-person visits or online communication—after any change in their psychotropic drug regimen; as a general rule, the lowest effective dosages of psychotropic agents should be utilized.

As mentioned previously (see section "Impulsive-Compulsive Syndrome of Parkinson's Disease" earlier in this chapter), Parkinson's disease is associated with three characteristic psychiatric syndromes: apathy, impulsive-compulsive behavior linked to dopamine agonist therapy, and Parkinson's disease psychosis. Apathy, distinguishable from depression (it is not associated with a negative mood and pessimistic thoughts unless depression is also present) and measurable with the AES, can be treated with a dopamine agonist such as pramipexole, a monoamine oxidase B inhibitor such as rasagiline, a stimulant, or modafinil. While all of these agents have a rationale, none has been established as a standard of care.

Impulsive-compulsive behavioral syndromes, distinguishable from hypomania (no euphoria) and from primary behavioral addictions (timing and severity linked to dopamine agonist dosage), can be identified using the QUIP as a screening tool. The QUIP can be used subsequently to measure the response of the impulsive-compulsive syndrome to changes in drug therapy or to behavioral therapy or environmental interventions. Treatment of impulsive-compulsive syndromes involves reduction in the dosage of dopamine agonists together with behavior therapy or environmental modification.

Parkinson's disease psychosis is a distinctive condition of gradual onset in patients with long-term Parkinson's disease. It comprises some combination of delusions, visual hallucinations, illusions, and a false sense of presence (e.g., feeling that one is not alone when in fact one is) in the absence of delirium or a primary psychotic disorder. Insight into the psychosis is variable; some individuals remain fully aware that their hallucinations and illusions are false. The FDA-approved treatment specific for Parkinson's disease psychosis is pimavanserin, a $5\text{-}HT_{2A}$ receptor inverse agonist. Pimavanserin does not block dopamine receptors or worsen the motor symptoms of Parkinson's disease. It is given at a fixed dosage of 34 mg/day. It takes 4–6 weeks to have its full therapeutic effect. Not all patients with Parkinson's disease psychosis respond to pimavanserin, and the outcome may not be clear for at least 4 weeks. The drug prolongs the QT interval and is metabolized by CYP3A4; both of these characteristics must be considered when the patient has multiple comorbid medical conditions and is on several other drugs. The other treatment for Parkinson's disease psychosis supported by multiple controlled studies is clozapine, which is initiated at the low dosage of 6.25 mg/day and titrated up slowly as tolerated. Clozapine may show some antipsychotic effects sooner than pimavanserin, but the time needed for dosage titration makes the time to improvement comparable. Patients may respond to one drug and not to the other, and there is no way to know in advance which drug would work better for a given patient (Black 2017).

Second-generation antipsychotic drugs, especially quetiapine and olanzapine, are sometimes used to treat Parkinson's disease psychosis. No atypical antipsychotic drug other than clozapine has been demonstrated to be superior to placebo in treating psychosis associated with Parkinson's disease, and all of these drugs can worsen motor function and/or increase mortality risk. Notwithstanding, quetiapine at the low dosage of 25 mg/day often is given first for Parkinson's disease psychosis because of the high cost of pimavanserin and the burdensome monitoring associated with clozapine (Chen et al. 2019; Moreno et al. 2018; Zhang et al. 2019).

Essential tremor was once regarded as an isolated motor syndrome without neuropsychiatric accompaniments. It is now known to be associated with an increased risk of MDD—with about one-third of affected patients having moderate or severe depression (Louis et al. 2016)—as well as an increased risk of mild cognitive impairment or progressive dementia when it occurs in older people (Lee et al. 2015). Essential tremor can significantly impair function, with spilled drinks and illegible handwriting being two examples, and it is an unpleasant subjective experience. In a study comparing the experience of essential tremor patients with that of Parkinson's disease patients, the former experienced themselves as being tremulous for a median of 10 hours a day, in contrast to the latter, who experienced themselves as being tremulous for a median of 3 hours a day (Louis 2016). In patients with essential tremor, depression is more closely associated with embarrassment over the tremor than with the severity of the tremor (Louis et al. 2016).

The first-line treatments for essential tremor are propranolol, a β-blocker; primidone, a barbiturate; and topiramate, an antiepileptic drug. Both β-blockers and barbiturates are associated with depression as an adverse effect as well as with risks for respiratory difficulties in individuals with risk factors or in the case of barbiturate abuse. Sedation and fatigue are related symptoms of psychiatric relevance. These symptoms are less likely to occur if the treatment is begun at a low dosage and gradually increased. Several other drugs are used off-label to treat essential tremor. While benzodiazepines can give partial relief for many patients, sedation and adverse effects on balance and cognition are problematic, especially for older patients with mild cognitive impairment or increased fall risk. Devices worn on the forearm that counteract the tremor are used to improve function in patients with moderate to severe tremor who obtain insufficient relief from medications. In the most severe cases, essential tremor can be reduced by unilateral thalamotomy. This ablative procedure can be performed noninvasively using MRI-guided ultrasound focused on the ventral intermediate nucleus (Health Quality Ontario 2018).

Many of the antidepressant drugs that might be used to treat depression in patients with essential tremor can worsen the tremor. Nonpharmacological treatments such as one of the psychotherapies, brain stimulation therapies such as TMS or ECT, or nutritional therapies might be better tolerated. If the patient has bipolar disorder, an antiepileptic drug such as valproate might be better tolerated than lithium for mood stabilization. Of note, psychiatrists treating patients with essential tremor should be aware that patients who are embarrassed by the condition, continually aware of their involuntary movements, and functionally compromised—for example, unable to eat or drink without spilling—can be very distressed, and that marked improvement in essential tremor with neurosurgery can be life changing.

References

Al-Diwani A, Handel A, Townsend L, et al: The psychopathology of NMDAR-antibody encephalitis in adults: a systematic review and phenotypic analysis of individual patient data. Lancet Psychiatry 6(3):235–246, 2019 30765329

American Psychiatric Association: Diagnostic and Statistical Manual of Mental Disorders, 5th Edition. Arlington, VA, American Psychiatric Association, 2013

Angst J, Adolfsson R, Benazzi F, et al: The HCL-32: towards a self-assessment tool for hypomanic symptoms in outpatients. J Affect Disord 88(2):217–233, 2005 16125784

Artemiadis AK, Anagnostouli MC, Alexopoulos EC: Stress as a risk factor for multiple sclerosis onset or relapse: a systematic review. Neuroepidemiology 36(2):109–120, 2011 21335982

Baldassari LE, Fox RJ: Therapeutic advances and challenges in the treatment of progressive multiple sclerosis. Drugs 78(15):1549–1566, 2018 30255442

Barker-Collo S, Jones K, Theadom A, et al; BIONIC Research Group: Neuropsychological outcome and its correlates in the first year after adult mild traumatic brain injury: a population-based New Zealand study. Brain Inj 29(13–14):1604–1616, 2015 26382561

Bear DM: Temporal lobe epilepsy—a syndrome of sensory-limbic hyperconnection. Cortex 15(3):357–384, 1979 540509

Bear DM, Fedio P: Quantitative analysis of interictal behavior in temporal lobe epilepsy. Arch Neurol 34(8):454–467, 1977 889477

Berkovich RR: Acute multiple sclerosis relapse. Continuum (Minneap Minn) 22(3):799–814, 2016 27261683

Bernitsas E, Khan O, Razmjou S, et al: Cerebrospinal fluid humoral immunity in the differential diagnosis of multiple sclerosis. PLoS One 12(7):e0181431, 2017 28727770

Bezzini D, Pepe P, Profili F, et al: Multiple sclerosis spatial cluster in Tuscany. Neurol Sci 38(12):2183–2187, 2017 29019004

Bharucha T, Manji H: "Montezuma's revenge": neurological disorders in the returning traveller. Pract Neurol 18(5):359–368, 2018 30042219

Bieniek KF, Ross OA, Cormier KA, et al: Chronic traumatic encephalopathy pathology in a neurodegenerative disorders brain bank. Acta Neuropathol 130(6):877–889, 2015 26518018

Bikson M, Grossman P, Thomas C, et al: Safety of transcranial direct current stimulation: evidence-based update 2016. Brain Stimul 9(5):641–661, 2016 27372845

Bivard A, Lillicrap T, Krishnamurthy V, et al: MIDAS (modafinil in debilitating fatigue after stroke): a randomized, double-blind, placebo-controlled, cross-over trial. Stroke 48(5):1293–1298, 2017 28404841

Black KJ: Treatment of Parkinson's disease psychosis. Med Int Rev 27(109):266–271, 2017 30140115

Blanchet P, Frommer GP: Mood change preceding epileptic seizures. J Nerv Ment Dis 174(8):471–476, 1986 3734769

Blumer D, Montouris G, Davies K: The interictal dysphoric disorder: recognition, pathogenesis, and treatment of the major psychiatric disorder of epilepsy. Epilepsy Behav 5(6):826–840, 2004 15582829

Boylan LS, Flint LA, Labovitz DL, et al: Depression but not seizure frequency predicts quality of life in treatment-resistant epilepsy. Neurology 62(2):258–261, 2004 14745064

Brola W, Sobolewski P, Zak M, et al: Profile of Polish patients with primary progressive multiple sclerosis. Mult Scler Relat Disord 33:33–38, 2019 31146082

Buranee K, Teeradej S, Chusak L, et al: Epilepsy-related psychoses and psychotic symptoms are significantly reduced by resective epilepsy surgery and are not associated with surgery outcome or epilepsy characteristics: a cohort study. Psychiatry Res 245:333–339, 2016 27573056

Buse DC, Manack AN, Fanning KM, et al: Chronic migraine prevalence, disability, and sociodemographic factors: results from the American Migraine Prevalence and Prevention Study. Headache 52(10):1456–1470, 2012 22830411

Buse DC, Silberstein SD, Manack AN, et al: Psychiatric comorbidities of episodic and chronic migraine. J Neurol 260(8):1960–1969, 2013 23132299

Buss AH, Perry M: The aggression questionnaire. J Pers Soc Psychol 63(3):452–459, 1992 1403624

Buysse DJ, Reynolds CF 3rd, Monk TH, et al: The Pittsburgh Sleep Quality Index: a new instrument for psychiatric practice and research. Psychiatry Res 28(2):193–213, 1989 2748771

Callesen MB, Weintraub D, Damholdt MF, Møller A: Impulsive and compulsive behaviors among Danish patients with Parkinson's disease: prevalence, depression, and personality. Parkinsonism Relat Disord 20(1):22–26, 2014 24090948

Camara-Lemarroy CR, Ibarra-Yruegas BE, Rodriguez-Gutierrez R, et al: The varieties of psychosis in multiple sclerosis: a systematic review of cases. Mult Scler Relat Disord 12:9–14, 2017 28283114

Centers for Disease Control and Prevention: Report to Congress on Traumatic Brain Injury in the United States: Epidemiology and Rehabilitation. Atlanta, GA, National Center for Injury Prevention and Control; Division of Unintentional Injury Prevention, 2015. Available at: https://www.cdc.gov/traumaticbraininjury/pdf/TBI_Report_to_-Congress_Epi_and_Rehab-a.pdf. Accessed September 29, 2018.

Centers for Disease Control and Prevention: Traumatic Brain Injury & Concussion (web page). Page last reviewed: March 4, 2019. Atlanta, GA, Centers for Disease Control and Prevention, National Center for Injury Prevention and Control. Available at: https://www.cdc.gov/traumaticbraininjury/. Accessed November 1, 2019.

Chan D, Binks S, Nicholas JM, et al: Effect of high-dose simvastatin on cognitive, neuropsychiatric, and health-related quality-of-life measures in secondary progressive multiple sclerosis: secondary analyses from the MS-STAT randomised, placebo-controlled trial. Lancet Neurol 16(8):591–600, 2017 28600189

Chan P, Brew BJ: HIV associated neurocognitive disorders in the modern antiviral treatment era: prevalence, characteristics, biomarkers, and effects of treatment. Curr HIV/AIDS Rep 11(3):317–324, 2014 24966139

Chen B, Choi H, Hirsch LJ, et al: Psychiatric and behavioral side effects of antiepileptic drugs in adults with epilepsy. Epilepsy Behav 76:24–31, 2017 28931473

Chen JJ, Hua H, Massihi L, et al: Systematic literature review of quetiapine for the treatment of psychosis in patients with parkinsonism. J Neuropsychiatry Clin Neurosci 31(3):188–195, 2019 30848989

Christensen J, Vestergaard M, Mortensen PB, et al: Epilepsy and risk of suicide: a population-based case-control study. Lancet Neurol 6(8):693–698, 2007 17611160

Ciotti JR, Cross AH: Disease modifying treatment in progressive multiple sclerosis. Curr Treat Options Neurol 20(5):12, 2018 29627873

Clarke DE, Ko JY, Kuhl EA, et al: Are the available apathy measures reliable and valid? A review of the psychometric evidence. J Psychosom Res 70(1):73–97, 2011 21193104

Clifford DB: HIV-associated neurocognitive disorder. Curr Opin Infect Dis 30(1):117–122, 2017 27798498

Cummings JL, Mega M, Gray K, et al: The Neuropsychiatric Inventory: comprehensive assessment of psychopathology in dementia. Neurology 44(12):2308–2314, 1994 7991117

Dallmeier JD, Meysami S, Merrill DA, Raji CA: Emerging advances of in vivo detection of chronic traumatic encephalopathy and traumatic brain injury. Br J Radiol 92(1101):20180925, 2019 31287716

Dalmau J, Lancaster E, Martinez-Hernandez E, et al: Clinical experience and laboratory investigations in patients with anti-NMDAR encephalitis. Lancet Neurol 10(1):63–74, 2011 21163445

Devinsky O, Abramson H, Alper K, et al: Postictal psychosis: a case control series of 20 patients and 150 controls. Epilepsy Res 20(3):247–253, 1995 7796797

Dias Alves M, Micoulaud-Franchi JA, Simon N, et al: Electroencephalogram modifications associated with atypical strict antipsychotic monotherapies. J Clin Psychopharmacol 38(6):555–562, 2018 30247179

Diaz-Olavarrieta C, Cummings JL, Velazquez J, et al: Neuropsychiatric manifestations of multiple sclerosis. J Neuropsychiatry Clin Neurosci 11(1):51–57, 1999 9990556

Druschky K, Bleich S, Grohmann R, et al: Seizure rates under treatment with antipsychotic drugs: data from the AMSP project. World J Biol Psychiatry, 2018 [Epub ahead of print] 30058414

Dubey D, Pittock SJ, Kelly CR, et al: Autoimmune encephalitis epidemiology and a comparison to infectious encephalitis. Ann Neurol 83(1):166–177, 2018a 29293273

Dubey D, Toledano M, McKeon A: Clinical presentation of autoimmune and viral encephalitides. Curr Opin Crit Care 24(2):80–90, 2018b 29401173

Ducharme S, Murray ED, Seiner SJ, et al: Retrospective analysis of the short-term safety of ECT in patients with neurological comorbidities: a guide for pre-ECT neurological evaluations. J Neuropsychiatry Clin Neurosci 27(4):311–321, 2015 25658682

Eggers C, Arendt G, Hahn K, et al: HIV-1-associated neurocognitive disorder: epidemiology, pathogenesis, diagnosis, and treatment. J Neurol 264(8):1715–1727, 2017 28567537

Ehlers DK, Fanning J, Salerno EA, et al: Replacing sedentary time with physical activity or sleep: effects on cancer-related cognitive impairment in breast cancer survivors. BMC Cancer 18(1):685, 2018 29940894

Eliasen A, Dalhoff KP, Horwitz H: Neurological diseases and risk of suicide attempt: a case-control study. J Neurol 265(6):1303–1309, 2018 29564603

Erga AH, Alves G, Larsen JP, et al: Impulsive and compulsive behaviors in Parkinson's disease: the Norwegian ParkWest study. J Parkinsons Dis 7(1):183–191, 2017 27911342

Eriksson M, Glader E-L, Norrving B, et al: Poststroke suicide attempts and completed suicides: a socioeconomic and nationwide perspective. Neurology 84(17):1732–1738, 2015 25832661

Everson-Rose SA, Roetker NS, Lutsey PL, et al: Chronic stress, depressive symptoms, anger, hostility, and risk of stroke and transient ischemic attack in the multi-ethnic study of atherosclerosis. Stroke 45(8):2318–2323, 2014 25013018

First MB, Spitzer RL, Gibbon M, Williams JBW: Structured Clinical Interview for DSM-IV Clinical Version (SCID-I/CV). Washington, DC, American Psychiatric Press, 1997

Folstein MF, Folstein SE, McHugh PR: "Mini-mental state." A practical method for grading the cognitive state of patients for the clinician. J Psychiatr Res 12(3):189–198, 1975 1202204

Fregni F, Schachter SC, Pascual-Leone A: Transcranial magnetic stimulation treatment for epilepsy: can it also improve depression and vice versa? Epilepsy Behav 7(2):182–189, 2005 16054872

Friedman DE, Kung DH, Laowattana S, et al: Identifying depression in epilepsy in a busy clinical setting is enhanced with systematic screening. Seizure 18(6):429–433, 2009 19409813

Gandy M, Sharpe L, Perry KN, et al: Assessing the efficacy of 2 screening measures for depression in people with epilepsy. Neurology 79(4):371–375, 2012 22786594

Gasim M, Bernstein CN, Graff LA, et al; CIHR team "Defining the burden and managing the effects of psychiatric comorbidity in chronic inflammatory disease": Adverse psychiatric effects of disease-modifying therapies in multiple sclerosis: a systematic review. Mult Scler Relat Disord 26:124–156, 2018 30248593

Geschwind N: Personality changes in temporal lobe epilepsy. Epilepsy Behav 15(4):425–433, 2009 19643670

Gholamzad M, Ebtekar M, Ardestani MS, et al: A comprehensive review on the treatment approaches of multiple sclerosis: currently and in the future. Inflamm Res 68(1):25–38, 2019 30178100

Gill SJ, Lukmanji S, Fiest KM, et al: Depression screening tools in persons with epilepsy: a systematic review of validated tools. Epilepsia 58(5):695–705, 2017 28064446

Grand'Maison F, Yeung M, Morrow SA, et al: Sequencing of high-efficacy disease-modifying therapies in multiple sclerosis: perspectives and approaches. Neural Regen Res 13(11):1871–1874, 2018 30233054

Graus F, Titulaer MJ, Balu R, et al: A clinical approach to diagnosis of autoimmune encephalitis. Lancet Neurol 15(4):391–404, 2016 26906964

Grover S, Somani A, Sahni N, et al: Effectiveness of electroconvulsive therapy (ECT) in parkinsonian symptoms: a case series. Innov Clin Neurosci 15(1–2):23–27, 2018 29497576

Hadidi NN, Huna Wagner RL, Lindquist R: Nonpharmacological treatments for post-stroke depression: an integrative review of the literature. Res Gerontol Nurs 10(4):182–195, 2017 28556875

Harrison RA, Field TS: Post stroke pain: identification, assessment, and therapy. Cerebrovasc Dis 39(3–4):190–201, 2015 25766121

Hayter AL, Salkovskis PM, Silber E, et al: The impact of health anxiety in patients with relapsing remitting multiple sclerosis: misperception, misattribution and quality of life. Br J Clin Psychol 55(4):371–386, 2016 26806805

Health Quality Ontario: Magnetic resonance-guided focused ultrasound neurosurgery for essential tremor: a health technology assessment. Ont Health Technol Assess Ser 18(4):1–141, 2018 29805721

Hermetter C, Fazekas F, Hochmeister S: Systematic review: syndromes, early diagnosis, and treatment in autoimmune encephalitis. Front Neurol 9:706, 2018 30233481

Hesdorffer DC, Ishihara L, Mynepalli L, et al: Epilepsy, suicidality, and psychiatric disorders: a bidirectional association. Ann Neurol 72(2):184–191, 2012 22887468

Hirschfeld RM, Williams JB, Spitzer RL, et al: Development and validation of a screening instrument for bipolar spectrum disorder: the Mood Disorder Questionnaire. Am J Psychiatry 157(11):1873–1875, 2000 11058490

Hoang H, Laursen B, Stenager EN, et al: Psychiatric co-morbidity in multiple sclerosis: the risk of depression and anxiety before and after MS diagnosis. Mult Scler 22(3):347–353, 2016 26041803

Hou Y, Jia Y, Hou J: Natural course of clinically isolated syndrome: a longitudinal analysis using a Markov model. Sci Rep 8(1):10857, 2018 30022111

Igra MS, Paling D, Wattjes MP, et al: Multiple sclerosis update: use of MRI for early diagnosis, disease monitoring and assessment of treatment related complications. Br J Radiol 90(1074):20160721, 2017 28362522

Isenberg-Grzeda E, Huband H, Lam H: A review of cognitive screening tools in cancer. Curr Opin Support Palliat Care 11(1):24–31, 2017 28009651

Johansson S, Kottorp A, Lee KA, et al: Can the Fatigue Severity Scale 7-item version be used across different patient populations as a generic fatigue measure? A comparative study using a Rasch model approach. Health Qual Life Outcomes 12:24, 2014 24559076

Judge BS, Rentmeester LL: Antidepressant overdose-induced seizures. Neurol Clin 29(3):565–580, 2011 21803210

Kalincik T: Multiple sclerosis relapses: epidemiology, outcomes and management. A systematic review. Neuroepidemiology 44(4):199–214, 2015 25997994

Kanner AM: Depression in epilepsy: prevalence, clinical semiology, pathogenic mechanisms, and treatment. Biol Psychiatry 54(3):388–398, 2003 12893113

Kanner AM, Trimble M, Schmitz B: Postictal affective episodes. Epilepsy Behav 19(2):156–158, 2010 20817613

Kappos L, Kuhle J, Multanen J, et al: Factors influencing long-term outcomes in relapsing-remitting multiple sclerosis: PRISMS-15. J Neurol Neurosurg Psychiatry 86(11):1202–1207, 2015 26374702

Katz DI, Cohen SI, Alexander MP: Mild traumatic brain injury. Handb Clin Neurol 127:131–156, 2015 25702214

Kaufer DI, Cummings JL, Ketchel P, et al: Validation of the NPI-Q, a brief clinical form of the Neuropsychiatric Inventory. J Neuropsychiatry Clin Neurosci 12(2):233–239, 2000 11001602

King NS, Crawford S, Wenden FJ, et al: The Rivermead Post Concussion Symptoms Questionnaire: a measure of symptoms commonly experienced after head injury and its reliability. J Neurol 242(9):587–592, 1995 8551320

Kingwell E, Marriott JJ, Jetté N, et al: Incidence and prevalence of multiple sclerosis in Europe: a systematic review. BMC Neurol 13:128, 2013 24070256

Kivilcim Y, Altintas M, Domac FM, et al: Screening for bipolar disorder among migraineurs: the impact of migraine-bipolar disorder comorbidity on disease characteristics. Neuropsychiatr Dis Treat 13:631–641, 2017 28280345

Korngold C, Farrell HM, Fozdar M: The National Football League and chronic traumatic encephalopathy: legal implications. J Am Acad Psychiatry Law 41(3):430–436, 2013 24051597

Krishnamoorthy ES, Trimble MR: Forced normalization: clinical and therapeutic relevance. Epilepsia 40 (suppl 10):S57–S64, 1999 10609605

Krivoy A, Stubbs B, Balicer RD, et al: Low adherence to antidepressants is associated with increased mortality following stroke: a large nationally representative cohort study. Eur Neuropsychopharmacol 27(10):970–976, 2017 28886897

Kroenke K, Spitzer RL, Williams JB: The PHQ-9: validity of a brief depression severity measure. J Gen Intern Med 16(9):606–613, 2001 11556941

Krupp LB, LaRocca NG, Muir-Nash J, et al: The fatigue severity scale. Application to patients with multiple sclerosis and systemic lupus erythematosus. Arch Neurol 46(10):1121–1123, 1989 2803071

La Mantia L, Munari LM, Lovati R: Glatiramer acetate for multiple sclerosis. Cochrane Database Syst Rev (5):CD004678, 2010 20464733

Laakso SM, Viitala M, Kuusisto H, et al: Multiple sclerosis in Finland 2018—data from the national register. Acta Neurol Scand 140(5):303–311, 2019 31271648

Lascano AM, Lalive PH, Hardmeier M, et al: Clinical evoked potentials in neurology: a review of techniques and indications. J Neurol Neurosurg Psychiatry 88(8):688–696, 2017 28235778

Lee SM, Kim M, Lee HM, et al: Nonmotor symptoms in essential tremor: comparison with Parkinson's disease and normal control. J Neurol Sci 349(1–2):168–173, 2015 25641389

Lee T, Lee HB, Ahn MH, et al: Increased suicide risk and clinical correlates of suicide among patients with Parkinson's disease. Parkinsonism Relat Disord 32:102–107, 2016 27637284

Leo RJ, Singh J: Migraine headache and bipolar disorder comorbidity: a systematic review of the literature and clinical implications. Scand J Pain 11:136 145, 2016 28850455

Leocani L, Comi G: Clinical neurophysiology of multiple sclerosis. Handb Clin Neurol 122:671–679, 2014 24507539

Leray E, Moreau T, Fromont A, Edan G: Epidemiology of multiple sclerosis. Rev Neurol (Paris) 172(1):3–13, 2016 26718593

Lindsley CW: Chronic traumatic encephalopathy (CTE): a brief historical overview and recent focus on NFL players. ACS Chem Neurosci 8(8):1629–1631, 2017 28810748

Lo Fermo S, Barone R, Patti F, et al: Outcome of psychiatric symptoms presenting at onset of multiple sclerosis: a retrospective study. Mult Scler 16(6):742–748, 2010 20350959

Loder F, Rizzoli P: Pharmacologic prevention of migraine: a narrative review of the state of the art in 2018. Headache 58 (suppl 3):218–229, 2018 30137671

Louis ED: Essential tremor. Handb Clin Neurol 100:433–448, 2011 21496600

Louis ED: More time with tremor: the experience of essential tremor versus Parkinson's disease patients. Mov Disord Clin Pract (Hoboken) 3(1):36–42, 2016 27430000

Louis ED, Ottman R: How many people in the USA have essential tremor? Deriving a population estimate based on epidemiological data. Tremor Other Hyperkinet Mov (N Y) 4:259, 2014 25157323

Louis ED, Cosentino S, Huey ED: Depressive symptoms can amplify embarrassment in essential tremor. J Clin Mov Disord 3:11, 2016 27429787

Lovell MR, Collins MW: Neuropsychological assessment of the college football player. J Head Trauma Rehabil 13(2):9–26, 1998 9575253

Lunde ME, Lee EK, Rasmussen KG: Electroconvulsive therapy in patients with epilepsy. Epilepsy Behav 9(2):355–359, 2006 16876485

Marin RS, Biedrzycki RC, Firinciogullari S: Reliability and validity of the Apathy Evaluation Scale. Psychiatry Res 38(2):143–162, 1991 1754629

Marrie RA, Reingold S, Cohen J, et al: The incidence and prevalence of psychiatric disorders in multiple sclerosis: a systematic review. Mult Scler 21(3):305–317, 2015 25583845

Matsos A, Loomes M, Zhou I, et al: Chemotherapy-induced cognitive impairments: white matter pathologies. Cancer Treat Rev 61:6–14, 2017 29073552

McCrae RR, Costa PT Jr: NEO Inventories For The NEO Personality Inventory–3 (NEO-PI-3), NEO Five-Factor Inventory–3 (NEO-FFI-3), NEO Personality Inventory–Revised (NEO PI-R): Professional Manual. Lutz, FL, Psychological Assessment Resources, 2010

McKee AC, Cairns NJ, Dickson DW, et al: The first NINDS/NIBIB consensus meeting to define neuropathological criteria for the diagnosis of chronic traumatic encephalopathy. Acta Neuropathologica 131(1):75–86, 2016 26667418

Mendez MF, Grau R, Doss RC, et al: Schizophrenia in epilepsy: seizure and psychosis variables. Neurology 43(6):1073–1077, 1993 8170544

Miller A, Pratt H, Schiffer RB: Pseudobulbar affect: the spectrum of clinical presentations, etiologies and treatments. Expert Rev Neurother 11(7):1077–1088, 2011 21539437

Miller AE, de Seze J, Hauser SL, et al: The Effect of Ocrelizumab on Cognitive Functioning in Relapsing Multiple Sclerosis: Analysis of the Phase III IFN Beta-1a-Controlled OPERA Studies. Presented at 2017 Annual Meeting of Consortium of Multiple Sclerosis Centers. New Orleans, LA, May 24–27, 2017

Minen MT, Begasse De Dhaem O, Kroon Van Diest A, et al: Migraine and its psychiatric comorbidities. J Neurol Neurosurg Psychiatry 87(7):741–749, 2016 26733600

Mitchell AJ, Sheth B, Gill J, et al: Prevalence and predictors of post-stroke mood disorders: a meta-analysis and meta-regression of depression, anxiety and adjustment disorder. Gen Hosp Psychiatry 47:48–60, 2017 28807138

Mohammad D, Ellis C, Rau A, et al: Psychometric properties of apathy scales in dementia: a systematic review. J Alzheimers Dis 66(3):1065–1082, 2018 30400094

Montalban X, Comi G, O'Connor P, et al: Oral fingolimod (FTY720) in relapsing multiple sclerosis: impact on health-related quality of life in a phase II study. Mult Scler 17(11):1341–1350, 2011 21727148

Moore SR, Gresham LS, Bromberg MB, et al: A self-report measure of affective lability. J Neurol Neurosurg Psychiatry 63(1):89–93, 1997 9221973

Moreno GM, Gandhi R, Lessig SL, et al: Mortality in patients with Parkinson disease psychosis receiving pimavanserin and quetiapine. Neurology 91(17):797–799, 2018 30258020

Mortensen JK, Johnsen SP, Andersen G: Prescription and predictors of post-stroke antidepressant treatment: a population-based study. Acta Neurol Scand 138(3):235–244, 2018 29691834

Murphy R, O'Donoghue S, Counihan T, et al: Neuropsychiatric syndromes of multiple sclerosis. J Neurol Neurosurg Psychiatry 88(8):697–708, 2017 28285265

Nasreddine ZS, Phillips NA, Bédirian V, et al: The Montreal Cognitive Assessment, MoCA: a brief screening tool for mild cognitive impairment. J Am Geriatr Soc 53(4):695–699, 2005 15817019

Negro A, Martelletti P: Chronic migraine plus medication overuse headache: two entities or not? J Headache Pain 12(6):593–601, 2011 21938457

Newman CW, Jacobson GP, Spitzer JB: Development of the Tinnitus Handicap Inventory. Arch Otolaryngol Head Neck Surg 122(2):143–148, 1996 8630207

Nicholas R, Rashid W: Multiple sclerosis. BMJ Clin Evid 2012:1202, 2012 22321967

Orlova Y, Rizzoli P, Loder E: Association of coprescription of triptan antimigraine drugs and selective serotonin reuptake inhibitor or selective norepinephrine reuptake inhibitor antidepressants with serotonin syndrome. JAMA Neurol 75(5):566–572, 2018 29482205

Ortiz A, Cervantes P, Zlotnik G, et al: Cross-prevalence of migraine and bipolar disorder. Bipolar Disord 12(4):397–403, 2010 20636637

Paolucci S: Advances in antidepressants for treating post-stroke depression. Expert Opin Pharmacother 18(10):1011–1017, 2017 28535081

Peña E, Mata M, López-Manzanares L, et al: Antidepressants in Parkinson's disease: recommendations by the movement disorder study group of the Neurological Association of Madrid. Neurologia 33(6):395–402, 2018 27004670

Perini GI: Emotions and personality in complex partial seizures. Psychother Psychosom 45(3):141–148, 1986 3823358

Peterlin BL, Tietjen GE, Brandes JL, et al: Posttraumatic stress disorder in migraine. Headache 49(4):541–551, 2009 19245387

Pfeiffer RF: Non-motor symptoms in Parkinson's disease. Parkinsonism Relat Disord 22 (suppl 1):S119–S122, 2016 26372623

Philbin M, Niewoehner J, Wan GJ: Clinical and economic evaluation of repository corticotropin injection: a narrative literature review of treatment efficacy and healthcare resource utilization for seven key indications. Adv Ther 34(8):1775–1790, 2017 28660550

Pioro EP: Current concepts in the pharmacotherapy of pseudobulbar affect. Drugs 71(9):1193–1207, 2011 21711063

Postuma RB, Berg D, Stern M, et al: MDS clinical diagnostic criteria for Parkinson's disease. Mov Disord 30(12):1591–1601, 2015 26474316

Quinn DK, Mayer AR, Master CL, et al: Prolonged postconcussive symptoms. Am J Psychiatry 175(2):103–111, 2018 29385828

Radakovic R, Harley C, Abrahams S, Starr JM: A systematic review of the validity and reliability of apathy scales in neurodegenerative conditions. Int Psychogeriatr 27(6):903–923, 2015 [Erratum in: Int Psychogeriatr 27(6):925, 2015] 25355282

Rai D, Kerr MP, McManus S, et al: Epilepsy and psychiatric comorbidity: a nationally representative population-based study. Epilepsia 53(6):1095–1103, 2012 22578079

Raimo S, Trojano L, Spitaleri D, et al: Apathy in multiple sclerosis: a validation study of the apathy evaluation scale. J Neurol Sci 347(1–2):295–300, 2014 25455303

Rao AS, Scher AI, Vieira RV, et al: The impact of post-traumatic stress disorder on the burden of migraine: results from the National Comorbidity Survey–Replication. Headache 55(10):1323–1341, 2015 26473981

Reijnders JS, Ehrt U, Weber WE, et al: A systematic review of prevalence studies of depression in Parkinson's disease. Mov Disord 23(2):183–189, quiz 313, 2008 17987654

Rivera Bonet CN, Hermann B, Cook CJ, et al: Neuroanatomical correlates of personality traits in temporal lobe epilepsy: findings from the Epilepsy Connectome Project. Epilepsy Behav 98(Pt A):220–227, 2019 31387000

Rocca MA, Amato MP, De Stefano N, et al: Clinical and imaging assessment of cognitive dysfunction in multiple sclerosis. Lancet Neurol 14(3):302–317, 2015 25662900

Rosen N, Pearlman E, Ruff D, et al: 100% response rate to galcanezumab in patients with episodic migraine: a post hoc analysis of the results from phase 3, randomized, double-blind, placebo-controlled EVOLVE-1 and EVOLVE-2 studies. Headache 58(9):1347–1357, 2018 30341990

Royall DR, Mahurin RK, Gray KF: Bedside assessment of executive cognitive impairment: the executive interview. J Am Geriatr Soc 40(12):1221–1226, 1992 1447438

Royall DR, Lauterbach EC, Kaufer D, et al: The cognitive correlates of functional status: a review from the Committee on Research of the American Neuropsychiatric Association. J Neuropsychiatry Clin Neurosci 19(3):249–265, 2007 17827410

Ruscheweyh R, Müller M, Blum B, Straube A: Correlation of headache frequency and psychosocial impairment in migraine: a cross-sectional study. Headache 54(5):861–871, 2014 23980919

Salter A, Thomas NP, Tyry T, et al: A contemporary profile of primary progressive multiple sclerosis participants from the NARCOMS Registry. Mult Scler 24(7):951–962, 2018 28524746

Satzer D, Bond DJ: Mania secondary to focal brain lesions: implications for understanding the functional neuroanatomy of bipolar disorder. Bipolar Disord 18(3):205–220, 2016 27112231

Schiffer R, Pope LE: Review of pseudobulbar affect including a novel and potential therapy. J Neuropsychiatry Clin Neurosci 17(4):447–454, 2005 16387982

Schmitz B: The effects of antiepileptic drugs on behavior, in The Neuropsychiatry of Epilepsy, 2nd Edition. Edited by Trimble MR, Schmitz B. Cambridge, UK, Cambridge University Press, 2011, pp 133–143

Shen K, Xu Y, Guan H, et al: Paraneoplastic limbic encephalitis associated with lung cancer. Sci Rep 8(1):6792, 2018 29717222

Sigurdardottir S, Andelic N, Roe C, et al: Post-concussion symptoms after traumatic brain injury at 3 and 12 months post-injury: a prospective study. Brain Inj 23(6):489–497, 2009 19484622

Singerman J, Lee L: Consistency of the Babinski reflex and its variants. Eur J Neurol 15(9):960–964, 2008 18637037

Sinha A, Shariq A, Said K, et al: Medical comorbidities in bipolar disorder. Curr Psychiatry Rep 20(5):36, 2018 29732528

Sinita E, Coghill D: The use of stimulant medications for non-core aspects of ADHD and in other disorders. Neuropharmacology 87:161–172, 2014 24951855

Smitherman TA, Burch R, Sheikh H, et al: The prevalence, impact, and treatment of migraine and severe headaches in the United States: a review of statistics from national surveillance studies. Headache 53(3):427–436, 2013 23470015

Solomon G: Chronic traumatic encephalopathy in sports: a historical and narrative review. Dev Neuropsychol 43(4):279–311, 2018 29533096

Spina E, Pisani F, de Leon J: Clinically significant pharmacokinetic drug interactions of antiepileptic drugs with new antidepressants and new antipsychotics. Pharmacol Res 106:72–86, 2016 26896788

Stankevich Y, Lueken U, Balzer-Geldsetzer M, et al: Psychometric properties of an abbreviated version of the Apathy Evaluation Scale for Parkinson Disease (AES-12PD). Am J Geriatr Psychiatry 26(10):1079–1090, 2018 30082208

Stovner LJ, Hagen K, Jensen R, et al: The global burden of headache: a documentation of head-ache prevalence and disability worldwide. Cephalalgia 27(3):193–210, 2007 17381554

Sun Y, Liang Y, Jiao Y, et al: Comparative efficacy and acceptability of antidepressant treatment in poststroke depression: a multiple-treatments meta-analysis. BMJ Open 7(8):e016499, 2017 28775189

Tanaka K, Wada-Isoe K, Nakashita S, et al: Impulsive compulsive behaviors in Japanese Parkin-son's disease patients and utility of the Japanese version of the Questionnaire for Impul-sive-Compulsive Disorders in Parkinson's disease. J Neurol Sci 331(1–2):76–80, 2013 23735774

Taylor-Rowan M, Momoh O, Averbe L, et al: Prevalence of pre-stroke depression and its asso-ciation with post-stroke depression: a systematic review and meta-analysis. Psychol Med 49(4):685–696, 2019 30107864

Teasdale G, Jennett B: Assessment of coma and impaired consciousness: a practical scale. Lan-cet 2(7872):81–84, 1974 4136544

Terwindt PW, Hubers AA, Giltay EJ, et al: Screening for cognitive dysfunction in Huntington's disease with the clock drawing test. Int J Geriatr Psychiatry 31(9):1013–1020, 2016 26766850

Titulaer MJ, McCracken L, Gabilondo I, et al: Treatment and prognostic factors for long-term outcome in patients with anti-NMDA receptor encephalitis: an observational cohort study. Lancet Neurol 12(2):157–165, 2013 23290630

Tse T, Douglas J, Lentin P, et al: Reduction in retained activity participation is associated with depressive symptoms 3 months after mild stroke: an observational cohort study. J Rehabil Med 49(2):120–127, 2017 28121336

Tu J, Wang LX, Wen HF, et al: The association of different types of cerebral infarction with post-stroke depression and cognitive impairment. Medicine (Baltimore) 97(23):e10919, 2018 29879031

Tysnes OB, Storstein A: Epidemiology of Parkinson's disease. J Neural Transm (Vienna) 124(8):901–905, 2017 28150045

Villa RF, Ferrari F, Moretti A: Post-stroke depression: mechanisms and pharmacological treat-ment. Pharmacol Ther 184:131–144, 2018 29128343

Wade BJ: Spatial analysis of global prevalence of multiple sclerosis suggests need for an up-dated prevalence scale. Mult Scler Int 2014:124578, 2014 24693432

Wang SB, Wang YY, Zhang QE, et al: Cognitive behavioral therapy for post-stroke depression: a meta-analysis. J Affect Disord 235:589–596, 2018 29704854

Warren N, Siskind D, O'Gorman C: Refining the psychiatric syndrome of anti-N-methyl-d-aspartate receptor encephalitis. Acta Psychiatr Scand 138(5):401–408, 2018 29992532

Waxman SG, Geschwind N: The interictal behavior syndrome of temporal lobe epilepsy. Arch Gen Psychiatry 32(12):1580–1586, 1975 1200777

Webster GD, Dewall CN, Pond RS Jr, et al: The brief aggression questionnaire: psychometric and behavioral evidence for an efficient measure of trait aggression. Aggress Behav 40(2):120–139, 2014 24115185

Weintraub D, Mamikonyan E, Papay K, et al: Questionnaire for Impulsive-Compulsive Disor-ders in Parkinson's Disease–Rating Scale. Mov Disord 27(2):242–247, 2012 22134954

World Health Organization: International Statistical Classification of Diseases and Related Health Problems, 10th Revision. Geneva, World Health Organization, 1992

Wuerfel J, Krishnamoorthy ES, Brown RJ, et al: Religiosity is associated with hippocampal but not amygdala volumes in patients with refractory epilepsy. J Neurol Neurosurg Psychia-try 75(4):640–642, 2004 15026516

Yi J, Padalino DJ, Chin LS, et al: Chronic traumatic encephalopathy. Curr Sports Med Rep 12(1):28–32, 2013 23314081

Zaborowski MP, Spaczynski M, Nowak-Markwitz E, et al: Paraneoplastic neurological syn-dromes associated with ovarian tumors. J Cancer Res Clin Oncol 141(1):99–108, 2015 24965744

Zhang G, Zhang Z, Liu L, et al: Impulsive and compulsive behaviors in Parkinson's disease. Front Aging Neurosci 6:318, 2014 25452726

Zhang H, Wang L, Fan Y, et al: Atypical antipsychotics for Parkinson's disease psychosis: a systematic review and meta-analysis. Neuropsychiatr Dis Treat 15:2137–2149, 2019 31551655

Zigmond AS, Snaith RP: The hospital anxiety and depression scale. Acta Psychiatr Scand 67(6):361–370, 1983 6880820

Zuckerman SL, Brett BL, Jeckell A, et al: Chronic traumatic encephalopathy and neurodegeneration in contact sports and American football. J Alzheimers Dis 66(1):37–55, 2018 30223396

Cancer

Psychiatric Care of the Oncology Patient

Carlos G. Fernandez-Robles, M.D., M.B.A.
Sean P. Glass, M.D.

Over the past two decades, refinement of chemotherapy protocols, emergence of new treatment options including targeted and biological therapies, and advancements in radiological and surgical techniques have transformed cancer care. With both incidence rates and survival rates on the rise, cancer is more common. No longer a death sentence for many patients, cancer is a chronic condition that affects a person physically, mentally, and socially. Psychiatrists work collaboratively with oncologists, offering expertise in the diagnosis and management of psychiatric symptoms that may result from the psychological burden or neuropsychiatric manifestations of cancer or from exacerbations of preexisting psychiatric conditions. In this chapter, we review the most frequently occurring neuropsychiatric disorders, and their treatment, in patients with cancer.

Mood Disorders

Mood disorders are common during cancer and its treatment, ranging from mild dysphoria and irritability to major depressive episodes and mania. Monitoring for mood disorders should be part of the routine psychiatric evaluation, and providers should be attuned to the broad range of psychological and organic contributors.

Depression

Epidemiology

The occurrence of depression in people with cancer has been documented extensively. General epidemiological prevalence data indicate that the prevalence of depressive disorders is two to three times higher in cancer patients than in the general population (Caruso et al. 2017). Cancer could be a risk factor for developing depression, but depression is not necessarily an inevitable consequence of cancer. The mean prevalence of depression in cancer patients ranges from 8% to 24% (Krebber et al. 2014). This wide range can be attributed to heterogeneity in methodology and population samples (Walker et al. 2013). For instance, depression has been found to be highly associated with brain, oropharyngeal, breast, lung, and pancreatic cancers but is less prevalent in genitourinary and colorectal malignancies and in lymphoma (Massie 2004; Walker et al. 2014). Prevalence is also influenced by treatment stage and type of treatment received, with higher rates of depression in patients who are in the posttreatment stage (Watts et al. 2014) and in those who have been treated with chemotherapy (Fann et al. 2008). Patients with a history of major depressive disorder (MDD) are more vulnerable to developing depressive symptoms following a cancer diagnosis (Kadan-Lottick et al. 2005). Depression may predict mortality (but not disease progression) in cancer patients, with an estimated 26% higher mortality rate over 5 years among patients with depressive symptoms and a 39% higher mortality rate over 5 years among those with a diagnosis of MDD (Satin et al. 2009).

Pathophysiology

No single pathway for the occurrence of depression has been elucidated; however, in addition to common psychological factors (e.g., anxiety, poor coping strategies, limited social support), several biological factors have been hypothesized to contribute to the greater rates of depression among cancer patients. These factors include alterations in the inflammatory system, altered stress response mechanisms, and genetic susceptibility.

Increased proinflammatory cytokine levels, which are seen in cancer patients, are thought to precipitate depressive symptoms by several mechanisms. Studies in cancer patients prior to treatment have found elevated levels of circulating interleukin (IL)-1β, IL-6, IL-8, and tumor necrosis factor (TNF)-α that correlate positively with both depression and anxiety (Oliveira Miranda et al. 2014). Adding to these abnormalities, chemotherapy and radiation lead to an increase in peripheral cytokines and subsequent activation of central cytokines that has been correlated with neurovegetative symptoms (Mills et al. 2005). The end result of this increase in proinflammatory factors is a depletion of tryptophan, a subsequent reduction in overall serotonin levels, and an increase in glutamatergic activity.

Cancer patients with MDD exhibit a significant reduction in the relative diurnal variance of cortisol, suggesting perturbation in the hypothalamic-pituitary-adrenal (HPA) axis (Jehn et al. 2010).

Genetic factors contribute to an increased risk for mood disorders in the general population. Studies have linked polymorphisms in brain-derived neurotrophic factor (BDNF) genes to the development of depressive symptomatology in breast cancer and leukemia patients (Kim et al. 2012; Romanowicz et al. 2012). In contrast, the serotonin transporter–linked polymorphic region, extensively associated with depression vulnerability after stressful life events, has not been found to be a determinant in cancer patients (Suppli et al. 2015). Increased levels of proinflammatory cytokines and direct toxicity of certain chemotherapeutic agents can lead to alterations in DNA methylation, histone acetylation, and chromatin structure, resulting in changes in gene expression.

Alterations in BDNF methylation status have been associated with increased incidence and severity of depressive symptoms in women with breast cancer that are independent of genotype variability (Kang et al. 2015). Structural damage to the central nervous system (CNS) caused by tumors and their treatment often results in a variety of neuropsychiatric manifestations; depressive symptoms have been predominantly associated with lesions in the anterior left hemisphere (Seddighi et al. 2015).

Diagnosis

Accurately diagnosing MDD in people with cancer can be challenging. In daily clinical practice, relying on the diagnostic criteria listed in the fifth edition of the *Diagnostic and Statistical Manual of Mental Disorders* (DSM-5; American Psychiatric Association 2013) is helpful, yet the overlap between somatic symptoms seen in depression and those seen in cancer and its treatment forces practitioners to assess each case individually, with particular attention to cognitive and mood-related symptoms. In an attempt to address this difficulty, the Endicott criteria for depression in the medically ill were proposed; in these criteria, nonsomatic symptoms are provided to use in place of the DSM somatic symptoms of depression (which overlap with cancer symptoms) (Endicott 1984; Table 13–1).

Screening instruments have been extensively studied and validated in cancer populations. Ultrashort methods (e.g., single-item screening question, distress thermometer) are modestly effective in screening for mood disorders. Although such instruments should not be used alone to diagnose depression, anxiety, or distress in cancer patients, they may be considered a first-stage screening tool (Mitchell 2007). The Hospital Anxiety and Depression Scale, a 14-item questionnaire focused more on emotional than on somatic symptoms, is the most extensively studied tool (Vodermaier and Millman 2011). Its depression subscale is particularly helpful in advanced cancer. Other useful tools include the Beck Depression Inventory, which is more generalizable across cancer types and disease stages and possesses good indices for screening and case finding, and the Center for Epidemiologic Studies Depression Scale, which has been found to be the best-weighted to measure depression specifically, particularly in older and terminally ill patients (Wakefield et al. 2015).

Consideration of possible medical causes in the differential diagnosis is critical when evaluating depressed cancer patients. Pain, metabolic alterations, hypothyroidism, and medications (e.g., corticosteroids, alpha interferon [IFN], pemetrexed, taxane drugs) may contribute to depression. Hypoactive delirium is often erroneously labeled as depression, but key features—such as impairment of attention and cognition, symptoms that wax and wane in severity, and a disturbance of the sleep-wake cycle—differentiate it from depression. Cancer-related fatigue is often incorrectly mislabeled as depression; the presence of sad mood and anhedonia and of diurnal variation in symptoms helps to distinguish the two (Reuter and Harter 2003).

Treatment

The treatment of depression in cancer patients, as in the general population, consists of antidepressant medications and psychotherapy. In the most severe cases, electroconvulsive therapy can rapidly relieve symptoms and enhance quality of life.

Despite the impact of depression on people with cancer, available studies on the use of antidepressants are scarce and of low quality. A meta-analysis found that anti-

TABLE 13–1.   Endicott substitution criteria for depression in medically ill persons

DSM criteria for MDD	Substituted criteria
Changes in appetite or weight	Tearful; appears depressed
Changes in sleep	Withdrawn; not talkative
Anergia	Broods; is pessimistic; engages in self-pity
Trouble thinking, concentrating, or making decisions	Mood not reactive

Note. MDD=major depressive disorder.
Source. Endicott 1984.

depressant treatment improved depressive symptoms more than placebo, even in patients with subsyndromal depressive symptoms (Laoutidis and Mathiak 2013). Considering the lack of head-to-head data, antidepressant use should be considered on an individual basis (Ostuzzi et al. 2015); previous response, side effects, and drug interactions should be taken into account when choosing an agent (Thekdi et al. 2015). Serotonin-norepinephrine reuptake inhibitors (SNRIs) and tricyclic antidepressants (TCAs) are excellent choices in patients with neuropathic pain; bupropion helps patients burdened by fatigue and poor concentration and those trying to stop smoking tobacco. Depressed cancer patients with insomnia and low appetite can benefit from mirtazapine. Stimulants (e.g., methylphenidate, dextroamphetamine) can rapidly lift mood, can paradoxically enhance appetite, and can ameliorate cognitive difficulties and fatigue in the medically ill and are an option for depressed cancer patients despite limited evidence to support their use (Hardy 2009).

Several studies have confirmed the efficacy of psychosocial interventions. Patients recently diagnosed with cancer with mild to moderate depression can benefit from psychoeducation, cognitive-behavioral therapy (CBT), relaxation strategies, and problem-solving approaches. Patients with advanced disease may benefit from supportive-expressive psychotherapy that focuses on processing fears associated with death and other existential concerns (Li et al. 2012). Pilot studies in the use of psilocybin to treat anxiety, depression, and existential concerns in patients with advanced disease are of interest but will require broader replication (Griffiths et al. 2016; Ross et al. 2016).

Mania

While the incidence of mania in cancer populations is similar to that in the general population, certain considerations should be taken into account in this group. Frequently used in cancer treatment, steroids can trigger manic symptoms; prednisone dosages of 40 mg/day or higher are thought to confer a larger risk (Brown and Suppes 1998). IFN-α2b, used in the treatment of melanoma and other malignancies, is well known to alter mood; mania is particularly associated with dosage reductions or pauses in IFN treatment (Greenberg et al. 2000). Although mania is not a common presentation of cerebral tumors, reports have associated it with frontal or temporal lesions, particularly in the right hemisphere (Brooks and Hoblyn 2005). As in patients with primary bipolar disorder, manic symptoms can be treated with lithium, mood-stabilizing anticonvulsants, and antipsychotics. The ability of lithium to cause leuko-cytosis has led to concern that it may also stimulate leukemic cells; however, epidemi-ological studies and in vivo data do not substantiate this association (Volf and Crismon 1991).

Anxiety Disorders and Posttraumatic Stress Disorder

The differential diagnosis of anxiety symptoms in cancer patients is broad; clinicians need to consider tumor-related, treatment-related, and primary psychiatric causes. Anxiousness may be considered normal in response to a dreaded situation (e.g., re-ceiving a diagnosis of cancer, undergoing cancer treatment). Distinguishing this non-clinical anxiousness from clinically significant anxiety, present in more than one-third of cancer patients (Brintzenhofe-Szoc et al. 2009), is key. While patients often experi-ence symptoms of posttraumatic stress, especially around the time of cancer diagno-sis, these symptoms resolve rapidly, and the occurrence of full-blown posttraumatic stress disorder (PTSD) is rare (Voigt et al. 2017).

Patients may be acutely aware of the possibility of pain, nausea, vomiting, disfig-urement, loss of function, cancer relapse, and other feared outcomes of cancer and its treatment. Associative learning through classical conditioning may result in signifi-cant anticipatory anxiety related to tests, treatments, and doctors' appointments. Sig-nificant anxiety while awaiting tumor marker and imaging results may be a harbinger of ongoing anxiety or depression if disease progresses (Fertig and Hayes 2001).

Phobic syndromes or responses may appear in various forms during cancer treat-ment. Claustrophobia with repeated magnetic resonance imaging (MRI) and needle phobia are two common clinical scenarios that cause significant distress and may lead to avoidance of treatment. CBT and pretreatment with rapid desensitization are effec-tive in treating phobic symptoms in cancer populations (Fernandes 2003; Hofmann et al. 2012).

Because clinical factors related to cancer and its treatment may be directly anxio-genic, possible medical causes of anxiety need to be considered in cancer patients. Structural brain lesions in brain areas modulating fear and anxiety may result in clin-ically relevant symptoms. Seizures in temporolimbic areas may manifest as panic at-tacks or anxiety (Plotnik et al. 2009). Pulmonary effusions, edema, or embolism or hypoxia associated with structural CNS lesions can trigger acute stress responses and anxiety (Dudgeon and Lertzman 1998). Metabolic derangements may cause anxiety in cancer patients (Cryer 1999). Finally, side effects from corticosteroids, antiemetics (due to akathisia and other side effects), and chemotherapeutic agents can lead to clinically significant anxiety in cancer patients.

Judicious use of psychotropic medications should be considered in cancer patients. Primary psychiatric disorders, whether related to comorbid medical causes or not, should be managed with standard treatments, including selective serotonin reuptake inhibitors (SSRIs), psychotherapy, mind-body medicine approaches, and other evi-dence-based therapies.

Psychosomatic Symptoms in Cancer

Cancer-Related Fatigue

Fatigue is the most commonly reported symptom in people with cancer, is described as more distressing than pain, and has the most debilitating impact on functioning (Williams et al. 2016). A meta-analysis examining the frequency of various cancer symptoms among older patients in palliative care found that fatigue (2 studies; $N=149$) had a pooled prevalence of nearly 80% (Van Lancker et al. 2014). Despite this high prevalence, most patients and providers report that the symptom of fatigue is rarely addressed during oncological visits (Passik et al. 2002).

Pathophysiology

Several mechanisms underlie the occurrence of cancer-related fatigue. Similar to depression, cancer-related fatigue has been associated with increased circulating pro-inflammatory cytokines, altered diurnal cortisol secretion, and a blunted cortisol response to stress (Miller et al. 2008). The abnormal serotonin secretion and altered synaptic clearance that occur in cancer and follow its treatment have been linked to the occurrence of fatigue through dysregulation of hypothalamic receptors and reduction of pituitary responsiveness (Ryan et al. 2007). Other studies have suggested a role for dysregulation of the autonomic system in the genesis of cancer-related fatigue, because reduced parasympathetic activity (measured by resting heart rate variability) was found to be associated with higher levels of fatigue, independent of inflammation (Crosswell et al. 2014). Finally, disturbances in circadian rhythm seen in cancer patients can disrupt a variety of physiological mechanisms related to fatigue (Ancoli-Israel et al. 2001).

Definition and Evaluation

Cancer-related fatigue is identified primarily by asking about the presence and severity of symptoms. The National Comprehensive Cancer Network (NCCN) clinical practice guidelines for cancer-related fatigue define *fatigue* as "a distressing, persistent, subjective sense of physical, emotional, and/or cognitive tiredness or exhaustion related to cancer or cancer treatment that is not proportional to recent activity and interferes with usual functioning" (Berger et al. 2015, p. 1012). The single-item Functional Assessment of Chronic Illness Therapy–Fatigue (FACIT-F; Cella et al. 2011) scale can be used to identify high-risk patients. According to the NCCN guidelines, a FACIT-F score of 4 or greater should prompt the clinician to conduct a further evaluation to identify other, possibly modifiable conditions that might be contributing to a patient's fatigue, including medical, emotional, and pharmacological factors (Berger et al. 2015).

Treatment

Abundant evidence supports aerobic exercise as beneficial for individuals with cancer-related fatigue during and after cancer therapy (Cramp and Byron-Daniel 2012). The American Society of Clinical Oncology recommended that patients engage in moderate levels of physical activity, including moderate aerobic exercise (150 minutes per week) and strength training (two or three times weekly) (Bower et al. 2014). Exercise routines and setting should be tailored to the patient's functional status and physical limitations.

Behavioral interventions (e.g., CBT, energy conservation) may be beneficial as both primary and adjunctive treatments for fatigue in cancer patients; such techniques emphasize managing fatigue rather than curing it (Gielissen et al. 2006). Cost-effective interventions such as web-based CBT programs can improve access for severely deconditioned patients (Abrahams et al. 2015). Finally, while somewhat controversial, current evidence supports the use of psychostimulants for cancer-related fatigue (Minton et al. 2010), and NCCN guidelines have recommended their use, although only after other, nonpharmacological approaches have failed (Berger et al. 2015). Risks and side effects should be considered carefully before recommending use of psychostimulants for cancer-related fatigue.

Anticipatory Nausea and Vomiting

Fifty percent of cancer patients will battle nausea or vomiting during the course of their disease (Warr 2008). Chemotherapeutic agents are toxic to the enterochromaffin cells lining the gastrointestinal mucosa, causing these cells to release neurotransmitters (e.g., dopamine, serotonin, substance P, acetylcholine, histamine, γ-aminobutyric acid [GABA]) that bind to receptors on abdominal vagal afferents. These stimuli are conducted to the dorsal vagal complex, which consists of the vomiting center, the chemoreceptor trigger zone in the area postrema, and the nucleus of the solitary tract (Darmani and Ray 2009). Chemotherapy-induced nausea and vomiting (CINV) often leads to anticipatory nausea and vomiting (ANV), which occurs when the vomiting center is activated by stimuli generated by personal thoughts, feelings, or sensory stimuli associated with chemotherapy (e.g., smells and sights associated with the treatment). ANV can persist for several months after completion of chemotherapy (Duigon 1986). This process is thought to occur in a Pavlovian classical conditioning fashion; anxious young patients are the population most severely affected (Kamen et al. 2014). Nausea and vomiting can start even before arriving at the infusion unit and can lead to complications, including anxiety, insomnia, and aversion to treatment. Controlling CINV is the single best intervention against ANV (Aapro et al. 2005). Aggressive management with a combination of drug classes is the standard of care for CINV. The addition of neurokinin-1 receptor antagonists to 5-hydroxytryptamine type 3 (5-HT$_3$) receptor antagonists or steroids significantly reduces the occurrence of CINV (Di Maio et al. 2013). Benzodiazepines, alone or in combination with other antiemetic agents, reduce the incidence of ANV as well as that of acute and delayed emesis (Malik et al. 1995). Anecdotal reports suggest a role for cannabinoids in the treatment of ANV, although further research is needed to evaluate their effectiveness in clinical settings (Parker et al. 2011). Nonpharmacological interventions—including systematic desensitization, hypnosis, biofeedback, imagery, and relaxation techniques—and complementary alternative interventions—including acupuncture and herbal products—all can help control ANV (Kamen et al. 2014).

Sleep Disruption

Sleep disturbances are common among cancer patients and significantly affect patients' quality of life. In a study involving 300 women who had been treated with radiotherapy for nonmetastatic breast cancer, 19% met criteria for an insomnia syndrome, and 58% reported that cancer that cancer either caused or aggravated their sleep problems (Savard et al. 2001). In comparison with noncancer patients, patients with breast cancer were found to have longer daytime total nap times, worse sleep quality, and greater disruption of circadian rhythms (Ancoli-Israel et al. 2014). Furthermore, actigraphy data, an objective measure of circadian function, demonstrated that patients with lung cancer experienced higher-than-expected levels of wakefulness during typical sleeping times and, surprisingly, extensive sleeping during typical awake times (Levin et al. 2005). Management of sleep disorders in cancer patients should be no different from that in noncancer populations. Sleep hygiene and behavioral interventions should be exhausted before pharmacological interventions are considered.

Neurocognitive and Neuropsychiatric Complications of Cancer and Its Treatment

Cancer and its treatment cause cognitive and psychiatric impairment by a variety of direct and indirect mechanisms. Depending on the type and location of structural lesions in the CNS, these impairments may be global in nature (as with delirium) or may affect specific cognitive, behavioral, or affective domains. Often, such problems go unnoticed by patients and caregivers and are recognized only with focused questioning or direct clinical testing. Patients who report cognitive dysfunction often describe general and vague symptoms that are difficult to verify and validate with neurocognitive testing. Difficulties in processing speed, attention, memory, and executive functions are among the most commonly reported difficulties across studies in patients treated for non-CNS solid tumors with chemotherapy (Wefel et al. 2015). Patients in whom cognitive and psychiatric deficits stem from acute drug reactions, paraneoplastic syndromes, brain metastases, and other severe disturbances usually manifest with a constellation of behavioral, affective, motor, and cognitive changes. The frequent presence of various complicating clinical factors in cancer patients often renders pinpointing the etiology of cognitive dysfunction elusive. Fatigue, concomitant use of anxiolytics or opioids, anemia, seizure disorders, and the stress associated with undergoing various treatments and procedures all can cause cognitive decline. Furthermore, premorbid risk factors (e.g., lower levels of educational or vocational achievement, substance use) may weigh heavily in producing deficits in some patients. In the following sections we discuss cognitive and psychiatric dysfunction associated with cancer-related delirium; specific cancer treatments, including chemotherapy, radiation, and stem cell transplantation; and specific cancer types, including primary brain tumors, brain metastases, leptomeningeal disease, and paraneoplastic syndromes.

Cancer-Related Delirium

Delirium is a frequent complication in cancer patients and should be suspected in any patient who shows even subtle changes in cognition, mood, or behavior. Delirium rates greater than 40% are seen in hospitalized cancer patients; in terminally ill patients, rates rise to 85% (Centeno et al. 2004; Massie et al. 1983; Şenel et al. 2017). Delirium rates increase with severity of illness, number of comorbidities, and presence of baseline risk factors (Inouye and Charpentier 1996). Risk factors for delirium include infection, medications (especially anticholinergics, benzodiazepines, and opioids), hypoxia, metabolic disarray, pain, constipation, and urinary retention (Lawlor et al. 2000). Elderly patients, patients with baseline sensory deprivation (e.g., vision or hearing impairment), immobilized patients, patients with preexisting cognitive impairment or structural brain disease, and patients with other end-organ dysfunction are more highly predisposed to delirium. In most cases, multiple factors contribute to delirium's emergence; in fact, the average number of precipitating factors is three (Lawlor et al. 2000). Inattention is the core cognitive deficit in delirium, regardless of motoric subtype (i.e., hyperactive, hypoactive, or mixed), and should be tested by history gathering and validated screens such as recitation of the months of the year backward (O'Regan et al. 2014). Inattention or changes in arousal will negatively affect other cognitive domains, including memory, language, and executive functions. Hypoactive delirium may be easily mistaken for depression, apathy, or volitional nonparticipation in care.

As in the general medical population, treatment of delirium consists of correcting all contributing factors. Adequate prevention and management of sleep deprivation, pain, constipation, immobility, sensory impairment, and dehydration are essential for prevention and management of delirium, particularly in elderly patients (Flaherty et al. 2010). Antipsychotics are used to treat agitation, hallucinations, and sleep-wake cycle disruptions and have been demonstrated to be useful in cancer populations (Breitbart and Alici 2012). While some clinicians have recommended the use of stimulants in the treatment of hypoactive delirium, evidence is still limited, and risk of agitation and exacerbation of psychotic symptoms precludes the routine use of these agents, whose use should be determined on a case-by-case basis. Melatonin can help normalize disruptions in the sleep-wake cycle, and it may play a role in the treatment of delirium through direct antioxidant and anti-inflammatory activity (Al-Aama et al. 2011).

Complications Associated With Cancer Treatments

Chemotherapy and Radiation

Chemotherapy-related cognitive dysfunction.   The effect of chemotherapy on cognitive function has long been a topic of study and debate among oncologists and psychiatrists. Symptoms are commonly reported yet challenging to document in office and formal examinations of cognitive function. In cancer survivors previously treated with chemotherapy, only one-third of cognitive complaints reported by patients had corresponding findings on objective testing (Hutchinson et al. 2012). A thorough understanding of cognitive impairment in various cancer populations has been impeded by lack of consistency among studies, due to lack of a standard definition for cognitive impairment, high variability in study methodologies and neuropsychological tests used, differences in statistical analyses, nonlongitudinal nature of studies, lack of control groups, heterogeneity in patient populations with different core pathologies, and heterogeneity in baseline clinical and demographic characteristics (Vardy and Tannock 2007; Wefel et al. 2011). Another challenge is that patient performance on office tests in a quiet, stress-free setting does not necessarily accurately reflect functioning in real-life circumstances. To address these problems, a task force—the International Cognition and Cancer Task Force (ICCTF)—was created to help guide researchers and clinicians in defining, assessing, and tracking cognitive problems in patients with chemotherapy-related cognitive dysfunction (CRCD) (Wefel et al. 2011). Learning and memory, processing speed, and executive functions such as planning and multitasking were identified as the most commonly affected processes. The task force recommended not using general cognitive testing tools (e.g., the Mini-Mental State Examination) but instead utilizing tests that examine these cognitive skills specifically (e.g., Hopkins Verbal Learning Test–Revised, Trail Making Test, Controlled Oral Word Association of the Multilingual Aphasia Examination).

Cancer patients may be vulnerable to cognitive dysfunction; longitudinal studies demonstrate that 20%–30% of patients had lower-than-expected cognitive performance before treatment (Wefel et al. 2011). CRCD-related changes persist beyond the completion of treatment. Chemotherapy-treated breast cancer survivors show consistent patterns of hypoactivation in prefrontal and parietal brain regions during executive tasks that can persist for 5–10 years after completion of adjuvant chemotherapy (de Ruiter and Schagen 2013; de Ruiter et al. 2011).

At present, much of the data on cognitive abnormalities in cancer patients comes from studies in chemotherapy-treated breast cancer or hematological cancer patients. The underlying mechanisms for non-CNS tumor–induced or peripheral chemotherapy–induced cognitive changes are heterogeneous and differ across therapeutic agents. Only a few chemotherapeutic agents cross the blood-brain barrier significantly (Table 13–2); moreover, direct toxic effects on brain parenchyma have been documented with an even smaller number of agents (e.g., methotrexate and fluorouracil damage white matter, resulting in both acute and chronic cognitive difficulties) (Han et al. 2008; Vezmar et al. 2003). CRCD is not limited to this direct effect; other mechanisms are thought to be responsible for a larger portion of cases. Evidence for these putative biological mechanisms includes changes in inflammatory cytokines, deficits in DNA repair mechanisms, and low-efficiency drug efflux pumps (Ahles and Saykin 2007). Other potential mechanisms include disruptions in the blood-brain barrier, increased oxidative stress, hormonal and HPA axis changes, epigenetic changes (including histone deacetylation), and alterations in neurogenesis and gliogenesis (Seigers and Fardell 2011; Seigers et al. 2013).

Other sources of information about the effects of chemotherapy on cognition are radiological studies of changes in brain structure and function. CRCD has been correlated with both short- and long-term global reductions in white and gray matter volume (Kaiser et al. 2014; McDonald et al. 2013; Simó et al. 2013). Diffusion tensor imaging (DTI) studies show decreased white matter integrity that correlates with poorer attention and working memory (Deprez et al. 2013). Prospective voxel-based morphometry studies in women with breast cancer receiving chemotherapy versus not receiving chemotherapy showed that the treatment group developed bilateral gray matter reductions in the frontal and medial temporal lobes and the cerebellum (McDonald and Saykin 2013; McDonald et al. 2013). Functional neuroimaging has demonstrated altered activation patterns in key brain regions and networks that correlate with abnormal cognitive processing. For instance, breast cancer patients receiving chemotherapy showed lower prefrontal cortex activation during memory encoding in comparison with control subjects (Kesler et al. 2009). A subset of these patients continued to show frontal cortex hypoactivation even years after treatment (Simó et al. 2013).

TABLE 13–2.   **Chemotherapeutic agents that penetrate the blood-brain barrier**

Busulfan	Irinotecan
Carmustine	Lenalidomide
Cisplatin (minimally)	Leuprolide
Cyclophosphamide (limited extent)	Lomustine
Cytarabine (infusion > intravenous push)	Mercaptopurine
Dacarbazine (limited extent)	Methotrexate
Erlotinib	Procarbazine
Estramustine	Sunitinib (in animal models)
Etoposide (minimally)	Temozolomide
Fludarabine	Teniposide (minimally)
Fluorouracil	Thiotepa
Goserelin	Topotecan
Hydroxyurea	Vinblastine (minimally)
Ifosfamide (subtherapeutic amounts)	Vorinostat

While several treatment options have been proposed for CRCD, no gold standard exists. Nonpharmacological options include standardized, progressive exercise programs geared toward reducing inflammation (Mustian et al. 2015), neurofeedback (Alvarez et al. 2013), and cognitive-behavioral management and rehabilitation (Ferguson et al. 2007). Medications such as modafinil and methylphenidate have proven useful (Moore 2014), and recent trials have suggested a role for donepezil (Lim et al. 2016).

Leukoencephalopathy.   Brain irradiation and certain chemotherapeutic agents (notably methotrexate) may damage white matter tracts, causing a leukoencephalopathy that results in various cognitive and neuropsychiatric deficits. The frontal lobes are the most frequently affected region, although smaller fibers may be damaged and result in region- and domain-specific cognitive deficits (Rimkus et al. 2014). The most common cognitive complaints involve dysfunction in the fronto-striatal-thalamo-frontal cortical-subcortical circuits that mediate executive functions and motivation/reward systems. Thus, difficulties with processing speed, sustained attention, and other executive functions are commonly seen. Depression, apathy, anxiety, irritability, and other neuropsychiatric changes also are possible, as are delirium and dementia in more severe cases. MRI findings are usually very prominent and include confluent intensities in white matter tracts on T2-weighted and fluid-attenuated inversion recovery (FLAIR) sequences.

Stem Cell Transplantation

Hematopoietic stem cell transplantation (HSCT) may be a significant cause of cognitive dysfunction; up to half of patients have mild, and roughly one-quarter have moderate long-term effects (Jim et al. 2012). As with CRCD, memory and executive function difficulties are common. Cumulative risks for long-term cognitive impairment include baseline cognitive impairment, multiple courses of standard-dosage chemotherapy, cranial or total-body irradiation, intrathecal chemotherapy, allogeneic rather than autologous transplantation, having an unrelated donor, and longer duration of hospitalization (Greenberg 2015; Jim et al. 2012).

Severe complications affecting cognition and other domains are not infrequent in patients undergoing HSCT. Posterior reversible encephalopathy syndrome (PRES) has been documented and linked to immunosuppressive drugs used for prophylaxis of graft-versus-host disease (Bhatt et al. 2015; Won et al. 2009). Monitoring and control of blood pressure are key. This approach, along with discontinuation of the offending drug, often suffices for effective reversal of symptoms.

Delirium rates have been noted to approach 50% shortly after HSCT, most often in the first 2 weeks after transplantation (Fann et al. 2011). Patients should be monitored for other signs of graft rejection, including rash, diarrhea, fever, edema, and dysfunction of the lungs, kidneys, and liver. Risk factors include high dosages of opioid medications, preexisting cognitive dysfunction, and elevated blood urea nitrogen and alkaline phosphatase (Weckmann et al. 2012). Finally, although rare, delirium has been described during the period of engraftment of allogeneic stem cell transplantation.

Complications Associated With Specific Cancer Types

Primary Brain Tumors, Brain Metastases, and Leptomeningeal Disease

Primary CNS tumors, metastatic brain lesions, and other structural defects such as cerebral edema can directly cause cognitive deficits by compressive or invasive means. Rates of cognitive dysfunction in patients with a history of brain tumors are as high as 90% (Ahles and Saykin 2007). Metastatic brain lesions are most likely to occur in non-small-cell and small-cell lung cancer (NSCLC and SCLC), breast cancer, and melanoma (Nayak et al. 2012). Brain metastases are known to occur with a variety of other peripheral cancers, including sarcoma and thyroid, pancreatic, bladder, prostate, testicular, uterine, and ovarian cancers. Cranial irradiation may be a viable option for individuals with brain metastases that have responded well to systemic chemotherapy. Surgical resection is another option for patients with debilitating neuropsychiatric and cognitive changes secondary to tumor burden.

Carcinomatous meningitis—encephalopathy and marked cognitive dysfunction with leptomeningeal disease—is seen in cancers of the lung and breast, melanoma, and non-Hodgkin's lymphoma (Balm and Hammack 1996). Symptoms and signs are associated with increased intracranial pressure such as headache, nausea, vomiting, and mental status changes or are related to the infiltration of nerves producing local neurological deficits (Pavlidis 2004). Abnormal findings on brain MRI (e.g., subarachnoid mass, parenchymal volume loss, sulcal/dural enhancement, hydrocephalus without a mass) and the presence of malignant cells in the cerebrospinal fluid (CSF) are diagnostic; however, the diagnosis may remain elusive. Lumbar puncture has a sensitivity of only 45%–55%; therefore, it is recommended that multiple CSF samples (i.e., at least two) and large sample volumes (e.g., at least 10.5 mL) be obtained (Chamberlain et al. 2009). MRI may not yield an accurate diagnosis in up to 76% of cases (Ko et al. 2019).

Primary brain tumors or brain metastases are expected to cause cognitive or behavioral deficits as a function of their location. Thus, lesions in the frontal lobes and their subcortical white matter tracts and specific highly connected subcortical regions would be expected to affect executive functioning, attention, processing speed, motivation, inhibition of inappropriate spontaneous behavior, and motor planning and execution (Bonelli and Cummings 2007). Post illness, cancer patients with frontal lesions had significantly greater problems with executive functions, disinhibition, and apathy than did cancer patients with cerebral lesions outside the frontal lobes (Gregg et al. 2014). Patients with nonfrontal lesions still had clinically significant levels of apathy and executive dysfunction, indicating the likely diffuse cortical-subcortical networks underlying these cognitive domains. Cancerous lesions in the temporal lobes can affect language processing, episodic and semantic memory, naming, object recognition, and auditory processing, among other functions with important temporal lobe hubs (Mesulam 2000). Parietal lobe lesions may affect visuospatial orientation and functioning, somatosensory processing, praxis, executive functioning, and working memory (Baldo and Dronkers 2006; Critchley 1953; Mesulam 2000). Cerebellar lesions could result in the cerebellar cognitive affective syndrome, in which executive dysfunction, inattention, and other cognitive problems traditionally associated with cerebral dysfunction occur as a result of core cerebellar or cerebrocerebellar dysfunction (Schmahmann and Sherman 1998).

Paraneoplastic Syndromes

Paraneoplastic limbic encephalitis is caused by cell-mediated autoimmune responses against specific neuronal antigens. Onconeuronal antibodies target *intracellular* neuronal proteins. Autoantibodies that target antigens *on the cell surface* are more likely in noncancerous etiologies, although underlying tumors may be the cause in some cases. Small-cell lung cancer is the most common cancer associated with paraneoplastic syndromes; other cancerous culprits include Hodgkin's lymphoma, thymoma, and cancers of the thyroid, breast, stomach, colon, kidneys, testes, ovaries, or uterus (Foster and Caplan 2009). Cognitive changes, including short-term memory deficits, are a hallmark. The most prominent neuropsychiatric features include psychosis, agitation, seizures, and delirium. For patients who present with acute or subacute neuropsychiatric and cognitive changes, consideration of common causes of delirium is a vital first step. The workup should include neuroimaging (MRI is preferred), electroencephalography, and serum and CSF analysis of autoimmune markers, infectious agents, and paraneoplastic antibodies. A search for underlying malignancies is also essential. Treatment includes removal of underlying tumors (if identified), immunotherapy, and adjunctive medications based on symptoms (e.g., anticonvulsants, antipsychotics). Primary immunotherapy includes steroids, intravenous immunoglobulin, and plasmapheresis. Secondary immunotherapy (e.g., with rituximab or cyclophosphamide) may be necessary. *N*-methyl-D-aspartate receptor (NMDAR)–associated limbic encephalitis most commonly occurs in young women and often manifests as new-onset psychotic illness. It is typically but not always associated with ovarian teratomas (Dalmau et al. 2007, 2011; see Chapter 8, "Inflammatory Diseases and Their Psychiatric Manifestations," for additional discussion).

Cancer-related ectopic production of corticotropin or corticotropin-releasing hormone (CRH) may induce cognitive and other neuropsychiatric effects, most typically mood-related symptoms due to the development of Cushing's syndrome. Approximately 10%–15% of cases of Cushing's syndrome are attributable to cancer, most commonly SCLC and less commonly neuroendocrine or gastroenteropancreatic tumors (Ferone and Albertelli 2014; Ilias et al. 2005). Treatment includes surgery and pharmacotherapy with somatostatin analogues.

Hyponatremia due to the syndrome of inappropriate antidiuretic hormone (SIADH) secretion can cause various cognitive and neurobehavioral changes in cancer patients; therefore, routine monitoring of serum sodium is required in cancer patients. While SCLC is the most common cancer-related cause, the differential diagnosis for SIADH is very broad, and other potential etiologies should be excluded (Adrogué and Madias 2000). Treatment involves increasing serum sodium by fluid restriction at rates no greater than 0.5 mEq/L per hour and by no more than 10–12 mEq/L in the first 24 hours in order to prevent osmotic demyelination syndrome (e.g., central pontine myelinolysis). More aggressive sodium correction (e.g., by using hypertonic saline) may be indicated in more acute or severe cases. For chronic, asymptomatic cases, vasopressin type 2 receptor antagonists or diuretics may be tried.

Pharmacological Considerations in Psycho-Oncology

Several medications used to treat cancer have neuropsychiatric side effects (Table 13–3). These effects can be the result of direct toxicity to the brain or of indirect effects on organ function, metabolic balance, hormones, proinflammatory cytokines, and the vascular system. Knowledge of these side effects can guide care decisions and help patients and family members understand the complexities of cancer care and make mindful choices among psychopharmacological agents to treat complications they may not have been expecting.

Pharmacokinetic interactions between psychiatric medications and agents used in the treatment of cancer are common. Bupropion and some of the SSRIs can affect the hepatic metabolism of chemotherapeutic agents by inhibition of cytochrome P450 (CYP) 2D6 enzymes. Tamoxifen—used to reduce the risk of breast cancer recurrence in premenopausal women—is metabolized by the CYP2D6 enzyme group to a more potent compound called endoxifen; strong inhibitors of this metabolic step (e.g., fluoxetine, fluvoxamine, paroxetine) were feared to reduce tamoxifen's therapeutic effect (Desmarais and Looper 2009). More recently, large cohort studies have failed to demonstrate a real increased risk for breast cancer recurrence as a result of this interaction, yet it remains prudent to avoid strong inhibitor antidepressants when selecting a new treatment for women who are taking tamoxifen (Haque et al. 2015). Most chemotherapeutic agents are metabolized by the CYP3A4 enzyme group, and although some psychotropic agents affect this system, those agents are not as widely used as antidepressants (Table 13–4). Antidepressant and antipsychotic medications can have significant effects on cardiac conduction, particularly QTc prolongation. Although no monitoring is recommended in routine practice, additive effects when combined with other agents that can prolong the QTc interval can significantly increase the risk of cardiac arrhythmias (Table 13–5). Finally, when choosing a psychotropic medication, avoidance of uncomfortable side effects in patients who are already burdened by the effects of cancer medications is critically important. Anticholinergic and gastrointes-

TABLE 13–3. Selected neuropsychiatric complications of agents used in cancer treatment

Agent	Neuropsychiatric complications
Hormonal agents	
Antiestrogens (tamoxifen, anastrozole)	Depression, mood swings, insomnia/fatigue, hot flashes
Androgen blockade (leuprolide)	Mood disturbances, fatigue, hot flashes
Biologicals	
Interferon-α	Depression, anxiety, cognitive impairment
Interleukin-2	Delirium, psychosis
Monoclonal antibodies	
Bevacizumab, rituximab, trastuzumab	Anxiety, PRES
Pembrolizumab	Delirium, insomnia
Nitrogen mustards	
Cyclophosphamide	Delirium, PRES, cognitive dysfunction
Ifosfamide	Delirium, parkinsonism
Chlorambucil	Hallucinations
Nitrosourea compound	
Carmustine	Asthenia, depression
Platinum-based agent	
Cisplatin	Delirium, PRES
Nonclassical alkylating agent	
Procarbazine	Serotonin syndrome, delirium, mania
Antimetabolites	
5-Fluorouracil	Hyperammonemic encephalopathy, leukoencephalopathy
Cytarabine	Delirium, seizures (with high dosages)
Gemcitabine	Fatigue, PRES
Hydroxyurea	Delirium, hallucinations
Methotrexate	Delirium, leukoencephalopathy, seizures, coma
Pemetrexed	Mood disturbances
Mitotic inhibitors	
Vinca alkaloids (vincristine, vinblastine)	Irritability, depression
Docetaxel, paclitaxel	Depression, alcohol intoxication (secondary to ethanol content)
Etoposide	PRES
Other agents	
Asparaginase	Depression, agitation, hallucinations, PRES
Inhibitors of kinase signaling enzymes (imatinib, dasatinib, erlotinib)	Agitated depression
Immunosuppressants (cyclosporine, tacrolimus, everolimus)	Depression, anxiety, panic attacks, insomnia, delusions, hallucinations, delirium

Note. PRES=posterior reversible encephalopathy syndrome.

TABLE 13–4.	QTc-prolonging drugs used in cancer treatment	
Bortezomib	Granisetron	Sunitinib
Bosutinib	Lapatinib	Tacrolimus
Crizotinib	Methadone	Tamoxifen
Dabrafenib	Ondansetron	Vandetanib
Dasatinib	Nilotinib	Vemurafenib
Dolasetron	Pazopanib	Vorinostat
Fluconazole	Sorafenib	

TABLE 13–5.	Cytochrome P450 (CYP) 3A4 substrates	
Substrates of CYP3A4		
Anastrozole	Gefitinib	Sunitinib
Cyclophosphamide	Ifosfamide	Tacrolimus
Cyclosporine	Imatinib	Tamoxifen
Docetaxel	Irinotecan	Teniposide
Doxorubicin	Paclitaxel	Vinblastine
Erlotinib	Sirolimus	Vincristine
Etoposide	Sorafenib	
Relevant medications with potential interactions		
Butalbital	Modafinil	Phenytoin
Carbamazepine	Oxcarbazepine	St. John's wort
Fluvoxamine	Phenobarbital	Topiramate

tinal effects can worsen preexisting conditions or side effects from cancer medications; SSRIs can cause SIADH; and SNRIs can worsen hypertension. Immediate-release bupropion can lower the seizure threshold and should be used cautiously in patients with preexisting risk due to brain lesions.

Conclusion

Psychiatrists can help guide the management of mood, behavioral, cognitive, and physical symptoms associated with cancer and its treatment and can provide thoughtful consultations that can help clarify the etiology and best management options. Working closely with medical, surgical, and radiation oncologists, neurologists, and other clinicians, psychiatrists can help ensure that potential medical, psychiatric, and psychosocial causes of neuropsychiatric distress are carefully assessed and identified.

References

Aapro MS, Molassiotis A, Olver I: Anticipatory nausea and vomiting. Support Care Cancer 13(2):117–121, 2005 15599779

Abrahams HJ, Gielissen MF, Goedendorp MM, et al: A randomized controlled trial of web-based cognitive behavioral therapy for severely fatigued breast cancer survivors (CHANGE-study): study protocol. BMC Cancer 15:765, 2015 26500019

Adrogué HJ, Madias NE: Hyponatremia. N Engl J Med 342(21):1581–1589, 2000 10824078

Ahles TA, Saykin AJ: Candidate mechanisms for chemotherapy-induced cognitive changes. Nat Rev Cancer 7(3):192–201, 2007 17318212

Al-Aama T, Brymer C, Gutmanis I, et al: Melatonin decreases delirium in elderly patients: a randomized, placebo-controlled trial. Int J Geriatr Psychiatry 26(7):687–694, 2011 20845391

Alvarez J, Meyer FL, Granoff DL, et al: The effect of EEG biofeedback on reducing postcancer cognitive impairment. Integr Cancer Ther 12(6):475–487, 2013 23584550

American Psychiatric Association: Diagnostic and Statistical Manual of Mental Disorders, 5th Edition. Arlington, VA, American Psychiatric Association, 2013

Ancoli-Israel S, Moore PJ, Jones V: The relationship between fatigue and sleep in cancer patients: a review. Eur J Cancer Care (Engl) 10(4):245–255, 2001 11806675

Ancoli-Israel S, Liu L, Rissling M, et al: Sleep, fatigue, depression, and circadian activity rhythms in women with breast cancer before and after treatment: a 1-year longitudinal study. Support Care Cancer 22(9):2535–2545, 2014 24733634

Baldo JV, Dronkers NF: The role of inferior parietal and inferior frontal cortex in working memory. Neuropsychology 20(5):529–538, 2006 16938015

Balm M, Hammack J: Leptomeningeal carcinomatosis. Presenting features and prognostic factors. Arch Neurol 53(7):626–632, 1996 8929170

Berger AM, Mooney K, Alvarez-Perez A, et al; National Comprehensive Cancer Network: Cancer-Related Fatigue, Version 2.2015: Clinical Practice Guidelines in Oncology. J Natl Compr Canc Netw 13(8):1012–1039, 2015 26285247

Bhatt VR, Balasetti V, Jasem JA, et al: Central nervous system complications and outcomes after allogeneic hematopoietic stem cell transplantation. Clin Lymphoma Myeloma Leuk 15(10):606–611, 2015 26184063

Bonelli RM, Cummings JL: Frontal-subcortical circuitry and behavior. Dialogues Clin Neurosci 9(2):141–151, 2007 17726913

Bower JE, Bak K, Berger A, et al: Screening, assessment, and management of fatigue in adult survivors of cancer: an American Society of Clinical oncology clinical practice guideline adaptation. J Clin Oncol 32(17):1840–1850, 2014 24733803

Breitbart W, Alici Y: Evidence-based treatment of delirium in patients with cancer. J Clin Oncol 30(11):1206–1214, 2012 22412123

Brintzenhofe-Szoc KM, Levin TT, Li Y, et al: Mixed anxiety/depression symptoms in a large cancer cohort: prevalence by cancer type. Psychosomatics 50(4):383–391, 2009 19687179

Brooks JO 3rd, Hoblyn JC: Secondary mania in older adults. Am J Psychiatry 162(11):2033–2038, 2005 16263839

Brown ES, Suppes T: Mood symptoms during corticosteroid therapy: a review. Harv Rev Psychiatry 5(5):239–246, 1998 9493946

Caruso R, Nanni MG, Riba M, et al: Depressive spectrum disorders in cancer: prevalence, risk factors and screening for depression: a critical review. Acta Oncol 56(2):146–155, 2017 28140731

Cella D, Lai JS, Stone A: Self-reported fatigue: one dimension or more? Lessons from the Functional Assessment of Chronic Illness Therapy—Fatigue (FACIT-F) questionnaire. Support Care Cancer 19(9):1441–1450, 2011 20706850

Centeno C, Sanz A, Bruera E: Delirium in advanced cancer patients. Palliat Med 18(3):184–194, 2004 15198131

Chamberlain MC, Glantz M, Groves MD, Wilson WH: Diagnostic tools for neoplastic meningitis: detecting disease, identifying patient risk, and determining benefit of treatment. Semin Oncol 36 (4 suppl 2):S35–S45, 2009 19660682

Cramp F, Byron-Daniel J: Exercise for the management of cancer-related fatigue in adults. Cochrane Database Syst Rev (11):CD006145, 2012 23152233

Critchley M: The Parietal Lobes. New York, Hafner Press, 1953

Crosswell AD, Lockwood KG, Ganz PA, et al: Low heart rate variability and cancer-related fatigue in breast cancer survivors. Psychoneuroendocrinology 45:58–66, 2014 24845177

Cryer PE: Symptoms of hypoglycemia, thresholds for their occurrence, and hypoglycemia unawareness. Endocrinol Metab Clin North Am 28(3):495–500, v–vi, 1999 10500927

Dalmau J, Tüzün E, Wu HY, et al: Paraneoplastic anti-N-methyl-D-aspartate receptor encephalitis associated with ovarian teratoma. Ann Neurol 61(1):25–36, 2007 17262855

Dalmau J, Lancaster E, Martinez-Hernandez E, et al: Clinical experience and laboratory investigations in patients with anti-NMDAR encephalitis. Lancet Neurol 10(1):63–74, 2011 21163445

Darmani NA, Ray AP: Evidence for a re-evaluation of the neurochemical and anatomical bases of chemotherapy-induced vomiting. Chem Rev 109(7):3158–3199, 2009 19522506

Deprez S, Billiet T, Sunaert S, et al: Diffusion tensor MRI of chemotherapy-induced cognitive impairment in non-CNS cancer patients: a review. Brain Imaging Behav 7(4):409–435, 2013 23329357

de Ruiter MB, Schagen SB: Functional MRI studies in non-CNS cancers. Brain Imaging Behav 7(4):388–408, 2013 23934234

de Ruiter MB, Reneman L, Boogerd W, et al: Cerebral hyporesponsiveness and cognitive impairment 10 years after chemotherapy for breast cancer. Hum Brain Mapp 32(8):1206–1219, 2011 20669165

Desmarais JE, Looper KJ: Interactions between tamoxifen and antidepressants via cytochrome P450 2D6. J Clin Psychiatry 70(12):1688–1697, 2009 20141708

Di Maio M, Bria E, Banna GL, et al: Prevention of chemotherapy-induced nausea and vomiting and the role of neurokinin 1 inhibitors: from guidelines to clinical practice in solid tumors. Anticancer Drugs 24(2):99–111, 2013 23165435

Dudgeon DJ, Lertzman M: Dyspnea in the advanced cancer patient. J Pain Symptom Manage 16(4):212–219, 1998 9803048

Duigon A: Anticipatory nausea and vomiting associated with cancer chemotherapy. Oncol Nurs Forum 13(1):35–40, 1986 3632858

Endicott J: Measurement of depression in patients with cancer. Cancer 53 (10 suppl):2243–2249, 1984 6704912

Fann JR, Thomas-Rich AM, Katon WJ, et al: Major depression after breast cancer: a review of epidemiology and treatment. Gen Hosp Psychiatry 30(2):112–126, 2008 18291293

Fann JR, Hubbard RA, Alfano CM, et al: Pre- and post-transplantation risk factors for delirium onset and severity in patients undergoing hematopoietic stem-cell transplantation. J Clin Oncol 29(7):895–901, 2011 21263081

Ferguson RJ, Ahles TA, Saykin AJ, et al: Cognitive-behavioral management of chemotherapy-related cognitive change. Psychooncology 16(8):772–777, 2007 17152119

Fernandes PP: Rapid desensitization for needle phobia. Psychosomatics 44(3):253–254, 2003 12724508

Ferone D, Albertelli M: Ectopic Cushing and other paraneoplastic syndromes in thoracic neuroendocrine tumors. Thorac Surg Clin 24(3):277–283, 2014 25065928

Fertig DL, Hayes DF: Considerations in using tumor markers: what the psycho-oncologist needs to know. Psychooncology 10(5):370–379, 2001 11536415

Flaherty JH, Steele DK, Chibnall JT, et al: An ACE unit with a delirium room may improve function and equalize length of stay among older delirious medical inpatients. J Gerontol A Biol Sci Med Sci 65(12):1387–1392, 2010 20679073

Foster AR, Caplan JP: Paraneoplastic limbic encephalitis. Psychosomatics 50(2):108–113, 2009 19377018

Gielissen MF, Verhagen S, Witjes F, et al: Effects of cognitive behavior therapy in severely fatigued disease-free cancer patients compared with patients waiting for cognitive behavior therapy: a randomized controlled trial. J Clin Oncol 24(30):4882–4887, 2006 17050873

Greenberg D: Brain tumors, in Psychiatric Care of the Medical Patient. Edited by Fogel BS, Greenberg DB. New York, Oxford University Press, 2015, pp 1034–1045

Greenberg DB, Jonasch E, Gadd MA, et al: Adjuvant therapy of melanoma with interferon-alpha-2b is associated with mania and bipolar syndromes. Cancer 89(2):356–362, 2000 10918166

Gregg N, Arber A, Ashkan K, et al: Neurobehavioural changes in patients following brain tumour: patients and relatives perspective. Support Care Cancer 22(11):2965–2972, 2014 24865878

Griffiths RR, Johnson MW, Carducci MA, et al: Psilocybin produces substantial and sustained decreases in depression and anxiety in patients with life-threatening cancer: a randomized double-blind trial. J Psychopharmacol 30(12):1181–1197, 2016 27909165

Han R, Yang YM, Dietrich J, et al: Systemic 5-fluorouracil treatment causes a syndrome of delayed myelin destruction in the central nervous system. J Biol 7(4):12, 2008 18430259

Haque R, Shi J, Schottinger JE, et al: Tamoxifen and antidepressant drug interaction in a cohort of 16,887 breast cancer survivors. J Natl Cancer Inst 108(3):djv337, 2015 26631176

Hardy SE: Methylphenidate for the treatment of depressive symptoms, including fatigue and apathy, in medically ill older adults and terminally ill adults. Am J Geriatr Pharmacother 7(1):34–59, 2009 19281939

Hofmann SG, Asnaani A, Vonk IJ, et al: The efficacy of cognitive behavioral therapy: a review of meta-analyses. Cognit Ther Res 36(5):427–440, 2012 23459093

Hutchinson AD, Hosking JR, Kichenadasse G, et al: Objective and subjective cognitive impairment following chemotherapy for cancer: a systematic review. Cancer Treat Rev 38(7):926–934, 2012 22658913

Ilias I, Torpy DJ, Pacak K, et al: Cushing's syndrome due to ectopic corticotropin secretion: twenty years' experience at the National Institutes of Health. J Clin Endocrinol Metab 90(8):4955–4962, 2005 15914534

Inouye SK, Charpentier PA: Precipitating factors for delirium in hospitalized elderly persons. Predictive model and interrelationship with baseline vulnerability. JAMA 275(11):852–857, 1996 8596223

Jehn CF, Kühnhardt D, Bartholomae A, et al: Association of IL-6, hypothalamus-pituitary-adrenal axis function, and depression in patients with cancer. Integr Cancer Ther 9(3):270–275, 2010 20702499

Jim HS, Small B, Hartman S, et al: Clinical predictors of cognitive function in adults treated with hematopoietic cell transplantation. Cancer 118(13):3407–3416, 2012 22139882

Kadan-Lottick NS, Vanderwerker LC, Block SD, et al: Psychiatric disorders and mental health service use in patients with advanced cancer: a report from the coping with cancer study. Cancer 104(12):2872–2881, 2005 16284994

Kaiser J, Bledowski C, Dietrich J: Neural correlates of chemotherapy-related cognitive impairment. Cortex 54:33–50, 2014 24632463

Kamen C, Tejani MA, Chandwani K, et al: Anticipatory nausea and vomiting due to chemotherapy. Eur J Pharmacol 722:172–179, 2014 24157982

Kang HJ, Kim JM, Kim SY, et al: A longitudinal study of BDNF promoter methylation and depression in breast cancer. Psychiatry Investig 12(4):523–531, 2015 26508964

Kesler SR, Bennett FC, Mahaffey ML, et al: Regional brain activation during verbal declarative memory in metastatic breast cancer. Clin Cancer Res 15(21):6665–6673, 2009 19843664

Kim JM, Kim SW, Stewart R, et al: Serotonergic and BDNF genes associated with depression 1 week and 1 year after mastectomy for breast cancer. Psychosom Med 74(1):8–15, 2012 22210241

Ko Y, Gwak HS, Park EY, et al: Association of MRI findings with clinical characteristics and prognosis in patients with leptomeningeal carcinomatosis from non-small cell lung cancer. J Neurooncol 143(3):553–562, 2019 31089925

Krebber AM, Buffart LM, Kleijn G, et al: Prevalence of depression in cancer patients: a meta-analysis of diagnostic interviews and self-report instruments. Psychooncology 23(2):121–130, 2014 24105788

Laoutidis ZG, Mathiak K: Antidepressants in the treatment of depression/depressive symptoms in cancer patients: a systematic review and meta-analysis. BMC Psychiatry 13:140, 2013 23679841

Lawlor PG, Gagnon B, Mancini IL, et al: Occurrence, causes, and outcome of delirium in patients with advanced cancer: a prospective study. Arch Intern Med 160(6):786–794, 2000 10737278

Levin RD, Daehler MA, Grutsch JF, et al: Circadian function in patients with advanced non-small-cell lung cancer. Br J Cancer 93(11):1202–1208, 2005 16265345

Li M, Fitzgerald P, Rodin G: Evidence-based treatment of depression in patients with cancer. J Clin Oncol 30(11):1187–1196, 2012 22412144

Lim I, Joung HY, Yu AR, et al: PET evidence of the effect of donepezil on cognitive performance in an animal model of chemobrain. BioMed Res Int 2016:6945415, 2016 27556039

Malik IA, Khan WA, Qazilbash M, et al: Clinical efficacy of lorazepam in prophylaxis of anticipatory, acute, and delayed nausea and vomiting induced by high doses of cisplatin. A prospective randomized trial. Am J Clin Oncol 18(2):170–175, 1995 7900711

Massie MJ: Prevalence of depression in patients with cancer. J Natl Cancer Inst Monogr 32(32):57–71, 2004 15263042

Massie MJ, Holland J, Glass E: Delirium in terminally ill cancer patients. Am J Psychiatry 140(8):1048–1050, 1983 6869591

McDonald BC, Saykin AJ: Alterations in brain structure related to breast cancer and its treatment: chemotherapy and other considerations. Brain Imaging Behav 7(4):374–387, 2013 23996156

McDonald BC, Conroy SK, Smith DJ, et al: Frontal gray matter reduction after breast cancer chemotherapy and association with executive symptoms: a replication and extension study. Brain Behav Immun 30 (suppl):S117–S125, 2013 22613170

Mesulam M-M: Principles of Behavioral and Cognitive Neurology, 2nd Edition. New York, Oxford University Press, 2000

Miller AH, Ancoli-Israel S, Bower JE, et al: Neuroendocrine-immune mechanisms of behavioral comorbidities in patients with cancer. J Clin Oncol 26(6):971–982, 2008 18281672

Mills PJ, Parker B, Dimsdale JE, et al: The relationship between fatigue and quality of life and inflammation during anthracycline-based chemotherapy in breast cancer. Biol Psychol 69(1):85–96, 2005 15740827

Minton O, Richardson A, Sharpe M, et al: Drug therapy for the management of cancer-related fatigue. Cochrane Database Syst Rev (7):CD006704, 2010 20614448

Mitchell AJ: Pooled results from 38 analyses of the accuracy of distress thermometer and other ultra-short methods of detecting cancer-related mood disorders. J Clin Oncol 25(29):4670–4681, 2007 17846453

Moore HC: An overview of chemotherapy-related cognitive dysfunction, or "chemobrain." Oncology (Williston Park) 28(9):797–804, 2014 25224480

Mustian KM, Janelsins MC, Peppone LK, et al: EXCAP exercise effects on cognitive impairment and inflammation: a URCC NCORP RCT in 479 cancer patients. J Clin Oncol 33(15 suppl):9504, 2015. Available at: https://ascopubs.org/doi/abs/10.1200/jco.2015.33.15_suppl.9504. Accessed April 6, 2019.

Nayak L, Lee EQ, Wen PY: Epidemiology of brain metastases. Curr Oncol Rep 14(1):48–54, 2012 22012633

Oliveira Miranda D, Soares de Lima TA, Ribeiro Azevedo L, et al: Proinflammatory cytokines correlate with depression and anxiety in colorectal cancer patients. BioMed Res Int 2014:739650, 2014 25309921

O'Regan NA, Ryan DJ, Boland E, et al: Attention! A good bedside test for delirium? J Neurol Neurosurg Psychiatry 85(10):1122–1131, 2014 24569688

Ostuzzi G, Matcham F, Dauchy S, et al: Antidepressants for the treatment of depression in people with cancer. Cochrane Database Syst Rev 6(6):CD011006, 2015 26029972

Parker LA, Rock EM, Limebeer CL: Regulation of nausea and vomiting by cannabinoids. Br J Pharmacol 163(7):1411–1422, 2011 21175589

Passik SD, Kirsh KL, Donaghy K, et al: Patient-related barriers to fatigue communication: initial validation of the fatigue management barriers questionnaire. J Pain Symptom Manage 24(5):481–493, 2002 12547048

Pavlidis N: The diagnostic and therapeutic management of leptomeningeal carcinomatosis. Ann Oncol 15 (suppl 4):iv285–iv291, 2004 15477323

Plotnik AN, Carney P, Schweder P, et al: Seizures initially diagnosed as panic attacks: case series. Aust N Z J Psychiatry 43(9):878 882, 2009 19670064

Reuter K, Harter M: Fatigue and/or depression? Examination of the construct validity of CRF. Psychooncology 12(suppl):S259–S260, 2003

Rimkus CdeM, Andrade CS, Leite CdaC, et al: Toxic leukoencephalopathies, including drug, medication, environmental, and radiation-induced encephalopathic syndromes. Semin Ultrasound CT MR 35(2):97–117, 2014 24745887

Romanowicz M, Ehlers S, Walker D, et al: Testing a diathesis-stress model: potential genetic risk factors for development of distress in context of acute leukemia diagnosis and transplant. Psychosomatics 53(5):456–462, 2012 22652301

Ross S, Bossis A, Guss J, et al: Rapid and sustained symptom reduction following psilocybin treatment for anxiety and depression in patients with life-threatening cancer: a randomized controlled trial. J Psychopharmacol 30(12):1165–1180, 2016 27909164

Ryan JL, Carroll JK, Ryan EP, et al: Mechanisms of cancer-related fatigue. Oncologist 12 (suppl 1):22–34, 2007 17573453

Satin JR, Linden W, Phillips MJ: Depression as a predictor of disease progression and mortality in cancer patients: a meta-analysis. Cancer 115(22):5349–5361, 2009 19753617

Savard J, Simard S, Blanchet J, et al: Prevalence, clinical characteristics, and risk factors for insomnia in the context of breast cancer. Sleep 24(5):583–590, 2001 11480655

Schmahmann JD, Sherman JC: The cerebellar cognitive affective syndrome. Brain 121 (Pt 4):561–579, 1998 9577385

Seddighi A, Seddighi AS, Nikouei A, et al: Psychological aspects in brain tumor patients: a prospective study. Hell J Nucl Med 18 (suppl 1):63–67, 2015 26665213

Seigers R, Fardell JE: Neurobiological basis of chemotherapy-induced cognitive impairment: a review of rodent research. Neurosci Biobehav Rev 35(3):729–741, 2011 20869395

Seigers R, Schagen SB, Van Tellingen O, et al: Chemotherapy-related cognitive dysfunction: current animal studies and future directions. Brain Imaging Behav 7(4):453–459, 2013 23949877

Şenel G, Uysal N, Oguz G, et al: Delirium frequency and risk factors among patients with cancer in palliative care unit. Am J Hosp Palliat Care 34(3):282–286, 2017 26722008

Simó M, Rifà-Ros X, Rodriguez-Fornells A, et al: Chemobrain: a systematic review of structural and functional neuroimaging studies. Neurosci Biobehav Rev 37(8):1311–1321, 2013 23660455

Suppli NP, Bukh JD, Moffitt TE, et al: 5-HTTLPR and use of antidepressants after colorectal cancer including a meta-analysis of 5-HTTLPR and depression after cancer. Transl Psychiatry 5:e631, 2015 26327689

Thekdi SM, Trinidad A, Roth A: Psychopharmacology in cancer. Curr Psychiatry Rep 17(1):529, 2015 25417593

Van Lancker A, Velghe A, Van Hecke A, et al: Prevalence of symptoms in older cancer patients receiving palliative care: a systematic review and meta-analysis. J Pain Symptom Manage 47(1):90–104, 2014 23764109

Vardy J, Tannock I: Cognitive function after chemotherapy in adults with solid tumours. Crit Rev Oncol Hematol 63(3):183–202, 2007 17678745

Vezmar S, Becker A, Bode U, et al: Biochemical and clinical aspects of methotrexate neurotoxicity. Chemotherapy 49(1–2):92–104, 2003 12714818

Vodermaier A, Millman RD: Accuracy of the Hospital Anxiety and Depression Scale as a screening tool in cancer patients: a systematic review and meta-analysis. Support Care Cancer 19(12):1899–1908, 2011 21898134

Voigt V, Neufeld F, Kaste J, et al: Clinically assessed posttraumatic stress in patients with breast cancer during the first year after diagnosis in the prospective, longitudinal, controlled COGNICARES study. Psychooncology 26(1):74–80, 2017 26898732

Volf N, Crismon ML: Leukemia in bipolar mood disorder: is lithium contraindicated? DICP 25(9):948–951, 1991 1949974

Wakefield CE, Butow PN, Aaronson NA, et al: Patient-reported depression measures in cancer: a meta-review. Lancet Psychiatry 2(7):635–647, 2015 26303561

Walker J, Holm Hansen C, Martin P, et al: Prevalence of depression in adults with cancer: a systematic review. Ann Oncol 24(4):895–900, 2013 23175625

Walker J, Hansen CH, Martin P, et al: Prevalence, associations, and adequacy of treatment of major depression in patients with cancer: a cross-sectional analysis of routinely collected clinical data. Lancet Psychiatry 1(5):343–350, 2014 26360998

Warr DG: Chemotherapy-and cancer-related nausea and vomiting. Curr Oncol 15 (suppl 1):S4–S9, 2008 18231647

Watts S, Leydon G, Birch B, et al: Depression and anxiety in prostate cancer: a systematic review and meta-analysis of prevalence rates. BMJ Open 4(3):e003901, 2014 24625637

Weckmann MT, Gingrich R, Mills JA, et al: Risk factors for delirium in patients undergoing hematopoietic stem cell transplantation. Ann Clin Psychiatry 24(3):204–214, 2012 22860240

Wefel JS, Vardy J, Ahles T, et al: International Cognition and Cancer Task Force recommendations to harmonise studies of cognitive function in patients with cancer. Lancet Oncol 12(7):703–708, 2011 21354373

Wefel JS, Kesler SR, Noll KR, et al: Clinical characteristics, pathophysiology, and management of noncentral nervous system cancer-related cognitive impairment in adults. CA Cancer J Clin 65(2):123–138, 2015 25483452

Williams LA, Bohac C, Hunter S, et al: Patient and health care provider perceptions of cancer-related fatigue and pain. Support Care Cancer 24(10):4357–4363, 2016 27207616

Won SC, Kwon SY, Han JW, et al: Posterior reversible encephalopathy syndrome in childhood with hematologic/oncologic diseases. J Pediatr Hematol Oncol 31(7):505–508, 2009 19564746

CHAPTER 14

Dermatology

Psychiatric Considerations in the Medical Setting

Katherine Taylor, M.D.

Janna Gordon-Elliott, M.D.

Philip R. Muskin, M.D., M.A.

Skin conditions are highly prevalent, affecting an estimated one in three of all patients in general medical settings, and are a common reason for presentation for care (Lowell et al. 2001). Psychiatric disorders and psychological distress are common in patients seeking help for dermatological complaints. The prevalence of psychiatric disorders in patients with skin disease is estimated to be approximately 30%–60% (Gupta and Gupta 2014; Korabel et al. 2008). Emotional and behavioral factors, psychiatric conditions, and psychotropic medications influence the skin; reciprocally, dermatological issues can negatively affect mental health. The relationships among stress, psychiatric illness, and the skin can confuse or complicate the assessment and management of patients presenting with dermatological concerns. In addition, several medical disorders that can have psychiatric symptoms—for example, psychosis in systemic lupus erythematosus, postinfectious manifestations of syphilis, and Lyme disease—can also have skin lesions.

In this chapter, we review two general categories of patient presentations:

1. Patients with primary dermatological conditions that are influenced by psychiatric symptoms and disorders. These patients have dermatological disorders that to the provider may appear to be "all in their head" or that may be clinically misunderstood because they manifest psychiatric or psychological features.
2. Patients with primary psychiatric disorders that present with secondary skin manifestations. These patients have atypical dermatological signs and symptoms that are the direct result of a psychiatric disorder.

In addition, we review pharmacological interactions between psychiatric and dermatological medications and special considerations in management.

Dermatological Conditions Influenced by Psychiatric Symptoms and Disorders

Clinical Vignette

Mr. S is a 49-year-old married man, employed as a tax accountant, with a history of asthma, eczema, generalized anxiety disorder (GAD), irritable bowel syndrome, and fibromyalgia, who presents to the primary care clinic with complaints of generalized itching and diarrhea. He is well known to clinic staff due to his frequent phone calls and visits, most often with bowel-related complaints. Multiple past gastrointestinal work-ups have been negative. Findings from the physical examination are unremarkable. The primary care physician suspects that his patient's complaints are related to increased stress at work.

The Biological Interaction Between Stress and the Skin

Psychiatric conditions and treatments—through biological, emotional, and behavioral factors—influence the presentation and course of dermatological disease. Emotional and behavioral issues, or preexisting psychiatric conditions, may confound the presentation and can easily lead to the assumption that the dermatological complaint is a function of the psychiatric condition rather than an independent disorder influenced by the patient's mental state.

Thirty percent of those with a dermatological condition have clinically significant levels of psychological distress (Gupta and Gupta 2014), which may be related to the effect of the condition on the individual's appearance, interpersonal functioning, or general well-being. Emotional and functional consequences of dermatological diseases often do not correlate directly with the objective severity of disease (Fried et al. 2005). Stress related to the dermatological condition, as well as to anxiety, depression, or other issues, will affect the skin disorder. The effect of stress may be mediated through a host of neurobiological factors that affect skin function or through behaviors that affect the skin. A vicious cycle may be established wherein a dermatological condition contributes to psychological stress that, in turn, further aggravates the skin condition.

Psychological stress has a direct impact on skin barrier function and on a wide range of immune parameters that can directly affect the skin. The brain and the skin have the same ectodermal origin and are affected by similar hormones and neurotransmitters (Koblenzer 1983). The so-called neuro-immuno-cutaneous system (Misery 1996) uses mediators similar to those involved in the hypothalamic-pituitary-adrenal axis and is similarly regulated by feedback inhibition. Thus, the skin functions as both a target and a source of key stress mediators, including corticotropin-releasing hormone and the proopiomelanocortin-derived neuropeptides α-melanocyte–stimulating hormone, β-endorphin, and adrenocorticotropic hormone (Slominski 2005).

The skin appears to respond differently to acute versus chronic stress. In acute stress, the skin shows enhanced immune function, with increased intracutaneous migration of immunocompetent cells and increased mast cell activation with degranulation and release of histamine. The mast cell is an important regulator of neurogenic inflammation during the stress response and plays an important role in stress-mediated dermatoses. In contrast, chronic stress correlates with decreased cutaneous immunity. People with chronic stress show worse initial inflammatory responses to wounds, with reduced proinflammatory cytokines and suppressed neutrophil transcriptome, prolonged inflammatory states via persistent neutrophil trafficking to the wound, and slowed wound healing (Walburn et al. 2009). In many inflammatory skin conditions (e.g., psoriasis, atopic dermatitis, acne, rosacea, eczema, lichen simplex chronicus, nodular prurigo, chronic urticaria, seborrheic dermatitis), there is a clear and chronological association between patient stress and exacerbation of dermatological symptoms. This relationship is thought to be mediated by the effects of stress on immune functioning (Gupta and Levenson 2005).

The Psychological Impact of Skin Disorders

Emotional and behavioral factors influence the presentation and course of dermatological disease (Table 14–1). Distress related to a skin condition may lead to social isolation or avoidance of health care providers. Indeed, the term *stigma,* used currently to refer to discrimination or social isolation frequently linked to mental disorders, derives from the word's original use to designate a mark on the skin often associated with illness or disgrace. Difficulty accessing treatment because of educational or socioeconomic deficits may lead to missed appointments with physicians or nonadherence to medications. Personality traits, anxiety, and depression influence an individual's ability to trust health care providers, contributing to lapses in treatment. The converse is also true—that is, similar problems might lead to excessive help seeking or dependence on providers. These behaviors can start a maladaptive dynamic in which escalating demands lead to reduced responsiveness on the part of the provider, such that the patient's complaints begin to be dismissed or invalidated.

In the clinical vignette, Mr. S presents as having an emotionally mediated symptom of itching, which could be dismissed as being "all in his head," at least in part, because of the patient's frequent complaints. Another way of conceptualizing this patient would be to consider the pathophysiology of pruritus and the so-called *itch-scratch cycle,* which has been hypothesized to be mediated by both peripheral (e.g., histamine, proteinases, substance P, opioid peptides, neurotrophins) and central nervous system factors. The perception of pruritus, irrespective of etiology, can be modulated by psychological factors, with stressful life events, psychiatric symptoms, and mental distress correlating with an increased likelihood of experiencing itching (Dalgard et al. 2007). Mr. S might be helped by a thorough evaluation of possible contributors to pruritus, including medical factors, medications, and behaviors, with psychoeducation about how responses—both emotional (anxiety and distress) and behavioral (repeated scratching)—may perpetuate and aggravate symptoms related to his skin condition. Addressing any underlying medical cause of the pruritus, prescribing appropriate pharmacotherapy (see "Treatment" subsection under "Evaluation and Management of Co-Occurring Depression and Anxiety" below), and encouraging him to learn techniques for managing his stress and habitual scratching (e.g., through a referral for psychotherapy or relaxation training) could support the patient and also lead to

TABLE 14–1.   **Common dermatological conditions influenced by psychological factors**

Mediated via stress	
Inflammatory skin disorders	Hair disorders
Psoriasis	Alopecia areata
Atopic dermatitis	Telogen effluvium
Acne	
Rosacea	Viral infections of the skin
Eczema	Viral warts (human papillomavirus)
Lichen simplex chronicus	Shingles (varicella-zoster virus)
Nodular prurigo	Oral/genital blisters (herpes simplex virus)
Seborrheic dermatitis	
Urticaria	Immunologically mediated skin disorders
Angioedema	Vitiligo
Attenuated physiological response	
Hyperhidrosis	Blushing

improvement in the dermatological condition. In the case of Mr. S, the primary care physician is surprised when the liver function panel returns with abnormal findings; this information leads to an appropriate workup and a diagnosis of primary biliary cirrhosis.

Management Strategies for the Primary Care Setting

Evaluation and Management of Co-Occurring Depression and Anxiety

Assessment of psychiatric and psychosocial comorbidity is an important component of the clinical evaluation and management plan. Untreated symptoms of depression and anxiety may contribute to a number of adverse outcomes, such as the use of poor coping strategies, engagement in maladaptive behaviors (e.g., substance use), nonadherence to medical treatment, increased suicide risk, and diminished social functioning (Dixon et al. 2016).

Screening.   Self-assessment scales such as the Hospital Anxiety and Depression Scale (Zigmond and Snaith 1983), the 9-item Patient Health Questionnaire (PHQ-9) for depression (Kroenke et al. 2001), and the Generalized Anxiety Disorder 7-item (GAD-7) scale for anxiety (Spitzer et al. 2006) are validated for use in primary care medical settings. Use of these tools can be a time-efficient strategy, given that these instruments are based on self-report and can be administered in the waiting room. After screening, definitive diagnosis relies on further clinical interview and a mental status examination, including assessment of level of distress and functional impairment (American Psychiatric Association 2013). A suicide risk assessment should be promptly conducted in patients who respond positively to PHQ-9 item number 9, "Thoughts that you would be better off dead or of hurting yourself in some way" (see

"Indications for Urgent Referral" section later in this chapter for a further discussion of suicide risk assessment).

Treatment.   If a patient meets criteria for a depressive or anxiety disorder, it is appropriate to initiate pharmacological treatment. Serotonin reuptake inhibitors (SRIs), including selective serotonin reuptake inhibitors (SSRIs) and serotonin-norepinephrine reuptake inhibitors (SNRIs), are efficacious in the treatment of both major depressive disorder (MDD) and GAD. No one subclass of SRIs has been found to be more efficacious than another (Gelenberg et al. 2010). Initial selection of an SRI medication should be based on the tolerability, safety, and cost of the medication as well as on patient preference, history of prior medication treatment, and potential for drug-drug interactions. For MDD, other medications that may be considered as first-line treatments include bupropion and mirtazapine. Other medications for SRI partial responders or for acute anxiety during the period before an SRI takes effect include buspirone, hydroxyzine, and pregabalin. Benzodiazepines, while effective for acute anxiety symptoms, should be used with great caution, given their significant risk of causing physiological dependence (Bandelow et al. 2008).

Referral.   Referral for adjunctive psychotherapies may be considered. Evidence-based treatments for depression include cognitive-behavioral therapy (CBT), interpersonal psychotherapy, behavioral psychotherapies (e.g., behavioral activation), and psychodynamic psychotherapy (Gelenberg et al. 2010). CBT has the strongest evidence for efficacy in the treatment of anxiety (Cuijpers et al. 2014). Mindfulness-based stress reduction and other relaxation-focused treatments (e.g., progressive muscle relaxation, biofeedback, guided imagery) also may be helpful.

Evaluation and Management of Associated Psychological Distress

A patient's skin condition may cause significant psychological distress and impaired functioning even in the absence of a diagnosable depressive or anxiety disorder.

Screening.   Signs that should trigger further inquiry into psychological factors include significant distress related to the symptom(s), frequent presentation for medical care, worse-than-expected response to treatment, or greater-than-expected frequency of relapse (Gordon-Elliott and Muskin 2013). Dermatology-specific diagnostic tools that measure psychological distress and functional impairment associated with a patient's dermatological condition include quality of life (QOL) assessment tools such as the Dermatology Life Quality Index (Finlay and Khan 1994) and Skindex (Chren et al. 1996) and disease-specific tools such as the Cardiff Acne Disability Index (Motley and Finlay 1992) and the Salford Psoriasis Index (Kirby et al. 2000). Gupta and Gupta (2013a) recommended that clinicians inquire specifically about the impact of the skin condition on the patient's interpersonal and sexual relationships, self-perception, occupational functioning, and sleep. Pediatric and adolescent patients should be asked about appearance-related teasing and bullying (Magin 2013).

Treatment.   Interventions should be aimed at identifying and reducing stressors, improving the patient's ability to cope with stressors that cannot be reduced or removed, and developing emotional states and support systems that enhance adaptation and coping. Psychoeducation about lifestyle modifications to enhance self-care should be provided, such as counseling about diet, exercise, and sleep hygiene. Patients may benefit from use of online apps that target stress reduction and healthy lifestyle choices. For some patients, the use of self-monitoring or an online app can be especially helpful if the behavior is viewed as part of the treatment plan, with clear goals and monitoring of progress.

Dermatological Manifestations of Psychiatric Disorders

Clinical Vignette

Ms. B is a 58-year-old single woman, now homeless, who presents to the dermatology clinic asking for help with "my bug issue," which she believes has worsened over the past 4 years. She shows the clinician marks on her skin and has brought in a jar containing dirt, pieces of dried skin, and scabs, as further "proof" of her infection. Ms. B has been staying in shelters or sleeping on park benches for the past year, after abandoning her apartment because of fears that it had become infested. When the clinician asks her whether she has had past interactions with psychiatric care providers or psychiatric treatment, Ms. B angrily replies, "Of course not, and what does that have to do with my current problem?"

Approach to the Patient With a Suspected Primary Psychiatric Disorder

Physicians presume that a patient will seek medical help for a definable disease—a condition with an identifiable etiology and (in most cases) an available treatment. The expectation is that the patient will present with signs and symptoms related to an underlying pathophysiological process (be it allergic, inflammatory, infectious, neoplastic, or otherwise) and will defer to the doctor's expertise. In actual practice, there can exist a significant discrepancy between what the patient and the doctor believe to be the problem. Such a discrepancy is experienced when a patient seeks medical attention for a skin concern believed to be a dermatological condition that the clinician suspects is psychiatric or behavioral in origin. The clinical care of patients like these can be complicated by patient factors, such as aberrant reporting of the history of the present illness or emotional difficulties. Clinical care can additionally be complicated by physician factors, including subtle or unconscious biases or limited experience in evaluating patients with overlapping psychiatric and dermatological presentations. Because of such complexities, the practitioner must approach a patient with a suspected primary psychiatric disorder in the same way as he or she would approach any other patient with a medical or dermatological complaint.

Provide a Comprehensive Medical Workup

It is vital that every patient receive a comprehensive evaluation and medical workup, even if a primary psychiatric disorder is suspected. Given the high rate of medical comorbidity in patients with psychiatric symptoms, a thorough evaluation ensures that no medical conditions are missed and serves to document and treat (if possible) any underlying disease, even if that disease is distinct from the patient's chief complaint. Studies have demonstrated that despite having high levels of medical comorbidity, patients with psychiatric disorders receive worse medical care overall in comparison with patients without psychiatric disorders, and their medical diagnoses are more likely to be missed. In a study of 47 patients with a diagnosis of delusional parasitosis who were referred to a psychiatrist, 11% were found to have an undiagnosed medical condition contributing to their disease, and 17% had obsessive-compulsive traits but had no true delusions (Reichenberg et al. 2013). Patients are much more likely to share their psychosocial concerns with health care providers if they feel that their physical concerns are being addressed.

Inquire About Psychological Factors

Given the limited time available in general medical settings, it can be helpful to point out to the patient at the outset that additional appointments may be required to complete the assessment. The patient should be made aware that skin problems can substantially impact psychological well-being, and that the evaluation therefore will include both medical and psychological factors. Many patients with primary psychiatric illness who present with medical complaints will have experienced being dismissed and rejected by medical professionals. The primary care physician should attempt to fully hear the individual's story, including any associated feelings of frustration or anger, and validate the concerns and distress while neither agreeing with the specific beliefs nor using direct confrontation. By eliciting patients' beliefs regarding the etiology of their symptoms, the physician can begin to assess whether patients have insight into the psychiatric aspects of their skin condition.

Obtain Collateral Information if Available

If family members or friends are available, it is helpful to ask these people to corroborate the history of the present illness, to report whether any changes in the patient's behavior have been observed (e.g., delirium, dementia, the onset of a new psychiatric disorder or episode of illness), and to list any medications or other substances the patient is taking or using. These collateral sources can also provide useful information about the patient's personality style and whether the current presentation is meaningfully different from the patient's baseline. Patients should be asked for a list of all health care providers (including psychiatrists) who have treated them in the past few years, and records should be requested for a comprehensive review.

Limit Excessive Testing

After the patient has received a comprehensive workup (as described above) and any reasonable treatments indicated by the symptoms and evaluation (e.g., a low-dose topical corticosteroid that is deemed to have a chance of improving the symptoms, even if an underlying behavioral health issue is suspected to be contributing to the pathogenesis of—or the distress induced by—the skin finding), the clinician should consider providing the patient and any other clinicians on the patient s health care team with documentation of the assessment, the treatment given, and (if relevant) the response to the treatment. Provision of such documentation can help to improve communication and may minimize unnecessary repeated interventions, which contribute to health care costs and increase the risk of harm to the patient through the direct effects of invasive or toxic interventions. Importantly, if the patient has demonstrated a tendency to engage in excessive help-seeking for the same problem and this behavior is thought to be driven by psychiatric issues, communicating with the patient's other providers and giving the patient a written summary of the encounter may help reduce the negative psychological effects for the patient of repeated evaluations and the vicious cycle of distress, help-seeking, disappointment, and further distress and help-seeking.

Dermatological Manifestations and Issues in Selected Psychiatric Disorders

Skin-related concerns, distress, and behaviors can present in the context of psychiatric disorders. Patients may seek the help of primary care providers for a wide range of troubles, from excessive worries about the skin despite the lack of evident dermatological pathology to significant skin injury due to behaviors driven by the psychiatric condition. In the following sections, we review prototypical examples of psychiatric disorders that manifest with dermatological signs and symptoms (summarized in Table 14–2).

Psychotic Disorders

Delusional parasitosis. *Clinical features.*   Delusional parasitosis—a nondiagnostic term that in DSM-5 (American Psychiatric Association 2013) would be categorized as a delusional disorder, somatic type—is a condition characterized by a fixed, false belief that one is infested with parasites, insects, or bugs. A similar condition is described in the literature as Morgellons disease (Pearson et al. 2012). Patients most commonly describe a perception that there are parasites crawling upon or burrowing into their skin, which is sometimes accompanied by a crawling and pinpricking sensation ("formication"). Impairment is usually confined to this specific belief, and additional delusions or disorders of thought typical of other psychotic disorders are absent. Patients are characteristically focused on proving the existence of the bugs, presenting to the doctor with detailed descriptions of the behavior and biology of the bugs (Koblenzer 2010; Koo and Gambla 1996). They may bring containers holding pieces of dried skin, lint, and dust to show the physician as evidence of the "parasites"—a characteristic behavior known as "the matchbox sign" (Lee 1983). Despite the limited focus of their delusion, these patients often experience significant secondary effects from their beliefs. These patients often cause severe secondary damage to their skin through applying noxious substances or even burning the skin in attempts to be rid of the "parasites." They experience significant functional impairment, losing jobs, homes, and social connections because of their preoccupation with the parasites and the sense that others do not understand their problem. Individuals with delusional parasitosis are distinguished from individuals with schizophrenia or other psychotic disorders by the lack of other significant psychotic symptoms, such as hallucinations or more pervasive delusional systems. Patients with delusional parasitosis may or may not have maladaptive personality traits such as rigidity and deficits in interpersonal relatedness. In an estimated 10% of cases, delusional parasitosis has been reported to lead to what has been referred to as *folie à deux* (also classically

TABLE 14–2. Primary psychiatric disorders that manifest dermatologically

Category	Disorder	Clinical features	Dermatological manifestation
Psychotic disorders Schizophrenia spectrum and other psychotic disorders Bipolar and related disorders Depressive disorders	Delusional disorder Schizophrenia Bipolar I disorder with psychotic features Major depressive disorder with psychotic features	Somatic delusions	Distorted beliefs or delusions about the appearance of, sensations related to, or conditions occurring in the skin (e.g., delusional parasitosis, delusional bromhidrosis, rigidly held concerns about perceived irregularities)
Obsessive-compulsive and related disorders	Obsessive-compulsive disorder	Presence of obsessions or compulsions	Dermatitis due to frequent hand washing
	Body dysmorphic disorder	Preoccupation with perceived defects or flaws in physical appearance that are not observable or appear slight to others	Complaints related to skin (perceived acne, scars, lines, wrinkles, paleness) Complaints related to hair ("thinning" hair, "excessive" body hair)
	Trichotillomania	Recurrent behavior that leads to physical consequence (hair loss, skin lesions) and causes distress or functional impairment	
	Excoriation (skin-picking) disorder		Acne excoriée
Somatic symptom and related disorders	Somatic symptom disorder	Experience of being ill: Physical symptoms cause distress or impairment in excess of what would be expected, may or may not identify underlying medical cause	"Psychogenic pruritus" or chronic idiopathic pruritus "Psychogenic purpura"
	Illness anxiety disorder	Fear of being ill: Preoccupation with having or acquiring a serious, undiagnosed medical illness, high general anxiety about health and disease	Variable (e.g., belief that a benign mole is cancer, or a macule in genital area is untreatable sexually transmitted disease)

TABLE 14–2. Primary psychiatric disorders that manifest dermatologically (continued)

Category	Disorder	Clinical features	Dermatological manifestation
Somatic symptom and related disorders (continued)	Factitious disorder	Deceptive falsification of symptoms in the absence of obvious external rewards	Dermatitis artefacta
Substance use disorders	Stimulant use disorder (cocaine, amphetamines, pseudoephedrine)	Acute intoxication	Excessive sweating Pruritus Formication: Sensation of insects crawling on (or under) skin, commonly causes itchiness, tingling, pins and needles, pain
		Chronic use	Skin picking Scarring and infections from excessive scratching
	Alcohol use disorder	Acute intoxication	Transient facial flushing
		Withdrawal	Paroxysmal sweats Pruritus secondary to formication (see above)
		Chronic use	Skin manifestations of liver disease (e.g., jaundice, easy bruising, spider angiomas, palmar erythema) Exacerbation of rosacea and psoriasis
	Opioid use disorder (heroin, morphine, synthetic opiates)	Chronic use	Skin infections related to injection use (e.g., ulcers, abscesses, cellulitis)

TABLE 14–2. Primary psychiatric disorders that manifest dermatologically *(continued)*

Category	Disorder	Clinical features	Dermatological manifestation
Personality disorders, maladaptive traits	Borderline personality disorder	Self-harm behaviors related to persistently unstable self-image and unstable moods, may be associated with suicidal acts or threats	Self-cutting Self-burning
	Other personality disorders/ traits Narcissistic Histrionic Obsessive-compulsive	May have psychological issues related to body image, difficulty adapting to changes in cutaneous body image such as skin changes related to aging or a chronic skin condition	Excessive pursuit of cosmetic or surgical procedures

known as *shared psychotic disorder*), in which the patient's belief of infestation comes to be shared by the patient's significant other (Trabert 1999).

Management.   As described earlier, patients with delusional parasitosis are difficult to manage due to their lack of insight and resistance to psychiatric referral. Collaboration between psychiatrists and other medical providers is vital. It is important to rule out secondary forms of delusional parasitosis, which may be due to another primary psychiatric disorder, a medical or neurological disorder, substance intoxication or withdrawal, or side effects of medications or supplements the patient may be taking. Primary psychiatric disorders that may manifest with similar somatic delusions include schizophrenia, bipolar I disorder with psychotic features, MDD with psychotic features, personality disorders, and neurocognitive disorders. In addition to having delusions of parasitic infestation, individuals with somatic delusions may believe that their bodies are rotting, emitting a foul odor, or not functioning properly.

Treatment with antipsychotic medication is recommended; there is no evidence to suggest that any one antipsychotic is more effective than another. Second-generation antipsychotics (SGAs) such as risperidone and olanzapine have shown efficacy in delusional parasitosis (Lepping et al. 2007). The first-generation antipsychotic (FGA) pimozide was considered the first-line treatment for many decades; however, there is no evidence of pimozide's superiority over other antipsychotics. Pimozide has a notable QT-prolonging effect, and its use should be avoided in older patients, patients with cardiac disease, and patients taking other medications that prolong the QT interval.

Obsessive-Compulsive and Related Disorders

Obsessive-compulsive disorder.   *Clinical features.*   The diagnosis of obsessive-compulsive disorder (OCD) is based on the presence of obsessions, compulsions, or both (American Psychiatric Association 2013). Patients with OCD often experience secondary dermatological effects caused by chronic compulsive behavior, such as dermatitis secondary to frequent hand washing in response to a contamination obsession.

Management.   OCD can be effectively treated with SSRIs, SNRIs, or clomipramine, as well as with CBT or behavioral treatments (e.g., exposure and response prevention). Management frequently warrants psychiatric referral.

Body dysmorphic disorder.   *Clinical features.*   The diagnosis of body dysmorphic disorder (BDD) is based on a preoccupation with perceived defects or flaws in a person's physical appearance that are not observable or appear slight to others. Patients commonly present with complaints related to their skin (e.g., perceived acne, scars, lines, vascular markings, wrinkles, paleness or redness of the complexion), hair (e.g., "thinning" hair or "excessive" body or facial hair), or nose (e.g., shape, size). The preoccupation may involve multiple bodily regions (e.g., genitals, breasts, buttocks, abdomen, upper and lower extremities, overall body size, body build, muscularity) in addition to the skin. These preoccupations are intrusive, unwanted, time consuming (occurring, on average, 3–8 hours per day), and difficult to resist or control (American Psychiatric Association 2013). Patients engage in repetitive behaviors or mental acts in response to the preoccupation, which include excessive grooming (e.g., combing, styling, plucking, or pulling hair), seeking reassurance (potentially from the clinician) about how the perceived flaws look, or attempting to change their appearance (e.g., excessive tanning, excessive use of skin products, recurrent cosmetic surgical and dermatological procedures). These patients may also engage in compulsive skin picking intended to improve perceived skin defects, which can cause skin damage, infections, or ruptured blood vessels (Gupta and Gupta 2013b). Patients have varying degrees of insight regarding their beliefs, ranging from good to absent or delusional. Regardless of the level of insight, the high degree of distress and dissatisfaction related to the perceived flaw(s) commonly perpetuates their search for relief through medical treatment; patients may avoid or resist psychiatric treatment because they do not believe that it will directly address their problem (i.e., improvement of the perceived flaw). The risk of suicide in patients with BDD is high; up to 25% attempt suicide at some point, and the rate of completed suicide among individuals with BDD may be twice that of individuals with other serious psychiatric disorders (e.g., MDD) (Phillips et al. 2005).

Management.   BDD may occur alone or in addition to other dermatological disorders. If BDD is not addressed, the patient is likely to remain dissatisfied with dermatological treatment outcomes. Treatments for BDD include SSRIs and CBT (Grant and Phillips 2005). Suicidality should always be assessed. These patients are particularly reluctant to see their conditions as psychiatric in nature, but their core pathology is best managed by referral to a psychiatrist or other experienced mental health care provider.

Trichotillomania.   *Clinical features.*   The essential feature of the trichotillomania diagnosis is recurrent pulling out of one's own hair, resulting in hair loss, with repeated attempts to decrease or stop hair pulling and related clinically significant distress or functional impairment (American Psychiatric Association 2013). Patients may describe an increasing sense of tension before the action of hair pulling and a sense of relief or pleasure after pulling out the hair. Patients may present to primary care physicians for treatment of patches of alopecia or infections at the site of hair follicles. Trichotillomania has been associated with a history of psychological trauma and posttraumatic stress disorder, high dissociation scores, and depression. It may also be a feature of intellectual disabilities, eating disorders, and personality disorders associated with dissociation (Gupta and Levenson 2005).

Management.   Habit-reversal therapy and clomipramine are the recommended treatments (Bloch et al. 2007). There may be a role for the SGA olanzapine and for mood stabilizers (Gupta and Levenson 2005). Treatment for trichotillomania is best offered by a trained mental health care provider.

Excoriation (skin-picking) disorder.   *Clinical features.*   The diagnosis of excoriation disorder is based on the presence of recurrent skin picking, resulting in skin lesions, with repeated attempts to stop or decrease the picking and related clinically significant distress or functional impairment (American Psychiatric Association 2013). Patients are aware of the self-inflicted nature of their lesions. In contrast to factitious disorder, they are not attempting to feign dermatological illness but are damaging their skin because of skin sensations or an attempt to remove a skin defect. Lesions are often located on easily reached areas and may be precipitated or exacerbated by an underlying dermatological condition. *Acne excoriée* is a subtype of excoriation disorder in which patients excessively pick their acne pimples, often causing further lesions and scarring (Gupta and Gupta 1996).

Management.   Other systemic and local causes of pruritus should be investigated. There is limited evidence for the efficacy of serotonergic antidepressants (SSRIs, clomipramine, doxepin), SGAs (olanzapine, aripiprazole), and naltrexone. Supportive psychotherapy also may be helpful (Gupta and Levenson 2005).

Somatic Symptom and Related Disorders

Somatic symptom disorder.   *Clinical features.*   The diagnosis of somatic symptom disorder is based on the presence of persistent somatic symptoms (typically for 6+ months) that are either very distressing or result in a significant disruption of functioning, along with excessive or disproportionate thoughts, feelings, and behaviors in response to these symptoms. Instead of focusing on medically unexplained symptoms (after appropriate medical evaluation), the diagnosis of somatic symptom disorder emphasizes recognition of the presence of physical symptoms and related distress, with minimal attention to whether or not there is an identifiable "cause" of the symptoms.

One condition that is not a formal psychiatric disorder but could be categorized as somatic symptom disorder is *chronic idiopathic pruritus*. Whereas pruritus is a common symptom of many dermatological and systemic diseases, chronic idiopathic pruritus does not have an identifiable etiology and causes significant distress. This form of pruritus is usually experienced on a daily basis; worse at night, it frequently disrupts sleep. It may manifest as generalized pruritus, most commonly involving the arms, legs, and back, or as focal pruritus, most commonly involving the genitals. It is important for the primary care physician to thoroughly review and consider all potential medical comorbidities (e.g., neurological disorders, chronic renal failure, cholestasis, systemic infections, malignancies, endocrine disorders, medication side effects) and to be aware that psychological factors may influence itch perception and can complicate chronic itch even in the presence of a medical comorbidity. An association among chronic pruritus, low self-esteem, and problems in managing aggression has been reported (Yosipovitch and Samuel 2008). Emotional distress appears to have an effect on itch threshold and the intensity and duration of histamine-induced pruritus (Fjellner et al. 1985). Not all patients with idiopathic pruritus have psychopathology or high stress levels.

Management.   For patients with somatic symptom disorder, the clinician is encouraged to focus on the presence of features (i.e., distress and dysfunction) rather than focusing on the absence of features (i.e., a medical explanation for symptoms). Patients with somatic symptom disorder are usually best managed within the medical setting, because they are particularly reluctant to consider themselves as having mental health problems. They are prone to experience alienation and to increase their maladaptive help-seeking behavior when they sense, rightly or wrongly, that they are being "dismissed" when psychiatric treatment is recommended. Clinicians can improve the care they offer to such patients by scheduling frequent routine visits and offering a set period of time at the start of each visit for reviewing medical complaints or concerns. Clinicians should additionally be judicious with medical testing and interventions. Patients can sometimes be encouraged to see a mental health care provider for "help managing stress," especially if the mental health care can be proposed as an adjunct to, not a replacement for, treatment with the primary provider.

For chronic idiopathic pruritus, as with somatic symptom disorder, it is helpful to target the psychological distress associated with symptoms, even if the medical workup is ongoing. Pharmacological agents commonly prescribed include antihistamines, antidepressants (especially those with antihistaminic properties, such as tricyclic antidepressants [TCAs], mirtazapine, and paroxetine) (Zylicz et al. 2003), opiate receptor antagonists (e.g., naltrexone, naloxone), and anticonvulsants (e.g., gabapentin, pregabalin, carbamazepine) (Gupta 2013; Matsuda et al. 2016). Behavioral treatments, including CBT and habit-reversal training to target interruption of the itch-scratch cycle, may be helpful.

Illness anxiety disorder. *Clinical features.* Patients with illness anxiety disorder have a preoccupation with having or acquiring a serious, undiagnosed medical illness as well as more general anxiety about health and disease. These patients engage in excessive health-related behaviors (repeated visits to doctors, repeated checking of their bodies for signs of illness, excessive Internet researching of their suspected disease), but their concerns about undiagnosed disease are not alleviated by appropriate medical reassurance, negative diagnostic tests, or benign course. Illness concerns assume a prominent place in the individual's life, affecting daily activities and potentially resulting in significant disability (American Psychiatric Association 2013). Dermatological concerns are frequent (e.g., worries that a benign mole represents undiagnosed skin cancer or that a macule in the genital area represents an untreatable sexually transmitted infection).

Management. The primary goal in managing illness anxiety disorder is to improve patients' coping with health fears and to discourage the adoption of the sick role. A key part of management is to schedule regular outpatient primary care visits that are not contingent upon active health concerns. Regular visits allow patients to voice their concerns without feeling the need to make telephone calls or emergency visits. It is important to recognize and treat any co-occurring anxiety or depressive disorders, which are common. CBT is recommended as the first-line treatment for illness anxiety disorder (Tyrer et al. 2014). Pharmacotherapy with SSRIs or SNRIs also may be helpful, either in combination with psychotherapy or as monotherapy if psychotherapy is unavailable or refused.

Factitious skin disorder (dermatitis artefacta). *Clinical features.* The diagnosis of factitious disorder is based on a patient's deceptive falsification of medical or psychological signs or symptoms, in the absence of obvious external rewards, with the objective of causing others to view him or her as ill or impaired (American Psychiatric Association 2013). The disorder can lead to excessive clinical intervention. It is hypothesized that the sick-role behavior associated with factitious disorder is a means of establishing or stabilizing one's identity, maintaining relationships with others, and addressing emotional dysregulation and unmet needs. In factitious skin disorder, or dermatitis artefacta, the patient classically focuses on self-induced skin lesions or exacerbates an existing skin problem to assume the sick role, which serves as a coping mechanism. The lesions may have various appearances (e.g., linear tears, bruises, cuts, purpura, blisters, ulcers, erythema, nodules), depending on the means employed to create them. Thus, they may mimic a wide range of other cutaneous disorders. The lesions might be distinguished from primary dermatoses based on their presence on accessible skin areas (where the patient can reach); having sharp, geometric borders with normal-appearing skin outside the lesion; or having an otherwise abnormal appearance not consistent with known skin disease. Full-thickness skin loss or severe scarring from self-inflicted lesions may necessitate extensive plastic surgery or lead to complications such as infection or even death. The patient's history is typically vague, dramatic, and sometimes inconsistent; external motivations for the behavior, such as economic gain or other reasons for malingering, are absent. A common feature of these patients is a connection with some aspect of health care, such as past employment in a health care field. The condition often appears in the setting of severe psychosocial stress or trauma. Dermatitis artefacta is more common in women than in men (by a ratio of at least 3:1), with the highest incidence seen in the late teens or early twenties (Koblenzer 1996). These patients often aggressively seek medical care and invasive interventions, with frequent visits to multiple providers or emergency departments. They are at risk for significant morbidity, not only due to their self-harming behaviors but also secondary to the excessive testing and interventions they undergo, often due to the sincere attempts of their providers to "get to the bottom of" the issue (Gordon-Elliott and Muskin 2013).

Management. Early diagnosis is important to help prevent unnecessary surgery and chronic morbidity. It is helpful to have one clinician oversee patient management (in the inpatient setting, this would be the attending of record; in the outpatient setting, this would be the primary care physician). Psychiatry should be consulted, and all members of the patient's treatment team should be informed of the diagnosis and treatment plan. In engaging the patient, the clinician's goals include offering appropriate care and minimizing escalation of the patient's behaviors. Instead of directly confronting the patient or attempting to persuade the patient to admit the self-inflicted nature of the lesions, treatment should focus on the following principles: 1) emphasize that the patient needs help; 2) avoid expressing anger, acting judgmentally, and taking punitive or retaliatory actions; 3) provide assurances that general medical care and support are available; and 4) minimize humiliation and help the patient "save face." To minimize humiliation, it can be helpful to discuss the entire differential diagnosis, not just factitious disorder, and to offer therapies that are unlikely to cause harm (e.g., progressive relaxation, self-hypnosis) so as to allow the patient to relinquish the factitious symptoms without acknowledging the disorder. Modalities such as supportive psychotherapy or CBT are often suggested, although evidence to support use of these modalities is limited, and likelihood of clinical improvement in symptoms is generally low (Koblenzer 1996).

Personality Disorders

Personality disorders are characterized by persistent, inflexible, maladaptive patterns of subjective experience and behavior that cause emotional distress and interfere with interpersonal relationships and social functioning. The prevalence of personality disorders is estimated at 9.1% in the general population (Lenzenweger et al. 2007) and is higher (estimated at 25% [Tyrer et al. 2015]) in primary care populations. Patients with narcissistic, histrionic, or obsessive-compulsive personality disorders/traits may have particular difficulty adjusting to a change in their appearance due to a skin condition or aging. The possibility of an underlying personality disorder should be considered in patients who present with frequent complaints but who are nonadherent to prescribed treatments.

Borderline personality disorder. *Clinical features.* Patients with borderline personality disorder commonly engage in self-mutilating acts (e.g., cutting, burning) related to persistently unstable self-image and unstable moods. The self-mutilating acts may be associated with suicidal acts or threats and are precipitated by threats of separation/rejection or by expectations that the individual should assume increased responsibility (American Psychiatric Association 2013).

Management. Psychotherapy—including psychodynamic individual/group therapies as well as CBT or dialectical behavioral therapy—is generally regarded as the first-line treatment for patients with borderline personality disorder (Oldham 2005). In primary care and psychiatric medication management, the patient-clinician relationship is facilitated by establishing appropriate patient expectations (discussing what the treatment will encompass, setting realistic goals for treatment, correcting false assumptions or unrealistic ideas) and taking a nonjudgmental stance toward patients (especially in regard to their history of behavioral problems, which are often a source of shame). When used as augmentation to psychotherapy in personality disorders, pharmacotherapy is generally targeted toward addressing co-occurring psychiatric conditions (e.g., depressive, anxiety, or substance use disorders) or problematic behaviors (e.g., impulsivity, irritability, or aggressive behavior toward self or others), although evidence for its effectiveness in resolving symptoms is limited. Care should be taken to avoid polypharmacy, and medications should not be changed at times of crisis. It is important to fully discuss the risks and benefits of medications with patients and to establish expectations for any requested dermatological or cosmetic interventions.

Dermatological Considerations in Psychopharmacotherapy

Clinical Vignette

Ms. A is a 26-year-old graduate student with no past medical history who presents to a primary care clinic with the chief complaint that "I think I have strep throat." She describes experiencing fever, fatigue, and diffuse myalgias for the past 3 days, and reports having woken up this morning with redness/itching in both eyes and pain on swallowing. The examination is notable for fever of 101.5°F and diffuse erythema on the patient's face, neck, and trunk. On further inquiry, the primary care physician discovers that the patient takes lamotrigine 400 mg/day for bipolar disorder. Ms. A reports that she forgot to bring the medication with her on a recent vacation but restarted it right away when she returned 10 days earlier.

Dermatological Reactions to Psychotherapeutic Agents

Reactions involving the skin are the most frequent adverse events in patients receiving pharmacological treatments of all types, with higher rates associated with psychotropic medications (Bliss and Warnock 2013). Psychotropic medications are among the most highly prescribed medications in the United States (Gu et al. 2010); therefore, all

providers should be prepared to identify adverse dermatological reactions to psychotropic agents and—after assessing severity and patient needs—either initiate medical
management or transfer the patient to a setting that provides the appropriate level of
care. Most skin-related adverse events associated with psychotropic medications are
benign and easily treated, although they may be bothersome. Antidepressants, mood
stabilizers, antipsychotic medications, and sedative-hypnotic/anxiolytic medications
(e.g., benzodiazepines and barbiturates) have been associated with emergence of pruritus, hyperpigmentation and photosensitivity, alopecia, and exanthematous drug
eruptions and fixed drug eruptions; antidepressants are known to induce hyperhidrosis (Bliss and Warnock 2013; Bond and Yee 1980; Harth and Rapoport 1996; Korkij
and Soltani 1984; Ming et al. 1999; Mufaddel et al. 2013). Psychiatric medications can
also be associated with serious dermatological adverse events, including drug reaction
with eosinophilia and systemic symptoms (DRESS), erythroderma, Stevens-Johnson
syndrome (SJS)/toxic epidermal necrolysis (TEN), and erythema multiforme (Bliss
and Warnock 2013; Camisa and Grines 1983; Evrensel and Ceylan 2015; Knowles et
al. 2012; Litt 2004; Mehta et al. 2014; Milionis et al. 2000; Mitkov et al. 2014; Mufaddel
et al. 2013; Purcell and Valmana 1996; Raz et al. 2001; Schlienger et al. 1998; Wernicke
1985; Wu et al. 2015). Although infrequent, these potentially life-threatening conditions should be suspected if adequate evidence is present in the clinical context, especially if the presumptive causative agent is an antiepileptic mood stabilizer and the
dermatological reaction appears soon after medication initiation or a dosage change
leading to an effective increase in medication serum level.

Factors that increase the risk of dermatological adverse events, benign and serious,
include a higher total number of medications taken, recent viral infection, older age,
and female gender. Individual genetic variations in the metabolism of a drug and human leukocyte antigen–associated drug hypersensitivity will also influence the development of adverse events.

Physicians should carefully weigh the decision to discontinue a possibly offending
agent, with consideration for the seriousness of the adverse event, the severity of the
patient's psychiatric illness, and the risk of relapse. For common adverse events, it
may be appropriate to continue the medication, with monitoring, reassurance, and
symptomatic treatment. For example, in the case of a patient's noticing mild hair thinning after starting an antidepressant medication, the provider might—following appropriate evaluation of any contributing medical factors (e.g., hypothyroidism),
nutrient (e.g., iron) deficiencies, or other nonpsychiatric medication potential culprits—encourage the patient to optimize her zinc and selenium intake (through food
or supplementation) and develop a plan with the patient for monitoring for any worsening of hair loss, including parameters for deciding when to discontinue the medication. For a patient with hyperhidrosis related to an SSRI, it might be appropriate to
consider a small dosage reduction to see if that eased the side effect without negatively impacting the antidepressant effect of the medication; alternatively, an antidote, such as a low dose of an alpha-adrenergic agent, could be tried, which might
modulate the autonomic hyperactivity leading to the excessive sweating.

By contrast, in most cases of a suspected serious adverse event, the causative medication should be immediately discontinued and hospital-level medical care should be
sought emergently. Dermatological and psychiatric consultation can assist with eval-

uation of appropriate options to consider after medication discontinuation, particularly in a patient with severe mental illness. It is important to recognize that a relapse of mania or severe depression poses a serious risk of morbidity and even mortality.

In the clinical vignette, Ms. A did not initially disclose her bipolar disorder diagnosis to the physician. When questioned about this omission, she reported that she did not consider it relevant when she was asked about "past medical problems." The primary care physician's high clinical suspicion for an adverse event led to a more detailed review of the patient's history and correct identification of the early signs and symptoms of Stevens-Johnsons syndrome (SJS). By immediately discontinuing the offending agent and escalating care to a hospital setting, the physician provided the necessary supportive medical interventions that allowed Ms. A to recover from this potentially life-threatening syndrome. Lamotrigine should not be readministered after SJS is identified, because symptoms can occur rapidly with reexposure during the recovery period. A retrial of lamotrigine could be considered in the future, following full recovery of the patient from SJS. The decision about whether a rechallenge at a later date would be prudent should involve consultation with a dermatologist and may include utilization of the ALDEN tool (algorithm of drug causality for epidermal necrolysis), which yields information about the causality and severity of an episode of SJS/TEN (Sassolas et al. 2010). A retrial of lamotrigine could be undertaken very cautiously (and only after careful consideration) for patients who previously experienced lamotrigine-associated rash without escalation to SJS.

Drug-Induced Exacerbation of a Primary Dermatological Disorder

Numerous primary dermatological disorders, including acne, psoriasis, seborrheic dermatitis, hyperhidrosis, and porphyria, may be triggered or exacerbated by psychotropic medications.

Acne has been associated with almost all antidepressants, as well as with the mood stabilizers lithium, topiramate, lamotrigine, gabapentin, and oxcarbazepine and the antipsychotics quetiapine and haloperidol (Bliss and Warnock 2013; Litt 2004). Acneiform eruptions typically occur on the face, chest, and upper back and consist of folliculocentric pustules, usually without comedones. Topical benzoyl peroxide generally is effective in managing the eruption and may allow for continuation of the agent. Retinoids are often less helpful, given that they are generally more effective for treatment of comedonal acne (Leyden et al. 2017).

It is well recognized that lithium can precipitate or exacerbate psoriasis. Lithium-induced psoriasis may manifest as an exacerbation of preexisting psoriasis or as de novo psoriasis, pustular psoriasis, nail changes, or psoriatic arthropathy (Jafferany 2008; Koo and Khera 2005). Psoriatic lesions may appear even at normal therapeutic serum lithium levels. The latency period for the development of psoriatic lesions is variable and can extend from months to the first few years of treatment; lesions can appear anywhere from a few weeks to a few months after treatment initiation. Lithium-induced psoriasis is often resistant to conventional treatment modalities, and some cases may require dosage reduction or discontinuation of lithium treatment. Because lithium is the mainstay of treatment in bipolar disorder, it is helpful for physicians to monitor the patient closely for lithium's potential dermatological side effects. Early recognition and management can be beneficial in minimizing issues that could lead to nonadherence or further deterioration of mood symptoms secondary to skin disfigurement. Anticonvulsants, SGAs, and SSRIs have been less commonly reported to precipitate or exacerbate psoriasis (Gupta and Gupta 1996).

Seborrheic dermatitis is common in patients on long-term phenothiazine FGAs (e.g., chlorpromazine, prochlorperazine, perphenazine, thioridazine) and also has been reported with other antipsychotics and mood stabilizers. Hyperhidrosis, often a cause of night sweats, is commonly reported with SSRIs, SNRIs, bupropion, and monoamine oxidase inhibitors (MAOIs). Although sweating is mediated by sympathetic cholinergic innervation of eccrine sweat glands, the more anticholinergic antidepressants (e.g., TCAs) also cause hyperhidrosis, so a switch may not necessarily be helpful. Porphyria, which manifests with acute dermatological, neuropsychiatric, and abdominal pain symptoms, may be exacerbated by carbamazepine, valproic acid, and many anxiolytic/sedative-hypnotic agents (especially barbiturates).

Psychiatric Consequences of Dermatological Medications

Numerous medications prescribed for dermatological disorders are known to have neuropsychiatric side effects (Table 14–3). Isotretinoin, a medication used to treat severe acne, has been studied extensively in connection with reports of depression, psychosis, and suicidal and aggressive behaviors arising during treatment. Warnings were issued by the U.S. Food and Drug Administration in 1998 and 2002 to make practitioners aware of these potential side effects. The association between isotretinoin and mood symptoms remains unclear, given the mixed data and lack of high-quality evidence (i.e., placebo-controlled clinical trials) (Gupta and Levenson 2005; Zaenglein et al. 2016). Current guidelines recommend asking about psychiatric history in the patient and family prior to initiation of treatment, as well as screening patients for depressive symptoms, mood disturbance, and suicidal ideation at each visit to determine whether further evaluation may be necessary (Zaenglein et al. 2016).

Systemic steroids (glucocorticoids) are commonly prescribed medications with potentially serious neuropsychiatric side effects, including mania, psychosis, delirium, and suicidal behavior. In a 2012 epidemiological study, patients who received glucocorticoids were seven times as likely to attempt suicide compared with age- and illness-matched control subjects (Fardet et al. 2012). Individuals younger than 30 years were at particular risk for suicide attempts, women were at increased risk for depression, and men were at increased risk for mania and delirium. Higher medication dosages were linked to overall greater risks for adverse outcomes (Fardet et al. 2012).

Special Topics in Management

Working With the Patient With Delusions or Limited Insight

Some patients will be open to discussion of the psychosocial impact of their disorder and the idea of a psychiatric referral; other patients (often those with delusional dis-

TABLE 14–3. **Dermatological medications with possible neuropsychiatric consequences**

Dermatological medication	Neuropsychiatric side effects
Antihistamines	Depression, extrapyramidal syndromes, delirium
Dapsone	Psychosis
Co-cyprindiol	Depression, anxiety, irritability
Isotretinoin	Depression, suicidal ideation, aggression
Methotrexate	Mood changes, mood disorders
Minocycline	Lupus erythematosus–like syndrome that may include psychiatric features
Psoralen ultraviolet A and ultraviolet B	Mood changes, euphoria
Systemic corticosteroids	Depression, suicidal ideation, mania/euphoria, psychosis, delirium

Source. Mitkov et al. 2014.

orders, BDD, or somatic symptom disorder) may be hostile or resistant to such suggestions. Clinical management of these patients involves unique challenges. It is sometimes helpful to include a discussion of psychological factors or referral to psychiatric consultation as part of the overall treatment plan. If a psychiatric referral is made, emphasizing that the relationship to the primary care physician will remain primary is crucial. Pursuing the psychiatric assessment or consultation too soon can be detrimental to therapeutic rapport. In patients with delusional disorders, treatment with antipsychotic agents can be presented as a means of decreasing distress. The patient may never be completely "cured." The goal of treatment should be to decrease patients' preoccupation with problematic beliefs in the hope of improving their social and occupational functioning.

Indications for Urgent Referral

Even given time constraints in a medical practice, at a minimum, physicians should ask patients how their problems are affecting their life and mood, and whether they are experiencing any thoughts about harming themselves or others. If a patient admits having thoughts about harming self or others, it is mandatory that the clinician explore those thoughts and make some assessment of how likely it is that the patient will act on them. A useful evidence-based screening tool for suicide risk assessment is the Columbia–Suicide Severity Rating Scale (Oquendo et al. 2003). If there is concern that the patient is a danger to self or others, the patient should be escorted to an emergency department, even without the patient's consent. Patients at particularly high risk for suicide include those with BDD, borderline personality disorder, active mood symptoms (especially hopelessness, insomnia, or anxiety), or active psychotic symptoms (especially paranoia or command auditory hallucinations) (Oquendo et al. 2003).

Strategies to Manage Countertransference

There are various types of patients who commonly engender strong, often negative, emotional reactions from physicians. Awareness of one's negative reactions to certain patients—also known as negative countertransference—is essential to maintain a therapeutic alliance and to provide appropriate medical care.

The Self-Harming Patient

Patients who self-inflict skin lesions and conditions include patients with factitious dermatitis, psychogenic excoriation, and trichotillomania. There are individuals who self-injure as part of borderline personality disorder. These patients can be difficult for the physician to care for and to understand. Doctors, trained to relieve suffering and cure disease, are inherently more comfortable treating patients who agree with their medical advice and cooperate with the treatment, and who are viewed as "innocent victims" of a disease. Patients who do not follow this pattern (e.g., who are nonadherent or interpersonally challenging, or who are somehow "causing" their medical presentations) commonly arouse negative or otherwise maladaptive responses in their providers, such as frustration, resentment, anger, helplessness, or a sense of futility. As a result, providers may overreact (e.g., lose patience with the patient, inappropriately discharge or refer the patient) or underreact (e.g., avoid interactions with the patient, fail to set appropriate limits). It can be useful for providers to be aware of how they normally engage with most patients so that they can notice deviations from these patterns when they occur. Such deviations may signal that factors related to the patient or to the patient-provider interaction—perhaps due to activation of implicit biases or countertransference responses—are influencing the provider's behavior. Patients who do not follow the standards implicitly set for them (e.g., those who are poorly adherent or who behave in ways that cause or aggravate their medical issues) are nonetheless still suffering; in fact, their behaviors may be manifestations of their emotional struggles. In such cases, the patient's distress (helplessness, anger, or other intolerable feelings) is passed on to, and experienced by, the provider. The emotional toll on the provider can be significant, and the patient may receive suboptimal care. Seeking guidance from an experienced colleague or mental health care specialist may allow the provider to better understand what is occurring, reduce the emotional burden of the situation, and develop more adaptive ways of responding to and engaging with the patient.

The Patient Who Is "in Denial"

Patients who are experienced as being "in denial" may reject their diagnosis, minimize their symptoms, be poorly compliant with prescribed treatment, or avoid or outright refuse treatment. Denial, a defense mechanism that is used to protect oneself from overwhelming anxiety in the face of a frightening reality, is not uncommon in people coping with medical illness (Strauss et al. 1990). It can sometimes be adaptive consciously to put aside one's fear in the setting of acute illness so as to move forward with treatment; however, significant problems arise when a patient's denial interferes with needed treatment. Treating the patient with a history of melanoma who does not come in for skin examinations, avoids the doctor's phone calls, and minimizes others' concerns by saying that he or she is "just fine" can be terrifying and even enraging to the physician. In working with these patients, it is important that the clinician keep in mind the goal of containing the patient's anxiety while promoting necessary treatment and minimizing risk. Confronting a patient's denial is rarely useful, but encouraging a conversation about what the patient is afraid of, while maintaining a nonthreatening and supportive stance, can help the patient and the doctor to move past the impasse (Gordon-Elliott and Muskin 2013). Notably, when considering a patient "in denial," it is essential to first exclude a psychotic disorder or cognitive distortions due to a severe mood disorder. Psychiatric consultation may be indicated to assist in assessment or to help the provider gain insight into the patient's resistance and, in turn, help to promote patient self-care. It can be helpful to emphasize to the patient that the psychiatric consultation will function as a supplement to, not a replacement for, the primary therapeutic relationship with the patient's physician.

The Pessimistic Patient

Patients who appear pessimistic or negative may be expressing anger or resentment related to previous experiences of feeling invalidated or misunderstood by physicians. These patients may evoke negative feelings in the provider, such as frustration, helplessness, or even a wish to avoid treating the patient due to fears that the patient will become demanding or direct anger toward the provider in the future. In this scenario, the provider should first listen to and validate the patient's concerns and inquire about past treatments and relationships with the health care system. Where relevant, it can be helpful to remind the patient that the new treatment relationship is an opportunity for a "fresh start" and that the patient will be included in shared treatment planning.

Conclusion

The skin, at the interface between the self and the rest of the world, can be a mode of communication, a cause of suffering, and a focal point of attention. Patients will present to their primary care providers with issues related to their skin that may be influenced by psychiatric disorders, or dermatological issues that negatively impact their mental health, or both. Given the complexity of how these reciprocal processes occur, the provider assessing and managing skin complaints and conditions has the daunting task of teasing out causes, contributing factors, and effects, often in the midst of great distress in the patient or uncomfortable responses in the provider. These challenging clinical encounters can be navigated more effectively, and with more ease, when the provider has adequate knowledge about the common mental health conditions and issues that influence, and are influenced by, dermatological presentations; confidence in one's ability to gather a useful history and engage the patient; and resources at one's disposal to serve the patient best, from psychiatric referral for the patient to supervision or support for the provider. Even the most difficult situations, such as patients who self-harm, or fabricate conditions, or excessively utilize the primary care system because of unmet psychiatric needs, can be improved in modest ways, perhaps by helping them to gain more insight into their behaviors, or by providing them with an opportunity to develop a trusting relationship with a provider, or by minimizing additional harm by limiting interventions and offering alternatives. As in all of medicine, elimination of disease may not be the outcome, and cannot always be the objective, but reducing suffering and enhancing well-being is often a reachable goal.

References

American Psychiatric Association: Diagnostic and Statistical Manual of Mental Disorders, 5th Edition. Arlington, VA, American Psychiatric Association, 2013

Bandelow B, Zohar J, Hollander E, et al: World Federation of Societies of Biological Psychiatry (WFSBP) guidelines for the pharmacological treatment of anxiety, obsessive-compulsive and post-traumatic stress disorders—first revision. World J Biol Psychiatry 9(4):248–312, 2008 18949648

Bliss SA, Warnock JK: Psychiatric medications: adverse cutaneous drug reactions. Clin Dermatol 31(1):101–109, 2013 23245981

Bloch MH, Landeros-Weisenberger A, Dombrowski P, et al: Systematic review: pharmacological and behavioral treatment for trichotillomania. Biol Psychiatry 62(8):839–846, 2007 17727824

Bond WS, Yee GC: Ocular and cutaneous effects of chronic phenothiazine therapy. Am J Hosp Pharm 37(1):74–78, 1980 6102438

Camisa C, Grines C: Amoxapine: a cause of toxic epidermal necrolysis? Arch Dermatol 119(9):709–710, 1983 6614956

Chren MM, Lasek RJ, Quinn LM, et al: Skindex, a quality-of-life measure for patients with skin disease: reliability, validity, and responsiveness. J Invest Dermatol 107(5):707–713, 1996 8875954

Cuijpers P, Sijbrandij M, Koole S, et al: Psychological treatment of generalized anxiety disorder: a meta-analysis. Clin Psychol Rev 34(2):130–140, 2014 24487344

Dalgard F, Svensson A, Holm J, et al: Self-reported itch and mental health. A Norwegian survey among adults (conference abstract). Journal of Investigative Dermatology 125(4):854, 2007. Available at: https://www.sciencedirect.com/journal/journal-of-investigative-dermatology/vol/125/issue/4. Accessed April 6, 2019.

Dixon LJ, Lee AA, Viana AG, et al: Anxiety sensitivity in dermatological patients. Psychosomatics 57(5):498–504, 2016 27137710

Evrensel A, Ceylan ME: Bupropion-induced erythema multiforme. Ann Dermatol 27(3):334–335, 2015 26082597

Fardet L, Petersen I, Nazareth I: Suicidal behavior and severe neuropsychiatric disorders following glucocorticoid therapy in primary care. Am J Psychiatry 169(5):491–497, 2012 22764363

Finlay AY, Khan GK: Dermatology Life Quality Index (DLQI)—a simple practical measure for routine clinical use. Clin Exp Dermatol 19(3):210–216, 1994 8033378

Fjellner B, Arnetz BB, Eneroth P, et al: Pruritus during standardized mental stress. Relationship to psychoneuroendocrine and metabolic parameters. Acta Derm Venereol 65(3):199–205, 1985 2411074

Fried RG, Gupta MA, Gupta AK: Depression and skin disease. Dermatol Clin 23(4):657–664, 2005 16112442

Gelenberg AJ, Freeman MP, Markowitz JC, et al: Practice Guidelines for the Treatment of Patients with Major Depressive Disorder, 3rd Edition. Arlington, VA, American Psychiatric Association, 2010

Gordon-Elliott JS, Muskin PR: Managing the patient with psychiatric issues in dermatologic practice. Clin Dermatol 31(1):3–10, 2013 23245968

Grant JE, Phillips KA: Recognizing and treating body dysmorphic disorder. Ann Clin Psychiatry 17(4):205–210, 2005 16402752

Gu Q, Dillon CF, Burt VL: Prescription drug use continues to increase: U.S. prescription drug data for 2007–2008. NCHS Data Brief (42):1–8, 2010 20854747

Gupta MA: Emotional regulation, dissociation, and the self-induced dermatoses: clinical features and implications for treatment with mood stabilizers. Clin Dermatol 31(1):110–117, 2013 23245982

Gupta MA, Gupta AK: Psychodermatology: an update. J Am Acad Dermatol 34(6):1030–1046, 1996 8647969

Gupta MA, Gupta AK: A practical approach to the assessment of psychosocial and psychiatric comorbidity in the dermatology patient. Clin Dermatol 31(1):57–61, 2013a 23245974

Gupta MA, Gupta AK: Cutaneous body image dissatisfaction and suicidal ideation: mediation by interpersonal sensitivity. J Psychosom Res 75(1):55–59, 2013b 23751239

Gupta MA, Gupta AK: Current concepts in psychodermatology. Curr Psychiatry Rep 16(6):449, 2014 24740235

Gupta MA, Levenson JL: Dermatology, in The American Psychiatric Publishing Textbook of Psychosomatic Medicine. Edited by Levenson JL. Arlington, VA, American Psychiatric Publishing, 2005, pp 667–690

Harth Y, Rapoport M: Photosensitivity associated with antipsychotics, antidepressants and anxiolytics. Drug Saf 14(4):252–259, 1996 8713693

Jafferany M: Lithium and psoriasis: what primary care and family physicians should know. Prim Care Companion J Clin Psychiatry 10(6):435–439, 2008 19287551

Kirby B, Fortune DG, Bhushan M, et al: [The Salford Psoriasis Index: an holistic measure of psoriasis severity]. Br J Dermatol 142(4):728–732, 2000 10792223

Knowles SR, Dewhurst N, Shear NH: Anticonvulsant hypersensitivity syndrome: an update. Expert Opin Drug Saf 11(5):767–778, 2012 22794330

Koblenzer CS: Psychosomatic concepts in dermatology. A dermatologist-psychoanalyst's viewpoint. Arch Dermatol 119(6):501–512, 1983 6859891

Koblenzer CS: Neurotic excoriations and dermatitis artefacta. Dermatol Clin 14(3):447–455, 1996 8818554

Koblenzer CS: The current management of delusional parasitosis and dermatitis artefacta. Skin Therapy Lett 15(9):1–3, 2010 20945052

Koo J, Gambla C: Delusions of parasitosis and other forms of monosymptomatic hypochondriacal psychosis. General discussion and case illustrations. Dermatol Clin 14(3):429–438, 1996 8818552

Koo J, Khera P: Update on the mechanisms and efficacy of biological therapies for psoriasis. J Dermatol Sci 38(2):75–87, 2005 15862940

Korabel H, Dudek D, Jaworek A, et al: [Psychodermatology: psychological and psychiatrical aspects of dermatology]. Przegl Lek 65(5):244–248, 2008 18853651

Korkij W, Soltani K: Fixed drug eruption. A brief review. Arch Dermatol 120(4):520–524, 1984 6231004

Kroenke K, Spitzer RL, Williams JB: The PHQ-9: validity of a brief depression severity measure. J Gen Intern Med 16(9):606–613, 2001 11556941

Lee WR: Matchbox sign. Lancet 2(8347):457–458, 1983 6135941

Lenzenweger MF, Lane MC, Loranger AW, et al: DSM-IV personality disorders in the National Comorbidity Survey Replication. Biol Psychiatry 62(6):553–564, 2007 17217923

Lepping P, Russell I, Freudenmann RW: Antipsychotic treatment of primary delusional parasitosis: systematic review. Br J Psychiatry 191:198–205, 2007 17766758

Leyden J, Stein-Gold L, Weiss J: Why topical retinoids are mainstay for therapy for acne. Dermatol Ther (Heidelb) 7(3):293–304, 2017 28585191

Litt JZ: Litt's Drug Eruption Reference Manual Including Drug Interactions. New York, Taylor & Francis, 2004

Lowell BA, Froelich CW, Federman DG, et al: Dermatology in primary care: prevalence and patient disposition. J Am Acad Dermatol 45(2):250–255, 2001 11464187

Magin P: Appearance-related bullying and skin disorders. Clin Dermatol 31(1):66–71, 2013 23245976

Matsuda KM, Sharma D, Schonfeld AR, et al: Gabapentin and pregabalin for the treatment of chronic pruritus. J Am Acad Dermatol 75(3):619–625.e6, 2016 27206757

Mehta M, Shah J, Khakhkhar T, et al: Anticonvulsant hypersensitivity syndrome associated with carbamazepine administration: case series. J Pharmacol Pharmacother 5(1):59–62, 2014 24554914

Milionis HJ, Skopelitou A, Elisaf MS: Hypersensitivity syndrome caused by amitriptyline administration. Postgrad Med J 76(896):361–363, 2000 10824052

Ming ME, Bhawan J, Stefanato CM, et al: Imipramine-induced hyperpigmentation: four cases and a review of the literature. J Am Acad Dermatol 40(2 Pt 1):159–166, 1999 10025739

Misery L: [Neuro-immuno-cutaneous system (NICS)]. Pathol Biol (Paris) 44(10):867–874, 1996 9157366

Mitkov MV, Trowbridge RM, Lockshin BN, et al: Dermatologic side effects of psychotropic medications. Psychosomatics 55(1):1–20, 2014 24099686

Motley RJ, Finlay AY: Practical use of a disability index in the routine management of acne. Clin Exp Dermatol 17(1):1–3, 1992 1424249

Mufaddel A, Osman O, Almugaddam F: Adverse cutaneous effects of psychotropic medications. Expert Review of Dermatology 8(6):681–692, 2013. Available at: https://www.tandfonline.com/doi/abs/10.1586/17469872.2013.846515. Accessed October 14, 2019.

Oldham JM: Guideline Watch: Practice Guideline for the Treatment of Patients With Borderline Personality Disorder. Arlington, VA, American Psychiatric Association, 2005. Available at: https://psychiatryonline.org/pb/assets/raw/sitewide/practice_guidelines/guidelines/bpd-watch.pdf. Accessed August 24, 2019.

Oquendo MA, Halberstam B, Mann JJ: Risk factors for suicidal behavior: utility and limitations of research instruments, in Standardized Evaluation in Clinical Practice. Edited by First MB (Review of Psychiatry Series, Vol 22; Oldham JM and Riba MB, series eds). Arlington, VA, American Psychiatric Publishing, 2003, pp 103–130

Pearson ML, Selby JV, Katz KA, et al: Clinical, epidemiologic, histopathologic and molecular features of an unexplained dermopathy. PLoS One 7(1):e29908, 2012 22295070

Phillips KA, Coles ME, Menard W, et al: Suicidal ideation and suicide attempts in body dysmorphic disorder. J Clin Psychiatry 66(6):717–725, 2005 15960564

Purcell P, Valmana A: Toxic epidermal necrolysis following chlorpromazine ingestion complicated by SIADH. Postgrad Med J 72(845):186–189, 1996 8731716

Raz A, Bergman R, Eilam O, et al: A case report of olanzapine-induced hypersensitivity syndrome. Am J Med Sci 321(2):156–158, 2001 11217818

Reichenberg JS, Magid M, Jesser CA, et al: Patients labeled with delusions of parasitosis compose a heterogeneous group: a retrospective study from a referral center. J Am Acad Dermatol 68(1):41–46, 46.e1–46.e2, 2013 23058734

Sassolas B, Haddad C, Mockenhaupt M, et al: ALDEN, an algorithm for assessment of drug causality in Stevens-Johnson syndrome and toxic epidermal necrolysis: comparison with case-control analysis. Clin Pharmacol Ther 88(1):60–68, 2010 20375998

Schlienger RG, Shapiro LE, Shear NH: Lamotrigine-induced severe cutaneous adverse reactions. Epilepsia 39 (suppl 7):S22–S26, 1998 9798758

Slominski A: Neuroendocrine system of the skin. Dermatology 211(3):199–208, 2005 16205064

Spitzer RL, Kroenke K, Williams JB, et al: A brief measure for assessing generalized anxiety disorder: the GAD-7. Arch Intern Med 166(10):1092–1097, 2006 16717171

Strauss DH, Spitzer RL, Muskin PR: Maladaptive denial of physical illness: a proposal for DSM-IV. Am J Psychiatry 147(9):1168–1172, 1990 2133370

Trabert W: Shared psychotic disorder in delusional parasitosis. Psychopathology 32(1):30–34, 1999 9885397

Tyrer P, Cooper S, Salkovskis P, et al: Clinical and cost-effectiveness of cognitive behaviour therapy for health anxiety in medical patients: a multicentre randomised controlled trial. Lancet 383(9913):219–225, 2014 24139977

Tyrer P, Reed GM, Crawford MJ: Classification, assessment, prevalence, and effect of personality disorder. Lancet 385(9969):717–726, 2015 25706217

Walburn J, Vedhara K, Hankins M, et al: Psychological stress and wound healing in humans: a systematic review and meta-analysis. J Psychosom Res 67(3):253–271, 2009 19686881

Wernicke JF: The side effect profile and safety of fluoxetine. J Clin Psychiatry 46(3 Pt 2):59–67, 1985 3156126

Wu MK, Chung W, Wu CK, et al: The severe complication of Stevens-Johnson syndrome induced by long-term clozapine treatment in a male schizophrenia patient: a case report. Neuropsychiatr Dis Treat 11:1039–1041, 2015 25914536

Yosipovitch G, Samuel LS: Neuropathic and psychogenic itch. Dermatol Ther 21(1):32–41, 2008 18318883

Zaenglein AL, Pathy AL, Schlosser BJ, et al: Guidelines of care for the management of acne vulgaris. J Am Acad Dermatol 74(5):945–73.e33, 2016 26897386

Zigmond AS, Snaith RP: The hospital anxiety and depression scale. Acta Psychiatr Scand 67(6):361–370, 1983 6880820

Zylicz Z, Krajnik M, Sorge AA, et al: Paroxetine in the treatment of severe non-dermatological pruritus: a randomized, controlled trial. J Pain Symptom Manage 26(6):1105–1112, 2003 14654262

Women's Mental Health and Reproductive Psychiatry

Marcela Almeida, M.D.

Kara Brown, M.D.

Leena Mittal, M.D.

Margo Nathan, M.D.

Hadine Joffe, M.D., M.Sc.

On par with the increasing visibility of women in various domains of contemporary life, the field of women's mental health has attracted special interest over the past few decades as growing knowledge has expanded our understanding of gender differences and unique characteristics pertaining to biological, cultural, and psychosocial aspects of a woman's life. The need for a chapter dedicated to these issues comes as a natural consequence of that trend.

Epidemiological studies have consistently shown a higher prevalence of mood and anxiety disorders among women compared with men. Lifetime rates of major depressive disorder (MDD) are twice as high among women as they are among men (National Institute of Mental Health 2016). Comparable statistics apply to posttraumatic stress disorder (PTSD), in part because women are subjected to more trauma and abuse (sexual, physical, and emotional) than are men (Karam et al. 2014). Similarly, the prevalence of any anxiety disorder is substantially higher among females than among males (30.5% vs. 19.2%) (Ford and Erlinger 2004; McLean et al. 2011). An overwhelming majority of eating disorders (85%–90%) occur in women (Smink et al. 2012).

The fact that rates of depression by sex diverge at puberty and are less divergent after menopause, with increased manifestations around periods of hormonal flux such as the perimenstrual, postpartum, and perimenopausal periods, suggests a biological contribution to the onset or worsening of psychiatric symptoms. The first observations of this connection focused on the influence of estrogen on serotonergic neurotransmission, as well as on the dopaminergic, γ-aminobutyric acid (GABA)-ergic, and glutamatergic systems, as potentially accounting for at least part of this observed gender difference (Bäckström et al. 2015; Borrow and Cameron 2014; Coates et al. 2010).

The close relationship between the serotonergic system and gonadal hormones was identified early on, and serotonergic agents have historically been used in the treatment of hormonally linked mood and anxiety disorders. More recently, emphasis has been given to the role of allopregnanolone (3α-hydroxy-5α-pregnan-20-one [ALLO]) as a positive reproductive steroid modulator of GABA type A (GABA$_A$) receptors and the hypothalamic-pituitary-adrenal (HPA) axis, potentially contributing to stress and depression, including hormonally linked depression episodes (Joffe et al. 2007).

These observations have led to important advancements in the field of women's mental health and reproductive psychiatry, and we now have robust biological evidence that the neuroendocrine system, neurotrophic factors, and inflammation have neuropsychiatric implications that contribute to mood and anxiety disorders (Borrow and Cameron 2014).

In this chapter, we examine how these commonly accepted medical and biological models contribute to differences in the gender expression of psychiatric illness. We also explore important physiological characteristics that influence the epidemiology, symptomatology, course, and management of psychiatric disorders in women. Finally, no discussion of women's mental health would be complete if it failed to mention some of the difficult cultural, psychological, and social challenges that women face. These include discrepancies in gender roles and social expectations, exposure to trauma and abuse, lower wages and accumulation of duties, disadvantaged social status, and gender discrimination. Each of these issues has a direct impact on how mental health and mental illness manifest throughout a woman's life. Awareness and understanding of these issues and problems on the part of clinicians can enhance the quality of care provided and can lead to improved strategies for treatment.

Psychiatric Disorders Associated With the Pubertal Transition and Menarche

There are important gender differences in the manifestations of nearly all psychiatric disorders, suggesting a potential role for gonadal hormones in their pathophysiology. This variance becomes particularly clear around puberty, a process characterized by dramatic hormonal changes, triggered by alterations in excitatory and inhibitory inputs to gonadotropin-releasing hormone neurons in the pituitary. The pubertal transition is a process that unfolds over time, driven by a progressive series of hormonal changes and gradual development of secondary sexual characteristics. In girls, puberty typically begins with breast development between the ages of 8 and 13 years and ends with menarche, or the first menstrual period. It is around menarche that mental illness becomes more prevalent among girls than boys. In addition to neuroendocrine-mediated changes, girls who mature earlier than their peers appear to have a more emotional and conflict-laden transition, which puts them at increased risk for depression, substance use, and early sexual activity (Graber 2013). Early menarche is also associated with higher rates of antisocial behaviors that persist into adulthood (Graber 2013; Mendle et al. 2018).

Environmental triggers, such as peer pressure and social roles, should be evaluated and addressed accordingly for girls presenting with mental disorders during the peripubertal period. The risk of psychiatric illness in this age group is also influenced by socioeconomic status, with children from lower-income families experiencing higher rates of depression (Mendle et al. 2015).

Treatment of psychiatric disorders during puberty must take into account the specific nature of this developmental and reproductive transition. Treatment encompasses psychotherapy, behavioral interventions, and psychotropic medications. Various psychotherapy approaches addressing the biopsychosocial stressors of adolescence can be beneficial for conflict resolution or alleviation of symptoms. Family therapy sessions are often recommended if there is significant family conflict, if the family has distorted schemata about the teenager's behavior, or if there are communication barriers that could improve with professional guidance and psychoeducation. Through an empathetic, nonjudgmental attitude, the clinician can obtain a careful sexual history, including a history of trauma and abuse, because teenagers are a particularly vulnerable population. Contraceptive methods should be discussed where applicable. Finally, it is crucial to obtain a detailed history of alcohol and drug use.

Psychiatric Disorders Associated With the Menstrual Cycle

Many psychiatric symptoms can be exacerbated during times of hormonal flux across the menstrual cycle. Anxiety, irritability, anger, dysphoria, mood lability, tearfulness, and personality changes, among other symptoms, can be transiently intensified or manifested exclusively during the luteal phase of the menstrual cycle, with resolution during the few days after the onset of menses. These psychiatric and psychological symptoms are usually accompanied by physical symptoms such as breast tenderness, bloating, decreased energy, and cravings for certain food (particularly carbohydrates).

The spectrum of mood symptoms associated with the menstrual cycle includes premenstrual dysphoric disorder (PMDD), premenstrual syndrome (PMS), and premenstrual exacerbation of a depressive disorder (PME-DD). PME-DD occurs in about 40% of women with an underlying unipolar depressive disorder (Peters et al. 2017). Approximately 65% of women with bipolar disorder reported a worsening of mood symptoms in the days leading up to their period (Sit et al. 2011).

A leading theory about the pathogenesis of premenstrual mood disorders posits that these symptoms represent an abnormal response to normal hormonal changes (Smith et al. 2006), because affected women do not have abnormal levels of reproductive hormones or some type of hormonal dysregulation, but rather an increased sensitivity to normative physiological cyclical hormones, which may affect the modulation of the serotonergic, noradrenergic, and dopaminergic pathways. The $GABA_A$ receptor agonist ALLO, a progesterone metabolite involved in the stress response, has been implicated in the pathogenesis of both PMS and PMDD (Li et al. 2012; Schüle et al. 2014; Vigod et al. 2009). ALLO has anxiolytic, anesthetic, and sedative properties. ALLO levels increase in the luteal phase and quickly decrease around the time of menses. Fluctuating levels of ALLO, in combination with rapid withdrawal of ovarian hormones, may be a key factor in the etiology of PMDD (Schüle et al. 2014). Animal studies demonstrate that withdrawal from physiological doses of progesterone causes social withdrawal, anxiety, and anhedonia, symptoms characteristic of PMDD (Li et al. 2012). It is possible that women with PMDD have developed tolerance to the arousal-reducing and $GABA_A$-enhancing effects of ALLO. ALLO's impact on GABAergic tone may be an important avenue for the development of PMDD treatments (Vigod et al. 2009). Roles for the opioid and adrenergic systems have also been proposed, but their mechanisms remain unclear. Brexanolone, a positive allosteric modulator of $GABA_A$ receptors that has been studied in recent trials for postpartum depression, is thought to operate via a mechanism consistent with this theory (Meltzer-Brody et al. 2018).

The fifth edition of the *Diagnostic and Statistical Manual of Mental Disorders* (DSM-5; American Psychiatric Association 2013) introduced a change from the previous edition and now recognizes PMDD as an independent depressive disorder that affects 2%–6% of premenopausal women (Vigod et al. 2009). PMDD often develops in the second or the beginning of the third decade of life, and its typical presentation includes prominent mood lability and reactivity, with predominantly irritable affect. Risk factors include a personal or family history of mood and anxiety disorders (heritability of these disorders ranges between 30% and 80%, according to DSM-5), a family and personal history of postpartum depression, stress, low socioeconomic status, and cigarette smoking (Turner et al. 2019). A diagnosis of PMDD also increases the risk of perinatal depression and of depression during the menopausal transition.

PMS, on the other hand, is a very common (30%–80% [Winer and Rapkin 2006]) and milder condition involving physical, emotional, and behavioral symptoms that last for a week or two prior to menses and subside with the onset of menses. It is important to distinguish between PMDD and PMS, because PMDD involves more profound social and occupational impairment and disruption of function.

Table 15–1 lists the DSM-5 diagnostic criteria for PMDD.

In contrast to women with the menstrually confined condition of PMDD, some women have an underlying depressive disorder with superimposed worsening of psychiatric symptoms in the perimenstrual period (PME-DD). PMDD and PME-DD can be diagnosed by using prospective mood charting over the course of two menstrual cycles. Several mobile applications have been developed for that purpose. The clinician may use the Structured Clinical Interview for PMDD (SCID-PMDD; First et al. 2016) instrument, preferably over two appointments at different stages of the menstrual cycle, to diagnose these disorders.

Treatment of premenstrual mood disorders involves both pharmacological and nonpharmacological approaches. First-line pharmacological options for PMDD are the selective serotonin reuptake inhibitor (SSRI) class of medications, which have a high response rate (>70%) (Casper and Yonkers 2019). There are three dosing strategies for SSRIs with an evidence base for the treatment of perimenstrual mood disorders—continuous dosing, luteal-phase dosing, and symptom-onset dosing. Fluoxetine, sertraline, and paroxetine are all U.S. Food and Drug Administration (FDA) approved for the treatment of PMDD and have been shown in randomized, placebo-controlled studies to alleviate both physical and psychological symptoms (Casper and Yonkers 2019). SSRIs are well tolerated and highly effective for PMDD, even in

| TABLE 15–1. | DSM-5 diagnostic criteria for premenstrual dysphoric disorder |

A. In the majority of menstrual cycles, at least five symptoms must be present in the final week before the onset of menses, start to improve within a few days after the onset of menses, and become minimal or absent in the week postmenses.

B. One (or more) of the following symptoms must be present:

1. Marked affective lability (e.g., mood swings; feeling suddenly sad or tearful, or increased sensitivity to rejection).

2. Marked irritability or anger or increased interpersonal conflicts.

3. Marked depressed mood, feelings of hopelessness, or self-deprecating thoughts.

4. Marked anxiety, tension, and/or feelings of being keyed up or on edge.

C. One (or more) of the following symptoms must additionally be present, to reach a total of five symptoms when combined with symptoms from Criterion B above:

1. Decreased interest in usual activities (e.g., work, school, friends, hobbies).

2. Subjective difficulty in concentration.

3. Lethargy, easy fatigability, or marked lack of energy.

4. Marked change in appetite; overeating; or specific food cravings.

5. Hypersomnia or insomnia.

6. A sense of being overwhelmed or out of control.

7. Physical symptoms such as breast tenderness or swelling, joint or muscle pain, a sensation of "bloating," or weight gain.

Note: The symptoms in Criteria A–C must have been met for most menstrual cycles that occurred in the preceding year.

D. The symptoms are associated with clinically significant distress or interference with work, school, usual social activities, or relationships with others (e.g., avoidance of social activities; decreased productivity and efficiency at work, school, or home).

E. The disturbance is not merely an exacerbation of the symptoms of another disorder, such as major depressive disorder, panic disorder, persistent depressive disorder (dysthymia), or a personality disorder (although it may co-occur with any of these disorders).

F. Criterion A should be confirmed by prospective daily ratings during at least two symptomatic cycles. (**Note:** The diagnosis may be made provisionally prior to this confirmation.)

G. The symptoms are not attributable to the physiological effects of a substance (e.g., a drug of abuse, a medication, other treatment) or another medical condition (e.g., hyperthyroidism).

Source. Reprinted from American Psychiatric Association: *Diagnostic and Statistical Manual of Mental Disorders,* 5th Edition, Arlington, VA, American Psychiatric Association, 2013, p. 311. Copyright © 2013 American Psychiatric Association. Used with permission.

the first menstrual cycle of use and when taken intermittently during the luteal phase only. As an alternative dosing strategy for perimenstrual disorders, SSRIs may be prescribed at symptom onset, with instructions limiting its use to the days when the patient is symptomatic. For PME-DD, SSRIs should be used continuously across the cycle and increased transiently during the luteal phase to prevent premenstrually linked exacerbation of mood symptoms.

An alternative to SSRI pharmacotherapy for PMDD is estrogen plus progestin combined hormonal contraceptive therapy. Risks and benefits of hormonal therapy should be assessed, taking into consideration the patient's smoking status and the potential for vascular and thromboembolic events, as well as cancer risk factors. An FDA-approved contraceptive option is the birth control pill that includes estradiol with the progestin drospirenone, which has antimineralocorticoid properties. Limited evidence suggests that hormonal contraceptives can be used to augment SSRIs in women with PME-DD (Joffe et al. 2003, 2007; Peters et al. 2017), but their use for this purpose warrants further study. Other agents with minimal testing that have been used include spironolactone and finasteride, as well as benzodiazepines (prescribed as a brief course to be taken during days of more severe symptoms). Induction of medical menopause using gonadotropin-releasing hormone agonist hormones is highly effective and can be used for refractory PMDD if symptoms are not responsive to other therapies and cause significant distress or impairment, but this option requires estrogen and progesterone add-back therapy to protect against osteoporosis if treatment is prolonged. Because of its irreversibility, surgical menopause induced by bilateral oophorectomy in premenopausal women should be considered only in rare cases. It should be noted that hormonal contraceptives have no adverse effects on mood in more than two-thirds of women, even among those with a history of depression (Joffe et al. 2003). However, results of recent large studies indicate that hormonal contraceptives may carry a heightened risk for future depression for women without a history of depression, especially younger women and teenagers (Skovlund et al. 2016).

Nonpharmacological options to improve premenstrual mood disturbance include lifestyle modifications such as regular aerobic exercise on most days and optimization of sleep hygiene (Maharaj and Trevino 2015). It is important to identify and manage sources of stress, particularly during the premenstrual period. Dietary changes—such as limiting alcohol, caffeine, salt, chocolate, and red meat and eating smaller, more frequent meals with complex carbohydrates—can be helpful for milder PMS symptoms. The scientific evidence regarding the efficacy of certain vitamins and dietary supplements is not consistent, and these supplements may carry risks; for example, vitamin B_6 supplementation offers no demonstrated benefit in PMDD and may lead to peripheral neuropathy at high dosages. Calcium supplementation, dosed at 1,200 mg daily, has been shown to ameliorate PMS symptoms (Shobeiri et al. 2017). Soy and chasteberry (*vitex agnus-castus*) may be helpful for physical but not mood symptoms in women with PMS.

Other therapeutic modalities that have been considered in the treatment of PMDD, PMS, and PME-DD include group or individual psychotherapy, acupuncture, yoga, and bright light therapy. There is little research evidence available for most of these treatments, although bright light therapy has shown some promise (Maharaj and Trevino 2015).

Psychiatric Disorders During Pregnancy and the Postpartum Period

Psychiatric Disorders During Pregnancy

Contrary to what has historically been proposed, pregnancy is not a state of emotional well-being that confers a protective effect against mood disorders. Instead, pregnancy represents a period of increased risk and vulnerability for women; it is estimated that between 15% and 29% of women suffer from a psychiatric disorder during their pregnancy (Gaynes et al. 2005; Vesga-López et al. 2008). Depression is the leading cause of disease-related disability in women, and pregnant women are at even higher risk for such disability. Furthermore, untreated depression during pregnancy is linked with profound consequences for both mother and child, including prematurity, preeclampsia, low birth weight or intrauterine growth restriction, and risky or maladaptive behaviors (e.g., poor nutrition and poor prenatal care, use of alcohol, tobacco, and illicit substances), as well as difficulties with maternal bonding and attachment, decreased social interactions, and other emotional difficulties (Engelstad et al. 2014). Studies have also shown a correlation between antenatal depression and increased risk of depression in adolescence in the offspring (Pawlby et al. 2009).

Combined point prevalence estimates of depression during pregnancy range from 3.1% to 4.9%, and approximately 14.5% of pregnant women experience a new episode of MDD or subsyndromal depression during pregnancy (Gaynes et al. 2005). Prevalence rates of other serious psychiatric disorders—including bipolar disorder, schizophrenia, and other psychotic disorders—are considerable (e.g., as high as 16% for anxiety disorders) (Siu et al. 2016). Approximately half of women with schizophrenia become mothers, and half of their pregnancies are unplanned. A significant number of these women will ultimately lose custody of their child.

Numerous studies have shown that the rates of recurrent mood episodes during pregnancy are significantly higher among women who discontinued versus maintained their preconception antidepressant medications (68% vs. 26%) or mood stabilizers (86% vs. 37%) (Cohen et al. 2006a; Viguera et al. 2007). According to one study, women who discontinued their mood stabilizer spent more than 40% of the time during pregnancy in an illness episode, versus only 9% of the time during pregnancy among women who maintained mood stabilizer use (Viguera et al. 2007).

The risks of psychiatric deterioration are even more marked during the postpartum period than during pregnancy (Viguera et al. 2007). The greatest risk factor for psychiatric destabilization during the postpartum period is the presence of psychiatric symptoms during pregnancy. It is therefore crucial to identify and treat mood, anxiety, and psychotic disorders during pregnancy to minimize the occurrence of puerperal psychiatric illness. The most serious postpartum condition is postpartum psychosis, a major psychiatric emergency that warrants hospitalization to ensure the protection of mother and child, because the potential for suicide and infanticide are important concerns in this postpartum population.

Screening of Pregnant and Postpartum Women

Early diagnosis and treatment of postpartum depression is a major public health imperative, and efforts to identify this disorder have increased worldwide. In the United States, screening for postpartum depression is now required by law in several states, and other states have funded initiatives to increase screening efforts (Rhodes and Segre 2013; Siu et al. 2016). In 2016, the U.S. Preventive Services Task Force expanded its general screening recommendations for depression to include screening of pregnant and postpartum women (Siu et al. 2016). The American College of Obstetricians and Gynecologists has recommended screening "at least once during the perinatal period for depression and anxiety symptoms using a standardized, validated tool" (American College of Obstetricians and Gynecologists 2018; Earls and Committee on Psychosocial Aspects of Child and Family Health, American Academy of Pediatrics 2010), and in its Bright Futures guidelines, the American Academy of Pediatrics recommended screening of all new mothers, noting that pediatricians were uniquely positioned to provide such screening because they are in contact with mothers routinely for well-baby visits (Liberto 2012). Still, establishing the optimal timing and frequency of perinatal screens, devising consistent strategies for implementing interventions, and determining who should be responsible for screening perinatal women are topics of ongoing debate. Research focused on integration of mental health care into obstetric and pediatric settings is emerging (Cox and Holden 2013).

The most widely used screening tools for perinatal depression are the Edinburgh Postnatal Depression Scale (EPDS) and the 9-item Patient Health Questionnaire (PHQ-9) for depression. The EPDS is a 10-item self-report scale assessing symptoms over the past 7 days (Cox and Holden 2013). It has the advantages of being brief, free, easily scored, and available in several languages (Gibson et al. 2009). The recommended cutoff scores for the EPDS are ≥10 for treatment settings with clinical resources to assess women with positive screens and ≥13 for settings with limited clinical capacity for postscreening evaluation (Cox and Holden 2013). The American Academy of Pediatrics suggested an EPDS cutoff of ≥10 for assessing risk of postpartum depression, a cutoff that would provide increased sensitivity in capturing at-risk women; however, many primary care clinicians use the more conservative cutoff of ≥13 to consume fewer postscreening resources for false-positive screens (Cox and Holden 2013).

The other widely used screening survey for postpartum depression is the PHQ-9, which consists of nine questions examining mood symptoms over a 2-week period (Kroenke et al. 2001). The PHQ-9 has the same advantages as the EPDS and is already in wide use by providers in numerous specialties (Wisner et al. 2013). One disadvantage of the PHQ-9 is its emphasis on neurovegetative symptoms, such as fatigue and disrupted sleep, that are common in pregnancy and the postpartum; this may result in overestimating peripartum depression. The PHQ-9 also does not capture anxiety symptoms, which tend to be highly correlated with perinatal mood disorders (Heron et al. 2008).

Regardless of which screening instrument is used to identify perinatal depression, the tool alone should not dictate clinical care. This is particularly important in primary care settings, where treatment may be initiated on the basis of a positive EPDS screen. Rather, a careful mental health assessment is needed to correctly identify the psychiatric disorder. A careful screening for previous episodes of mania or hypomania is also extremely important, because a substantial proportion of women (20%) who experience a postpartum depressive episode actually have bipolar disorder (Wisner et al. 2013). Similarly, a bipolar disorder diagnosis should be considered for any woman who experiences postpartum psychosis (Bergink et al. 2016; Clark et al. 2015). In these women with a unrecognized propensity for bipolar illness, unopposed antidepressant pharmacotherapy increases the risk of exacerbating the illness and prolonging its course due to treatment nonresponse. Screening with the Mood Disorder Questionnaire (MDQ) by primary care providers can improve diagnostic accuracy, and psychiatric referral is indicated for a positive MDQ screen (Clark et al. 2015).

Treatment Decision Making in Pregnancy

Treatment during pregnancy involves a careful and individual assessment of the risks and benefits of available treatment options, including pharmacological and nonpharmacological approaches. The decision of whether to treat psychiatric disorders must also include careful consideration of the consequences of not treating these disorders. Untreated mental health problems are associated with risks to the woman, her pregnancy, and her baby, and these risks should be considered alongside any risks associated with treatment. The decision of which treatments to use involves an assessment of the history of the illness, the history of prior treatment, the level of severity of—and debilitation from—symptoms, the patient's access to treatment, and the patient's preference.

Many nonpharmacological treatment options are evidence based and, when optimized, can be highly effective alone or in combination with medications. Such options include behavioral modification therapy, cognitive-behavioral therapy (CBT), and interpersonal therapy, as well as approaches emphasizing physical exercise, mindfulness meditation, and social support.

Psychopharmacotherapy During Pregnancy

When a clinician is considering medication treatment, the first thing to assess is whether the patient is currently taking a psychotropic agent and whether this medication has been effective. If so, the preference is always to maximize and optimize the current treatment to avoid additional exposures during pregnancy. If the patient is not on a medication and the decision is made to start pharmacological treatment, use of an agent with known prior efficacy for the patient is favored barring specific concerns about teratogenicity. Throughout pregnancy and lactation, the preference is always to minimize switching and to favor monotherapy, or the fewest medications possible, to limit total exposures to the fetus and baby. Generally, dosing during pregnancy does not differ from dosing outside of pregnancy, because it is always important to use the most effective dosage of a medication. It is also important to counsel women on the possibility that dosages may need to be increased as pregnancy advances and the physiological changes of pregnancy lead to increased metabolism and excretion of medication, potentially resulting in lower levels and reduced efficacy.

Of note, in 2015, the FDA replaced the letter system (A, B, C, D, X) with a more detailed system incorporating expanded summaries of potential maternal and fetal risks and supporting clinical data. The previous system could at times be perceived as confusing, simplistic, or misleading, and it did not incorporate updated information about drug safety and risk profiles in pregnancy and lactation. The new labeling system has separate sections for pregnancy and lactation, each with three main components: risk summary, clinical considerations, and analysis of data (animal vs. human) (Becker at al. 2009). The new model offers clearer and more comprehensive guidance for the treatment decision-making process.

In the following subsections, we provide an overview of currently available data on the reproductive safety of the main psychotropic classes.

Selective serotonin reuptake inhibitor antidepressants.　　SSRI antidepressants are the most frequently prescribed psychotropics and are used to treat many conditions, but they are most commonly used for depressive and anxiety disorders. Antidepressant use during pregnancy is not uncommon; for example, in a cohort study of 1,106,757 pregnancies in 47 American states, it was found that nearly 1 in 12 women used an antidepressant during pregnancy (Huybrechts et al. 2013). SSRI use during pregnancy has been investigated extensively in many observational studies with very large populations.

The most common adverse neonatal outcome associated with SSRI use in pregnancy is the poor neonatal adaptation syndrome or neonatal adaptation syndrome. This syndrome is characterized by respiratory distress, tremor, irritability, sleep disturbance, and feeding difficulties, although definitions in the literature are heterogeneous. The syndrome is mild, transient, and self-limited, generally requiring only supportive care; it does not require medication treatment or extended care in the hospital (Grigoriadis et al. 2013). Most reassuring, however, is the consistent finding in the literature that exposure to SSRIs with or without subsequent poor neonatal adaptation after birth does not appear to be associated with lasting cognitive or developmental consequences (El Marroun et al. 2017; Klinger et al. 2011).

In 2006, concerns were raised about an association between use of SSRIs in pregnancy and increased risk of persistent pulmonary hypertension of the newborn (PPHN) (Chambers et al. 2006). However, over time, the strength of the association was called into question, because most additional studies showed a more modest increase in risk. In the largest study to date, the odds ratio for PPHN associated with antidepressant exposure was 1.28 after adjustment for maternal illness and use of propensity scoring (Huybrechts et al. 2015). Furthermore, antidepressant exposure was not found to be associated with a risk of severe PPHN requiring procedures or special interventions for respiratory assistance (e.g., use of ventilators).

Numerous studies have examined the effects of antidepressant medication use on pregnancy outcomes, including preterm birth, although these studies vary with respect to size and quality as well as adjustment for confounding, including maternal diagnosis and severity. SSRIs have been associated with increased risk for earlier delivery and lower birth weight, although the magnitude of the absolute risk is generally low, and untreated maternal depression has been associated with the same findings (Huybrechts et al. 2014; Ross et al. 2013).

Concerns have been raised about a possible association between autism spectrum disorder (ASD) and SSRI exposure. The literature is complicated by studies lacking in appropriate adjustment for confounders. The majority of studies, especially those that do control for confounds, have not confirmed this association (Lusskin et al. 2018).

The issue of whether SSRIs are associated with structural congenital anomalies is fraught with contradictory literature and an absence of randomized controlled trials due to the challenges of conducting such studies in pregnant women. The studies that remain are challenged by the limitations of retrospective database and case-control study designs. This literature is notable for the large number of studies describing a variety of malformations associated with SSRIs. However, the majority of studies are large database studies that suffer from methodological flaws, including the risk of multiple queries and the lack of appropriate controls for confounding by indication. The most important finding is that these studies have not yielded consistent evidence of malformations associated with any single agent or with the class as a whole. Prospective, controlled cohort studies and meta-analyses have demonstrated no increased risk from SSRIs (Ban et al. 2014b). Although there was an early finding of an association between paroxetine and cardiac malformations, this association was not replicated in large cohort studies (Boukhris et al. 2016; Huybrechts et al. 2014) in which potential confounders (e.g., depression severity, maternal medical illness, use of other medications) were taken into account.

Other antidepressants. Among the serotonin-norepinephrine reuptake inhibitors (SNRIs), the majority of data available for use in pregnancy are for venlafaxine. Venlafaxine and duloxetine are not associated with structural teratogenicity (Lassen et al. 2016). Similar to SSRIs, SNRIs are associated with small increases in risk for pregnancy-associated complications as well as for poor neonatal adaptation (Grigoriadis et al. 2013; Ross et al. 2013).

Among the tricyclic antidepressants (TCAs), most studies have focused on nortriptyline, desipramine, imipramine, and amitriptyline. Differences among TCAs are difficult to discern because studies have been small, with limited data identified for elevated obstetrical or neonatal risks (Pearson et al. 2007).

Monoamine oxidase inhibitors are used much less frequently than other classes, although they may be important for individuals with treatment-refractory depression. Few data exist for their use in pregnancy outside of case reports and animal data; however, these data are not suggestive of risk for teratogenicity (Bauer et al. 2017).

Mood stabilizers. Options for mood stabilization in pregnancy include lithium, lamotrigine, and second-generation antipsychotics (SGAs).

Lithium remains the gold standard mood stabilizer after more than six decades. It is effective in preventing postpartum psychosis when used prophylactically in the third trimester, and it has antisuicidal properties. Important considerations include the risk of Ebstein's cardiac malformation, which affects 1–2 per 1,000 infants with first-trimester exposure to lithium (Patorno et al. 2017). Folate supplementation is advised to decrease risk. Additionally, lithium is not associated with cognitive or developmental abnormalities. Maternal complications of lithium use during pregnancy may include polyuria, polydipsia, nausea, and goiter. Possible neonatal complications include diabetes insipidus, nephrotoxicity, hypothyroidism, arrhythmias, and floppy baby syndrome. It is important to keep in mind that the glomerular filtration rate increases during pregnancy; therefore, the lithium dosage may need to be adjusted as the pregnancy advances. The clinician can check lithium levels at 8–12 weeks' gestational age and again in the second and third trimesters to monitor and maintain therapeutic levels and efficacy. To reduce the risk of delivery complications, lithium should be discontinued 24–48 hours prior to the scheduled delivery or at the onset of labor. Close monitoring of infant and mother serum levels after delivery is recommended, with attention to fluid shifts and dehydration.

Among anticonvulsants, studies have found that lamotrigine represents a relatively safe and effective option for mood stabilization in pregnancy, particularly for the maintenance stage of bipolar depression. Recent studies found no association between lamotrigine exposure during pregnancy and major malformations (Dolk et al. 2016). Lamotrigine has also been shown to be effective in preventing puerperal mood episodes when used during pregnancy (Wesseloo et al. 2017). In their study comparing rates of congenital malformations among children exposed to various anticonvulsants during the first trimester, Bromley et al. (2017) found that lamotrigine and levetiracetam were associated with the lowest rates and valproate was associated with the highest rates.

Valproic acid is a well-known teratogen and has been associated with a 3%–5% risk of neural tube defects in infants exposed to the drug during the first trimester, as well as other major malformations, including hypospadias and cardiac defects (Koren et al. 2006). This risk is greater for infants of women who take valproic acid for bipolar disorder than for infants of women who take the drug for epilepsy, suggesting a dosage-dependent effect (given that treatment of bipolar disorder typically requires higher dosages than that of epilepsy). Valproic acid may also be associated with ASD and neurocognitive deficits that persist throughout infancy and early childhood (Bromley et al. 2017; Meador et al. 2009). In July 2017, the government of France banned the use of valproic acid for bipolar disorder in women of reproductive age (Casassus 2017), a decision that is expected to be followed by 27 other European countries.

It is recommended that valproic acid be avoided for the entire pregnancy if possible, unless all other options are contraindicated or have been ineffective. When the drug is prescribed for women of reproductive potential, concurrent reliable contraception should be started and documented. If a fetus has been exposed to valproic acid, careful evaluation of the extent of and gestational age/period of the exposure is important to determine the nature of the teratogenic risks. A supplemental dosage of folate (4 mg/day) is also indicated to decrease the risk of neural tube defects and other malformations.

Antipsychotics.   First-generation antipsychotics (FGAs) have a long record of use in pregnancy, occasionally for off-label indications such as hyperemesis gravidarum (Coughlin et al. 2015; Huybrechts et al. 2016). However, over the past decade, SGAs have become more widely used by women of childbearing age and are now much more commonly prescribed than FGAs. This increase is in part due to these agents' wider spectrum of indications and uses for both psychotic and mood disorders.

The literature examining antipsychotic use during pregnancy focuses more on SGAs than on FGAs. Antipsychotics are often grouped together in studies, which can make determining unique risk profiles more difficult, and the newest antipsychotics have not yet been sufficiently studied to produce evidence to guide risk-benefit decisions about their use. This lack of data can lead to difficulties for clinicians who need current information on the risk and adverse-effect profiles of available antipsychotics in order to select the best agent for a given patient. A small study that compared rates of placental passage among haloperidol, risperidone, olanzapine, and quetiapine found that quetiapine had the lowest rate (Newport et al. 2007). While fetal exposure may be lower with quetiapine, making it seem an attractive option for use in a pregnant patient, it is worth emphasizing that exposure is not zero, and there is still risk associated with its use. Antipsychotics that increase prolactin levels as a side effect (e.g., risperidone) may suppress ovulation and reduce the likelihood of conception. The risk of miscarriage with antipsychotic use has not been well studied. A careful risk-benefit analysis—weighing both the perinatal risks and the health risks related to anovulation, hypoestrogenism, and subfertility—must be conducted to inform selection of antipsychotics for women of childbearing potential.

Current evidence indicates that FGAs and SGAs do not pose significant teratogenic risk. While some older studies (e.g., Iqbal et al. 2005) showed an association between antipsychotic use in the first trimester and risk of cardiac abnormalities, more recent studies with large sample sizes and good control for confounders have not observed this risk (Cohen et al. 2016). In comparison with FGAs, SGAs are associated with a higher incidence of metabolic side effects, including diabetes and dyslipidemia, in all patients who take them; pregnant women using antipsychotics have been shown to develop gestational diabetes at higher rates than their counterparts who do not take antipsychotics, just as in the nonpregnant patient population. While weight gain during pregnancy in women taking SGAs has not been clearly demonstrated to be greater than that in women not taking these medications, women taking SGAs may enter pregnancy with a higher body mass index, which can increase their risks of complications during pregnancy (Freeman et al. 2018).

Antipsychotic use during pregnancy is associated with preterm labor and fetal growth restriction (i.e., small-for-gestational-age birth) as well as neonatal intensive care unit (NICU) admissions (Bodén et al. 2012). However, evidence also suggests that pregnant women with bipolar disorder and schizophrenia may be at higher risk of adverse birth outcomes, independent of exposure to medications (Coughlin et al. 2015; Huybrechts et al. 2016). In 2011, the FDA issued a warning regarding the potential risks of extrapyramidal symptoms (EPS) or withdrawal symptoms in newborns whose mothers had been treated with antipsychotic drugs during the third trimester of pregnancy. This warning was based on 69 spontaneously reported cases of neonatal EPS or withdrawal symptoms—including increased or decreased muscle tone, tremor, sleepiness, severe difficulty breathing, and difficulty feeding—associated with exposure to antipsychotics (either FGAs or SGAs) during the third trimester of pregnancy. The symptoms were often mild, transient, and self-limited and did not incur a need for specialized treatments or procedures. The FDA counseled health care providers to monitor newborns carefully for resolution of symptoms, because in rare cases, newborns may require longer hospitalizations to ensure stabilization. Longitudinal data regarding the impact of antipsychotics on developmental and cognitive outcomes are lacking, although active research is ongoing in this area (Galbally et al. 2014).

Anxiolytics. Antidepressants can also be beneficial in the treatment of perinatal anxiety disorders. Many antidepressants (including those in the SSRI and TCA classes, among others) are well studied and have been shown to be relatively safe during pregnancy, therefore constituting a reasonable first choice for management of perinatal anxiety disorders.

Benzodiazepines are commonly used to treat anxiety disorders; however, their relative safety in pregnancy is less well characterized than that of antidepressants. Early studies suggested a possible increased risk of cleft lip and palate associated with first-trimester exposure to benzodiazepines (Dolovich et al. 1998); however, more recent studies, including a large population-based cohort study that analyzed data from almost 400,000 British women over the course of two decades, have not confirmed that association (Ban et al. 2014a). Apart from this unconfirmed association with cleft lip and palate, benzodiazepine use during the first trimester has in general not been linked to other congenital malformations.

Some studies have linked benzodiazepine use during late pregnancy with preterm delivery and low birth weight. However, it is unclear whether these associations are related to medication use or to the conditions for which these medications are prescribed (e.g., anxiety and mood disorders), given that such disorders have independently been associated with these neonatal outcomes.

Neonatal exposure to benzodiazepines (particularly near delivery) can be associated with withdrawal or toxicity symptoms in the neonate. For this reason, collaboration between the obstetrics and pediatrics teams is particularly important, because newborns exposed to benzodiazepines in utero may need additional monitoring and support following delivery. At present, the long-term effects of neonatal benzodiazepine exposure on child development are not fully known.

Nonpharmacological treatment strategies—in particular, CBT—can also be effective in the treatment of mild to moderate perinatal anxiety.

Stimulants.   Stimulants are typically used to manage attention-deficit/hyperactivity disorder (ADHD) or to augment antidepressant treatment in mood disorders. Decisions about stimulant use during pregnancy require a careful assessment that takes into account the potential risks of the illnesses these medications are being used to treat in addition to the risks of the medications themselves, as well as the potential risks to the fetus. In mild to moderate ADHD, behavioral therapy may be sufficient to control symptoms. In more severe cases in which untreated illness can lead to safety concerns or functional impairment (e.g., occupational difficulty), there may be a need to initiate or continue pharmacological treatment.

In general, there are limited data on the safety of stimulant use during pregnancy. Available studies rarely separate patients who use stimulants for therapeutic indications from those who abuse stimulants. Most studies that examined stimulant use during the first trimester have not shown a link between these medications and an increased risk of congenital malformations (Dideriksen et al. 2013; Huybrechts et al. 2018; Louik et al. 2015). Some studies have shown a higher rate of miscarriages in women taking stimulants, particularly methylphenidate (Diav-Citrin et al. 2016). Additionally, there is evidence that third-trimester exposure to stimulants may increase the risks for low birth weight, preterm birth, growth retardation, and neonatal withdrawal symptoms, but those findings are based on very small studies with several confounding limitations (Golub et al. 2005).

Alternative pharmacological treatment options for ADHD include TCAs, bupropion, and clonidine, all of which have reasonable evidence to support their safety in pregnancy.

In conclusion, the data on use of stimulant medications in pregnancy do not allow for definite conclusions regarding their safety. Available data for amphetamines suggest no increase in the risk of malformations, while infants might have slightly lower birth weights and lower Apgar scores (Huybrechts et al. 2018). Whenever possible, attempts can be made to manage ADHD symptoms through use of nonpharmacological strategies, through treatment of comorbidities (e.g., mood and anxiety symptoms, sleep difficulties, alcohol and substance use) that may aggravate ADHD symptoms, or through use of alternative pharmacological treatments for ADHD that have more supporting evidence in pregnancy.

Treatment of Insomnia During Pregnancy

Virtually all pregnant women will experience sleep difficulties at some point during their pregnancy. Pregnancy-related risk factors for sleep problems include alterations in sleep architecture, physical discomfort, higher incidence of restless legs syndrome and obstructive sleep apnea, nocturia or increased urinary frequency due to anatomic changes, and depression and anxiety. Improved sleep hygiene, CBT, and other nonpharmacological options (e.g., physical exercise, yoga, meditation) can be effective in the treatment of insomnia in pregnancy and should be encouraged to the extent possible.

Some women, however, have persistent and debilitating insomnia that interferes with their ability to function and may require pharmacological treatment for management. Identifying and treating an underlying psychiatric disorder that can manifest with sleep disturbances, such as depression or anxiety, and initiating treatment accordingly is crucial.

Most epidemiological studies have found no congenital malformations from first-trimester exposure to sedative-hypnotics (e.g., zolpidem, eszopiclone, zaleplon) (Ban et al. 2014a), although some studies have suggested that these agents may increase the risk of adverse obstetrical outcomes such as preterm birth, low birth weight, or small-for-gestational-age infants (Calderon-Margalit et al. 2009; Chaudhry and Susser 2018) (for information on benzodiazepine use in pregnancy, see the "Anxiolytics" subsection earlier in this chapter).

Antihistamines are used frequently in the treatment of insomnia during pregnancy and are considered to be reasonably safe and effective (Gilboa et al. 2014). A review of antihistamines' safety in pregnancy found no clear association between first-trimester antihistamine exposure and birth defects (Gilboa et al. 2014). More research exists for older histamine 1 (H_1) receptor blockers such as diphenhydramine, promethazine, and hydroxyzine, which are commonly used for sleep disturbance in pregnancy, and there are good data for their safety in pregnancy (Gilboa et al. 2014).

Psychiatric Disorders During the Postpartum Period

Postpartum psychiatric syndromes comprise three major clusters of symptom domains—that is, postpartum depression (PPD; to be differentiated from postpartum blues or "baby blues"), postpartum psychosis, and postpartum obsessive-compulsive disorder (OCD). While baby blues is the most common of these syndromes, it is PPD that has garnered the most attention in recent years and that will be the primary focus of our discussion.

Postpartum Depression

PPD is a public health concern, with an estimated cost of $192,000,000 per year (Ko et al. 2017). It is defined as a major depressive episode that has its onset in the first year after giving birth. PPD has an estimated prevalence of one in nine women, according to the Centers for Disease Control and Prevention (Ko et al. 2017), although other large population studies have cited prevalence rates as high as one in seven women. Active psychiatric illness during pregnancy is one of the most important risk factors for a postpartum mood episode. Similarly, the occurrence of a postpartum depressive episode is associated with a fourfold increase in the risk of future episodes in subsequent pregnancies (Viguera et al. 2011). Other risk factors for PPD include having a history of a mood disorder, of pregnancy complications (e.g., preterm delivery, infertility, multiple gestation), of a teen pregnancy, of substance use, or of trauma; belonging to a racial or ethnic minority group; and being of lower socioeconomic status.

PPD must be distinguished from postpartum blues, and there are many differences that can be used to help discern between the two. One of the main differences is that the predominant moods in postpartum blues are happiness and joy, whereas in PPD they are pervasive sadness, depression, and anhedonia. Baby blues is extremely common, occurring in approximately 75% of women (American Pregnancy Association 2015) during the first few days after giving birth and lasting up to 2 weeks; by contrast, PPD can occur at any time during the postpartum period (and often begins during pregnancy, as previously mentioned) and typically lasts much longer than a few weeks (Manjunath et al. 2011).

In addition to the usual symptoms of depression, PPD may also include increased tearfulness; prominent anxiety; feelings of anger, numbness, or disconnection from the baby; intense or excessive worries about harming the baby; and feelings of guilt about being an inadequate mother. The consequences of untreated mood symptoms during the postpartum period can include decreased rates of seatbelt use and other child safety measures and difficulty in adhering to well-child visit schedules and keeping postpartum appointments. While difficult to study, untreated depression also negatively affects mother-child bonding and attachment. The exact mechanism of this effect is unknown but may relate to the mother's decreased responsiveness to the infant's needs and distress, less healthy lifestyle habits, and low drive to provide enrichment activities for the baby.

Primary care physicians (e.g., internists, pediatricians, family doctors) and obstetrical providers have a pivotal role in diagnosing postpartum depression because they have regular opportunities to screen and engage women in treatment. It is important that these providers perform routine screening with instruments such as the EPDS and the PHQ-9 (see "Screening of Pregnant and Postpartum Women" section earlier in chapter) in order to identify patients who should be referred to a specialist and to rule out other medical illnesses that may be contributing to depression (e.g., thyroid disease, iron deficiency anemia, vitamin D deficiency). Treatment options for women with PPD are similar to those for pregnant women with depression, although with medications, the risk of potential fetal exposure is replaced with concern for transmission through breast milk; as always, a careful risk-benefit analysis should be done with the mother. In March 2019, brexanolone, a positive allosteric modulator of $GABA_A$ receptors, became the first drug to receive FDA approval specifically for treatment of PPD.

Postpartum Psychosis

Postpartum psychosis is a major psychiatric emergency that affects 1 in 1,000 women (VanderKruik et al. 2017). As with PPD, the greatest risk factor for postpartum psychosis is a prior episode of postpartum psychosis. A diagnosis of bipolar disorder is an important risk factor as well. Any woman who develops postpartum psychosis should be carefully screened for previous episodes of mania or hypomania and should be assumed to have bipolar disorder—and receive treatment appropriate for that diagnosis—unless proven otherwise. Postpartum psychosis is characterized not only by psychotic symptoms (e.g., delusion, hallucination) but also by a fluctuating sensorium reminiscent of delirium; insomnia and agitation may also be present. Onset is rapid, usually within the first few days after giving birth, although onset during the first 3 months following delivery can occur. Hallucinations may be nontraditional in nature (i.e., involving senses other than hearing), and delusions frequently center on the baby. The 4% risk of infanticide associated with postpartum psychosis (Brockington 2017), along with the increased risk of maternal suicide, makes this disorder an emergency; inpatient hospitalization is warranted, and treatment with antipsychotic medications should be initiated to ensure the safety of mother and baby. Despite its name, postpartum psychosis is often associated with an underlying diagnosis of bipolar disorder. For women who have no prior psychiatric history, this is an important consideration, because treatment of prominent mood symptoms may require a mood stabilizer instead of an antidepressant, in addition to an antipsychotic. In addition to medication, psychotherapy and sleep protection are also recommended treatments that may have important implications for breastfeeding. In women with a history of postpartum psychosis who are contemplating a future pregnancy, evidence supports the use of lithium therapy as prophylaxis against recurrence.

Postpartum Obsessive-Compulsive Disorder

OCD is another psychiatric disorder that may worsen during the postpartum period. A longitudinal study in a cohort of 461 postpartum women found a prevalence of 11% at 2 weeks and 6 months postpartum, compared with a lifetime prevalence of 2%–3% in the general population (Miller et al. 2013). Most notably, up to 90% of women in the general population experience "mild, transient intrusive thoughts" during the postpartum period that are less intense than the intrusive thoughts experienced in OCD (Miller at al. 2015). Intrusive, ego-dystonic thoughts are common, as are unwanted images of harming the newborn child and pervasive fears about making wrong decisions or being a bad mother in such a way that the baby may be inadvertently harmed. These intrusive images can sometimes be quite bizarre (e.g., throwing the baby down the stairs, placing the baby in a microwave) and therefore are both embarrassing and a source of great shame. Patients may not disclose these experiences unless asked directly about them and reassured that such experiences are common in postpartum OCD. Well-intentioned providers may be confused and greatly concerned about the possibility of postpartum psychosis when a postpartum mother describes intrusive thoughts about harming her infant. The key distinction between postpartum OCD and postpartum psychosis is that in postpartum OCD, the thoughts are ego-dystonic and highly distressing to the mother. Nevertheless, these characteristics can be complicated to untangle, and they require a thorough assessment. Postpartum OCD carries no increased risk of harming the baby (Hudak and Wisner 2012). Common compulsive behaviors include avoidance of certain aspects of baby care due to fears about harming the baby, repeatedly asking family members for reassurance that no harm to or abuse of the baby has occurred, performing repeated and excessive checking on a baby as he or she sleeps, and having a pervasive preoccupation with germs. Approximately 70% of women with postpartum OCD experience comorbid PPD and should be treated for both conditions when present (Miller et al. 2013). Correct diagnosis of postpartum OCD is important, because its treatment differs from that for other postpartum psychiatric illnesses—for example, patients with OCD typically require higher dosages of SSRIs than those used to treat depression, and they tend to respond well to medication augmentation with CBT. Postpartum OCD is frequently misdiagnosed as PPD due to the high comorbidity of the two disorders and a lack of clinician familiarity with postpartum OCD.

Other Relevant Obstetrical Conditions

The effect of high-risk obstetrical conditions on the development of psychiatric issues has become an area of active research over the past several years, generating increasing evidence that dysregulation of the immune and neuroendocrine systems may represent a predisposing factor for the development of perinatal psychiatric disorders (Osborne and Monk 2013), particularly first-onset postpartum disorders (Bergink et al. 2013, 2015b).

Depression, an independent risk factor for cardiovascular disease, was found to be associated with an increased risk of preeclampsia, a severe immunological disorder (Abedian et al. 2015; Hoedjes et al. 2011; Qiu et al. 2007), and this finding has been replicated in at least one large population study (Bergink et al. 2015b). Furthermore, it has been proposed that severe forms of preeclampsia have a higher correlation with postpartum mood symptoms than do milder forms, although that observation appears likely to be due to the consequences of severe disease, such as admission to the NICU or neonatal death.

Recent studies have reported an increased incidence in new-onset psychiatric symptoms, often including psychosis, in patients, most typically but not exclusively young women. The onset of psychiatric symptoms in young female patients, particularly those without a prior psychiatric history, at times associated with nonspecific neurological symptoms, should raise suspicion for anti–N-methyl-D-aspartate receptor (NMDAR) encephalitis. Ovarian teratoma has been associated with the development of this syndrome, although anti-NMDAR encephalitis can also occur in men and in association with other disorders. For presentations that warrant a high level of suspicion, evaluation for the presence of anti-NMDAR autoantibodies should be considered (Bergink et al. 2015a). This topic is reviewed in greater detail elsewhere in this volume (see Chapter 8, "Inflammatory Diseases and Their Psychiatric Manifestations," and Chapter 17, "Psychotic Disorders Due to Medical Illnesses").

Given the risks that obesity confers on a woman and her developing fetus, and the increasing use of SGAs in women of reproductive age, it has been postulated that SGA use during pregnancy might be associated with increased weight gain. However, studies investigating this issue have found no such association (Freeman et al. 2018; Miller et al. 2016). (It was noted, however, that women who were prescribed SGAs entered their pregnancies at a higher body mass index in comparison with nonexposed women).

In regard to the inflammatory role of depression, there is now evidence that prepregnancy diabetes (but not gestational diabetes) is associated with the development of PPD (but not antenatal depression) (Freeman et al. 2018; Katon et al. 2011).

Hyperemesis gravidarum, a condition that affects approximately 0.3%–2.0% of pregnancies, is likewise considered a predisposing risk factor for depression, anxiety, and emotional distress during pregnancy (Annagür et al. 2013; Kjeldgaard et al. 2017) as well as up to 18 months following delivery (Mitchell-Jones et al. 2017), with greater severity of hyperemesis gravidarum symptoms correlating with more serious emotional symptoms.

Psychotropic Medications in Lactating Mothers

The decision to breast-feed a child may be complex for some, but for women with psychiatric illness, the decision becomes even more complex if they are taking psychotropic medications postpartum. Factors to consider in weighing the risks and benefits of breast feeding while taking psychotropic medications include the known and unknown risks of the infant's exposure to the medication and the benefits associated with breast feeding, including health benefits to the infant and to the mother as well as enhanced mother-infant bonding, in part through increased skin-to-skin contact (Grummer-Strawn and Rollins 2015). Pregnant women have a range of expectations about breast feeding, at times holding a strong preference for either breast feeding or formula feeding. The decision to breast-feed is based on many factors and can be influenced by health considerations as well as by social aspects, such as family and cultural attitudes toward breast feeding, personal experience with breast feeding, body image concerns, or a history of trauma.

Successful breast feeding is possible for women with psychiatric illness. It is essential for women in the early postpartum period to be supported in their chosen feeding method.

For women with mental disorders, the benefits of breast feeding must be balanced against the risks to the infant from exposure to medications. Women who are taking psychotropic medication should have a conversation with their provider regarding the use of medications during lactation. When weighing a medication's risk, the amount of drug passed into breast milk and the impact of the exposure on the infant must be considered. Most psychiatric medications are present only in very low amounts in breast milk, are often not detected in the baby's plasma, and have not been linked to acute health problems in the infant (Kronenfeld et al. 2017). An extensive literature search (Berle and Spigset 2011; Lanza di Scalea and Wisner 2009) performed to develop clinical guidelines for antidepressant use during breast feeding concluded that the SSRIs sertraline and paroxetine and the TCA nortriptyline were generally the preferred antidepressants in lactation because levels are rarely detectable in infant plasma, although these antidepressants are typically detected at very low levels in breast milk. There have been no reports of short-term adverse effects associated with their use during breastfeeding. However, limited data are available regarding potential long-term effects of exposure to psychotropic agents during the newborn period.

Exclusive breast feeding markedly disrupts sleep, which has important implications for the course of postpartum psychiatric disorders, which can be significantly impacted by sleep disruption. While sleep disruption can cause serious problems for most women with mood disorders, its impact can be devastating for women with bipolar spectrum illness. It is important to work closely with the patient to consider the potential impacts of breast feeding on her risk for decompensation in the postpartum period and to evaluate the resources available to mitigate this risk. Preserving sleep by arranging for assistance with nighttime care and feeding is a key element of post-partum psychiatric illness management.

Psychiatric Symptoms and Disorders in Perimenopause

The menopausal transition represents a period of reproductive aging and is character-ized by changes in length of the menstrual cycle as well as by more marked fluctuation in and eventually sustained suppression of gonadal steroid hormones (Bromberger et al. 2007). This reproductive transition is divided into phases delineated by the Stages of Reproductive Aging Workshop (STRAW) criteria, which are used both clinically and for research (Harlow et al. 2012). Hot flashes are the most common symptom re-ported during the menopausal transition, although this is also a period of increased risk for subthreshold depressive symptoms, major depressive episodes, sleep distur-bance, and insomnia.

Depression

Women have a twofold increased cumulative lifetime risk for MDD compared with men (Bromberger and Kravitz 2011; Bromberger et al. 2007). Longitudinal studies have shown an increased risk of depressive symptoms among women during the menopausal transition (or perimenopause) (Table 15–2; Bromberger and Kravitz 2011; Bromberger et al. 2015). Mood symptoms are most commonly subsyndromal and may not meet full criteria for a major depressive episode. A prior history of MDD has been linked to an increased risk for recurrence of MDD and emergence of subsyn-dromal depressive symptoms during this time (Cohen et al. 2006b; Freeman et al. 2006). Women without a history of MDD are at risk for perimenopause-associated de-pressive symptoms, while evidence indicating their risk for a first lifetime onset of a major depressive episode is less consistent (Bromberger et al. 2016; Woods et al. 2008).

Hot Flashes

Vasomotor symptoms (hot flashes and night sweats) are the most common symptoms experienced during the menopausal transition, with as many as 85% of women expe-riencing these symptoms at some point during midlife (Gold et al. 2006; Mitchell and Woods 2015). Symptoms are described as intense heat along with flushing and sweat-ing, generally localized to the head and trunk. Vasomotor symptoms are linked with sleep disturbance, mood symptoms, and reduced quality of life (de Zambotti et al. 2014; Ensrud et al. 2009; Kravitz et al. 2008). Furthermore, they are a primary reason that women seek medical treatment during the menopausal transition (Murphy and Campbell 2007; Timur and Sahin 2009; Williams et al. 2007). Nocturnal hot flashes, but not daytime symptoms, are linked with depressive mood changes. Vasomotor symptoms may precede or follow the onset of depressive symptoms. Additionally, the presence of anxiety both prior to the onset of vasomotor symptoms and during the menopausal transition has been linked to more frequent and intense vasomotor symptoms (Freeman et al. 2005).

TABLE 15–2. **Risk factors for mood symptoms during perimenopause**

Age—Younger age at onset of the menopausal transition has been linked to increased risk for depressive symptoms during this time period (Dennerstein et al. 2000; Epperson et al. 2017; Williams et al. 2007).

Hormone changes—Greater variability in estradiol levels has been linked with depressive symptoms (Freeman et al. 2004).

Hot flashes—Nocturnal hot flashes especially have been linked to increased risk for depressive symptoms during the menopausal transition (Freeman et al. 2009; Joffe et al. 2016). Hot flashes have not been linked to perimenopausal major depressive disorder (MDD).

Sleep disturbance—Sleep interruption and poor sleep quality have been linked to perimenopausal MDD and subsyndromal depressive symptoms.

Adverse life experiences—Exposure to stress in midlife and to traumatic events in early life, particularly events that occurred after puberty, is associated with increased risk for perimenopausal mood symptoms (Avis et al. 2003).

History of premenstrual syndrome—A history of mood symptoms prior to menses— suggesting hormonal sensitivity—has been associated with both depressive symptoms and risk for a major depressive episode during the menopausal transition (Freeman et al. 2004).

Health conditions—Experiencing health problems before menopause increases the risk of MDD during perimenopause (Williams et al. 2007).

Sleep Disruption

Around 30%–60% of women experience insomnia symptoms during the menopausal transition (Kravitz et al. 2003). Sleep disruption during the menopausal transition most commonly results from hot flashes (Joffe et al. 2013, 2016), although not universally. There is an increased risk for sleep disturbance during this period even in the absence of hot flashes (Timur and Sahin 2009), suggesting that there is likely a hormonal basis for the onset of insomnia symptoms during this time period (Joffe et al. 2016). The risk of obstructive sleep apnea also increases markedly at menopause. Menopause-related sleep disruption has been linked to increased health care utilization, reduced quality of life, mood symptoms, and reduced functioning (Williams et al. 2007).

Interplay Among Depression, Hot Flashes, and Sleep Disruption

It was previously thought that hot flashes triggered poor sleep and that this sleep disruption precipitated depressive symptoms during the menopausal transition. However, more recent research has shown that nighttime hot flashes are independently linked to the onset of depressive symptoms, even in the absence of sleep disturbance (Joffe et al. 2016).

Bipolar Disorder

Women with bipolar disorder are at increased risk of mood exacerbations, particularly depressive symptoms, during the menopausal transition (Perich et al. 2017).

Anxiety Disorders

Some studies have shown that panic attacks are more common after menopause than before, and postmenopausal panic attacks have been linked to an increased risk of cardiovascular disease (Smoller et al. 2003).

Treatment

Pharmacological

Multiple studies have shown that SSRIs and SNRIs are beneficial in the treatment of depressive symptoms (in addition to the treatment of hot flashes) during the menopausal transition. Hormone therapy (estrogen plus a progestin) has also been shown to be helpful for depressive symptoms during perimenopause, particularly when used in conjunction with antidepressants.

Nonpharmacological

Although not well studied, CBT has been shown to have some benefit for depressive symptoms that emerge during the menopausal transition. Limited data are available to support the use of other behavioral therapies for mood disturbance associated specifically with the menopausal transition, but data from depressed midlife populations in general can be used to support the use of such strategies.

Substance Use Disorders

According to findings from the 2016 National Survey on Drug Use and Health, substance use disorders are more common in men than in women (National Institute on Drug Abuse 2018). However, because of the biological and psychosocial factors associated with sex and gender, the presentation, course, impact, and management of substance use disorders in women can differ from those in men.

The course and natural history of substance use disorders carry notable differences in women as compared with men. In comparison with men, women have a later onset of severe use and a more rapid decline between first use and impairment—a phenomenon called *telescoping,* seen in women who use alcohol, tobacco, or opioids (Hernandez-Avila et al. 2004). For women to a greater degree than for men, interpersonal relationships heavily influence use of substances and maintenance of sobriety. For example, retaining custody of children can be highly motivating in maintaining sobriety, and having a partner who is using substances can be destabilizing to a greater degree for women than for men (Greenfield et al. 2010).

Biological differences between women and men have an impact on the effects and sequelae of substance use as well as the response to intervention. In addition, the fluctuations of hormonal states in the luteal and follicular phases of the menstrual cycle can cause differences in subjective experiences of intoxication in women who use cocaine, amphetamines, or tobacco (Substance Abuse and Mental Health Services Administration 2009). Sex differences in the expression of alcohol dehydrogenase are reflected in the separate definitions of at-risk drinking for women and men (National Institute on Alcohol Abuse and Alcoholism 2005).

In pregnancy and lactation, ongoing substance use and substance abuse treatments carry significant risks to both the mother and the fetus, and these risks need to be weighed when considering the appropriate treatment plan. However, pregnancy also offers a unique treatment opportunity, often serving as a strong motivator for change. Women with substance use disorders commonly present later to prenatal care, thus narrowing the window of time in which treatment providers can assess and engage them in discussions about treatment. It is essential that providers be aware of the legal standards regarding reports to social services regarding maternal substance use when issues of custody and parenting are raised.

In regard to treatment of substance use disorders in this setting, cessation of substances that pose significant health risks for a woman and her pregnancy, such as alcohol, tobacco, cocaine, and opioids, should be prioritized. Differences in treatment approach for pregnant versus nonpregnant women are most notable in the context of opioid use disorder. During pregnancy, the standard of care is to recommend that women be maintained on agonist therapy with methadone or buprenorphine, while also receiving psychosocial support services, including residential treatment, counseling, and parenting support. Primary care and obstetric providers are encouraged to screen all women for substance use disorders to identify problematic use and assess the need for treatment early and to increase the likelihood of engagement in treatment.

Psychological, Social, and Cultural Aspects of Women's Mental Health

Finally, a chapter on women's mental health would not be complete without mentioning the myriad cultural, psychological, and social forces that shape women's lives, many times in the form of chronic, ingrained disadvantages. These imbalances pervade many aspects of life, including economic status, employment rates, access to resources, and family roles, among others, and can erode mental health, leading to depression, anxiety, medication nonadherence, and reduced access to care. According to the United Nations, women around the world ages 15–44 years are more at risk from rape and domestic violence than from cancer, car accidents, war, and malaria (World Health Organization 2017). Global estimates published by the World Health Organization indicate that about 1 in 3 women (35%) worldwide has experienced physical or sexual intimate-partner violence or nonpartner sexual violence in their lifetime. One in five women on U.S. college campuses has experienced sexual assault (World Health Organization 2017). Female genital mutilation affects more than 125 million girls and women alive today and is recognized internationally as a human rights violation. Four out of five victims of human trafficking are girls (World Health Organization 2017).

A little over half of the world's working-age women are in the labor force, compared with 70% of working-age men. Women with full-time jobs are still paid only about 77% of their male counterparts' earnings for equivalent work, according to the latest U.S. Census statistics, and the gap is significantly wider for women of color, with African American women earning 64 cents and Latina women earning 56 cents for every dollar earned by a Caucasian man (Women's Bureau, U.S. Department of Labor 2019).

The United States is one of three countries, along with Oman and Papua New Guinea, that do not offer paid maternity leave. Maternity leave has a direct impact on the health of both child and mother. Studies have concluded that an additional week of maternity leave in industrialized countries reduces infant mortality rates by 0.5 deaths per 1,000 live births (Avendano et al. 2015; Burtle and Bezruchka 2016). Mothers who receive maternity leave benefits are able to breast-feed on a regular schedule, conferring on their babies protection against a variety of infections, as well as asthma, obesity, and sudden infant death syndrome (American Academy of Pediatrics 2019). Moreover, there is considerable evidence that maternal care is especially crucial during the first 2 months of life, when bonding and attachment are initially established, and that such bonding has long-lasting consequences for the infant's neurocognitive development.

Women on maternity leave are often required to return to work prematurely, adding an additional layer of stress and further responsibilities to their already delicate transition to motherhood, and after they return to work, these mothers typically must take sole responsibility for finding a balance between their personal and professional roles. Mothers who return to work soon after the birth of a child are more likely to become depressed than are mothers who have more time for maternity leave (Avendano et al. 2015; Burtle and Bezruchka 2016).

Despite significant advances in the field of women's mental health and reproductive psychiatry, it is important that these societal factors be adequately addressed and that effective policies be implemented to ensure that women's mental health needs are properly addressed.

Summary and Conclusions

Diagnosis and treatment of psychiatric disorders across women's reproductive years should be done with close attention to the medical, biological, and psychosocial factors affecting women's physical and mental health. It is important for clinicians to take special consideration of periods of hormonal flux (i.e., puberty and menarche, the monthly cycle, pregnancy, and menopause); clinicians also must remain aware of the psychosocial inequalities that shape women's lives, such as those affecting gender roles and societal expectations, as well as those conveying greater vulnerability to trauma, abuse, and domestic violence.

References

Abedian Z, Soltani N, Mokhber N, et al: Depression and anxiety in pregnancy and postpartum in women with mild and severe preeclampsia. Iran J Nurs Midwifery Res 20(4):454–459, 2015 26257800

Alwan S, Reefhuis J, Rasmussen SA, et al: Patterns of antidepressant medication use among pregnant women in a United States population. J Clin Pharmacol 51(2):264–270, 2011 20663997

American Academy of Pediatrics: Benefits of Breastfeeding (web page). 2019. Available at: https://www.aap.org/en-us/advocacy-and-policy/aap-health-initiatives/Breastfeeding/Pages/Benefits-of-Breastfeeding.aspx. Accessed October 23, 2019.

American College of Obstetricians and Gynecologists: ACOG Committee Opinion No. 757 Summary: Screening for Perinatal Depression. Obstet Gynecol 132(5):1314–1316, 2018 30629563

American Pregnancy Association: Baby Blues: Birth & Beyond (web page). Last updated: August 2015. Available at: https://americanpregnancy.org/first-year-of-life/baby-blues/. Accessed September 20, 2019.

American Psychiatric Association: Diagnostic and Statistical Manual of Mental Disorders, 5th Edition. Arlington, VA, American Psychiatric Association, 2013

Annagür BB, Tazegül A, Gündüz S: Do psychiatric disorders continue during pregnancy in women with hyperemesis gravidarum: a prospective study. Gen Hosp Psychiatry 35(5):492–496, 2013 23810464

Avendano M, Berkman LF, Brugiavini A, et al: The long-run effect of maternity leave benefits on mental health: evidence from European countries. Soc Sci Med 132:45–53, 2015 25792339

Avis NE, Ory M, Matthews KA, et al: Health-related quality of life in a multiethnic sample of middle-aged women: Study of Women's Health Across the Nation (SWAN). Med Care 41(11):1262–1276, 2003 14583689

Bäckström T, Bixo M, Strömberg J: GABAA receptor-modulating steroids in relation to women's behavioral health. Curr Psychiatry Rep 17(11):92–98, 2015 26396092

Ban L, West J, Gibson JE, et al: First trimester exposure to anxiolytic and hypnotic drugs and the risks of major congenital anomalies: a United Kingdom population-based cohort study. PLoS One 9(6):e100996, 2014a 24963627

Ban L, Gibson JE, West J, et al: Maternal depression, antidepressant prescriptions, and congenital anomaly risk in offspring: a population-based cohort study. BJOG 121(12):1471–1481, 2014b 24612301

Bauer RL, Orfei J, Wichman CL: Use of transdermal selegiline in pregnancy and lactation: a case report. Psychosomatics 58(4):450–452, 2017 28501290

Becker MA, Mayor GF, Elisabeth JS: Psychotropic medications and breastfeeding. Primary Psychiatry 16(3):42–51, 2009. Available at: http://primarypsychiatry.com/psychotropic-medications-and-breastfeeding/. Accessed April 6, 2019.

Bergink V, Burgerhout KM, Weigelt K, et al: Immune system dysregulation in first-onset postpartum psychosis. Biol Psychiatry 73(10):1000–1007, 2013 23270599

Bergink V, Armangue T, Titulaer MJ, et al: Autoimmune encephalitis in postpartum psychosis. Am J Psychiatry 172(9):901–908, 2015a 26183699

Bergink V, Laursen TM, Johannsen BM, et al: Pre-eclampsia and first-onset postpartum psychiatric episodes: a Danish population-based cohort study. Psychol Med 45(16):3481–3489, 2015b 26243040

Bergink V, Rasgon N, Wisner KL: Postpartum psychosis: madness, mania, and melancholia in motherhood. Am J Psychiatry 173(12):1179–1188, 2016 27609245

Berle JO, Spigset O: Antidepressant use during breastfeeding. Curr Womens Health Rev 7(1):28–34, 2011 22299006

Bodén R, Lundgren M, Brandt L, et al: Antipsychotics during pregnancy: relation to fetal and maternal metabolic effects. Arch Gen Psychiatry 69(7):715–721, 2012 22752236

Borrow AP, Cameron NM: Estrogenic mediation of serotonergic and neurotrophic systems: implications for female mood disorders. Prog Neuropsychopharmacol Biol Psychiatry 54:13–25, 2014 24865152

Boukhris T, Sheehy O, Mottron L, et al: Antidepressant use during pregnancy and the risk of autism spectrum disorder in children. JAMA Pediatr 170(2):117–124, 2016 26660917

Brockington I: Suicide and filicide in postpartum psychosis. Arch Womens Ment Health 20(1):63–69, 2017 27778148

Bromberger JT, Kravitz HM: Mood and menopause: findings from the Study of Women's Health Across the Nation (SWAN) over 10 years. Obstet Gynecol Clin North Am 38(3):609–625, 2011 21961723

Bromberger JT, Matthews KA, Schott LL, et al: Depressive symptoms during the menopausal transition: the Study of Women's Health Across the Nation (SWAN). J Affect Disord 103(1–3):267–272, 2007 17331589

Bromberger JT, Schott L, Kravitz HM, et al: Risk factors for major depression during midlife among a community sample of women with and without prior major depression: are they the same or different? Psychol Med 45(8):1653–1664, 2015 25417760

Bromberger JT, Kravitz HM, Youk A, et al: Patterns of depressive disorders across 13 years and their determinants among midlife women: SWAN mental health study. J Affect Disord 206:31–40, 2016 27455356

Bromley RL, Weston J, Marson AG: Maternal use of antiepileptic agents during pregnancy and major congenital malformations in children. JAMA 318(17):1700–1701, 2017 29114815

Burtle A, Bezruchka S: Population health and paid parental leave: what the United States can learn from two decades of research. Healthcare (Basel) 4(2):30, 2016 27417618

Calderon-Margalit R, Qiu C, Ornoy A, et al: Risk of preterm delivery and other adverse peri-natal outcomes in relation to maternal use of psychotropic medications during pregnancy. Am J Obstet Gynecol 201(6):579.e1–579.e8, 2009 19691950

Casassus B: France bans sodium valproate use in case of pregnancy. Lancet 390(10091):217, 2017 28721869

Casper RF, Yonkers KA: Treatment of premenstrual syndrome and premenstrual dysphoric dis-order. Barbieri RL, Crowley WF, section eds. Last updated October 9, 2019. Waltham, MA, Up-ToDate Inc. Available at: https://www.uptodate.com/contents/treatment-of-premenstrual-syndrome-and-premenstrual-dysphoric-disorder?topicRef=2159&source=see_link. Accessed October 23, 2019.

Chambers CD, Hernandez-Diaz S, Van Marter LJ, et al: Selective serotonin-reuptake inhibitors and risk of persistent pulmonary hypertension of the newborn. N Engl J Med 354(6):579–587, 2006 16467545

Chaudhry SK, Susser LC: Considerations in treating insomnia during pregnancy: a literature review. Psychosomatics 59(4):341–348, 2018 29706359

Clark CT, Sit DK, Driscoll K, et al: Does screening with the MDQ and EPDS improve identifi-cation of bipolar disorder in an obstetrical sample? Depress Anxiety 32(7):518–526, 2015 26059839

Coates JM, Gurnell M, Sarnyai Z: From molecule to market: steroid hormones and financial risk-taking. Philos Trans R Soc Lond B Biol Sci 365(1538):331–343, 2010 20026470

Cohen LS, Altshuler LL, Harlow BL, et al: Relapse of major depression during pregnancy in women who maintain or discontinue antidepressant treatment. JAMA 295(5):499–507, 2006a 16449615

Cohen LS, Soares CN, Vitonis AF, et al: Risk for new onset of depression during the meno-pausal transition: the Harvard study of moods and cycles. Arch Gen Psychiatry 63(4):385–390, 2006b 16585467

Cohen LS, Viguera AC, McInerney KA, et al: Reproductive safety of second-generation anti-psychotics: current data from the Massachusetts General Hospital National Pregnancy Registry for Atypical Antipsychotics. Am J Psychiatry 173(3):263–270, 2016 26441156

Coughlin CG, Blackwell KA, Bartley C, et al: Obstetric and neonatal outcomes after antipsy-chotic medication exposure in pregnancy. Obstet Gynecol 125(5):1224–1235, 2015 25932852

Cox J, Holden J: Perinatal Mental Health: A Guide to the Edinburgh Postnatal Depression Screening Scale. Glasgow, Scotland, Bell & Bain Ltd, 2013

de Zambotti M, Colrain IM, Javitz HS, et al: Magnitude of the impact of hot flashes on sleep in perimenopausal women. Fertil Steril 102(6):1708–1715, 2014 25256933

Dennerstein L, Dudley EC, Hopper JL, et al: A prospective population-based study of meno-pausal symptoms. Obstet Gynecol 96(3):351–358, 2000 10960625

Diav-Citrin O, Shechtman S, Arnon J, et al: Methylphenidate in pregnancy: a multicenter, pro-spective, comparative, observational study. J Clin Psychiatry 77(9):1176–1181, 2016 27232650

Dideriksen D, Pottegård A, Hallas J, et al: First trimester in utero exposure to methylphenidate. Basic Clin Pharmacol Toxicol 112(2):73–76, 2013 23136875

Dolk H, Wang H, Loane M, et al: Lamotrigine use in pregnancy and risk of orofacial cleft and other congenital anomalies. Neurology 86(18):1716–1725, 2016 27053714

Dolovich LR, Addis A, Vaillancourt JM, et al: Benzodiazepine use in pregnancy and major malformations or oral cleft: meta-analysis of cohort and case-control studies. BMJ 317(7162):839–843, 1998 9748174

Earls MF, Committee on Psychosocial Aspects of Child and Family Health, American Academy of Pediatrics: Incorporating recognition and management of perinatal and postpartum depression into pediatric practice. Pediatrics 126(5):1032–1039, 2010 20974776

El Marroun H, White TJ, Fernandez G, et al: Prenatal exposure to selective serotonin reuptake inhibitors and non-verbal cognitive functioning in childhood. J Psychopharmacol 31(3):346–355, 2017 27624153

Engelstad HJ, Roghair RD, Calarge CA, et al: Perinatal outcomes of pregnancies complicated by maternal depression with or without selective serotonin reuptake inhibitor therapy. Neonatology 105(2):149–154, 2014 24356332

Ensrud KE, Stone KL, Blackwell TL, et al: Frequency and severity of hot flashes and sleep disturbance in postmenopausal women with hot flashes. Menopause 16(2):286–292, 2009 19002015

Epperson CN, Sammel MD, Bale TL, et al: Adverse childhood experiences and risk for first-episode major depression during the menopause transition. J Clin Psychiatry 78(3):e298–e307, 2017 28394509

First MB, Williams JBW, Karg RS, Spitzer RL: Structured Clinical Interview for DSM-5® Disorders—Clinician Version (SCID-5-CV). Arlington, VA, American Psychiatric Association, 2016

Ford DE, Erlinger TP: Depression and C-reactive protein in US adults: data from the Third National Health and Nutrition Examination Survey. Arch Intern Med 164(9):1010–1014, 2004 15136311

Freeman EW, Sammel MD, Rinaudo PJ, et al: Premenstrual syndrome as a predictor of menopausal symptoms. Obstet Gynecol 103(5 Pt 1):960–966, 2004 15121571

Freeman EW, Sammel MD, Lin H, et al: The role of anxiety and hormonal changes in menopausal hot flashes. Menopause 12(3):258–266, 2005 15879914

Freeman EW, Sammel MD, Lin H, et al: Associations of hormones and menopausal status with depressed mood in women with no history of depression. Arch Gen Psychiatry 63(4):375–382, 2006 16585466

Freeman EW, Sammel MD, Lin H: Temporal associations of hot flashes and depression in the transition to menopause. Menopause 16(4):728–734, 2009 19188849

Freeman MP, Sosinsky AZ, Goez-Mogollon L, et al: Gestational weight gain and pre-pregnancy body mass index associated with second-generation antipsychotic drug use during pregnancy. Psychosomatics 59(2):125–134, 2018 29078988

Galbally M, Snellen M, Power J: Antipsychotic drugs in pregnancy: a review of their maternal and fetal effects. Ther Adv Drug Saf 5(2):100–109, 2014 25083265

Gaynes BN, Gavin N, Meltzer-Brody S, et al: Perinatal depression: prevalence, screening accuracy, and screening outcomes. Evid Rep Technol Assess (Summ) (119):1–8, 2005 15760246

Gibson J, McKenzie-McHarg K, Shakespeare J, et al: A systematic review of studies validating the Edinburgh Postnatal Depression Scale in antepartum and postpartum women. Acta Psychiatr Scand 119(5):350–364, 2009 19298573

Gilboa SM, Ailes EC, Rai RP, et al: Antihistamines and birth defects: a systematic review of the literature. Expert Opin Drug Saf 13(12):1667–1698, 2014 25307228

Gold EB, Colvin A, Avis N, et al: Longitudinal analysis of the association between vasomotor symptoms and race/ethnicity across the menopausal transition: study of women's health across the nation. Am J Public Health 96(7):1226–1235, 2006 16735636

Golub M, Costa L, Crofton K, et al: NTP-CERHR Expert Panel Report on the reproductive and developmental toxicity of amphetamine and methamphetamine. Birth Defects Res B Dev Reprod Toxicol 74(6):471–584, 2005 16167346

Graber JA: Pubertal timing and the development of psychopathology in adolescence and beyond. Horm Behav 64(2):262–269, 2013 23998670

Greenfield SF, Back SE, Lawson K, et al: Substance abuse in women. Psychiatr Clin North Am 33(2):339–355, 2010 20385341

Grigoriadis S, VonderPorten EH, Mamisashvili L, et al: The effect of prenatal antidepressant ex-posure on neonatal adaptation: a systematic review and meta-analysis. J Clin Psychiatry 74(4):e309–e320, 2013

Grummer-Strawn LM, Rollins N: Summarising the health effects of breastfeeding. Acta Paediatr 104(467):1–2, 2015 26535930

Harlow SD, Gass M, Hall JE, et al: Executive summary of the Stages of Reproductive Aging Workshop + 10: addressing the unfinished agenda of staging reproductive aging. Menopause 19(4):387–395, 2012 22343510

Hernandez-Avila CA, Rounsaville BJ, Kranzler HR: Opioid-, cannabis- and alcohol-dependent women show more rapid progression to substance abuse treatment. Drug Alcohol Depend 74(3):265–272, 2004 15194204

Heron J, McGuinness M, Blackmore ER, et al: Early postpartum symptoms in puerperal psychosis. BJOG 115(3):348–353, 2008 18190371

Hoedjes M, Berks D, Vogel I, et al: Postpartum depression after mild and severe preeclampsia. J Womens Health (Larchmt) 20(10):1535–1542, 2011 21815820

Hudak R, Wisner KL: Diagnosis and treatment of postpartum obsessions and compulsions that involve infant harm. Am J Psychiatry 169(4):360–363, 2012 22476676

Huybrechts KF, Palmsten K, Avorn J, et al: Antidepressant use in pregnancy and the risk of cardiac defects. N Engl J Med 370(25):2397–2407, 2014 24941178

Huybrechts KF, Palmsten K, Mogun H, et al: National trends in antidepressant medication treatment among publicly insured pregnant women. Gen Hosp Psychiatry 35(3):265–271, 2013 23374897

Huybrechts KF, Bateman BT, Palmsten K, et al: Antidepressant use late in pregnancy and risk of persistent pulmonary hypertension of the newborn. JAMA 313(21):2142–2151, 2015 26034955

Huybrechts KF, Hernández-Díaz S, Patorno E, et al: Antipsychotic use in pregnancy and the risk for congenital malformations. JAMA Psychiatry 73(9):938–946, 2016 27540849

Huybrechts KF, Bröms G, Christensen LB, et al: Association between methylphenidate and amphetamine use in pregnancy and risk of congenital malformations: a cohort study from the International Pregnancy Safety Study Consortium. JAMA Psychiatry 75(2):167–175, 2018 29238795

Iqbal MM, Aneja A, Rahman A, et al: The potential risks of commonly prescribed antipsychotics: during pregnancy and lactation. Psychiatry (Edgmont) 2(8):36–44, 2005 21152171

Joffe H, Cohen LS, Harlow BL: Impact of oral contraceptive pill use on premenstrual mood: predictors of improvement and deterioration. Am J Obstet Gynecol 189(6):1523–1530, 2003 14710055

Joffe H, Petrillo LF, Viguera AC, et al: Treatment of premenstrual worsening of depression with adjunctive oral contraceptive pills: a preliminary report. J Clin Psychiatry 68(12):1954–1962, 2007 18162029

Joffe H, Crawford S, Economou N, et al: A gonadotropin-releasing hormone agonist model demonstrates that nocturnal hot flashes interrupt objective sleep. Sleep (Basel) 36(12):1977–1985, 2013 24293774

Joffe H, Crawford SL, Freeman MP, et al: Independent contributions of nocturnal hot flashes and sleep disturbance to depression in estrogen-deprived women. J Clin Endocrinol Metab 101(10):3847–3855, 2016 27680875

Karam EG, Friedman MJ, Hill ED, et al: Cumulative traumas and risk thresholds: 12-month PTSD in the World Mental Health (WMH) surveys. Depress Anxiety 31(2):130–142, 2014 23983056

Katon JG, Russo J, Gavin AR, et al: Diabetes and depression in pregnancy: is there an association? J Womens Health (Larchmt) 20(7):983–989, 2011 21668382

Kjeldgaard HK, Eberhard-Gran M, Benth JŠ, et al: Hyperemesis gravidarum and the risk of emotional distress during and after pregnancy. Arch Women Ment Health 20(6):747–756, 2017 28842762

Klinger G, Frankenthal D, Merlob P, et al: Long-term outcome following selective serotonin reuptake inhibitor induced neonatal abstinence syndrome. J Perinatol 31(9):615–620, 2011 21311497

Ko JY, Rockhill KM, Tong VT, et al: Trends in postpartum depressive symptoms—27 states, 2004, 2008, and 2012. MMWR Morb Mortal Wkly Rep 66(6):153–158, 2017 28207685

Koren G, Nava-Ocampo AA, Moretti ME, et al: Major malformations with valproic acid. Can Fam Physician 52:441–442, 444, 447, 2006 16639967

Kravitz HM, Ganz PA, Bromberger J, et al: Sleep difficulty in women at midlife: a community survey of sleep and the menopausal transition. Menopause 10(1):19–28, 2003 12544673

Kravitz HM, Zhao X, Bromberger JT, et al: Sleep disturbance during the menopausal transition in a multi-ethnic community sample of women. Sleep 31(7):979–990, 2008 18652093

Kroenke K, Spitzer RL, Williams JB: The PHQ-9: validity of a brief depression severity measure. J Gen Intern Med 16(9):606–613, 2001 11556941

Kronenfeld N, Berlin M, Shaniv D, et al: Use of psychotropic medications in breastfeeding women. Birth Defects Res 109(12):957–997, 2017 28714610

Lanza di Scalea T, Wisner KL: Antidepressant medication use during breastfeeding. Clin Obstet Gynecol 52(3):483–497, 2009 19661763

Lassen D, Ennis ZN, Damkier P: First-trimester pregnancy exposure to venlafaxine or duloxetine and risk of major congenital malformations: a systematic review. Basic Clin Pharmacol Toxicol 118(1):32–36, 2016 26435496

Li Y, Pehrson AL, Budac DP, et al: A rodent model of premenstrual dysphoria: progesterone withdrawal induces depression-like behavior that is differentially sensitive to classes of antidepressants. Behav Brain Res 234(2):238–247, 2012 22789402

Liberto TL: Screening for depression and help-seeking in postpartum women during well-baby pediatric visits: an integrated review. J Pediatr Health Care 26(2):109–117, 2012 22360930

Louik C, Kerr S, Kelley KE, et al: Increasing use of ADHD medications in pregnancy. Pharmacoepidemiol Drug Saf 24(2):218–220, 2015 25630904

Lusskin SI, Khan SJ, Ernst C, et al: Pharmacotherapy for perinatal depression. Clin Obstet Gynecol 61(3):544–561, 2018 29561284

Maharaj S, Trevino K: A comprehensive review of treatment options for premenstrual syndrome and premenstrual dysphoric disorder. J Psychiatr Pract 21(5):334–350, 2015 26352222

Manjunath NG, Venkatesh G, Rajanna: Postpartum blue is common in socially and economically insecure mothers. Indian J Community Med 36(3):231–233, 2011 22090680

McLean CP, Asnaani A, Litz BT, et al: Gender differences in anxiety disorders: prevalence, course of illness, comorbidity and burden of illness. J Psychiatr Res 45(8):1027–1035, 2011 21439576

Meador KJ, Baker GA, Browning N, et al: Cognitive function at 3 years of age after fetal exposure to antiepileptic drugs. N Engl J Med 360(16):1597–1605, 2009 19369666

Meltzer-Brody S, Colquhoun H, Riesenberg R, et al: Brexanolone injection in post-partum depression: two multicentre, double-blind, randomised, placebo-controlled, phase 3 trials. Lancet 392(10152):1058–1070, 2018 [Erratum in: Lancet 392(10153):1116, 2018] 30177236

Mendle J, Moore SR, Briley DA, et al: Puberty, socioeconomic status, and depression in girls: evidence for gene x environment interactions. Clin Psychol Sci 4(1):3–16, 2015. Available at: https://journals.sagepub.com/doi/abs/10.1177/2167702614563598. Accessed April 6, 2019.

Mendle J, Ryan RM, McKone KMP: Age at menarche, depression, and antisocial behavior in adulthood. Pediatrics 141(1):e20171703, 2018 29279324

Miller ES, Chu C, Gollan J, et al: Obsessive-compulsive symptoms during the postpartum period. A prospective cohort. J Reprod Med 58(3–4):115–122, 2013 23539879

Miller ES, Hoxha D, Wisner KL, Gossett DR: Obsessions and compulsions in postpartum women without obsessive compulsive disorder. J Womens Health (Larchmt) 24(10):825–830, 2015 26121364

Miller ES, Peri MR, Gossett DR: The association between diabetes and postpartum depression. Arch Women Ment Health 19(1):183–186, 2016 26184833

Mitchell ES, Woods NF: Hot flush severity during the menopausal transition and early postmenopause: beyond hormones. Climacteric 18(4):536–544, 2015 25748168

Mitchell-Jones N, Gallos I, Farren J, et al: Psychological morbidity associated with hyperemesis gravidarum: a systematic review and meta-analysis. BJOG 124(1):20–30, 2017 27418035

Murphy PJ, Campbell SS: Sex hormones, sleep, and core body temperature in older postmenopausal women. Sleep 30(12):1788–1794, 2007 18246988

National Institute of Mental Health: Major Depression (web page). Bethesda, MD, National Institute of Mental Health, 2016. Available at: https://www.nimh.nih.gov/health/statistics/major-depression.shtml. Accessed April 6, 2019.

National Institute on Alcohol Abuse and Alcoholism: Helping Patients Who Drink Too Much: A Clinician's Guide. Bethesda, MD, National Institute on Alcohol Abuse and Alcoholism, 2005. Available at: https://pubs.niaaa.nih.gov/publications/practitioner/cliniciansguide2005/guide.pdf. Accessed October 23, 2019.

National Institute on Drug Abuse: Substance Use in Women: Sex and Gender Differences in Substance Use. Page last updated July 2018. Available at: https://www.drugabuse.gov/publications/research-reports/substance-use-in-women/sex-gender-differences-in-substance-use. Accessed October 23, 2019.

Newport DJ, Calamaras MR, DeVane CL, et al: Atypical antipsychotic administration during late pregnancy: placental passage and obstetrical outcomes. Am J Psychiatry 164(8):1214–1220, 2007 17671284

Osborne LM, Monk C: Perinatal depression—the fourth inflammatory morbidity of pregnancy? Theory and literature review. Psychoneuroendocrinology 38(10):1929–1952, 2013 23608136

Patorno E, Huybrechts KF, Bateman BT, et al: Lithium use in pregnancy and the risk of cardiac malformations. N Engl J Med 376(23):2245–2254, 2017 28591541

Pawlby S, Hay DF, Sharp D, et al: Antenatal depression predicts depression in adolescent offspring: prospective longitudinal community-based study. J Affect Disord 113(3):236–243, 2009 18602698

Pearson KH, Nonacs RM, Viguera AC, et al: Birth outcomes following prenatal exposure to antidepressants. J Clin Psychiatry 68(8):1284–1289, 2007 17854255

Perich T, Ussher J, Meade T: Menopause and illness course in bipolar disorder: a systematic review. Bipolar Disord 19(6):434–443, 2017 28796389

Peters W, Freeman MP, Kim S, et al: Treatment of premenstrual breakthrough of depression with adjunctive oral contraceptive pills compared with placebo. J Clin Psychopharmacol 37(5):609–614, 2017 28816924

Qiu C, Sanchez SE, Lam N, et al: Associations of depression and depressive symptoms with preeclampsia: results from a Peruvian case-control study. BMC Womens Health 7:15, 2007 17900360

Rhodes AM, Segre LS: Perinatal depression: a review of US legislation and law. Arch Women Ment Health 16(4):259–270, 2013 23740222

Ross LE, Grigoriadis S, Mamisashvili L, et al: Selected pregnancy and delivery outcomes after exposure to antidepressant medication: a systematic review and meta-analysis. JAMA Psychiatry 70(4):436–443, 2013 23446732

Schüle C, Nothdurfter C, Rupprecht R: The role of allopregnanolone in depression and anxiety. Prog Neurobiol 113:79–87, 2014 24215796

Shobeiri F, Araste FE, Ebrahimi R, et al: Effect of calcium on premenstrual syndrome: a double-blind randomized clinical trial. Obstet Gynecol Sci 60(1):100–105, 2017 28217679

Sit D, Seltman H, Wisner KL: Menstrual effects on mood symptoms in treated women with bipolar disorder. Bipolar Disord 13(3):310–317, 2011 21676134

Siu AL, U.S. Preventive Services Task Force, Bibbins-Domingo K, et al: Screening for depression in adults: US Preventive Services Task Force recommendation statement. JAMA 315(4):380–387, 2016 26813211

Skovlund CW, Mørch LS, Kessing LV, et al: Association of hormonal contraception with depression. JAMA Psychiatry 73(11):1154–1162, 2016 27680324

Smink FRE, van Hoeken D, Hoek HW: Epidemiology of eating disorders: incidence, prevalence and mortality rates. Curr Psychiatry Rep 14(4):406–414, 2012 22644309

Smith SS, Ruderman Y, Frye C, et al: Steroid withdrawal in the mouse results in anxiogenic effects of 3alpha,5beta-THP: a possible model of premenstrual dysphoric disorder. Psychopharmacology (Berl) 186(3):323–333, 2006 16193334

Smoller JW, Pollack MH, Wassertheil-Smoller S, et al: Prevalence and correlates of panic attacks in postmenopausal women: results from an ancillary study to the Women's Health Initiative. Arch Intern Med 163(17):2041–2050, 2003 14504117

Substance Abuse and Mental Health Services Administration: Substance Abuse Treatment: Addressing the Specific Needs of Women. Treatment Improvement Protocol (TIP) Series, No. 51. HHS Publication No. (SMA) 13–4426. Rockville, MD, Substance Abuse and Mental Health Services Administration, 2009

Timur S, Sahin NH: Effects of sleep disturbance on the quality of life of Turkish menopausal women: a population-based study. Maturitas 64(3):177–181, 2009 19815356

Turner E, Jones M, Vaz LR, et al: Systematic review and meta-analysis to assess the safety of bupropion and varenicline in pregnancy. Nicotine Tob Res 21(8):1001–1010, 2019 29579233

VanderKruik R, Barreix M, Chou D, et al; Maternal Morbidity Working Group: The global prevalence of postpartum psychosis: a systematic review. BMC Psychiatry 17(1):272, 2017 28754094

Vesga-López O, Blanco C, Keyes K, et al: Psychiatric disorders in pregnant and postpartum women in the United States. Arch Gen Psychiatry 65(7):805–815, 2008 18606953

Vigod SN, Ross LE, Steiner M: Understanding and treating premenstrual dysphoric disorder: an update for the women's health practitioner. Obstet Gynecol Clin North Am 36(4):907–924, 2009 19944308

Viguera AC, Whitfield T, Baldessarini R, et al: Risk of recurrence in women with bipolar disorder during pregnancy: prospective study of mood stabilizer discontinuation. Am J Psychiatry 164(12):1817–1824, quiz 1923, 2007 18056236

Viguera AC, Tondo L, Koukopoulos AE, et al: Episodes of mood disorders in 2,252 pregnancies and postpartum periods. Am J Psychiatry 168(11):1179–1185, 2011 21799064

Wesseloo R, Liu X, Clark CT, et al: Risk of postpartum episodes in women with bipolar disorder after lamotrigine or lithium use during pregnancy: a population-based cohort study. J Affect Disord 218:394–397, 2017 28501739

Williams RE, Kalilani L, DiBenedetti DB, et al: Healthcare seeking and treatment for menopausal symptoms in the United States. Maturitas 58(4):348–358, 2007 17964093

Winer SA, Rapkin AJ: Premenstrual disorders: prevalence, etiology and impact. J Reprod Med 51 (4 suppl):339–347, 2006 16734317

Wisner KL, Sit DK, McShea MC, et al: Onset timing, thoughts of self-harm, and diagnoses in postpartum women with screen-positive depression findings. JAMA Psychiatry 70(5):490–498, 2013 23487258

Women's Bureau, U.S. Department of Labor: Women's earnings by race and ethnicity as a percentage of White, non-Hispanic men's earnings (graph; data from 1987–2018 Annual Social and Economic Supplements, Current Population Survey, U.S. Census Bureau). 2019. Available at: https://www.dol.gov/wb/stats/NEWSTATS/facts/earn_earnings_ratio.htm#earn-race-percent. Accessed October 23, 2019.

Woods NF, Smith-DiJulio K, Percival DB, et al: Depressed mood during the menopausal transition and early postmenopause: observations from the Seattle Midlife Women's Health Study. Menopause 15(2):223–232, 2008 18176355

World Health Organization: Violence Against Women (web page). Geneva, Switzerland, World Health Organization, November 29, 2017. Available at: http://www.who.int/mediacentre/factsheets/fs239/en/. Accessed April 6, 2019.

PART III

Medical Considerations in Psychiatric Disorders

CHAPTER 16

Neurodevelopmental Disorders

Aaron Hauptman, M.D.

Sheldon Benjamin, M.D.

Individuals with neurodevelopmental disorders are commonly seen by psychiatrists and other physicians. Neurodevelopmental disorders may be missed in childhood, and an alert clinician may be the first to make the diagnosis. Correct diagnosis is important for several reasons:

1. Individuals with neurodevelopmental disabilities can present with, or continue to experience, comorbid psychiatric symptoms in adulthood.
2. The medical and neurological issues associated with neurodevelopmental disorders may need to be managed concurrently with psychiatric symptoms by psychiatrists, neurologists, or others.
3. The physician, ideally in concert with a specialist from the relevant discipline, may need to engage in further diagnostic evaluation when an underlying neurodevelopmental or pediatric condition is suspected to be involved in the adult patient's current psychiatric presentation.
4. Condition-specific behavioral and psychiatric management is sometimes required, and awareness of appropriate treatment paradigms is always crucial to maintaining the safety of individuals with neurodevelopmental disabilities.

A vast range of conditions may be associated with intellectual, neurodevelopmental, and specific learning disabilities. Some of these have been characterized into syndromes, such as Angelman syndrome and fragile X syndrome (FXS). Other conditions have specific medical and neurological comorbidities, such as Alzheimer's disease in Down syndrome or cardiac abnormalities in velocardiofacial syndrome. In addition, there are several disorders that can cause symptoms closely resembling autism spectrum disorder. These are listed in Table 16–1. Physicians should be familiar with the most common neurodevelopmental disorders and should be able to evaluate individuals with neurodevelopmental disabilities. Experience in the neuropsychiatric evaluation of people with neurodevelopmental disabilities is seldom included in general psychiatric residency training and even less so in internal medicine or family medicine training. This chapter presents a summary of the more common neurodevelopmental disorders of interest to general psychiatrists, internists, pediatricians and other clinicians.

Approach to the Patient

The neuropsychiatric evaluation of an individual with a neurodevelopmental disability includes a comprehensive developmental, psychiatric, medical, social, and family history, followed by observation for the presence of dysmorphic and neurocutaneous features. Table 16–2 provides a structured inventory of common dysmorphic features. Because there is an extremely wide range of appearance variations in neurotypical adults, such findings do not always signal an underlying syndrome or specific developmental disability. Also, many intellectual disabilities are not associated with identified syndromes. Nonetheless, the presence of dysmorphic features may point the clinician toward an identified syndrome. A complete neurological examination, including a search for neurological soft signs (Table 16–3) as well as focal neurological deficits, should be conducted to determine the need for neurodiagnostic evaluation. Neurological soft signs are often seen in neurodevelopmental disorders, schizophrenia, bipolar disorder, substance use disorders, obsessive-compulsive disorder (OCD), and antisocial personality disorder, as well as in prematurity, malnutrition, and low birth weight. These signs generally occur without demonstrable abnormalities on structural neuroimaging but are thought to represent subtle brain dysfunction. Cardiac auscultation is included to seek evidence of cardiac comorbidity, while cutaneous examination is included to identify common forms of neurocutaneous disorders.

In the setting of aggression, withdrawal, or self-injurious or other behaviors that represent a clear change from the historical baseline, underlying medical illness should be considered. Common medical comorbidities that can manifest with behavioral change or aggression in nonverbal or developmentally disabled individuals are listed in Table 16–4. Consideration should also be given to aging-related complaints common to all older adults, such as presbyopia, arthritis, dizziness, and cataracts. Because developmentally disabled individuals often have communication difficulties, they may not be able to verbally express or localize their discomfort; therefore, the clinician must conduct a careful physical and laboratory investigation. Once a specific illness is identified, it will generally be treated as it would be in neurotypical populations.

The differential diagnosis of behavioral presentations in developmentally disabled individuals is broad, and symptoms are often overlapping. For example, it is important to be able to differentiate the repetitive behaviors and restricted interests seen in autism spectrum disorder (ASD) from the symptoms of a separate, superimposed neuropsychiatric condition such as a tic disorder, OCD, or an anxiety disorder. Once the clinician determines that a given symptom is due either to the underlying neurodevelopmental condition or to a comorbid neuropsychiatric condition, treatment appropriate for that symptom should be pursued, keeping in mind the elevated medication

TABLE 16–1.   **Medical etiologies of autism spectrum disorder**

Adrenoleukodystrophies (e.g., X-linked adrenoleukodystrophy)

Amino acidopathies (e.g., phenylketonuria)

Central nervous system infections (e.g., congenital rubella)

Copy number variations (e.g., Angelman, Klinefelter, Prader-Willi, Turner, velocardiofacial syndromes)

Gangliosidoses

Hormonal abnormalities (e.g., hypothyroidism)

Lipofuscinoses

Metachromatic leukodystrophy

Mitochondrial disorders

Monogenetic syndromes (e.g., fragile X syndrome, *MECP2*, tuberous sclerosis)

Neuroimmunological conditions (e.g., anti-*N*-methyl-D-aspartate receptor encephalitis)

Seizure disorders and syndromes (e.g., Landau-Kleffner, Lennox-Gastaut)

TABLE 16–2.   **Structured observation for dysmorphic features**

Stature/head size	Mouth and lips
Hair growth pattern	Teeth
Ear structure, size, placement	Hand size
Nose size	Fingers and thumbs
Face size and structure	Nails
Philtrum	Foot structure and size

Source.   Adapted from Benjamin and Lauterbach 2018.

TABLE 16–3.   **Neurological soft signs**

Dysarthria	Slow or irregular fine finger movements
Inability to move eyes without moving head	Bradykinesia
Dysphagia	Motor impersistence
Nystagmus	Overflow/mirror movements
Drooling	Dystonic posturing
Asymmetry of face or extremities	Nonsustained clonus
Clumsiness, incoordination	Asymmetric reflexes, hyperreflexia
Hypotonia	Astereognosis
Ataxia	Agraphesthesia
Slow or irregular rapid alternating movements	Extinction to visual/tactile double simultaneous stimulation

Source.   Adapted from Benjamin and Lauterbach 2018.

sensitivity that may occur in developmental disorders. Discrimination between a manifestation of the underlying disorder and a comorbid neuropsychiatric disorder may be challenging and can require detailed assessment to arrive at the appropriate diagnoses.

TABLE 16–4.   **Common medical etiologies of aggressive behavior**

Pain or physiological change

  Dental pain

  Headache

  Gastrointestinal distress (e.g., cramps, reflux, gastroesophagitis)

  Constipation or diarrhea

  Dysmenorrhea

  Sensory changes (e.g., visual problems, hearing loss, neuropathy)

  Metabolic abnormality

Infection

  Urinary tract infection

  Otitis media

  Dental abscess

  Skin breakdown or infection

  Occult infection

Substance or side effect

  Medication or illicit drug effect

  Substance or medication withdrawal

  Medication side effect (e.g., akathisia, tardive dyskinesia, dystonia, rapid appetite change)

Psychiatric comorbidity

  Mood disorder

  Anxiety

  Psychotic disorder

  Premenstrual dysphoric disorder

  Personality disorders or traits

Neurological condition

  Seizure

  Traumatic brain injury (known or unknown)

  Neurocognitive disorders (e.g., superimposed dementia)

Cerebral Palsy

Cerebral palsy refers to static motor deficits caused by prenatal, perinatal, or postnatal brain insults, which occur in about 2.0%–2.5% of births (Koman et al. 2004). The five commonly recognized forms of cerebral palsy are spastic hemiplegia, spastic diplegia, spastic quadriplegia, extrapyramidal (or choreoathetoid), and ataxic cerebral palsy, with about 70%–75% of affected individuals having one of the spastic subtypes, 10%–15% having the choreoathetoid type, and less than 5% having the ataxic type (Rana et al. 2017). Cerebral palsy occurs most often in premature and very-low-birthweight infants (<1.5 kg [3 lb, 5 oz]) and is associated with periventricular leukomalacia. Rates of comorbid intellectual disability and epilepsy vary among the different types of cerebral palsy: 95% of individuals with mixed cerebral palsy, 75% of those with spastic quadriplegic cerebral palsy, 50% of those with spastic hemiplegic cerebral palsy, 25% of those with spastic diplegic cerebral palsy, and 10% of those with extrapyramidal cerebral palsy have comorbid intellectual disability or epilepsy (Kaufman and Milstein 2013). Seventy-five percent of individuals with combined cerebral palsy and epilepsy have intellectual disability (Vukojević et al. 2017).

Among non–intellectually disabled individuals with cerebral palsy, depression has been found to occur in 25% (14/56), chronic pain in 75% (42/56), and fatigue in 41% (23/56) (Van Der Slot et al. 2012). A pediatric study in 451 children with cerebral palsy demonstrated co-occurring ASD in 6.9% and epilepsy in 41% (Christensen et al. 2014).

Middle-aged (ages 40–60 years) individuals with cerebral palsy have high rates of multimorbidity (defined as the presence of multiple chronic diseases), with certain disease combinations being especially prevalent; for example, in a cohort of 435 middle-aged patients with cerebral palsy, the overall prevalence of multimorbidity was 60%, and the most common disease combinations were elevated blood pressure plus decreased bone density, osteoarthritis plus decreased bone density, and elevated blood pressure plus asthma (Cremer et al. 2017). Risks for secondary health concerns increase with sedentary behavior, weakness, and decreased muscle mass (Cremer et al. 2017).

Fragile X Syndrome

FXS is an X-linked, trinucleotide-repeat disorder caused by disruption of *FMR1* gene expression. It is the most common single-gene cause of ASD, occurring in about 1 in 4,000 males and about 1 in 6,000–4,000 females (Erickson et al. 2017). The typical male phenotype includes macrocephaly, long face, square chin, prominent brow, high-arched palate, prominent floppy ears, hyperextensible finger joints, flat feet, pectus excavatum, and macro-orchidism (Belmonte and Bourgeron 2006; Erickson et al. 2017). The phenotype may be subtle in females.

The typical pattern of neurocognitive symptoms involves moderate to severe intellectual disability with hyperactivity and deficits in attention, speech, and language. The majority of individuals with FXS have at least one symptom of ASD, with 25%–52% meeting full DSM-5 criteria for ASD. Certain differences from idiopathic ASD are notable, such as less prominent irritability (Erickson et al. 2017; Lee et al. 2016).

Seizures are present in about 25%–40% of males with FXS. Females with the *FMR1* mutation also are at increased risk of seizures. The *FMR1* mutation increases the risk of tremor ataxia syndrome, a neurodegenerative disorder characterized by neurocognitive and executive function decline, parkinsonism, gait ataxia, kinetic tremor, and neuropathy (Hall and Berry-Kravis 2018). Female carriers of the *FMR1* mutation are at higher risk of primary ovarian insufficiency (Sullivan et al. 2005). Other medical complications include aortic root dilatation, mitral valve prolapse, sleep disorders, gastrointestinal issues, obesity, strabismus, and chronic recurrent otitis media (Hall and Berry-Kravis 2018).

Down Syndrome

Down syndrome is one of the most common intellectual disabilities, with a prevalence of about 1 in 700 live births (Parker et al. 2010). Down syndrome results from an extra copy of chromosome 21, either by trisomy or, more rarely, from mosaicism or Robertsonian translocation. Associated physical characteristics include microcephaly with small ears and mouth; upward slanting eyes; Brushfield spots (small light-colored spots on the periphery of the iris); short neck; single palmar crease; wide, short hands; short fingers; and decreased muscle tone (Devlin and Morrison 2004; Lyle et al. 2009; Sinet et al. 1994).

ASD occurs 17–20 times more frequently in individuals with Down syndrome than in the general population (DiGuiseppi et al. 2010). Anxiety and mood disorders occur frequently in adults with Down syndrome, although depression may be no more frequent in Down syndrome than in other forms of intellectual disability (Mantry et al. 2008). In one study, adolescents and young adults with Down syndrome had an increased risk of psychosis in comparison with age-matched control subjects with intellectual disability (Mantry et al. 2008). Catatonia risk also is elevated in Down syndrome, while the risk of impulse-control disorders and bipolar disorder is lower in Down syndrome than in nonsyndromic intellectual disability (Mantry et al. 2008). Data from community populations indicate that rates of impulsivity, aggression, and disruptive behaviors are typically low in Down syndrome (Mantry et al. 2008; Melville et al. 2008). Dementia is well known to occur at high rates in Down syndrome, with prevalences of 3.4%, 10.3%, and 40%, respectively, in the fourth, fifth, and sixth decades of life (Holland et al. 1998). Alzheimer's disease occurs at particularly high rates in Down syndrome due to the location of the gene for amyloid precursor protein on chromosome 21. Variability in baseline intellectual function and in other factors often complicates and delays diagnosis and contributes to atypical dementia presentations. Common medical comorbidities present in Down syndrome are listed in Table 16–5 (Kinnear et al. 2018; Wisniewski et al. 1982).

Chromosomal Number Variations (Klinefelter and Turner Syndromes)

Klinefelter Syndrome

Klinefelter syndrome is a condition in which a male has one or more additional X chromosomes. Its prevalence is 1 in 670 live-born males (Bojesen et al. 2003). Klinefelter syndrome is associated with tall stature, hypogonadism, sparse body hair, possible gynecomastia, and developmental delay.

The intelligence quotient (IQ) in Klinefelter syndrome is about 1 standard deviation (10 points) below average. The neurocognitive profile of Klinefelter syndrome is particularly notable for deficits in verbal reasoning; a deficit in some aspect of language processing, such as receptive or expressive language, is present in 80% of males with Klinefelter syndrome (Boone et al. 2001). In some individuals with the syndrome, the neurocognitive profile improves over time, perhaps due to development of compensatory skills (Gravholt et al. 2018). A number of studies suggest that rates of attention-deficit/hyperactivity disorder (ADHD), ASD, bipolar disorder, and schizophrenia may be elevated in Klinefelter syndrome (Cederlöf et al. 2014).

Klinefelter syndrome is associated with hypogonadism (hypotestosteronism) in the setting of elevated luteinizing hormone (Aksglaede et al. 2007). In addition to high rates of infertility, common medical comorbidities include gynecomastia (38%–75%), metabolic syndrome (44%), osteopenia (5%–40%), and osteoporosis (10%) with asso-

TABLE 16–5.	**Common medical comorbidities in Down syndrome**
Congenital heart disease	Dermatitis, eczema
Obesity	Musculoskeletal pain
Hypothyroidism	Ataxia, gait disorders
Visual impairment	Oral/dental disease
Atlantoaxial instability	Dyspnea
Hearing impairment	Epilepsy
Nail disorders	Osteoporosis
Basal ganglia calcifications	Leukemia
Chronic constipation	Gonadal deficiency with male infertility
Fungal infection	

Source.   Kinnear et al. 2018; Wisniewski et al. 1982.

ciated fracture risk, as well as an increased risk of breast and mediastinal cancers (Groth et al. 2013).

Turner Syndrome

Turner syndrome occurs in 1 in 2,500–2,000 female births and is defined by absence or less-than-complete presence of the second X chromosome (Nielsen and Wohlert 1991). Turner syndrome is classically associated with characteristic morphological features including webbed neck, narrow palate, micrognathia, down-slanted palpebral fissures with epicanthal folds, and low-set ears. Delayed puberty, left-sided cardiac abnormality, unexplained short stature, and infertility also are classic features (Shankar and Backeljauw 2018).

Turner syndrome is associated with superior language skills but deficits across a range of other neurocognitive domains, including executive and visuospatial functioning. Rates of ADHD and ASD are elevated, and intellectual disability is seen in 10% of women with Turner syndrome (Shankar and Backeljauw 2018; Temple and Shephard 2012).

The most serious health risk associated with Turner syndrome in adult women is aortic dissection. Risk factors associated with dissection include hypertension, bicuspid aortic valve, and aortic root dilatation (Carlson and Silberbach 2009). Thyroid abnormalities occur in about 24%–28% of women with Turner syndrome (El-Mansoury et al. 2005). Ninety percent of women with Turner syndrome experience ovarian failure. Rates of dyslipidemia, glucose intolerance, diabetes, and osteoporosis are high; celiac disease is seen in 4%–6% of individuals with Turner syndrome (Bondy and Turner Syndrome Study Group 2007; Conway et al. 2010). Turner syndrome is associated with a threefold greater risk of mortality compared with the general population (Schoemaker et al. 2008).

Microdeletion Syndromes

Prader-Willi syndrome (PWS) and Angelman syndrome are genomic imprinting disorders that result from lack of expression of the genes on chromosome 15q11.2–q13.

When the chromosomal deletion is paternally inherited, PWS results; when the chromosomal deletion is inherited from the mother, Angelman syndrome occurs.

Prader-Willi Syndrome

PWS has a prevalence ranging from 1 in 30,000 to 1 in 10,000. The syndrome initially manifests in infancy with hypotonia and failure to thrive, requiring prolonged intensive care. In later infancy and early childhood, a distinct phenotypic pattern emerges, characterized by decreased growth rate, hyperphagia and excessive weight gain, an average IQ of 65, skin-picking and self-injurious behavior with a high pain threshold, and autistic features. Classic morphological features include almond-shaped palpebral fissures, thin vermilion border of the upper lip, down-turned mouth, small hands and feet, central adiposity, and hypogonadism (Angulo et al. 2015).

Disruptive behaviors, skin-picking or rectal gouging, and obsessive-compulsive features are common. Adults with PWS have high rates of psychiatric comorbidities: in a cohort study of 53 adolescents and adults with PWS, 89% had at least one psychiatric diagnosis, with the most common being disruptive behavior disorders, found in 68%; OCD, found in 45%; and excoriation (skin-picking) disorder, found in 35% (Shriki-Tal et al. 2017). Another study also found high rates of psychiatric comorbidities among adults (N=73 participants) living in a specialized PWS group home system, with anxiety disorders in 38%, excoriation (skin-picking) disorder in 33%, intermittent explosive disorder in 30%, and psychosis in 23% (Manzardo et al. 2018a). In a pediatric PWS study, nearly one-third of the participants were found to meet criteria for ASD (Bennett et al. 2017).

In adults with PWS, complications and sequelae of obesity are the primary cause of morbidity and mortality. One-quarter of adults with PWS have been reported to have type 2 diabetes mellitus; obstructive sleep apnea is also common (Angulo et al. 2015; Butler et al. 2018). Cardiorespiratory failure, pulmonary embolism, and sequelae of hyperphagia-related behaviors, such as aspiration and gastrointestinal perforation, are frequent contributors to morbidity and mortality in this population (Manzardo et al. 2018b). Decreased gastrointestinal motility and poor gag reflex in combination with hyperphagic behavior can result in significant risk. In a study examining mortality data from 152 individuals with PWS, choking episodes were the cause of death for 8% of the individuals (Stevenson et al. 2007). Excessive daytime sleepiness occurs in 70%–100% of adults with PWS (Angulo et al. 2015). A range of endocrine problems are common in PWS, including growth hormone and adrenal insufficiency, osteoporosis, and hypothyroidism (Angulo et al. 2015).

Angelman Syndrome

Angelman syndrome has an estimated prevalence ranging from about 1 in 20,000 to about 1 in 12,000. It is associated with motor delay, hypotonia, microcephaly, hyperreflexia, and seizures. The characteristic gait in Angelman syndrome is sometimes described as "marionette-like," with around 10% of individuals requiring a wheelchair because of extensive motor impairment (Buiting et al. 2016). Individuals with Angelman syndrome have characteristic features, which include microcephaly, protruding tongue, skin and hair hypopigmentation, prognathism, excessive drooling, and widely spaced teeth; some of these features become more pronounced as the individual ages (Pelc et al. 2008; Thibert et al. 2013).

Individuals with Angelman syndrome have severe neurodevelopmental difficulties. They tend to have profound expressive language deficits with greater preservation of receptive and nonverbal communication domains. A common behavioral phenotype in Angelman syndrome involves emotional excitability; a happy-seeming affect; repetitive, autistic-like behaviors such as hand-flapping; and intensely exploratory and motorically excited behavior. Individuals with Angelman syndrome often have sleep disturbances, including decreased need for sleep, abnormal sleep-wake cycles, early awakenings, sleep apnea, and sleep-related movement disorders. Ritualistic and repetitive behaviors are common, as are aggressive behaviors. Given these individuals' expressive language deficits, manifestations of anxiety, pain, or other medical symptoms can be very challenging to separate from dysregulated behaviors (Thibert et al. 2013).

In adulthood, common challenges faced by individuals with Angelman syndrome include seizures, motor limitations that can include progressive scoliosis, chronic gastrointestinal problems, and obesity. Status epilepticus, including nonconvulsive status, can occur. With age, adults with Angelman syndrome develop worsening gait, balance disorders, and muscle rigidity, and the majority experience ataxia and tremor that can manifest as jerking movements or lurching gait (Thibert et al. 2013). Mortality tends to cluster in early childhood and later adulthood. Pediatric mortality is most often related to seizures or accidents due to the combination of increased exploratory behavior and intellectual and expressive language disability (Buiting et al. 2016).

22q11.2 Deletion Syndrome

22q11.2 deletion syndrome (22qDS)—also called velocardiofacial syndrome, conotruncal anomaly face syndrome, and DiGeorge syndrome—is the most common microdeletion syndrome, estimated to affect between 1 in 4,000 and 1 in 2,000 live births (Swillen and McDonald-McGinn 2015). It involves a classic triad of features: conotruncal cardiac anomalies, hypocalcemia, and thymic hypoplasia. 22qDS is the most common cause of schizophrenia secondary to an identifiable genetic etiology that can currently be found by genetic testing. Phenotypic features in 22qDS-associated schizophrenia differ in some ways from features in idiopathic schizophrenia—in particular, physical features consistent with the syndrome and lower IQ are found in the 22qDS disorder (Bassett et al. 2011). Common morphological features include hooded eyelids, upslanted palpebral fissures, a range of often-subtle ear and nose abnormalities, and micrognathia (McDonald-McGinn and Sullivan 2011; McDonald-McGinn et al. 2015).

22qDS carries high rates of psychiatric (35%) and neurocognitive (90%) comorbidity (Vorstman et al. 2015). The syndrome may be uncovered in childhood or during adolescence or adulthood in the setting of psychiatric and behavioral symptoms associated with characteristic findings on the history and physical examination (McDonald-McGinn et al. 2015; Swillen and McDonald-McGinn 2015). In a cross-sectional study of 112 patients with 22q11DS (Tang et al. 2014), 79% met criteria for one or more psychiatric disorders. Mood disorders and anxiety disorders were present in 14% and 34% of these patients, respectively (Tang et al. 2014). Learning disabilities can be very common, and IQs generally range from 70 to 84 (Swillen and McDonald-McGinn 2015).

The medical comorbidities most commonly associated with 22qDS are conotruncal cardiac defects (present in about 60% of individuals with 22qDS) (McDonald-McGinn and Sullivan 2011). These defects are recognized in early childhood and are either cyanotic (interrupted aortic arch, truncus arteriosus, tetralogy of Fallot) or acyanotic (atrial septal defect, ventricular septal defect, vascular ring) and often require surgical intervention (McDonald-McGinn and Sullivan 2011). Hypocalcemia is present in about 60% of individuals with 22qDS and often presents during infancy, manifesting with tetany, elevated serum phosphorus, and low parathyroid hormone levels (Bassett et al. 2011; McDonald-McGinn et al. 2015). In adults, these symptoms may occur in the setting of emotional and physical stressors. The thymus may be partially or fully absent, resulting in immunocompromise and recurrent infections. High rates of allergies, autoimmune disease, and endocrine, genitourinary, gastrointestinal, central nervous system, palatal, and other disorders may be found (McDonald-McGinn et al. 2015; Staple et al. 2005).

Neurocutaneous Syndromes

Neurocutaneous syndromes are congenital disorders that affect the central and peripheral nervous systems and other tissues of ectodermal origin, such as skin and eyes. Some can affect mesodermal- and endodermal-derived structures as well. Many neurocutaneous syndromes share a propensity to cause tumors, seizures, intellectual disability, and other symptoms. The neurocutaneous syndromes most commonly associated with psychiatric conditions are neurofibromatosis type 1 (NF1) and tuberous sclerosis.

Tuberous Sclerosis

Tuberous sclerosis is estimated to occur in between 1 in 10,000 and 1 in 6,000 births. Affected individuals have a wide range of multiorgan manifestations, including dermatological (hypomelanotic "ash-leaf" lesions, angiofibromas, shagreen patches, facial angiofibromas), ocular (astrocytic hamartoma, achromic retinal lesions), renal (renal angiolipomas), cardiac (cardiac rhabdomyomas), pulmonary (lymphangioleiomyomatosis), and neurological manifestations (Islam and Roach 2015).

The most common neuropsychiatric symptom in tuberous sclerosis is epilepsy, present in more than 80% (Nabbout et al. 2018). Seizure types depend on age; in adults, generalized tonic-clonic and complex partial seizures are the most common (Islam and Roach 2015). Individuals with tuberous sclerosis also have high rates of ASD and intellectual disability. Ninety percent will experience behavioral, neuropsychiatric, or neurocognitive symptoms over the life course (de Vries et al. 2015). Intellectual disability is present in about 50% and severity correlates inversely with degree of seizure control (Islam and Roach 2015; Winterkorn et al. 2007). The prevalence of ASD in tuberous sclerosis is estimated at 25%–50% (Hunt and Shepherd 1993). Other commonly associated diagnoses include ADHD (prevalence of 30%–50%) and depression and anxiety (prevalence of 30%–60%) (de Vries et al. 2015). A study that retrospectively assessed psychiatric symptoms in 241 children and adults with tuberous sclerosis found high rates of mood disorders (27%), ADHD (30%), and aggressive or disruptive behavior disorders (28%) (Muzykewicz et al. 2007).

In addition to the syndrome's neuropsychiatric risks, tuberous sclerosis results in abnormal cellular proliferation in the majority of organs. The most common cause of death in adults with tuberous sclerosis is renal disease associated with angiolipomas (Shepherd et al. 1991). Pulmonary disease also carries a high risk of mortality, particularly in adult women with tuberous sclerosis (Islam and Roach 2015).

Neurofibromatosis Type 1

NF1 is an autosomal dominant disorder affecting between 1 in 3,000 and 1 in 2,500 people (Huson et al. 1989; "Neurofibromatosis" 1988). It is characterized by neurofibromas and predisposition to other tumors; skin manifestations, including cafe-au-lait spots and freckling in skin folds; and Lisch nodules in the iris (Ferner et al. 2007; Radtke et al. 2007). A diagnosis of NF1 requires the presence of two of the following six findings: 1) six or more cafe-au-lait spots, 2) two ore more neurofibromas or one plexiform neurofibroma, 3) axillary or inguinal freckling, 4) optic glioma, 5) two or more Lisch nodules, and 6) specific bony lesions or a first-degree relative with NF1 ("Neurofibromatosis" 1988). Individuals with NF1 are at increased risk for a range of other benign and malignant tumors (Williams et al. 2009).

Whereas IQs in children with NF1 are in the normal range or perhaps slightly lower in comparison with IQs in siblings (Hyman et al. 2005), psychiatric comorbidities are common in this population and most often involve behavioral and cognitive disorders. In a study examining cognitive performance in 81 children with NF1, 81% were found to have moderate to severe impairment in one or more neurocognitive domains, including 20% with specific learning disorder, 63% with deficits in sustained attention, 38% meeting criteria for ADHD, and 51% with poor performance in reading, mathematics, or spelling (Hyman et al. 2005). Nearly 11% of children with NF1 have ASD, and a considerably higher proportion have subclinical ASD symptoms (Eijk et al. 2018).

Medical comorbidities of NF1 generally are related to sequelae of neurofibromas, such as weakness and visual and auditory impairment associated with neurofibroma burden. Chronic pain and physical disfigurement can result directly from neurofibromas or surgical excisions.

Nonverbal Learning Disorder

Nonverbal learning disorder (NVLD) is a term widely used in behavioral neurology and neuropsychology to describe individuals with deficits specific to nonverbal learning domains and with otherwise intact neurocognitive functioning. NVLD has been estimated to account for 10%–15% of all learning disorders (Volden 2013). On neuropsychological investigation, individuals with NVLD show stronger verbal intelligence skills and weaker visuospatial and tactile perceptual skills. As described by Pelletier et al. (2001), core characteristics in children with NVLD include tactile perception errors, finger agnosia, Wide Range Achievement Test reading test scores at least 8 points above arithmetic subtest standard scores, a 10-point split between Verbal IQ and Performance IQ on the Wechsler Intelligence Scale for Children, among others.

NVLD is hypothesized to develop due to underlying neurological vulnerabilities that result in deficits in processing of tactile and visual information during key developmental states. These deficits, in turn, cause decreased environmental exploration during critical periods, ultimately resulting in difficulties with complex problem solving, hypothesis testing, and higher-order concept formation (Rourke 1995; Volden 2013). There is controversy as to how the syndrome might arise, but one hypothesis commonly discussed is that NVLD results from developmental deficits in right-hemisphere white matter connectivity, resulting in functional connectivity anomalies that cause an abnormal pattern of left-sided lateralization (Rourke 1995). NVLD overlaps with the congenital right-hemisphere deficit syndrome described by Weintraub and Mesulam (1983). This syndrome includes indicators of congenital right-hemisphere dysfunction such as asymmetric left-sided posturing with stressed gait or left-sided motor slowing, deficient arithmetic skills, verbal greater than performance IQ, nonverbal memory deficits greater than verbal memory deficits, emotional aprosodia, and a tendency toward diminished eye contact, shyness, diminished social skills, and depression (Voeller 1995; Weintraub and Mesulam 1983). The congenital right-hemisphere deficit syndrome tends to be diagnosed when evidence of right-hemisphere pathology is found. NVLD is more often diagnosed when such evidence is not uncovered.

NVLD may manifest in childhood with poor performance in mathematics but strong facility in subjects such as spelling and text decoding (Rourke 1995). Individuals with NVLD are thought to be highly verbal and expressive, but over time, they may begin to struggle with nuance in conversation (Rourke and Tsatsanis 1996). Social difficulties are thought to result from problems with interpretation of nonverbal communicative information such as gestures, figurative language, and humor. They may struggle with interpersonal relationships as a result. There is controversy as to whether NVLD constitutes a unique learning disability—and, if so, what the boundaries are that differentiate it from other conditions, particularly given some overlap with symptoms of other neurodevelopmental conditions, such as ASD, ADHD, and specific learning disabilities, among others (Volden 2013).

There is some evidence that individuals with a history of NVLD in childhood are at risk for social and emotional sequelae throughout life. In particular, there has been some evidence suggesting high risk for internalizing psychopathologies, including anxiety and depression, and an increased risk for suicidality later in life (Volden 2013).

Exposures: Fetal Alcohol Syndrome

A wide range of intrauterine chemical exposures can affect neurocognitive development. The most common of these is alcohol. Fetal alcohol spectrum disorder (FASD) is an overarching term that encompasses fetal alcohol syndrome, partial fetal alcohol syndrome, alcohol-related neurodevelopmental disorder, neurobehavioral disorder associated with prenatal alcohol exposure, and alcohol-related birth defects (Bertrand et al. 2005; Stratton et al. 1996; Weber et al. 2002). Characteristic morphological features of FASD are short palpebral fissures, flattened philtrum, thin vermilion border of the upper lip, and microcephaly (Hagan et al. 2016). Importantly, many individuals with neurocognitive sequelae related to prenatal alcohol exposure may not demonstrate all, or even some, of these morphological features. While there is no single set of universally accepted criteria for FASD, a number of different sets of criteria have been proposed. In the Section III chapter "Conditions for Further Study," DSM-5 introduced criteria for a new diagnosis: neurobehavioral disorder associated with prenatal alcohol exposure (American Psychiatric Association 2013; Hoyme and Coles 2016). Differences exist among FASD consensus criteria, although all criteria sets agree on the core features of facial dysmorphia and central nervous system involvement (Astley and Clarren 2000; Cook et al. 2016; Hoyme et al. 2016; Weber et al. 2002).

Studies have found that approximately three-quarters of individuals with FASD have one or more psychiatric disorders (54% ADHD, 9% oppositional defiant disorder, 7% posttraumatic stress disorder, 5% major depressive disorder), and up to 70% have difficulties functioning socially (Astley 2010). Executive dysfunction is very common in this population and can manifest as poor impulse control, sexual acting out, and poor judgment. In a study of 415 patients (ages 6–51 years) with FASD, lifetime prevalences of sexually inappropriate behaviors, alcohol or drug problems, and legal trouble among adolescents and adults were 52%, 46%, and 60%, respectively (Streissguth et al. 2004). Individuals with FASD tend to have difficulties with instrumental and basic activities of daily living. Dependence on others may result in problems with social functioning, employment, or establishing adult independence (Spohr et al. 2007; Streissguth et al. 1991). Individuals with FASD may also be especially vulnerable to abuse and bullying (Streissguth et al. 1991, 2004).

Comorbid conditions commonly present (i.e., in 50%–91%) in individuals with FAS include abnormalities of the peripheral nervous system and special senses; conduct disorder; receptive or expressive language disorders; and chronic serous otitis media (Popova et al. 2016).

Conclusion

The neurodevelopmental disorders discussed in this chapter merit the attention of all psychiatrists because they are frequently encountered in clinical practice. The standard approach to assessment should include a gestational, developmental, social, medical, and psychiatric history followed by a neurological examination that includes neurodevelopmental soft signs and physical examination for cardiac and skin abnormalities. Knowledge of the psychiatric comorbidities commonly present in patients with neurodevelopmental disorders may facilitate diagnosis. In daily practice, clinicians may see patients with dysmorphic features or medical comorbidities not included among the disorders reviewed in this chapter. When faced with unfamiliar presentations, clinicians are encouraged to consult online resources such as Online Mendelian Inheritance in Man (www.omim.org), Orphanet (www.orpha.net), and Face2Gene (www.face2gene.com), as well as standard references such as the *Oxford Desk Reference: Clinical Genomics and Genetics* (Firth and Hurst 2017).

References

Aksglaede L, Andersson AM, Jørgensen N, et al: Primary testicular failure in Klinefelter's syndrome: the use of bivariate luteinizing hormone-testosterone reference charts. Clin Endocrinol (Oxf) 66(2):276–281, 2007 17223999

American Psychiatric Association: Diagnostic and Statistical Manual of Mental Disorders, 5th Edition. Arlington, VA, American Psychiatric Association, 2013

Angulo MA, Butler MG, Cataletto ME: Prader-Willi syndrome: a review of clinical, genetic, and endocrine findings. J Endocrinol Invest 38(12):1249–1263, 2015 26062517

Astley SJ: Profile of the first 1,400 patients receiving diagnostic evaluations for fetal alcohol spectrum disorder at the Washington State Fetal Alcohol Syndrome Diagnostic and Prevention Network. Can J Clin Pharmacol 17(1):e132–e164, 2010 20335648

Astley SJ, Clarren SK: Diagnosing the full spectrum of fetal alcohol-exposed individuals: introducing the 4-digit diagnostic code. Alcohol Alcohol 35(4):400–410, 2000 10906009

Bassett AS, McDonald-McGinn DM, Devriendt K, et al: Practical guidelines for managing patients with 22q11.2 deletion syndrome. J Pediatr 159(2):332–339, 2011 21570089

Belmonte MK, Bourgeron T: Fragile X syndrome and autism at the intersection of genetic and neural networks. Nat Neurosci 9(10):1221–1225, 2006 17001341

Benjamin S, Lauterbach MD: The neurological examination adapted for neuropsychiatry. CNS Spectr 23(3):219–227, 2018 29789033

Bennett JA, Hodgetts S, Mackenzie ML, et al: Investigating autism-related symptoms in children with Prader-Willi syndrome: a case study. Int J Mol Sci 18(3):E517, 2017 28264487

Bertrand J, Floyd LL, Weber MK: Guidelines for identifying and referring persons with fetal alcohol syndrome. MMWR Recomm Rep 54(RR-11):1–14, 2005 16251866

Bojesen A, Juul S, Gravholt CH: Prenatal and postnatal prevalence of Klinefelter syndrome: a national registry study. J Clin Endocrinol Metab 88(2):622–626, 2003 12574191

Bondy CA, Turner Syndrome Study Group: Care of girls and women with Turner syndrome: a guideline of the Turner Syndrome Study Group. J Clin Endocrinol Metab 92(1):10–25, 2007 17047017

Boone KB, Swerdloff RS, Miller BL, et al: Neuropsychological profiles of adults with Klinefelter syndrome. J Int Neuropsychol Soc 7(4):446–456, 2001 11396547

Buiting K, Williams C, Horsthemke B: Angelman syndrome—insights into a rare neurogenetic disorder. Nat Rev Neurol 12(10):584–593, 2016 27615419

Butler MG, Kimonis V, Dykens E, et al: Prader-Willi syndrome and early onset morbid obesity NIH rare disease consortium: a review of natural history study. Am J Med Genet A 176(2):368–375, 2018 29271568

Carlson M, Silberbach M: Dissection of the aorta in Turner syndrome: two cases and review of 85 cases in the literature. BMJ Case Rep 2009:bcr0620091998, 2009 21731587

Cederlöf M, Ohlsson Gotby A, Larsson H, et al: Klinefelter syndrome and risk of psychosis, autism and ADHD. J Psychiatr Res 48(1):128–130, 2014 24139812

Christensen D, Van Naarden Braun K, Doernberg NS, et al: Prevalence of cerebral palsy, co-occurring autism spectrum disorders, and motor functioning—Autism and Developmental Disabilities Monitoring Network, USA, 2008. Dev Med Child Neurol 56(1):59–65, 2014 24117446

Conway GS, Band M, Doyle J, et al: How do you monitor the patient with Turner's syndrome in adulthood? Clin Endocrinol (Oxf) 73(6):696–699, 2010 20718775

Cook JL, Green CR, Lilley CM, et al: Fetal alcohol spectrum disorder: a guideline for diagnosis across the lifespan. CMAJ 188(3):191–197, 2016 26668194

Cremer N, Hurvitz EA, Peterson MD: Multimorbidity in middle-aged adults with cerebral palsy. Am J Med 130(6):744.e9–744.e15, 2017 28065772

de Vries PJ, Whittemore VH, Leclezio L, et al: Tuberous sclerosis associated neuropsychiatric disorders (TAND) and the TAND Checklist. Pediatr Neurol 52(1):25–35, 2015 25532776

Devlin L, Morrison PJ: Accuracy of the clinical diagnosis of Down syndrome. Ulster Med J 73(1):4–12, 2004 15244118

DiGuiseppi C, Hepburn S, Davis JM, et al: Screening for autism spectrum disorders in children with Down syndrome: population prevalence and screening test characteristics. J Dev Behav Pediatr 31(3):181–191, 2010 20375732

Eijk S, Mous SE, Dieleman GC, et al: Autism spectrum disorder in an unselected cohort of children with neurofibromatosis type 1 (NF1). J Autism Dev Disord 48(7):2278–2285, 2018 29423604

El-Mansoury M, Bryman I, Berntorp K, et al: Hypothyroidism is common in Turner syndrome: results of a five-year follow-up. J Clin Endocrinol Metab 90(4):2131–2135, 2005 15623818

Erickson CA, Davenport MH, Schaefer TL, et al: Fragile X targeted pharmacotherapy: lessons learned and future directions. J Neurodev Disord 9:7, 2017 28616096

Ferner RE, Huson SM, Thomas N, et al: Guidelines for the diagnosis and management of individuals with neurofibromatosis 1. J Med Genet 44(2):81–88, 2007 17105749

Firth HV, Hurst JA: Oxford Desk Reference: Clinical Genetics and Genomics, 2nd Edition. Oxford, UK, Oxford University Press, 2017

Gravholt CH, Chang S, Wallentin M, et al: Klinefelter syndrome: integrating genetics, neuropsychology, and endocrinology. Endocr Rev 39(4):389–423, 2018 29438472

Groth KA, Skakkebæk A, Høst C, et al: Clinical review: Klinefelter syndrome—a clinical update. J Clin Endocrinol Metab 98(1):20–30, 2013 23118429

Hagan JF Jr, Balachova T, Bertrand J, et al: Neurobehavioral disorder associated with prenatal alcohol exposure. Pediatrics 138(4):e20151553, 2016 27677572

Hall DA, Berry-Kravis E: Fragile X syndrome and fragile X-associated tremor ataxia syndrome. Handb Clin Neurol 147:377–391, 2018 29325626

Holland AJ, Hon J, Huppert FA, et al: Population-based study of the prevalence and presentation of dementia in adults with Down's syndrome. Br J Psychiatry 172:493–498, 1998 9828989

Hoyme HE, Coles CD: Alcohol-related neurobehavioral disabilities: need for further definition and common terminology. Pediatrics 138(4):e20161999, 2016 27677571

Hoyme HE, Kalberg WO, Elliott AJ, et al: Updated clinical guidelines for diagnosing fetal alcohol spectrum disorders. Pediatrics 138(2):e20154256, 2016 27464676

Hunt A, Shepherd C: A prevalence study of autism in tuberous sclerosis. J Autism Dev Disord 23(2):323–339, 1993 8331050

Huson SM, Compston DA, Clark P, Harper PS: A genetic study of von Recklinghausen neurofibromatosis in south east Wales, I: prevalence, fitness, mutation rate, and effect of parental transmission on severity. J Med Genet 26(11):794–711, 1989 2511318

Hyman SL, Shores A, North KN: The nature and frequency of cognitive deficits in children with neurofibromatosis type 1. Neurology 65(7):1037–1044, 2005 16217056

Islam MP, Roach ES: Tuberous sclerosis complex. Handb Clin Neurol 132:97–109, 2015 26564073

Kaufman DM, Milstein MJ: Congenital cerebral impairments, in Kaufman's Clinical Neurology for Psychiatrists, 7th Edition. New York, Saunders Elsevier, 2013, p 288

Kinnear D, Morrison J, Allan L, et al: Prevalence of physical conditions and multimorbidity in a cohort of adults with intellectual disabilities with and without Down syndrome: cross-sectional study. BMJ Open 8(2):e018292, 2018 29431619

Koman LA, Smith BP, Shilt JS: Cerebral palsy. Lancet 363(9421):1619–1631, 2004 15145637

Lee M, Martin GE, Berry-Kravis E, et al: A developmental, longitudinal investigation of autism phenotypic profiles in fragile X syndrome. J Neurodev Disord 8:47, 2016 28050218

Lyle R, Béna F, Gagos S, et al: Genotype-phenotype correlations in Down syndrome identified by array CGH in 30 cases of partial trisomy and partial monosomy chromosome 21. Eur J Hum Genet 17(4):454–466, 2009 19002211

Mantry D, Cooper SA, Smiley E, et al: The prevalence and incidence of mental ill-health in adults with Down syndrome. J Intellect Disabil Res 52 (Pt 2):141–155, 2008 18197953

Manzardo AM, Weisensel N, Ayala S, et al: Prader-Willi syndrome genetic subtypes and clinical neuropsychiatric diagnoses in residential care adults. Clin Genet 93(3):622–631, 2018a 28984907

Manzardo AM, Loker J, Heinemann J, et al: Survival trends from the Prader-Willi Syndrome Association (USA) 40-year mortality survey. Genet Med 20(1):24–30, 2018b 28682308

McDonald-McGinn DM, Sullivan KE: Chromosome 22q11.2 deletion syndrome (DiGeorge syndrome/velocardiofacial syndrome). Medicine (Baltimore) 90(1):1–18, 2011 21200182

McDonald-McGinn DM, Sullivan KE, Marino B, et al: 22q11.2 deletion syndrome. Nat Rev Dis Primers 1:15071, 2015 27189754

Melville CA, Cooper SA, Morrison J, et al: The prevalence and incidence of mental ill-health in adults with autism and intellectual disabilities. J Autism Dev Disord 38(9):1676–1688, 2008 18311512

Muzykewicz DA, Newberry P, Danforth N, et al: Psychiatric comorbid conditions in a clinic population of 241 patients with tuberous sclerosis complex. Epilepsy Behav 11(4):506–513, 2007 17936687

Nabbout R, Belousova E, Benedik MP, et al; TOSCA Consortium and TOSCA Investigators: Epilepsy in tuberous sclerosis complex: findings from the TOSCA study. Epilepsia Open 4(1):73–84, 2018 30868117

Neurofibromatosis: Conference statement. National Institutes of Health Consensus Development Conference. Arch Neurol 45(5):575–578, 1988 3128965. Available at: https://consensus.nih.gov/1987/1987Neurofibramatosis064html.htm. Accessed September 6, 2019.

Nielsen J, Wohlert M: Chromosome abnormalities found among 34,910 newborn children: results from a 13-year incidence study in Arhus, Denmark. Hum Genet 87(1):81–83, 1991 2037286

Parker SE, Mai CT, Canfield MA, et al: Updated national birth prevalence estimates for selected birth defects in the United States, 2004–2006. Birth Defects Res A Clin Mol Teratol 88(12):1008–1016, 2010 20878909

Pelc K, Cheron G, Dan B: Behavior and neuropsychiatric manifestations in Angelman syndrome. Neuropsychiatr Dis Treat 4(3):577–584, 2008 18830393

Pelletier PM, Ahmad SA, Rourke BP: Classification rules for basic phonological processing disabilities and nonverbal learning disabilities: formulation and external validity. Child Neuropsychol 7(2):84–98, 2001 11935416

Popova S, Lange S, Shield K, et al: Comorbidity of fetal alcohol spectrum disorder: a systematic review and meta-analysis. Lancet 387(10022):978–987, 2016 26777270

Radtke HB, Sebold CD, Allison C, et al: Neurofibromatosis type 1 in genetic counseling practice: recommendations of the National Society of Genetic Counselors. J Genet Couns 16(4):387–407, 2007 17636453

Rana M, Upadhyay J, Rana A, et al: A systematic review on etiology, epidemiology, and treatment of cerebral palsy. International Journal of Nutrition, Pharmacology, Neurological Diseases 7(4):76–83, 2017

Rourke BP: Syndrome of Nonverbal Learning Disabilities: Neurodevelopmental Manifestations. New York, Guilford Press, 1995

Rourke BP, Tsatsanis K: Syndrome of nonverbal learning disabilities: psycholinguistic assets and deficits. Top Lang Disord 16(2):30–44, 1996

Schoemaker MJ, Swerdlow AJ, Higgins CD, et al: Mortality in women with Turner syndrome in Great Britain: a national cohort study. J Clin Endocrinol Metab 93(12):4735–4742, 2008 18812477

Shankar RK, Backeljauw PF: Current best practice in the management of Turner syndrome. Ther Adv Endocrinol Metab 9(1):33–40, 2018 29344338

Shepherd CW, Gomez MR, Lie JT, et al: Causes of death in patients with tuberous sclerosis. Mayo Clin Proc 66(8):792–796, 1991 1861550

Shriki-Tal L, Avrahamy H, Pollak Y, et al: Psychiatric disorders in a cohort of individuals with Prader-Willi syndrome. Eur Psychiatry 44:47–52, 2017 28545008

Sinet PM, Théophile D, Rahmani Z, et al: Mapping of the Down syndrome phenotype on chromosome 21 at the molecular level. Biomed Pharmacother 48(5–6):247–252, 1994 7999986

Spohr HL, Willms J, Steinhausen HC: Fetal alcohol spectrum disorders in young adulthood. J Pediatr 150(2):175–179, 2007 17236896

Staple L, Andrews T, McDonald-McGinn D, et al: Allergies in patients with chromosome 22q11.2 deletion syndrome (DiGeorge syndrome/velocardiofacial syndrome) and patients with chronic granulomatous disease. Pediatr Allergy Immunol 16(3):226–230, 2005 15853951

Stevenson DA, Heinemann J, Angulo M, et al: Deaths due to choking in Prader-Willi syndrome. Am J Med Genet A 143A(5):484–487, 2007 17036318

Stratton KR, Howe CJ, Battaglia FC, et al: Fetal Alcohol Syndrome: Diagnosis, Epidemiology, Prevention, and Treatment. Washington, DC, National Academies Press, 1996

Streissguth AP, Aase JM, Clarren SK, et al: Fetal alcohol syndrome in adolescents and adults. JAMA 265(15):1961–1967, 1991 2008025

Streissguth AP, Bookstein FL, Barr HM, et al: Risk factors for adverse life outcomes in fetal alcohol syndrome and fetal alcohol effects. J Dev Behav Pediatr 25(4):228–238, 2004 15308923

Sullivan AK, Marcus M, Epstein MP, et al: Association of FMR1 repeat size with ovarian dysfunction. Hum Reprod 20(2):402–412, 2005 15608041

Swillen A, McDonald-McGinn D: Developmental trajectories in 22q11.2 deletion. Am J Med Genet C Semin Med Genet 169(2):172–181, 2015 25989227

Tang SX, Yi JJ, Calkins ME, et al: Psychiatric disorders in 22q11.2 deletion syndrome are prevalent but undertreated. Psychol Med 44(6):1267–1277, 2014 24016317

Temple CM, Shephard EE: Exceptional lexical skills but executive language deficits in school starters and young adults with Turners syndrome: implications for X chromosome effects on brain function. Brain Lang 120(3):345–359, 2012 22240237

Thibert RL, Larson AM, Hsieh DT, et al: Neurologic manifestations of Angelman syndrome. Pediatr Neurol 48(4):271–279, 2013 23498559

Van Der Slot WM, Nieuwenhuijsen C, Van Den Berg-Emons RJ, et al: Chronic pain, fatigue, and depressive symptoms in adults with spastic bilateral cerebral palsy. Dev Med Child Neurol 54(9):836–842, 2012 22809436

Voeller KK: Clinical neurologic aspects of the right-hemisphere deficit syndrome. J Child Neurol 10 (suppl 1):S16–S22, 1995 7751549

Volden J: Nonverbal learning disability. Handb Clin Neurol 111:245–249, 2013 23622171

Vorstman JA, Breetvelt EJ, Duijff SN, et al: Cognitive decline preceding the onset of psychosis in patients with 22q11.2 deletion syndrome. JAMA Psychiatry 72(4):377–385, 2015 25715178

Vukojević M, Cvitković T, Splavski B, et al: Prevalence of intellectual disabilities and epilepsy in different forms of spastic cerebral palsy in adults. Psychiatr Danub 29 (suppl 2):111–117, 2017 28492217

Weber MK, Floyd RL, Riley EP, et al: National Task Force on Fetal Alcohol Syndrome and Fetal Alcohol Effect: defining the national agenda for fetal alcohol syndrome and other prenatal alcohol-related effects. MMWR Recomm Rep 51(RR-14):9–12, 2002 12572781

Weintraub S, Mesulam MM: Developmental learning disabilities of the right hemisphere. Emotional, interpersonal, and cognitive components. Arch Neurol 40(8):463–468, 1983 6870605

Williams VC, Lucas J, Babcock MA, et al: Neurofibromatosis type 1 revisited. Pediatrics 123(1):124–133, 2009 19117870

Winterkorn EB, Pulsifer MB, Thiele EA: Cognitive prognosis of patients with tuberous sclerosis complex. Neurology 68(1):62–64, 2007 17200495

Wisniewski KE, French JH, Rosen JF, et al: Basal ganglia calcification (BGC) in Down's syndrome (DS)—another manifestation of premature aging. Ann N Y Acad Sci 396:179–189, 1982 6185033

CHAPTER 17

Psychotic Disorders Due to Medical Illnesses

Hannah E. Brown, M.D.

Shibani Mukerji, M.D., Ph.D.

Oliver Freudenreich, M.D.

Because many medical illnesses can cause psychosis, a targeted yet thorough medical workup is necessary for new-onset psychotic symptoms. The medical evaluation has three main goals: 1) to differentiate between primary psychosis (due to a psychiatric disorder) and secondary psychosis (due to a medical condition or a toxic exposure); 2) to expedite treatment of an underlying medical illness; and 3) to establish a medical baseline for patients with a primary psychotic illness, because many will require long-term care (Freudenreich et al. 2009).

Overview of Medical Evaluation

The diagnosis of any psychiatric disorder with prominent psychosis (e.g., schizophrenia spectrum and related disorders; bipolar I disorder, manic episode, with psychotic features) is one primarily of exclusion; potential medical causes for the putative psychiatric syndrome must be ruled out. Findings from the complete history and physical examination should guide the workup and should include an evaluation of the illness course and its consistency with typical presentations of psychotic disorders. In general, the following should be obtained: details regarding the onset, duration, and character of psychotic symptoms; an evaluation for delirium; information on current or past drug use (including illicit substances and nonprescribed medications); and a detailed medical history that guides the medical evaluation.

While many medical illnesses can manifest with psychotic symptoms, screening for all of them would be inefficient, costly, and unnecessary. When considering potential medical or toxic causes of psychosis, the clinician must consider the prevalence of the illness, the sensitivity and specificity of diagnostic tests obtained, and the causal attribution when a test result is positive (Freudenreich et al. 2009). There exists a hierarchy of possibilities:

- Common neuropsychiatric conditions in which psychotic symptoms are diagnostically necessary (e.g., schizophrenia, drug-induced psychosis)
- Common medical conditions that potentially can—but do not typically—cause psychotic symptoms (e.g., systemic lupus erythematosus [SLE])
- Uncommon conditions (of which the clinician may be unaware) that commonly cause psychotic symptoms
- Rare conditions that only atypically manifest with psychosis (e.g., adult-onset Niemann-Pick disease)

When selecting laboratory tests, the clinician must consider the prevalence of the illness, because screening without clinical suspicion for a rare disease is likely to yield false-positive results. A test with high *specificity* (i.e., a low rate of false-positives) should be ordered to confirm a medical illness, whereas a test with high *sensitivity* (i.e., a low rate of false-negatives) helps to exclude a medical illness. Finally, when a medical condition is diagnosed, the clinician must determine whether that illness is actually *causing* the psychotic symptoms.

Although there is no consensus on the proper evaluation of the underlying causes of psychotic symptoms, a broad laboratory screening coupled with additional tests based on the history and physical examination is prudent (Table 17–1).

Among patients (of all ages) with new-onset psychosis without neurological findings, neither brain computed tomography (CT) nor magnetic resonance imaging (MRI) is likely to reveal an underlying medical cause for the psychosis; rates of incidental findings are similar for patients with first-episode psychosis and healthy control subjects (Albon et al. 2008; Khandanpour et al. 2013). MRI should be pursued only for individuals with a relevant clinical history (i.e., an atypical presentation of schizophrenia) or with focal findings suggestive of a neurological process (e.g., a space-occupying lesion). Normal results from neuroimaging can reassure patients that a neurological cause has been excluded and allow prompt treatment of psychiatric disorders. A "spot" electroencephalogram (EEG)—that is, one taken at a random time point when the patient is not seizing (and one would not expect to see seizure activity)—is neither sensitive nor specific. A sleep-deprived EEG, however, is warranted for a patient who has a history of seizures, a clinical history consistent with ictal episodes, or a history of traumatic brain injury (Freudenreich et al. 2009).

Because it would be impractical to review all medical conditions that can cause psychosis, our approach in this chapter is to highlight broad categories and to discuss specific presentations and workups for specific diseases. Some other potentially relevant illnesses and exposures not discussed here are listed in Table 17–2.

TABLE 17–1. **Recommended initial workup for secondary psychosis**

Thorough medical and psychiatric history, including detailed history of psychotic symptoms and evaluation for delirium

Vital signs

Physical examination, including neurological examination

Screening tests: CBC, CMP, LFTs, ESR, ANA, UTS

Tests to exclude treatable conditions: HIV, FTA-ABS, TSH, B_{12}, folate, ceruloplasmin

Tests to consider if clinically indicated: Head CT, brain MRI, EEG, LP

Note. ANA=antinuclear antibodies; CBC=complete blood count; CMP=comprehensive metabolic panel; CT=computed tomography; EEG=electroencephalogram; ESR=erythrocyte sedimentation rate; FTA-ABS=fluorescent treponemal antibody absorbed; LFTs=liver function tests; LP=lumbar puncture; MRI=magnetic resonance imaging; TSH=thyroid-stimulating hormone; UTS=urine toxicology screen.

TABLE 17–2. **Other medical illnesses and medications that can cause psychosis**

Genetic disorders	**Endocrine conditions**
Prader-Willi syndrome	Pheochromocytoma
Metabolic syndromes	**Medications**
Metachromatic leukodystrophy	Antimalarial drugs: mefloquine
X-linked adrenoleukodystrophy	Antituberculosis drugs: D-cycloserine,
Mitochondrial disorders	ethambutol, isoniazid
Tay-Sachs disease	Antibiotics: ciprofloxacin
Niemann-Pick disease	Antivirals: efavirenz, acyclovir
Infectious diseases	**Neurological conditions**
Viral: varicella zoster virus, cytomegalovirus, John Cunningham virus	Tuberous sclerosis
Abscess	Stroke

Medical Conditions That Can Cause Psychosis

Delirium

Delirium has many potential causes. Untreated, delirium causes significant morbidity and mortality; therefore, a delirious process must be excluded early in the medical workup (Salluh et al. 2015). Key clinical features of delirium include acute onset (hours to days) with fluctuating attention and awareness, disruption in the sleep-wake cycle, and impaired cognitive functioning. There must be evidence that the delirium is due to an underlying medical condition or to substance intoxication or withdrawal. Psychosis is present in about half of patients with delirium and is characterized by disorganized thinking, hallucinations (usually visual, auditory, or tactile), and delusions (Webster and Holroyd 2000). Factors that differentiate delirium from a primary psychotic disorder include a relatively acute onset, a fluctuating course, the presence of inattention, and vital sign abnormalities. Treatment of delirium requires quick identification and reversal of the underlying medical cause of the delirium. Antipsychotic medication may be indicated if agitation interferes with treatment, even if frank psychotic symptoms are absent. First-generation antipsychotics (FGAs) and second-generation antipsychotics (SGAs) are equally effective in treating the behavioral symptoms associated with delirium (Bourne et al. 2008; Cook 2004). Psychosocial and environmental interventions can also be used (Caplan et al. 2016). If antipsychotic medications are used, dosages should be reduced gradually and ultimately discontinued after the delirium resolves.

Autoimmune Conditions

Systemic Lupus Erythematosus

SLE is an inflammatory autoimmune disease with multiorgan involvement. Depending on the disease definition used, between 37% and 95% of patients with SLE develop neuropsychiatric symptoms (Govoni et al. 2016). SLE is associated with autoantibodies, a subset of which has been associated with neuropsychiatric SLE, including psychosis. In a systematic review, elevated titers of antiribosomal protein antibodies were found to be associated with lupus psychosis; however, testing for these antibodies was neither sensitive enough nor specific enough to predict or confirm the diagnosis (Sciascia et al. 2014). In a small sample of patients with neuropsychiatric manifestations of SLE, the Rab guanosine diphosphate dissociation inhibitor, a neuronal protein that regulates synaptic vesicle exocytosis, was present in the sera of 4 of 5 patients with psychosis, compared with 0 of 13 patients without psychosis. The psychosis was treated successfully with immunosuppressive therapy (Kimura et al. 2010). Psychotic symptoms are present during active disease in approximately 3% of patients; this percentage increases to 30%–39% in patients taking high-dosage corticosteroids (often a mainstay of treatment) (Pego-Reigosa and Isenberg 2008). Psychotic symptoms often occur early in the disease course, and in rare cases, psychotic symptoms may be the first presentation of SLE (Pego-Reigosa and Isenberg 2008). SLE psychosis typically appears in conjunction with cutaneous (e.g., malar rash) and hematological systemic manifestations (Pego-Reigosa and Isenberg 2008). Treatment with immunosuppressive therapy is indicated for neuropsychiatric SLE (including psychotic symptoms). Symptomatic treatment with antipsychotic medication also may be considered if the psychosis persists. There is a lack of evidence regarding whether any one antipsychotic agent is superior to any other in the treatment of SLE psychosis. In a retrospective study in a cohort of patients with SLE, the most commonly used antipsychotic medications were the FGAs chlorpromazine and haloperidol (Pego-Reigosa and Isenberg 2008). Most patients achieved long-term remission from psychotic symptoms after immunosuppressive therapy and ultimately discontinued antipsychotic medication.

Hashimoto's Encephalopathy

Hashimoto's encephalopathy is characterized by an encephalopathic clinical picture in the setting of autoimmune thyroiditis. It is often divided into two subtypes: one with an acute onset, with episodes of cerebral ischemia, and one that is more diffuse and progressive, with cognitive deficits and psychiatric (including psychotic and affective) symptoms (Chong et al. 2003). Both types may have accompanying stupor, tremor, myoclonus, and ataxia (Wilcox et al. 2008). Psychotic symptoms such as visual and auditory hallucinations and paranoid delusions are present in up to 36% of patients with Hashimoto's encephalopathy (Chong et al. 2003). Clinical diagnosis is facilitated by characteristic EEG findings (diffuse slowing in 90% of patients), the presence in serum of antibodies against thyroid peroxidase and thyroglobulin, and a high protein concentration in cerebrospinal fluid (CSF) (seen in 71% of patients) (de Holanda et al. 2011; Wilcox et al. 2008). Thyroid function is not a clinical predictor, because patients may be hypothyroid or euthyroid. About 80% of patients are women (Wilcox et al. 2008). Hashimoto's encephalopathy is highly responsive to corticosteroids, and prompt treatment results in full resolution of symptoms. In many case series, psychotic symptoms resolved after treatment with glucocorticoids (Chong et al. 2003). Time-limited antipsychotic treatment also may be beneficial.

Paraneoplastic Limbic Encephalitis

Paraneoplastic limbic encephalitis (PLE) is an autoimmune syndrome resulting from an antibody response to a tumor—not in the central nervous system (CNS)—that causes inflammation of limbic structures. PLE can manifest with a constellation of neuropsychiatric symptoms including psychosis, depression, anxiety, confusion, memory deficits, and seizures. PLE is frequently associated with small-cell lung cancer but may also occur in lymphoma and malignancies of the breast, thyroid, ovaries, or testes. Among patients with PLE, 50%–60% of have antibodies against onconeural antigens, which are categorized by whether the target antigen is located on the neuronal cell membrane or inside the cell (Foster and Caplan 2009). Antibodies are present in both serum and CSF, but only CSF antibody confirmation is critical for diagnosis. MRI findings include unilateral or bilateral mesial temporal lobe abnormalities; EEG findings are nonspecific. Of note, psychotic symptoms can precede the actual oncological diagnosis in up to 70% of cases, and PLE may not be immediately recognized if there is no known malignancy (Foster and Caplan 2009). Treatment of the underlying malignancy coupled with immunotherapy (e.g., corticosteroids, cyclophosphamide) will resolve the psychotic symptoms (Foster and Caplan 2009). Antipsychotic medications may be used temporarily if the psychotic symptoms are bothersome; whether any one antipsychotic medication is superior for symptomatic treatment is unknown.

Anti–*N*-Methyl-D-Aspartate Receptor Encephalitis

Anti–*N*-methyl-D-aspartate receptor (NMDAR) encephalitis is characterized by the presence (in CSF or serum) of antibodies against the GluN1 subunit of the NMDAR (Kuppuswamy et al. 2014). Antibodies may be present with or without a known underlying tumor. Close to 80% of patients with anti-NMDAR encephalitis are female, and an ovarian teratoma is the primary cause of paraneoplastic anti-NMDAR encephalitis in women (Dalmau et al. 2007; Titulaer et al. 2013).

Patients with anti-NMDAR encephalitis may present with a viral prodrome (in up to 70% of cases [Warren et al. 2018]) of fever, fatigue, and headache and within weeks may develop psychotic symptoms, including delusions, auditory and visual hallucinations, and bizarre or aggressive behavior. The illness may soon progress to cognitive impairment, seizures, catatonia, hemiparesis, and autonomic instability (Kuppuswamy et al. 2014), which often require intensive care. In a systematic literature review and analysis of 464 cases of anti-NMDAR encephalitis by Al-Diwani et al. (2019), the most common psychiatric symptoms were agitation, aggression, depressed mood, mood instability, hallucinations, delusions, mutism, and irritability. When these symptoms were grouped into higher-level categories, five categories accounted for the greatest proportion of patient symptoms: behavioral disturbances (present in 68% of patients), psychosis (67%), mood symptoms (47%), catatonia (30%), and sleep disturbances (21%). This mixed presentation—and especially the overlap of mood and psychosis symptoms—were distinctive findings in this study (Al-Diwani et al. 2019). In a literature review of published cases of anti-NMDAR encephalitis by Warren et al. (2018), the most commonly reported behavioral disturbances were severe agitation and aggression, abnormal speech, and catatonia, and these symptoms were often accompanied by neurological symptoms, including movement abnormalities, short-term memory impairment, and confusion as the disease progressed. In the Al-Diwani et al. (2019) study, the neurological abnormalities that most commonly developed over time were movement disorders, including choreoathetoid movements; seizures; and hyporesponsive states (i.e., a reduced level of consciousness).

Anti-NMDAR encephalitis should be considered primarily, but not exclusively, in young women who present with a relatively rapid onset of psychotic illness that often seems discontinuous from prior clinical history. Similarly, the presence of neurological signs and symptoms in any patient with new-onset psychosis should raise suspicion for this disease. Analysis of CSF for the presence of NMDAR antibodies is necessary to confirm the diagnosis, given that NMDAR antibody testing is more sensitive in CSF (100%) than in serum (86%) (Dalmau et al. 2011; Graus et al. 2016; Gresa-Arribas et al. 2014). Higher CSF antibody titers correlate with greater severity of psychiatric symptoms. Lymphocytic pleocytosis also may be present in CSF (Kayser et al. 2013). Nonspecific slowing and disorganized activity, or extreme delta brush, are found on EEG in up to 90% of patients with anti-NMDAR encephalitis (Dalmau et al. 2011; Titulaer et al. 2013). Brain MRI reveals T2 signal hyperintensity in limbic structures, cerebral or cerebellar cortex, basal ganglia, or brain stem in only 33%–50% of patients (Dalmau et al. 2011; Kuppuswamy et al. 2014; Wandinger et al. 2011). In the Al-Diwani et al. (2019) study, 257 (62%) of the 464 patients had abnormal EEG scans, and 135 (32%) had abnormal findings on brain MRI.

Treatment is focused on resection of the underlying tumor and immunotherapy (e.g., corticosteroids or plasma exchange) (Kuppuswamy et al. 2014). Early treatment with immunotherapy has been reported to be beneficial. Although most patients recover fully after timely treatment, delay in treatment prolongs the illness course and increases the risk of relapse (Titulaer et al. 2013). Antipsychotic treatment is indicated to treat the psychosis. While case reports describe the use of both FGAs and SGAs, high-potency FGAs (e.g., haloperidol) can cause extrapyramidal symptoms (EPS) and may worsen comorbid dyskinesias. Other antipsychotics used in case reports have included the SGAs clozapine, aripiprazole, and ziprasidone and the FGA chlorpromazine (Kuppuswamy et al. 2014).

NMDAR hypofunction has been hypothesized to play a role in the pathophysiology of schizophrenia. A case-control study that investigated whether NMDAR serum antibodies could be detected in patients with first-episode psychosis at higher rates than in healthy control subjects found that such antibodies were indeed more prevalent in the patients (Lennox et al. 2017). However, no major differences in clinical characteristics were noted between antibody-positive and antibody-negative patients, a finding that highlights the need for further research to clarify their precise pathogenicity in regard to psychosis (Lennox et al. 2017).

Chromosomal Abnormalities

Chromosome 22q11.2 deletion syndrome, or velocardiofacial syndrome (VCFS), is caused by a microdeletion on the long arm of chromosome 22; in the United States, it affects close to 1 in 3,000 infants (Kobrynski and Sullivan 2007). Features of the syndrome include cleft palate, velopharyngeal insufficiency, conotruncal cardiac defects, abnormal facies, hypoparathyroidism, and hypocalcemia. Motor and language skills are often delayed in those with the syndrome (Ebert et al. 2016). The combination of physical stigmata and developmental difficulties should alert clinicians to the need for genetic testing for this syndrome. The rate of psychotic illness in adults with VCFS is 30%, and the rate of schizophrenia is between 20% and 25% (Monks et al. 2014). Psychotic illness in VCFS may occur at a later age, and patients with VCFS-related psychosis may have fewer negative symptoms and milder illness in comparison with patients with non-VCFS schizophrenia (Monks et al. 2014; Murphy et al. 1999). Maintenance treatment with an antipsychotic medication is necessary in most cases.

Neuroendocrine Conditions

Hypothyroidism

"Myxedema madness," a late-stage (i.e., after months or years) manifestation of hypothyroidism, is characterized by a range of psychotic symptoms, including hallucinations (auditory and visual), paranoid delusions, and thought disorder (Heinrich and Grahm 2003). These psychotic symptoms may be preceded or accompanied by other clinical features of hypothyroidism, such as fatigue, weight gain, cold intolerance, dry skin, and delayed deep tendon reflexes. "Myxedema" refers to nonpitting edematous tissue changes caused by infiltration of glycosaminoglycans and water in the skin. It is estimated that 5%–15% of patients with myxedema have psychosis (Heinrich and Grahm 2003). Thyroid replacement is the mainstay of treatment, and most case reports note improvement of psychotic symptoms over weeks to months, although symptom resolution may occur more rapidly in some cases (Moeller et al. 2009). A short course of antipsychotic medication may be indicated until the thyroid abnormality is corrected. Risperidone and haloperidol are effective, but quetiapine should be avoided, because it can cause hypothyroidism (Hynicka 2015).

Thyrotoxicosis

Thyrotoxicosis refers to an excess of circulating thyroid hormone that may be caused by antibodies against the thyroid gland (Graves' disease), toxic multinodular goiter, thyroiditis, or exogenous thyroid hormone ingestion. A radioiodine study can help in distinguishing among these possible causes. Older literature suggested that psychotic symptoms may occur in 10%–20% of patients with hyperthyroidism, but these percentages may have been inflated, and the actual incidence may be closer to 1% (Benvenga et al. 2003; Brownlie et al. 2000). A retrospective review of 18 patients with thyrotoxicosis complicated by psychosis demonstrated primarily affective psychoses, with mania occurring as frequently as depression (Brownlie et al. 2000). Other symptoms of hyperthyroidism include weight loss, tremor, palpitations, insomnia, and anxiety. Treatment is focused on correcting the underlying cause of the thyroid hormone excess by decreasing production, blocking release, or reducing peripheral action of thyroid hormone. Antipsychotic medication and mood stabilizers may be used concomitantly until the thyroid abnormality is corrected.

Adrenal Insufficiency

Adrenal insufficiency may be either primary (as in Addison's disease) or secondary (e.g., due to infection or exposure to excess glucocorticoids). Diagnosis is made on the basis of low plasma cortisol, elevated adrenocorticotropic hormone (ACTH), and blood levels of cortisol before and after an ACTH stimulation test. Symptoms of adrenal insufficiency include weakness, fatigue, weight loss, nausea, vomiting, myalgias, and hyperpigmentation of the skin and mucosae. Mood and behavioral symptoms are the most common psychiatric presentations; psychosis occurs rarely and in more extreme cases (e.g., Addisonian crisis with hypotension) and is usually present prior to treatment (i.e., it is not due to steroid replacement) (Anglin et al. 2006). Hyponatremia in the setting of adrenal insufficiency may cause delirium, which can include psychotic symptoms among its manifestations. Glucocorticoids are the mainstay of treatment.

Hypercortisolism

A syndrome of chronic and excessive exposure to glucocorticoids, hypercortisolism can be caused by adrenal hypersecretion of cortisol due to a tumor, ectopic production of ACTH from a pituitary adenoma (Cushing's disease) or a nonpituitary malignancy (Cushing's syndrome), or continual exposure to medications such as corticosteroids. Physical symptoms include the classic "cushingoid" presentation characterized by "moon facies," truncal obesity, abdominal striae, peripheral wasting, and hirsutism. Urinary free cortisol and ACTH are elevated. In some cases of hypercortisolism, presenting symptoms have included psychosis, irritability, depressed mood, mania, or cognitive impairment. The clinician must consider the entire clinical picture if psychosis is present; in most case series, there has been physical evidence of glucocorticoid excess (Rasmussen et al. 2015). Removal of the underlying cause of the glucocorticoid excess usually leads to resolution of the psychosis.

Infectious Diseases

HIV

New-onset psychosis occurs in 0.2%–15% of patients with HIV; these individuals often have a CD4 count <200 (Owe-Larsson et al. 2009; Watkins and Treisman 2012). Psychotic symptoms may be caused by primary CNS involvement of the virus or comorbid viral infections, such as cytomegalovirus (CMV), Epstein-Barr virus (EBV), herpes simplex virus (HSV), and John Cunningham (JC) virus. Psychosis in the setting of HIV infection can appear suddenly, without a prodromal period, and commonly manifests with delusions (persecutory, grandiose, and somatic), hallucinations, psychomotor retardation, apathy, and withdrawal (Beckett et al. 1987; Dolder et al. 2004; Harris et al. 1991). Because illicit drug use is a common comorbidity in patients with HIV, with lifetime rates of 40%–50%, substance use must be excluded as a potential cause of psychosis in this population (Owe-Larsson et al. 2009). Stimulant misuse is the most likely culprit for development of psychosis. Psychosis may also occur in the setting of HIV-associated dementia; although symptoms are variable, they can include delusions (persecutory, grandiose, and somatic) and hallucinations (auditory and visual) (Owe-Larsson et al. 2009). Treatment of HIV psychosis involves initiation of antiretroviral therapy and of antipsychotic medication to address the psychotic symptoms. Some antiretroviral medications—including zidovudine, nevirapine, and efavirenz—can cause psychosis (Foster et al. 2003). Because sensitivity to EPS and risk for tardive dyskinesia are increased in individuals with HIV, high-potency FGAs should be avoided if possible (Freudenreich et al. 2012; Singh and Goodkin 2007). If the patient requires long-term antipsychotic treatment, the clinician must also consider the metabolic side effects of both SGAs and antiretroviral medications, because both drug classes promote cardiometabolic derangements and can lead to insulin insensitivity, dyslipidemia, renal dysfunction, and cardiovascular disease. Antipsychotics should be started at low dosages and increased slowly to minimize side effects.

Neurosyphilis

The number of cases of syphilis in the United States has steadily increased since 2000; in 2017, the total number of cases (both primary and secondary) was 30,644, the highest recorded since 1992 (Centers for Disease Control and Prevention 2018). Rates are highest among men, particularly men who have sex with men, among whom the majority are co-infected with HIV. Thus, a medical workup of psychosis should always include screening for both syphilis and HIV. Without treatment, up to 40% of syphilis-infected patients can develop neurosyphilis, which can manifest at any time during infection (Rahman et al. 2011). Early neurosyphilis can affect the meninges and blood vessels, while late forms occur years to decades after the primary infection and can affect the brain and spinal cord parenchyma. The diagnosis of neurosyphilis is confirmed with the Venereal Disease Research Laboratory (VDRL) CSF test; a reactive test shows the presence of CSF lymphocytic pleocytosis and high protein concentration. Neurosyphilis may be indistinguishable from a primary psychotic illness. Psychotic symptoms may include delusions and hallucinations and may be accompanied by cognitive impairment (Friedrich et al. 2014). Treatment includes both aqueous crystalline penicillin G and antipsychotic medication. It is not known whether any one antipsychotic agent is superior to any other in the treatment of psychotic symptoms associated with neurosyphilis (Friedrich et al. 2014).

Viral Encephalitis

Typical features of viral encephalitis include fever, headache, confusion, and an altered sensorium. HSV is the most common sporadic viral encephalitis, affecting approximately 1 in 2,000 adults in the United States, with tropism for the temporal and orbitofrontal lobes (Beck and Tompkins 2016). Although most cases of herpes simplex encephalitis (HSE) are caused by HSV-1, HSE due to HSV-2 is common in neonates and can be observed in immunocompromised patients. HSE may manifest with personality changes, mood lability, bizarre behavior, gustatory or olfactory hallucinations, and ultimately seizures (Kennedy and Chaudhuri 2002). Brain MRI findings are abnormal in more than 90% of cases, typically demonstrating T2-weighted fluid-attenuated inversion recovery (T2-FLAIR) hyperintensity in the anterior and mesial temporal lobes, inferior frontal lobes, and insular cortex (Rabinstein 2017). EEGs may show nonspecific slowing or, in later stages of illness, periodic lateralizing epileptiform discharges. CSF typically shows lymphocytic pleocytosis, normal glucose, and increased protein. An HSV-1 or HSV-2 polymerase chain reaction assay can confirm the diagnosis with 95% specificity (Kennedy and Chaudhuri 2002). Acyclovir is the first-line treatment; antipsychotic medication may be used symptomatically (Guaiana and Markova 2006).

Creutzfeldt-Jakob Disease

Creutzfeldt-Jakob disease (CJD) is a rapidly progressive and fatal spongiform disease caused by abnormal conformation (i.e., misfolding) and accumulation of prion proteins in the brain. Most cases (~85%) are sporadic; the remainder are familial (Imran and Mahmood 2011). In very rare cases (<1%), the disease is acquired from contact with infected tissue (acquired CJD) or from ingestion of meat products from animals infected with bovine spongiform encephalopathy (variant CJD) (Martindale et al. 2003). Onset of sporadic CJD typically occurs in the sixth to eighth decade (Imran and Mahmood 2011). MRI abnormalities in sporadic CJD involve increased signal in cortex, thalamus, and striatum on T2- and diffusion-weighted images. The EEG shows periodic sharp wave complexes. Clinical features of sporadic CJD include rapid cognitive decline, myoclonus, cerebellar ataxia, EPS, and akinetic mutism. In a case series of 126 patients with sporadic CJD, psychotic symptoms (including disorganized speech and thinking and visual and auditory hallucinations) were present in 42% of patients; most psychotic symptoms occurred within the first 3 months of illness, but only rarely as the presenting symptom (Wall et al. 2005). Only symptomatic treatment is possible for CJD.

Metabolic Conditions

Wilson's Disease

Wilson's disease is an autosomal recessive disease of impaired copper metabolism, leading to copper accumulation in the brain, liver, bones, and kidneys. Diagnosis is based on the presence of Kayser-Fleischer rings and low serum ceruloplasmin levels; other findings include low serum copper levels, increased urinary copper excretion, elevated transaminases, and hemolytic anemia. In one systematic review, the most common psychiatric presentation of Wilson's disease was psychotic symptoms (e.g., delusions, disorganized thinking) in 36% of patients, followed by depression and personality changes; the average time between onset of psychotic symptoms and diagnosis was nearly 2.5 years (Zimbrean and Schilsky 2014). This time lag between symptom onset and diagnosis is substantially longer than that for neurological Wilson's disease or hepatic Wilson's disease, indicating that clinicians frequently miss the diagnosis of Wilson's disease when psychosis is the primary presenting symptom. Treatment involves chelation therapy or zinc supplementation, either of which can ameliorate the psychotic symptoms. While antipsychotic medications also may be indicated for the treatment of psychotic symptoms, patients with Wilson's disease are particularly sensitive to the side effects of FGAs. One study reported effective treatment with use of quetiapine (with slow dosage titration) as the initial treatment (Zimbrean and Schilsky 2014). No evidence is available regarding the appropriate duration of antipsychotic treatment, but clinicians may consider tapering the antipsychotic dosage as disease markers normalize (Zimbrean and Schilsky 2014).

Acute Intermittent Porphyria

Acute intermittent porphyria (AIP) is an autosomal dominant metabolic disorder characterized by a deficiency in porphobilinogen deaminase, which regulates heme biosynthesis, resulting in an accumulation of porphobilinogen and δ-aminolevulinic acid (ALA). AIP occurs in approximately 1 in 10,000 people (Demily and Sedel 2014). Onset is usually after puberty and is characterized by acute attacks that cause abdominal pain, tachycardia, hypertension, and peripheral neuropathy, as well as psychiatric symptoms including anxiety and psychosis. Attacks may be triggered by infection; medications such as hormones, barbiturates, and sulfonamides; or consumption of alcohol. Diagnosis is based on the finding of elevated urine porphobilinogen and ALA levels; urine is often dark-colored. Psychotic symptoms occur in a remitting-relapsing pattern and are temporally related to the physical symptoms and signs (Kumar 2012). Hematin, a form of heme, may be given to suppress the rate-limiting enzyme in the heme biosynthetic pathway, resulting in a decrease in porphyrin (González-Arriaza and Bostwick 2003). Porphyrogenic (i.e., able to precipitate porphyria) medications such as carbamazepine and barbiturates should be avoided. Antipsychotic medication may be indicated for symptomatic treatment.

Neurocognitive Disorders

Alzheimer's Dementia

Accounting for 60%–80% of all dementias (Gatchel et al. 2016), Alzheimer's disease is the most common form of progressive dementia. Onset is most commonly in the eighth and ninth decades, and memory loss is progressive. CT and MRI demonstrate atrophy in the medial temporal lobes and parietal convexities (Gatchel et al. 2016). Diagnosis is confirmed postmortem by identification of characteristic neurofibrillary tangles and neuritic plaques. In addition to cognitive decline, neuropsychiatric symptoms are present in the early phases of the illness; psychotic symptoms (including delusions of persecution and of misidentification in 30%–40% of patients and hallucinations in 5%–20%) occur later in the illness (Koppel and Greenwald 2014). Treatment of Alzheimer's disease focuses on behavioral strategies, including environmental cueing, continual reorienting, and reassurance. Pharmacological treatment includes cholinesterase inhibitors and NMDAR antagonists. If psychotic symptoms distress the patient or lead to violent or dangerous behavior, antipsychotic medication should be considered. Of note, although antipsychotic medications may be indicated for relief of psychotic symptoms in the context of dementia, there have been reports of small, but clinically relevant, increases in all-cause mortality associated with the use of FGAs and SGAs in elderly patients with dementia (Gill et al. 2007; Schneider et al. 2005). Thus, the clinician must carefully weigh the risks and benefits of prescribing antipsychotic medication in these patients. If antipsychotic medication is used, the lowest effective dosage should be used; if after 4 weeks there is no significant clinical response, the medication should be tapered and discontinued (Reus et al. 2016). The SGAs olanzapine, quetiapine, and aripiprazole are more efficacious than placebo in treating behavioral disturbances in Alzheimer's disease and are generally favored over FGAs because they are less likely to cause EPS (Ma et al. 2014). Data are lacking for a robust effect of specific SGAs in the treatment of psychotic symptoms, but olanzapine and risperidone may have some benefit (Koppel and Greenwald 2014; Sultzer et al. 2008).

Frontotemporal Dementia

Frontotemporal dementia (FTD) is characterized by degeneration in the frontal and temporal lobes and includes Pick's disease, primary progressive aphasia, and fronto-temporal lobar degeneration (Gatchel et al. 2016). FTD occurs at a younger age than other dementias, with onset between 45 and 64 years (Seltman and Matthews 2012). Onset may be gradual, with progressive impairment in judgment accompanied by disinhibited behavior, social inappropriateness, inappropriate affect, and impulsivity. CT and MRI may show atrophy in frontotemporal areas. Among patients with patho-logically confirmed FTD, psychotic symptoms occurred in 32%; paranoid ideas (i.e., clinically significant irrational suspiciousness or distrust) were the most common psychotic symptom, followed by hallucinations (most frequently visual and audi-tory) and delusions (most commonly persecutory) (Landqvist Waldö et al. 2015). There is a paucity of evidence on the treatment of psychosis in FTD. As with Alzhei-mer's disease, high-potency FGAs should be avoided because of the risk of EPS; as with other dementing illnesses, supportive care is the mainstay of treatment.

Dementia With Lewy Bodies

A significant cause of dementia, dementia with Lewy bodies (DLB) is characterized by progressive cognitive impairment in multiple realms, impaired attention, parkin-sonism (occurring within 1 year of cognitive deficits), rapid eye movement sleep dis-turbance, and visual hallucinations (McKeith et al. 2017). Lewy bodies (primarily composed of α-synuclein and β-amyloid cortical depositions) are the hallmark neu-ropathological finding. Visual hallucinations occur in up to 90% of patients with DLB and frequently involve animals or humans (Dudley et al. 2019). Up to 41% of patients with DLB experience delusions, and approximately 10% of patients experience audi-tory hallucinations (Snowden et al. 2012). These psychotic symptoms may be present even in the early stages of the illness. Evidence is limited regarding the benefit of anti-psychotic treatment, but it is thought that FGAs and even some SGAs cause signifi-cant EPS in patients with DLB (Dodel et al. 2008). Clozapine or quetiapine (which has a lower anticholinergic burden than clozapine) are rational antipsychotic choices in these patients (Dodel et al. 2008).

Brain Tumors

Most brain tumors manifest with neurological findings due to mass effect; it is rare for either primary or metastatic brain tumors to cause psychosis as an initial present-ing symptom. In case series, pituitary tumors and temporal lobe tumors were found to be the most common brain tumors associated with psychotic symptoms (Madhu-soodanan et al. 2010, 2015). Psychotic symptoms associated with brain tumors in-clude auditory and visual hallucinations and persecutory delusions. Peduncular hallucinosis is associated with focal midbrain (peduncular) or cerebellar tumors. Ad-ditionally, some drugs used in the treatment of brain tumors (e.g., dopamine agonists for prolactinomas, corticosteroids for vasogenic edema) can exacerbate psychotic symptoms.

Seizure Disorders

Psychosis can occur transiently during ictal, postictal, and interictal periods. Ictal psychosis has been described during status epilepticus, most commonly with partial complex status. Seizure activity is most often seen in the temporal region (Williamson and Spencer 1986). Brief interictal psychosis can last anywhere from days to weeks, and paranoid delusions and auditory hallucinations are common (Sachdev 1998). Chronic interictal psychosis is difficult to differentiate from schizophrenia itself. Postictal psychosis is the most commonly occurring psychosis in patients with seizure disorders and can last for days to weeks after the seizure (and in rare cases can last even longer) (Adachi et al. 2007). Common symptoms of postictal psychosis include persecutory and grandiose delusions, referential thinking, and hallucinations. Postictal psychotic symptoms often resolve spontaneously (Farooq and Sherin 2015). There is a higher rate of psychosis in individuals with epilepsy than in the general population; the converse is also true (Clarke et al. 2012; Gaitatzis et al. 2004). Evidence is lacking regarding the use of specific antipsychotic medications to treat psychotic symptoms in the context of seizure disorder; however, some antipsychotic medications (in particular, clozapine) can lower the seizure threshold (Farooq and Sherin 2015).

Diseases of the Basal Ganglia

Parkinson's Disease

Parkinson's disease is a neurodegenerative disorder characterized by resting tremor, rigidity, bradykinesia, and impaired postural reflexes. Although mood and anxiety symptoms are more common, psychosis occurs in 20%–40% of Parkinson's disease patients and is characterized by hallucinations (primarily visual), delusions (grandiose, religious, and infidelity themes), and disorganized thinking (Zahodne and Fernandez 2008). Psychotic symptoms initially occur in the presence of a clear sensorium and intact insight (i.e., without delirium or dementia); over time, however, insight may diminish. Psychotic symptoms usually occur years after the initial diagnosis (Ravina et al. 2007). Psychotic symptoms are considered to be due to the underlying illness and to dopaminergic antiparkinsonism medications. Treatment of psychotic symptoms in Parkinson's disease includes dosage reductions for antiparkinsonism medications (if clinically appropriate) and treatment with a short-acting formulation of levodopa (Zahodne and Fernandez 2008). SGAs are preferred over FGAs, given the latter's greater propensity to cause parkinsonian symptoms. Clozapine and quetiapine have the most favorable side-effect profiles; however, clozapine requires strict blood monitoring, and quetiapine has not been found to reduce psychotic symptoms significantly in comparison with placebo (Desmarais 2016; Zahodne and Fernandez 2008). Although experience with pimavanserin, a selective serotonin type 2A (5-HT$_{2A}$) receptor inverse agonist, is limited, it is now approved by the U.S. Food and Drug Administration for treatment of hallucinations and delusions associated with Parkinson's disease psychosis (Tampi et al. 2019).

Huntington's Disease

Huntington's disease is an autosomal dominant progressive neurodegenerative illness characterized by chorea, cognitive decline, and neuropsychiatric symptoms. Onset is usually in the fourth or fifth decade, and the disease is diagnosed on the basis of family history, clinical findings, and genetic testing. In one-third of patients with Huntington's disease, neuropsychiatric symptoms can occur up to a decade prior to the classic motor symptoms of the disease (Epping et al. 2016). Psychotic symptoms (mainly delusions and hallucinations) occur in 3%–11% of patients with Huntington's disease (Ding and Gadit 2014). In the initial phase of the disease, psychotic symptoms and chorea can be treated with FGAs; later, when dystonia and rigidity are present, SGAs such as quetiapine or clozapine, which are associated with a lower risk of EPS, may be better tolerated (Flaherty and Ivkovic 2016). Risperidone also may be used (Ding and Gadit 2014).

Multiple Sclerosis

Multiple sclerosis (MS) is a chronic, episodic multifocal inflammatory demyelinating illness of the CNS that can involve the entire neuraxis (brain and spinal cord). The illness is two to three times more prevalent in women, and onset is usually between the ages of 20 and 40 years (Gilberthorpe et al. 2017). Presenting symptoms include weakness, paresthesias, ataxia, visual disturbances (e.g., vision loss, nystagmus, diplopia), bladder dysfunction, and sensory abnormalities. Brain MRI may show focal lesions consistent with demyelination (hyperintensities on T2-weighted images); the presence of oligoclonal bands in CSF confirms the diagnosis. Most patients experience psychiatric symptoms (most typically fatigue, depression, and anxiety), and the prevalence of psychosis in MS is only about 4% (Marrie et al. 2015). In a small study of 13 patients with confirmed cases of MS with psychosis, the median age at onset of psychosis was 39 years; in 3 patients, psychotic symptoms first appeared 7–11 years prior to the diagnosis of MS (Gilberthorpe et al. 2017). The most common psychotic symptoms were persecutory delusions (87%); delusions of reference (53%); and auditory hallucinations, grandiose delusions, and passivity phenomena (27%) (Gilberthorpe et al. 2017). There is a dearth of literature regarding antipsychotic treatment in MS patients with psychosis. FGAs are usually avoided because of their propensity to cause EPS. Case reports suggest that clozapine, ziprasidone, and aripiprazole may be tolerable, reasonable choices (Muzyk et al. 2010).

Vitamin Deficiencies

Vitamin B₁₂ (Cobalamin)

Often caused by malabsorption (through lack of intrinsic factor or poor nutrition), vitamin B_{12} deficiency is associated with a range of neurological features, including paresthesias, ataxia, autonomic dysregulation, and loss of proprioception, vibration sense, and sphincter function. Psychosis may be the presenting symptom and is characterized by persecutory and religious delusions, auditory or visual hallucinations, and disorganized thinking (Hutto 1997). Laboratory findings include macrocytic anemia, low serum cobalamin levels, and elevated serum methylmalonic acid and homocysteine levels. The mainstay of treatment is B_{12} replacement either orally or (if absorption is impaired) intramuscularly.

Vitamin B₁ (Thiamine)

In resource-rich settings (e.g., where vitamin fortification occurs), 90% of thiamine deficiency is caused by chronic alcohol use (Isenberg-Grzeda et al. 2012). Wernicke-

Korsakoff syndrome (WKS) is a feared neuropsychiatric consequence of thiamine deficiency and is characterized by encephalopathy, ophthalmoplegia, and ataxia; both visual and auditory hallucinations may occur in WKS (Greenberg and Lee 2001). The encephalopathy can progress to Korsakoff amnestic syndrome, characterized by anterograde and retrograde amnesia, apathy, confusion, and confabulation. Confabulation may be responsible for the "psychotic" component of so-called Korsakoff psychosis. WKS occurs at higher rates in individuals with alcohol use disorder (12.5%), AIDS (10%), or bone marrow transplants (5.5%) in comparison with the general population (Isenberg-Grzeda et al. 2012). Aggressive treatment with thiamine, either intramuscularly or intravenously, is indicated. When treating a malnourished alcoholic patient, it is important to administer thiamine prior to glucose, because administration of glucose prior to thiamine can worsen WKS.

Drugs and Toxins That Can Cause Psychosis

Because a wide range of toxins have been associated with psychotic symptoms, it is critical that patients be asked about all drugs they are taking (including over-the-counter drugs, supplements, and illicit substances). In this section we focus on selected offending agents for which causation of psychosis is fairly well established.

Corticosteroids

There is a 5.7% incidence of psychosis in patients who have elevated endogenous steroid levels or who are being treated with exogenous steroids (Ross and Cetas 2012). While development of psychotic symptoms is dosage related, psychotic symptoms can occur even at low dosages (Ross and Cetas 2012). Most psychotic symptoms (primarily hallucinations and delusions) appear within days of treatment initiation. Ideally, treatment of psychotic symptoms involves tapering the steroid; however, if tapering is not clinically feasible, antipsychotic medication may be necessary. Olanzapine and risperidone are efficacious antipsychotic medications in this clinical setting (Ross and Cetas 2012). Psychotic symptoms resolve quickly after antipsychotic treatment is initiated (Dubovsky et al. 2012).

Stimulants

Stimulants (e.g., methylphenidate, dextroamphetamine) rarely cause psychotic symptoms (Kraemer et al. 2010). One review estimated that the risk of psychotic symptoms in children taking stimulants was 0.25% (Ross 2006). In most cases of stimulant-induced psychosis, symptoms resolve within days after withdrawal of the medication (Ross 2006; Spear and Alderton 2003); therefore, antipsychotic medication is not usually indicated.

Methamphetamine or cocaine intoxication can result in psychotic symptoms. Symptoms include hypervigilance, auditory hallucinations, referential thinking, and paranoid delusions. Up to 46% of chronic methamphetamine users and between 43% and 88% of cocaine users report experiencing at least transient psychotic symptoms during intoxication (Grant et al. 2012; Roncero et al. 2013). Psychotic symptoms may resolve within hours or can last for weeks to months, depending on the amount and chronicity of use (Grant et al. 2012; Roncero et al. 2014). Accompanying physical symptoms include tachycardia, hypertension, pupillary dilation, and diaphoresis. Because methamphetamine or cocaine intoxication can result in cardiac arrhythmias, dystonic movements, and seizures, benzodiazepine treatment should be initiated before antipsychotic medications, which may exacerbate these effects. Olanzapine, quetiapine, risperidone, and aripiprazole effectively ameliorate psychotic symptoms. Haloperidol also is effective but may be more likely to cause EPS (Farnia et al. 2014; Shoptaw et al. 2009; Verachai et al. 2014).

Interferon

Interferon (along with ribavirin) is the mainstay of treatment for hepatitis C virus (HCV) infection. While depressive symptoms are commonly associated with interferon treatment, psychotic symptoms are rare, with an incidence of less than 1% (Budhram and Cebrian 2014). Psychotic symptoms include hallucinations and delusions and can occur at any point in treatment, even days after treatment is completed (Silverman et al. 2010). Both discontinuation of interferon and initiation of antipsychotic medication may be considered. The benefit of prophylactic or symptomatic treatment with antipsychotic medication is unknown (Silverman et al. 2010).

Anticholinergic Medications

Anticholinergic medications are antagonists at muscarinic receptors; they increase dopamine in the snaptic cleft, and this dopamine increase is thought to cause psychotic symptoms at higher dosages (Gulsun et al. 2006). Elderly patients may be particularly vulnerable to the psychotic side effects of anticholinergic medications. Polypharmacy is a major cause of anticholinergic burden; many of the medications commonly prescribed in the elderly population have anticholinergic effects (Cancelli et al. 2009). Common anticholinergic medications include oxybutynin, diphenhydramine, and benztropine. Psychotic symptoms may include hallucinations (usually visual), delusions, and agitation. Psychotic symptoms may also occur in the setting of anticholinergic delirium, with physical symptoms including dry skin and mouth, skin flushing, mydriasis, tachycardia, constipation, and urinary retention. Treatment of anticholinergic delirium involves supportive care and withdrawal of the anticholinergic medication.

Alcohol

Alcohol can cause psychotic symptoms during periods of intoxication and withdrawal. Psychosis during intoxication is characterized by agitation, aggressive behavior, visual hallucinations, and delusions; patients may have no recollection of the intoxication episode. Symptoms typically last for several hours. Alcohol withdrawal syndrome (AWS) occurs hours to days after alcohol consumption ceases (or, in chronic drinkers, is reduced). AWS may include auditory or visual hallucinations or other perceptual disturbances (Mirijello et al. 2015). Alcohol withdrawal delirium usually develops about 2–3 days after onset of withdrawal symptoms. The delirium associated with alcohol withdrawal is generally accompanied by hypertension, tachycardia, and agitation, a feature that differentiates alcohol withdrawal from alcoholic hallucinosis or alcohol-induced psychotic disorder, which is characterized by acute onset of auditory, visual, or tactile hallucinations or persecutory delusions within a clear sensorium (i.e., without delirium) (Perälä et al. 2010). Treatment of AWS includes benzodiazepines or barbiturates and correction of the autonomic instability. If alcohol withdrawal with psychotic symptoms is present (e.g., as in alcohol withdrawal delirium), antipsychotic medications are used in addition to benzodiazepines or barbiturates. Thiamine should be given to prevent Wernicke's encephalopathy.

Cannabis

Cannabis intoxication can cause a range of transient psychotic symptoms, including paranoid and grandiose delusions, suspiciousness, feelings of "unreality," referential thinking, and disorganized thinking (D'Souza et al. 2004, 2009). Psychotic symptoms may last minutes to hours, but there are case reports of symptoms persisting up to weeks (D'Souza et al. 2009). Other physical symptoms of cannabis intoxication include increased appetite, conjunctival injection, and dry mouth. In comparison with nonusers and users of lower-potency cannabis, users of high-potency cannabis (i.e., containing higher levels of tetrahydrocannabinol [THC]) are more likely to develop psychotic symptoms (Murray et al. 2016). A standard urine toxicology screen will detect cannabis up to 10 days after use (longer in chronic users). Treatment involves discontinuing use of cannabis. The antipsychotic medications haloperidol and olanzapine are equally effective in treating cannabis-induced psychosis; however, haloperidol is associated with a greater risk of EPS (Bui et al. 2015).

Hallucinogens and Dissociative Agents

Lysergic acid diethylamide (LSD) and N,N-dimethyltryptamine (DMT) are hallucinogens that act as a partial agonist and an agonist at the 5-HT_{2A} receptor, respectively. These compounds can cause derealization, depersonalization, and hallucinations in multiple sensory modalities (Passie et al. 2008; Strassman et al. 1994). LSD's effects last between 12 and 72 hours, depending on the dosage ingested. Psychotic symptoms after inhalation of DMT are transient (minutes), with longer effects after it is used intravenously or intramuscularly. Phencyclidine (PCP), a dissociative agent, acts through blockade of the NMDAR and causes auditory and visual hallucinations, "out of body" sensations, and altered time perception. Aggressive behavior also is frequently observed with PCP use. In a standard urine toxicology screen, LSD is detectable for 2–4 days after use (its metabolites potentially longer), DMT is not detectable, and PCP may be detectable for weeks in chronic users. Several medications (e.g., diphenhydramine, dextromethorphan, tramadol) can cause false-positive results for PCP.

New Psychoactive Substances

Synthetic cathinones ("bath salts") cause a range of psychotic symptoms, including auditory and visual hallucinations and paranoid delusions. Depending on the cathinone used, the effects can occur within minutes and can last for hours. Like PCP, synthetic cathinones may cause significant agitation and aggression accompanying the psychotic symptoms. Not all synthetic cathinones are detectable on a urine toxicology screen. Synthetic cannabinoids (e.g., "Spice" or "K2") are agonists at the cannabinoid subtype 1 receptor. Synthetic cannabinoids can cause paranoia, auditory and visual hallucinations, and disorganized behavior (Fattore 2016). Synthetic cannabinoids are detectable only on newer, more sensitive, and specific urine assays (Spinelli et al. 2015).

Treatment of Psychosis Induced by Hallucinogens, Dissociative Agents, and New Psychoactive Substances

Treatment of psychotic symptoms associated with hallucinogens, dissociative agents, and new psychoactive substances focuses on keeping the patient and those around the patient safe (e.g., physical restraints if necessary in the setting of agitation) and discontinuation of the offending agent. Antipsychotic medications with benzodiazepines may be used for acute agitation.

Conclusion

Examining potential secondary causes of psychosis is important to guide clinical management and understand the prognosis of a patient presenting with psychotic symptoms. Unfortunately, no pathognomonic signs differentiate primary from secondary psychotic illnesses. Psychotic symptoms may be the first presentation of a medical condition, and a detailed history and examination help guide the subsequent workup. Treatable conditions (e.g., vitamin B_{12} deficiency, neurosyphilis) must always be excluded. Clinicians should look for patterns that may or may not be consistent with a primary psychiatric disorder; longitudinal follow-up often clarifies the diagnosis. The decision of whether to treat symptoms with an antipsychotic medication will depend on the cause of the secondary psychosis, the duration of the psychotic symptoms, and the risk of side effects. Often, treatment of the underlying illness will ameliorate the psychotic symptoms.

References

Adachi N, Ito M, Kanemoto K, et al: Duration of postictal psychotic episodes. Epilepsia 48(8):1531–1537, 2007 17386048

Albon E, Tsourapas A, Frew E, et al: Structural neuroimaging in psychosis: a systematic review and economic evaluation. Health Technol Assess 12(18):iii–iv, ix–163, 2008 18462577

Al-Diwani A, Handel A, Townsend L, et al: The psychopathology of NMDAR-antibody encephalitis in adults: a systematic review and phenotypic analysis of individual patient data. Lancet Psychiatry 6(3):235–246, 2019 30765329

Anglin RE, Rosebush PI, Mazurek MF: The neuropsychiatric profile of Addison's disease: revisiting a forgotten phenomenon. J Neuropsychiatry Clin Neurosci 18(4):450–459, 2006 17135373

Beck BJ, Tompkins KT: Mental disorders due to another medical condition, in Comprehensive Clinical Psychiatry, 2nd Edition. Edited by Stern T, Fava M, Wilens TE, et al. New York, Elsevier, 2016, pp 205–228

Beckett A, Summergrad P, Manschreck T, et al: Symptomatic HIV infection of the CNS in a patient without clinical evidence of immune deficiency. Am J Psychiatry 144(10):1342–1344, 1987 3661770

Benvenga S, Lapa D, Trimarchi F: Don't forget the thyroid in the etiology of psychoses. Am J Med 115(2):159–160, 2003 12893408

Bourne RS, Tahir TA, Borthwick M, et al: Drug treatment of delirium: past, present and future. J Psychosom Res 65(3):273–282, 2008 18707951

Brownlie BE, Rae AM, Walshe JW, et al: Psychoses associated with thyrotoxicosis—"thyrotoxic psychosis." A report of 18 cases, with statistical analysis of incidence. Eur J Endocrinol 142(5):438–444, 2000 10802519

Budhram A, Cebrian C: Paranoid psychosis and cognitive impairment associated with hepatitis C antiviral therapy. Gen Hosp Psychiatry 36(1):126.e3–126.e5, 2014 24210465

Bui QM, Simpson S, Nordstrom K: Psychiatric and medical management of marijuana intoxication in the emergency department. West J Emerg Med 16(3):414–417, 2015 25987916

Cancelli I, Beltrame M, Gigli GL, et al: Drugs with anticholinergic properties: cognitive and neuropsychiatric side-effects in elderly patients. Neurol Sci 30(2):87–92, 2009 19229475

Caplan JP, Cassem NH, Murray GB, et al: Delirium, in Comprehensive Clinical Psychiatry, 2nd Edition. Edited by Stern T, Fava M, Wilens TE, et al. New York, Elsevier, 2016, pp 173–183

Centers for Disease Control and Prevention: Sexually Transmitted Disease Surveillance 2017, Table 1: Sexually Transmitted Diseases—Reported Cases and Reported Cases per 100,00 Population, United States, 1941–2017. Last updated July 24, 2018. Division of STD Prevention, National Center for HIV/AIDS, Viral Hepatitis, STD, and TB Prevention, Centers for Disease Control and Prevention. Available at: https://www.cdc.gov/std/stats17/tables/1.htm. Accessed September 1, 2019.

Chong JY, Rowland LP, Utiger RD: Hashimoto encephalopathy: syndrome or myth? Arch Neurol 60(2):164–171, 2003 12580699

Clarke MC, Tanskanen A, Huttunen MO, et al: Evidence for shared susceptibility to epilepsy and psychosis: a population-based family study. Biol Psychiatry 71(9):836–839, 2012 22365727

Cook IA: Guideline Watch: Practice Guideline for the Treatment of Patients With Delirium. Arlington, VA, American Psychiatric Association, 2004

D'Souza DC, Perry E, MacDougall L, et al: The psychotomimetic effects of intravenous delta-9-tetrahydrocannabinol in healthy individuals: implications for psychosis. Neuropsychopharmacology 29(8):1558–1572, 2004 15173844

D'Souza DC, Sewell RA, Ranganathan M: Cannabis and psychosis/schizophrenia: human studies. Eur Arch Psychiatry Clin Neurosci 259(7):413–431, 2009 19609589

Dalmau J, Tüzün E, Wu HY, et al: Paraneoplastic anti-N-methyl-D-aspartate receptor encephalitis associated with ovarian teratoma. Ann Neurol 61(1):25–36, 2007 17262855

Dalmau J, Lancaster E, Martinez-Hernandez E, et al: Clinical experience and laboratory investigations in patients with anti-NMDAR encephalitis. Lancet Neurol 10(1):63–74, 2011 21163445

de Holanda NC, de Lima DD, Cavalcanti TB, et al: Hashimoto's encephalopathy: systematic review of the literature and an additional case. J Neuropsychiatry Clin Neurosci 23(4):384–390, 2011 22231308

Demily C, Sedel F: Psychiatric manifestations of treatable hereditary metabolic disorders in adults. Ann Gen Psychiatry 13:27, 2014 25478001

Desmarais P, Massoud F, Filion J, et al: Quetiapine for psychosis in Parkinson disease and neurodegenerative parkinsonian disorders: a systematic review. J Geriatr Psychiatry Neurol 29(4):227–236, 2016 27056066

Ding J, Gadit AM: Psychosis with Huntington's disease: role of antipsychotic medications. BMJ Case Rep 2014:bcr2013202625, 2014 25139915

Dodel R, Csoti I, Ebersbach G, et al: Lewy body dementia and Parkinson's disease with dementia. J Neurol 255 (suppl 5):39–47, 2008 18787881

Dolder CR, Patterson TL, Jeste DV: HIV, psychosis and aging: past, present and future. AIDS 18 (suppl 1):S35–S42, 2004 15075496

Dubovsky AN, Arvikar S, Stern TA, et al: The neuropsychiatric complications of glucocorticoid use: steroid psychosis revisited. Psychosomatics 53(2):103–115, 2012 22424158

Dudley R, Aynsworth C, Mosimann U, et al: A comparison of visual hallucinations across disorders. Psychiatry Res 272:86–92, 2019 30579187

Ebert DH, Finn CT, Smoller JW: Genetics and psychiatry, in Comprehensive Clinical Psychiatry, 2nd Edition. Edited by Stern T, Fava M, Wilens TE, et al. New York, Elsevier, 2016, pp 677–702

Epping EA, Kim JI, Craufurd D, et al; PREDICT-HD Investigators and Coordinators of the Huntington Study Group: Longitudinal psychiatric symptoms in prodromal Huntington's disease: a decade of data. Am J Psychiatry 173(2):184–192, 2016 26472629

Farnia V, Shakeri J, Tatari F, et al: Randomized controlled trial of aripiprazole versus risperidone for the treatment of amphetamine-induced psychosis. Am J Drug Alcohol Abuse 40(1):10–15, 2014 24359506

Farooq S, Sherin A: Interventions for psychotic symptoms concomitant with epilepsy. Cochrane Database Syst Rev (12):CD006118, 2015 26690687

Fattore L: Synthetic cannabinoids: further evidence supporting the relationship between cannabinoids and psychosis. Biol Psychiatry 79(7):539–548, 2016 26970364

Flaherty AW, Ivkovic AI: Movement disorders, in Comprehensive Clinical Psychiatry, 2nd Edition. Edited by Stern T, Fava M, Wilens TE, et al. New York, Elsevier, 2016, pp 871–882

Foster AR, Caplan JP: Paraneoplastic limbic encephalitis. Psychosomatics 50(2):108–113, 2009 19377018

Foster R, Olajide D, Everall IP: Antiretroviral therapy-induced psychosis: case report and brief review of the literature. HIV Med 4(2):139–144, 2003 12702135

Freudenreich O, Schulz SC, Goff DC: Initial medical work-up of first-episode psychosis: a conceptual review. Early Interv Psychiatry 3(1):10–18, 2009 21352170

Freudenreich O, Basgoz N, Fernandez-Robles C, et al: Case records of the Massachusetts General Hospital. Case 5–2012. A 39-year-old man with a recent diagnosis of HIV infection and acute psychosis. N Engl J Med 366(7):648–657, 2012 22335743

Friedrich F, Aigner M, Fearns N, et al: Psychosis in neurosyphilis—clinical aspects and implications. Psychopathology 47(1):3–9, 2014 23711816

Gaitatzis A, Trimble MR, Sander JW: The psychiatric comorbidity of epilepsy. Acta Neurol Scand 110(4):207–220, 2004 15355484

Gatchel JR, Wright CI, Falk WE, et al: Dementia, in Comprehensive Clinical Psychiatry, 2nd Edition. Edited by Stern T, Fava M, Wilens TE, et al. New York, Elsevier, 2016, pp 184–197

Gilberthorpe TG, O'Connell KE, Carolan A, et al: The spectrum of psychosis in multiple sclerosis: a clinical case series. Neuropsychiatr Dis Treat 13:303–318, 2017 28203081

Gill SS, Bronskill SE, Normand SL, et al: Antipsychotic drug use and mortality in older adults with dementia. Ann Intern Med 146(11):775–786, 2007 17548409

González-Arriaza HL, Bostwick JM: Acute porphyrias: a case report and review. Am J Psychiatry 160(3):450–459, 2003 12611823

Govoni M, Bortoluzzi A, Padovan M, et al: The diagnosis and clinical management of the neuropsychiatric manifestations of lupus. J Autoimmun 74:41–72, 2016 27427403

Grant KM, LeVan TD, Wells SM, et al: Methamphetamine-associated psychosis. J Neuroimmune Pharmacol 7(1):113–139, 2012 21728034

Graus F, Titulaer MJ, Balu R, et al: A clinical approach to diagnosis of autoimmune encephalitis. Lancet Neurol 15(4):391–404, 2016 26906964

Greenberg DM, Lee JW: Psychotic manifestations of alcoholism. Curr Psychiatry Rep 3(4):314–318, 2001 11470038

Gresa-Arribas N, Titulaer MJ, Torrents A, et al: Antibody titres at diagnosis and during follow-up of anti-NMDA receptor encephalitis: a retrospective study. Lancet Neurol 13(2):167–177, 2014 24360484

Guaiana G, Markova I: Antipsychotic treatment improves outcome in herpes simplex encephalitis: a case report. J Neuropsychiatry Clin Neurosci 18(2):247, 2006 16720808

Gulsun M, Pinar M, Sabanci U: Psychotic disorder induced by oxybutynin: presentation of two cases. Clin Drug Investig 26(10):603–606, 2006 17163294

Harris MJ, Jeste DV, Gleghorn A, et al: New-onset psychosis in HIV-infected patients. J Clin Psychiatry 52(9):369–376, 1991 1894589

Heinrich TW, Grahm G: Hypothyroidism presenting as psychosis: myxedema madness revisited. Prim Care Companion J Clin Psychiatry 5(6):260–266, 2003 15213796

Hutto BR: Folate and cobalamin in psychiatric illness. Compr Psychiatry 38(6):305–314, 1997 9406735

Hynicka LM: Myxedema madness: a case for short-term antipsychotics? Ann Pharmacother 49(5):607–608, 2015 25870443

Imran M, Mahmood S: An overview of human prion diseases. Virol J 8:559, 2011 22196171

Isenberg-Grzeda E, Kutner HE, Nicolson SE: Wernicke-Korsakoff syndrome: under-recognized and under-treated. Psychosomatics 53(6):507–516, 2012 23157990

Kayser MS, Titulaer MJ, Gresa-Arribas N, et al: Frequency and characteristics of isolated psychiatric episodes in anti–N-methyl-d-aspartate receptor encephalitis. JAMA Neurol 70(9):1133–1139, 2013 23877059

Kennedy PG, Chaudhuri A: Herpes simplex encephalitis. J Neurol Neurosurg Psychiatry 73(3):237–238, 2002 12185148

Khandanpour N, Hoggard N, Connolly DJ: The role of MRI and CT of the brain in first episodes of psychosis. Clin Radiol 68(3):245–250, 2013 22959259

Kimura A, Kanoh Y, Sakurai T, et al: Antibodies in patients with neuropsychiatric systemic lupus erythematosus. Neurology 74(17):1372–1379, 2010 20421581

Kobrynski LJ, Sullivan KE: Velocardiofacial syndrome, DiGeorge syndrome: the chromosome 22q11.2 deletion syndromes. Lancet 370(9596):1443–1452, 2007 17950858

Koppel J, Greenwald BS: Optimal treatment of Alzheimer's disease psychosis: challenges and solutions. Neuropsychiatr Dis Treat 10:2253–2262, 2014 25473289

Kraemer M, Uekermann J, Wiltfang J, et al: Methylphenidate-induced psychosis in adult attention-deficit/hyperactivity disorder: report of 3 new cases and review of the literature. Clin Neuropharmacol 33(4):204–206, 2010 20571380

Kumar B: Acute intermittent porphyria presenting solely with psychosis: a case report and discussion. Psychosomatics 53(5):494–498, 2012 22902088

Kuppuswamy PS, Takala CR, Sola CL: Management of psychiatric symptoms in anti-NMDAR encephalitis: a case series, literature review and future directions. Gen Hosp Psychiatry 36(4):388–391, 2014 24731834

Landqvist Waldö M, Gustafson L, Passant U, et al: Psychotic symptoms in frontotemporal dementia: a diagnostic dilemma? Int Psychogeriatr 27(4):531–539, 2015 25486967

Lennox BR, Palmer-Cooper EC, Pollak T, et al: Prevalence and clinical characteristics of serum neuronal cell surface antibodies in first-episode psychosis: a case-control study. Lancet Psychiatry 4(1):42–48, 2017 27965002

Ma H, Huang Y, Cong Z, et al: The efficacy and safety of atypical antipsychotics for the treatment of dementia: a meta-analysis of randomized placebo-controlled trials. J Alzheimers Dis 42(3):915–937, 2014 25024323

Madhusoodanan S, Opler MG, Moise D, et al: Brain tumor location and psychiatric symptoms: is there any association? A meta-analysis of published case studies. Expert Rev Neurother 10(10):1529–1536, 2010 20925469

Madhusoodanan S, Ting MB, Farah T, Ugur U: Psychiatric aspects of brain tumors: a review. World J Psychiatry 5(3):273–285, 2015 26425442

Marrie RA, Reingold S, Cohen J, et al: The incidence and prevalence of psychiatric disorders in multiple sclerosis: a systematic review. Mult Scler 21(3):305–317, 2015 25583845

Martindale JL, Geschwind MD, Miller BL: Psychiatric and neuroimaging findings in Creutzfeldt-Jakob disease. Curr Psychiatry Rep 5(1):43–46, 2003 12686001

McKeith IG, Boeve BF, Dickson DW, et al: Diagnosis and management of dementia with Lewy bodies: fourth consensus report of the DLB Consortium. Neurology 89(1):88–100, 2017 28592453

Mirijello A, D'Angelo C, Ferrulli A, et al: Identification and management of alcohol withdrawal syndrome. Drugs 75(4):353–365, 2015 25666543

Moeller KE, Goswami R, Larsen LM: Myxedema madness rapidly reversed with levothyroxine. J Clin Psychiatry 70(11):1607–1608, 2009 20031108

Monks S, Niarchou M, Davies AR, et al: Further evidence for high rates of schizophrenia in 22q11.2 deletion syndrome. Schizophr Res 153(1–3):231–236, 2014 24534796

Murphy KC, Jones LA, Owen MJ: High rates of schizophrenia in adults with velo-cardio-facial syndrome. Arch Gen Psychiatry 56(10):940–945, 1999 10530637

Murray RM, Quigley H, Quattrone D, et al: Traditional marijuana, high-potency cannabis and synthetic cannabinoids: increasing risk for psychosis. World Psychiatry 15(3):195–204, 2016 27717258

Muzyk AJ, Christopher EJ, Gagliardi JP, et al: Use of aripiprazole in a patient with multiple sclerosis presenting with paranoid psychosis. J Psychiatr Pract 16(6):420–424, 2010 21107148

Owe-Larsson B, Säll L, Salamon E, et al: HIV infection and psychiatric illness. Afr J Psychiatry (Johannesbg) 12(2):115–128, 2009 19582313

Passie T, Halpern JH, Stichtenoth DO, et al: The pharmacology of lysergic acid diethylamide: a review. CNS Neurosci Ther 14(4):295–314, 2008 19040555

Pego-Reigosa JM, Isenberg DA: Psychosis due to systemic lupus erythematosus: characteristics and long-term outcome of this rare manifestation of the disease. Rheumatology (Oxford) 47(10):1498–1502, 2008 18658205

Perälä J, Kuoppasalmi K, Pirkola S, et al: Alcohol-induced psychotic disorder and delirium in the general population. Br J Psychiatry 197(3):200–206, 2010 20807964

Rabinstein AA: Herpes virus encephalitis in adults: current knowledge and old myths. Neurol Clin 35(4):695–705, 2017 28962808

Rahman S, Trimzi I, Centers N, et al: Neurosyphilis and organic psychosis. Del Ned J 83(10):313–315, 2011 22359842

Rasmussen SA, Rosebush PI, Smyth HS, et al: Cushing disease presenting as primary psychiatric illness: a case report and literature review. J Psychiatr Pract 21(6):449–457, 2015 26554329

Ravina B, Marder K, Fernandez HH, et al: Diagnostic criteria for psychosis in Parkinson's disease: report of an NINDS, NIMH work group. Mov Disord 22(8):1061–1068, 2007 17266092

Reus VI, Fochtmann LJ, Eyler AE, et al: The American Psychiatric Association practice guideline on the use of antipsychotics to treat agitation or psychosis in patients with dementia. Am J Psychiatry 173(5):543–546, 2016 27133416

Roncero C, Daigre C, Gonzalvo B, et al: Risk factors for cocaine-induced psychosis in cocaine-dependent patients. Eur Psychiatry 28(3):141–146, 2013 22118812

Roncero C, Daigre C, Grau-López L, et al: An international perspective and review of cocaine-induced psychosis: a call to action. Subst Abus 35(3):321–327, 2014 24927026

Ross DA, Cetas JS: Steroid psychosis: a review for neurosurgeons. J Neurooncol 109(3):439–447, 2012 22763760

Ross RG: Psychotic and manic-like symptoms during stimulant treatment of attention deficit hyperactivity disorder. Am J Psychiatry 163(7):1149–1152, 2006 16816217

Sachdev P: Schizophrenia-like psychosis and epilepsy: the status of the association. Am J Psychiatry 155(3):325–336, 1998 9501741

Salluh JI, Wang H, Schneider EB, et al: Outcome of delirium in critically ill patients: systematic review and meta-analysis. BMJ 350:h2538, 2015 26041151

Schneider LS, Dagerman KS, Insel P: Risk of death with atypical antipsychotic drug treatment for dementia: meta-analysis of randomized placebo-controlled trials. JAMA 294(15):1934–1943, 2005 16234500

Sciascia S, Bertolaccini ML, Roccatello D, et al: Autoantibodies involved in neuropsychiatric manifestations associated with systemic lupus erythematosus: a systematic review. J Neurol 261(9):1706–1714, 2014 24952022

Seltman RE, Matthews BR: Frontotemporal lobar degeneration: epidemiology, pathology, diagnosis and management. CNS Drugs 26(10):841–870, 2012 22950490

Shoptaw SJ, Kao U, Ling W: Treatment for amphetamine psychosis. Cochrane Database Syst Rev (1):CD003026, 2009 19160215

Silverman BC, Kim AY, Freudenreich O: Interferon-induced psychosis as a "psychiatric contraindication" to hepatitis C treatment: a review and case-based discussion. Psychosomatics 51(1):1–7, 2010 20118434

Singh D, Goodkin K: Choice of antipsychotic in HIV-infected patients. J Clin Psychiatry 68(3):479–480, 2007 17388720

Snowden JS, Rollinson S, Lafon C, et al: Psychosis, C9ORF72 and dementia with Lewy bodies. J Neurol Neurosurg Psychiatry 83(10):1031–1032, 2012 22832738

Spear J, Alderton D: Psychosis associated with prescribed dexamphetamine use. Aust N Z J Psychiatry 37(3):383, 2003 12780481

Spinelli E, Barnes AJ, Young S, et al: Performance characteristics of an ELISA screening assay for urinary synthetic cannabinoids. Drug Test Anal 7(6):467–474, 2015 25167963

Strassman RJ, Qualls CR, Uhlenhuth EH, et al: Dose-response study of N,N-dimethyltryptamine in humans, II: subjective effects and preliminary results of a new rating scale. Arch Gen Psychiatry 51(2):98–108, 1994 8297217

Sultzer DL, Davis SM, Tariot PN, et al: Clinical symptom responses to atypical antipsychotic medications in Alzheimer's disease: phase 1 outcomes from the CATIE-AD effectiveness trial. Am J Psychiatry 165(7):844–854, 2008 18519523

Tampi RR, Tampi DJ, Young JJ, et al: Evidence for using pimavanserin for the treatment of Parkinson's disease psychosis. World J Psychiatry 9(3):47–54, 2019 31211112

Titulaer MJ, McCracken L, Gabilondo I, et al: Treatment and prognostic factors for long-term outcome in patients with anti-NMDA receptor encephalitis: an observational cohort study. Lancet Neurol 12(2):157–165, 2013 23290630

Verachai V, Rukngan W, Chawanakrasaesin K, et al: Treatment of methamphetamine-induced psychosis: a double-blind randomized controlled trial comparing haloperidol and quetiapine. Psychopharmacology (Berl) 231(16):3099–3108, 2014 24535654

Wall CA, Rummans TA, Aksamit AJ, et al: Psychiatric manifestations of Creutzfeldt-Jakob disease: a 25-year analysis. J Neuropsychiatry Clin Neurosci 17(4):489–495, 2005 16387988

Wandinger KP, Saschenbrecker S, Stoecker W, et al: Anti-NMDA-receptor encephalitis: a severe, multistage, treatable disorder presenting with psychosis. J Neuroimmunol 231(1–2):86–91, 2011 20951441

Warren N, Siskind D, O'Gorman C: Refining the psychiatric syndrome of anti-N-methyl-d-aspartate receptor encephalitis. Acta Psychiatr Scand 138(5):401–408, 2018 29992532

Watkins CC, Treisman GJ: Neuropsychiatric complications of aging with HIV. J Neurovirol 18(4):277–290, 2012 22644745

Webster R, Holroyd S: Prevalence of psychotic symptoms in delirium. Psychosomatics 41(6):519–522, 2000 11110116

Wilcox RA, To T, Koukourou A, Frasca J: Hashimoto's encephalopathy masquerading as acute psychosis. J Clin Neurosci 15(11):1301–1304, 2008 18313925

Williamson PD, Spencer SS: Clinical and EEG features of complex partial seizures of extratemporal origin. Epilepsia 27 (suppl 2):S46–S63, 1986 3720713

Zahodne LB, Fernandez HH: Pathophysiology and treatment of psychosis in Parkinson's disease: a review. Drugs Aging 25(8):665–682, 2008 18665659

Zimbrean PC, Schilsky ML: Psychiatric aspects of Wilson disease: a review. Gen Hosp Psychiatry 36(1):53–62, 2014 24120023

Zimbrean PC, Schilsky ML: The spectrum of psychiatric symptoms in Wilson's disease: treatment and prognostic considerations. Am J Psychiatry 172(11):1068–1072, 2015 26575449

CHAPTER 18

Catatonia in the Medically Ill Patient

Scott R. Beach, M.D.
Gregory L. Fricchione, M.D.

Catatonia is a syndrome of motor, behavioral, and affective symptoms that can result from a variety of psychiatric and medical illnesses. Although classically conceptualized as a psychiatric disorder and frequently associated with mood disorders or schizophrenia spectrum disorders, up to half of all cases of catatonia may be caused by an underlying neuromedical etiology, and features of catatonia are not uncommon in older patients referred for psychiatric consultation (Jaimes-Albornoz and Serra-Mestres 2013). Physicians who care for patients with medical and neurological illnesses must be well versed in the diagnosis and treatment of catatonia and related syndromes in order to recognize subtle symptoms and signs and manage them effectively. In this chapter, we describe the syndrome of catatonia, review neuromedical causes, discuss the differential diagnosis and diagnostic assessment, provide evidence-based management and treatment recommendations, and consider related syndromes, including neuroleptic malignant syndrome and serotonin syndrome.

Phenomenology

Catatonia is best thought of as a syndrome or constellation of associated symptoms and signs rather than a specific diagnosis. From a motor perspective, patients with catatonia demonstrate features consistent with increased muscle tone (e.g., catalepsy). Behaviorally, patients engage in repetitive, perseverative speech and movements and are prone to becoming stuck and indecisive. Affectively, catatonia is accompanied by an intense sense of fear or anxiety.

All symptoms of catatonia occur on a spectrum; although physicians often picture extreme forms of a given symptom when they think of a catatonic patient, symptoms often take much subtler forms. For example, mutism may be represented by the complete absence of speech but also may manifest as decreased speech production, reduced volume of voice, increased latency, or an odd speech pattern in which the volume trails off at the end. Some symptoms of catatonia may have overlapping presentations; for example, the patient who resists having his eyes manually opened by the examiner is almost certainly exhibiting negativism but also may be demonstrating *Gegenhalten* (Table 18–1).

The exact definition of catatonia remains controversial. According to the fifth edition of the *Diagnostic and Statistical Manual of Mental Disorders* (DSM-5; American Psychiatric Association 2013), catatonia is defined by the presence of 3 or more of 12 symptoms and can be further classified as catatonia associated with another mental disorder, catatonic disorder due to another medical condition, or unspecified catatonia. By contrast, the Bush-Francis Catatonia Rating Scale (BFCRS; see Table 18–1), the instrument most widely used to diagnose and assess the severity of catatonia, requires the presence of only 2 of 14 symptoms for diagnosis and lists 23 symptoms for rating severity (Bush et al. 1996). Some researchers have contended that even one cardinal symptom has as much diagnostic utility as the presence of three or more of such symptoms (Taylor 1990).

Subtypes

When told that a patient may have features of catatonia, most clinicians picture hypoactive, or stuporous catatonia, characterized by immobility, mutism, staring, catalepsy, and waxy flexibility. This most common subtype of catatonia causes patients to appear "slowed down." However, some patients exhibit hyperactive, or excited catatonia, displaying impulsivity, frenzied movements, increased speech marked by echolalia or verbigeration, and repetitive movements including stereotypies and mannerisms. This excessive motor activity may be misdiagnosed as mania, psychosis, or hyperactive delirium. A subset of patients with excited catatonia may also have delirious mania. A small subset of patients may alternate between stuporous and excited catatonia in a recurrent cycle, typically starting in adolescence. Historically described as periodic catatonia and particularly challenging to treat, this pattern has a chronic course, often with residual symptoms between discrete episodes. Finally, some patients display a malignant or lethal catatonia, accompanied by severe muscle rigidity, elevated creatine phosphokinase (CPK), hyperthermia, or autonomic instability. Malignant features can be seen in either the stuporous or the excited variant and often constitute a psychiatric emergency requiring immediate treatment to prevent morbidity and mortality. Neuroleptic malignant syndrome is a subtype of malignant catatonia.

Etiologies

Neuromedical etiologies of catatonia should be considered early in the assessment. Catatonia is too frequently assumed to be psychiatric or behavioral in nature, with the result that a thorough medical workup is not pursued. In a focused review of the lit-

TABLE 18–1. **Symptoms and signs of catatonia: the Bush-Francis Catatonia Rating Scale**

Symptom or sign	Description
1. Excitement/agitation	Constant non-goal-directed movement, not influenced by external stimuli or attributed to akathisia
2. Immobility/stupor	Slowed or absent movement; minimal response
3. Mutism	Reduced or absent speech output, markedly slowed speech, or marked reduction of volume of speech
4. Staring	Fixed gaze or decreased blink rate
5. Catalepsy/posturing	Spontaneous maintenance of posture, including mundane
6. Grimacing	Maintenance of or repeated odd facial expressions, often conveying discomfort
7. Echopraxia/echolalia	Mimicking of others' movements or speech
8. Stereotypy	Repetitive, non-goal-directed motor activity
9. Mannerisms	Repetitive purposeful movements done in odd or bizarre manner
10. Verbigeration	Nonpurposeful repetition of the patient's own words
11. Rigidity	Maintenance of a rigid position despite efforts to be moved; increased muscle tone
12. Negativism	Apparently motiveless resistance or opposition to instructions or external stimuli
13. Waxy flexibility	Initial resistance before acceptance of repositioning, with slowed return to original position
14. Withdrawal	Refusal to eat, drink, or make eye contact
15. Impulsivity	Sudden inappropriate behaviors without provocation
16. Automatic obedience	Exaggerated cooperation with the examiner's request, including potentially painful ones
17. *Mitgehen*	Arm raising in response to light pressure, despite instructions to the contrary
18. *Gegenhalten*	Resistance to passive movement proportional to the strength of the stimulus
19. Ambitendency	The appearance of being "stuck" in indecisive, hesitant movement in the setting of contradictory commands
20. Grasp reflex	Involuntarily grasping of fingers when palm is stroked
21. Perseveration	Repetition of speech or movements
22. Combativeness	Aggression toward others in an undirected, often purposeless manner
23. Autonomic abnormality	Abnormal temperature, pulse, respiratory rate, or blood pressure; diaphoresis

Note. The presence of 2 or more of the first 14 items for at least 24 hours reaches the threshold for catatonia. The severity score is determined by rating each of the 23 items on a scale of 0–3.
Source. Modified from Bush et al. 1996.

erature examining the proportion of catatonia cases attributable to medical etiologies in various hospital settings (including psychiatric units), medical causes were found in 20% of cases across all general hospital settings and in more than 50% of cases in acute medical and surgical settings (Oldham 2018). The most frequent causes were central nervous system (CNS) inflammation, most typically encephalitis, neurological injury or structural CNS pathology, epilepsy, or toxin or medication effects.

Substance-Related Causes

Substances, both illicit and prescribed, should be considered as a possible etiology in all cases of catatonia (Table 18–2). Intoxication with phencyclidine, ecstasy, and (more recently) cathinones ("bath salts") has been linked to excited catatonia. Synthetic marijuana has been described as causing stuporous catatonia (Khan et al. 2016). Withdrawal from alcohol or benzodiazepines represents another significant risk factor for the development of catatonia. Acute cessation of illicit drugs with strong dopaminergic activity (e.g., cocaine, methamphetamine) also has been linked to catatonia.

Among prescribed medications, those leading to decreased dopamine levels carry the highest risk of catatonia. Dopamine antagonists—including all antipsychotics as well as the antiemetics metoclopramide and prochlorperazine—are frequently associated with catatonia. These medications can trigger malignant catatonia or neuroleptic malignant syndrome and can also cause nonmalignant catatonia, which may be more difficult to recognize. Use of medications that deplete dopamine (e.g., tetrabenazine) or abrupt cessation of prodopaminergic medications (e.g., bupropion, pramipexole, ropinirole) also may lead to the development of catatonia. Somewhat paradoxically, abrupt cessation of clozapine, in addition to causing a rebound psychosis, can lead to a rapidly developing catatonia (Bastiampillai et al. 2009).

Tacrolimus has been associated with several cases of catatonia, usually, although not always, occurring in the setting of elevated serum levels (Chopra et al. 2012). Disulfiram and baclofen also have been implicated in several reports (Pauker and Brown 1986; Weddington et al. 1980). Other medications that may carry risk for inducing catatonia are dexamethasone, pegylated interferon alfa-2b, ribavirin, cyclosporine, and certain antibiotics (including macrolides and fluoroquinolones).

Neurological Causes

Catatonia has been linked to multiple neuromedical etiologies (Table 18–3). CNS neoplasms and cerebrovascular accidents—particularly those occurring in the basal ganglia, medial temporal lobe, posterior parietal cortex, and cerebellum—can cause catatonic syndromes (Fishman et al. 2017). However, focal neurological injuries involving the same regions do not consistently cause catatonia, suggesting that such injuries may function as contributors in a cumulative risk model. Catatonia also may occur in the setting of traumatic or anoxic brain injury and may be particularly challenging to treat in those circumstances (Quinn and Abbott 2014). Posterior reversible encephalopathy syndrome and multiple sclerosis have been described as causative in several case reports (Klingensmith et al. 2017; Mendez 1999; Spiegel and Varnell 2011). Wernicke's encephalopathy is increasingly being recognized as a potential etiology of catatonia (Oldham 2018). Systemic lupus erythematosus has been linked to catatonia in dozens of cases, not all of which have shown evidence of lupus cerebritis (Grover et al. 2013).

CNS infections can potentially cause catatonia. Classically, patients with viral encephalitides (e.g., those caused by the herpes virus) or bacterial meningoencephaliti-

TABLE 18–2.	Substance-related causes of catatonia
Use of medications	**Abrupt cessation of medications**
Typical antipsychotics	Carbidopa-levodopa
Atypical antipsychotics	Pramipexole
Tricyclic antidepressants	Cabergoline
Monoamine oxidase inhibitors	Bromocriptine
Metoclopramide	Ropinirole
Prochlorperazine	Bupropion
Promethazine	Amantadine
Tetrabenazine	Benzodiazepines
Carbamazepine	Barbiturates
Primidone	Stimulants
Aspirin	
Disulfiram	**Intoxication with substances**
Baclofen	Mescaline
Macrolides	Phencyclidine
Fluoroquinolones	Lysergic acid diethylamide
Steroids	Cathinones
Tacrolimus	Synthetic cannabinoids
Cyclosporine	
Dexamethasone	**Withdrawal from substances**
Interferon	Alcohol
Ribavirin	Cannabinoids
Lithium	Amphetamines
Morphine	Cocaine

des were described as exhibiting signs of catatonia (Ryali et al. 2017; Saini et al. 2013). Over the past decade, autoimmune, infectious, and paraneoplastic limbic encephalitides have come to be recognized as one of the most frequent causes of catatonia, particularly in children and adolescents (Espinola-Nadurille et al. 2019; Oldham 2018). In fact, *N*-methyl-D-aspartate (NMDA) receptor antibody–related encephalitis (anti-NMDA receptor encephalitis) is now considered by some to represent a prototypical catatonia syndrome (Espinola-Nadurille et al. 2019). The typical course begins as a viral-like illness, with headache, upper respiratory and gastrointestinal symptoms, and fever lasting up to 2 weeks. Anxiety commonly follows, often with new-onset panic attacks, leading many patients to seek psychiatric treatment. Catatonic symptoms emerge later in the course, frequently accompanied by delirium, psychosis, behavioral disturbances, autonomic instability, and seizures (Kruse et al. 2014).

Several neurological illnesses with a strong genetic basis, particularly those causing autism spectrum disorder or intellectual disability, also are highly associated with catatonic features. Prader-Willi syndrome, a genetic disorder due to lack of gene expression from paternal chromosome 15q11–q13, is highly associated with catatonia (Dhossche et al. 2005). Catatonia also has been associated with fragile X and DiGeorge syndromes.

TABLE 18–3.   **Neuromedical etiologies of catatonia**

Neurological causes	
AIDS	Multiple sclerosis
Alzheimer's disease	Paraneoplastic/autoimmune limbic encephalitis
Anoxic brain injury	Parkinson's disease
Bacterial meningoencephalitis	Postencephalitic states
Central nervous system neoplasm	Posterior reversible encephalopathy syndrome
Cerebellar degeneration	Progressive multifocal leukoencephalopathy
Cerebromacular degeneration	Seizure disorder
Cerebrovascular accident	Subacute sclerosing panencephalitis
Creutzfeldt-Jakob disease	Syphilis
Dementia with Lewy bodies	Traumatic brain injury
Frontotemporal dementia	Tuberous sclerosis
Huntington's disease	Viral encephalitides
Hydrocephalus	Wernicke's encephalopathy
Malaria	

General medical causes	
Acute intermittent porphyria	Idiopathic hyperadrenergic state
Addison's disease	Iron deficiency anemia
Bacterial sepsis	Mononucleosis
Cushing's disease	Pellagra
Delirium	Systemic lupus erythematosus
Diabetic ketoacidosis	Thrombocytopenic purpura
Glucose-6-phosphate dehydrogenase deficiency	Tuberculosis
	Typhoid fever
Hepatic dysfunction	Uremia
Hereditary coproporphyria	Vitamin B_{12} deficiency
Homocystinuria	Viral hepatitis
Hyperparathyroidism	Wilson's disease

General Medical Causes

Deficiency syndromes of several vitamins, including niacin (pellagra) and vitamin B_{12}, have been linked to catatonia. Iron deficiency is a significant risk factor not only for development of catatonia but also for development of malignant features in a patient who is already catatonic (Carroll and Goforth 1995). Glucose-6-phosphate dehydrogenase deficiency appears to confer a vulnerability to catatonia. Endocrinological abnormalities that have been associated with catatonia include Cushing's disease, Addison's disease, and hyperparathyroidism. Other systemic illnesses, including Wilson's disease and acute intermittent porphyria, also have been described as causes of catatonia.

Of particular importance to consultation psychiatrists is the relationship between catatonia and delirium. According to DSM-5, the presence of delirium precludes a diagnosis of catatonia, and catatonia cannot be diagnosed if the disturbance occurs exclusively in the context of delirium (American Psychiatric Association 2013). In clinical practice, the relationship between the two conditions is far more complicated, and there is no obvious empirical basis for this exclusion. In fact, catatonic features— most commonly mutism, posturing, withdrawal, and immobility—are common in delirium; in one study, such features were observed in 37% of delirious patients (Francis and Lopez-Canino 2009). Furthermore, delirium is very frequently comorbid with catatonia when there is a neuromedical etiology (Oldham and Lee 2015). Delirious patients who manifest catatonia are more likely to be female and to have the hypoactive form of delirium (Grover et al. 2014). The diagnostic and therapeutic implications of this overlap warrant further study.

Differential Diagnosis

The differential diagnosis of catatonia involves relatively few conditions but includes several entities whose exclusion is important (Table 18–4). Malignant hyperthermia, a severe adverse reaction to certain anesthetics (e.g., halothane, sevoflurane), can cause a clinical syndrome that appears nearly identical to malignant catatonia or neuroleptic malignant syndrome, with rigidity, fever, autonomic instability, and elevated CPK. A review of administered medications and the timing of administration relative to the onset of symptoms will likely lead to identification of the cause. Additionally, malignant hyperthermia tends to develop over minutes to hours, whereas malignant catatonia develops over hours to days (Keck et al. 1995).

Locked-in syndrome may manifest with mutism, immobility, and increased muscle tone. This syndrome can be caused by lesions in the midbrain or pons, or by overly rapid repletion of sodium in a patient with hyponatremia, leading to osmotic demyelination syndrome. One distinguishing feature of locked-in syndrome is preservation of eye movements, with patients demonstrating the ability to track the movements of others and to communicate by means of eye movements or blinking. This behavior is distinct from behavior seen in catatonia, in which most patients do not attempt to communicate and often do not track individuals who are present, but instead stare straight ahead. Neuroimaging may be useful in revealing a lesion consistent with locked-in syndrome (Beach and Stern 2011).

Minimally conscious and persistent vegetative states, often caused by diffuse cortical damage, are characterized by lack of alertness, absence of speech output, and lack of purposeful motor responses. Occasionally, patients in these states will exhibit cycles of eye opening and closure. Isolated reports of awakenings with zolpidem, an agent that has also shown some benefit in relieving catatonia, raise questions about the diagnosis in some cases (Georgiopoulos et al. 2010).

Akinetic mutism is a neurological syndrome occurring in the setting of a defined lesion, typically a cerebrovascular or space-occupying lesion involving damage to the frontal lobe, basal ganglia, or mesencephalothalamic regions (Nagaratnam et al. 2004). Patients show a lack of responsiveness, with a deficit in spontaneous initiation of voluntary movements and speech in spite of preserved awareness. Akinetic mutism is thought to be on a spectrum with abulia and amotivational syndrome. It has many features in common with catatonia, and some researchers consider it to be a related syndrome. For example, both patients with catatonia and patients with akinetic

TABLE 18–4.	Differential diagnosis of catatonia	
Malignant hyperthermia	Seizure
Locked-in syndrome	Parkinsonism
Minimally conscious and persistent vegetative states	Factitious disorder
Akinetic mutism	Malingering

mutism may exhibit the "telephone sign" (i.e., they are mute when attempts are made to engage them in a face-to-face conversation, but when a telephone rings at bedside, they pick up the phone and carry on a perfectly normal conversation). Akinetic mutism is somewhat distinct from catatonia in that patients tend to lack certain affective and behavioral components that are common in catatonia (e.g., intense fear; repetitive, purposeless behaviors) and are less likely to show catalepsy and waxy flexibility. Dopaminergic agents (e.g., amantadine) can be helpful for akinetic mutism (Arciniegas et al. 2004).

Patients in nonconvulsive complex partial status epilepticus exhibit repetitive behaviors and speech and increased muscle tone and thus resemble catatonic patients in some respects. In addition, catatonia may emerge as both an ictal and a postictal phenomenon. If the clinical history or the presence of impaired consciousness or aura suggests seizures, electroencephalography (EEG) may be useful. Patients with epilepsy do not recall their seizures, whereas patients with catatonia typically remember being in that state. Some researchers have even speculated that catatonia may be a form of limbic epilepsy, with subtle ictal events in the prefrontal cortex and the basal ganglia causing the symptoms and signs of the catatonic syndrome (Fink and Taylor 2009). Proponents of this hypothesis point out that the treatments—including benzodiazepines, anticonvulsants, and electroconvulsive therapy (ECT)—for the two conditions are the same.

Patients with parkinsonism, whether due to medication or to idiopathic Parkinson's disease, demonstrate features that overlap with catatonia, including immobility, ambitendency, and rigidity. The rigidity of parkinsonism is typically of a cogwheel nature, with a superimposed resting tremor, as opposed to the *Gegenhalten* of catatonia. Although patients with parkinsonism may exhibit posturing, they rarely hold their limbs in raised positions for extended periods of time. Parkinson's disease is slowly progressive, and most patients do not exhibit features of catatonia until the disease's latter stages.

Finally, some patients may feign catatonic symptoms, either consciously (as in the case of malingering or factitious disorder) or unconsciously (as in the case of conversion disorder). One example occasionally seen by emergency personnel is that of a prisoner pretending to be unresponsive in order to be taken to the hospital. Given the lay public's lack of familiarity with catatonia, many such cases are detected because of inconsistencies in presentation. In extreme cases, in which the patient is suspected of feigning but the examination findings are equivocal, the late senior psychiatrist at Massachusetts General Hospital, George B. Murray, S.J., M.D., advocated initiating a loud conversation at the bedside regarding the possible need for an extreme procedure (e.g., vigorous palpation of the testes), noting that such a discussion often proves diagnostic if the patient decides that the risk of continued manipulation is too great.

As a caveat, because of the sometimes-fluctuating nature of catatonia and the bizarre symptoms associated with the syndrome, it is not uncommon for physicians and nurses who are unfamiliar with catatonia to believe that a genuinely catatonic patient is "playing possum" and feigning the behavior.

Diagnosis

The evaluation of catatonia should be targeted toward both ruling out other entities on the differential diagnosis and determining the etiology of the catatonic syndrome. In ruling out potential mimics of catatonia, magnetic resonance imaging (MRI) and EEG are likely to have the highest yield. Once the diagnosis of catatonia is made and the patient has been examined with a standardized assessment instrument (e.g., the BFCRS [see Table 18–1]), further tests may be ordered to determine the etiology of the catatonia. Standard laboratory tests useful for this purpose include a metabolic panel, a complete blood count, and serum and urine toxicologies (see Chapter 5, "Toxicological Exposures and Nutritional Deficiencies in the Psychiatric Patient"). CPK levels should be ordered for all patients with catatonia to monitor for the emergence of malignant catatonia. Iron studies are recommended for all patients, given that low serum iron represents a risk factor for catatonia and for development of malignant catatonia (Carroll and Goforth 1995). Depending on clinical suspicion, other studies might also be done, such as an infectious disease workup (HIV antibody and rapid plasma reagin testing) and an autoimmune screening (i.e., erythrocyte sedimentation rate, C-reactive protein, antinuclear antibodies, paraneoplastic panel). Finally, in addition to helping to rule out other syndromes, EEG may point to a neuromedical etiology if it demonstrates diffuse background slowing consistent with delirium.

When catatonic symptoms are associated with delirium and vital sign changes, limbic encephalitis must be considered as a potential cause. In such cases, MRI may show enhancement in the limbic regions but is often normal (Ali et al. 2008). The clinician should strongly consider cerebrospinal fluid analysis rather than peripheral blood screening for detection of paraneoplastic antibodies, because absence of antibodies in the cerebrospinal fluid is the only way to rule out this potential etiology. If suspicion for limbic encephalitis is high and abdominal and pelvic imaging do not reveal a tumor, consideration should be given to full-body positron emission tomography to locate a possible tumor.

Pathophysiology

The pathophysiology of catatonia is complex and involves multiple brain regions and neurotransmitter systems. Although early work took a top-down approach to understanding the mechanistic underpinnings, more recent work suggests that a bottom-up approach is equally important (Fricchione 2002). Attention has largely been directed toward the basal ganglia–thalamocortical loop systems. Various symptoms of catatonia align with dysfunction in components of these circuits; for example, mutism is likely related to disruption of the anterior cingulate–medial orbitofrontal circuit, whereas repetitive behaviors likely reflect dysfunction in the lateral orbitofrontal circuit (Caroff et al. 2007). From a neurotransmitter perspective, catatonia appears to represent a state of hypodopaminergia in these circuits, with reduced dopamine flow in the medial forebrain bundle, nigrostriatal tract, and tuberoinfundibular tract. This hypodopaminergic state is consistent with the role of dopamine-blocking agents in causing catatonia. Reduced γ-aminobutyric acid (GABA) receptor subtype A (GABA$_A$) inhibition of GABA receptor subtype B (GABA$_B$) interneurons in the substantia nigra and ventral tegmental area interneurons may lead to reduced dopamine activity in the dorsal and ventral striatum and paralimbic cortex. This reduced GABA$_A$ activity is supported by the observations that GABA$_A$ receptor agonists (e.g., benzodiazepines) improve catatonia and that catatonic patients can tolerate high doses of these medications without experiencing sedation. Reduced GABA$_A$ receptor inhibition of frontal corticostriatal tracts also may lead to NMDA changes in the ventral and dorsal striata; these changes may account for the beneficial effects of the NMDA receptor antagonists memantine and amantadine in catatonia. The contribution of serotonergic excess to catatonia is less well-defined than the relative contributions of other chemical pathways.

Management and Treatment

In cases of catatonia secondary to neuromedical etiologies, primary treatment should be targeted toward the underlying etiology. Catatonia due to clozapine withdrawal, for example, is best treated with reinstitution of clozapine (Hung et al. 2006). Similarly, the literature contains many cases of catatonia due to systemic lupus erythematosus that were treated successfully with steroids or anti-inflammatory agents and of catatonia due to posterior reversible encephalopathy syndrome that were treated by normalization of blood pressure (Grover et al. 2013).

In many cases of secondary catatonia, the catatonia will not fully resolve or will continue to recur until the underlying illness is addressed. This persistence in the absence of treatment of the underlying illness appears to be especially relevant in cases of catatonia due to paraneoplastic limbic encephalitis, although ECT has been used with success in such cases (Jones et al. 2015). If a causative tumor is present, its removal is often curative, and immunosuppressive therapies also are commonly used to treat paraneoplastic limbic encephalitis.

Although primary treatment should be directed toward the underlying cause, efforts should be made to treat the symptoms of catatonia with traditional approaches. In cases in which treatment of the underlying etiology must be delayed, benzodiazepines and ECT can reduce symptoms remarkably. Even in situations in which catatonia is due to a fixed lesion in the brain, benzodiazepines and ECT can lead to significant improvement. One study demonstrated that 8 of 12 patients with catatonia due to a CNS abnormality responded to treatment with lorazepam (Rosebush et al. 1990).

Benzodiazepines

Regardless of the cause of the catatonia, benzodiazepines should be used to reverse the symptoms. Intravenous lorazepam is generally preferred over other agents and routes of administration because of its ease of administration, quick onset of action, and longer effective duration of action (Greenblatt and Shader 1978). Despite having a shorter elimination half-life than some other benzodiazepines, lorazepam administered intravenously has a longer duration of effective clinical activity because tissue distribution is less rapid and extensive, making more of the drug available at the $GABA_A$ receptor, to which lorazepam preferentially binds. If intravenous access is unavailable, intramuscular or sublingual routes are preferred over oral administration, although repeated intramuscular administration may exacerbate the patient's fear response. A dose of 2 mg is generally recommended as a *challenge* or test dose so as to avoid an equivocal response. Although patients with catatonia have a higher threshold for sedation with benzodiazepines, sedation following a challenge dose of lorazepam does not rule out catatonia, because patients may later awaken with improvement in their symptoms.

Once a positive response to lorazepam has been established, or if suspicion for the diagnosis remains high despite a negative response, lorazepam should be instituted in a standing regimen, generally at a dosage of 2 mg every 6–8 hours (Fricchione et al. 2018). Because catatonia has a very high likelihood of recurrence as lorazepam wears off, nursing staff should be instructed to administer the scheduled medication dose even if the patient is asleep and to hold the dose only if signs of respiratory depression are present. Regular doses of lorazepam generally maintain the therapeutic effect, and standing benzodiazepines are recommended for at least the first 24–48 hours. If improvement is significant over that time, consideration can be given to a slow taper of benzodiazepines, on the order of a 10%–25% decrease in the total daily dosage each day (Fricchione et al. 2018). Maintenance benzodiazepines should be considered in all cases of catatonia but may be particularly important when a neuromedical etiology exists, because the underlying illness may cause an ongoing vulnerability. If lorazepam does not produce improvement within 5 days or if symptoms of malignant catatonia emerge, ECT should be considered.

Electroconvulsive Therapy

ECT remains the definitive treatment for catatonia and should be considered when lorazepam fails to achieve full resolution of symptoms. ECT is successful in up to 90% of cases of catatonia, with most patients showing some response after the first two or three treatment sessions (Leroy et al. 2018). A course of 4–6 sessions is typically sufficient to mitigate the risk of relapse, although some patients require up to 20 sessions. No absolute medical contraindications to ECT exist, and patients with symptoms due to neuromedical etiologies frequently experience substantial benefit from ECT. The safety of ECT has been demonstrated as early as 4 weeks after a cerebrovascular accident and in patients with increased intracranial pressure, provided that appropriate pretreatment and consultations are pursued (Murray et al. 1986). Cases of catatonia associated with anti-NMDA receptor encephalitis have been successfully treated with ECT, both as monotherapy and as an adjunct to immune-targeted therapies (Jones et al. 2015).

Other Agents (Third-Line Treatments)

Other agents are increasingly being used to treat catatonia, and these alternatives may have particular utility in cases with neuromedical causes. Antiglutamatergic agents, including memantine and amantadine, are the most widely used alternative agents, and there are several case reports of their use in nonpsychiatric etiologies (Carroll et al. 2007). These agents may be particularly beneficial in cases of catatonia comorbid with delirium, given that antipsychotics used to treat delirium may worsen catatonia, and benzodiazepines used to treat catatonia may worsen delirium. In contrast, memantine and amantadine may treat catatonia effectively without leading to worsened cognition. Carbamazepine (Kritzinger and Jordaan 2001) and olanzapine (Spiegel and Klaiber 2013) each have been reported to be effective in treating catatonia with a neuromedical etiology. Caution should be used when administering atypical antipsychotics to patients with catatonia, given the potential risk for worsening of catatonic features or transitioning to malignant catatonia. Atypical antipsychotics of relatively lower potency (e.g., olanzapine, aripiprazole) are preferred and should always be combined with benzodiazepines to minimize risk.

Prognosis and Complications

The prognosis for catatonia is generally good; most patients recover with treatment over a period of days to weeks. Patients with an acute onset, a symptom duration of less than 1 month, a diagnosis of depression, or a family history of depression have a better prognosis (Carroll et al. 2007). The prognosis tends to be more variable, however, for patients with neuromedical etiologies, depending largely on the prognosis of the underlying cause. Cases of malignant catatonia tend to have a worse prognosis and frequently require more aggressive treatment.

Because of the immobility frequently associated with catatonia, potential complications are myriad (Philbrick and Rummans 1994). Among these, respiratory infections and deep vein thrombosis are two of the more commonly encountered complications, and steps should be taken to guard against them, particularly in medically ill patients.

Related Syndromes

Neuroleptic Malignant Syndrome

Neuroleptic malignant syndrome (NMS) is a form of malignant catatonia that by definition is caused either by the administration of an antidopaminergic agent or by the abrupt cessation of a prodopaminergic agent. As with other malignant catatonias, patients with NMS exhibit features of catatonia accompanied by severe muscle rigidity, fever, autonomic instability, and elevated CPK. Most commonly, NMS develops over a few days, often beginning with rigidity and mental status changes followed by signs of hypermetabolism. Various criteria for NMS have been proposed over the years, but the 2011 International Expert Consensus (IEC) diagnostic criteria, which emphasize rigidity, hyperthermia, mental status changes, and elevated CPK (at least four times the upper limit of normal), are currently the most widely accepted (Gurrera et al. 2011; 2017).

Risk factors for NMS include a history of catatonia or NMS, male sex and young age, presence of dehydration, and use of a high-potency antipsychotic (Gurrera 2017). Basal ganglia disorders are thought to enhance risk, and patients with low serum iron in the context of catatonia may be at increased risk for NMS if given dopamine antagonist medications.

NMS can occur with the use of atypical antipsychotics. Although some researchers have suggested that NMS associated with atypical antipsychotic use may lack common core features, the vast majority of patients with NMS caused by such use will present with all of the typical features of NMS (Trollor et al. 2009). In comparison with patients with NMS due to other agents, patients with clozapine-induced NMS may be less likely to exhibit rigidity, and patients with NMS secondary to aripiprazole may have a less severe fever (Belvederi Murri et al. 2015). Many cases of atypical antipsychotic–induced NMS reported in the literature are likely cases of nonmalignant catatonia.

Treatment of NMS relies on cessation of the offending agent (in use-related cases) or reinstitution of the prodopaminergic agent (in cases caused by abrupt cessation). High-dose benzodiazepines should be administered to reduce rigidity and to treat associated symptoms of catatonia. The syndrome's course is usually self-limited, lasting days to weeks after dopamine antagonists have been stopped and supportive measures have been instituted. ECT is frequently required in cases of NMS, is often curative, and should be considered very early in the course. Persistent cases of NMS are usually secondary to the use of depot antipsychotics, and ECT is highly effective in these cases. Although bromocriptine is a theoretical treatment for NMS because of its dopamine agonism, the efficacy of this agent is disputed, and it significantly increases the risk for emerging or worsening psychosis; therefore, bromocriptine should be used sparingly and with caution (Rosebush et al. 1991). NMS continues to carry a mortality risk of approximately 6%; acute respiratory failure appears to be the strongest predictor of mortality in patients with NMS (Modi et al. 2016).

Rechallenging a patient who has experienced NMS with an antipsychotic carries a significant risk for NMS recurrence but is sometimes necessary. Recommendations (Pelonero et al. 1985) suggest that antipsychotics should not be restarted until at least 2 weeks after the episode of NMS has resolved and that rechallenge should be with an agent of lower potency than the one that caused the episode.

Serotonin Syndrome

Patients with serotonin syndrome commonly present with symptoms and signs of serotonergic excess, including tremor, hyperreflexia, clonus, mydriasis, increased bowel sounds, delirium, diaphoresis, and tachycardia. The syndrome ranges from mild to severe, with mildly affected patients showing restlessness, tremor, tachycardia, shivering, diaphoresis, and mild hyperreflexia. Patients with moderately severe symptoms show tachycardia, hypertension, and fever (sometimes as high as 40°C [104°F]). Patients with serotonin syndrome will also display symptoms of catatonia, which can manifest as either stupor or excitement. Serotonergic excess may lead to downstream dopamine depletion in certain brain regions, which could lead to the emergence of catatonia.

Historically, the most common cause of serotonin syndrome was use of a monoamine oxidase inhibitor (MAOI) in combination with another serotonergic medication. In recent years, cases occur far more frequently in the setting of polypharmacy with multiple serotonergic agents or overdose on serotonergic agents. It is estimated that about 15% of patients who overdose on selective serotonin reuptake inhibitors develop serotonin syndrome (Isbister et al. 2004). Although most providers recognize that antidepressants have strong serotonergic properties, they may not be aware that many other agents and classes of medications, including lithium, tramadol, and atypical antipsychotics, also act on serotonergic receptors.

Two sets of diagnostic criteria for serotonin syndrome have been proposed: the Sternbach criteria and the Hunter criteria. The Sternbach criteria are less specific, requiring the presence of 3 out of 10 symptoms (mental status changes, agitation, myoclonus, hyperreflexia, diaphoresis, hyperthermia, shivering, tremor, diarrhea, and incoordination), many of which overlap with symptoms of other toxidromes, including sympathomimetic excess and anticholinergic toxicity (Sternbach 1991). The Hunter criteria are more specific, providing an algorithm for diagnosis based on one sign or a combination of signs (Dunkley et al. 2003). Although more widely accepted than the Sternbach criteria, the Hunter criteria may miss cases of mild to moderate serotonin syndrome because of their lower sensitivity.

Leukocytosis, rhabdomyolysis, and liver function test abnormalities all have been reported in patients with serotonin syndrome. Notably, certain secreting tumors (e.g., carcinoid tumor; small-cell carcinoma) have been associated with serotonin syndrome, and imaging of the chest and abdomen may sometimes be helpful in the workup.

Following recognition and removal of the offending agents, treatment of serotonin syndrome is largely supportive. Most cases resolve within 24 hours. Supportive measures can be used to prevent complications. For example, antipyretics and cooling blankets can reduce hyperthermia; intravenous hydration may prevent renal failure; and antihypertensive agents can help correct elevated blood pressure. Dantrolene was classically recommended for its muscle-relaxant properties, but benzodiazepines often work equally well, reduce mortality, and have the added bonus of treating any catatonic features that may be present. Physical restraints should be avoided if possible, because muscle stress can lead to lactic acidosis and elevated temperature. Cyproheptadine, a serotonin antagonist, is sometimes used to treat serotonin syndrome but often is not needed, because most cases resolve with proper hydration in a matter of days. Although prognosis is generally good, potential complications can include disseminated intravascular coagulation, generalized seizures, and acute kidney injury secondary to myoglobinuria.

Because of the potential risk for serotonin syndrome associated with use of an MAOI in combination with any other medicine with serotonergic properties, a 2-week washout interval after discontinuation of an MAOI is required before starting any serotonergic medication. In the case of discontinuation of fluoxetine, which has a very long half-life, the washout period should be at least 5 weeks.

Delirious Mania

Delirious mania is a somewhat controversial syndrome that overlaps significantly with excited catatonia and is commonly described as occurring mainly in young women (Karmacharya et al. 2008). Patients with this syndrome exhibit features of mania that begin abruptly and wax and wane over the course of hours to days, co-occurring with elements of delirium, including inattention, disorientation, and executive dysfunction (Jacobowski et al. 2013). Other commonly described features include an obsession with water, inappropriate toileting, and disrobing (Karmacharya et al.

2008). Many patients with delirious mania also exhibit features of excited catatonia, including excitement, verbigeration, stereotypies, and mannerisms. For this reason, some clinicians consider delirious mania to be a subtype of excited catatonia, whereas others argue that it represents a separate entity that occasionally includes catatonic features (Fink and Taylor 2001). Patients with delirious mania often exhibit malignant features, and this presentation is thus considered to be a psychiatric emergency, with high rates of complications and death. Lithium and dopamine antagonists may worsen the catatonic symptoms and lead to NMS. Treatment relies on high-dose benzodiazepines and often ECT. Although most patients with delirious mania have bipolar disorder, cases caused by neuromedical illness have been described (Washinsky and Quinn 2013).

Conclusion

It is important for clinicians to be aware of the varied presentations of catatonia and the potential influences of neuromedical illness on the development and course of the syndrome. As many as half of cases of catatonia seen in the general hospital setting may have a nonpsychiatric cause. A variety of illnesses may mimic catatonia, and an even greater number of maladies have been etiologically associated with the syndrome. Although much is still unknown about the pathophysiology of catatonia, an awareness of the underlying cause and any comorbidities present may be helpful in guiding treatment choices. Clinicians should also be on the lookout for related syndromes, such as NMS, serotonin syndrome, and delirious mania, which may manifest with catatonic features and may potentially represent medical and psychiatric emergencies.

References

Ali S, Welch CA, Park LT, et al: Encephalitis and catatonia treated with ECT. Cogn Behav Neurol 21(1):46–51, 2008 18327024

American Psychiatric Association: Diagnostic and Statistical Manual of Mental Disorders, 5th Edition. Arlington, VA, American Psychiatric Association, 2013

Arciniegas DB, Frey KL, Anderson CA, et al: Amantadine for neurobehavioural deficits following delayed post-hypoxic encephalopathy. Brain Inj 18(12):1309–1318, 2004 15666573

Bastiampillai T, Forooziya F, Dhillon R: Clozapine-withdrawal catatonia. Aust N Z J Psychiatry 43(3):283–284, 2009 19230235

Beach SR, Stern TA: "Playing possum:" differential diagnosis, work-up, and treatment of profound interpersonal withdrawal. Psychosomatics 52(6):560–562, 2011 22054626

Belvederi Murri M, Guaglianone A, Bugliani M, et al: Second-generation antipsychotics and neuroleptic malignant syndrome: systematic review and case report analysis. Drugs R D 15(1):45–62, 2015 25578944

Bush G, Fink M, Petrides G, et al: Catatonia, I: rating scale and standardized examination. Acta Psychiatr Scand 93(2):129–136, 1996 8686483

Caroff SN, Mann SC, Francis A, et al: Catatonia: From Psychopathology to Neurobiology, Washington, DC, American Psychiatric Publishing, 2007

Carroll BT, Goforth HW: Serum iron in catatonia. Biol Psychiatry 38(11):776–777, 1995 8580236

Carroll BT, Goforth HW, Thomas C, et al: Review of adjunctive glutamate antagonist therapy in the treatment of catatonic syndromes. J Neuropsychiatry Clin Neurosci 19(4):406–412, 2007 18070843

Chopra A, Das P, Rai A, et al: Catatonia as a manifestation of tacrolimus-induced neurotoxicity in organ transplant patients: a case series. Gen Hosp Psychiatry 34(2):209.e9–209.e11, 2012 21937118

Dhossche DM, Song Y, Liu Y: Is there a connection between autism, Prader-Willi syndrome, catatonia, and GABA? Int Rev Neurobiol 71:189–216, 2005 16512352

Dunkley EJ, Isbister GK, Sibbritt D, et al: The Hunter serotonin toxicity criteria: simple and accurate diagnostic decision rules for serotonin toxicity. QJM 96(9):635–642, 2003 12925718

Espinola-Nadurille M, Flores-Rivera J, Rivas-Alonso V, et al: Catatonia in patients with anti-NMDA receptor encephalitis. Psychiatry Clin Neurosci 73(9):574–580, 2019 31115962

Fink M, Taylor MA: The many varieties of catatonia. Eur Arch Psychiatry Clin Neurosci 251 (suppl 1):I8–I13, 2001 11776271

Fink M, Taylor MA: The catatonia syndrome: forgotten but not gone. Arch Gen Psychiatry 66(11):1173–1177, 2009 19884605

Fishman D, Beach S, Quinn D, et al: Special Interest Group-sponsored Updates in Psychosomatics (SIG-UPs): understanding the pathophysiology of catatonia through associated neurological insults (Neuropsychiatry SIG). Psychosomatics 58(1):90–91, 2017 28010749

Francis A, Lopez-Canino A: Delirium with catatonic features: a new subtype? Psychiatric Times 26(7):32, 2009. Available at: https://www.psychiatrictimes.com/delirium-catatonic-features-new-subtype. Accessed May 9, 2019.

Fricchione G: Catatonia: a disorder of motivation and movement. Behav Brain Sci 25(5):584–585, 2002

Fricchione GL, Beach SR, Gross AF, et al: Catatonia, neuroleptic malignant syndrome, and serotonin syndrome, in Massachusetts General Handbook of General Hospital Psychiatry, 7th Edition. Edited by Stern TA, Freudenreich O, Smith FA, et al. New York, Elsevier, 2018, pp 253–266

Georgiopoulos M, Katsakiori P, Kefalopoulou Z, et al: Vegetative state and minimally conscious state: a review of the therapeutic interventions. Stereotact Funct Neurosurg 88(4):199–207, 2010 20460949

Greenblatt DJ, Shader RI: Prazepam and lorazepam, two new benzodiazepines. N Engl J Med 299(24):1342–1344, 1978 30899

Grover S, Parakh P, Sharma A, et al: Catatonia in systemic lupus erythematosus: a case report and review of literature. Lupus 22(6):634–638, 2013 23690443

Grover S, Ghosh A, Ghormode D: Do patients of delirium have catatonic features? An exploratory study. Psychiatry Clin Neurosci 68(8):644–651, 2014 24521083

Gurrera RJ: A systematic review of sex and age factors in neuroleptic malignant syndrome diagnosis frequency. Acta Psychiatr Scand 135(5):398–408, 2017 28144982

Gurrera RJ, Caroff SN, Cohen A, et al: An international consensus study of neuroleptic malignant syndrome diagnostic criteria using the Delphi method. J Clin Psychiatry 72(9):1222–1228, 2011 21733489

Gurrera RJ, Mortillaro G, Velamoor V, Caroff SN: A validation study of the international consensus diagnostic criteria for neuroleptic malignant syndrome. J Clin Psychopharmacol 37(1):67–71, 2017 28027111

Hung YY, Yang PS, Huang TL: Clozapine in schizophrenia patients with recurrent catatonia: report of two cases. Psychiatry Clin Neurosci 60(2):256–258, 2006 16594953

Isbister GK, Bowe SJ, Dawson A, et al: Relative toxicity of selective serotonin reuptake inhibitors (SSRIs) in overdose. J Toxicol Clin Toxicol 42(3):277–285, 2004 15362595

Jacobowski NL, Heckers S, Bobo WV: Delirious mania: detection, diagnosis, and clinical management in the acute setting. J Psychiatr Pract 19(1):15–28, 2013 23334676

Jaimes-Albornoz W, Serra-Mestres J: Prevalence and clinical correlations of catatonia in older adults referred to a liaison psychiatry service in a general hospital. Gen Hosp Psychiatry 35(5):512–516, 2013 23684045

Jones KC, Schwartz AC, Hermida AP, et al: A case of anti-NMDA receptor encephalitis treated with ECT. J Psychiatr Pract 21(5):374–380, 2015 26348805

Karmacharya R, England ML, Ongür D: Delirious mania: clinical features and treatment response. J Affect Disord 109(3):312–316, 2008 18191210

Keck PE Jr, Caroff SN, McElroy SL: Neuroleptic malignant syndrome and malignant hyperthermia: end of a controversy? J Neuropsychiatry Clin Neurosci 7(2):135–144, 1995 7626956

Khan M, Pace L, Truong A, et al: Catatonia secondary to synthetic cannabinoid use in two patients with no previous psychosis. Am J Addict 25(1):25–27, 2016 26781357

Klingensmith KE, Sanacora G, Ostroff R: Co-occurring catatonia and posterior reversible encephalopathy syndrome responsive to electroconvulsive therapy. J ECT 33(3):e22, 2017 28383349

Kritzinger PR, Jordaan GP: Catatonia: an open prospective series with carbamazepine. Int J Neuropsychopharmacol 4(3):251–257, 2001 11602030

Kruse JL, Jeffrey JK, Davis MC, et al: Anti-N-methyl-D-aspartate receptor encephalitis: a targeted review of clinical presentation, diagnosis, and approaches to psychopharmacologic management. Ann Clin Psychiatry 26(2):111–119, 2014 24501734

Leroy A, Naudet F, Vaiva G, et al: Is electroconvulsive therapy an evidence-based treatment for catatonia? A systematic review and meta-analysis. Eur Arch Psychiatry Clin Neurosci 268(7):675–687, 2018 28639007

Mendez MF: Multiple sclerosis presenting as catatonia. Int J Psychiatry Med 29(4):435–441, 1999 10782426

Modi S, Dharaiya D, Schultz L, et al: Neuroleptic malignant syndrome: complications, outcomes, and mortality. Neurocrit Care 24(1):97–103, 2016 26223336

Murray GB, Shea V, Conn DK: Electroconvulsive therapy for poststroke depression. J Clin Psychiatry 47(5):258–260, 1986 3700345

Nagaratnam N, Nagaratnam K, Ng K, et al: Akinetic mutism following stroke. J Clin Neurosci 11(1):25–30, 2004 14642361

Oldham MA: The probability that catatonia in the hospital has a medical cause and the relative proportions of its causes: a systematic review. Psychosomatics 59(4):333–340, 2018 29776679

Oldham MA, Lee HB: Catatonia vis-à-vis delirium: the significance of recognizing catatonia in altered mental status. Gen Hosp Psychiatry 37(6):554–559, 2015 26162545

Pauker SL, Brown R: Baclofen-induced catatonia. J Clin Psychopharmacol 6(6):387–388, 1986 3805341

Pelonero AL, Levenson JL, Silverman JJ: Neuroleptic therapy following neuroleptic malignant syndrome. Psychosomatics 26(12):946–947, 1985 4089133

Philbrick KL, Rummans TA: Malignant catatonia. J Neuropsychiatry Clin Neurosci 6(1):1–13, 1994 7908547

Quinn DK, Abbott CC: Catatonia after cerebral hypoxia: do the usual treatments apply? Psychosomatics 55(6):525–535, 2014 25262046

Rosebush PI, Hildebrand AM, Furlong BG, Mazurek MF: Catatonic syndrome in a general psychiatric inpatient population: frequency, clinical presentation, and response to lorazepam. J Clin Psychiatry 51(9):357–362, 1990 2211547

Rosebush PI, Stewart T, Mazurek MF: The treatment of neuroleptic malignant syndrome. Are dantrolene and bromocriptine useful adjuncts to supportive care? Br J Psychiatry 159:709–712, 1991 1843801

Ryali V, Banerjee A, John MJ, Rathod J: Herpes simplex encephalitis presenting with catatonia. Med J Armed Forces India 53(4):317–318, 1997 28769525

Saini SM, Eu CL, Wan Yahya WN, Abdul Rahman AH: Malignant catatonia secondary to viral meningoencephalitis in a young man with bipolar disorder. Asia Pac Psychiatry 5 (suppl 1):55–58, 2013 23857838

Spiegel DR, Klaiber N: A case of catatonia status-post left middle cerebral artery cerebrovascular accident, treated successfully with olanzapine. Clin Neuropharmacol 36(4):135–137, 2013 23783004

Spiegel DR, Varnell C Jr: A case of catatonia due to posterior reversible encephalopathy syndrome treated successfully with antihypertensives and adjunctive olanzapine. Gen Hosp Psychiatry 33(3):302.e3–302.e5, 2011 21601735

Sternbach H: The serotonin syndrome. Am J Psychiatry 148(6):705–713, 1991 2035713

Taylor MA: Catatonia: a review of a behavioral neurologic syndrome. Cognitive and Behavioral Neurology 3(1):48–72, 1990. Available at: https://journals.lww.com/cogbehavneurol/Abstract/1990/00310/Catatonia__A_Review_of_a_Behavioral_Neurologic.6.aspx. Accessed May 12, 2019.

Trollor JN, Chen X, Sachdev PS: Neuroleptic malignant syndrome associated with atypical antipsychotic drugs. CNS Drugs 23(6):477–492, 2009 19480467

Washinsky M, Quinn DK: Delirious mania associated with Bardet-Biedl syndrome, an inherited ciliopathy. Psychosomatics 54(5):484–487, 2013 23352051

Weddington WW Jr, Marks RC, Verghese JP: Disulfiram encephalopathy as a cause of the catatonia syndrome. Am J Psychiatry 137(10):1217–1219, 1980 7416268

CHAPTER 19

Mood Disorders Due to Medical Illnesses

Sivan Mauer, M.D., M.S.

John Querques, M.D.

Paul Summergrad, M.D.

Mood describes how a person feels, the summation of his or her internal milieu of thoughts, emotions, and bodily sensations in interaction with the external world. Mood normally fluctuates over the course of a day, simply on the basis of the passage of time and depending on the person's thoughts, circumstances, and interactions with other people and the environment. A *distinct* period of *persistent* alteration in mood that is *distinguishable* from an individual's usual demeanor and from normal, everyday fluctuations defines an abnormal mood state. Abnormal mood states—either depressive or manic—can be caused by a major depressive, bipolar, or schizoaffective disorder, but also by a variety of medical illnesses, substances of abuse (or withdrawal from them), and medications. In addition, medical conditions can precipitate states that resemble, and that can be confused with, depressive and manic episodes. In this chapter we review the definition, medical differential diagnosis, and principles of treatment of abnormal mood states.

Definition of Abnormal Mood States

Because no laboratory or radiological studies have been proven diagnostic of mood disorders, these conditions are defined by consensus criteria codified in the fifth edition of the *Diagnostic and Statistical Manual of Mental Disorders* (DSM-5; American Psychiatric Association 2013). A depressive episode is characterized by at least a 2-week period of persistent dysphoria or anhedonia associated with sleep or appetite disturbance; fatigue or anergia; difficulty thinking, concentrating, or making decisions; feeling worthless or guilty; psychomotor slowing or agitation; and thoughts of death or suicide. One can be depressed, sad, down, blue, or any of the myriad descriptors for dysphoria and not be in the throes of a depressive episode (Horwitz and Wakefield 2007). That is, one can have a certain *mood* without having a mood *disorder,* just as one can have a cough without having pneumonia, or chest pain without a myocardial infarction. The key distinction is the persistence of the mood over at least 2 weeks, with associated features, causing distress or impairment in functioning. Recognizing that one can be sad or unhappy without having a depressive disorder is particularly relevant in working with patients with medical and surgical illnesses. Many of the diagnostic criteria for mood disorders were established in patients without other major medical disorders and include symptoms such as fatigue or sleep disturbances that can also be due to primary medical conditions. For this reason, clinicians must remain attentive to atypical presentations of mood disorders, including unexplained symptoms or nonresponsiveness to standard therapies.

A manic episode is defined as a period lasting at least 1 week (or any duration if hospitalization is required) characterized by the presence of "abnormally and persistently elevated, expansive, or irritable mood and…increased goal-directed activity or energy" associated with reduced need for sleep, racing thoughts, talkativeness, distractibility, injudicious behavior, and grandiosity or an elevation in self-esteem (American Psychiatric Association 2013, p. 124). Impairment is severe, hospitalization is required, or psychosis is present. A hypomanic episode has similar characteristics but by definition involves a shorter period—at least 4 days—and is not severe enough to cause marked impairment or require hospitalization. Although manic and hypomanic states differ in their severity (compare manic and hypomanic diagnostic criteria in DSM-5, pp. 124–125), in this chapter we will use the term *manic* to refer to both states. People unfamiliar with the diagnostic definitions may think that being bipolar simply means having mood swings—that is, rapid fluctuations in mood throughout the day that may or may not coincide with prevailing circumstances. However, mild mood fluctuations would not qualify for a diagnosis of bipolar disorder, and the "up" periods during such transient fluctuations would not reach the level of severity seen in a manic episode or a depressive episode with mixed features (see DSM-5, p. 150).

Etiological, Pathophysiological, and Genetic Factors

While much is known about various circumstances that can induce a depressive or a manic state, the underlying etiology and pathophysiology that specifically explain and describe how those factors precipitate abnormal mood states are unknown. Various theories—involving monoaminergic neurotransmission; the endocrine system, especially the hypothalamic-pituitary-adrenal (HPA) and hypothalamic-pituitary-thyroid (HPT) axes; abnormalities in neurocircuitry or neuroanatomy; and neuroplasticity—have been posited, but none has proven definitive or fully explanatory of all of the dimensions of affective illness. Recently, the roles of genetics and inflammation in causing or contributing to abnormal mood states have been the subjects of intense investigation (Bui et al. 2017; Grande et al. 2016; Misiak et al. 2018; Otte et al. 2016; Vieta et al. 2018). Both major depressive disorder (MDD) and bipolar disorder are known to be heritable, likely polygenic, and best explained by gene-environment interactions. From several lines of evidence, both depressive and manic states are thought to be potentially related to inflammation and immune dysfunction. For example, treatment with interleukin (IL)-2 or interferon-γ can precipitate depressive symptoms, and microglial activation and elevations in serum levels of C reactive protein and the proinflammatory cytokines IL-6 and tumor necrosis factor-α occur in some patients with MDD. Still, no diagnostic inflammatory, immune, or other biomarkers have yet emerged.

Medical Conditions Causing Abnormal Mood States

Clues that an abnormal mood episode is not due to a primary psychiatric illness but is secondary to a medical condition include first occurrence at a later age than is usual in primary illness; onset after the start of a medical condition; atypical features; atypical—or lack of—response to standard treatment; and absence of a family history of affective disturbance. Discerning whether a given symptom is due to a psychiatric disorder or secondary to another condition can be challenging in patients with medical illnesses, especially in the case of somatic or neurovegetative symptoms, because often there is overlap (e.g., fatigue in a depressed cancer patient can be due to MDD, cancer, or both). While it is possible and important to ask a medically ill patient what his mood is like, determining whether his response truly reflects his mood state or simply a momentary state of well-being or comfort is critical. Failure to assess mood accurately can result in incorrect diagnoses, especially of depressive states.

That manic states can have medical, neurological, pharmacological, and substance-related causes has been long recognized (Brooks and Hoblyn 2005; Krauthammer and Klerman 1978; Satzer and Bond 2016; Taylor et al. 2018). In addition, patients with bipolar disorder are at elevated risk of obesity, diabetes mellitus, cardiovascular disease, and autoimmune disorders; these risks may be mediated by inflammatory and immune mechanisms (SayuriYamagata et al. 2017). A Danish registry analysis of more than 3.5 million persons born between 1945 and 1976 found that risk of a hospital diagnosis of a mood disorder was increased in persons with a previous hospital contact for an infectious or autoimmune disease. The incidence rate ratios (IRRs) for autoimmune disorders and infectious disorders were 1.45 and 1.62, respectively, with infections being far more common than autoimmune conditions (Benros et al. 2013).

Neurological Conditions

Neoplasm

More than half of people with brain tumors experience psychiatric symptoms, with 44% experiencing depressive symptoms and 15% experiencing manic symptoms (Madhusoodanan et al. 2010; Satzer and Bond 2016). The polarity of mood symptoms (i.e., whether they are depressive or manic) depends on the brain area affected (Madhusoodanan et al. 2010). In a meta-analysis, tumors of the frontal lobe were most often associated with mood symptoms, with depressive symptoms more commonly associated with left frontal tumors and manic symptoms more commonly associated with right frontal tumors (Madhusoodanan et al. 2010, 2015). In a retrospective study, psychiatric symptoms were the only presenting symptoms in nearly one-quarter of cases in patients in the fifth decade of life (Gupta and Kumar 2004). In many cases, long-tract neurological symptoms are absent.

While history and physical examination may be of value in diagnosis, particularly with onset of a mood disorder later in life, many tumors, particularly those in the frontal lobe, may not produce localizing neurological findings. Magnetic resonance imaging (MRI) is more sensitive than computed tomography (CT) in detecting tumors, in part because of its better ability to distinguish abnormalities in close proximity to bone.

Traumatic Brain Injury and Chronic Traumatic Encephalopathy

Traumatic brain injury (TBI) and chronic traumatic encephalopathy (CTE) are brain conditions found in individuals (e.g., athletes, soldiers) with a history of repetitive brain trauma, including symptomatic concussions and asymptomatic subconcussive blows to the head. Both conditions have important psychiatric aspects, including depression, mania, aggression, and rage, as well as a strong association with posttraumatic stress disorder, especially in military settings. Concussions that occur even in the absence of a blow to the head (e.g., a blow elsewhere in the body whose force is transmitted to the head) can be associated with an elevated risk of depression (Radhakrishnan et al. 2016).

TBI is triggered by head trauma, single or recurrent; this type of injury (often caused by improvised explosive devices) is commonly seen in veterans of the Iraq and Afghanistan wars. TBI can produce depression, mania, memory impairment, executive dysfunction, impulsivity, and aggression. TBI is a broad category that encompasses many kinds of brain injury. One specific subtype of TBI is CTE, a progressive degenerative disease of the brain (McKee et al. 2009). Since the 1920s, CTE has been known to affect boxers; in recent years, high rates of neuropathologically confirmed CTE have been reported in retired professional football players and other athletes with a history of repetitive brain trauma (Lehman et al. 2012). CTE is associated with progressive degeneration of the brain and widespread deposition of hyperphosphorylated tau (p-tau) protein (McKee et al. 2013; Mez et al. 2017; Stein et al. 2014). These changes can begin months, years, or even decades after the last brain trauma or cessation of active athletic involvement (Stein et al. 2014). CTE is associated with memory loss, confusion, impaired judgment, diminished impulse control, aggression, depression, and eventually progressive dementia (Lehman et al. 2012; McKee et al. 2009; Stern et al. 2013).

Among people with TBI, depressive symptoms are most common; manic symptoms are less frequent (Ponsford et al. 2018). Estimates of the frequency of depressive symptoms as a complication of TBI have ranged from 25% to 50% in the first year after TBI, with lifetime rates of 26%–64% (Jorge and Arciniegas 2014). In a study of nearly 100,000 adults older than 65 years, the presence of TBI was found to increase the risk of depression, especially in men (Albrecht et al. 2015).

TBI is an important risk factor for mania and mixed affective symptoms (Perry et al. 2016). Manic symptoms affect around 9% of patients with TBI and usually involve right ventral frontal or basotemporal injury. There is no relationship between the occurrence of manic symptoms and family history of bipolar disorder (Jorge and Arciniegas 2014). Mixed states—that is, states with both depressive and manic features—are important, because TBI has a close relationship with suicidal ideation, and mixed affective symptoms are important established risk factors for suicide (Balázs et al. 2006; Mackelprang et al. 2014; Rihmer et al. 2008). In a retrospective cohort study of a sample of 1,877 people who committed suicide, TBI was found in 103 (5.5%) of the victims, 20% of whom had brain lesions and 80% of whom had experienced concussions (Mainio et al. 2007).

In a brain autopsy study of 202 football players, CTE was diagnosed in 177 players (Mez et al. 2017). Depressive symptoms were found in 67% and manic symptoms in 22% of patients with CTE. Suicide was the cause of death in 27% of this sample (Mez et al. 2017).

Cerebrovascular Disease

Depression is highly prevalent in patients with hypertension and vascular dementia and is a well-known outcome of strokes, most commonly those involving left anterior locations (Alexopoulos et al. 1997; Hackett et al. 2014; Robinson and Jorge 2016; Robinson et al. 1984). Cerebrovascular burden, especially small-vessel disease, could be a factor in the pathogenesis of late-onset depressive episodes. Introducing the concept of vascular depression in the 1990s, Alexopoulos et al. (1997) defined its cardinal features as the presence of vascular disease (or vascular risk factors) and late-onset depression (or change in the course of early-onset depression after the onset of vascular disease).

In elderly individuals, the clinical manifestations of vascular depression may be distinct from those of nonvascular depression. The clinical presentation of vascular depression is characterized by apathy, psychomotor slowing, lack of initiative, a history of hypertension, and absence of a family history of mood disorders (Aizenstein et al. 2016). Abulia, incontinence, and gait disturbance are common symptoms, as are cognitive decline and progression to dementia. The depression is often treatment resistant, and there is a poor prognosis. The hallmark of MRI-defined vascular depression is the presence of extensive white matter lesions identified as white matter hyperintensities (WMH), especially in and around the centrum semiovale and extending from the lateral ventricles into deep white matter (Taylor et al. 2013). A recent meta-analysis of studies in patients 40 years of age or older found an increased risk of depression in patients with cerebral infarctions or WMH (van Agtmaal et al. 2017).

Mania also has been associated with vascular disease and stroke, and the term *vascular mania* has been proposed to describe this condition. Its main features are mania onset after age 50 years, mania occurring in the context of clinical or neuroimaging evidence of cerebrovascular disease (including WMH or gray matter hyperintensities), cognitive impairment, and absence of a family history of affective illness (Steffens and Krishnan 1998). The evidentiary basis for the concept of vascular mania is not robust, however, because the majority of papers that have reported manic symptoms occurring in patients with cerebrovascular burden are case reports or case series and lack reliable prevalence data (Wijeratne and Malhi 2007). One study found that silent cerebral infarction was more common in patients with late-onset mania than in patients with early-onset mania (Fujikawa et al. 1995).

Neurodegenerative Disorders

Huntington's disease.   A triad of symptoms—motor disturbance, cognitive impairment, and psychiatric manifestations—characterizes Huntington's disease, a hereditary neurodegenerative disorder caused by abnormal expansion of a trinucleotide CAG repeat in the huntingtin (*HTT*) gene on chromosome 4. Psychiatric manifestations occur even in the prodromal period and do not fully track with the motor and cognitive aspects (Epping et al. 2016). Part of the phenomenology since the disease's first description, depressive symptoms normally precede motor manifestations. The lifetime prevalence of depression in patients with Huntington's disease is about 30%–40%, with a suicide rate six to seven times higher than that in the general population (Rosenblatt 2007). Suicide risk is highest in the early stages of the disorder. The mechanism responsible for depression in Huntington's disease is unclear. Low expression of brain-derived neurotrophic factor in various brain regions may be contributory (Pla et al. 2014).

The lifetime prevalence of manic syndromes in Huntington's disease is 5%–10% (Rosenblatt 2007). Patients may present with irritability, impulsiveness, hypersexuality, and grandiosity. The main treatments are anticonvulsants or antipsychotics, although the latter can worsen extrapyramidal symptoms (Rosenblatt 2007). Manic states often precede chorea.

Parkinson's disease.   Parkinson's disease affects 1% of older adults (Tysnes and Storstein 2017). One of the most common neurodegenerative disorders, Parkinson's disease is characterized by tremor, rigidity, and bradykinesia. Many patients experience neuropsychiatric symptoms, including depression, anxiety, and, less frequently, mania. In fact, depression is one of the most frequently reported neuropsychiatric disturbances in Parkinson's disease, occurring in 40%–50% of patients (Katunina and Titova 2017). The underlying mechanism of depression in Parkinson's disease remains unknown. The onset and natural history of depressive syndromes do not parallel the course of motor disturbance (Marsh 2013). A multivariate analysis found that greater depression at baseline, older age, and longer duration of Parkinson's disease were associated with a lower likelihood of depression remission (Aarsland et al. 2011).

There may be a neurobiological association between mood disorders and Parkinson's disease, such that mood disorders in Parkinson's disease do not represent comorbidities but rather are part of the illness (Mørkeberg Nilsson 2012). Manic symptoms are not well characterized in Parkinson's disease and are more related to dopamine replacement therapy (DRT) than to Parkinson's disease. In one case-control study, 18 of 108 patients (16.7%) had mania or hypomania with DRT (Maier et al. 2014).

Frontotemporal dementia.   Accounting for 10%–50% of dementia cases in patients younger than 65 years at onset, frontotemporal dementia (FTD) encompasses behavioral-variant FTD, non-fluent-variant primary progressive aphasia, and semantic-variant primary progressive aphasia (Bang et al. 2015). The features of the behavioral variant include progressive changes in mood and personality (Woolley et al. 2011). Disinhibition leading to indiscretions can be mistaken for mania; apathy can be mistaken for depression. A meta-analysis of 29 studies (total *N*=870 patients with FTD) found an event rate of 33% for depressed mood in FTD (Chakrabarty et al. 2015).

In comparison with patients with other types of dementia, patients with FTD are twice as likely to be diagnosed with bipolar illness (Satzer and Bond 2016). FTD is associated with a later (after age 40–45 years) and more insidious onset; a family history of dementia; a progressive and continuous course; progressive cognitive impairment; genetic and neuroimaging evidence of FTD, including prominent frontal atrophy; and poor response to psychiatric treatment (Galimberti et al. 2015).

Alzheimer's disease.   In addition to cognitive decline, neuropsychiatric symptoms—such as depression, mania, and psychomotor agitation—are common in people with Alzheimer's disease. Clinical and epidemiological studies have found that 75%–95% of patients experience at least one psychiatric symptom of any severity over the course of the disease, with resulting poor prognosis (Charernboon and Phanasathit 2014). Neuropsychiatric symptoms are more prevalent in people diagnosed with mild cognitive impairment (MCI) (Geda et al. 2008). Depression or mania/agitation can also occur as a prodrome of Alzheimer's disease.

Depression is found in 16% of Alzheimer's patients in population-based studies and in 44% of these patients in hospital-based studies (Lanctôt et al. 2017). Also common in MCI, depression is a predictor of progression from normal cognitive functioning to MCI to dementia. Several risk factors for depression in Alzheimer's disease have been described, including a family history of mood disorders in first-degree relatives, a prior personal history of depression, female gender, and a younger age at onset of Alzheimer's disease (Lyketsos and Olin 2002). Potential mechanisms include neurodegeneration in frontal limbic circuits and disruption of frontal-subcortical pathways due to either volumetric change in prefrontal gray matter or changes (e.g., WMH or lacunae) in the basal ganglia. Another mechanism may be HPA axis dysfunction resulting in neurodegeneration through overrelease of glucocorticoids, occurring in both patients with depressive disorders and patients with Alzheimer's disease (Chi et al. 2014).

Differentiating depression from apathy in Alzheimer's disease is critical. Apathy is characterized by akinesia, decreased initiative, lack of motivation, and emotional indifference. The most common neuropsychiatric symptom in Alzheimer's disease, apathy is a primary cause of caregiver distress. In neuroimaging studies in individuals with preclinical or prodromal Alzheimer's disease, apathy has been found to be associated with cortical dysfunction in the posterior cingulate or inferior temporal cortex, as well as general cortical atrophy and hypometabolism (Lanctôt et al. 2017).

Agitation and manic-like symptoms occur frequently in Alzheimer's disease. In a small case-control study involving 19 patients with Alzheimer's disease and 13 healthy control subjects, agitation was reported in 31.6% of patients and elation in 5.2% (Tascone et al. 2017). Agitation—defined as excessive motor activity or verbal or physical aggression associated with emotional distress or disability—increases as disease severity increases and is often accompanied by anxiety, psychosis, and disinhibition. Agitation is associated with structural and functional abnormalities in brain regions associated with emotional regulation (e.g., amygdala, hippocampus) (Lanctôt et al. 2017).

Multiple Sclerosis

Multiple sclerosis (MS) is an autoimmune demyelinating disease of the central nervous system that may lead to severe neurological disability in early to middle adulthood. Common clinical features include weakness, fatigue, vertigo, visual disturbance, swallowing difficulties, gait disturbance, and urinary problems. Neuropsychiatric symptoms are common and may be the first manifestation of MS (Koutsouraki et al. 2010).

Depression is the most common neuropsychiatric illness found in MS, with a point prevalence of nearly 30% in ambulatory clinic patients; increased rates of epilepsy and stroke are also found (Viguera et al. 2018). Findings from hospital-based clinics reveal that approximately one-quarter to one-half of patients with MS develop depression over the course of their lives, a rate two to three times higher than that in the general population (Feinstein et al. 2014). Certain prominent risk factors for depression—younger age, female gender, and family history of depression—are less consistently associated with depression in MS than they are in the general population (Patten et al. 2017). Depression is less common early in MS than in later stages, but fluctuations in mood may correlate with disease relapse (Feinstein et al. 2014). Etiological factors that may contribute to comorbid depression in MS include unpredictable disease course, severe physical disability, HPA axis dysfunction, and medication used to treat MS (e.g., steroids) (Murphy et al. 2017).

Bipolar disorder is twice as common in MS patients as it is in the general population, and mania in MS is often attributed to steroid treatment (Hotier et al. 2015; Paparrigopoulos et al. 2010). A Turkish study found high scores for cyclothymic and dysthymic temperament in patients with MS (Özkan et al. 2016). A Swedish cohort study found that bipolar patients had an increased risk of MS (Johansson et al. 2014).

Pathological laughing and crying (PLC) and euphoria sclerotica (described below) can be misdiagnosed as mania. PLC occurs in approximately 10% of patients with MS, often in advanced stages (Murphy et al. 2017). PLC (also referred to as pseudobulbar affect or emotional incontinence) is characterized by frequent, sudden outbursts of uncontrolled crying or laughing that are disproportionate to or incongruent with underlying mood or external triggers. PLC has traditionally been considered to represent a disconnection syndrome resulting from loss of cortical or brain stem inhibition of a putative center of laughing and crying; this loss of inhibition is possibly due to lesions in the cerebropontocerebellar pathways involved in appropriate adjustment to social contexts (Murphy et al. 2017; Paparrigopoulos et al. 2010).

Euphoria sclerotica refers to a fixed mental state of unusual cheerfulness and optimism about the future despite the presence of significant neurological disability. Prevalence rates of up to 25% have been reported in patients with MS (Patten et al. 2003). Euphoria sclerotica has been associated with cognitive impairment, disease progression, and extensive neuropathological lesions, particularly in the frontal lobe (Murphy et al. 2017; Paparrigopoulos et al. 2010). The euphoria in this condition is not associated with the speech disturbance and psychomotor agitation that are central to the diagnosis of mania.

Epilepsy

Psychiatric symptoms are common in patients with epilepsy. The prevalence of depressive symptoms is estimated as more than 30% in community-based epilepsy samples and as 20%–55% in specialist epilepsy clinic samples (Gilliam et al. 2006; Viguera et al. 2018). The frequency of depression depends on the severity of the epilepsy and the location of the epileptogenic focus (Schmitz 2005). Epilepsy is a risk factor for depression, and a history of depression is associated with a four- to sixfold greater risk of developing epilepsy, a finding corroborating the bidirectional relationship Hippocrates identified centuries ago: "Melancholics ordinarily become epileptics, and epileptics, melancholics" (Kanner 2003; Kanner and Ribot 2016).

Among patients with epilepsy in a community-based sample, 30%–50% experienced depressive episodes with mixed features, including euphoria, irritability, and anxiety (Kanner and Ribot 2016). These episodes tended to follow a chronic course with recurrent symptom-free periods (Kanner and Ribot 2016). Preictal symptoms of depression typically manifest as dysphoria that may extend for hours or even days before a seizure (Kanner and Ribot 2016). Although postictal symptoms of depression have been recognized for decades, only one study (Kanner et al. 2004) has investigated the prevalence and characteristics of postictal symptoms of depression in a systematic manner. In this study, which used a standardized questionnaire to assess postictal psychiatric symptoms in 100 patients with refractory epilepsy, depression— experienced by 43%—was one of the most common symptoms (Kanner et al. 2004). These symptoms occurred after more than half of seizures, and their duration ranged from 0.5 to 108 hours; in some cases, they persisted for up to 2 weeks.

Manic symptoms in epilepsy have been considered less common than depressive symptoms, with the exception of two specific circumstances: postictal symptoms and post–epilepsy surgery symptoms. Manic symptoms are reported in 22% of postictal patients (Mula 2016), often in association with psychotic phenomena; are long-lasting; and recur more frequently in the presence of postictal psychosis and nondominant hemisphere involvement (Mula 2016; Schmitz 2005).

A possible link among temporal lobe epilepsy, seizure activity, and mania is illustrated by the high incidence of manic episodes after temporal lobectomies in patients whose seizures are refractory to medical management. After surgery, manic episodes occur in around 10% of patients (Schmitz 2005). Episodes may begin with excessive feelings of gratitude toward the surgeon and progress to socially inappropriate behavior, feeling emotionally close to distant people, and finally, classic symptoms of mania. These episodes occur weeks after surgery. Postsurgical mania is associated with poor seizure outcome. Patients who undergo right temporal lobectomies have a higher risk of postoperative mania, as do patients with bilateral abnormalities (Mula 2016; Schmitz 2005).

Cardiovascular Conditions

Depressed individuals are more likely to develop heart disease, and patients with heart disease are more likely to become depressed. Mild forms of depression are found in up to two-thirds of patients in the hospital after acute myocardial infarction, with clinical depression generally found in 17%–44% (Khawaja et al. 2009). This prevalence is two to three times that found in the general population (Hare et al. 2014). Although there are some inconsistencies in the literature, risk factors for depression in cardiac patients include younger age, female gender, and a premorbid history of depression (Huffman et al. 2013). Thirty-eight percent of patients with depression have comorbid anxiety, a presentation most commonly found among patients with acute coronary syndrome (Huffman et al. 2013). Depression is common in patients with heart failure, is associated with both its development and its progression, and portends worse outcomes (Celano et al. 2018). In relation to mania, only one study has suggested that mania may elevate the risk of cardiovascular disease; in comparison with patients without a history of mood episodes, patients with a history of mania were three times more likely to have cardiovascular disease (Ramsey et al. 2010).

Endocrine and Metabolic Conditions

Thyroid Dysfunction

Thyroid hormones are important for the development, maturation, and functioning of the brain. Thyroid hormones influence brain gene expression. The association of thyroid function with mood symptoms was first described more than 200 years ago; thyroid hormone dysfunction in adults can cause mania and depression (Bunevičius and Prange 2010). In a large meta-analytic study, patients with autoimmune thyroiditis (broadly defined) were at elevated risk of developing depressive symptoms or depressive disorders, as well as anxiety disorders (Siegmann et al. 2018). Both excess and insufficient thyroid hormones can cause mood abnormalities; classically, mania is associated with hyperthyroidism and depression with hypothyroidism. However, recent literature has shown that this relation is not so straightforward.

The prevalence of depressive symptoms in hypothyroidism has been reported to be as high as 60%, while the prevalence of hypothyroidism in psychiatric patients has been estimated to be 0.5%–8% (Talaei et al. 2017). A substantial number of patients with hyperthyroidism exhibit features of depression (Hu et al. 2013). The occurrence of depression in hyperthyroidism has especially been reported in older patients, who may have what is termed *apathetic hyperthyroidism*. These patients are often described as withdrawn and may have an increased likelihood of cardiac symptoms, including arrhythmia (Wu et al. 2010).

The vast majority of patients with depression do not have biochemical evidence of thyroid dysfunction. When thyroid abnormalities do exist, they consist mainly of elevated thyroxine (T_4), low triiodothyronine (T_3), and a blunted thyroid-stimulating hormone (TSH) response to thyrotropin-releasing hormone (TRH) (Hage and Azar 2012). TSH levels may correlate with the severity of depressive symptoms.

Patients being treated for hypothyroidism, and even those with subclinical hypothyroidism (i.e., TSH levels at the high end of normal with normal thyroid hormone levels) who are being treated for depression but have residual depressive symptoms, may benefit from achieving a TSH level below 2.5 µIU/mL (Cohen et al. 2018).

Mania is more typically associated with hyperthyroidism than is depression. A Taiwanese case-control study involving more than 40,000 subjects found a higher incidence of bipolar illness in patients with hyperthyroidism than in control subjects (Hu et al. 2013). A few case reports have described mania with hypothyroidism. One study involving 18 case reports, the majority of them with female patients, described manic symptoms in hypothyroid patients after T_4 replacement therapy (Josephson and Mackenzie 1980).

Cushing's Syndrome

Cushing's syndrome is the term used to describe a set of symptoms associated with hypercortisolism. When these symptoms are due to a hypophyseal microadenoma secreting excess adrenocorticotropic hormone (ACTH), the condition is called *Cushing's disease*. In the majority of cases, ACTH-independent endogenous hypercortisolism is caused by adrenal gland tumors, while the most common exogenous cause of Cushing's syndrome is glucocorticoid supplementation (Bratek et al. 2015). Obesity, hypertension, and edema are the most common manifestations of Cushing's syndrome (Bruno 2011).

Harvey Cushing was a pioneer in identifying a relationship between endocrine diseases and psychiatric symptoms. Hypothesizing a pathogenic role for stressful life events, he recognized the occurrence of organic affective disorders and the effects of chronic states of glandular over- and underactivity on the psyche and the nervous system (Sonino et al. 2010).

Mood symptoms are the most common psychiatric presentation of Cushing's syndrome. Depression occurs in more than half of patients, and it appears in the prodromal phase in about 25% of patients (Sonino et al. 2010). The features of depression in Cushing's syndrome are irritability, hyperphagia, hypersomnia, and increased fatigability (Bratek et al. 2015; Sonino et al. 2010). Risk factors include female gender, advanced age, and undetected pituitary tumors (Sonino et al. 2010).

Mania also has been reported in Cushing's syndrome; about one-third of patients have manic episodes during the course of the illness (Sonino et al. 2010). In fact, manic symptoms may be among the early manifestations of the illness.

Vitamin B_{12} (Cobalamin) Deficiency

Vitamin B_{12} deficiency is a common cause of psychiatric symptoms in elderly patients (Lachner et al. 2012). People who eat vegetarian and vegan diets also have this problem because most dietary sources of vitamin B_{12}—including meat, dairy products, and eggs—are derived from animals. The elderly population is especially at risk for cobalamin deficiency, given the higher prevalence of atrophic gastritis and other gastrointestinal pathology in this population, as well as the use of medications that can interfere with B_{12} absorption or metabolism. Definitions of vitamin B_{12} deficiency vary and usually rely on population statistics (normal range, 180–900 pg/mL). Vitamin B_{12} is associated with macrocytic anemia, and a finding of macrocytic anemia on a routine complete blood count is often a clue to the presence of B_{12} deficiency. Vitamin B_{12} is also associated with the production of dopamine and serotonin. The prevalence of vitamin B_{12} deficiency among older adults has been estimated at 3%–40% (Lachner et al. 2012). The relationship between vitamin B_{12} deficiency and cognitive impairment is well established, and a growing body of evidence suggests a role for vitamin B_{12} deficiency in mood symptoms (Kapoor et al. 2017; Lachner et al. 2012).

A cross-sectional study of community-dwelling persons older than 55 years with depressive symptoms found that B_{12} deficiency was independently associated with depression (Tiemeier et al. 2002). A Canadian study involving 1,368 subjects with a mean age of 74 years found that men in the highest tertile of dietary B_{12} intake had a decreased risk of depression (Gougeon et al. 2016). A meta-analysis of nine B_{12}-related studies (involving 6,308 individuals) observed an increased risk for depression in subjects with low vitamin B_{12} levels (Petridou et al. 2016).

Symptoms of mania have been described in the presence of vitamin B_{12} deficiency in a few case reports. In a review of 89 published case studies of vitamin B_{12} deficiency, a manic or mixed episode was present in at least five cases (Rusher and Pawlak 2013).

Infections

HIV

In 2018, there were 1.7 million new HIV infections and 770,000 deaths due to AIDS (Joint United Nations Programme on HIV/AIDS 2019). Since the late 1990s, highly active antiretroviral therapy has transformed HIV into a manageable chronic disease (Nanni et al. 2015). A consequence of this change is an increase in comorbidities. Depression and mania are common complications in HIV-infected patients.

Depression is prevalent among HIV patients, with rates of approximately 20% among larger community-based samples (Rabkin 2008). The etiology of depression in HIV involves biological factors (alterations in cerebral white matter, HPT axis dysfunction) and psychological factors (stigma, isolation, occupational disability, body image changes, debilitation), as well as a history of or comorbidity with psychiatric illness (Arseniou et al. 2014). The clinical manifestations of depression in patients with HIV are generally the same as those in patients without HIV; however, the presence of HIV-related MCI or of overt dementia can also complicate the clinical picture and evaluation, because subcortical dementia secondary to HIV can be associated with apathy or withdrawal. Severe depression is associated with low body mass index and low CD4 count (<200 cells/mm^3) (Nanni et al. 2015; Zoungrana et al. 2017).

Mania also has been noted with progression of HIV infection. In the early stages of infection, 1%–2% of patients experience manic episodes (Dubé et al. 2005). However, after the onset of AIDS, 4%–8% of patients appear to experience mania. Symptoms in these patients are sometimes different from those in patients not infected with HIV. Irritability is more prominent than euphoria in HIV patients (Dubé et al. 2005). In a study in Uganda, patients with mania secondary to HIV were older than patients with primary mania (35 vs. 21 years) and did not have a family history of mood disorders. HIV patients with secondary mania were more likely than those without mania to be immunologically compromised (Nakimuli-Mpungu et al. 2006).

Syphilis

Neurosyphilis is caused by the spirochete *Treponema pallidum*, first identified in 1905. Historically, patients with syphilis accounted for 5%–15% of psychiatric admissions. Although neurosyphilis became far less common with the advent of penicillin, it can manifest with psychiatric illness (Mirsal et al. 2007). In the HIV era, neurosyphilis remains a part of the differential diagnosis for a wide variety of psychiatric syndromes, including mood disorders. The contemporary literature lacks comprehensive epidemiological data on the incidence of psychiatric presentations of neurosyphilis; however, about 27% of patients with primary psychiatric manifestations of neurosyphilis present with depression characterized by melancholia, psychomotor retardation, and suicidal ideation (Cubala and Czarnowska-Cubala 2008).

Mania accounts for 5.5% of mood disorder cases in neurosyphilis (Barbosa et al. 2012). As with depression, patients with mania secondary to neurosyphilis present with a late-onset mood disorder (in the sixth decade), often without any family history of psychiatric illnesses. Cognitive decline is more rapid in patients with secondary mania than in patients with a primary mood disorder (Barbosa et al. 2012).

Autoimmune and Inflammatory Conditions

Limbic Encephalitis

Encephalitides from an array of antibody-mediated causes are now recognized, some associated with antibodies against intracellular neuronal antigens—causing neuron loss by cytotoxic T-cell mechanisms—and others with antibodies against cell-surface proteins—causing reversible neuronal injury (Dalmau and Graus 2018). Limbic encephalitis from either of these etiologies is characterized by subacute development of short-term memory loss, depression, irritability, disrupted sleep, hallucinations, and seizures (Tüzün and Dalmau 2007). Paraneoplastic limbic encephalitis is most common in small-cell lung cancer and involves anti-Hu (type 1 anti-neuronal-nuclear) antibodies (Foster and Caplan 2009). Mood changes are also seen with antiamphiphysin and anti-Ma2 (also known as anti-Ta) antibodies.

Systemic Lupus Erythematosus

A systemic autoimmune disease that affects nearly every organ system, systemic lupus erythematosus (SLE) can cause or contribute to focal neurological conditions (e.g., stroke, neuropathies) as well as mood disturbances, psychosis, and delirium (Calabrese and Stern 1995). Neuropsychiatric complications in SLE are thought to be related to both brain-specific and systemic autoantibodies (most commonly anticardiolipin antibodies), as well as to direct vasculopathy, choroid-plexus injury, immune complexes, and cytokines (Calabrese and Stern 1995; Lisnevskaia et al. 2014). Clinically, it can be difficult to determine whether mood disturbances are related to SLE, in part because corticosteroids, frequently part of SLE treatment, also can cause neuropsychiatric phenomena (see section "Medications Associated With Abnormal Mood States" later in chapter).

Inflammatory Bowel Disease

Inflammatory bowel disease (IBD) encompasses Crohn's disease and ulcerative colitis, both chronic diseases involving genetic and environmental factors, the intestinal microbiome, and innate and adaptive immune responses (Abraham and Cho 2009; Torres et al. 2017). In a retrospective study of 432 IBD patients, nearly 45% reported anxiety, depression, or both; in comparison with patients not reporting anxiety or depression, patients reporting these symptoms had more emergency department visits, hospitalizations, prescriptions for steroids, and nonadherence to follow-up (Navabi et al. 2018).

Cancer

Cancer can cause or contribute to depressive and manic states through direct involvement as well as through metastasis and paraneoplastic limbic encephalitis (most prominently in small-cell lung and pancreatic malignancies); in addition, cancer has psychological ramifications that can lead to dysphoria or to more developed depressive states in many patients. Depending on the screening instrument used, cancer type, and treatment phase, prevalence estimates for depression in cancer vary widely, with reported figures ranging from 8% to 24% (Krebber et al. 2014). A diagnosis of cancer raises the specter of mortality, and the experience of undergoing invasive procedures, operations, and other treatments can stimulate issues around physical appearance and attractiveness, bodily integrity, and sexual function. In some circumstances, the need for isolation (e.g., after a stem cell transplant) can exacerbate the feeling that one is shouldering the burden alone.

Medications Associated With Abnormal Mood States

Table 19–1 lists medications that have been associated with depressive and manic states. When considering these associations in planning treatment, clinicians should bear in mind several caveats. It is often difficult to establish whether a specific medication causes, or even contributes to, a specific outcome ("Drugs That May Cause Psychiatric Symptoms" 2008). The evidence for these associations is mostly at the level of case reports. Despite these caveats, the iatrogenic contribution of medications to depression may be consequential, given that the overall prevalence of the use of potentially depressogenic medications is estimated to approach 40% (Qato et al. 2018).

Exogenous Corticosteroids

Exogenous corticosteroids can cause a host of neuropsychiatric phenomena, including depression and mania. In a review of 13 uncontrolled studies (N=2,555) of corticosteroid treatment in various medical illnesses (Lewis and Smith 1983, as reported by Warrington and Bostwick 2006), *severe* psychiatric side effects—defined as a constellation of major symptoms consistent with a diagnosable psychiatric condition—were found in 5.7% of patients, with euphoria and hypomania being the most common early symptoms and depression developing with longer treatment (Warrington and Bostwick 2006). Psychiatric side effects tended to appear early in treatment, with corticosteroid dosage being the strongest risk factor for symptom development (Warrington and Bostwick 2006). Another review found that among patients who developed psychiatric symptoms during corticosteroid treatment, more than 80% did so within 5 days of corticosteroid initiation (Ciriaco et al. 2013).

Principles of Treatment of Abnormal Mood States

Treatments for both depressive and manic states include medications, psychotherapy, electroconvulsive therapy, and transcranial magnetic stimulation—and also, where possible, treatment of underlying medical disorders. Here we focus on the mainstay of these treatments: medications.

Classes of antidepressants include selective serotonin reuptake inhibitors (SSRIs), serotonin-norepinephrine reuptake inhibitors (SNRIs), tricyclic antidepressants (TCAs), and monoamine oxidase inhibitors (MAOIs). The so-called atypical antidepressants (bupropion, mirtazapine, vortioxetine, vilazodone) do not fit neatly into any of these classes. Because TCAs and MAOIs are difficult to use and take and have abundant side effects, the first-line treatments are SSRIs, SNRIs, and atypical antidepressants.

When a depressive syndrome is caused by a medical or a neurological condition, treatment for both disorders is often necessary, and the treatments can proceed in parallel. Starting with a low dosage and increasing it slowly is recommended, but caution to the point of prescribing homeopathic dosages is not warranted. It is likewise necessary to give attention to the potential pharmacokinetic interactions and adverse effects

TABLE 19–1. Medications associated with depressive and manic states

Depression		
Analgesics	Cardiovascular agents	Neurological agents
NSAIDs	Antihypertensives	Amantadine
Opioids	ACE inhibitors	Anticonvulsants
	Acetazolamide	Carbamazepine
Antibiotics	β-Blockers	Phenytoin
Antibacterials	Calcium channel blockers	Primidone
Cycloserine	Clonidine	Baclofen
Dapsone	Hydralazine	Levodopa
Ethionamide	Methyldopa	
Fluoroquinolones	Thiazide diuretics	Oncological agents
Isoniazid	Digoxin	Asparaginase
Metronidazole	Disopyramide	Vinblastine
Sulfonamides	Phenylephrine	Vincristine
Antifungals		
Antimalarials	Endocrine agents	Psychiatric agents
Chloroquine	Anabolic steroids	Barbiturates
Mefloquine	Bromocriptine	Benzodiazepines
Antivirals	Contraceptives	Gabapentin
Abacavir	Corticosteroids	Prazosin
Acyclovir	Thyroid hormones	Ramelteon
Efavirenz		Zaleplon
Interferon-α	Gastrointestinal agents	
Nevirapine	Histamine-2 blockers	Miscellaneous
Valganciclovir	Metoclopramide	Isotretinoin
	Proton pump inhibitors	Procaine derivatives
		Varenicline
Mania		
Antibiotics	Endocrine agents	Oncological agents
Antibacterials	Androgens	Procarbazine
Dapsone	Corticosteroids	
Fluoroquinolones		Psychiatric agents
Isoniazid	Gastrointestinal agents	Antidepressants
Macrolides	Histamine-2 blockers	Atomoxetine
Antivirals	Metoclopramide	Modafinil
Interferon-α		Ramelteon
	Neurological agents	
	Amantadine	Miscellaneous
Cardiovascular agents	Anticonvulsants	Procaine derivatives
Antihypertensives	Baclofen	Sildenafil
ACE inhibitors	Levodopa	Theophylline
Calcium channel blockers	Selegiline	
Digoxin		
Propafenone		
Sympathomimetics		

Note. ACE=angiotensin-converting enzyme; NSAID=nonsteroidal anti-inflammatory drug.
Source. Data from "Drugs That May Cause Psychiatric Symptoms" 2008; Geringer et al. 2018; Kraut-hammer and Klerman 1978; Lambrichts et al. 2017; Qato et al. 2018; Taylor et al. 2018; Vieta et al. 2018.

of the chosen medication that may be additive to those of other agents or that may exacerbate the symptoms of the underlying illness. However, some side effects can be used to advantage; for example, a depressed patient with cancer-related anorexia may benefit from the appetite-promoting effects of mirtazapine. Drug-drug interactions are best checked by using electronic resources to ensure accurate and current information, bearing in mind that some interactions are only theoretical or based only on a few case reports.

Mood-stabilizing medications used for the treatment of mania include lithium and various anticonvulsants, including valproic acid, carbamazepine, oxcarbazepine, and lamotrigine. These medications are more useful in preventing future mood episodes than in controlling acute symptoms, although their sedating effects may be useful acutely. Because these medications have effects on electrolytes, platelets, liver enzymes, and thyroid and renal function, their use in patients with acute medical illnesses warrants caution. For patients who are acutely manic, antipsychotic agents, especially those that also have mood-stabilizing properties, may be preferable to anticonvulsants.

Conclusion

Mood disorders—both major depressive and bipolar disorder—are common and disabling conditions. While mood states and mood disorders can occur in reaction to the impairment and life-threatening nature of medical and neurological disorders, a wide variety of medical conditions can directly cause or significantly exacerbate depression or other disorders. In this chapter we have highlighted a number of medical conditions that are commonly associated with mood disorders, and this list is by no means exhaustive. As always, clinical vigilance and attention to medical comorbidity is required to accurately diagnose and treat patients with these complex presentations.

References

Aarsland D, Påhlhagen S, Ballard CG, et al: Depression in Parkinson disease—epidemiology, mechanisms and management. Nat Rev Neurol 8(1):35–47, 2011 22198405

Abraham C, Cho JH: Inflammatory bowel disease. N Engl J Med 361(21):2066–2078, 2009 19923578

Aizenstein HJ, Baskys A, Boldrini M, et al: Vascular depression consensus report—a critical update. BMC Med 14(1):161, 2016 27806704

Albrecht JS, Kiptanui Z, Tsang Y, et al: Depression among older adults after traumatic brain injury: a national analysis. Am J Geriatr Psychiatry 23(6):607–614, 2015 25154547

Alexopoulos GS, Meyers BS, Young RC, et al: "Vascular depression" hypothesis. Arch Gen Psychiatry 54(10):915–922, 1997 9337771

American Psychiatric Association: Diagnostic and Statistical Manual of Mental Disorders, 5th Edition. Arlington, VA, American Psychiatric Association, 2013

Arseniou S, Arvaniti A, Samakouri M: HIV infection and depression. Psychiatry Clin Neurosci 68(2):96–109, 2014 24552630

Balázs J, Benazzi F, Rihmer Z, et al: The close link between suicide attempts and mixed (bipolar) depression: implications for suicide prevention. J Affect Disord 91(2–3):133–138, 2006 16458364

Bang J, Spina S, Miller BL: Frontotemporal dementia. Lancet 386(10004):1672–1682, 2015 26595641

Barbosa IG, Vale TC, de Macedo DL, et al: Neurosyphilis presenting as mania. Bipolar Disord 14(3):309–312, 2012 22548904

Benros ME, Waltoft BL, Nordentoft M, et al: Autoimmune diseases and severe infections as risk factors for mood disorders: a nationwide study. JAMA Psychiatry 70(8):812–820, 2013 23760347

Bratek A, Koźmin-Burzyńska A, Górniak E, et al: Psychiatric disorders associated with Cushing's syndrome. Psychiatr Danub 27 (suppl 1):S339–S343, 2015 26417792

Brooks JO 3rd, Hoblyn JC: Secondary mania in older adults. Am J Psychiatry 162(11):2033–2038, 2005 16263839

Bruno OD: Clinical features of Cushing's syndrome, in Cushing's Syndrome: Pathophysiology, Diagnosis and Treatment. Edited by Bronstein MD. New York, Humana Press, 2011, pp 53–64

Bui M, Mufson M, Gitlin D: The relationships between depression and medical illness, in Depression in Medical Illness. Edited by Barsky AJ, Silbersweig DA. New York, McGraw-Hill, 2017, pp 3–13

Bunevičius R, Prange AJ: Thyroid-brain interactions in neuropsychiatric disorders, in Neuropsychiatric Disorders. Edited by Miyoshi K, Morimura Y, Maeda K. Tokyo, Springer Japan, 2010, pp 17–32

Calabrese LV, Stern TA: Neuropsychiatric manifestations of systemic lupus erythematosus. Psychosomatics 36(4):344–359, 1995 7652137

Celano CM, Villegas AC, Albanese AM, et al: Depression and anxiety in heart failure: a review. Harv Rev Psychiatry 26(4):175–184, 2018 29975336

Chakrabarty T, Sepehry AA, Jacova C, et al: The prevalence of depressive symptoms in frontotemporal dementia: a meta-analysis. Dement Geriatr Cogn Disord 39(5–6):257–271, 2015 25662033

Charernboon T, Phanasathit M: Prevalence of neuropsychiatric symptoms in Alzheimer's disease: a cross-sectional descriptive study in Thailand. J Med Assoc Thai 97(5):560–565, 2014 25065098

Chi S, Yu J-T, Tan M-S, et al: Depression in Alzheimer's disease: epidemiology, mechanisms, and management. J Alzheimers Dis 42(3):739–755, 2014 24946876

Ciriaco M, Ventrice P, Russo G, et al: Corticosteroid-related central nervous system side effects. J Pharmacol Pharmacother 4 (suppl 1):S94–S98, 2013 24347992

Cohen BM, Sommer BR, Vuckovic A: Antidepressant-resistant depression in patients with comorbid subclinical hypothyroidism or high-normal TSH levels. Am J Psychiatry 175(7):598–604, 2018 29961367

Cubala WJ, Czarnowska-Cubala M: Neurosyphilis presenting with depressive symptomatology: is it unusual? Acta Neuropsychiatrica 20(2):110, 2008. Available at: https://www.cambridge.org/core/journals/acta-neuropsychiatrica/article/neurosyphilis-presenting-with-depressive-symptomatology-is-it-unusual/FFD1F06FDB232CD00FB52D4F0F2D0ED2. Accessed April 6, 2019.

Dalmau J, Graus F: Antibody-mediated encephalitis. N Engl J Med 378(9):840–851, 2018 29490181

Drugs that may cause psychiatric symptoms. Med Lett Drugs Ther 50(1301–1302):100–103, quiz 2, 104, 2008 19078866

Dubé B, Benton T, Cruess DG, et al: Neuropsychiatric manifestations of HIV infection and AIDS. J Psychiatry Neurosci 30(4):237–246, 2005 16049567

Epping EA, Kim JI, Craufurd D, et al: Longitudinal psychiatric symptoms in prodromal Huntington's disease: a decade of data. Am J Psychiatry 173(2):184–192, 2016 26472629

Feinstein A, Magalhaes S, Richard J-F, et al: The link between multiple sclerosis and depression. Nat Rev Neurol 10(9):507–517, 2014 25112509

Foster AR, Caplan JP: Paraneoplastic limbic encephalitis. Psychosomatics 50(2):108–113, 2009 19377018

Fujikawa T, Yamawaki S, Touhouda Y: Silent cerebral infarctions in patients with late-onset mania. Stroke 26(6):946–949, 1995 7762043

Galimberti D, Dell'Osso B, Altamura AC, et al: Psychiatric symptoms in frontotemporal dementia: epidemiology, phenotypes, and differential diagnosis. Biol Psychiatry 78(10):684–692, 2015 25958088

Geda YE, Roberts RO, Knopman DS, et al: Prevalence of neuropsychiatric symptoms in mild cognitive impairment and normal cognitive aging: population-based study. Arch Gen Psychiatry 65(10):1193–1198, 2008 18838636

Geringer ES, Querques J, Kolodziej MS, et al: Diagnosis and treatment of depression in the intensive care unit patient, in Irwin and Rippe's Intensive Care Medicine, 8th Edition. Philadelphia, PA, Wolters Kluwer, 2018, pp 1428–1439

Gilliam FG, Barry JJ, Hermann BP, et al: Rapid detection of major depression in epilepsy: a multicentre study. Lancet Neurol 5(5):399–405, 2006 16632310

Gougeon L, Payette H, Morais JA, et al: Intakes of folate, vitamin B6 and B12 and risk of depression in community-dwelling older adults: the Quebec Longitudinal Study on Nutrition and Aging. Eur J Clin Nutr 70(3):380–385, 2016 26648330

Grande I, Berk M, Birmaher B, et al: Bipolar disorder. Lancet 387(10027):1561–1572, 2016 26388529

Gupta RK, Kumar R: Benign brain tumours and psychiatric morbidity: a 5-years retrospective data analysis. Aust N Z J Psychiatry 38(5):316–319, 2004 15144507

Hackett ML, Köhler S, O'Brien JT, et al: Neuropsychiatric outcomes of stroke. Lancet Neurol 13(5):525–534, 2014 24685278

Hage MP, Azar ST: The link between thyroid function and depression. J Thyroid Res 2012:590648, 2012 22220285

Hare DL, Toukhsati SR, Johansson P, et al: Depression and cardiovascular disease: a clinical review. Eur Heart J 35(21):1365–1372, 2014 24282187

Horwitz AV, Wakefield JC: The Loss of Sadness: How Psychiatry Transformed Normal Sorrow Into Depressive Disorder. New York, Oxford University Press, 2007

Hotier S, Maltete D, Bourre B, et al: A manic episode with psychotic features improved by methylprednisolone in a patient with multiple sclerosis. Gen Hosp Psychiatry 37(6):621.e1–621.e2, 2015 26321022

Hu LY, Shen CC, Hu YW, et al: Hyperthyroidism and risk for bipolar disorders: a nationwide population-based study. PLoS One 8(8):e73057, 2013 24023669

Huffman JC, Celano CM, Beach SR, et al: Depression and cardiac disease: epidemiology, mechanisms, and diagnosis. Cardiovasc Psychiatry Neurol 2013:695925, 2013 23653854

Johansson V, Lundholm C, Hillert J, et al: Multiple sclerosis and psychiatric disorders: comorbidity and sibling risk in a nationwide Swedish cohort. Mult Scler 20(14):1881–1891, 2014 25013151

Joint United Nations Programme on HIV/AIDS: UNAIDS Data 2019. Geneva, Joint United Nations Programme on HIV/AIDS (UNAIDS), 16 July 2019. Available at: https://www.unaids.org/sites/default/files/media_asset/2019-UNAIDS-data_en.pdf. Accessed August 14, 2019.

Jorge RE, Arciniegas DB: Mood disorders after TBI. Psychiatr Clin North Am 37(1):13–29, 2014 24529421

Josephson AM, Mackenzie TB: Thyroid-induced mania in hypothyroid patients. Br J Psychiatry 137:222–228, 1980 7437657

Kanner AM: Depression in epilepsy: prevalence, clinical semiology, pathogenic mechanisms, and treatment. Biol Psychiatry 54(3):388–398, 2003 12893113

Kanner AM, Ribot R: Depression, in Neuropsychiatric Symptoms of Epilepsy. Edited by Mula M. Basel, Switzerland, Springer, 2016, pp 25–41

Kanner AM, Soto A, Gross-Kanner H: Prevalence and clinical characteristics of postictal psychiatric symptoms in partial epilepsy. Neurology 62(5):708–713, 2004 15007118

Kapoor A, Baig M, Tunio SA, et al: Neuropsychiatric and neurological problems among vitamin B12 deficient young vegetarians. Neurosciences (Riyadh) 22(3):228–232, 2017 28678220

Katunina E, Titova N: The epidemiology of nonmotor symptoms in Parkinson's disease (cohort and other studies). Int Rev Neurobiol 133:91–110, 2017 28802941

Khawaja IS, Westermeyer JJ, Gajwani P, et al: Depression and coronary artery disease: the association, mechanisms, and therapeutic implications. Psychiatry (Edgmont Pa) 6(1):38–51, 2009 19724742

Koutsouraki E, Costa V, Baloyannis S: Epidemiology of multiple sclerosis in Europe: a review. Int Rev Psychiatry 22(1):2–13, 2010 20233110

Krauthammer C, Klerman GL: Secondary mania: manic syndromes associated with antecedent physical illness or drugs. Arch Gen Psychiatry 35(11):1333–1339, 1978 757997

Krebber AMH, Buffart LM, Kleijn G, et al: Prevalence of depression in cancer patients: a meta-analysis of diagnostic interviews and self-report instruments. Psychooncology 23(2):121–130, 2014 24105788

Lachner C, Steinle NI, Regenold WT: The neuropsychiatry of vitamin B12 deficiency in elderly patients. J Neuropsychiatry Clin Neurosci 24(1):5–15, 2012 22450609

Lambrichts S, Van Oudenhove L, Sienaert P: Antibiotics and mania: a systematic review. J Affect Disord 219:149–156, 2017 28550767

Lanctôt KL, Amatniek J, Ancoli-Israel S, et al: Neuropsychiatric signs and symptoms of Alzheimer's disease: new treatment paradigms. Alzheimers Dement (N Y) 3(3):440–449, 2017 29067350

Lehman EJ, Hein MJ, Baron SL, et al: Neurodegenerative causes of death among retired National Football League players. Neurology 79(19):1970–1974, 2012 22955124

Lewis DA, Smith RE: Steroid-induced psychiatric syndromes. A report of 14 cases and a review of the literature. J Affect Disord 5(4):319–332, 1983 6319464

Lisnevskaia L, Murphy G, Isenberg D: Systemic lupus erythematosus. Lancet 384(9957):1878–1888, 2014 24881804

Lyketsos CG, Olin J: Depression in Alzheimer's disease: overview and treatment. Biol Psychiatry 52(3):243–252, 2002 12182930

Mackelprang JL, Bombardier CH, Fann JR, et al: Rates and predictors of suicidal ideation during the first year after traumatic brain injury. Am J Public Health 104(7):e100–e107, 2014 24832143

Madhusoodanan S, Opler MGA, Moise D, et al: Brain tumor location and psychiatric symptoms: is there any association? A meta-analysis of published case studies. Expert Rev Neurother 10(10):1529–1536, 2010 20925469

Madhusoodanan S, Ting MB, Farah T, et al: Psychiatric aspects of brain tumors: a review. World J Psychiatry 5(3):273–285, 2015 26425442

Maier F, Merkl J, Ellereit AL, et al: Hypomania and mania related to dopamine replacement therapy in Parkinson's disease. Parkinsonism Relat Disord 20(4):421–427, 2014 24467817

Mainio A, Kyllönen T, Viilo K, et al: Traumatic brain injury, psychiatric disorders and suicide: a population-based study of suicide victims during the years 1988–2004 in Northern Finland. Brain Inj 21(8):851–855, 2007 17676442

Marsh L: Depression and Parkinson's disease: current knowledge. Curr Neurol Neurosci Rep 13(12):409, 2013 24190780

McKee AC, Cantu RC, Nowinski CJ, et al: Chronic traumatic encephalopathy in athletes: progressive tauopathy after repetitive head injury. J Neuropathol Exp Neurol 68(7):709–735, 2009 19535999

McKee AC, Stern RA, Nowinski CJ, et al: The spectrum of disease in chronic traumatic encephalopathy. Brain 136(Pt 1):43–64, 2013 23208308

Mez J, Daneshvar DH, Kiernan PT, et al: Clinicopathological evaluation of chronic traumatic encephalopathy in players of American football. JAMA 318(4):360–370, 2017 28742910

Mirsal H, Kalyoncu A, Pektaş Ö, et al: Neurosyphilis presenting as psychiatric symptoms: an unusual case report. Acta Neuropsychiatr 19(4):251–253, 2007 26952892

Misiak B, Beszłej JA, Kotowicz K, et al: Cytokine alterations and cognitive impairment in major depressive disorder: from putative mechanisms to novel treatment targets. Prog Neuropsychopharmacol Biol Psychiatry 80(Pt C):177–188, 2018 28433456

Mørkeberg Nilsson F: Parkinson's disease and affective disorder: the temporal relationship. Open Journal of Psychiatry 2(2):96–109, 2012. Available at: https://www.scirp.org/Journal/PaperInformation.aspx?PaperID=18478. Accessed April 6, 2019.

Mula M: Mania and elation, in Neuropsychiatric Symptoms of Epilepsy. Edited by Mula M. Basel, Switzerland, Springer, 2016, pp 43–51

Murphy R, O'Donoghue S, Counihan T, et al: Neuropsychiatric syndromes of multiple sclerosis. J Neurol Neurosurg Psychiatry 88(8):697–708, 2017 28285265

Nakimuli-Mpungu E, Musisi S, Mpungu SK, et al: Primary mania versus HIV-related secondary mania in Uganda. Am J Psychiatry 163(8):1349–1354, quiz 1480, 2006 16877646

Nanni MG, Caruso R, Mitchell AJ, et al: Depression in HIV infected patients: a review. Curr Psychiatry Rep 17(1):530, 2015 25413636

Navabi S, Gorrepati VS, Yadav S, et al: Influences and impact of anxiety and depression in the setting of inflammatory bowel disease. Inflamm Bowel Dis 24(11):2303–2308, 2018 29788469

Otte C, Gold SM, Penninx BW, et al: Major depressive disorder. Nat Rev Dis Primers 2:16065, 2016 27629598

Özkan A, Altinbaş K, Koç ER, et al: Affective temperament profiles in patients with multiple sclerosis: association with mood disorders. Noro Psikiyatri Arsivi 53(4):311–316, 2016 28360804

Paparrigopoulos T, Ferentinos P, Kouzoupis A, et al: The neuropsychiatry of multiple sclerosis: focus on disorders of mood, affect and behaviour. Int Rev Psychiatry 22(1):14–21, 2010 20233111

Patten SB, Beck CA, Williams JVA, et al: Major depression in multiple sclerosis: a population-based perspective. Neurology 61(11):1524–1527, 2003 14663036

Patten SB, Marrie RA, Carta MG: Depression in multiple sclerosis. Int Rev Psychiatry 29(5):463–472, 2017 28681616

Perry DC, Sturm VE, Peterson MJ, et al: Association of traumatic brain injury with subsequent neurological and psychiatric disease: a meta-analysis. J Neurosurg 124(2):511–526, 2016 26315003

Petridou ET, Kousoulis AA, Michelakos T, et al: Folate and B12 serum levels in association with depression in the aged: a systematic review and meta-analysis. Aging Ment Health 20(9):965–973, 2016 26055921

Pla P, Orvoen S, Saudou F, et al: Mood disorders in Huntington's disease: from behavior to cellular and molecular mechanisms. Front Behav Neurosci 8:135, 2014 24795586

Ponsford J, Alway Y, Gould KR: Epidemiology and natural history of psychiatric disorders after TBI. J Neuropsychiatry Clin Neurosci 30(4):262–270, 2018 29939106

Qato DM, Ozenberger K, Olfson M: Prevalence of prescription medications with depression as a potential adverse effect among adults in the United States. JAMA 319(22):2289–2298, 2018 29896627

Rabkin JG: HIV and depression: 2008 review and update. Curr HIV/AIDS Rep 5(4):163–171, 2008 18838056

Radhakrishnan R, Garakani A, Gross LS, et al: Neuropsychiatric aspects of concussion. Lancet Psychiatry 3(12):1166–1175, 2016 27889010

Ramsey CM, Leoutsakos J-M, Mayer LS, et al: History of manic and hypomanic episodes and risk of incident cardiovascular disease: 11.5 year follow-up from the Baltimore Epidemiologic Catchment Area Study. J Affect Disord 125(1–3):35–41, 2010 20570367

Rihmer A, Gonda X, Balazs J, et al: The importance of depressive mixed states in suicidal behaviour. Neuropsychopharmacol Hung 10(1):45–49, 2008 18771019

Robinson RG, Jorge RE: Post-stroke depression: a review. Am J Psychiatry 173(3):221–231, 2016 26684921

Robinson RG, Kubos KL, Starr LB, et al: Mood disorders in stroke patients. Importance of location of lesion. Brain 107(Pt 1):81–93, 1984 6697163

Rosenblatt A: Neuropsychiatry of Huntington's disease. Dialogues Clin Neurosci 9(2):191–197, 2007 17726917

Rusher DR, Pawlak R: A review of 89 published case studies of vitamin B12 deficiency. Journal of Human Nutrition & Food Science 1(2):1008, 2013

Satzer D, Bond DJ: Mania secondary to focal brain lesions: implications for understanding the functional neuroanatomy of bipolar disorder. Bipolar Disord 18(3):205–220, 2016 27112231

SayuriYamagata A, Brietzke E, Rosenblat JD, et al: Medical comorbidity in bipolar disorder: the link with metabolic-inflammatory systems. J Affect Disord 211:99–106, 2017 28107669

Schmitz B: Depression and mania in patients with epilepsy. Epilepsia 46 (suppl 4):45–49, 2005 15938709

Siegmann E-M, Müller HHO, Luecke C, et al: Association of depression and anxiety disorders with autoimmune thyroiditis: a systematic review and meta-analysis. JAMA Psychiatry 75(6):577–584, 2018 29800939

Sonino N, Fallo F, Fava GA: Psychosomatic aspects of Cushing's syndrome. Rev Endocr Metab Disord 11(2):95–104, 2010 19960264

Steffens DC, Krishnan KRR: Structural neuroimaging and mood disorders: recent findings, implications for classification, and future directions. Biol Psychiatry 43(10):705–712, 1998 9606523

Stein TD, Alvarez VE, McKee AC: Chronic traumatic encephalopathy: a spectrum of neuropathological changes following repetitive brain trauma in athletes and military personnel. Alzheimers Res Ther 6(1):4, 2014 24423082

Stern RA, Daneshvar DH, Baugh CM, et al: Clinical presentation of chronic traumatic encephalopathy. Neurology 81(13):1122–1129, 2013 23966253

Talaei A, Rafee N, Rafei F, et al: TSH cut off point based on depression in hypothyroid patients. BMC Psychiatry 17(1):327, 2017 28882111

Tascone LDS, Payne ME, MacFall J, et al: Cortical brain volume abnormalities associated with few or multiple neuropsychiatric symptoms in Alzheimer's disease. PLoS One 12(5):e0177169, 2017 28481904

Taylor JB, Prager LM, Quijije NV, et al: Case 21–2018: a 61-year-old man with grandiosity, impulsivity, and decreased sleep. N Engl J Med 379(2):182–189, 2018 29996076

Taylor WD, Aizenstein HJ, Alexopoulos GS: The vascular depression hypothesis: mechanisms linking vascular disease with depression. Mol Psychiatry 18(9):963–974, 2013 23439482

Tiemeier H, van Tuijl HR, Hofman A, et al: Vitamin B12, folate, and homocysteine in depression: the Rotterdam Study. Am J Psychiatry 159(12):2099–2101, 2002 12450964

Torres J, Mehandru S, Colombel J-F, et al: Crohn's disease. Lancet 389(10080):1741–1755, 2017 27914655

Tüzün E, Dalmau J: Limbic encephalitis and variants: classification, diagnosis and treatment. Neurologist 13(5):261–271, 2007 17848866

Tysnes OB, Storstein A: Epidemiology of Parkinson's disease. J Neural Transm (Vienna) 124(8):901–905, 2017 28150045

van Agtmaal MJM, Houben AJHM, Pouwer F, et al: Association of microvascular dysfunction with late-life depression: a systematic review and meta-analysis. JAMA Psychiatry 74(7):729–739, 2017 28564681

Vieta E, Berk M, Schulze TG, et al: Bipolar disorders. Nat Rev Dis Primers 4:18008, 2018 29516993

Viguera AC, Fan Y, Thompson NR, et al: Prevalence and predictors of depression among patients with epilepsy, stroke, and multiple sclerosis using the Cleveland Clinic Knowledge Program within the Neurological Institute. Psychosomatics 59(4):369–378, 2018 29580558

Warrington TP, Bostwick JM: Psychiatric adverse effects of corticosteroids. Mayo Clin Proc 81(10):1361–1367, 2006 17036562

Wijeratne C, Malhi GS: Vascular mania: an old concept in danger of sclerosing? A clinical overview. Acta Psychiatr Scand Suppl 116(434):35–40, 2007 17688461

Woolley JD, Khan BK, Murthy NK, et al: The diagnostic challenge of psychiatric symptoms in neurodegenerative disease: rates of and risk factors for prior psychiatric diagnosis in patients with early neurodegenerative disease. J Clin Psychiatry 72(2):126–133, 2011 21382304

Wu W, Sun Z, Yu J, et al: A clinical retrospective analysis of factors associated with apathetic hyperthyroidism. Pathobiology 77(1):46–51, 2010 20185967

Zoungrana J, Dembélé JP, Sako FB, et al: Depression and HIV: epidemiological and clinical aspects at the Bamako University Hospital (Mali). Med Sante Trop 27(2):186–189, 2017 28655681

CHAPTER 20

Anxiety and Related Disorders

Manifestations in the General Medical Setting

Charles Hebert, M.D.

David Banayan, M.D., M.Sc., FRCPC

Fernando Espi-Forcen, M.D., Ph.D.

Kathryn Perticone, A.P.N., M.S.W.

Sameera Guttikonda, M.D.

Mark Pollack, M.D.

Physicians frequently encounter patients with acute anxiety in general medical settings. While many patients may have only episodic anxiety, some patients present with recurrent symptoms that may be representative of a formal anxiety disorder. Such cases often require a substantial investment of time and attention from clinicians as well as from the health care system. Generalized anxiety disorder (GAD) and panic disorder are among the most common anxiety disorders described in the fifth edition of the *Diagnostic and Statistical Manual of Mental Disorders* (DSM-5; American Psychiatric Association 2013). Obsessive-Compulsive and Related Disorders, including obsessive-compulsive disorder (OCD), and Trauma- and Stressor-Related Disorders, including posttraumatic stress disorder (PTSD), are now classified independently of Anxiety Disorders in DSM-5; however, they are of relevance in the general medical setting. The DSM-5 criterion requiring that individuals experience "clinically significant distress or impairment in social, occupational, or other important areas of functioning" as a result of their symptoms is a unifying criterion for all mental disorders. While the level of impairment that anxiety produces for patients is sometimes quite transparent to primary care providers, the etiology of a patient's anxious distress may be less readily identified. Given that anxiety disorder presentations may include physical as well as cognitive signs and symptoms, practitioners often face the conundrum of determining whether a patient's anxious distress represents a primary psychiatric diagnosis or is induced by an underlying medical condition. Discriminating which of these etiologies is more likely may be especially challenging in patients with long-standing comorbid medical conditions.

In this chapter, we focus on the aforementioned psychiatric disorders, with particular attention to medical signs and symptoms that might overlap with their presentations. We also discuss common physical symptoms that are often coincident with anxiety disorders but might escape clinical attention, and we review treatment strategies.

Panic Disorder

Panic attacks are characterized by an abrupt surge of intense fear or discomfort that rapidly ascends to peak intensity within seconds to minutes. Physical symptoms of distress associated with panic attacks include heart pounding or palpitations, tachycardia, diaphoresis, tremors, chest pain, nausea, dizziness (presyncope or a feeling of disorientation), feeling faint, and paresthesias. It is important to note that a *panic attack* is not itself a codable psychiatric diagnosis; rather, *panic disorder* is defined as recurrent panic attacks that lead to either 1) persistent worry about potential future attacks or the consequences thereof or 2) maladaptive changes in behavior aimed at mitigating future attacks (American Psychiatric Association 2013).

The lifetime prevalence of panic disorder in adults in the United States is estimated to be 6.8%. The 12-month prevalence has been estimated at 2.4%, based on DSM-IV-TR diagnostic criteria (American Psychiatric Association 2000; Kessler et al. 2012). A significant portion of cases (up to 49%) are classified as being severe (Kessler et al. 2005). Because of the intense physical presentation of panic attacks, primary care clinicians are frequently tasked with discerning what aspects of a patient's presentation are due to possible panic disorder or to a general medical condition. A wide range of pathophysiological processes can produce symptoms of panic with varied degrees of intensity. However, the symptoms may not be easily recognizable as being due to a general medical condition. Understandably, misattribution of symptoms to panic disorder or a related psychiatric problem occurs commonly (van Loon et al. 2011). As with all approaches to proper diagnosis and management, the process begins with a complete patient history and detailed but targeted physical examination. Knowledge about the various medical causes of panic attacks helps the provider establish a differential diagnosis that can be further refined by tests or investigations. Table 20–1 lists physiological causes of panic attacks and symptoms of anxiety attacks, organized by bodily system. This list is not exhaustive; rather, it is intended to highlight both common and selected rare etiologies of panic and anxiety presentations that may be encountered by primary care clinicians.

Tachyarrhythmias

One of the more challenging diagnoses to make is an anxiety state provoked by a nonsustained tachyarrhythmia, such as paroxysmal supraventricular tachycardia (PSVT) (Frommeyer et al. 2013; McCrank et al. 1998). PSVT is caused by conduction signal re-

TABLE 20–1. **Medical causes of anxiety and panic attacks**

Cardiovascular	**Nutritional**
Tachyarrhythmias (PSVT, AFib with RVR)	B$_{12}$ deficiency
Orthostatic hypotension	
Dysautonomia	**Recreational drugs/substance use**
Mitral valve prolapse syndrome	Alcohol withdrawal
Angina pectoris	Sedative-hypnotic withdrawal
Congestive heart failure	Benzodiazepines
Paroxysmal nocturnal dyspnea	Barbiturates
	Caffeine intoxication
Respiratory	LSD, cannabis, MDMA, PCP
Chronic obstructive pulmonary disease	
Asthma	**Pharmacological**
Exercised-induced acute bronchospasm	Albuterol
Flash pulmonary edema	Salmeterol
	Systemic steroids
Hematological	Abrupt cessation of an adrenergic inhibitor
Severe hypoproliferative anemia	
	Drug interaction: MAOI + tyramine
Endocrinological	Stimulants
Hyperthyroidism	Methylphenidate
Adrenal insufficiency/crisis	Dextroamphetamine
Thyrotoxicosis	Antiarrhythmics (e.g., flecainide, propafenone)
Hypothyroidism	
Pheochromocytoma	Akathisia
Pancreatic islet cell tumors	Antipsychotic medications
Insulinoma	SSRIs/SNRIs
VIPoma	
Neuroendocrine tumors	
Carcinoid syndrome	

Note. AFib=atrial fibrillation; LSD=lysergic acid diethylamide; MAOI=monoamine oxidase inhibitor; MDMA=methylenedioxymethamphetamine; PCP=phencyclidine; PSVT=paroxysmal supraventricular tachycardia; RVR=rapid ventricular response; SNRI=serotonin-norepinephrine reuptake inhibitor; SSRI=selective serotonin reuptake inhibitor; VIP=vasoactive intestinal peptide.

entry into the atrioventricular node or by aberrant conduction between the atria and ventricles, often by way of an accessory pathway (McCrank et al. 1998). Both panic attacks and PSVT share the same subjective symptom of racing heartbeat. Not surprisingly, PSVT can also induce chest pain, dyspnea, feelings of lightheadedness, presyncope or syncope, diaphoresis, and difficulty concentrating—all of which are prominent features of panic attacks.

The duration of a PSVT event can vary greatly. Attacks of PSVT that are of short duration pose significant challenges for making the correct diagnosis. The arrhythmia has frequently resolved by the time the patient has arrived at the emergency department. Unless there are cardinal electrocardiogram (ECG) findings (e.g., short PR interval or a delta wave associated with Wolff-Parkinson-White syndrome), the underlying cardiac etiology may go undetected. In a single-center retrospective survey of 107 patients with PSVT who were referred for electrophysiological evaluation, 67% of patients met DSM-IV (American Psychiatric Association 1994) diagnostic criteria for panic disorder, and 55.5% of patients were incorrectly diagnosed by nonpsychiatrist physicians after the initial medical evaluation (Lessmeier et al. 1997). Physicians most commonly ascribed patients' complaints to panic, stress, anxiety, mitral valve prolapse, or excess caffeine consumption. The median time to correct diagnosis of PSVT was 3.3 years (Lessmeier et al. 1997). Women were more likely than men to receive a misdiagnosis of panic disorder rather than PSVT. Patients who had ECG signs of ventricular preexcitation remained misdiagnosed for almost 3.5 years. Use of Holter monitoring detected PSVT in only 6 of 64 (9%) patients, whereas use of an event recorder detected PSVT in 8 of 17 (47%) patients. Of the patients diagnosed with PSVT, 81% underwent catheter ablation; in 86% of these patients, complete recovery was noted, with no further panic attacks (Lessmeier et al. 1997).

It is not possible to make a correct diagnosis of PSVT from physical examination alone. ECG, Holter, or event monitoring are necessary steps for a thorough evaluation. Even though the number of patients appropriately diagnosed through the use of such techniques may be fairly small, detecting such cases is of clear importance, because electrophysiological ablation is quite effective in reducing the number of recurrent events. The ongoing challenge of making a correct diagnosis can confuse both physicians and patients. Thus, patients with tachyarrhythmia may not receive the correct treatment, and the identified "panic disorder" may be classified as "treatment resistant" by a psychiatrist. Consequently, the patient with a tachyarrhythmia may not be referred to a cardiologist, with resultant delays in care.

Paroxysmal Nocturnal Dyspnea

A common clinical symptom observed in patients with congestive heart failure, paroxysmal nocturnal dyspnea (PND) should be considered not only in elderly individuals but also in all patients with major risk factors for heart disease or known myocardial dysfunction. PND is caused by failure of cardiac contractility, which impairs forward flow, resulting in pulmonary edema due to venous congestion in the lungs. Fluid accumulation in the lung parenchyma impairs oxygen and carbon dioxide gas exchange, resulting in hypoxia. Patients with PND typically describe having suddenly awoken from sleep with intense shortness of breath, needing to sit upright or stand, and not uncommonly seeking an open window to "get more air." Individuals who describe such symptoms may incorrectly be diagnosed as having panic attacks that are exclusively nocturnal. Primary care clinicians should remain cognizant of the likelihood that these moments of "panic" may represent undiagnosed congestive heart failure in patients with underlying cardiac risk factors and should consider appropriate workup. An echocardiogram can definitively determine whether a patient has impaired myocardial contractility and can help gauge the severity of that impairment.

Wheezing

Wheezing is a common symptom encountered by primary care practitioners in patients with obstructive lung disease, including chronic obstructive pulmonary disease

(COPD) and asthma. Primary care clinicians are often tasked with managing both of these illnesses either independently or in conjunction with a pulmonologist. The comorbidity of panic disorder and COPD has been well described, and the prevalence of panic disorder in patients with COPD may be as much as 10 times the prevalence in the general population (approximately 1.5%–3.5%) (Centers for Disease Control and Prevention 2005; Smoller et al. 1996). Estimates of the prevalence of panic disorder in COPD vary widely and range from 6% to as high as 67% (Kunik et al. 2005; Pollack et al. 1996). A systematic review examining the prevalence of comorbid anxiety disorders in patients with a diagnosis of COPD found that the prevalence of panic disorder (with and without agoraphobia) among inpatients ranged from zero to 41%, whereas the prevalence among outpatients ranged from 8% to 21% (Willgoss and Yohannes 2013). Among inpatients with COPD, 10%–55% had a clinical diagnosis of some form of anxiety disorder (generalized anxiety disorder, panic disorder, specific phobia, social phobia), whereas outpatients had a somewhat lesser prevalence, ranging from 13% to 46% (Willgoss and Yohannes 2013). In another study conducted at a Veterans Affairs Medical Center, a large sample of patients ($N=1,134$) with chronic breathing disorders (i.e., not exclusively COPD) were screened for depression and anxiety (Kunik et al. 2005). Among the subset of patients with confirmed COPD who underwent a structured clinical interview ($n=204$), 65% received a diagnosis of anxiety and/or depression; among these patients, only 31% were receiving psychiatric care at the time of assessment (Kunik et al. 2005).

COPD is characterized by destruction of the lung parenchyma and effacement of the normal architecture of the terminal bronchioles and the alveolar-vascular air-exchange interface. These structural abnormalities result in decreased efficiency of air exchange as well as trapping of carbon dioxide. The resulting hypoxia and hypercapnia trigger a central nervous system–mediated response, including physical symptoms and signs of anxiety frequently mimicking panic—hypertension, tachycardia, palpitations, hyperventilation, paresthesias, dizziness, lightheadedness, air hunger, shortness of breath, and presyncope. Similarly, acute asthma exacerbations resulting from recurrent bronchoconstriction produce a sympathetic response elicited by both lack of adequate oxygenation and a subjective sense of air hunger, smothering, and fear of death by asphyxiation. Many of the cardinal symptoms of asthma can appear at night, and physicians often include frequency of nighttime symptoms in the overall assessment as a marker for control of illness (Colice 2004).

Both COPD and asthma can elicit the physiological response of panic, and panic disorder is often comorbid with these chronic respiratory conditions (Smoller et al. 2003). The presence of wheezing should raise suspicion for the presence of pulmonary disease, because wheezing is neither pathognomonic nor a common feature of a panic attack. Patients who present with panic characterized by wheezing, especially if the wheezing is associated with a prolonged expiratory phase or use of accessory respiratory muscles, should undergo further evaluation for comorbid respiratory disease. Although a history of tobacco use is particularly relevant, pulmonary function tests (e.g., spirometry) and chest X ray (looking for barrel chest, overinflated lungs, or emphysema) may be helpful in identifying patients with COPD and asthma. More invasive tests, such as arterial blood gas analysis, should be undertaken only if the results of noninvasive testing, such as ambulatory oximetry, are inconclusive or equivocal.

Short-acting β_2 adrenergic receptor agonists such as albuterol play an important role in relieving acute bronchoconstriction associated with exacerbations of COPD and asthma. These agents have positive chronotropic and inotropic effects on myocardium, which can simulate some of the core symptoms of a panic attack. Side effects from medications in this class include dizziness or sensations of presyncope, which also occur in panic disorder. Detailed inquiry about use of both short-acting (e.g., albuterol) and long-acting (e.g., formoterol, salmeterol) β_2 receptor agonists is important to create a temporal outline of the frequency and timing of attacks and should be part of any primary care assessment.

Tremor

Tremor, a fairly nonspecific symptom, is a common finding among patients with anxiety disorders, including panic disorder. DSM-5 includes trembling and shaking among the physical symptoms experienced during a panic attack; however, clinicians should maintain vigilance for medical etiologies of tremor (American Psychiatric Association 2013).

Key among potential medical etiologies for tremor are endocrinological causes, such as pheochromocytoma and hyperthyroidism, diagnoses that are frequently accompanied by anxious symptoms. Pheochromocytoma is characterized by the development of a catecholamine-secreting tumor derived from chromaffin cells of the adrenal medulla or a tumor of the sympathetic ganglia. The average annual incidence rate of pheochromocytoma has been estimated at approximately 0.8 cases per 100,000 person-years (Beard et al. 1983). Prevalence estimates for comorbid panic disorder in patients with pheochromocytoma approach 40% (Beard et al. 1983; Fishman et al. 2004). The classic triad of symptoms seen in pheochromocytoma is episodic headache, sweating, and tachycardia (Stein and Black 1991). A fine tremor of the hands may also be apparent. Symptom presentation varies, and the symptoms noted here cannot be relied on alone for diagnosis (Kudva et al. 1999). In addition to tremors, a number of other signs and symptoms are common to both the hyperadrenergic spells of pheochromocytoma and the panic attacks of panic disorder; these include nonexertional palpitations, diaphoresis, tremor, and headache. Like panic attacks, the symptoms of adrenergic surge seen in pheochromocytoma are periodic, unpredictable (i.e., no identifiable trigger), and generally self-limited. Clues that point toward a diagnosis of pheochromocytoma include onset of hypertension at a young age, presence of "treatment-resistant" hypertension, and family history of pheochromocytoma—in particular, the genetic syndromes of multiple endocrine neoplasia type 2 (MEN-2), neurofibromatosis type 1 (NF-1), or von Hippel–Lindau (VHL) disease (Young 2016a, 2016b). Workup consists of 24-hour urinary catecholamine and metanephrine collection. Because many psychotropic agents modulate adrenergic tone as their mechanism of action, tricyclic antidepressants (TCAs), selective serotonin reuptake inhibitors (SSRIs), and serotonin norepinephrine reuptake inhibitors (SNRIs) should be discontinued for at least 2 weeks prior to such diagnostic testing, because they can falsely elevate results.

Hyperthyroidism may also be a medical etiology of tremor and should be excluded in individuals who present with signs and symptoms of panic disorder. In addition to tremulousness (usually a fine intention tremor of the hands), typical symptoms of hyperthyroidism include palpitations, heat intolerance, proximal muscle weakness, emotional lability, and unintentional weight loss. Physical examination often reveals tachycardia, diaphoresis, warm skin, hair loss, intense gaze (stare) and lid lag, and proptosis. In patients with hyperthyroidism due to Graves' disease, exophthalmos and pretibial myxedema can also be present. Palpation of the thyroid may reveal nodules or uniform enlargement of the gland. Neurological examination may reveal hyperreflexia. Initial laboratory workup consists of serum thyroid-stimulating hormone (TSH) and free thyroxine (T_4) levels. Free T_4 will be elevated, whereas TSH will be low (suppressed by elevated levels of thyroxine) in primary hyperthyroidism. In some cases, patients will have normal free T_4 levels and only triiodothyronine (T_3) will be elevated (Fishman et al. 2004).

In a systematic review of the literature and meta-analysis of 19 studies involving more than 36,000 patients with autoimmune thyroiditis, Hashimoto's thyroiditis, or subclinical or overt hypothyroidism, increased hazard ratios for depressive disorders (3.56) or anxiety disorders (2.32) were found in patients compared with healthy control subjects (Siegmann et al. 2018).

Additional discussion of thyroid disorders can be found elsewhere in this volume (see Chapter 7, "Endocrine Disorders and Their Psychiatric Manifestations," and Chapter 8, "Inflammatory Diseases and Their Psychiatric Manifestations").

Generalized Anxiety Disorder

The hallmark feature of GAD is an excessive and persistent sense of worry that is difficult to control (American Psychiatric Association 2013). Like many psychiatric illnesses, GAD causes significant distress for individuals, and the chronic nature of the condition—which is often marked by periodic exacerbations—can result in longstanding disability. Distinct from "fear," which represents the physiological and emotional response to an overt external threat, the worries associated with GAD are instead grounded in a *perceived* threat that does not have an external correlate. GAD permeates all spheres of the patient's life and includes even the more mundane aspects of daily life (i.e., worrying excessively about the weather forecast or traffic delays). Many patients report extreme difficulty in putting aside certain concerns when more pressing matters arise (Schneider and Levenson 2008).

With a lifetime prevalence of approximately 4%–7%, GAD is frequently found in community and primary care settings (American Psychiatric Association 2013; Schneider and Levenson 2008). It is the most common anxiety disorder encountered in primary care clinics and accounts for high utilization of health care resources (Munk-Jørgensen et al. 2006; Hoge et al. 2012). The disorder is often comorbid with other psychiatric conditions, including other anxiety disorders and mood disorders (American Psychiatric Association 2013; Schneider and Levenson 2008).

Symptom onset often occurs in late adolescence or early adulthood, and a 2:1 female-to-male predominance has been observed (Schneider and Levenson 2008; Wittchen et al. 2002).

The DSM-5 diagnosis of GAD rests on identification of a combination of cognitive and somatic symptoms (American Psychiatric Association 2013). Cognitive symptoms include a feeling of excessive or uncontrollable worry occurring more days than not, irritability, and an internal feeling of being "keyed up" or "on edge" for a period of at least 6 months. Somatic symptoms include fatigue, impairment in concentration, muscle tension, and disturbed sleep.

The underpinnings of the somatic symptoms are rooted in a well-established mind-body interface. The Hungarian-American psychoanalyst and physician Franz Alexander was among the first to point out that mental states such as anger, fear, sadness, and frustration can manifest as physical symptoms and that such symptoms can be multiple (Alexander 1943). Many patients with GAD initially present to primary care clinicians for evaluation of their physical complaints instead of seeking mental health care for their anxiety. Although somatic symptoms are typically "front and center" for clinicians, the underlying emotional states responsible for a patient's physical distress often elude detection and may not become fully apparent until later in a patient's course. Clinicians may attempt multiple treatments in the interim, only to find that the usual interventions targeting patients' apparent general medical complaints do not result in meaningful subjective or objective improvement in daily functioning or quality of life. These patients' recurrent presentations for care of ongoing symptoms and physical concerns can lead to frustration on the part of clinicians as well as a tendency to perceive such patients as "chronic complainers" (Stuart and Lieberman 2008).

While DSM-5 specifies some concrete physical symptoms frequently encountered among GAD patients in clinical practice, recognition of GAD in primary care settings is nonetheless limited by significant variability of patient presentation. Patients may seek care for disabling physical complaints that are sometimes distinct from the formal GAD diagnostic criteria. Patients may also manifest only subsyndromal signs of illness, which may make recognition of anxious distress difficult (Schneider and Levenson 2008). In the latter case, symptoms may intensify during periods of increased psychosocial duress (i.e., an upcoming work presentation or deadline) or in response to a major life change (i.e., relocation to a new city, birth of a child, divorce). Patients may not independently recognize or be willing to consider the influence of their level of anxiety on physical symptoms, which can lead to a faulty clinical diagnosis and premature closure by providers. In such cases, the clinician's proposed plan of care runs the risk of neglecting unmet psychiatric needs and also of introducing unnecessary risk via other medical treatments (e.g., side effects of analgesics used for neck pain or of bronchodilators used for shortness of breath). Close attention and vigilance to the pattern and periodicity of a patient's physical symptoms are necessary. In many patients, acute worsening in symptom frequency or severity concurrent with a change in psychosocial circumstances can serve as a valuable clue to the clinician to consider psychiatric etiologies as possible and likely contributors to patient complaints (Schneider and Levenson 2008).

As described, the broad range of symptoms with which patients present makes prompt detection of GAD challenging for many physicians. Patients report a variety of symptoms, including headaches, tremors, shortness of breath, diaphoresis, palpitations, dizziness, chest pain, neck pain, and nausea. Patients may present for evaluation of a single symptom or several symptoms. Symptom severity may likewise vary, with one complaint predominating over others in intensity at any given point in time (Wittchen et al. 2002). Such symptoms may be representative of GAD in their own right; however, clinicians should take note that ongoing, untreated GAD can also influence the severity of comorbid physical illnesses that drive a patient's physical complaints (Niles et al. 2015; Wittchen et al. 2002). In both scenarios, the cognitive distortion of catastrophizing plays a central role. *Catastrophizing* refers to an irrational thought process in which a person imagines the worst conceivable outcome of a situation, without any evidence to support such a likelihood, and then comes to expect that "worst case" outcome. This style of thinking has been linked to a number of anxiety disorders, including GAD, and is closely intertwined with physical symptoms experienced by patients.

Although not included in the DSM-5 diagnostic criteria for GAD, headache and back pain have an important relationship with catastrophic cognitions.

Headache

Substantial comorbidity exists between primary headache disorders and GAD. In some samples, as many as 37% of patients with headache met formal criteria for GAD (Lucchetti et al. 2013; Niles et al. 2015). Importantly, subsyndromal symptoms of anxiety (i.e., symptoms that do not meet formal diagnostic criteria for GAD but lead to distress and impaired functioning in daily life) have been linked to development of headache symptomatology. Lucchetti et al. (2013) observed that among patients with primary headache disorders, subsyndromal anxiety was associated with a more than twofold increased risk of developing migraine headaches. Maladaptive pain-coping strategies, including catastrophizing, significantly contribute to this association. Other authors have demonstrated that catastrophizing predicts development of migraine headaches, of longer-duration migraine attacks, and of chronic migraines (Bond et al. 2015).

Back Pain

Low back pain is a common and frequent reason for presentation to general physicians. Pain complaints may take many forms, including muscle spasm, neuropathic (i.e., sciatic or radicular) pain, weakness of an extremity, soreness, or self-reported muscle "tension." Back pain may be localized to the lumbosacral regions but can also be more widespread, with involvement of the shoulders and neck. Symptoms of pain may lead to severe physical debility, resulting in significant reductions in quality of life and in work productivity, as well as ongoing high utilization of medical services (Bair et al. 2008).

The frequent co-occurrence of chronic low back pain with anxious distress has been well described (Gore et al. 2012; Means-Christensen et al. 2008). The physiological and autonomic arousal response of highly anxious states seen in patients with GAD frequently leads to muscle tension that affects paraspinal muscles, resulting in pain. The experience of such pain is not purely a cognitive construct; rather, it is the consequence of a known neurophysiological process by which the state of being anxious results in increased motor unit activation of skeletal muscles (Burns et al. 2009). There is electrophysiological evidence that unmitigated catastrophic cognitions adversely affect this process (Pakzad et al. 2016). For example, in patients with low back pain, it has been observed that altered trunk muscle activation (which is believed to contribute to symptom severity) is more strongly associated with the degree of patient catastrophizing than with the intensity of the applied pain stimuli, resulting in higher rates of perceived discomfort than would be anticipated for a given pain stimulus (Pakzad et al. 2016).

Given that the catastrophic attributional style common in GAD patients can manifest with somatic symptoms and can worsen preexisting physical ailments (Uniyal et al. 2017), prompt recognition of GAD is critical in primary care settings. While some patients report feelings of excessive worry that lead a clinician to consider GAD, many patients do not report such symptoms. A high index of suspicion is necessary to recognize anxious distress among such patients, who often complain only of physical symptoms. Screening tools such as the Generalized Anxiety Disorder seven-item scale (GAD-7; Spitzer et al. 2006) have been developed for this purpose and can be implemented easily in an outpatient setting. A score of 7 or greater on the GAD-7 is generally accepted as indicative of a clinically significant degree of anxiety that warrants further investigation and possible intervention (Schneider and Levenson 2008).

Although psychiatric scales and inventories are in widespread use, they should not serve as a substitute for a thorough and deliberate clinical interview. Clinicians should ask patients directly if they have difficulty "shutting their mind off" or controlling their level of worry. Questioning patients about the impressions of others who are close to them also yields valuable information about whether a patient's level of anxiety causes meaningful distress with interpersonal relationships (Schneider and Levenson 2008). Many patients reveal clues suggestive of possible untreated GAD or other anxiety disorders when primary care providers inquire empathically. Primary care clinicians should not dismiss a patient's anxious worries as being simply part of daily life. Concerns about whether the bus will arrive in order for a patient reliant on public transportation to get to work on time may seem clinically negligible on the surface. Such "everyday hassles" are unlikely to produce physical symptoms in the vast majority of patients, but the co-occurrence of excessive mundane worries and physical symptoms should prompt clinicians to explore GAD as a possibility (American Psychiatric Association 2013; Schneider and Levenson 2008). Importantly, the broader and more widespread a patient's worries are, the greater the likelihood that the patient has GAD (American Psychiatric Association 2013).

Other historical clues to the diagnosis include engaging in maladaptive behaviors to self-manage co-occurring physical symptoms. Increasing use of substances—in particular, alcohol—is one such strategy among GAD patients. Patients may turn to alcohol as an aid to dampen the cognitive symptoms of GAD or to relieve the insomnia or muscle tension that commonly coexist (American Psychiatric Association 2013; Schneider and Levenson 2008). Clinicians should be aware that the severity of insomnia is strongly correlated with the severity of GAD (Ferre Navarette et al. 2017). Therefore, screening patients for frequency of alcohol use can identify those who may have undiagnosed GAD.

Additional patient features that may prompt consideration of GAD come from the physical examination. Often the severity of a patient's complaint will not correlate with the physical examination findings. In such cases, there is often just cause to conduct a formal assessment for anxiety. For example, patients complaining of severe headache who have a benign neurological examination may benefit from a discussion about associated anxious distress and concurrent psychosocial stressors. Patients reporting severe back pain who have no alarming features on physical examination (i.e., no saddle anesthesia, lower-extremity weakness, or focal tenderness to palpation) may benefit from a similar screen for GAD as a complement to or before consideration of diagnostic spine imaging.

General physicians are frequently on the front lines of diagnosis and management of GAD. Although many patients report feelings of uncontrollable worry or hypervigilance, a significant proportion communicate their distress by bringing uncomfortable physical symptoms to clinical attention for redress. Careful investigation of a patient's physical complaints, including a comprehensive clinical history with attention to catastrophic thinking and apparent worsening of physical symptoms with coincident worsening of psychosocial distress, can point clinicians toward GAD as a contributor to or cause of patient distress. Patients who endorse severe intensity of their chronic physical complaints (i.e., severe headache or back pain) but for whom physical examination is reassuring also should be evaluated for GAD. When GAD is considered and identified, appropriate evaluation includes screening for depression as well as for excessive alcohol or other substance use, which frequently co-occur and portend greater chronicity and poorer prognosis of anxious symptoms (Kessler et al. 2008). Keen attention to recognition and treatment of GAD in this manner is essential to both improve patient quality of life and limit patient exposure to the risks of unnecessary medical interventions.

Specific Phobia

DSM-5 defines *specific phobia* as a clinical condition in which exposure to an object or situation provokes immediate and persistent fear or anxiety that is out of proportion to the actual danger posed (American Psychiatric Association 2013). The phobic object or situation is avoided completely by the patient or tolerated with high distress, and this fear, anxiety, or avoidance causes significant impairment in the patient's overall functioning. Distinct from panic disorder (in which panic attacks are initially unprovoked and unexpected) or agoraphobia (in which the fear is typically associated with concerns about having a panic attack in situations in which help is unavailable or easy escape is difficult), the fear response induced by a specific phobia is associated with a definite external trigger. The phobic stimulus is commonly situational or related to animals or the natural environment (i.e., insects, altitude). The lifetime prevalence of specific phobia in the U.S. population is estimated at 7%–9% (American Psychiatric Association 2013).

The condition is more common in women and in individuals of younger age and lower socioeconomic status (Stinson et al. 2007). An exception of particular relevance to the primary care setting is blood-injection-injury phobia, which is encountered with equal frequency in men and women (Stinson et al. 2007).

Blood-Injection-Injury Phobia

Blood-injection-injury phobias are variable in scope and are characterized by a pattern of fear and avoidance of blood, injury, needle injections, blood transfusions, or other medical care (American Psychiatric Association 2013). Potential situational triggers can include blood donation, routine phlebotomy for laboratory testing, invasive procedures, and needles. In a subset of patients with blood-injection-injury phobia, a diphasic response is triggered when the individual is exposed to the phobic stimulus. An initial increase in heart rate and blood pressure is followed by an abrupt deceleration of heart rate, with resultant hypotension leading to vasovagal syncope (Engel and Romano 1947; Graham et al. 1961; Ritz et al. 2013). The act of fainting can further reinforce the associated anxiety and avoidance, leading to medical neglect (Marks 1988).

Disclosure of phobic triggers by a patient to the doctor may not be routine. Clues to the presence of a blood-injection-injury phobia may include inability to follow through with recommended laboratory testing, which may be misconstrued as nonadherence rather than being recognized as phobic avoidance of a trigger. In such instances, a careful history often establishes the diagnosis. A blood-injection-injury phobia should also be suspected in a patient who experiences syncope or a vasovagal response only when confronted with blood products, phlebotomy, and injections.

Specific Phobia Related to Situations That May Lead to Choking or Vomiting

The specific phobia of choking, sometimes referred to as *pseudodysphagia* or *sitophobia*, is characterized by avoidance of food (particularly hard solids and chewy foods) and of swallowing pills. Individuals frequently complain of poor appetite, and malnutrition frequently results. Patients are often highly vigilant, or even refuse to eat, in social settings out of fear of experiencing a choking episode. Panic attacks may also occur as part of the disorder. The differential diagnosis for sitophobia includes a primary eating disorder, namely anorexia nervosa, which also often leads to profound malnutrition. A cardinal distinction between a choking phobia and anorexia nervosa is that swallowing is the phobic stimulus that triggers food avoidance in the former. Distinct from anorexia nervosa, the preoccupation with body image and weight is absent in sitophobia (American Psychiatric Association 2013).

Typically, patients present to the outpatient setting with complaints of choking or dysphagia, often prompting a workup for aspiration (e.g., a video fluoroscopic swallowing evaluation, flexible laryngoscopy, barium swallow, esophageal manometry). In some patients, the presentation may be more subtle, characterized only by unintentional weight loss or malnutrition driven by a patient's aversion to eating. The diagnosis of specific phobia should be considered in patients who complain of choking but in whom workup is unrevealing and in whom no accompanying aspiration event occurs despite repeated choking episodes. Proper diagnosis of sitophobia in these settings can limit delays in provision of needed psychiatric care and also prevent unnecessary expenditures related to an unduly extensive medical workup.

Social Anxiety Disorder

Social anxiety disorder is characterized by marked anxiety due to a disproportionate fear of excessive scrutiny or rejection by others when in social settings (American Psychiatric Association 2013). The anxiety and fear response are severe and cause significant distress and avoidance of social situations. Patients generally recognize their fear as being excessive. Epidemiological studies suggest a prevalence of 3%–13% for social phobia, with women more commonly affected than men (Sadock and Sadock 2007). While the exact etiology of social anxiety disorder has not yet been fully elucidated, multiple biological and psychosocial factors likely contribute to development of the disorder. For example, studies examining the use of sympatholytic drugs such as nonselective β-blockers (e.g., propranolol) in the treatment of performance phobia support the hypothesis that individuals who inherit a greater propensity for autonomic arousal may be more at risk for development of social phobia. Similarly, individuals with a genetic predisposition to intense vasodepressor responses also may be more likely to develop the condition. Psychosocial influences, such as chronic social stressors that induce the primary affects of shame and humiliation, likewise play a role. People experiencing such social stress may learn to incorporate these emotional states into their sense of identity, which in part accounts for the finding that the peak onset of the disorder occurs in the teenage years (Sadock and Sadock 2007).

For many patients with social anxiety disorder, worry about disapproval and rejection may result in physical symptoms of anxiety, such as tremor, blushing, increased heart rate, and stutter (American Psychiatric Association 2013). Patients with social anxiety disorder may be averse to discussing particularly sensitive topics (e.g., sexual history) and may also be unable to comply with procedures required for medical testing (e.g., provision of a urine sample by a patient whose social anxiety is so severe that he or she cannot urinate in a public lavatory) (American Psychiatric Association 2013). Primary care clinicians should take notice of such symptoms and should refer patients for appropriate psychiatric evaluation.

Obsessive-Compulsive Disorder

Obsessions are recurrent and persistent thoughts, urges, or images that are experienced as intrusive and unwanted, whereas *compulsions* are repetitive behaviors or mental acts that an individual feels driven to perform to relieve obsessional anxiety (American Psychiatric Association 2013). Although OCD has classically been considered to be an anxiety spectrum disorder, it is now placed in a distinct syndromal class—Obsessive-Compulsive and Related Disorders—in DSM-5. This new classification also includes related disorders such as body dysmorphic disorder, hoarding disorder, trichotillomania (hair-pulling disorder), and excoriation (skin-picking) disorder. Nonetheless, due to the historical correlation of OCD with the anxiety disorders and the high comorbidity and similar treatment, the physical manifestations of OCD may be encountered by primary care practitioners and are thus pertinent to this chapter (American Psychiatric Association 2013).

OCD is characterized by the presence of obsessions and/or compulsions. While the specific content of obsessions and compulsions varies among individuals, certain symptom dimensions are frequently seen in OCD: 1) contamination obsessions and cleaning compulsions; 2) obsessions with symmetry accompanied by repeating, ordering, or counting compulsions; 3) forbidden or taboo thoughts (i.e., intrusive aggressive or sexual thoughts and religious obsessions and compulsions); and 4) obsessions of potential harm (i.e., fears of harm to oneself or others, with related checking compulsions aimed at reduction of perceived harm). The 12-month prevalence of OCD ranges from 1.1% to 1.8%, and the lifetime prevalence approaches 3% (Cilliçilli et al. 2004). The mean onset age is 19.5 years (American Psychiatric Association 2013). Adult women are affected at a slightly higher rate than adult men; however, the childhood-onset form of OCD disproportionately affects males (Walitza et al. 2011). If untreated, OCD often becomes chronic, especially when the disease is of childhood onset (American Psychiatric Association 2013; Schneider and Levenson 2008).

The course of OCD is frequently complicated by other comorbid psychiatric disorders. Up to 76% of patients with OCD have a comorbid anxiety disorder such as GAD, panic disorder, social anxiety disorder, or specific phobia (American Psychiatric Association 2013; Pallanti et al. 2011). Furthermore, OCD is a common comorbidity in schizophrenia, occurring in as many as 12% of patients with schizophrenia (American Psychiatric Association 2013).

The pathophysiology of OCD is rooted in abnormal serotonergic and dopaminergic transmission. Whereas serotonin enhancers such as SSRIs can alleviate OCD symptoms, dopamine enhancers such as stimulants typically worsen symptoms (Sadock and Sadock 2007). Physicians in general medical settings may occasionally encounter new-onset compulsive behavior in patients taking prodopaminergic agents (i.e., amphetamines, pramipexole, ropinirole). The serotonergic and dopaminergic pathways that underlie OCD symptoms are an intense focus of investigation. Functional neuroimaging studies in OCD patients show increased activation of the orbitofrontal cortex, anterior cingulate gyrus, and basal ganglia, particularly the caudate and putamen (Higgins and George 2013; Husted et al. 2006). These areas may be overactive because of their connections within the cortico-striatal-thalamic-cortical circuit. The particular circuitry involved may depend on the exact ritual a patient experiences; washing, checking, and hoarding seem to activate slightly different brain regions (Higgins and George 2013). Likewise, treatment for OCD, whether psychotherapy or medications, decreases activity in the basal ganglia for patients who respond, a finding that further implicates the role of these brain regions in OCD pathogenesis (Higgins and George 2013).

In certain circumstances, OCD can manifest abruptly in children following a *Streptococcus* infection such as pharyngitis or impetigo. In this clinical setting, the child often presents with comorbid neurological abnormalities such as tics or myoclonus in addition to obsessive-compulsive behavior. The etiology of OCD in such cases is thought to be related to a systemic autoimmune reaction to the streptococcal infection as a result of molecular mimicry. For this reason, the syndrome is referred to as pediatric autoimmune neurological disorders associated with *Streptococcus* (PANDAS; National Institute of Mental Health 2017; Swedo et al. 1998). Initial management includes appropriate treatment of the suspected infection with antibiotics, which may lead to reduction in symptom severity, although residual symptoms may persist and require further management with immunotherapy.

Physical Manifestations of Obsessive-Compulsive Disorder

Among the more common physical manifestations of OCD and its related disorders are dermatological lesions such as excoriations and hair loss due to skin picking and hair pulling. Fear of contamination is a well-known obsession seen in OCD patients, and repetitive hand washing is the compulsion that most commonly accompanies this obsession. About 16% of patients with OCD have a hand-washing compulsion (Zhu et al. 2017). Excessive hand washing in OCD can result in irritant toxic dermatitis, lichen planus chronicus, and dry eczema. These complications may be more prevalent among individuals working in certain occupations, such as health care, cosmetic, and hairdressing professionals (Kouris et al. 2015; Zhu et al. 2017). These patients may delay formal treatment of their psychiatric condition for years and develop chronic hand eczema in the ensuing time (Zhu et al. 2017). Of key importance is the risk of superinfection of such lesions; excoriations from skin picking or compulsive hand washing frequently lead to skin and soft-tissue infections, including bacterial cellulitis caused by pathogens such as methicillin-resistant *Staphylococcus aureus* and others.

Some patients with OCD characterized by fears of contamination cover their hands in an effort to limit such contamination. Patients may wear latex, cotton, or wool gloves to prevent physical contact with potential pollutants or microbes. In severe cases of this behavior, paradoxical avoidance of appropriate hand hygiene may occur, with resultant increased risk of bacterial, viral, or even parasitic infections of the skin (Kouris et al. 2015).

When OCD escapes clinical attention, patients may present to physicians with recurrent bouts of cellulitis, often resulting in the prescription of sequential courses of antibiotics and a perceived need to work up a possible immunodeficiency syndrome. Close attention to signs and symptoms of OCD in patients with the features described here can help establish a proper diagnosis and prevent unnecessary costs and risks of repeated medical treatments. To limit the chance of missing a diagnosis of OCD, primary care clinicians should routinely screen patients for the disorder. Questions such as "Do you often have thoughts or impulses that come to mind even if you are not trying to have them?" can aid in the detection of bothersome obsessions. Practitioners should also ask direct questions about common compulsions (e.g., "Do you find yourself needing to check things all the time?" or "Do you feel dirty or have the compulsion to wash your hands often if you touch something dirty?"). Validated instruments for assessment of OCD in primary care settings—such as the self-reported Obsessive-Compulsive Inventory–Revised (Foa et al. 2002) and the Florida Obsessive-Compulsive Inventory (Storch et al. 2007)—are also valuable. Symptom severity and treatment response can be accurately monitored with the Yale-Brown Obsessive-Compulsive Scale (Goodman et al. 1989).

Treatment of Physical Manifestations

Patients with OCD often present to general physicians or dermatologists instead of to psychiatrists. Once a diagnosis of OCD is suspected, prompt referral of the patient to a psychiatrist or psychologist is indicated. Treatment of OCD includes psychotherapy such as exposure and response prevention therapy or cognitive-behavioral therapy (CBT) to address obsessions and compulsions. Exposure and response prevention, a protocol-based therapy that combines elements of cognitive therapy and behavioral therapy, helps patients to confront their obsessional anxiety and learn to delay or prevent the accompanying escape response. The protocol involves gradual desensitization aimed at abolishing the compulsive response to an obsessive thought. For example, if a patient has a compulsion to wash his or her hands every time an object is touched, then exposure and response prevention therapy will consist of having the patient practice touching perceived contaminated objects, with a graduated level of intensity, without washing his or her hands afterward. Psychotropic medications, including SSRIs or the TCA clomipramine, are often a critical component of effective treatment (American Psychiatric Association 2013; Kouris et al. 2015).

Treatment of dermatological lesions caused by excessive washing and cleaning includes lipid-replenishing creams and ointments applied for protection of broken skin. Zinc-containing ointments can be helpful for mild dermatitis lesions. Patients should not be prescribed gloves even if they request them, because doing so reinforces the pathology that requires treatment. In cases of severe eczema or lichen planus chronicus, topical steroids (i.e., hydrocortisone) also can be used. Intralesional steroid injections and occasionally oral steroids may be prescribed for the most severe cases (Mavrogiorgiu et al. 2015; Shab et al. 2008).

Posttraumatic Stress Disorder

PTSD is a well-known psychiatric disorder commonly encountered in psychiatry clinics and also in primary care practices. The diagnosis has garnered significant public attention in recent years, with increasing portrayals of PTSD in the news media, which has positioned this condition at the forefront of mental health. PTSD is highly prevalent among military veterans (Gates et al. 2012). PTSD also frequently occurs in the general population, in whom exposures to a variety of potentially traumatic events (i.e., accidents, assaults, sudden unexpected death of a loved one) are not uncommon. Given the variable manifestations of this disorder, screening and proper detection are important.

The DSM-5 diagnosis of PTSD requires direct or indirect exposure to actual or threatened death, serious injury, or sexual violation (American Psychiatric Association 2013). The exposure must result from a scenario in which the individual directly experiences a traumatic event, witnesses an event in person, learns that a traumatic event occurred to a close family member or friend (with the actual or threatened death being either violent or accidental), or experiences firsthand repeated or extreme exposure to aversive details of the traumatic event through means other than media, pictures, television, or movies (unless work related) (American Psychiatric Association 2013).

Both serious medical illness and traumatic brain injury can be associated with the development of PTSD. Regardless of the inciting trauma, a PTSD diagnosis requires that the disturbance cause clinically significant distress or impairment in the individual's social and interpersonal interactions, capacity to work, or other important areas of functioning. PTSD is also marked by intrusive symptoms, such as nightmares of the event, recurrent daytime memories of the event, and dissociative flashbacks. Avoidance of trauma-related stimuli (e.g., an airport for the survivor of a plane crash), negative alterations in cognitions and mood, and alterations in arousal and reactivity (e.g., pronounced startle response) also are present (American Psychiatric Association 2013).

Estimates of the overall prevalence of PTSD vary, with reported rates of 6%–7% among the general population (Pacella et al. 2013). It is estimated that about 25% of the general population will experience a traumatic event by midadulthood, although only about 20%–30% of those individuals will develop PTSD (Almli et al. 2014; Kilpatrick et al. 2013). Despite similar traumatic event exposure between the sexes, women are about twice as likely as men to develop PTSD. Unsurprisingly, the overall likelihood of developing PTSD increases with the number of successive traumatic exposures (Perrin et al. 2014). In addition to repeated traumatic exposures, genetic predisposition, alcohol use, and comorbid bipolar disorder also confer an increased risk of developing PTSD (Del Gaizo et al. 2011).

While many physicians are likely familiar with the psychological symptoms of PTSD, the physical symptoms of this disorder can easily be missed because they often mimic symptoms of other medical conditions. Common symptoms include insomnia and diffuse body pain or muscle tension (Pacella et al. 2013). Comorbid substance use is also common in PTSD patients, and such use, when identified in the clinic setting, should prompt further investigation. It is important for the primary care provider to accurately identify the physical symptoms as part of the larger syndrome of PTSD, which can then be adequately treated, rather than treating individual symptoms in isolation.

Insomnia

Patients with PTSD may present to primary care clinics with sleep disturbances without disclosing the traumatic event that provoked the sleep disruption. Nightmares, which are common in PTSD, are often vivid enough to wake patients from sleep (American Psychiatric Association 2013). Fear of recurrence of these nightmares often intensifies the hypervigilance already present in these patients. A common inclination among clinicians is to treat the patient's sleep problems with sedative or hypnotic medications, but providers must first assess the circumstances surrounding the sleep disturbance, because a comprehensive sleep history can aid in correct diagnosis and management. Does the patient's sleep difficulty involve sleep initiation or sleep maintenance? Are there early-morning awakenings? If there are nightmares, what is their content? How frequently do nightmares occur? Is there a precipitating factor? After a therapeutic alliance has been established, patients often answer these questions with little hesitation. Clinicians assessing patients with frequent, vivid nightmares, for example, should empathically engage in screening for history of trauma.

Substance Use

The concept of self-medication is familiar to many physicians. When they feel unable to cope with their distress, patients with PTSD may turn to alcohol, tobacco, or illicit substances to "treat" these overwhelming symptoms (Almli et al. 2014). Both tobacco use and alcohol use are more common among patients with PTSD than among the general population (Del Gaizo et al. 2011). In the course of a clinical encounter, primary care providers may identify patients who are consuming excessive amounts of alcohol. All such patients should be screened for trauma, because they are likely to turn to substances for relief of hyperarousal and hypervigilance. Appropriate recognition and treatment of the underlying cause of the patient's anxious distress can lead to meaningful harm reduction through decreased use of ethanol.

Diffuse Body Pain

Pain and PTSD frequently co-occur due to the physiological stress response of increased cortisol release and muscle tension that renders pain more acute (Barrett et al.

2002; Del Gaizo et al. 2011). Patients with both pain and PTSD may describe bodily locations of pain, including joints and back pain, but clinical evaluation for causative physical diagnoses is generally unrevealing. The lack of a discernible source of pain and corresponding negative workup may frustrate both the patient and the provider. Analgesic medications, including nonsteroidal anti-inflammatory drugs (NSAIDs), anticonvulsants (e.g., gabapentin), and opioids, are frequently prescribed in this situation. While such medications may provide acute relief, they also can lead to complications, including gastrointestinal bleeding, delirium, falls, or the development of opioid use disorders. In patients with PTSD, altered inflammatory responses can directly cause pain in their own right (Andreski et al. 1998). Evaluation for a history of trauma in such patients may lead them to a better understanding of the nature of the pain as well as a recognition of the need for psychiatric care. Failing to identify trauma as a potential contributor to a patient's pain may result in chronic and sometimes escalating use of pain medications, with significant adverse complications over time.

Screening for trauma may seem overwhelming for physicians and other clinicians. Discussions about past traumas can make patients feel vulnerable; assessments that are rushed or indelicate can exacerbate this feeling. Because trauma-exposed individuals often tend to be hypervigilant, ensuring a safe and comfortable environment is critical when this assessment is conducted. Speaking with the patient in a conversational tone, using nonjudgmental language, and giving patients the liberty to avoid discussion of distressing material until prepared to do so all are important. Telling patients, "I'd like to ask you some questions that might be difficult for you, but you don't have to talk about anything you don't wish to" may evoke a greater sense of ease and diminish the patient's sense of vulnerability. For those patients who do disclose a traumatic experience, an empathic stance must be maintained, because some patients feel an accompanying sense of shame. A similar approach is recommended when discussing treatment options. Patients should be given information about available treatment options, including both CBT and pharmacological management, with efforts to promote partnership in treatment selection and preserve agency and individual autonomy.

Approaches to Treatment

For most anxiety disorders, treatment can easily be initiated in the primary care setting. A necessary first step is an appropriate diagnostic evaluation for medical etiologies of anxiety or related medical comorbidities. Table 20–2 lists laboratory and diagnostic tests that are commonly ordered in the assessment of medical etiologies of anxiety. When an underlying medical etiology is identified, prompt treatment of the condition often provides substantial relief of the anxiety symptoms as well. Anxiety disorders such as GAD and panic disorder are frequently comorbid with medical illnesses and often influence the wide array of clinical manifestations of such illnesses. Effective management requires treatment of both conditions.

Many patients with anxiety disorders respond best to combined treatment with pharmacological and psychotherapeutic interventions (Sadock and Sadock 2007). SSRIs (e.g., citalopram, escitalopram, sertraline, paroxetine) are recommended as the first-line pharmacotherapy for many anxiety disorders. These agents are also of value

TABLE 20–2.   **Commonly ordered tests in the assessment of medical etiologies of anxiety**

Medical diagnosis	Test
Tachyarrhythmias	12-lead ECG Holter monitor Loop recorder
Orthostatic hypotension	Orthostatic vital signs
Angina pectoris; acute coronary syndrome	12-lead ECG Serum troponin
Congestive heart failure	Transthoracic echocardiogram
Chronic obstructive pulmonary disease; asthma	Chest X ray Pulmonary function testing
Anemia	Complete blood count Reticulocyte count Serum vitamin B_{12} level
Hyperthyroidism	Serum thyroid-stimulating hormone Serum free thyroxine Serum free triiodothyronine
Adrenal insufficiency	Serum morning cortisol
Cushing's syndrome	24-hour urinary cortisol
Pheochromocytoma	24-hour urinary catecholamines and metanephrines
Carcinoid syndrome	24-hour urinary 5-HIAA Serum chromogranin A

Note.   ECG=electrocardiogram; 5-HIAA=5-hydroxyindoleacetic acid.

in patients with comorbid major depressive disorder. Because of differences in side effects among the SSRIs, the choice of SSRI must be carefully tailored to the specific patient. Care should be taken to assess for potential drug-drug interactions in patients who are receiving other medications, because some SSRIs (e.g., paroxetine, fluoxetine, fluvoxamine) are known to inhibit the metabolism of cytochrome P450 isozymes, whereas other SSRIs (e.g., citalopram, escitalopram) are more inert. Titration to effective dosages of SSRIs often can be achieved within a matter of weeks, and patients should be reassessed after approximately 4–6 weeks for signs of therapeutic response to the selected agent (Sadock and Sadock 2007).

Given that onset of the therapeutic effects of SSRIs is delayed, many patients request benzodiazepines from their physicians. Benzodiazepines provide more rapid relief of anxiety symptoms, which often makes them an enticing choice among patients with debilitating symptoms. While the common practice of initially coprescribing a benzodiazepine and an SSRI for patients is reasonable, treatment of anxiety disorders with benzodiazepines as monotherapy is not recommended, because these agents are known to be habit-forming. Clinicians should slowly taper benzodiazepines within 3 months once SSRI therapy has been effective in controlling anxiety symptoms. Even in patients who do not develop a benzodiazepine use disorder from long-term use, the well-known side effects of benzodiazepines, such as cognitive disturbance and falls, can occur with even short-term use of these drugs. Patients should be advised to avoid use of alcohol and other agents with sedative potential (including antihistamines and hypnotics) while receiving benzodiazepines. Likewise, caution while driving and during other potentially hazardous activities is necessary.

Psychotherapeutic treatments of anxiety disorders are effective for the management of GAD, panic disorder, and phobias, as well as for OCD and PTSD. Although the full use of these interventions is more routinely practiced in mental health settings, clinicians in medical settings should feel comfortable addressing concerns and questions about therapeutic modalities raised by patients. CBT is the most common psychotherapy employed in the treatment of anxiety disorders. The process of CBT is manualized, with a set course of interventions—including homework assignments—utilized at key points during the treatment course. A principal focus of CBT is the interplay between thoughts or cognitions and emotional states. Homework frequently targets faulty cognitions—called "automatic thoughts"—which are irrational thoughts held as accurate by patients (Sadock and Sadock 2007).

CBT helps to elucidate how such automatic thoughts negatively influence mood states and engender anxiety. Patients who are able to limit perpetuation of cognitive distortions through this therapeutic process often experience corresponding relief from anxiety symptoms.

Conclusion

Anxiety is a common patient complaint in the general medical setting, and a comprehensive history and physical examination are critical to identify the etiology of a patient's symptoms. Whether symptoms are due to medical illness or to a comorbid psychiatric disorder, such as GAD, panic disorder, specific phobia, OCD, or PTSD, patients frequently look to their primary care providers for guidance on management of their anxious distress. The general medical setting is often well positioned for this purpose, and appropriate management includes use of both psychopharmacological and psychotherapeutic interventions. A dual treatment approach with similar management of associated medical comorbidities is recommended. When this approach to care is employed, physicians and other clinicians can bring meaningful relief to patients whose lives are significantly affected by these frequently encountered and disabling conditions.

References

Alexander F: Fundamental concepts of psychosomatic research: psychogenesis, conversion, specificity. Psychosomatic Medicine 5(3):205–210, 1943. Available at: https://insights.ovid.com/crossref?an=00006842-194307000-00001. Accessed April 29, 2019.

Almli LM, Fani N, Smith AK, et al: Genetic approaches to understanding post-traumatic stress disorder. Int J Neuropsychopharmacol 17(2):355–370, 2014 24103155

American Psychiatric Association: Diagnostic and Statistical Manual of Mental Disorders, 4th Edition. Washington, DC, American Psychiatric Association, 1994

American Psychiatric Association: Diagnostic and Statistical Manual of Mental Disorders, 4th Edition, Text Revision. Washington, DC, American Psychiatric Association, 2000

American Psychiatric Association: Diagnostic and Statistical Manual of Mental Disorders, 5th Edition. Arlington, VA, American Psychiatric Association, 2013

Andreski P, Chilcoat H, Breslau N: Post-traumatic stress disorder and somatization symptoms: a prospective study. Psychiatry Res 79(2):131–138, 1998 9705051

Bair MJ, Wu J, Damush TM, et al: Association of depression and anxiety alone and in combination with chronic musculoskeletal pain in primary care patients. Psychosom Med 70(8):890–897, 2008 18799425

Barrett DH, Doebbeling CC, Schwartz DA, et al: Posttraumatic stress disorder and self-reported physical health status among U.S. Military personnel serving during the Gulf War period: a population-based study. Psychosomatics 43(3):195–205, 2002 12075034

Beard CM, Sheps SG, Kurland LT, et al: Occurrence of pheochromocytoma in Rochester, Minnesota, 1950 through 1979. Mayo Clin Proc 58(12):802–804, 1983 6645626

Bond DS, Buse DC, Lipton RB, et al: Clinical pain catastrophizing in women with migraine and obesity. Headache 55(7):923–933, 2015 26087348

Burns JW, Quartana PJ, Bruehl S: Anger management style moderates effects of attention strategy during acute pain induction on physiological responses to subsequent mental stress and recovery: a comparison of chronic pain patients and healthy nonpatients. Psychosom Med 71(4):454–462, 2009 19251875

Centers for Disease Control and Prevention: Annual smoking-attributable mortality, years of potential life lost, and productivity losses—United States, 1997–2001. MMWR Morb Mortal Wkly Rep 54(25):625–628, 2005 15988406

Cilliçilli AS, Telcioglu M, A?kin R, et al: Twelve-month prevalence of obsessive-compulsive disorder in Konya, Turkey. Compr Psychiatry 45(5):367–374, 2004 15332200

Colice GL: Categorizing asthma severity: an overview of national guidelines. Clin Med Res 2(3):155–163, 2004 15931352

Del Gaizo AL, Elhai JD, Weaver TL: Posttraumatic stress disorder, poor physical health and substance use behaviors in a national trauma-exposed sample. Psychiatry Res 188(3):390–395, 2011 21481478

Engel CL, Romano J: Studies of syncope: biologic interpretation of vasodepressor syncope. Psychosom Med 9(5):288–294, 1947 18904528

Ferre Navarette F, Perez Paramo M, Fermin Ordono J, et al: Prevalence of insomnia and associated factors in outpatients with generalized anxiety disorder treated in psychiatric clinics. Behav Sleep Med 15(6):491–501, 2017 27167699

Fishman MC, Hoffman AR, Klausner RD, et al: Medicine, 5th Edition. Philadelphia, PA, Lippincott Williams & Wilkins, 2004

Foa EB, Huppert JD, Leiberg S, et al: The Obsessive-Compulsive Inventory: development and validation of a short version. Psychol Assess 14(4):485–496, 2002 12501574

Frommeyer G, Eckardt L, Breithardt G: Panic attacks and supraventricular tachycardias: the chicken or the egg? Neth Heart J 21(2):74–77, 2013 23179613

Gates MA, Holowka DW, Vasterling JJ, et al: Posttraumatic stress disorder in veterans and military personnel: epidemiology, screening, and case recognition. Psychol Serv 9(4):361–382, 2012 23148803

Goodman WK, Price LH, Rasmussen SA, et al: The Yale-Brown Obsessive Compulsive Scale, I: development, use, and reliability. Arch Gen Psychiatry 46(11):1006–1011, 1989 2684084

Gore M, Sadosky A, Stacey BR, et al: The burden of chronic low back pain: clinical comorbidities, treatment patterns, and health care costs in usual care settings. Spine 37(11):E668–E677, 2012 22146287

Graham DT, Kabler JD, Lunsford L Jr: Vasovagal fainting: a diphasic response. Psychosom Med 23:493–507, 1961 13901013

Higgins E, George M: The Neuroscience of Clinical Psychiatry. Philadelphia, PA, Wolters Kluwer/Lippincott Williams & Wilkins, 2013

Hoge EA, Ivkovic A, Friechione GL: Generalized anxiety disorder: diagnosis and treatment. BMJ 345:e7500, 2012 23187094

Husted DS, Shapira NA, Goodman WK: The neurocircuitry of obsessive-compulsive disorder and disgust. Prog Neuropsychopharmacol Biol Psychiatry 30(3):389–399, 2006 16443315

Kessler RC, Chiu WT, Demler O, et al: Prevalence, severity, and comorbidity of 12-month DSM-IV disorders in the National Comorbidity Survey Replication. Arch Gen Psychiatry 62(6):617–627, 2005 15939839

Kessler RC, Gruber M, Hettema JM, et al: Co-morbid major depression and generalized anxiety disorders in the National Comorbidity Survey follow-up. Psychol Med 38(3):365–374, 2008 18047766

Kessler RC, Petukhova M, Sampson NA, et al: Twelve-month and lifetime prevalence and life-time morbid risk of anxiety and mood disorders in the United States. Int J Methods Psychiatr Res 21(3):169–184, 2012 22865617

Kilpatrick DG, Resnick HS, Milanak ME, et al: National estimates of exposure to traumatic events and PTSD prevalence using DSM-IV and DSM-5 criteria. J Trauma Stress 26(5):537–547, 2013 24151000

Kouris A, Armyra K, Christodoulou C, et al: Quality of life, anxiety, depression and obsessive-compulsive tendencies in patients with chronic hand eczema. Contact Dermat 72(6):367–370, 2015 25693684

Kudva YC, Young WF Jr, Thompson GB, et al: Adrenal incidentaloma: an important component of the clinical presentation spectrum of benign sporadic adrenal pheochromocytoma. The Endocrinologist 9(2):77, 1999. Available at: https://journals.lww.com/theendocrinologist/Abstract/1999/03000/Adrenal_Incidentaloma__An_Important_Component_of.2.aspx. Accessed April 29, 2019.

Kunik ME, Roundy K, Veazey C, et al: Surprisingly high prevalence of anxiety and depression in chronic breathing disorders. Chest 127(4):1205–1211, 2005 15821196

Lessmeier TJ, Gamperling D, Johnson-Liddon V, et al: Unrecognized paroxysmal supraventricular tachycardia. Potential for misdiagnosis as panic disorder. Arch Intern Med 157(5):537–543, 1997 9066458

Lucchetti G, Peres MF, Lucchetti AL, et al: Generalized anxiety disorder, subthreshold anxiety and anxiety symptoms in primary headache. Psychiatry Clin Neurosci 67(1):41–49, 2013 23331287

Marks I: Blood-injury phobia: a review. Am J Psychiatry 145(10):1207–1213, 1988 3048117

Mavrogiorgiu P, Bader A, Stockfleth E, et al: Obsessive-compulsive disorder in dermatology. J Dtsch Dermatol Ges 13(10):991–999, 2015 26408459

McCrank E, Schurmans K, Lefcoe D: Paroxysmal supraventricular tachycardia misdiagnosed as panic disorder. Arch Intern Med 158(3):297, 1998 9472212

Means-Christensen AJ, Roy-Byrne PP, Sherbourne CD, et al: Relationships among pain, anxiety, and depression in primary care. Depress Anxiety 25(7):593–600, 2008 17932958

Munk-Jørgensen P, Allgulander C, Dahl AA, et al: Prevalence of generalized anxiety disorder in general practice in Denmark, Finland, Norway, and Sweden. Psychiatr Serv 57(12):1738–1744, 2006 17158488

National Institute of Mental Health: PANDAS: Questions and Answers (website). Bethesda, MD, National Institute of Mental Health, 2017. Available at: https://www.nimh.nih.gov/health/publications/pandas/index.shtml. Accessed June 2017.

Niles AN, Dour HJ, Stanton AL, et al: Anxiety and depressive symptoms and medical illness among adults with anxiety disorders. J Psychosom Res 78(2):109–115, 2015 25510186

Pacella ML, Hruska B, Delahanty DL: The physical health consequences of PTSD and PTSD symptoms: a meta-analytic review. J Anxiety Disord 27(1):33–46, 2013 23247200

Pakzad M, Fung J, Preuss R: Pain catastrophizing and trunk muscle activation during walking in patients with chronic low back pain. Gait Posture 49:73–77, 2016 27388960

Pallanti S, Grassi G, Sarrecchia ED, et al: Obsessive-compulsive disorder comorbidity: clinical assessment and therapeutic implications. Front Psychiatry 2:70, 2011 22203806

Perrin M, Vandeleur CL, Castelao E, et al: Determinants of the development of post-traumatic stress disorder, in the general population. Soc Psychiatry Psychiatr Epidemiol 49(3):447–457, 2014 24022753

Pollack MH, Kradin R, Otto MW, et al: Prevalence of panic in patients referred for pulmonary function testing at a major medical center. Am J Psychiatry 153(1):110–113, 1996 8540567

Ritz T, Meuret AE, Simon E: Cardiovascular activity in blood-injection-injury phobia during exposure: evidence for diphasic response patterns? Behav Res Ther 51(8):460–468, 2013 23747585

Sadock BJ, Sadock VA: Kaplan and Sadock's Synopsis of Clinical Psychiatry. Philadelphia, PA, Wolters Kluwer/Lippincott Williams & Wilkins, 2007

Schneider RK, Levenson JL: Psychiatry Essentials for Primary Care. Philadelphia, PA, American College of Physicians, 2008

Shab A, Matterne U, Diepgen TL, et al: Are obsessive-compulsive disorders and personality disorders sufficiently considered in occupational dermatoses? A discussion based on three case reports. J Dtsch Dermatol Ges 6(11):947–951, 2008 18761610

Siegmann EM, Müller HHO, Luecke C, et al: Association of depression and anxiety disorders with autoimmune thyroiditis: a systematic review and meta-analysis. JAMA Psychiatry 75(6):577–584, 2018 29800939

Smoller JW, Pollack MH, Otto MW, et al: Panic anxiety, dyspnea, and respiratory disease. Theoretical and clinical considerations. Am J Respir Crit Care Med 154(1):6–17, 1996 8680700

Smoller JW, Pollack MH, Wassertheil-Smoller S, et al: Prevalence and correlates of panic attacks in postmenopausal women: results from an ancillary study to the Women's Health Initiative. Arch Intern Med 163(17):2041–2050, 2003 14504117

Spitzer RL, Kroenke K, Williams JB, et al: A brief measure for assessing generalized anxiety disorder: the GAD-7. Arch Intern Med 166(10):1092–1097, 2006 16717171

Stein PP, Black HR: A simplified diagnostic approach to pheochromocytoma. A review of the literature and report of one institution's experience. Medicine (Baltimore) 70(1):46–66, 1991 1988766

Stinson FS, Dawson DA, Patricia Chou S, et al: The epidemiology of DSM-IV specific phobia in the USA: results from the National Epidemiologic Survey on Alcohol and Related Conditions. Psychol Med 37(7):1047–1059, 2007 17335637

Storch EA, Kaufman DA, Bagner D, et al: Florida Obsessive-Compulsive Inventory: development, reliability, and validity. J Clin Psychol 63(9):851–859, 2007 [Erratum in: J Clin Psychol 63(12):1265, 2007] 17674398

Stuart MR, Lieberman JA: The Fifteen Minute Hour: Therapeutic Talk in Primary Care, 4th Edition. New York, Radcliffe, 2008

Swedo SE, Leonard HL, Garvey M, et al: Pediatric autoimmune neuropsychiatric disorders associated with streptococcal infections: clinical description of the first 50 cases. Am J Psychiatry 155:264–271, 1998 9464208

Uniyal R, Paliwal VK, Tripathi A: Psychiatric comorbidity in new daily persistent headache: a cross-sectional study. Eur J Pain 21(6):1031–1038, 2017 28146324

van Loon IN, Lamberts J, Valk GD, et al: The evaluation of spells. Neth J Med 69(7):309–317, 2011 21934175

Walitza S, Melfsen S, Jans T, et al: Obsessive-compulsive disorder in children and adolescents. Dtsch Arztebl Int 108(11):173–179, 2011 21475565

Willgoss TG, Yohannes AM: Anxiety disorders in patients with COPD: a systematic review. Respir Care 58(5):858–866, 2013 22906542

Wittchen HU, Kessler RC, Beesdo K, et al: Generalized anxiety and depression in primary care: prevalence, recognition, and management. J Clin Psychiatry 63 (suppl 8):24–34, 2002 12044105

Young WF Jr: Clinical presentation and diagnosis of pheochromocytoma, in UpToDate (website). Edited by Martin KA. Alphen aan den Rijn, The Netherlands, Wolters Kluwer, 2016a. Available at: http://www.uptodate.com/contents/clinical-presentation-and-diagnosis-of-pheochromocytoma. Accessed March 2017.

Young WF Jr: Pheochromocytoma in genetic disorders, in UpToDate (website). Edited by Martin KA. Alphen aan den Rijn, The Netherlands, Wolters Kluwer, 2016b. Available at: http://www.uptodate.com/contents/pheochromocytoma-in-genetic-disorders?source=see_link. Accessed June 2017.

Zhu TH, Nakamura M, Farahnik B, et al: Obsessive-compulsive skin disorders: a novel classification based on degree of insight. J Dermatolog Treat 28(4):342–346, 2017 27658538

CHAPTER 21

Substance Use Disorders in the Medical Setting

Samata R. Sharma, M.D.

Saria El Haddad, M.D.

Joji Suzuki, M.D.

There is a significant presence of substance use disorders (SUDs) in the inpatient medical setting, with prevalence rates for SUDs in hospitalized patients ranging from 15% to 40% (Owens et al. 2018). Although SUDs are commonly seen in the hospital setting, most patients struggling with SUDs are not actively engaged in addiction treatment, despite the fact that many hospital admissions are due to medical complications from untreated SUDs. There is growing evidence pointing to the significant impact that early identification and treatment of SUDs can have on overall morbidity and mortality and associated health care costs. The inpatient hospital setting offers consultation-liaison (C-L) psychiatrists an opportunity to make a significant impact throughout the course of a patient's hospital stay. They can identify SUDs at the time of admission, start treatment during the course of the inpatient stay, and then ensure adequate linkage to ongoing outpatient treatment at the time of discharge.

The medical perspective has gradually shifted and now views SUDs as chronic diseases with specific maladaptive behavioral patterns. These patterns perpetuate ongoing substance use that interferes with both psychological and physiological well-being across multiple disease spectra. The C-L psychiatrist is uniquely positioned to address and treat this often underlying and unmet illness within the inpatient medical setting. So-called dual-diagnosis patients—patients with both a non-SUD mental disorder and an SUD—often have a more severe course of both disease processes, complicating treatment initiation and adherence. Anxiety and depression are reported in up to 40% of patients with alcohol use disorder (AUD), and alcohol use is found in up to 35% of patients with anxiety and depression (National Institute on Drug Abuse 2018a).

Beyond dual-diagnosis patients, high rates of SUDs co-occur and also can exacerbate certain medical and surgical comorbidities, including chronic pain, cancer, heart disease, and infectious diseases (through needle-borne transmission such as hepatitis C and HIV) (Table 21–1; El-Bassel et al. 2014; Klevens et al. 2012; Schulte and Hser 2014). Among patients admitted to trauma intensive care units (TICUs), up to 79% are found to have at least one co-occurring SUD (Zatzick et al. 2012). In 2006, the American College of Surgeons mandated provision of alcohol screening and brief interventions (consisting of education about risks associated with use, motivational interviewing to increase awareness and improve motivation to reduce use, and the offer of referral for treatment) across all level I and II TICUs (Zatzick et al. 2012). Patients with active SUDs also struggle with impaired medication and treatment adherence for their medical conditions, which may worsen the course of their medical illness (Schulte and Hser 2014).

There is strong evidence that SUD comorbidity confers significant increases in disease burden and 10-year overall mortality rates for several major medical illnesses (Bahorik et al. 2017; Substance Abuse and Mental Health Services Administration 2015; Young et al. 2015). However, most patients with SUDs do not actively seek treatment, or even believe that they need treatment.

C-L consultations in this patient population may arise secondary to behavioral exacerbations from acute intoxication, withdrawal, or decompensation of the patient's primary psychiatric illness. Nevertheless, in the absence of acute behavioral dysregulation or an SUD-associated chief complaint, patients hospitalized for a primary medical condition that may be both exacerbating and exacerbated by a comorbid SUD often do not receive any treatment for the SUD on the inpatient medical unit. This situation persists despite the fact that emergency department (ED) visits associated with SUDs continue to rise; the total number of drug-related ED visits increased 81% from 2004 (2.5 million) to 2009 (4.6 million) (Substance Abuse and Mental Health Services Administration 2010). ED visits involving nonmedical use of pharmaceuticals increased 98.4% over the same period, from 627,291 visits to 1,244,679 (Substance Abuse and Mental Health Services Administration 2010).

Although barriers loom large, as ED visits and hospitalizations associated with SUDs have increased, awareness has gradually begun to shift, with accompanying changes in the U.S. health care delivery system. The Mental Health Parity and Addiction Equity Act of 2008 and the Patient Protection and Affordable Care Act of 2010 have increased the number of people carrying insurance that covers addiction and mental health treatment. This increase has created an opening for greater clinician support and incentive to implement evidence-based practices for collaborative and integrated care for physical and mental disorders (National Institute on Drug Abuse 2018a).

Alcohol-Related Disorders in the Inpatient Medical Setting

Unhealthful alcohol use is common in patients admitted to medical settings and is estimated to be responsible for up to 40% of intensive care unit (ICU) admissions (Gentilello et al. 2005). The systemic effects of heavy alcohol use result in an increased risk of hospitalization and also predispose patients to multiple conditions and compli-

TABLE 21–1.   **Medical conditions commonly associated with substance use disorders**

Alcohol use disorder	Opioid use disorder
Cardiovascular diseases	Arthritis
Cancers	Chronic pain
Injuries	Headache
Stroke	Hepatitis C
Cirrhosis	Musculoskeletal disorders
	Infectious disorders
Cannabis use disorder	Opioid-related overdoses
Respiratory deficits	
Cardiovascular diseases	
Lung cancer	

Source.   Reprinted from National Institute on Drug Abuse: "Substance Use Disorders Are Associated With Major Medical Illnesses and Mortality Risk in a Large Integrated Health Care System." NIDA Notes (Sarlin E), October 24, 2017. National Institute on Drug Abuse website; available at: https://www.drugabuse.gov/news-events/nida-notes/2017/10/substance-use-disorders-are-associated-major-medical-illnesses-mortality-risk-in-large-integrated. Accessed May 19, 2019.

cations, including acute respiratory distress syndrome, septic shock, aspiration pneumonia, and nosocomial infections. Physicians often fail to recognize alcohol-related problems in patients admitted to the hospital.

There is evidence demonstrating that patients treated in TICUs who received brief interventions consumed nearly 15 fewer alcoholic beverages per week than did patients in the control group 12 months after discharge (Clark and Moss 2011). This reduced consumption was coupled with a 47% reduction in injuries in patients with risky alcohol use (Clark and Moss 2011). Additional studies have shown the efficacy of brief interventions in halving rates of instances of driving under the influence for patients in TICUs involved in motor vehicle collisions.

Diagnosis and Screening

The diagnoses of *alcohol abuse* and *alcohol dependence* that appeared in the fourth edition (and its text revision) of the *Diagnostic and Statistical Manual of Mental Disorders* (DSM-IV [DSM-IV-TR]; American Psychiatric Association 1994, 2000) were replaced by a single diagnosis, *alcohol use disorder* (AUD), in the fifth edition (DSM-5; American Psychiatric Association 2013) as part of the new edition's overall revision of the substance use disorder category. Various screening tools are available for detecting unhealthful alcohol use; here we focus on tools that can be used in the acute inpatient setting.

Developed by the World Health Organization, the Alcohol Use Disorders Identification Test (AUDIT) is a 10-question survey that has been validated in multiple languages and health care settings (Saunders et al. 1993). With use of a cutoff score of ≥8, the reported sensitivity values range from 50% to 90%, and specificity is approximately 80% for the identification of unhealthful alcohol use in men. In trauma patients, a cutoff of 5 for women yields a sensitivity and specificity similar to those produced with a cutoff of 8 for men (Neumann et al. 2004). The AUDIT-C is shorter than the original test and therefore more practical to use in the acute setting. It is composed of three items and also requires scoring.

Several laboratory tests—including blood alcohol concentration, liver function tests, mean corpuscular volume, γ-glutamyltransferase, and carbohydrate-deficient transferrin—may be abnormal in patients with AUD. These tests lack sufficient sensitivity and specificity to be used for screening and diagnostic purposes in ICU settings (Neumann and Spies 2003). Laboratory testing can be helpful when the patient is unconscious or cannot speak. In these cases, a blood alcohol level can be used as a reasonable proxy for problematic use.

Management and Treatment

Withdrawal

For patients with AUD in early abstinence, standardized measures should be used to assess the severity of the alcohol withdrawal syndrome (AWS). In medically ill, hospitalized patients (not in a specialized detoxification or SUD unit), most cases of AWS are mild to moderate and require symptom management. Complicated withdrawal is relatively rare (up to 10% of all patients with alcohol withdrawal); most patients with AUD experience mild withdrawal, with symptom resolution within 2–7 days of the last drink (Hall and Zador 1997; Schuckit 2009).

Manifestations of AWS may include insomnia, autonomic symptoms, increased hand tremors, nausea or vomiting, psychomotor agitation, anxiety, seizures, and hallucinations. Symptoms appear gradually and worsen progressively with increasing time since the last drink. A patient history of delirium tremens (DT), previous episodes of AWS, or co-occurring medical conditions all are commonly accepted as indications for inpatient medical supervision of alcohol withdrawal. The advantages of inpatient withdrawal management include having fewer medical and logistical concerns, allowing closer monitoring for AWS, providing complex addiction-focused medical management (e.g., cardiac monitoring, intravenous hydration) of AWS and co-occurring medical conditions, and having a higher likelihood of completion of the AWS management protocol. Depending on the medical complexity of the specific patient, withdrawal may be managed in either a general medical or an intensive care setting.

Standardized scales can aid in the diagnosis of withdrawal, can indicate the need for medications, and can help predict the severity of alcohol withdrawal and the need for intensive care. Use of such scales may improve patient safety by ensuring systematic assessment and symptom-guided administration of medication. The Clinical Institute Withdrawal Assessment for Alcohol–revised version (CIWA-Ar) is perhaps the most widely used standardized scale (Sullivan et al. 1989). CIWA-Ar is able to fulfill all three purposes of standardized withdrawal assessment: 1) studies have demonstrated its validity and interrater reliability in assessing the severity of alcohol withdrawal; 2) it is relatively quick to administer (about 1 minute for trained administrators); and 3) it can help to identify patients who are at risk for more complicated alcohol withdrawal. In addition, the use of the CIWA-Ar in determining the need for medication in symptom-triggered protocols is associated with lower total dosages of benzodiazepines and shorter hospital stays. Because it is used to determine the severity of the withdrawal symptoms as they are actively experienced, the CIWA-Ar does not predict risk for complicated alcohol withdrawal in patients before the onset of AWS.

The AUDIT was studied as a tool for predicting risk of developing AWS (Babor et al. 2001). It was shown to have a good positive predictive value, especially when combined with laboratory test results; however, it can overestimate the risk of developing AWS, thus leading to unnecessary prophylaxis in about half of patients screened.

The Prediction of Alcohol Withdrawal Severity Scale (PAWSS) was developed to help identify medically ill patients at risk of developing AWS before they begin to show signs of withdrawal. The PAWSS consists of three parts: 1) threshold criteria (one question to determine whether the patient consumed alcohol during the 30 days prior to admission *or* had a positive blood alcohol level on admission); 2) patient interview (seven yes/no questions from the patient interview about previous use, consequences, and treatment); and 3) clinical evidence (two questions about current clinical status used in assessing known risk factors for withdrawal) (Maldonado et al. 2014).

Guidelines that can help the clinician determine whether inpatient medically supervised withdrawal is advisable are summarized in Table 21–2 (U.S. Department of Veterans Affairs/Department of Defense 2015).

Laboratory tests commonly ordered on admission include blood alcohol level, complete blood count with differential, comprehensive metabolic panel, prothrombin time with international normalized ratio, and urine toxicology screens. Additional tests that can be considered include lipase, uric acid, ammonia, and a volatile panel (ethanol, methanol, isopropyl alcohol, and acetone). Cardiac telemetry is recommended for patients who have underlying cardiac disease.

Potential consultations to round out management may include a social work consultation for further assessment of psychosocial factors triggering alcohol use, information about additional resources, and referral to postdischarge abstinence programs; a nicotine dependency consultation (given high rates of co-occurrence of the two disorders); and a psychiatry consultation if the patient has an untreated comorbid psychiatric disorder or if there are concerns about psychiatric pharmacotherapy. A nutrition consultation can be considered if the patient reports significant weight loss or has signs of poor nutrition.

Management of Uncomplicated Withdrawal

Benzodiazepines. *Choice of agent.* Benzodiazepines are the most commonly used medications for treatment of moderate to severe alcohol withdrawal. Compared with placebo, benzodiazepines reduce severity of withdrawal, incidence of delirium, and incidence of withdrawal seizures (Holbrook et al. 1999). They are generally well tolerated, although some sedation can occur. Although all benzodiazepines seem to be equally effective in treating AWS, the choice of agent depends on the preferred pharmacokinetic properties in relation to patient characteristics, including presence of respiratory illness or liver disease. The most commonly used benzodiazepines for alcohol withdrawal treatment are chlordiazepoxide, diazepam (long-acting), lorazepam, and oxazepam (short- or intermediate-acting).

Long-acting agents are generally preferred because they can provide a smooth course of treatment, minimizing the need for repeated dosing and the risk of rebound symptoms. They are not recommended for use in patients with liver disease because they are metabolized through demethylation and hydroxylation metabolic pathways, which could result in accumulation of their active metabolites. Shorter-acting agents such as lorazepam are used in patients with severe liver disease and patients at risk of

TABLE 21–2. **Guidelines for determining advisability of inpatient medically supervised withdrawal management**

Inpatient management is recommended for patients with any of the following conditions:

History of delirium tremens or withdrawal seizures

Inability to tolerate oral medications

Co-occurring medical conditions that would pose serious risk for ambulatory withdrawal management (e.g., severe coronary artery disease, congestive heart failure, cirrhosis)

Severe alcohol withdrawal (i.e., CIWA-Ar score ≥20)

Risk of withdrawal from other substances in addition to alcohol (e.g., sedative-hypnotics)

Inpatient management is suggested for patients with symptoms of at least moderate alcohol withdrawal (i.e., CIWA-Ar score ≥10) and any of the following conditions:

Recurrent unsuccessful attempts at ambulatory withdrawal management

Reasonable likelihood that the patient will not complete ambulatory withdrawal management (e.g., due to homelessness)

Active psychosis or severe cognitive impairment

Medical conditions that could make ambulatory withdrawal management problematic (e.g., pregnancy, nephrotic syndrome, cardiovascular disease, lack of medical support system)

Note. CIWA-Ar=Clinical Institute Withdrawal Assessment for Alcohol–revised version (Sullivan et al. 1989).

Source. Reprinted from Recommendations 27 and 28 (pp. 28, 56–57), in *VA/DoD Clinical Practice Guideline for the Management of Substance Use Disorders,* December 2015. Washington, DC, U.S. Department of Veterans Affairs/Department of Defense, 2015. Available at: https://www.healthquality.va.gov/guidelines/MH/sud/VADoDSUDCPGRevised22216.pdf. Accessed May 19, 2019.

respiratory depression (e.g., the elderly, patients with severe lung disease) because they have no active metabolites and their metabolism does not primarily depend on the liver.

Benzodiazepine regimens. The two most commonly used pharmacotherapy strategies for managing AWS are predetermined fixed medication tapering schedule with additional medication as needed and CIWA-based symptom-triggered therapy. Generally, a CIWA-based symptom-triggered approach is preferred. One randomized double-blind trial of fixed-dosage versus symptom-triggered treatment found that the symptom-triggered group had a significantly shorter duration of treatment and required significantly less chlordiazepoxide during withdrawal (Saitz et al. 1994). The symptom-triggered approach ensures that the patient receives only the amount of the medication needed to manage alcohol withdrawal. However, this approach requires staff members that are comfortable administering the CIWA and using it to determine the severity of and subsequent management of withdrawal (Daeppen et al. 2002; Sullivan et al. 1991).

For patients with certain risk factors (e.g., history of severe withdrawal, altered mental status, high CIWA scores on initial assessment), a fixed-dosage approach may be preferred. In the fixed-dosage approach, medication is given in advance of the emergence of anticipated withdrawal signs and symptoms. This approach helps ensure that the patient will receive sufficient medication to prevent the emergence of alcohol withdrawal; the level of clinical monitoring needed may be somewhat less than with the symptom-triggered approach (Mayo-Smith and American Society of

Addiction Medicine Working Group on Pharmacological Management of Alcohol Withdrawal 1997). The disadvantage of this approach is that it is often difficult to estimate a fixed-dosage regimen, and the patient may consequently receive higher dosages of benzodiazepines than are required to control the withdrawal symptoms, which could cause more side effects. Patients with established DT will often require very high benzodiazepine dosages to control their illness.

Anticonvulsants. A few small randomized controlled trials have supported the efficacy of anticonvulsants (e.g., gabapentin, carbamazepine, valproic acid, vigabatrin) in the treatment of alcohol withdrawal (Asplund et al. 2004; Malcolm et al. 2001; Myrick et al. 1998; Reoux et al. 2001; Stuppaeck et al. 1992). These medications are worth considering for management of mild to moderate alcohol withdrawal in patients for whom the risks of benzodiazepines (e.g., inadequate monitoring available, abuse liability, allergy or adverse reactions) outweigh benefits.

The potential advantages of anticonvulsant medications include decreasing the seizure risk; reducing cravings; the lack of an abuse potential; and treating mood disorders, which share some symptoms with AWS, including depression, irritability, and anxiety. These medications also have less propensity to cause sedation as compared with benzodiazepines (Myrick and Anton 1998).

Adrenergic medications. α_2-Adrenergic agonists (clonidine) and β-adrenergic blockers (propranolol) can be used as adjunctive medications administered with benzodiazepines to improve autonomic symptoms by reducing elevated pulse and blood pressure. They are not recommended for use as the main agents to treat alcohol withdrawal, because there is no evidence that these medications can prevent or treat delirium or seizures (Saitz and O'Malley 1997).

Dexmedetomidine (Precedex) is an intravenous α_2-adrenergic agonist that has been investigated as a potential adjunct for treatment of AWS in the ICU setting. Its pharmacological characteristics, which include rapid onset, lack of respiratory depression, and short duration of action, make it a promising agent for treatment of AWS in medically ill persons, thus reducing the need for benzodiazepines (Linn and Loeser 2015).

Barbiturates. Barbiturates are used in some facilities, primarily in ICUs. These γ-aminobutyric acid medications have cross-tolerance with alcohol and can treat withdrawal symptoms effectively. Their narrow therapeutic index and toxicity limit their use (Saitz 1998). More recent studies suggest that phenobarbital is an effective alternative to benzodiazepines in the treatment of AWS in various clinical settings (Nelson et al. 2018; Phan 2018; Saukkonen et al. 2018).

Alcohol. Alcohol itself is used by some practitioners to treat AWS (Sattar et al. 2006). No solid evidence exists, other than clinical experience, to support this practice. One small randomized controlled trial conducted in an ICU compared two types of prophylactic treatment: an intravenous ethanol (alcohol) infusion and diazepam (Weinberg et al. 2008). No advantages were found for alcohol compared with diazepam, and more patients treated with alcohol exhibited inadequate sedation. One patient on the alcohol regimen failed to respond to this treatment and had to be protectively transferred to a diazepam regimen. Because alcohol has a very short duration of action, it is more likely than benzodiazepines to cause respiratory depression. Furthermore, it can have proconvulsant effects and is damaging to many organ systems.

No convincing rationale supports the use of alcohol to treat alcohol withdrawal, especially given that safer and more effective alternatives—benzodiazepines—are available.

Management of Complicated Withdrawal

The occurrence of seizures during AWS is indicative of complicated alcohol withdrawal. Patients who have a history of alcohol withdrawal seizures or who experience seizures during the current withdrawal episode should be given prophylactic lorazepam intravenously or intramuscularly (D'Onofrio et al. 1999). Lorazepam is used because it has a consistent plasma level distribution, unlike diazepam, which has a more extensive tissue distribution (Greenblatt and Divoll 1983).

Ideally, patients should be admitted and monitored for at least 36–48 hours. Detailed neurological examination, blood tests, and brain imaging may be performed to rule out alternative etiologies. Patients typically require high doses of benzodiazepines to prevent seizure recurrence and DT (Saitz and O'Malley 1997).

DT is a medical emergency that requires intensive care in most cases. Medical workup and a detailed neurological examination should be performed to rule out alternative etiologies for delirium, such as hypoglycemia, electrolyte abnormalities, infection, brain injury, and renal or hepatic failure. DT is treated symptomatically, with the goal of normalizing vital signs and keeping the patient calm. This goal is best achieved through the use of benzodiazepines, administered at short intervals via intramuscular or intravenous routes. Lorazepam is the agent of choice in patients with liver disease and in the elderly, in whom there are risks of oversedation and respiratory depression with diazepam (Clergue et al. 1981; Peppers 1996). In some cases, loading dosages of diazepam can be used. Centralized vital-sign monitoring is critically important and should be conducted continuously, especially for patients requiring higher-dosage medication.

Adjunctive Supplements

Chronic alcohol use can lead to depletion of thiamine (vitamin B_1) and magnesium. Thiamine deficiency can lead to the classical triad of ataxia, altered mental status, and ophthalmoplegia, better known as *Wernicke's encephalopathy*. Because all three of these signs may not be present in every case, diagnosis of Wernicke's encephalopathy is best achieved through use of the Caine criteria (Caine et al. 1997), which require the presence of two of the following four signs in an individual at high risk of thiamine depletion (e.g., a patient with AUD, a patient who has undergone gastric bypass surgery): 1) clinical evidence of malnutrition, 2) oculomotor abnormalities, 3) cerebellar dysfunction, and 4) either an altered mental state or mild memory impairment. Undiagnosed Wernicke's encephalopathy can lead to the severe amnestic syndrome known as *Korsakoff syndrome*.

Parenteral thiamine is essential for the prevention of Wernicke's encephalopathy. It is common practice to give thiamine before intravenous administration of glucose, because glucose can deplete thiamine stores and precipitate Wernicke's encephalopathy in thiamine-deficient patients. High-dosage thiamine is recommended both for the treatment of Wernicke's encephalopathy and for its prevention in patients who screen positive on the Caine criteria as being at risk for the disorder. The typical thiamine dosage range is 200–500 mg, administered intravenously three times daily for

3–5 consecutive days. Intravenous thiamine may be switched to the oral formulation after 3 days (or sooner if the patient is able to tolerate oral medications), and oral thiamine should be continued at 100 mg thrice daily. On hospital discharge, oral thiamine should be continued at a daily dosage of 100 mg for at least 30 days (Isenberg-Grzeda et al. 2012; Latt and Dore 2014).

Chronic alcohol use can also result in magnesium and niacin (vitamin B$_3$) depletion due to alterations in the metabolism and absorption of these nutrients. Hypomagnesemia can result in neuropathy and altered mental status. Magnesium repletion and intravenous multivitamins should be given to patients who show signs of deficiency and should be administered prophylactically to patients who have severe AWS (Sullivan et al. 1963).

Altered mental status can have one or multiple etiologies; the most common causes are alcohol withdrawal, alcohol hallucinosis, alcohol withdrawal seizures, DT, hepatic encephalopathy, Wernicke's encephalopathy, and Korsakoff syndrome. Distinctive symptoms associated with these etiologies can aid in diagnosis and guide treatment.

In *alcohol hallucinosis,* auditory or visual hallucinations occur in the presence of an intact sensorium, and hallucinations are more pronounced than delusions. In *alcohol withdrawal,* the patient may exhibit anxiety and irritability. Hallucinations, if present, will generally be transient and poorly formed. *Alcohol withdrawal seizures* can be associated with loss of consciousness and followed by postictal confusion, but hallucinations are not usually present. *DT* is the most common cause of psychotic symptoms in this patient population, and confusion or disorientation will be present. In *Wernicke's encephalopathy,* confusion is more likely than psychosis. *Korsakoff syndrome* is not a true psychosis but rather a confabulatory state wherein amnesia (both retrograde and anterograde) is a cardinal feature. The patient usually presents as alert and cooperative but might display frontal lobe signs such as apathy, inertia, and impaired insight (Wyszynski 2004).

Long-Term Maintenance Treatment

For patients with moderate to severe alcohol withdrawal, long-term medication treatment is recommended. Randomized controlled trials and meta-analyses have demonstrated the efficacy of acamprosate, disulfiram, and naltrexone in the treatment of AUD.

Acamprosate.   Acamprosate is believed to normalize central glutamatergic dysregulation in AUD, thereby targeting symptoms of protracted alcohol withdrawal. European trials (Jonas et al. 2014) have indicated that acamprosate can reduce drinking days, increase days of abstinence, and lengthen the time to relapse. Trials in the United States have shown discordant results, which may be due to differences in study design and population genetics. The thrice-daily dosing can be cumbersome for some patients and can have negative effects on adherence. Acamprosate is renally cleared, which makes it a good agent in patients with hepatic impairment. Its use should also be considered in patients who are taking opioids, for whom naltrexone is contraindicated. Acamprosate may be particularly effective in patients who are abstinent prior to initiation and can adhere to its dosing schedule (Jonas et al. 2014).

Disulfiram.   Disulfiram is an aversive agent and therefore does not directly influence motivation to drink. If the patient drinks when taking disulfiram, it can cause a toxic reaction by blocking the metabolism of alcohol by the enzyme acetaldehyde dehydrogenase, leading to the accumulation of acetaldehyde. Disulfiram is best suited for patients who have made an informed choice of this type of treatment, are highly compliant, and are under medical supervision. Because of the risk of significant toxicity, risks and benefits should be carefully considered, and disulfiram should be used only in patients for whom abstinence is the goal and only in conjunction with addiction-focused counseling.

Naltrexone.   Naltrexone is a μ opioid receptor antagonist available as a tablet for once-daily oral administration and as an extended-release suspension for once-monthly intramuscular injection. It works by modulating the mesolimbic system in the ventral tegmental area and projections to the nucleus accumbens. Naltrexone reduces alcohol craving and the euphoric effect of alcohol, thereby reducing the number of heavy-drinking days. The usual dosage of oral naltrexone is 50 mg/day. Oral naltrexone requires daily adherence to the medication. Injectable naltrexone (Vivitrol) should be considered for patients in whom medication adherence is a significant concern. Naltrexone is contraindicated for patients who have used opioids in the preceding 7 days or methadone in the preceding 10 days because of the risk of precipitating opioid withdrawal. It is also contraindicated in patients who have acute hepatitis or liver failure. Pretreatment abstinence from alcohol is not a requirement but can improve response.

Specific Populations and Special Considerations

Pregnancy

In addition to the aforementioned screening tools for AUD in the general population, more specific assessment instruments—such as TWEAK (five questions; Chan et al. 1993) and T-ACE (four questions; Sokol et al. 1989)—are available for screening pregnant women (Table 21–3).

Pregnancy poses a challenge in the treatment of AUD because most approved medications for relapse prevention are unsafe to use in pregnancy or in women who are breastfeeding. In pregnant women, pharmacological treatments are used only in treating acute alcohol withdrawal; the agents of choice are benzodiazepines (Reus et al. 2018). Psychosocial interventions aimed at promoting abstinence remain the mainstay of AUD treatment in pregnancy.

Summary of Alcohol-Related Disorders

Alcohol-related disorders and their associated medical comorbidities are the fourth leading cause of death in the United States and are commonly encountered in the inpatient medical setting. Effective treatment requires the timely management of acute withdrawal syndromes; it also requires early access to and initiation of maintenance medications and early linkage to outpatient treatment to reduce relapse rates and the risk of complications from comorbid disease processes.

Opioid-Related Disorders

Opioid-related hospitalizations and ED visits are increasing across the United States. Epidemiological data from the Agency for Healthcare Research and Quality (AHRQ)

TABLE 21–3. **T-ACE and TWEAK brief screening tools for alcohol use disorder in pregnant women**

T-ACE	TWEAK
T—Tolerance: How many drinks does it take to make you feel high?	T—Tolerance: How many drinks can you hold?
A—Have people Annoyed you by criticizing your drinking?	W—Have close friends or relatives Worried or complained about your drinking in the past year?
C—Have you ever felt you ought to Cut down on your drinking?	E—Eye opener: Do you sometimes take a drink in the morning when you get up?
E—Eye opener: Have you ever had a drink first thing in the morning to steady your nerves or get rid of a hangover?	A—Amnesia: Has a friend or family member ever told you about things you said or did while you were drinking that you could not remember?
	K(C)—Do you sometimes feel the need to Cut down on your drinking?
Note. T-ACE scoring: 2 points for a positive response to question T (>2 drinks); 1 point each for a positive response to question A, C, or E. A total score ≥2 indicates a positive outcome for pregnancy risk drinking.	*Note.* TWEAK scoring: 2 points each for a positive response to question T (>5 drinks) or W; 1 point each for a positive response to question E, A, or K. A total score of ≥2 indicates a positive outcome for pregnancy risk drinking.
Source. Sokol et al. 1989.	*Source.* Chan et al. 1993.

Healthcare Cost and Utilization Project (HCUP) revealed that between 2000 and 2014, annual deaths due to opioid overdose in the United States increased by 200% (Weiss et al. 2016). Hospitalizations related to opioid misuse and dependence spiked sharply as well, with the number of adult hospital inpatient stays per 100,000 population nearly doubling between 2000 and 2012 (Weiss et al. 2016) (Figure 21–1).

The significant increases in opioid use disorder (OUD)–associated overdoses, hospitalizations, and disease comorbidities led the U.S. Department of Health and Human Services (2017) to declare the opioid epidemic a public health emergency and to delineate a five-point strategy to combat the crisis:

1. Improve access to treatment and recovery services.
2. Promote use of overdose-reversing drugs.
3. Strengthen our understanding of the epidemic through better public health surveillance.
4. Provide support for cutting-edge research on pain and addiction.
5. Advance better practices for pain management.

The inpatient medical setting offers physicians, including psychiatrists, an opportunity to make a particular impact in the first strategy point (i.e., improve access) through assisting with patient screenings, brief interventions, early initiation of medication-assisted treatment, and linkages to outpatient treatment.

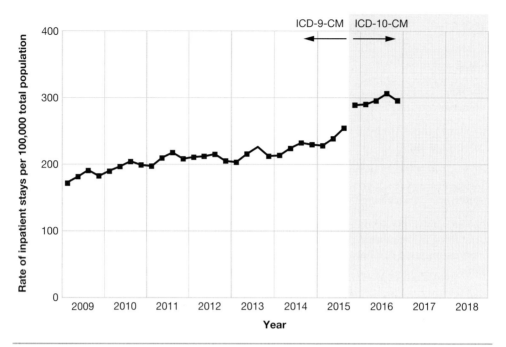

FIGURE 21–1. Opioid-related hospital use: rate of inpatient stays, Nationwide Inpatient Sample, 2009–2016.

Inpatient stays include those admitted through the emergency department.

Source. HCUP Fast Stats—Opioid-Related Hospital Use. Data from Agency for Healthcare Research and Quality, Healthcare Cost and Utilization Project, National (Nationwide) Inpatient Sample, 2009–2016 (all available data as of March 22, 2019). Public Domain. Available at: https://www.hcup-us.ahrq.gov/faststats/OpioidUseServlet. Accessed May 19, 2019.

Screening

Patients with OUD enter the hospital through various scenarios. Patients may self-present either requesting narcotics or voluntarily seeking detoxification. They may also come to medical attention after unintentional overdoses, in the context of acute or chronic comorbid psychiatric disorders, for reasons ancillary to prolonged maintenance on long-term opioid therapy for noncancer chronic pain, or because of infections secondary to intravenous drug use.

The majority of patients with underlying OUD do not voluntarily present for treatment. Screening of all patients in all circumstances, as part of a routine history and physical, may unearth an underlying diagnosis that would otherwise be missed. Screening should be implemented broadly and universally in both inpatient and outpatient medical settings. Within inpatient medical settings, simple initial screens may be conducted through use of the National Institute on Drug Abuse single-item drug use screen (NIDA-1; Smith et al. 2010) or the 10-item Drug Abuse Screening Test (DAST-10; Yudko et al. 2007). Certain populations are at higher risk for developing OUD, and automatic consultations for such patients should be considered a routine part of their inpatient admission.

Prescription opioid use has been linked to a distinct set of demographics: younger age (20–29 years), white ethnicity, and higher socioeconomic status, with fewer comorbid mental illnesses (Mendelson et al. 2008). In addition, high-risk populations that would benefit from automatic consultations may include the following:

- *Patients with known SUDs or a strong family history of SUDs*—Genetic influences are believed to contribute about 50% to the risk of developing an SUD (Ducci and Goldman 2012). The etiology is multifactorial, and associations with specific genes have been suggested; however, definitive evidence tailored to specific genes is still lacking.
- *Patients taking opioid medications for noncancer chronic pain management*—Chronic noncancer pain syndromes that are treated with long-term opioid therapy have also been linked to an increase in OUD in the United States (Zacny and Lichtor 2008). Chronic pain and associated emotional distress are thought to dysregulate the brain's stress and reward circuitry, increasing the risk for OUD. Among patients being treated with long-term opioid therapy, approximately 10% misuse these medications (Garland et al. 2013).
- *Patients presenting with common infections associated with intravenous drug use*—Common infections from intravenous drug use include cutaneous and subcutaneous abscesses ranging from cellulitis to deeper extension of infections into underlying fascia and muscle tissue. These infections lead to associated complications such as necrotizing fasciitis, myositis, endocarditis, pyomyositis, bacteremia, and sepsis.
- *Patients referred from the criminal justice system*—Estimates suggest that up to 45% of individuals in state and local prisons and jails struggle with dual diagnoses of mental illness and SUDs without adequate access to treatment services (James and Glaze 2006). Early recognition of underlying mental illness and SUDs in this patient population not only may reduce medical comorbidities but also may diminish the rate and frequency of criminal recidivism (James and Glaze 2006).
- *Psychiatric patients*—Patients with psychiatric disorders such as bipolar disorder, attention-deficit/hyperactivity disorder (ADHD), major depression, anxiety disorders, personality disorders, posttraumatic stress disorder, and psychosis have an increased risk of developing SUDs (Compton and Volkow 2006).
- *Patients admitted to level I or II TICUs*—Patients who undergo mandatory alcohol screens and would benefit from concomitant drug screens, which may be done as part of the initial admission process.
- *Pregnant female patients at high risk of OUD*—The American College of Obstetricians and Gynecologists recommends universal early screening for substance abuse in all pregnant women, taking place at the first prenatal visit; many times, an inpatient medical admission may provide the first opportunity for this screen (Committee on Obstetric Practice 2017).

Brief initial screening requires minimal time and effort on the part of clinicians during initial patient contact. Brief screening instruments include the NIDA-1 quick screen (Smith et al. 2010), the 4Ps Plus questionnaire for pregnant women (Chasnoff et al. 2005), and the CRAFFT Screening Test (questions relating to **c**ar, **r**elax, **a**lone, **f**orget, **f**riends, and **t**rouble) for adolescents (Knight et al. 1999). The CAGE Questions Adapted to Include Drug Use (CAGE-AID), a modification of the CAGE (**c**ut down, **a**nnoyed, **g**uilty, **e**ye opener) questionnaire, is a four-item screen that incorporates both alcohol and drug use; it is geared more toward identifying dependence than toward identifying general or risky use (Brown and Rounds 1995). The NIDA-1 remains the preferred instrument for initial screening for general substance use.

A positive finding on initial screens should prompt further investigation and more detailed assessments. Additional screening tools such as the DAST-10 (Yudko et al. 2007) may be used in conjunction with a more detailed history. The clinical interview is critical at this stage to further clarify the nature and extent of current use.

Laboratory tests may serve as an adjunct to the screening and clinical interview process in establishing a diagnosis and directing the clinician toward the appropriate interventions. The "drug screen 9" is a commonly used urine drug panel that tests for opiates (morphine, heroin, codeine), two opioids (hydromorphone and hydrocodone), cocaine, marijuana, benzodiazepines, phencyclidine, amphetamines, and barbiturates. Separate screens are required to test for the presence of oxycodone, buprenorphine, and synthetic opioids (including methadone and fentanyl).

A positive urine screen should be followed by a confirmatory urine test to rule out false-positive results. The opioid confirmation urine test by gas chromatography–mass spectrometry is highly specific and sensitive and will identify the specific opioid in the urine. Most opioids are detectable in the urine for 1–3 days. Methadone may be detected up to 7 days after last use.

Drugs can also be detected in other body fluids, and alternative tests include oral fluid tests and sweat or hair analyses. However, urine drug testing is currently the best-validated and most clinically acceptable method (Kapur 1993).

Diagnosis

The diagnosis of OUD is clinical; therefore, a thorough history and a careful psychiatric and medical examination, along with appropriate laboratory tests, are essential for making the diagnosis. In addition to establishing a diagnosis of OUD, it is important to identify any additional SUDs or medical and psychiatric problems. Diagnosis of OUD should be made according to DSM-5. Patients who are taking opioids solely under appropriate medical supervision are not considered to meet the tolerance and withdrawal portions of the DSM-5 diagnostic criteria for OUD.

Brief Interventions

Brief interventions can—and should—be provided before, as a part of, or after the diagnosis of substance use. Brief interventions for OUD include education around opioid use through nonjudgmental motivational interviewing based on open-ended questions aimed at creating an alliance with the patient, exploring patient ambivalence, and augmenting patient self-efficacy for behavior change. These interventions may be used in a targeted fashion in the inpatient hospital setting. Many patients with OUD are reluctant to discuss their opioid use in medical settings; a nonconfrontational, respectful, and empathic approach can significantly assist the interviewer in establishing trust and rapport, allowing the patient to disclose more freely without fear of stigma.

Clinical Presentation

Patients with OUD may present with chronic constipation, weight loss, or symptoms of either tolerance or withdrawal. Tolerance may manifest as either blunting to the pleasurable effects of opioids or adverse effects such as nausea and sedation. Tolerance can develop as soon as 3 days following continuous use of opioids, with patients seeking gradual dose escalation rather than decreasing doses over the first week even in prescribed amounts.

Clinical manifestations of opioid-related disorders may include the following:

- OUD—miosis; sedation; evidence of track or needle marks, scars, or skin necrosis at injection sites
- Opioid overdose—pinpoint pupils, reduced respiratory rate (<10 breaths per minute), reduced pulse rate (<40 beats per minute), apnea, stupor, unconsciousness
- Opioid withdrawal—dilated pupils; excessive perspiration or lacrimation; rhinorrhea; restlessness; piloerection; aggressive behavior; tachypnea or laborious breathing; hypertension; tachycardia, bradycardia, or other cardiac dysrhythmias. Neonates of opioid-dependent mothers can present with seizures during withdrawal, making withdrawal life-threatening to both mother and fetus (National Institute on Drug Abuse 2018d).

Treatment

There is extensive evidence to support the combination of pharmacotherapy and psychosocial treatment for optimal management of OUD. Although detoxification primarily involves judicious use of medications, psychosocial support and supervision also are helpful at this stage. For longer-term treatment, pharmacological maintenance therapies with adjunctive evidence-based psychosocial treatments are effective in retaining patients in treatment and suppressing illicit opioid use. An inpatient stay offers an opportune period for brief interventions and for early initiation of medication-assisted treatment, which has been demonstrated to improve patient linkage to and retention in outpatient treatment (Suzuki et al. 2015).

Intoxication

Risks of life-threatening intoxication and overdose are higher for patients who use opioids intravenously or who combine opioids with sedative-hypnotic agents. Clinicians should maintain a high index of suspicion for opioid overdose, and should immediately administer naloxone to a patient who presents with sedation, slurred speech, alterations in arousal, decreased respiratory rates, slowed pulse rates, or stupor. More than one dose of naloxone may be required to reverse overdoses in patients who have used large amounts of opioids or long-acting formulations. Naloxone administration in the field should always be accompanied by transport to the nearest ED. With the increasing use and high potency of fentanyl, rates of overdose have dramatically escalated. All patients presenting with a history of intravenous drug use should be provided with access to naloxone kits to help mitigate subsequent risks of overdose.

Withdrawal

Physiological dependence on opioids is maintained by the rewarding effect of opioids mediated through the mesolimbic dopamine system and the avoidance of aversive opioid withdrawal symptoms mediated through norepinephrine pathways. Neurochemicals (e.g., cortisol) and dysfunction in other brain areas (e.g., prefrontal cortex) also appear to play a role in the development of physiological dependence (Kosten and George 2002).

Symptoms of withdrawal generally develop from 12 to 72 hours after the last dose of opioid; the time of symptom emergence correlates with the specific opioid's half-life. The earliest symptoms may be anxiety, irritability, and cravings, and as withdrawal progresses, additional physical symptoms appear, such as sneezing, yawning, and restless sleep. More severe manifestations of withdrawal include nausea, vomiting, diarrhea, abdominal cramps, backache, muscle spasm, hot and cold flashes, and insomnia.

Symptom severity can be assessed with the Clinical Opioid Withdrawal Scale (COWS; Wesson and Ling 2003). Use of this scale can help guide initiation of medication-assisted treatment for both withdrawal management and maintenance, as described in the next section ("Buprenorphine").

Two evidence-based detoxification strategies are in use: 1) gradual opioid substitution and taper with an opioid agonist (i.e., buprenorphine or methadone) and 2) more rapid discontinuation with an α_2-adrenergic agonist (i.e., clonidine) used with or without naltrexone (Gowing et al. 2016).

Buprenorphine. Buprenorphine is a potent partial agonist at the μ opioid receptor and an antagonist at the κ opioid receptor. It is available in two formulations: 1) a sublingual tablet containing buprenorphine only, and 2) a sublingual tablet containing buprenorphine and naloxone. The latter formulation is preferred for most patients, because it decreases the likelihood of intravenous abuse of buprenorphine, given that parenteral administration of buprenorphine with naloxone can precipitate withdrawal. Initiation of buprenorphine therapy differs from initiation of methadone in that buprenorphine therapy can precipitate withdrawal symptoms if given too soon after an opioid agonist because of its partial rather than full agonist effects on the μ opioid receptor.

Moderate withdrawal symptoms (usually appearing about 12–24 hours after the last use) must be present prior to buprenorphine induction. In most cases, a COWS score of at least 8 is sufficient for initiation of buprenorphine; however, a COWS score of 15 is required in a patient transitioning from methadone. Detoxification protocols may begin with a 4-mg induction dose followed by subsequent 4 mg dosing every 4–6 hours until full symptomatic resolution; generally, patients will not require more than 16 mg within 24 hours (World Health Organization 2019). Reductions of 25% per day are common for dosage tapering in withdrawal management.

Methadone. Methadone is an alternative first-line option for detoxification. It is a synthetic full μ opioid agonist and an N-methyl-D-aspartate (NMDA) antagonist that has demonstrated safety and efficacy in withdrawal management. The total dosage should not exceed 40 mg in the first 24 hours; dosage reduction may proceed by 25% per day (World Health Organization 2019). There is evidence to suggest that a single intramuscular dose of 10 mg of methadone is effective in reducing withdrawal symptoms within 30 minutes for patients presenting to acute care in mild to moderate withdrawal (Su et al. 2018).

Currently, the federal methadone regulations restrict the use of methadone for treating opioid addiction to the following four situations: 1) a licensed narcotic treatment program; 2) a licensed, hospital-based, inpatient addiction treatment unit for detoxification from opioid addiction; 3) a hospital, for temporary maintenance or detoxification, when the admission is for an illness other than opioid addiction; and 4) an outpatient setting (hospital, private practice, clinic, or nursing home with a medical director and 24-hour nursing care) in which methadone is administered daily for a maximum of 3 days while the patient awaits admission into a methadone treatment program. The only circumstance in which methadone can be routinely prescribed and administered on an outpatient basis outside an officially registered narcotic treatment program is for the treatment of pain.

Patients who are already taking methadone when they present for care may be continued on their maintenance dosage, after confirmation with their methadone clinic, through the duration of their hospitalization. Prior to discharge, the patient's methadone clinic must be notified of the last inpatient hospital dose received and the anticipated discharge time to ensure that there are no interruptions to the outpatient dosing schedule. For patients with newly diagnosed OUD in the inpatient medical setting, a methadone taper can be used for relief of withdrawal symptoms. Patients may then be discharged to a methadone treatment program for continued treatment. If no resources are available for the patient on discharge, or if the patient is ready for discharge before his or her withdrawal protocol can be completed, a hospital may accommodate him or her by completing the withdrawal protocol on an outpatient basis. For a patient awaiting admission to a licensed narcotic treatment program, the hospital may maintain the patient on a maintenance dosage of methadone while in the inpatient medical setting until the patient is admitted by the program. In either case, methadone must be administered daily at the facility by a staff member licensed to handle and administer opioids. Patients should not be given prescriptions for methadone for this purpose on discharge from the hospital (Rettig and Yarmolinsky 1995).

Clonidine. Clonidine is an α_2-adrenergic receptor agonist that reduces symptoms of noradrenergic activation in opioid withdrawal. It is an effective supportive or primary agent in second-line treatment for the management of acute opioid withdrawal as well as for longer-term residual withdrawal effects that may persist for weeks after cessation of long-acting opioids such as methadone.

Supportive therapies. Adequate hydration and food intake should be ensured during withdrawal management and maintenance treatment. Ancillary medications in therapeutic doses may be required for symptomatic relief (e.g., loperamide for diarrhea, ondansetron for vomiting, dicyclomine for bowel cramps, ibuprofen for muscle pain). Benzodiazepines may be given in an inpatient setting on a time-limited basis for treatment of muscle cramps; they should not be used in conjunction with methadone- or buprenorphine-assisted withdrawal management.

Maintenance

Medications for relapse prevention include long-acting opioid agonists (i.e., methadone, buprenorphine) and opioid antagonists (i.e., injectable extended-release naltrexone). Treatment should be continued for the duration that the following criteria are met: the patient continues to benefit from treatment, wishes to remain in treatment, remains at risk for relapse, and has no serious adverse effects.

Continuing treatment after completion of detoxification is essential because of the high risk of relapse. Although this phase can be accomplished without the use of opioid agonists, substantial evidence indicates that medication treatment is essential for the majority of patients with OUD.

Buprenorphine and Buprenorphine-Naloxone

Evidence suggests that patients who are started and maintained on buprenorphine (Subutex) treatment in the inpatient medical setting have higher rates of successful linkage to outpatient treatment and higher numbers of total days abstinent at 3, 6, and 9 months' follow-up compared with patients who are not started on medication-assisted treatment in the inpatient medical setting. This window of opportunity for early initiation of medication-assisted treatment is critically underutilized, despite emerging evidence that initiation of buprenorphine treatment at the time of hospitalization for acute medical illness leads to significant improvements in patient linkage to, and retention in, outpatient treatment (C.S. Lee et al. 2017; Suzuki et al. 2015).

The greater flexibility in administration sites permitted with buprenorphine (inpatient medical settings, outpatient office settings) in comparison with methadone (specialized clinics only) makes buprenorphine an ideal option for early initiation of medication-assisted treatment. Properties that make it a good candidate for maintenance therapy include lower levels of physical dependence and lower severity of withdrawal symptoms compared with methadone. Because of a ceiling effect on respiratory depression and poor systemic bioavailability, buprenorphine has a reduced potential for lethality in overdose and has a prolonged duration of action (24–60 hours). Most patients will require maintenance dosages between 8 and 24 mg daily during early phases of treatment.

Additional formulations are available and include an implantable device that delivers a consistent dose of buprenorphine over 6 months (Probuphine) and a once-monthly injection (Sublocade).

Buprenorphine may also be used for patients wishing to undergo detoxification from methadone and transition to naltrexone or non-medication-assisted abstinence. In the inpatient setting, patients will generally go into withdrawal about 72 hours after the last dose of methadone; the COWS score must be greater than 15 prior to induction on buprenorphine. In the outpatient setting, patients should be tapered to 30 mg of methadone and maintained on that dosage for 1–2 weeks before cessation and transition to buprenorphine.

Methadone

Methadone is the first-line option for maintenance therapy, especially in patients with very-high-dose opioid addiction. Patients must present daily to a methadone clinic to obtain their medication. With ongoing treatment adherence, there is a gradual increase in the amount of medication they are able to take home. Ultimately, after a sustained period of abstinence, patients are able to progress to monthly take-home doses. Methadone produces strong physical dependence, and discontinuation of methadone maintenance treatment can cause a protracted withdrawal syndrome that can last more than 4 weeks. Only 10%–20% of patients who discontinue methadone are able to remain abstinent (Galanter and Kleber 2008).

Comparisons between buprenorphine and methadone at fixed medium or high doses show that the two agents have similar effectiveness in regard to treatment retention and suppression of illicit opioid use (Mattick et al. 2004). However, because methadone, even at low doses, has a relatively high risk (as compared with buprenorphine or other opioids) of elevating the QTc interval, caution and close monitoring should be used when initiating treatment with methadone. The risk increases with dosage elevation and with polypharmacy with medications that interfere with methadone's metabolism (Behzadi et al. 2018).

Naltrexone

Naltrexone is a pure μ opioid receptor antagonist that is nonaddictive and produces no euphoria. The lack of agonist effects may lead to poorer medication compliance and lower retention rates, which limits the efficacy of the oral formulation in clinical settings in the treatment of OUD specifically, although certain patient populations (nurses, physicians, prison populations) or highly motivated individuals may be successful. However, the development of longer-acting preparations of naltrexone may improve compliance as well as clinical efficacy across patient populations. A systematic Cochrane review found no benefit of oral formulations of naltrexone over placebo in decreasing side effects and relapse risk and increasing treatment retention (Minozzi et al. 2011). In contrast, recent studies have demonstrated similar outcomes between the longer-acting injectable formulation of naltrexone and sublingual buprenorphine in maintenance treatment for patients as long as either medication was initiated following a successful completion of detoxification (Jarvis et al. 2018; Lee et al. 2018). A naloxone challenge test should be conducted prior to initiation of naltrexone maintenance therapy.

Dihydrocodeine

Dihydrocodeine is a full opioid receptor agonist that has been used on a limited basis outside the United States as an alternative to methadone maintenance. Limited data indicate that it is equivalent to buprenorphine in terms of treatment retention (Wright et al. 2007). Clinical use of dihydrocodeine is limited because of the lack of standardized guidelines, and more supportive evidence must be obtained before its adoption in mainstream clinical use can be recommended.

Heroin Maintenance

There is some evidence suggesting the efficacy of controlled heroin administration to a subset of patients who have failed to benefit from first-line medication-assisted treatments (Uchtenhagen 2011). This approach has been adopted in certain European health care systems, with trials under way in the United Kingdom and Belgium. It is not used in clinical practice in the United States.

Supportive Therapies

Psychosocial interventions and urine drug screen monitoring, as well as assessment and treatment of comorbid medical and psychiatric conditions (e.g., depression, anxiety disorders, personality disorders), should be part of maintenance therapy. Monitoring of physical health problems (e.g., cardiovascular, respiratory, gastrointestinal) and HIV testing and counseling, as well as hepatitis C screening and referral for treatment, should be integrated into the maintenance program. Patients benefit from psychosocial treatments such as individual and group drug counseling, contingency management, cognitive therapy, supportive-expressive therapy, and 12-step-oriented groups such as Narcotics Anonymous or non-spiritual-based recovery groups such as SMART Recovery.

Specific Populations and Special Considerations

Adolescents

Because of its better safety profile, buprenorphine is generally preferred over methadone for treatment induction and maintenance in adolescent patients. For patients younger than 18 years of age, methadone treatment is considered only if the patient has failed to benefit from medication-assisted treatment with buprenorphine and has relapsed on opioids after at least two attempts at detoxification and short-term rehabilitation.

Pregnancy

Pregnant women with OUD experience increased obstetric and neonatal complications. Detoxification is generally not recommended during pregnancy because of the risk of fetal distress and premature birth. If absolutely necessary, detoxification should be done in the inpatient medical setting. For pregnant women, buprenorphine monotherapy rather than buprenorphine-naloxone formulations (Suboxone, Zubsolv, Bunavail) should be used for treatment induction and stabilization because of the potential dangers of precipitated withdrawal to both mother and fetus if the combination formulation is misused or injected. Maintenance treatment with either methadone or buprenorphine is preferred. Methadone has been the drug of choice for detoxification or maintenance therapy because of its larger evidence base. It has demonstrated efficacy in longer maternal drug abstinence; improved obstetrical care adherence; and reduction in associated risk behaviors when compared with no medication-assisted treatment. However, data have shown that buprenorphine has improved outcomes in neonatal abstinence syndromes when compared with methadone and has equal efficacy to methadone in maintenance treatment for the duration of pregnancy. Nevertheless, longitudinal data evaluating the impact of buprenorphine versus methadone on neonatal outcomes have been limited to neonatal abstinence syndrome and the neonatal period. Further research is needed to evaluate long-term health and developmental outcomes of children exposed to buprenorphine during pregnancy as well as to develop clinical guidelines and patient educational materials to guide patient and provider decision making regarding the most effective treatment for a particular patient during pregnancy (Krans et al. 2016).

HIV and Hepatitis C

The Centers for Disease Control and Prevention (2012) recommend hepatitis A and B vaccinations for persons who engage in intravenous drug use. Screening and referral for treatment of HIV, hepatitis C, tuberculosis, and sexually transmitted diseases also are recommended. Neither methadone nor buprenorphine is contraindicated in patients receiving antiretroviral therapies; however, emerging evidence suggests that buprenorphine is less likely than methadone to cause drug-drug interactions with antiretroviral treatments (Herron and Brennan 2015; Li et al. 2015).

Kratom

Recently recognized by the NIDA as an emerging drug of abuse but not yet currently regulated by the Controlled Substances Act, kratom is a tropical plant that has both stimulant and antinociceptive properties through activation of the descending mono-aminergic system and μ opioid receptors. It is being used as a substitute for opioids in misuse or as self-medication in withdrawal. Although most medical consequences are minor, rare fatalities have been reported (Fluyau and Revadigar 2017).

Chronic Pain

Buprenorphine in transdermal (Butrans) and buccal (Belbuca) formulations is currently approved for use in the treatment of chronic pain. It is less clear if buprenorphine is a suitable treatment for chronic pain that is comorbid with OUD. Further research is needed to better understand the patient demographics that would best predict successful transition to and maintenance on buprenorphine treatment within the chronic pain patient population (Roux et al. 2013; Suzuki et al. 2014).

Summary of Opioid-Related Disorders

OUD is a chronic disease, with relapse rates greater than 90% in untreated patients (McLellan et al. 2000). With effective treatment, relapse rates are similar to those in other well-characterized chronic medical illnesses, such as diabetes, hypertension, and asthma (McLellan et al. 2000). The treatment of OUD involves modifying deeply ingrained behaviors and associated stigmas; relapse does not equate with treatment failure. With each relapse, both patients and providers should evaluate the current treatment approach, identify gaps in treatment and adherence, and tailor the approach to specific patient profiles.

The American Society of Addiction Medicine (2015) consensus statement reports that the advent of buprenorphine and the passage of the Drug Addiction Treatment Act in 2000 have revolutionized the opioid treatment delivery system by granting physicians the ability to administer office-based opioid treatment, thereby giving patients greater access to treatment. Therapeutic outcomes for patients who self-select office-based treatment with buprenorphine are comparable to outcomes for patients in methadone programs. There are few absolute contraindications to the use of buprenorphine, although the experience and skill levels of treating physicians can vary considerably, as can access to the resources needed to treat comorbid medical or psychiatric conditions; all of these variables can affect outcomes. Psychiatrists and addiction medicine specialists are uniquely qualified to provide early access to medication-assisted treatment for patients in hospital-based settings, thereby reducing barriers to treatment and improving outcomes.

Tobacco-Related Disorders

Fewer people are smoking, yet smoking still remains the leading cause of all preventable deaths worldwide. The proportion of U.S. adults who smoke cigarettes declined from 20.9% in 2005 (45.1 million smokers) to 15.5% in 2016 (37.8 million smokers); however, cigarette smoking prevalence has remained steady since 2015 (Centers for Disease Control and Prevention 2016). Lower income and medically vulnerable populations continue to show disproportionately high smoking rates both in the United States and globally. Despite the downward trend in prevalence, smoking kills approximately 480,000 people per year in the United States. This number is 10 times higher than the number of annual deaths from opioid overdoses; it is also higher than the number of annual deaths from alcohol, drugs, AIDS, motor vehicle collisions, murders, and suicides *combined.*

Worldwide, the statistics are similarly grim: tobacco causes 6 million deaths annually. If current consumption rates continue, numbers are projected to increase to 8 million per year by 2030 and to total 1 billion deaths by the end of this century, despite the availability of low-cost, easily administered, and highly effective treatments. These statistics attest to the tenacity of the addiction and the critical need for more effective prevention and treatment interventions (Ziedonis et al. 2017).

A 2004 report from the U.S. Surgeon General concluded that epidemiological evidence was sufficient to link smoking with multiple diseases that commonly result in ICU admission (Office of the Surgeon General 2004). Similar statistics appear in studies linking smoking with an increased risk of any medical hospitalization, with the prevalence of smoking in ICU patients ranging from 22% to 46% in prospective studies where smoking rates are reported (Clark and Moss 2011). These studies reveal that acute medical care providers encounter current smokers at a higher rate than the general population and that current smokers are more likely to have more severe medical illness and prolonged hospitalizations from medical complications (Clark and Moss 2011). In addition, tobacco use disorders are two or three times more prevalent among patients with other psychiatric disorders, including anxiety, attention-deficit, mood, and other substance use disorders, with higher rates of tobacco-related mortality. Forty percent of all cigarettes smoked in the United States are consumed by smokers with mental illness or substance use disorders (Lipari and Van Horn 2017).

Studies have found that cigarette smoking increases the likelihood of relapse among people in recovery from any SUD. Cigarette smoking often accompanies illicit drug use, and cigarettes may serve as a drug cue, enhancing cravings for stimulants and opioids and triggering relapses. Assisting patients in quitting smoking may also improve their chances for sustained recovery from use of other drugs (Weinberger et al. 2017).

Major gaps in provider confidence, limits in time allotted to patient visits, and lack of awareness of the persistence of the problem all contribute to reduce the likelihood that patients will receive much-needed medical education on smoking cessation techniques and interventions or will be started on such treatment. One study revealed that smoking cessation counseling was received by only 48% of active smokers admitted to a large urban academic training hospital for a chronic obstructive pulmonary disease (COPD) exacerbation, despite the well-known body of evidence linking smoking cessation to a decreased rate of COPD exacerbation (Freund et al. 2009). A recent retrospective study found that among 36,675 smokers hospitalized for coronary heart disease, only 8,316 (22.7%) received nicotine replacement treatment (NRT) during their hospitalization (Pack et al. 2017). In the inpatient medical setting, brief interventions and NRTs are easy-to-use and ultimately lifesaving measures that can be routinely offered by the C-L psychiatrist.

Diagnosis and Identification

The National Health Interview Survey is used to estimate annual smoking rates in the United States; in this survey, a current smoker is defined as a person who has smoked more than 100 cigarettes in his or her lifetime and currently smokes every day or almost every day (National Center for Health Statistics 2017). Although a formal diagnosis of tobacco use disorder is based on DSM-5 criteria, any amount of smoking is considered detrimental to health, and all patients who are identified as smokers should be offered smoking cessation therapy. Smoking cessation therapy is crucial and highly underutilized; studies demonstrate that documented smoking histories are obtained in only 66%–75% of hospitalized patients, and only 20%–30% of smokers who make an attempt to quit use therapies that are proven to double or triple abstinence rates (Clark and Moss 2011).

Brief Interventions and Treatment

As noted earlier in chapter, brief interventions typically precede formal treatment and often are provided during the initial interview or as part of motivational interviewing to improve acceptance of and adherence to treatment. The brief interventions framed by the "5 A's" (ask, advise, assess, assist, arrange) model of treating tobacco use disorder are endorsed in guidelines from the U.S. Surgeon General (Fiore et al. 2008). The framework is most effective when coupled with intensive smoking cessation interventions consisting of both behavioral modification therapy and individualized pharmacotherapy. In a cohort of hospitalized cardiac patients ($N=209$) with high-risk smoking, an intensive intervention—consisting of 12 weeks of behavioral modification therapy plus individualized pharmacotherapy—resulted in smoking cessation rates that were significantly higher than rates with usual care in the hospital setting (i.e., brief counseling and printed educational material) (Mohiuddin et al. 2007). At 24 months, continuous-abstinence smoking cessation rates were 33% in the intensive-treatment group ($n=109$) and 9% in the usual-care group ($n=100$) (Mohiuddin et al. 2007). Secondary prevention may be particularly important in this population, because smoking cessation leads to a marked reduction in mortality for patients with coronary artery disease, including patients with left ventricular dysfunction following acute myocardial infarction (Clark and Moss 2011).

Additional studies have noted that beneficial effects of intensive counseling on smoking cessation persist regardless of admission diagnosis and are independent of the provision of pharmacotherapy. In addition to increasing the rate of smoking cessation, intensive interventions may also decrease the rate of rehospitalization and improve mortality (Rigotti et al. 2008).

Clinicians have an opportunity to influence treatment outcomes significantly by intervening in the hospital setting. Interventions may include motivational interviewing to improve self-efficacy in setting and adhering to a quit date and education focused on specific medication-assisted treatments and proper techniques for using NRTs.

There is strong evidence that combining psychosocial and pharmacological approaches is more effective than using either approach alone. However, in addition to, or in lieu of, medication, important psychosocial or community-based interventions can also be used, including individual and group counseling with behavioral therapy, phone counseling (quitlines) and text messaging interventions, and support groups such as Nicotine Anonymous, to assist patients in maintaining this behavior change following discharge from the hospital (Ziedonis et al. 2017).

Nicotine causes release of dopamine and upregulation of dopamine receptors, which over time results in nicotine dependence and craving, with a drive to return to consuming nicotine. Nicotine's short half-life means that withdrawal symptoms—including irritability, frustration, anxiety, difficulty concentrating, restlessness, depressed mood, insomnia, increased appetite, weight gain, and cravings—will begin within 1–2 hours after the last cigarette.

When individuals who are heavy smokers are admitted to a smoke-free facility and are forced to abstain, they develop changes that affect the metabolism of certain drugs (including caffeine). Therefore, hospitalized patients who are heavy smokers should be provided with specific education about the use of caffeine, and patients receiving atypical antipsychotics, specifically clozapine, should be monitored for the anticipated spikes in blood levels that occur in the absence of smoking. These effects are the result of interactions between chemicals in tobacco smoke and metabolism and are not related to nicotine itself. Initiation of NRT therefore will not prevent rising levels of clozapine, and close monitoring and dosage adjustments of clozapine will be necessary.

Seven medications have received U.S. Food and Drug Administration (FDA) approval for smoking cessation: the non-nicotine replacement pill options bupropion (Zyban) and varenicline (Chantix) and five nicotine-replacement therapies.

Varenicline appears to be the most effective medication in comparison with placebo, followed by bupropion and NRTs (Cahill et al. 2016). Varenicline is a partial agonist at the α4β2 neuronal nicotinic acetylcholine receptor; it relieves craving and withdrawal symptoms following smoking cessation and also reduces the reinforcing effects of nicotine by blocking dopaminergic stimulation (thereby providing less smoking reinforcement or reward).

Bupropion acts on dopaminergic, norepinephrine, and nicotinic-cholinergic receptors to decrease cravings and withdrawal symptoms. Studies suggest that bupropion has greater efficacy (as measured by sustained cessation rates) than NRTs, but less efficacy than varenicline (Cahill et al. 2013).

NRTs offer a steady, low-level delivery of nicotine, which provides consistent plasma levels to ameliorate cravings and withdrawal symptoms while also reducing the rewarding and reinforcing effects from the sharp nicotine spikes and drops that occur via inhalation of tobacco products. In addition to having slower delivery rates of nicotine in comparison with cigarettes, NRTs typically contain only 30%–75% of the total amount of nicotine found in consumer tobacco products.

Additional benefits of NRT in ICU patients may extend beyond smoking cessation. Prospective observational studies have demonstrated an association between current smoking and delirium or agitation in ICU patients that may potentially be mediated by nicotine withdrawal and its effects on acetylcholine receptors. Prospective randomized controlled trials are now examining whether the use of NRT in ICU patients can help prevent the development of delirium and agitation and improve smoking cessation rates in ICU survivors (Clark and Moss 2011).

Choice of medication depends on patient history, patient preference, medication cost, number of previous cessation attempts, and severity of dependence or withdrawal and breakthrough symptoms. Therapies are often more effective when used in combination. Concurrent pairings of a long-acting NRT—such as a nicotine patch or a long-acting medication (e.g., varenicline, bupropion—with a short-acting NRT—such as nicotine gum or lozenges—may be beneficial across patient populations.

Summary of Tobacco-Related Disorders

Smoking remains the leading cause of preventable deaths worldwide and contributes to high rates of morbidity and mortality across diseases of every organ system. Lower-income populations and patients with psychiatric illnesses have higher rates of smoking-associated morbidity and mortality, which create severe health disparities for particularly vulnerable populations.

Treatment of tobacco use disorder is optimized by the integration of evidence-based pharmacological and psychosocial treatments, as well as by effective implementation in real-world settings. Treatment can often begin in the hospital setting, thereby producing far-reaching benefits. C-L psychiatrists can facilitate patient education and access to medication treatment as well as provide guidance to colleagues on how to more effectively and universally implement screening and treatment initiation in this setting. On a systems level, increased advocacy for greater clinician and provider training, improved access to clinical and support tools, and wider availability of technical assistance may help address some of the current barriers to treatment.

Tobacco use is a global epidemic, but there has been a long tradition of ignoring the disease burden caused by this substance. Although clinical knowledge and the availability of effective treatment options have increased rapidly over the past 50 years, implementation of these options in clinical practice remains widely underutilized. The inpatient hospital setting offers an often-overlooked opportunity for starting treatment, with the potential to significantly alter the disease course and burden for current smokers.

Cannabis-Related Disorders

More than half of new users of illicit drugs begin with marijuana (National Institute on Drug Abuse 2015) (Figure 21–2).

The *Cannabis sativa* plant contains both cannabidiol (CBD), which is known to have antipsychotic properties, and delta-9-tetrahydrocannabinol (THC), which is known for its psychoactive properties. The term *medical marijuana* refers to use of the whole, unprocessed marijuana plant or its basic extracts to treat symptoms of illness and other conditions. The FDA has not recognized or approved the marijuana plant as medicine; however, scientific study of the chemicals in marijuana, called *cannabinoids*, has led to two FDA-approved medications that contain cannabinoid chemicals in pill form. Continued research may lead to more medications (National Institute on Drug Abuse 2019b). Thus, medications that act on cannabinoid receptors may be confused with medical marijuana, but they are not the same thing, and their effects are not interchangeable or broadly applicable. CBD has antipsychotic effects in humans; a recent study found evidence that these effects occur through partial normalization of the underlying functional alterations in regions critical to the pathophysiology of psychosis (i.e., the parahippocampal, striatal, and midbrain) in antipsychotic-naive individuals who are at clinically high risk for development of psychosis (Bhattacharyya et al. 2018). THC, by contrast, is a psychoactive compound that activates cannabinoid type 1 (CB_1) receptors, central nervous system receptors distributed throughout the frontal cortex and thalamus; over time, activation of CB_1 receptors is believed to affect down-

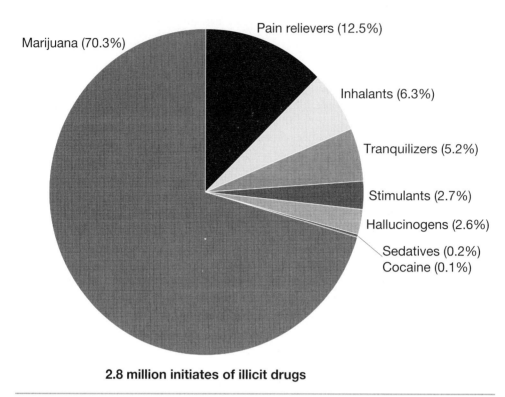

2.8 million initiates of illicit drugs

FIGURE 21–2. First specific drug associated with initiation of illicit drug use among past-year illicit drug initiates ages 12 years or older: 2013.

Note. Percentages do not add up to 100 either because of rounding or because a small number of respondents initiated multiple drugs on the same day. "First specific drug" refers to the one that was used on the occasion of first-time use of any illicit drug.
Source. Reprinted from Figure 5.1 (p. 59) in Substance Abuse and Mental Health Services Administration: "Results from the 2013 National Survey on Drug Use and Health: Summary of National Findings" (NSDUH Series H-48, HHS Publication No. SMA 14-4863). Rockville, MD, Substance Abuse and Mental Health Services Administration, 2014. Public Domain. Available at: https://www.samhsa.gov/data/sites/default/files/NSDUHresultsPDFWHTML2013/Web/NSDUHresults2013.pdf. Accessed May 19, 2019.

stream dopaminergic regulation in the mesolimbic pathway and nucleus accumbens, leading to the drug's psychoactive and addictive effects (Lazenka et al. 2017).

However, THC itself has proven medical benefits in particular formulations. The FDA has approved the THC-based medications dronabinol (Marinol) and nabilone (Cesamet), prescribed in pill forms, for use in treating nausea in patients undergoing cancer chemotherapy and for use in stimulating appetite in patients with wasting syndrome due to AIDS. In addition, several other marijuana-based medications have been approved or are undergoing clinical trials for use in a range of conditions, such as spasticity, neuropathic pain, and refractory epilepsy (including the severe childhood-onset forms of Dravet syndrome and Lennox-Gastaut syndrome) (National Institute on Drug Abuse 2018b).

To date, research examining the effects of cannabis on opioid use in pain patients has yielded mixed findings. Some data suggest that medical cannabis treatment may reduce the dosage of opioids required for pain relief (Wiese and Wilson-Poe 2018), whereas a National Institutes of Health–funded study found that cannabis use appeared to increase the risk of nonmedical use of prescription opioids and development of an OUD (Olfson et al. 2018). Although no single study has produced definitive evidence, research cumulatively suggests that medical marijuana products may play a role in reducing the amount of opioids needed to control pain, but also that these products do not come without risk. More research is needed to investigate the potential therapeutic role of marijuana, including its role as a treatment option for OUD and its ability to reduce specific types of pain (National Institute on Drug Abuse 2018b).

These findings, along with increased societal permissiveness around THC use, have fueled the emerging debate about the use of medical marijuana. A distinction is necessary here: clinical trials and THC-based medications use purified chemical analogues of the marijuana plant, not the whole marijuana plant or its extracts. To date, the FDA has not approved a marketing application for the medical use of marijuana for any indication. Yet a growing number of states have legalized the dispensing of marijuana or its extracts to people with a range of medical conditions. This practice continues to occur despite the lack of any evidence base supporting its efficacy and the limited amount of data available on the long-term effects of marijuana on various health outcomes, in both general and specific patient populations.

In particular, the lack of clinical data on how cannabis use may affect certain vulnerable populations (e.g., patients with cancer, AIDS, cardiovascular disease, multiple sclerosis, or other neurodegenerative diseases) should be noted when providing patient education. Research is needed to determine whether there are actual long-term health consequences of marijuana use, and if so, what these consequences may be (National Institute on Drug Abuse 2019a). Although societal attitudes and legal policies have become increasingly permissive regarding recreational marijuana use, regular use can lead to varying degrees of cognitive and behavioral impairment. The potential medical risks from prolonged use also should not be overlooked. Further research is needed to elucidate the long-term implications of cannabis use and the degree to which different use patterns may be associated with different long-term cognitive, behavioral, and physiological health outcomes.

Limited data suggest that cannabis use disorder (CUD) may be associated with certain long-term health consequences, including increased risk of further illicit substance use and multiple medical comorbidities from prolonged inhalation of cannabis smoke. Inhalation injury and prolonged cannabis use can damage various organ systems. Damage to the respiratory system can lead to chronic inflammation of the upper respiratory tract, bronchitis, and damage to cilia; damage to the cardiovascular system can occur through alterations in heart rate and elevations in blood pressure; and damage to the reproductive systems can lead to alterations in fertility in both sexes. Data on increased cancer risk associated with marijuana use are limited and remain equivocal. Case reports have suggested a potential association between marijuana and testicular cancer (Daling et al. 2009). No clear association has been found between marijuana and lung cancer, and both positive and negative associations have been reported with cancers of the head or neck, potentially with human papillomavirus infection being a mediating factor (Huang et al. 2015).

The Monitoring the Future study used latent class analysis to identify distinct patterns of marijuana use among nearly 10,000 participants as they progressed in age from 18 to 50 years. The study found that longer-term marijuana use (from age 18 years through the late 20s or beyond) was associated with an increased risk of self-reported health problems at age 50 years. Compared with nonuse of the drug, all use patterns were associated with a greater number of recent psychological visits and a greater number of lifetime psychiatric problems at age 50 years; a higher prevalence of lifetime drug problems; and higher rates of cognitive difficulties, physical illnesses, and lifetime alcohol problems at 50 years of age (Terry-McElrath et al. 2017).

Screening

Screening should be considered with every patient encounter, given escalating rates of recreational use. As of October 2019, 33 states and the District of Columbia have passed laws broadly legalizing marijuana in some form. With increasing legalization of the drug, the reported recreational use of marijuana has also increased. In 2015, the National Survey on Drug Use and Health estimated that 22.2 million Americans ages 12 years or older were consumers of cannabis, accounting for 8.3% of the total population; these percentages were significantly higher than those reported between 2002 and 2013 (Substance Abuse and Mental Health Services Administration 2016).

Clinical interviewing, screening tools, and urine toxicology screens all should be used in the screening for cannabis use. Given the progression toward decriminalization and stigma reduction, patients are likely to be more forthcoming regarding cannabis use in comparison with the use of other substances with abuse potential.

Diagnosis and Brief Intervention

The formal diagnosis of CUD is recognized in DSM-5; however, any amount of cannabis use, particularly use through inhalation, may carry adverse health consequences. Patients should be offered education and supportive treatment if and when opportunities arise, and where possible, patient ambivalence should be appropriately redirected toward increasing motivation to reduce use. Resolving patient ambivalence and increasing motivation to quit may be more challenging, specifically with cannabis use, given the common social perception that the substance is relatively harmless, despite growing evidence that contradicts this reputation (National Institute on Drug Abuse 2018b).

Clinical Presentation

Intoxication

Cannabis intoxication creates an almost immediate physiological effect, although the full neuropsychiatric effects may take up to 3 hours to manifest. The physiological signs of cannabis intoxication may include tachycardia, increased blood pressure or orthostatic hypotension, increased respiratory rate, conjunctival injection, increased appetite, nystagmus, ataxia, and slurred speech. Even intermittent use can carry serious cardiovascular consequences, including a fivefold increased risk for acute myocardial infarction within the first hour of smoking (J. Lee et al. 2017; Mittleman et al. 2001; Thomas et al. 2014).

Cannabis intoxication in adolescents and adults typically produces an initial "high" marked by euphoria and an increase in sociability, with a decrease in anxiety, alertness, and tension. Conversely, in certain population subsets (including first-time users and persons with underlying mood disorders), intoxication can produce anxiety, dysphoria, panic, and social withdrawal.

Cannabis use slows reaction time and impairs attention, concentration, short-term memory, motor coordination, and risk assessment. These effects are additive when cannabis is used in conjunction with other central nervous system depressants, and the psychomotor impairment may last significantly longer than the initial mood-altering properties of the substance. A meta-analysis of nine studies found an association between cannabis intoxication and an increased risk of a motor vehicle collision involving serious injury or death, with drivers using cannabis two to seven times more likely to cause accidents compared with drivers not using any drugs or alcohol (Rogeberg and Elvik 2016).

Perceptual changes from cannabis intoxication may include distortions in space and time orientation. More potent formulations may cause psychoactive changes, including mystical thinking, increased self-consciousness, and depersonalization, as well as transient grandiosity, paranoia, and other signs of psychosis.

There is growing interest in the relationship between cannabis and psychosis; however, although there is evidence to suggest a link, the relationship remains convoluted. The link between cannabis use and psychosis may be conceptualized as three distinct relationships: acute psychosis associated with cannabis intoxication, acute psychosis that lasts beyond the period of acute intoxication, and persistent post-exposure psychosis (D'Souza et al. 2016). Experimental studies reveal that cannabis, THC, and synthetic cannabinoids reliably produce transient positive, negative, and cognitive symptoms in healthy volunteers (Hasin 2018). The level of intoxication and potential for negative cognitive effects and psychosis increase in a dose-dependent manner, with high-potency synthetic cannabinoids carrying the greatest risk (Hasin 2018). Exposure to cannabis in adolescence is associated with an increased risk for psychotic disorder in adulthood; this association is consistent, somewhat specific, shows a dose-response relationship, and provides a biologically plausible environmental risk factor or component cause triggering the development of psychosis in a genetically vulnerable adolescent (D'Souza et al. 2016).

Withdrawal

Cannabis withdrawal is reported by up to one-third of regular users in the general population and by 50%–95% of heavy users in treatment or research studies (Bonnet and Preuss 2017). The clinical significance of cannabis withdrawal is demonstrated by reports of psychological, physiological, and functional impairment following cessation that is relieved by cannabis or other substances (Allsop et al. 2012); the associated risks of relapse secondary to this clinical syndrome (Budney et al. 2007; Copersino et al. 2006; Levin et al. 2010); and worse treatment outcomes without supportive interventions (Allsop et al. 2012; Chung et al. 2008; Cornelius et al. 2008). Symptoms of cannabis withdrawal include both physiological and psychological symptoms. In early stages, individuals may present with physiological symptoms such as sweating, tremor, chills, nausea, and gastrointestinal discomfort as well as neurovegetative symptoms such as diminished appetite, sleep, and fatigue. Psychological and behavioral symptoms may include irritability, anxiety, and depression; clinical presentations may mirror those in primary mood disorders.

Treatment

Some psychosocial interventions have a demonstrated ability to reduce cannabis use. Evidence suggests that the most clinically effective approach is a combination of motivational enhancement therapy and cognitive-behavioral therapy, preferably accompanied by a contingency management approach (National Institute on Drug Abuse 2018b).

There are no pharmacotherapies specifically approved for the treatment of CUD. Gabapentin, *N*-acetylcysteine, and certain CB_1 agonists have been shown to attenuate withdrawal symptoms of CUD in single studies, but these promising findings have not been replicated in subsequent controlled studies (Balter et al. 2014). Other classes of medications, including antidepressants and antipsychotics, have been unsuccessful in producing such effects. There is an urgent need for further clinical trials to develop more effective treatments for CUD (Gorelick 2016; Mason et al. 2012; Sabioni and Le Foll 2018).

Special Considerations in the Medical Setting

Synthetic Cannabinoids

In 2004, a synthetic class of cannabinoids became available through unregulated channels (Sweet et al. 2018). These products are a purported mixture of herbs or other plant-based blends of various ingredients and were designed to produce a marijuana-like effect when smoked. Referred to as *synthetic cannabinoids,* these products may be sold under street names such as spice, K2, space, dream, or genie and are available in herbal formulations (composed of random shredded plant materials that are sprayed with a variety of psychoactive chemicals) that are designed to be smoked and in liquid formulations that are designed to be heated, vaporized, or inhaled. There are growing data to suggest that these synthetic products may be associated with potentially dangerous physical and psychiatric health effects that are more serious than the effects reported with marijuana. These effects include acute behavioral and cognitive effects manifesting as aggression, confusion, or psychosis and potentially life-threatening physiological effects such as seizures, cardiac damage (including myocardial infarction), and renal impairment. Treatment is supportive until symptoms resolve (Sweet et al. 2018).

Testicular Cancer

A few studies have shown a link between marijuana use in adolescence and increased risk for an aggressive form of testicular cancer (nonseminomatous testicular germ cell tumor) that predominantly strikes young adult males (Daling et al. 2009). The early onset of testicular cancers compared with lung and most other cancers indicates that, whatever the nature of marijuana's contribution, it may accumulate over just a few years of use (Daling et al. 2009).

Hyperemesis Syndrome

Despite the well-established antiemetic properties of marijuana, there is increasing evidence of its paradoxical effects on the gastrointestinal tract and central nervous system. THC, CBD, and cannabigerol are three cannabinoids found in the cannabis plant with opposing effects on the emesis response. Studies have shown that in rare cases, chronic use of marijuana can lead to cannabinoid hyperemesis syndrome

(CHS)—a condition characterized by recurrent bouts of severe nausea, vomiting, and dehydration via an unknown mechanism. This syndrome has been found to occur in persons with a long history of marijuana use and often those younger than 50 years (Galli et al. 2011; Sorensen et al. 2017).

CHS is painful and incapacitating and can lead to frequent trips to the ED, but the syndrome may resolve when the person stops using marijuana. Knowledge of the epidemiology, pathophysiology, and natural course of CHS is limited, and further investigation is required. The clinical course of CHS may be divided into three phases: prodromal, hyperemetic, and recovery. The hyperemetic phase usually lasts for about 48 hours, and treatment involves supportive therapy with fluid replenishment and antiemetic medications. Patients often report that they are able to achieve temporary symptom relief by taking hot baths, and they may do this multiple times a day to reduce nausea, vomiting, and abdominal pain. The broad differential diagnosis of nausea and vomiting often leads to delay in making the diagnosis of CHS; inquiring about the use of hot baths may provide a distinct clinical clue to this diagnosis (Galli et al. 2011).

Summary of Cannabis-Related Disorders

For many people, cannabis use does not progress beyond mild recreational use. Despite widespread social acceptance and legal decriminalization of recreational marijuana use, deleterious health consequences from chronic use remain quite significant and should not be overlooked. Research continues on elucidating the potential medicinal effects of cannabinoids, particularly in relation to antinociceptive properties for chronic pain and treatment in refractory epileptic disorders.

In the medical setting, clinicians have an opportunity to inform patients about the physiological and cognitive risks associated with prolonged use of marijuana and the dangers of inhalation injury, as well as the risks associated with use of synthetic formulations of unregulated potency. Providing education on the potential deleterious effects of ongoing marijuana use while also clarifying the differences among medical marijuana, recreational use, and emerging CBD pharmacotherapies may allow patients to make better-informed decisions regarding continued use.

Stimulant-Related Disorders

Stimulants, whether illicit, prescribed, or available for general consumption, are the most widely used psychoactive drugs worldwide. In 2011, there were an estimated 17 million people using cocaine worldwide and 33.7 million users of prescription stimulants for nonmedical purposes (Gorelick 2017).

Stimulants enhance extracellular concentrations of monoamine neurotransmitters by disrupting the function of plasma membrane transporter proteins. Stimulants can be divided into two main classes on the basis of mechanism: transporter blockers and transporter substrates. Transporter blockers, such as cocaine, inhibit the reuptake of monoamine neurotransmitters (dopamine and norepinephrine) that have been previously released into synaptic spaces and thereby prolong the neurotransmitter effect. Transporter substrates, such as methamphetamine, act on intravesical monoamine transporters within the neuronal cytoplasm to trigger the efflux of large amounts of stored monoamines into the synapse. All stimulants exert an effect on the dopaminergic mesolimbic pathway (consisting of the ventral tegmental areas, prefrontal cortex, nucleus accumbens, and amygdala), and alterations in neuronal firing patterns along with fluctuations in levels of extracellular dopamine concentrations along this pathway mediate the rewarding and addictive effects of stimulants. Thus, all stimulants, including prescribed medications, have the potential for misuse and dependence.

Historically, stimulants were used to treat asthma, obesity, neurological disorders, and a variety of other ailments. As the potential of stimulants for misuse and addiction became more apparent, the number of conditions treated with these agents decreased. Today, stimulants are prescribed for the treatment of only a few health conditions, including ADHD, narcolepsy, and occasionally treatment-resistant depression (National Institute on Drug Abuse 2018c).

Commonly prescribed stimulants include the following:

- Dextroamphetamine (Dexedrine)
- Dextroamphetamine-amphetamine combination product (Adderall)
- Methylphenidate (Ritalin, Concerta)

Street names and slang terms for prescription stimulants include speed, uppers, and vitamin R (National Institute on Drug Abuse 2018c).

Illicitly used stimulants include the following:

- Cocaine (coke, snow, snow white, rock, powder, blow)
- Crack cocaine (crack, rock, base, sugar block, kryptonite)
- Methamphetamine (meth, crystal, crystal meth, ice, glass, speed, tina, chalk)
- Methylenedioxymethamphetamine (MDMA) (ecstasy, molly, E, X, XTC, ADAM, rolls)

Synthetic Cathinones ("Bath Salts")

Over the past few years, there has been an increase in the abuse of synthetic psychoactive substances known as *designer drugs*—also commonly called "bath salts"— which are intentionally manufactured to circumvent regulatory laws around the sale and use of controlled substances. This trend is expected to continue despite legislation passed by several countries, including the United States, to ban the sale, possession, and use of these substances (Baumann et al. 2014).

Synthetic cathinones activate the same monoamine neurotransmitter systems in the central nervous system and sympathetic nervous system that stimulants activate to produce amphetamine- or cocaine-like effects. Low recreational doses of bath salts produce the expected desirable effects. High doses or chronic exposure can lead to dangerous medical consequences, including psychosis, violent behaviors, tachycardia, hyperthermia, and, in rare cases, death. Identification, diagnosis, and treatment are similar to protocols used for more commonly encountered clinical scenarios involving stimulant use disorders.

Diagnosis

Stimulant use disorder is recognized under SUDs in DSM-5 and follows the same criteria outline. For patients on prescribed stimulants, misuse or diversion should be suspected in those who obtain or purchase stimulants via nonprescribed means, seek early refills, procure multiple prescriptions from multiple providers, take escalating dosages over a constrained period of time, or display acute alterations in baseline mood and behavior. All stimulants exert a similar range of physiological and psychological effects, with clinical presentation, intensity, and duration of effects varying according to potency, route of administration (oral, inhalation, and intravenous are most frequent), and duration of use.

Clinical Presentation

Intoxication

Common effects of stimulant ingestion include increased alertness, decreased fatigue, increased sociability, euphoria or restlessness, anxiety, increased reactivity, or aggression. Longer-term use and dosage escalations may result in repetitive behaviors; stereotypy; and symptoms of secondary psychosis such as paranoia, auditory hallucinations, tactile hallucinations (e.g., formication), and delusions.

In acute ingestion of large doses, particularly via inhalation or intravenously, stimulants may cause tremors; overactive reflexes; rapid, shallow breathing; confusion; agitation; nystagmus (both horizontal and vertical nystagmus may be seen with acute phencyclidine intoxication); hallucinations; panic states; abnormally increased fever; and rapid or irregular heartbeat. Overdoses may result in death through acute myocardial infarctions, seizures, or circulatory failure.

Withdrawal

Abrupt cessation of stimulants can result in an acute withdrawal syndrome in which patients may report extreme fatigue, exhaustion, either insomnia or hypersomnia, hyperphagia, depression, anhedonia, decreased motivation, and increased anxiety. With both prolonged use and abrupt cessation of stimulants, tactile sensations such as formication have been reported. Although not associated with acute medical emergencies, stimulant withdrawal symptoms often last several weeks and may cause functional impairment. The discomfort associated with the withdrawal syndrome may motivate patients to seek relief by ingesting alternative substances or relapsing to cocaine use.

Treatment

First-line treatment of behavioral symptoms in acute stimulant intoxication is generally supportive and includes placement of the patient in a secluded, darkened, quiet room to minimize sensory overload. Use of restraints should be avoided to the extent possible because of increased risk of rhabdomyolysis. As a rule, β-blockers also should be avoided because of the risk of systemic vasoconstriction through creation of unopposed α-adrenergic stimulation (although it should be noted that evidence to support this contraindication remains confined to case studies with inconsistent findings) (Richards et al. 2017). For agitation that requires pharmacological intervention, benzodiazepines are considered the first-line pharmacotherapy and should be used before antipsychotics. If agitation cannot be managed with benzodiazepines alone, an antipsychotic could be used, with selection limited to first-generation or high-potency second-generation agents to minimize anticholinergic effects in patients with already altered central nervous system ratios of reduced acetylcholine to increased dopamine levels.

There is no specific psychopharmacological treatment to facilitate stimulant withdrawal or to reduce craving and promote abstinence. Therefore, withdrawal interventions focus primarily on stabilizing sleep and treating underlying or comorbid mood symptoms that may emerge in the days to weeks following cessation of use. Current studies in preclinical stages suggest a possible role for serotonin antagonists or monoamine transporter inhibitors or releasers in reducing cravings as well as the frequency of stimulant use, but specific medications have not yet been identified (Howell and Cunningham 2015).

Special Considerations in the Medical Setting

Stimulants and Cardiovascular Risk

There is a known association between cocaine use and cardiovascular toxicity. Approximately 5%–10% of ED visits in the United States are attributed to acute cocaine toxicity, with chest pain being the most common symptom on presentation (Maraj et al. 2010). Cocaine can precipitate myocardial ischemia both in patients with coronary artery occlusion and in patients without coronary artery pathology. Histopathological findings on autopsy have included atherosclerosis, ventricular hypertrophy, cardiomegaly, myocarditis, and contraction band necrosis in almost one-third of cases of cocaine-associated deaths (Graziani et al. 2016).

A smaller but growing body of evidence has found risks of cardiovascular events associated with methamphetamine and prescription amphetamine stimulant use as well, including cases of left ventricular hypertrophy, left ventricular failure, and dilated cardiomyopathy, with some data suggesting a degree of reversibility with cessation of use (Won et al. 2013).

Summary of Stimulant-Related Disorders

Stimulants are the most widely used substances worldwide. In general, clinical presentations in the inpatient medical setting will involve acute alterations in mood, cognition, or behavior with potentially life-threatening neurological or cardiovascular complications. Treatment is often supportive; however, opportunities should be taken to increase patient awareness of the deleterious effects of prolonged stimulant use and to provide education through motivational-based approaches. Cardiovascular, neurological, or behavioral complications may occur with either acute or chronic stimulant use. Heightened awareness of these risks, or the experience of being hospitalized following one of these complications, may increase patients' willingness to engage in outpatient treatment, leading to improved decision making with regard to ongoing use.

Conclusion

SUDs remain a leading cause of major medical comorbidities and overall disease-associated morbidity both in the United States and worldwide. Despite the development of safe and effective treatments for SUDs, implementation of these treatments in the clinical setting remains highly underutilized. Psychiatrists and other trained physicians can play a significant and influential role in promoting practices that allow for broader and more comprehensive treatment implementation strategies. Advocating for wider use of patient screenings and earlier and more frequent use of routine consultations for high-risk patients should yield greater opportunities to engage patients in supportive counseling and to facilitate their access to treatment. Earlier interventions will create opportunities for earlier initiation of medication treatments in the inpatient setting and will subsequently lead to higher rates of successful outpatient links to, and retention in, treatment. In particular, earlier initiation of medication treatment for SUDs may fundamentally alter the underlying maladaptive behavioral patterns that drive relapse and rehospitalization, thereby profoundly improving overall disease burden and substance use–associated morbidity in multiple patient populations and across the spectrum of nearly all major medical conditions.

References

Allsop DJ, Copeland J, Norberg MM, et al: Quantifying the clinical significance of cannabis withdrawal. PLoS ONE 7(9):e44864, 2012 23049760

American Psychiatric Association: Diagnostic and Statistical Manual of Mental Disorders, 4th Edition. Washington, DC, American Psychiatric Association, 1994

American Psychiatric Association: Diagnostic and Statistical Manual of Mental Disorders, 4th Edition, Text Revision. Washington, DC, American Psychiatric Association, 2000

American Psychiatric Association: Diagnostic and Statistical Manual of Mental Disorders, 5th Edition. Arlington, VA, American Psychiatric Association, 2013

American Society of Addiction Medicine: The ASAM National Practice Guideline: For the Use of Medications in the Treatment of Addiction Involving Opioid Use. Rockville, MD, American Society of Addiction Medicine, 2015

Asplund CA, Aaronson JW, Aaronson HE: 3 regimens for alcohol withdrawal and detoxification. J Fam Pract 53(7):545–554, 2004 15251094

Babor TF, Higgins-Biddle JC, Saunders JB, et al: AUDIT: The Alcohol Use Disorders Identification Test: Guidelines for Use in Primary Health Care. Geneva, Switzerland, World Health Organization, 2001

Bahorik AL, Satre DD, Kline-Simon AH, et al: Alcohol, cannabis, and opioid use disorders, and disease burden in an integrated health care system. J Addict Med 11(1):3–9, 2017 27610582

Balter RE, Cooper ZD, Haney M: Novel pharmacologic approaches to treating cannabis use disorder. Curr Addict Rep 1(2):137–143, 2014 24955304

Baumann MH, Solis E Jr, Watterson LR, et al: Baths salts, spice, and related designer drugs: the science behind the headlines. J Neurosci 34(46):15150–15158, 2014 25392483

Behzadi M, Joukar S, Beik A: Opioids and cardiac arrhythmia: a literature review. Med Princ Pract 27(5):401–414, 2018 30071529

Bhattacharyya S, Wilson R, Appiah-Kusi E, et al: Effect of cannabidiol on medial temporal, midbrain, and striatal dysfunction in people at clinical high risk of psychosis: a randomized clinical trial. JAMA Psychiatry 75(11):1107–1117, 2018 30167644

Bonnet U, Preuss UW: The cannabis withdrawal syndrome: current insights. Subst Abuse Rehabil 8:9–37, 2017 28490916

Brown RL, Rounds LA: Conjoint screening questionnaires for alcohol and other drug abuse: criterion validity in a primary care practice. Wis Med J 94(3):135–140, 1995 7778330

Budney AJ, Roffman R, Stephens RS, et al: Marijuana dependence and its treatment. Addict Sci Clin Pract 4(1):4–16, 2007 18292704

Cahill K, Stevens S, Perera R, Lancaster T: Pharmacological interventions for smoking cessation: an overview and network meta-analysis. Cochrane Database Syst Rev (5):CD009329, 2013 23728690

Cahill K, Lindson-Hawley N, Thomas KH, et al: Nicotine receptor partial agonists for smoking cessation. Cochrane Database Syst Rev (5):CD006103, 2016 27158893

Caine D, Halliday GM, Kril JJ, Harper CG: Operational criteria for the classification of chronic alcoholics: identification of Wernicke's encephalopathy. J Neurol Neurosurg Psychiatry 62(1):51–60, 1997 9010400

Centers for Disease Control and Prevention: Integrated prevention services for HIV infection, viral hepatitis, sexually transmitted diseases, and tuberculosis for persons who use drugs illicitly: summary guidance from CDC and the U.S. Department of Health and Human Services. MMWR Recomm Rep 61(RR–5):1–40, 2012 23135062

Centers for Disease Control and Prevention: Opioid Overdose: Drug Overdose Deaths. Atlanta, GA, Centers for Disease Control and Prevention, 2016. Available at: www.cdc.gov/drugoverdose/data/statedeaths.html. Accessed September 13, 2017.

Chan AW, Pristach EA, Welte JW, et al: Use of the TWEAK test in screening for alcoholism/ heavy drinking in three populations. Alcohol Clin Exp Res 17(6):1188–1192, 1993 8116829

Chasnoff IJ, McGourty RF, Bailey GW, et al: The 4P's Plus screen for substance use in pregnancy: clinical application and outcomes. J Perinatol 25(6):368–374, 2005 15703775

Chung T, Martin CS, Cornelius JR, et al: Cannabis withdrawal predicts severity of cannabis involvement at 1-year follow-up among treated adolescents. Addiction 103(5):787–799, 2008 18412757

Clark BJ, Moss M: Secondary prevention in the intensive care unit: does intensive care unit admission represent a "teachable moment?" Crit Care Med 39(6):1500–1506, 2011 21494113

Clark N, Lintzeris N, Jolley D, et al: Transferring from high doses of methadone to buprenorphine: a randomized trial of three different buprenorphine schedules. Presented at College on the Problems of Drug Dependence, Scottsdale, AZ, June 2006

Clergue F, Desmonts JM, Duvaldestin P, et al: Depression of respiratory drive by diazepam as premedication. Br J Anaesth 53(10):1059–1063, 1981 6794583

Committee on Obstetric Practice: Committee opinion no. 711: opioid use and opioid use disorder in pregnancy. Obstet Gynecol 130(2):e81–e94, 2017 28742676

Compton WM, Volkow ND: Major increases in opioid analgesic abuse in the United States: concerns and strategies. Drug Alcohol Depend 81(2):103–107, 2006 16023304

Copersino ML, Boyd SJ, Tashkin DP, et al: Cannabis withdrawal among non-treatment-seeking adult cannabis users. Am J Addict 15(1):8–14, 2006 16449088

Cornelius JR, Chung T, Martin C, et al: Cannabis withdrawal is common among treatment-seeking adolescents with cannabis dependence and major depression, and is associated with rapid relapse to dependence. Addict Behav 33(11):1500–1505, 2008 18313860

Daeppen JB, Gache P, Landry U, et al: Symptom-triggered vs fixed-schedule doses of benzodiazepine for alcohol withdrawal: a randomized treatment trial. Arch Intern Med 162(10):1117–1121, 2002 12020181

Daling JR, Doody DR, Sun X, et al: Association of marijuana use and the incidence of testicular germ cell tumors. Cancer 115(6):1215–1223, 2009 19204904

D'Onofrio G, Rathlev NK, Ulrich AS, et al: Lorazepam for the prevention of recurrent seizures related to alcohol. N Engl J Med 340(12):915–919, 1999 10094637

D'Souza DC, Radhakrishnan R, Sherif M, et al: Cannabinoids and psychosis. Curr Pharm Des 22(42):6380–6391, 2016 27568729

Ducci F, Goldman D: The genetic basis of addictive disorders. Psychiatr Clin North Am 35(2):495–519, 2012 22640768

El-Bassel N, Shaw SA, Dasgupta A, et al: Drug use as a driver of HIV risks: re-emerging and emerging issues. Curr Opin HIV AIDS 9(2):150–155, 2014 24406532

Fiore MC, Jaén CR, Baker TB, et al: Treating Tobacco Use and Dependence: 2008 Update. Clinical Practice Guideline. Rockville, MD, U.S. Department of Health and Human Services, Public Health Service, May 2008. Available at: https://www.ahrq.gov/prevention/guidelines/tobacco/clinicians/update/index.html. Accessed October 23, 2019.

Fluyau D, Revadigar N: Biochemical benefits, diagnosis, and clinical risks evaluation of Kratom. Front Psychiatry 8:62, 2017 28484399

Freund M, Campbell E, Paul C, et al: Increasing smoking cessation care provision in hospitals: a meta-analysis of intervention effect. Nicotine Tob Res 11(6):650–662, 2009 19423696

Galanter M, Kleber HD (eds): The American Psychiatric Publishing Textbook of Substance Abuse Treatment. Washington, DC, American Psychiatric Publishing, 2008

Galli JA, Sawaya RA, Friedenberg FK: Cannabinoid hyperemesis syndrome. Curr Drug Abuse Rev 4(4):241–249, 2011 22150623

Garland EL, Froeliger B, Zeidan F, et al: The downward spiral of chronic pain, prescription opioid misuse, and addiction: cognitive, affective, and neuropsychopharmacologic pathways. Neurosci Biobehav Rev 37 (10 pt 2):2597–2607, 2013 23988582

Gentilello LM, Ebel BE, Wickizer TM, et al: Alcohol interventions for trauma patients treated in emergency departments and hospitals: a cost benefit analysis. Ann Surg 241(4):541–550, 2005 15798453

Gorelick DA: Pharmacological treatment of cannabis-related disorders: a narrative review. Curr Pharm Des 22(42):6409–6419, 2016 27549375

Gorelick DA: Cocaine use disorder in adults: epidemiology, pharmacology, clinical manifestations, medical consequences, and diagnosis, in UpToDate. Edited by Saxon AJ. Waltham, MA, UpToDate, 2017. Available at: https://www.uptodate.com/contents/cocaine-use-disorder-in-adults-epidemiology-pharmacology-clinical-manifestations-medical-consequences-and-diagnosis. Accessed May 10, 2019.

Gowing L, Farrell M, Ali R, et al: Alpha-adrenergic agonists for the management of opioid withdrawal. Cochrane Database Syst Rev (5):CD002024, 2016 27140827

Graziani M, Antonilli L, Togna AR, et al: Cardiovascular and hepatic toxicity of cocaine: potential beneficial effects of modulators of oxidative stress. Oxid Med Cell Longev 2016:8408479, 2016 26823954

Greenblatt DJ, Divoll M: Diazepam versus lorazepam: relationship of drug distribution to duration of clinical action. Adv Neurol 34:487–491, 1983 6131586

Hall W, Zador D: The alcohol withdrawal syndrome. Lancet 349(9069):1897–1900, 1997 9217770

Hasin DS: US epidemiology of cannabis use and associated problems. Neuropsychopharmacology 43(1):195–212, 2018 28853439

Herron AJ, Brennan TK (eds): The ASAM Essentials of Addiction Medicine, 2nd Edition. Rockville, MD, American Society of Addiction Medicine, 2015

Holbrook AM, Crowther R, Lotter A, et al: Meta-analysis of benzodiazepine use in the treatment of acute alcohol withdrawal. CMAJ 160(5):649–655, 1999 10101999

Howell LL, Cunningham KA: Serotonin 5-HT2 receptor interactions with dopamine function: implications for therapeutics in cocaine use disorder. Pharmacol Rev 67(1):176–197, 2015 25505168

Huang Y-HJ, Zhang Z-F, Tashkin DP, et al: An epidemiologic review of marijuana and cancer: an update. Cancer Epidemiol Biomarkers Prev 24(1):15–31, 2015 25587109

Isenberg-Grzeda E, Kutner HE, Nicolson SE: Wernicke-Korsakoff-syndrome: under-recognized and under-treated. Psychosomatics 53(6):507–516, 2012 23157990

James DJ, Glaze LE: Mental health problems of prison and jail inmates. Bureau of Justice Statistics Special Report, Washington, DC, Bureau of Justice Statistics, September 2006

Jarvis BP, Holtyn AF, Subramaniam S, et al: Extended-release injectable naltrexone for opioid use disorder: a systematic review. Addiction 113(7):1188–1209, 2018 29396985

Jonas DE, Amick HR, Feltner C, et al: Pharmacotherapy for adults with alcohol use disorders in outpatient settings: a systematic review and meta-analysis. JAMA 311(18):1889–1900, 2014 24825644

Jones RT: Cardiovascular system effects of marijuana. J Clin Pharmacol 42(S1 suppl):58S–63S, 2002 12412837

Kapur BM: Drug-testing methods and clinical interpretations of test results. Bull Narc 45(2):115–154, 1993 7920539

Klevens RM, Hu DJ, Jiles R, Holmberg SD: Evolving epidemiology of hepatitis C virus in the United States. Clin Infect Dis 55 (suppl 1):S3–S9, 2012 22715211

Knight JR, Shrier LA, Bravender TD, et al: A new brief screen for adolescent substance abuse. Arch Pediatr Adolesc Med 153(6):591–596, 1999 10357299

Kosten TR, George TP: The neurobiology of opioid dependence: implications for treatment. Sci Pract Perspect 1(1):13–20, 2002 18567959

Krans EE, Bogen D, Richardson G, et al: Factors associated with buprenorphine versus methadone use in pregnancy. Subst Abus 37(4):550–557, 2016 26914546

Latt N, Dore G: Thiamine in the treatment of Wernicke encephalopathy in patients with alcohol use disorders. Intern Med J 44(9):911–915, 2014 25201422

Lazenka MF, Kang M, De DD, et al: Delta-9-tetrahydrocannabinol experience influences delta-FosB and downstream gene expression in prefrontal cortex. Cannabis Cannabinoid Res 2(1):224–234, 2017 29082320

Lee CS, Liebschutz JM, Anderson BJ, et al: Hospitalized opioid-dependent patients: Exploring predictors of buprenorphine treatment entry and retention after discharge. Am J Addict 26(7):667–672, 2017 28324627

Lee J, Sharma N, Aponte CS, et al: Clinical characteristics and angiographic findings of myocardial infarction among marijuana users and non-users. Scifed J Cardiol 1(2):1000008, 2017 29795798

Lee JD, Nunes EV Jr, Novo P, et al: Comparative effectiveness of extended-release naltrexone versus buprenorphine-naloxone for opioid relapse prevention (X:BOT): a multicentre, open-label, randomised controlled trial. Lancet 391(10118):309–318, 2018 29150198

Levin KH, Copersino ML, Heishman SJ, et al: Cannabis withdrawal symptoms in non-treatment-seeking adult cannabis smokers. Drug Alcohol Depend 111(1–2):120–127, 2010 20510550

Li X, Shorter D, Stine SM, Kosten TR: Pharmacologic interventions for opioid dependence, in The ASAM Essentials of Addiction Medicine, 2nd Edition. Edited by Herron AJ, Brennan TK. Rockville, MD, American Society of Addiction Medicine, 2015, pp 294–300

Linn DD, Loeser KC: Dexmedetomidine for alcohol withdrawal syndrome. Ann Pharmacother 49(12):1336–1342, 2015 26400008

Lipari RN, Van Horn SL: Smoking and mental illness among adults in the United States. The CBHSQ Report: March 30, 2017. Rockville, MD, Center for Behavioral Health Statistics and Quality, Substance Abuse and Mental Health Services Administration. Available at: https://www.samhsa.gov/data/sites/default/files/report_2738/ShortReport-2738.html. Accessed October 23, 2019.

Malcolm R, Myrick H, Brady KT, Ballenger JC: Update on anticonvulsants for the treatment of alcohol withdrawal. Am J Addict 10(s1):s16–s23, 2001 11268817

Maldonado JR, Sher Y, Ashouri JF, et al: The "Prediction of Alcohol Withdrawal Severity Scale" (PAWSS): systematic literature review and pilot study of a new scale for the prediction of complicated alcohol withdrawal syndrome. Alcohol 48(4):375–390, 2014 24657098

Maraj S, Figueredo VM, Lynn Morris D: Cocaine and the heart. Clin Cardiol 33(5):264–269, 2010 20513064

Mason BJ, Crean R, Goodell V, et al: A proof-of-concept randomized controlled study of gabapentin: effects on cannabis use, withdrawal and executive function deficits in cannabis-dependent adults. Neuropsychopharmacology 37(7):1689–1698, 2012 22373942

Mattick RP, Breen C, Kimber J, et al: Buprenorphine maintenance versus placebo or methadone maintenance for opioid dependence. Cochrane Database Syst Rev (3):CD002207, 2004 15266465

Mayo-Smith MF; American Society of Addiction Medicine Working Group on Pharmacological Management of Alcohol Withdrawal: Pharmacological management of alcohol withdrawal: a meta-analysis and evidence-based practice guideline. JAMA 278(2):144–151, 1997 9214531

McLellan AT, Lewis DC, O'Brien CP, et al: Drug dependence, a chronic medical illness: implications for treatment, insurance, and outcomes evaluation. JAMA 284(13):1689–1695, 2000 11015800

Mendelson J, Flower K, Pletcher MJ, et al: Addiction to prescription opioids: characteristics of the emerging epidemic and treatment with buprenorphine. Exp Clin Psychopharmacol 16(5):435–441, 2008 18837640

Minozzi S, Amato L, Vecchi S, et al: Oral naltrexone maintenance treatment for opioid dependence. Cochrane Database Syst Rev (4):CD001333, 2011 21491383

Mittleman MA, Lewis RA, Maclure M, et al: Triggering myocardial infarction by marijuana. Circulation 103(23):2805–2809, 2001 11401936

Mohiuddin SM, Mooss AN, Hunter CB, et al: Intensive smoking cessation intervention reduces mortality in high-risk smokers with cardiovascular disease. Chest 131(2):446–452, 2007 17296646

Myrick H, Anton RF: Treatment of alcohol withdrawal. Alcohol Health Res World 22(1):38–43, 1998 15706731

Myrick H, Malcolm R, Brady KT: Gabapentin treatment of alcohol withdrawal. Am J Psychiatry 155(11):1632, 1998 9812141

National Center for Health Statistics: National Health Interview Survey: Adult Tobacco Use Information—Glossary (web page). Page last reviewed: August 29, 2017. Available at: https://www.cdc.gov/nchs/nhis/tobacco/tobacco_glossary.htm. Accessed October 23, 2019.

National Institute on Drug Abuse: Current Trends (Drug Facts). Rockville, MD, National Institute on Drug Abuse, 2015. Available at: https://www.drugabuse.gov/publications/drugfacts/nationwide-trends. Accessed October 23, 2019.

National Institute on Drug Abuse: Common Comorbidities With Substance Use Disorders (Research Report Series). Rockville, MD, National Institute on Drug Abuse, 2018a. Available at: https://www.drugabuse.gov/publications/research-reports/common-comorbidities-substance-use-disorders/introduction. Accessed June 2, 2019.

National Institute on Drug Abuse: Marijuana (Research Report Series). Rockville, MD, National Institute on Drug Abuse, 2018b. Available at: https://www.drugabuse.gov/publications/research-reports/marijuana/letter-director. Accessed June 2, 2019.

National Institute on Drug Abuse: Prescription Stimulants (Drug Facts). Rockville, MD, National Institute on Drug Abuse, 2018c. Available at: https://www.drugabuse.gov/publications/drugfacts/prescription-stimulants. Accessed October 23, 2019.

National Institute on Drug Abuse: Substance Use in Women (Research Report Series). Rockville, MD, National Institute on Drug Abuse, 2018d. Available at: https://www.drugabuse.gov/publications/research-reports/substance-use-in-women/summary. Accessed October 23, 2019.

National Institute on Drug Abuse: Marijuana (Drug Facts). Rockville, MD, National Institute on Drug Abuse, 2019a. Available at: https://www.drugabuse.gov/publications/drugfacts/marijuana. Accessed October 23, 2019.

National Institute on Drug Abuse: Marijuana as Medicine (Drug Facts). Rockville, MD, National Institute on Drug Abuse, 2019b. Available at: https://www.drugabuse.gov/publications/drugfacts/marijuana-medicine. Accessed October 23, 2019.

Nelson AC, Kaucher KA, Sankoff J, et al: Incorporating phenobarbital into your symptom-based benzodiazepine alcohol withdrawal protocol in the emergency department. Am J Emerg Med 36(11):2120–2121, 2018 29685362

Neumann T, Spies C: Use of biomarkers for alcohol use disorders in clinical practice. Addiction 98 (suppl 2):81–91, 2003 14984245

Neumann T, Neuner B, Gentilello LM, et al: Gender differences in the performance of a computerized version of the alcohol use disorders identification test in subcritically injured patients who are admitted to the emergency department. Alcohol Clin Exp Res 28(11):1693–1701, 2004 15547456

Office of the Surgeon General: The Health Consequences of Smoking: A Report of the Surgeon General. Atlanta, GA, Centers for Disease Control and Prevention, 2004 PMID: 20669512

Olfson M, Wall MM, Liu SM, Blanco C: Cannabis use and risk of prescription opioid use disorder in the United States. Am J Psychiatry 175(1):47–53, 2018 28946762

Owens PL, Heslin KC, Fingar KR, et al: Co-occurrence of Physical Health Conditions and Mental Health and Substance Use Conditions Among Adult Inpatient Stays, 2010 Versus 2014. Healthcare Cost and Utilization Project (HCUP) Statistical Brief #240. June 2018. Rockville,

MD, Agency for Healthcare Research and Quality. Available at: https://www.hcup-us.ahrq.gov/reports/statbriefs/sb240-Co-occurring-Physical-Mental-Substance-Conditions-Hospital-Stays.pdf. Accessed October 23, 2019.

Pack QR, Priya A, Lagu TC, et al: Smoking cessation pharmacotherapy among smokers hospitalized for coronary heart disease. JAMA Intern Med 177(10):1525–1527, 2017 28828485

Peppers MP: Benzodiazepines for alcohol withdrawal in the elderly and in patients with liver disease. Pharmacotherapy 16(1):49–57, 1996 8700792

Phan SV: Phenobarbital monotherapy for alcohol withdrawal syndrome in the non-intensive care unit setting: a review. Drugs & Therapy Perspectives 34(9):429–436, 2018. Available at: https://link.springer.com/article/10.1007/s40267-018-0523-1. Accessed May 10, 2019.

Reoux JP, Saxon AJ, Malte CA, et al: Divalproex sodium in alcohol withdrawal: a randomized double-blind placebo-controlled clinical trial. Alcohol Clin Exp Res 25(9):1324–1329, 2001 11584152

Rettig RA, Yarmolinsky A: Treatment standards and optimal treatment, in Federal Regulation of Methadone Treatment. Edited by Rettig RA, Yarmolinsky A. Washington, DC, National Academies Press, 1995, pp 185–216. Available at: www.ncbi.nlm.nih.gov/books/NBK232109. Accessed June 2, 2019.

Reus VI, Fochtmann LJ, Bukstein O, et al: The American Psychiatric Association practice guideline for the pharmacological treatment of patients with alcohol use disorder. Am J Psychiatry 175(1):86–90, 2018 29301420

Richards JR, Hollander JE, Ramoska EA, et al: Beta-blockers, cocaine, and the unopposed alpha-stimulation phenomenon. J Cardiovasc Pharmacol Ther 22(3):239–249, 2017 28399647

Rigotti NA, Munafo MR, Stead LF: Smoking cessation interventions for hospitalized smokers: a systematic review. Arch Intern Med 168(18):1950–1960, 2008 18852395

Rogeberg O, Elvik R: The effects of cannabis intoxication on motor vehicle collision revisited and revised. Addiction 111(8):1348–1359, 2016 26878835

Roux P, Sullivan MA, Cohen J, et al: Buprenorphine/naloxone as a promising therapeutic option for opioid abusing patients with chronic pain: reduction of pain, opioid withdrawal symptoms, and abuse liability of oral oxycodone. Pain 154(8):1442–1448, 2013 23707283

Sabioni P, Le Foll B: Psychosocial and pharmacological interventions for the treatment of cannabis use disorder. F1000 Res 7:173, 2018 29497498

Saitz R: Introduction to alcohol withdrawal. Alcohol Health Res World 22(1):5–12, 1998 15706727

Saitz R, O'Malley SS: Pharmacotherapies for alcohol abuse. Withdrawal and treatment. Med Clin North Am 81(4):881–907, 1997 9222259

Saitz R, Mayo-Smith MF, Roberts MS, et al: Individualized treatment for alcohol withdrawal: a randomized double-blind controlled trial. JAMA 272(7):519–523, 1994 8046805

Sattar SP, Qadri SF, Warsi MK, et al: Use of alcoholic beverages in VA medical centers. Subst Abuse Treat Prev Policy 1(1):30, 2006 17052353

Saukkonen JJ, Mekuria T, Ronan M, et al: Treatment of alcohol withdrawal syndrome with benzodiazepines or phenobarbital in the medical intensive care unit, a retrospective comparison. American Journal of Respiratory and Critical Care Medicine 197:A6049, 2018. Available at: https://www.atsjournals.org/doi/abs/10.1164/ajrccm-conference.2018.197.1_MeetingAbstracts.A6049. Accessed May 10, 2019.

Saunders JB, Aasland OG, Babor TF, et al: Development of the Alcohol Use Disorders Identification Test (AUDIT): WHO Collaborative Project on Early Detection of Persons With Harmful Alcohol Consumption—II. Addiction 88(6):791–804, 1993 8329970

Schuckit MA: Alcohol-use disorders. Lancet 373(9662):492–501, 2009 19168210

Schulte MT, Hser Y-I: Substance use and associated health conditions throughout the lifespan. Public Health Rev 35(2), 2014 28366975

Shibuya K, Ciecierski C, Guindon E, et al: WHO Framework Convention on Tobacco Control: development of an evidence based global public health treaty. BMJ 327(7407):154–157, 2003 12869461

Smith PC, Schmidt SM, Allensworth-Davies D, Saitz R: A single-question screening test for drug use in primary care. Arch Intern Med 170(13):1155–1160, 2010 20625025

Sokol RJ, Martier SS, Ager JW: The T-ACE questions: practical prenatal detection of risk-drinking. Am J Obstet Gynecol 160(4):863–868, discussion 868–870, 1989 2712118

Sorensen CJ, DeSanto K, Borgelt L, et al: Cannabinoid hyperemesis syndrome: diagnosis, pathophysiology, and treatment—a systematic review. J Med Toxicol 13(1):71–87, 2017 28000146

Stuppaeck CH, Pycha R, Miller C, et al: Carbamazepine versus oxazepam in the treatment of alcohol withdrawal: a double-blind study. Alcohol Alcohol 27(2):153–158, 1992 1524606

Su MK, Lopez JH, Crossa A, et al: Low dose intramuscular methadone for acute mild to moderate opioid withdrawal syndrome. Am J Emerg Med 26(11):1951–1956, 2018 29544903

Substance Abuse and Mental Health Services Administration: Highlights of the 2009 Drug Abuse Warning Network (DAWN) findings on drug-related emergency department visits. The DAWN Report. Rockville, MD, Center for Behavioral Health Statistics and Quality, Substance Abuse and Mental Health Services Administration, December 28, 2010

Substance Abuse and Mental Health Services Administration: Federal Guidelines for Opioid Treatment Programs. Rockville, MD, Substance Abuse and Mental Health Services Administration, 2015

Substance Abuse and Mental Health Services Administration: Reports and Detailed Tables From the 2015 National Survey on Drug Use and Health (NSDUH). Rockville, MD, Substance Abuse and Mental Health Services Administration, 2016

Sullivan JF, Lankford HG, Swartz MJ, et al: Magnesium metabolism in alcoholism. Am J Clin Nutr 13(5):297–303, 1963 14080503

Sullivan JT, Sykora K, Schneiderman J, et al: Assessment of alcohol withdrawal: the revised clinical institute withdrawal assessment for alcohol scale (CIWA-Ar). Br J Addict 84(11):1353–1357, 1989 2597811

Sullivan JT, Swift RM, Lewis DC: Benzodiazepine requirements during alcohol withdrawal syndrome: clinical implications of using a standardized withdrawal scale. J Clin Psychopharmacol 11(5):291–295, 1991 1684974

Suzuki J, Matthews ML, Brick D, et al: Implementation of a collaborative care management program with buprenorphine in primary care: a comparison between opioid-dependent patients and patients with chronic pain using opioids nonmedically. J Opioid Manag 10(3):159–168, 2014 24944066

Suzuki J, DeVido J, Kalra I, et al: Initiating buprenorphine treatment for hospitalized patients with opioid dependence: a case series. Am J Addict 24(1):10–14, 2015 25823630

Sweet G, Kim S, Martin S, et al: Psychiatric symptoms and synthetic cannabinoid use: information for clinicians. Ment Health Clin 7(4):156–159, 2018 29955515

Terry-McElrath YM, O'Malley PM, Johnston LD, et al: Longitudinal patterns of marijuana use across ages 18–50 in a US national sample: a descriptive examination of predictors and health correlates of repeated measures latent class membership. Drug Alcohol Depend 171:70–83, 2017 28024188

Thomas G, Kloner RA, Rezkalla S: Adverse cardiovascular, cerebrovascular, and peripheral vascular effects of marijuana inhalation: what cardiologists need to know. Am J Cardiol 113(1):187–190, 2014 24176069

Uchtenhagen AA: Heroin maintenance treatment: from idea to research to practice. Drug Alcohol Rev 30(2):130–137, 2011 21375613

U.S. Department of Health and Human Services: HHS Acting Secretary Declares Public Health Emergency to Address National Opioid Crisis. Press release, October 26, 2017. Available at: https://www.hhs.gov/about/news/2017/10/26/hhs-acting-secretary-declares-public-health-emergency-address-national-opioid-crisis.html. Accessed June 10, 2019.

U.S. Department of Veterans Affairs/Department of Defense: VA/DoD Clinical Practice Guideline for the Management of Substance Use Disorders, December 2015. Available at: https://www.healthquality.va.gov/guidelines/MH/sud/VADoDSUDCPGRevised22216.pdf. Accessed May 19, 2019.

Weinberg JA, Magnotti LJ, Fischer PE, et al: Comparison of intravenous ethanol versus diazepam for alcohol withdrawal prophylaxis in the trauma ICU: results of a randomized trial. J Trauma 64(1):99–104, 2008 18188105

Weinberger AH, Platt J, Esan H, et al: Cigarette smoking is associated with increased risk of substance use disorder relapse: a nationally representative, prospective longitudinal investigation. J Clin Psychiatry 78(2):e152–e160, 2017 28234432

Weiss AJ, Elixhauser A, Barrett ML, et al: Opioid-Related Inpatient Stays and Emergency Department Visits by State, 2009–2014. Healthcare Cost and Utilization Project (HCUP) Statistical Brief #219. December 2016. Rockville, MD, Agency for Healthcare Research and Quality. Available at: https://www.hcup-us.ahrq.gov/reports/statbriefs/sb219-Opioid-Hospital-Stays-ED-Visits-by-State.pdf. Accessed October 23, 2019.

Wesson DR, Ling W: The Clinical Opiate Withdrawal Scale (COWS). J Psychoactive Drugs 35(2):253–259, 2003 12924748

Wiese B, Wilson-Poe AR: Emerging evidence for cannabis' role in opioid use disorder. Cannabis Cannabinoid Res 3(1):179–189, 2018 30221197

Won S, Hong RA, Shohet RV, et al: Methamphetamine-associated cardiomyopathy. Clin Cardiol 36(12):737–742, 2013 24037954

World Health Organization: Withdrawal management, in Clinical Guidelines for Withdrawal Management and Treatment of Drug Dependence in Closed Settings. Geneva, World Health Organization, 2009, pp 29–50. Available at: https://www.ncbi.nlm.nih.gov/books/NBK310652/. Accessed October 23, 2019.

Wright NM, Sheard L, Tompkins CN, et al: Buprenorphine versus dihydrocodeine for opiate detoxification in primary care: a randomised controlled trial. BMC Fam Pract 8:3, 2007 17210079

Wyszynski AA: The patient with hepatic disease, alcohol dependence, and altered mental status, in Manual of Psychiatric Care for the Medically Ill. Edited by Wyszynski AA, Wyszynski B. Washington, DC, American Psychiatric Publishing, 2004, pp 27–47

Young JQ, Kline-Simon AH, Mordecai DJ, et al: Prevalence of behavioral health disorders and associated chronic disease burden in a commercially insured health system: findings of a case-control study. Gen Hosp Psychiatry 37(2):101–108, 2015 25578791

Yudko E, Lozhkina O, Fouts A: A comprehensive review of the psychometric properties of the Drug Abuse Screening Test. J Subst Abuse Treat 32(2):189–198, 2007 17306727

Zacny JP, Lichtor SA: Nonmedical use of prescription opioids: motive and ubiquity issues. J Pain 9(6):473–486, 2008 18342577

Zatzick D, Donovan D, Dunn C, et al: Substance use and posttraumatic stress disorder symptoms in trauma center patients receiving mandated alcohol screening and brief intervention. J Subst Abuse Treat 43(4):410–417, 2012 22999379

Ziedonis D, Das S, Larkin C: Tobacco use disorder and treatment: new challenges and opportunities. Dialogues Clin Neurosci 19(3):271–280, 2017 29302224

CHAPTER 22

Neurocognitive Disorders

Flannery Merideth, M.D.

Ipsit V. Vahia, M.D.

Dilip V. Jeste, M.D.

The neurocognitive disorders represent a group of conditions that are categorized and defined on the basis of their impact on cognition. This diagnostic category includes major neurocognitive disorder (also referred to as dementia) and delirium. While both of these conditions have been extensively studied and significant research is being conducted to identify a neuropathology and biomarkers, our primary focus in this chapter will be the psychiatric management of these conditions.

We begin by addressing dementia, first outlining the major clinical subtypes (based on both neuropathology and clinical presentation), then describing the neuropsychiatric sequelae, and finally reviewing the pharmacological and nonpharmacological approaches to treatment and management of this challenging condition. We then address delirium, describing its clinical subtypes and neuropsychiatric presentations, the process of assessment and clinical workup, and the approaches to prevention and management (both pharmacological and behavioral) of this condition.

Dementia

Dementia is a syndrome characterized by progressive cognitive decline in one or more domains (such as memory, executive function, or language) leading to significant functional impairment. As defined in the fifth edition of the *Diagnostic and Statistical Manual of Mental Disorders* (DSM-5; American Psychiatric Association 2013), dementia, now called major neurocognitive disorder, produces deficits that cannot exclusively be explained by another psychiatric illness or by concurrent delirium. Besides cognitive disturbance, dementias also cause a variety of disabling neuropsychiatric symptoms. The disease has a great impact on patients, their families, and the health care system; as the population ages, dementia is becoming a significant public health problem.

Using data from the U.S. Health and Retirement Study, Hurd et al. (2013) estimated that the prevalence of dementia of any kind among people age 70 years and older was 14.7%. Approximately 11% of Americans older than 65 years have Alzheimer's disease (AD) (Hebert et al. 2013; Hurd et al. 2013); however, these figures are likely to be underestimates. Only about half of community-dwelling elderly individuals who meet diagnostic criteria for a neurocognitive disorder are actually identified by a physician; illnesses on the dementia spectrum are significantly underdiagnosed and underreported (Bradford et al. 2009).

In 2010, more than $40,000 per patient per year was spent on dementia-related costs (Hurd et al. 2013). These costs include monetary estimates of informal caregiving, which is the unpaid assistance provided by patients' families and friends with activities such as dressing, toileting, managing finances, and grocery shopping. Moreover, these costs do not capture the emotional toll or psychological stress that caregiving can have on families with a loved one with dementia. Caregivers of patients with dementia exhibit significantly more stress than caregivers of chronically ill family members without dementia; this is due, in part, to the challenges of neuropsychiatric symptoms associated with dementia, including agitation (González-Salvador et al. 1999).

Major Subtypes of Dementia/Neurocognitive Disorder

Alzheimer's Disease

AD is the most common type of dementia. By the year 2050, the number of people in the United States living with AD is projected to reach 13.8 million, almost triple the number of those living with the disease in 2016 (Hebert et al. 2013). The disease is characterized by progressive episodic memory loss, deficits in executive function, word-finding difficulties, apraxia, visual processing deficits, and neuropsychiatric changes. The underlying cause of AD is still under debate, but common neuropathological findings on autopsy include amyloid-beta (Aβ) plaques, neurofibrillary tangles, and hyperphosphorylated tau protein.

There are several theories as to the etiology and pathogenesis of AD. The Aβ hypothesis postulates that amyloid precursor protein (APP) is cleaved by beta and gamma secretases, producing Aβ peptides that aggregate to form toxic Aβ oligomers, or plaques. These plaques subsequently bind to cellular prion protein on the neural membrane, triggering activation of Fyn, an intracellular tyrosine kinase. Fyn activation is related to a number of significant neuropathological events, including tau hyperphosphorylation, synaptic dysfunction, and disruptions in neuroplasticity. This theory is debated, because some patients who have been clinically diagnosed with AD do not have any evidence of Aβ accumulation on autopsy or neuroimaging. An alternative theory, the adaptive response hypothesis, suggests that Aβ may accumulate as an adaptive response to chronic stressors such as oxidative stress, metabolic dysregulation (e.g., hyperlipidemia, insulin resistance), genetic factors, and inflammation. Each of these stressors is capable of eliciting a response in which Aβ is produced, and it is the nature of that response, not the amount of Aβ that accumulates, that determines progression to AD (Castello et al. 2014). Many drug therapy trials have been based on the assumption that Aβ accumulation is the primary trigger for the development of AD, and several phase 3 clinical trials of monoclonal antibodies targeting Aβ (solanazumab, bapineuzumab) have failed to show clinical improvement (Doody et al. 2014; Salloway et al. 2014).

Genetics are a major risk factor for the development of AD. Patients with a first-degree relative with AD are more likely to develop it (Green et al. 2002). Specifically, autosomal-dominant inheritance of missense mutations on chromosomes 14 and 1 (presenilin 1 and 2 genes, respectively) contribute to early-onset AD, in which symptoms occur before the age of 65 years. Alterations on chromosome 21 (the APP associated with Down syndrome) also are strongly associated with development of the disease. Inheritance of the ε4 allele of apolipoprotein E (ApoE) is a risk factor for development of late-onset AD (Loy et al. 2014). Other established risk factors for cognitive decline and dementia include hypertension, brain trauma, cerebrovascular disease, and impaired glucose metabolism (Baumgart et al. 2015).

Vascular Dementia

Vascular dementia (VaD) is the second most common cause of dementia (O'Brien and Thomas 2015). Until the 1960s, all senile dementia (the then-prevalent term) was considered to be secondary to cerebrovascular disease, and Alzheimer's pathology was thought to account only for cases of presenile dementia. In the late 1960s and early 1970s, Alzheimer's pathology was found to be present in cases of senile dementia. It is difficult to differentiate the clinical presentation of VaD from that of AD, although VaD—particularly when linked to deep small-vessel arteriolar disease—has been categorized as a subcortical dementia because of the involvement of white matter tracts and deeper brain structures, such as the basal ganglia, as well as the associated prominent executive function difficulties, mood symptoms, or apathetic/abulic states. VaD is often described as having a stepwise progression; however, it can have a slower progression with subcortical illness. A "stepwise course" was a diagnostic requirement in DSM-III-R (American Psychiatric Association 1987), although major or mild vascular neurocognitive disorder in DSM-5 can be diagnosed by either cognitive deficits temporally associated with cerebrovascular events or decline associated with significant difficulties in complex attention, processing speed, and frontal executive function. There is often an abrupt onset of symptoms after a major cerebrovascular event. Motor symptoms and functional impairment are more common in VaD than in AD, with patients having gait disorders, incontinence, and parkinsonism. Disruption of cortical-subcortical circuits leaves these patients with prominent executive dysfunction, poor visuospatial skills, and language problems.

VaD can develop after a stroke has damaged a significant portion of the brain, or it can result from a collection of smaller strokes, lacunes, or chronic subcortical hypoxia (Dichgans and Leys 2017; Sachdev et al. 2014). The greatest risk factors for VaD are cerebrovascular disease, diabetes, hypertension, atrial fibrillation, and other heart disease. There are a few pure genetic forms of VaD. Cerebral autosomal dominant arteriopathy with subcortical infarcts and leukoencephalopathy (CADASIL) is a familial disorder of recurrent strokes (usually lacunar infarcts) occurring in the absence of vascular risk factors. Mitochondrial encephalopathy with lactic acidosis and stroke-like episodes (MELAS) can also lead to VaD. Cerebral amyloid angiopathy and sickle cell disease are other heritable conditions that confer risk for VaD.

Of note, cerebrovascular disease and vascular risk factors influence the progression of both vascular and Alzheimer's dementias, further complicating understanding of the relationship between these two dementing processes (Baumgart et al. 2015).

Dementia With Lewy Bodies and Parkinson's Disease Dementia

Eighty percent of patients with Parkinson's disease will develop dementia (Emre et al. 2007). Parkinson's disease dementia (PDD) typically emerges years after the onset of motor symptoms, but some patients develop mild cognitive impairment with the onset of Parkinson's disease, and full-blown dementia can occur as early as 1 year after motor symptoms begin. In Lewy body dementia (LBD), the dementia and the motor symptoms manifest simultaneously, although the cognitive symptoms can occur even before the emergence of parkinsonism. Both PDD and LBD are characterized by aggregates of Lewy bodies—collections of α-synuclein (a protein located at the presynaptic terminal of neurons)—within the brain. It is unclear to what extent Lewy bodies contribute to the overall clinical picture, however, because some individuals who have α-synuclein pathology on autopsy did not show symptoms of PDD or LBD in life. Most cases of these dementias are sporadic, but some autosomal-dominant inheritance has been reported, including mutations in *SNCA* and *LRRK2* genes (Walker et al. 2015). There is also overlap with the genetics of AD; some LBD patients have the *ApoE4* allele that confers risk for the development of late-onset AD.

Characteristic symptoms of LBD include well-formed visual hallucinations, spontaneous parkinsonism, and cognitive fluctuations. Periodic limb movement disorder also may be present. Both PDD and LBD are marked by executive, attentional, memory, and visuospatial deficits as well as sleep disturbance and autonomic dysfunction. PDD and LBD patients have more visuospatial/constructional impairment than do patients with AD or frontotemporal dementia (FTD) (Walker et al. 2015). Additionally, PDD is associated with anxiety, mood and behavior changes, visual hallucinations, and apathy. Psychotic symptoms may also be seen as a side effect of medications used to treat Parkinson's disease.

Frontotemporal Dementia

FTD is a progressive degeneration of the prefrontal and anterior temporal lobes. FTD often manifests in later middle age, with an average onset between the ages of 45 and 65 years (Olney et al. 2017). The disease was first described by Arnold Pick in 1892. Alois Alzheimer discovered that Pick bodies (aggregates of tau protein) were a pathological finding associated with the clinical presentation and gave this dementia variant the eponym "Pick's disease," although only some cases of FTD have Pick bodies (Bang et al. 2015). A family history of dementia is reported in up to 40% of cases of FTD; the three genes most commonly associated with an inherited diagnosis are *C9orf72, MAPT,* and *GRN.* Only 10% of cases have a clear autosomal-dominant inheritance pattern (Rohrer et al. 2009).

There are three distinct variants of FTD. The behavioral variant (bvFTD), which accounts for roughly 60% of all FTD cases, is associated with early behavioral change and executive function deficits (Olney et al. 2017). Common symptoms seen in bvFTD include disinhibition, apathy, lack of empathy, hyperorality, compulsions, and executive dysfunction. The second variant, primary progressive aphasia (PPA), is characterized by progressive deficits in speech, grammar, and language output. Finally, the semantic variant of PPA is a progressive disorder of semantic knowledge and naming.

In bvFTD, structural neuroimaging (with magnetic resonance imaging [MRI] or computed tomography [CT]) will show frontal lobe or anterior temporal lobe atrophy as well as hypometabolism of those same brain regions on positron emission tomography (PET) or single-photon emission computed tomography (SPECT). In PPA, neuroimaging may reveal more involvement of the anterior temporal lobe (Olney et al. 2017).

Huntington's Disease

Huntington's disease (HD) is one of the most common inherited neurodegenerative diseases. It occurs as the result of excessive CAG trinucleotide repeats in the huntingtin gene on chromosome 4, leading to a loss of γ-aminobutyric acid (GABA)-ergic neurons in the basal ganglia (chiefly affecting the caudate nucleus and putamen). It is autosomal dominant, but up to 10% of cases may represent new mutations (Tabrizi et al. 2013). Peak onset is between the ages of 35 and 44 years, but onset can occur earlier or later in life. The size of the CAG expansion is inversely correlated with both age at onset and symptom severity (Tabrizi et al. 2013), with smaller expansions leading to later development of HD and less severe symptoms.

The first motor symptom in HD is typically chorea, which progresses to difficulties with voluntary movement, including bradykinesia and rigidity. There is a wide range of psychiatric and cognitive symptoms in addition to the movement disorder. Cognitive impairment usually begins after the movement disorder and worsens with time. Patients with HD have prominent deficits in processing speed, verbal fluency, attention, and executive function (Pagan et al. 2017).

Neuropsychiatric Presentations of Dementia/ Neurocognitive Disorder

Psychosis

Roughly 41% of patients with AD will exhibit psychotic symptoms (Ropacki and Jeste 2005), including delusions, hallucinations, and misidentifications. For example, a patient with AD may misplace his keys but come to the delusional belief that his keys were stolen. Psychotic symptoms are associated with greater caregiver distress (Bédard et al. 1997) and predict earlier functional decline and institutionalization (Magni et al. 1996). Bizarre delusions such as thought broadcasting, thought insertion, and thought withdrawal are rare in dementia.

Whereas delusions are more common than hallucinations in AD, hallucinations are very prevalent in dementia associated with Lewy bodies, with about 80% of patients (McKeith et al. 2017) experiencing visual hallucinations, typically involving nondistressing content (e.g., animals or children). Hallucinations in LBD may not need any treatment beyond simple reassurance. Delusions and hallucinations are less common in VaD.

Agitation

Agitation in dementia is very common; nearly half of all patients with dementia experience symptoms monthly. Agitation is associated with poor quality of life, helplessness and anger in family members and caregivers, and nursing home admission (Livingston et al. 2014).

Agitation can be expressed in both physical and verbal ways, and not all agitation is aggressive. Behaviors such as wandering, disrobing, or hoarding are examples of nonaggressive physical agitation, while aggressive agitation may manifest as hitting, kicking, or resistance to care. Verbal agitation might include moaning/screaming or constant unwarranted requests for attention or help.

Agitation symptoms and their severity can be tracked and categorized with a number of research-validated tools. The Pittsburgh Agitation Scale, developed in 1994, provides a means for tracking the intensity of an agitated behavior as it is occurring (Rosen et al. 1994). The Cohen-Mansfield Agitation Inventory tracks the type of agitated behavior and its frequency (Cohen-Mansfield 1996). Finally, the Neuropsychiatric Inventory is a structured interview of the caregiver to determine the frequency and severity of 10 types of behavioral disturbance seen in dementia, including agitation, disinhibition, and aberrant motor activity, among others (Cummings 1997). Use of rating scales can help clinicians track the efficacy of behavioral and pharmacological interventions for agitation and thereby help shape treatment.

Depression

Having major depressive disorder (MDD) doubles an individual's risk for developing dementia (Ownby et al. 2006). Depression symptoms in late life can also be a prodrome of dementia (Gutzmann and Qazi 2015). It is difficult to distinguish depression symptoms from dementia symptoms because of overlap in their clinical presentations. The phenomenology of depression in late life is somewhat different from that of depression in younger people, with elderly individuals having more somatic symptoms, insomnia, cognitive complaints, and affective dysregulation (Hegeman et al. 2012). All of these symptoms can be seen in dementia without a co-occurring mood disorder. Apathy is also a frequent symptom in both depression and dementia.

Depression is relatively common in AD but is even more prevalent in VaD (Cummings 1988). Cerebrovascular disease may lead to, or worsen, geriatric depressive symptoms as a result of damage to frontal-subcortical circuits, leading to vascular depression. In vascular depression, a patient may not meet full DSM-5 criteria for MDD but will have significant cognitive problems, as would be expected with VaD (Aizenstein et al. 2016). Depression affects 40%–50% of patients with HD, and the rate of completed suicides in HD may be as high as 13% (Cummings 1995).

Insomnia

Sleep disorders are common among patients with dementia, and in some cases, sleep disturbance may appear before cognitive deficits emerge (Cipriani et al. 2015). These disturbances include insomnia, sleep-phase disorders, oversleeping, and restless leg syndrome. Patients with LBD or PDD may also struggle with periodic leg movements during sleep (PLMS) and rapid eye movement (REM) sleep behavior disorder.

In a sample of 205 community-dwelling individuals with AD, the most common sleep disturbance was oversleeping, reported for 40% of patients, followed by terminal insomnia, reported for 31%; however, the most distressing sleep behavior for caregivers was awakening in the middle of the night, which was reported for 24% of patients with AD (McCurry et al. 1999). Sleep disturbance can worsen cognitive functioning and lead to psychological distress and an increase in agitated behaviors during the day (Shin et al. 2014).

Diagnostic and Laboratory Findings in Dementia/ Neurocognitive Disorder

Standard Workup

The standard workup for dementia includes physical and neurological examinations, cognitive testing, neuroimaging, and laboratory data. These tests can be helpful to rule out delirium and reversible causes of dementia (e.g., normal-pressure hydrocephalus), to help delineate the underlying type of dementia, and to identify comorbidities that commonly occur in elderly persons with dementia. Structural brain imaging with MRI or CT is also recommended (Knopman et al. 2001).

Neuroimaging

Typical findings on MRI or CT in AD include widened sulci, enlarged lateral ventricles, and hippocampal/medial temporal lobe atrophy. New research studies are looking beyond structural imaging by using amyloid PET scans in patients with unexplained mild cognitive impairment or dementia of uncertain etiology to see if amyloid PET results will change management and outcomes for these patients (Herscovitch 2015). One such research study, "Imaging Dementia—Evidence for Amyloid Scanning," also known as the IDEAS study, began enrollment in 2016 and will finish data collection in 2019. Preliminary results from nearly 4,000 patients suggested that amyloid PET imaging was associated with a change in medical management for 67.8% of patients with mild cognitive impairment and 65.9% of patients with dementia (Alzheimer's Association 2017).

Unlike MRI studies in patients with AD, MRI studies in patients with LBD would be expected to show absent or minimal medial temporal lobe atrophy. In Lewy body disease, reduced dopamine transporter (DAT) uptake is seen in the basal ganglia on SPECT and PET, and occipital hypometabolism is seen on fluorodeoxyglucose (FDG)-PET (McKeith et al. 2017). In FTD, structural neuroimaging shows prominent atrophy of the frontal and temporal lobes, but in HD, there may not be any specific findings beyond generalized cortical atrophy or specific caudate atrophy. Hence, a definitive diagnosis of HD requires genetic testing for the CAG expansion (Pagan et al. 2017). In VaD, findings include white matter hyperintensities on T2-weighted fluid-attenuated inversion recovery (FLAIR) MRI as well as evidence of lacunar infarcts or other signs of poststroke damage.

Ruling Out Delirium or Reversible Cognitive Impairment

Much of the laboratory workup in dementia is focused on ruling out delirium or cognitive changes caused by a reversible medical condition. Evaluation includes complete blood count, basic metabolic panel, liver function tests, urine toxicology, and urinalysis.

Elderly persons, especially those with cognitive impairment, are at increased risk of hypothyroidism and cyanocobalamin (vitamin B_{12}) deficiency, both of which can worsen cognition. All patients should be screened for vitamin B_{12} deficiency and thyroid-stimulating hormone abnormalities (Knopman et al. 2001). Folate deficiency also can lead to or worsen cognitive impairment, and elderly individuals are at greater risk for folate deficiency due to malabsorption. We recommend routine screening with a serum folate level, especially if the patient has a megaloblastic macrocytic anemia. Vitamin D deficiency also has been associated with dementia and cognitive impairment and is simple to remedy with supplementation.

The U.S. Preventive Services Task Force has recommended that all adults up to age 64 years should be screened for HIV at least once, and that all adults 65 years and older with specific risk factors should also be screened (Chou et al. 2012). HIV should definitely be considered in the evaluation of cognitive impairment, given that HIV-associated neurocognitive disorders (HAND) can manifest as a dementing illness. Tests used to screen for syphilis (Venereal Disease Research Laboratory [VDRL], rapid plasma reagin, and fluorescent treponemal antibody), however, are nonspecific, and some published guidelines recommend screening only in patients who have evidence of prior syphilitic infection or who live in areas with a high prevalence of syphilis (Knopman et al. 2001).

Additional workup may be warranted, depending on physical examination findings. For example, a chest radiography may be needed to rule out pneumonia in a patient with cough and fever, or a lumbar puncture to evaluate for encephalitis in a patient with new neurological deficits. A variety of malignancies and antibody-mediated encephalitides can cause cognitive impairment (see Chapter 8, "Inflammatory Disease").

Treatment of Neuropsychiatric Syndromes in Dementia/Neurocognitive Disorder

Pharmacological Treatment

The physiological changes that occur in the older human body have consequential implications for drug metabolism. Pharmacokinetics are substantially changed: elderly persons have a lower volume of distribution, less albumin available to bind active drug, and an increase in elimination half-life. These changes mean that more active drug is available in the body for a longer period of time. Certain medications, especially those metabolized through the hepatic cytochrome P450 (CYP) system, can increase or decrease drug levels.

Older adults are also more sensitive to medications, and patients with dementia are especially sensitive. Usually, dosages need to be much lower for patients with dementia.

Cholinesterase inhibitors.   Cholinesterase inhibitors enhance cholinergic transmission by inhibiting the enzyme acetylcholinesterase. Cholinesterase inhibitors were developed for the treatment of the cognitive symptoms of dementia but also have some neuropsychiatric benefits. There is evidence that galantamine (a cholinesterase inhibitor that also modulates nicotinic acetylcholine receptors) can improve behavioral disturbance in AD (Wang et al. 2015). Donepezil has been shown to contribute to a small but significant reduction in behavioral and psychological symptoms of dementia (Dyer et al. 2018). Donepezil and rivastigmine have been shown to diminish apathy and reduce visual hallucinations and delusions in LBD (McKeith et al. 2017). Rivastigmine has been shown to ameliorate psychiatric symptoms in FTD, but other cholinesterase inhibitors have been of little benefit and have even worsened confusion in some trials (Buoli et al. 2017).

Antidepressants. Broadly, depression co-occurring with dementia can be treated with selective serotonin reuptake inhibitors (SSRIs), serotonin-norepinephrine reuptake inhibitors (SNRIs), and mirtazapine (a noradrenergic and serotonergic antidepressant), with overall choice depending on the individual patient's preference, history of prior medication trials, and tolerability. Antidepressants can also be used to treat agitation. Overall, while there is minimal evidence supporting the efficacy of SSRIs in treating depression in patients with dementia, the treatment appears to be safe (Gutzmann and Qazi 2015). Venlafaxine, an SNRI, has shown some evidence for treating depression in Parkinson's disease (Broen et al. 2016). Antidepressant medication may be helpful for treating agitation and is often used in geriatric psychiatry, despite the fact that not all antidepressants have been studied for this purpose. Citalopram at dosages between 10 mg and 30 mg/day has been shown to decrease agitation in patients with dementia, thereby reducing distress in their caregivers (Rabins et al. 2014). Trazodone is too sedating at antidepressant dosages to be a reasonable choice for treatment of depression in patients with dementia, but at low dosages it can be helpful for insomnia and agitation (Camargos et al. 2011).

Antipsychotics. Of the various medication classes investigated for effectiveness in the management of behavioral and psychological symptoms associated with neurocognitive disorders, antipsychotics have been the most extensively studied. The American Psychiatric Association practice guideline recommends that antipsychotics be used with caution in older adults with dementia, because these agents have been associated with severe adverse events and death (Reus et al. 2016). All antipsychotics carry a black-box warning regarding their use in patients with dementia. Antipsychotics should be used only if other interventions have failed. If used, they should be given at the lowest effective dosage and should be discontinued if symptoms do not improve. First-generation antipsychotics (FGAs; also called typical antipsychotics) should not be used in the management of dementia symptoms because of their higher risks for side effects and mortality as compared with second-generation antidepressants (SGAs; also called atypical antipsychotics) (Yohanna and Cifu 2017). Dopamine blockers should be avoided in LBD and PDD because of the risk of worsening parkinsonism. Clozapine at low dosages is helpful for psychosis in PDD and is less likely than other SGAs to worsen motor symptoms. Quetiapine at low dosages is safer than other SGAs for treating psychotic symptoms in LBD and PDD (Walker et al. 2015). Pimavanserin is a new atypical agent that was approved by the U.S. Food and Drug Administration (FDA) in 2016 for the treatment of PDD psychosis (Combs and Cox 2017).

Mood stabilizers. Although mood stabilizers may be helpful for mood dysregulation and agitation in dementia, these agents carry significant risks and have a limited evidence base. The use of carbamazepine is best supported, particularly for treatment of aggression (Yeh and Ouyang 2012). However, carbamazepine carries a risk for significant adverse effects (e.g., Stevens-Johnson syndrome) and has a higher potential for drug interactions, limiting its use. Several randomized controlled trials have concluded that valproate is not very effective for agitation in dementia, and some have demonstrated an increase in adverse events, including hepatotoxicity, associated with its use (Lonergan and Luxenberg 2009). Valproate should be avoided. Lithium at low dosages is being investigated for efficacy and safety in the treatment of behavioral symptoms of dementia (Devanand et al. 2018). Case series have shown some efficacy for gabapentin, lamotrigine, and topiramate in treating these symptoms, but more evidence is needed (Yeh and Ouyang 2012).

Anxiolytics.   Benzodiazepines should be avoided because of their propensity to cause delirium, cognitive decline, and falls and hip fractures in elderly patients (American Geriatrics Society 2015 Beers Criteria Update Expert Panel 2015). Anticholinergic and antihistaminergic drugs (e.g., hydroxyzine, diphenhydramine) also should be avoided in this population because these agents carry an increased risk of delirium and urinary retention. A retrospective study examining use of buspirone (a serotonin type 1A partial agonist) to treat behavioral disturbance in dementia showed moderate improvement in aggressive behavior (Santa Cruz et al. 2017).

Melatonin.   Melatonin is a hormone excreted by the pineal gland for the regulation of the sleep-wake cycle. Melatonin may help reduce sleep-related behavioral symptoms in dementia, but studies thus far have had very small samples (Dyer et al. 2018). Melatonin is not recommended (i.e., weak evidence against) for irregular circadian rhythm disorders in dementia. Light therapy is the treatment of choice for these disorders in elderly individuals with dementia (Auger et al. 2015).

Dronabinol.   There is evidence from one small open study that dronabinol may be an effective adjunct treatment for neuropsychiatric symptoms such as anxiety and agitation in dementia (Woodward et al. 2014).

Nonpharmacological (Including Behavioral) Treatments

Nonpharmacological treatments for neuropsychiatric disturbances in dementia are encouraged as first-line treatment, given the significant risks associated with psychotropic medication use in dementia (Fochtmann 2016). Nonpharmacological interventions are wide ranging and can be implemented in any setting (hospital, home, skilled nursing facility). Some techniques—such as reorientation, use of environmental cues (signs, color coding), and ensuring that hearing and vision are maximized with use of hearing aids and glasses—are very simple to implement and should be used routinely.

Music therapy.   Music therapy can be passive (e.g., listening to music alone, with a therapist, or in a group) or active (e.g., singing, dancing, or instrument playing). Music has been shown to reduce agitated behaviors and improve depressed mood, especially in the first 4–6 weeks of its use (Li et al. 2019). Several theories have been proposed to explain its efficacy. Music therapy may provide an emotional outlet for patients; can create opportunities for social interaction and communication that distract patients from stressful environmental or emotional cues; may help engage patients in meaningful activities that reduce stress and apathy; and may remind patients of life before the disease or life outside of their current living environment (Pedersen et al. 2017).

Behavior management techniques.   Techniques for managing behavior focus on improving communication, modifying the physical and social environment, training caregivers, and providing cognitive-behavioral-type therapies. One such technique is dementia care mapping, which involves observing and assessing each individual's behavior for agitation triggers as well as factors that increase well-being. These results are shared with caregivers, and changes are made to the environment to minimize triggers and increase well-being (Livingston et al. 2014). Although most primary studies of behavioral management techniques have been limited by small sample size, overall these techniques have been shown to be effective in reducing behavioral and psychiatric symptoms associated with dementia (Abraha et al. 2017).

Reminiscence therapy.   Reminiscence therapy involves discussion (or silent recall) of past activities, events, and experiences in a person's life with the aid of prompts, such as photographs, items from the past, or archived sound recordings. In a meta-analysis of 12 randomized controlled trials, reminiscence therapy was found to improve cognitive functioning significantly but did not have lasting, long-term effects (Huang et al. 2015). Similar findings were reported for reduction in depressive symptoms.

Delirium

Delirium, also referred to as encephalopathy and acute brain failure, is a disturbance in attention, awareness, and cognition that is a direct physiological consequence of another medical condition (First 2014). This disturbance represents a distinct change from the patient's baseline, has a rapid onset, and is characterized by symptoms that fluctuate throughout the day. Older patients are at higher risk of developing delirium, especially those with dementia, depression, or sensory impairment. Chronic use of medications with substantial effects on the central nervous system (e.g., opioids, benzodiazepines) also confers delirium risk (Vasilevskis et al. 2012). Delirium can be classified into three different motor subtypes: hyperactive, hypoactive, and mixed. These subtypes share the core diagnostic elements of delirium and have similar degrees of cognitive impairment but differ with regard to other, nonmotor symptoms; duration; underlying cause; and outcome.

Major Subtypes of Delirium

Hyperactive delirium includes symptoms of increased motor activity, loss of control of activity, restlessness, and wandering. In contrast, patients with hypoactive delirium show decreased motor activity, decreased speed of actions, reduced awareness of their surroundings, slowed speech, lethargy, and withdrawal (Meagher et al. 2008). Delirium tremens is a particularly aggressive form of hyperactive delirium that is associated with alcohol withdrawal and hypertension, tachycardia, and agitation as well as the other cardinal manifestations of delirium. If not adequately treated (including treatment of comorbid medical disorders), delirium tremens can be associated with high mortality.

Hyperactive

In addition to manifesting with impaired attention and awareness and with cognitive disturbance, hyperactive delirium is characterized by mood lability, delusions, and hallucinations (Grover et al. 2014). Patients with hyperactive delirium tend to be younger. Hyperactive delirium can be caused by any number of medical problems, but there is a greater propensity for it to be caused by medication side effects or toxicity or by intoxication or withdrawal from drugs or substances of abuse, such as alcohol. Patients with hyperactive delirium are more easily recognized because their symptoms cause greater difficulties with medical care. These patients are more likely than those with hypoactive delirium to end up in restraints.

Hypoactive

Patients with hypoactive delirium tend to be more withdrawn, with flat affect and language disturbance. They also have more thought-process abnormalities (e.g., slowed processing). Hypoactive delirium is the most common motor subtype among hospitalized older adults (Morandi et al. 2017). It can be difficult to recognize, because hypoactive patients tend to cause fewer problems in the hospital than do hyperactive patients. As a result, patients with hypoactive delirium may be undertreated (Grover et al. 2014). Hypoactive delirium can be confused with depression because the symptoms of prominent flat affect, withdrawal, and decreased oral intake mirror the neurovegetative symptoms of MDD. The underlying cause of hypoactive delirium is commonly a metabolic disturbance such as hypo- or hypernatremia or hepatic failure.

Mixed

Mixed delirium manifests with fluctuating symptoms of both hyper- and hypoactive subtypes. Patients with mixed delirium have more delusions and hallucinations than do hypoactive patients but more thought-process abnormalities than do patients with hyperactive delirium.

Neuropsychiatric Presentations in Delirium

Psychosis

Psychosis in delirium most commonly manifests as visual (rather than auditory) hallucinations, other perceptual disturbances, delusions, and thought-process abnormalities. Paranoid delusions often stem from disorientation and misunderstanding of environmental stimuli. For example, a patient may become convinced that she is being targeted and purposely harmed by her medical team. Psychotic symptoms are most prevalent in patients with the mixed motor subtype (Meagher et al. 2011).

Agitation

Like delusions of persecution, agitation also stems from misattributions and misunderstandings. Agitation can seriously inhibit a patient's care. Common symptoms seen with physical agitation include pulling on/removing medical equipment (e.g., intravenous catheters, electrocardiogram [ECG] leads, nasogastric tubes), attempting to get out of bed without assistance, and striking out at or being combative toward medical care providers or family members. Delirious patients may also demonstrate agitation verbally, with yelling and aggressive language. Agitation is significantly less common in hypoactive delirium than in the hyperactive subtype (Meagher et al. 2011; Morandi et al. 2017).

Depression/Abulia

Hypoactive delirium can mimic depression, so patients may be profoundly abulic, with social withdrawal, reduced oral intake, and decreased speech. Premorbid MDD is a risk factor for the development of delirium in elderly individuals (Inouye et al. 2014).

Insomnia

While insomnia does not cause delirium per se, it often accompanies delirium; sleep deprivation research has shown that lack of sleep can induce delirium symptoms (Weinhouse et al. 2009). Delirious patients may be very tired during the day, napping off and on, but wide awake at night. A small body of literature has also suggested that improving sleep in the hospital may help prevent delirium or improve its course (Flannery et al. 2016).

Diagnostic and Laboratory Findings in Delirium

Standard Workup

Delirium is a clinical diagnosis. In addition to a history (including history from an informed observer), an orientation assessment and a quick bedside test of attention should be performed (e.g., reciting the days of the week forward and backward, spelling the word "world" backward, digit span testing) for all patients (Inouye et al. 2014). Several screening instruments and delirium severity rating scales have been developed; the most widely used is the Confusion Assessment Method (CAM), an algorithm that has been employed in more than 4,500 published studies (Oh et al. 2017).

The workup for delirium should be driven by the history, the physical examination, and previous examination results. At the most basic level, the laboratory workup should include a complete metabolic panel to look for electrolyte derangements or liver function abnormalities, a complete blood count, a urinalysis, and an ECG (because myocardial infarction can manifest as delirium in octogenarians) (Inouye et al. 2014). Other tests should be performed on the basis of clinical suspicion. For example, a patient who has a history of falls or who is taking an anticoagulant should have a noncontrast head CT to rule out subdural or intracranial hemorrhage. A patient with a history of drug or alcohol use should receive a urine toxicology screen and measurement of blood alcohol levels. Chest radiography should be performed in a patient with a cough and fever. The mnemonic WWHHHHIMPS (Table 22–1) can be used to guide the differential diagnosis and to ensure that life-threatening causes of delirium are not overlooked.

Additional Studies

Electroencephalography is an area of special interest in delirium. The electroencephalogram (EEG) in delirium shows diffuse background slowing, with significant reductions in alpha waves and increased theta and delta slow-wave activity (Koponen et al. 1989). In addition to being potentially diagnostic of delirium, the EEG can be used to help determine whether seizures (including nonconvulsive status epilepticus) are contributing to the presentation. Researchers are using bispectral index monitors—small portable EEG monitors employed by anesthesiologists for intraoperative monitoring of patients' response to anesthesia—to detect delirium, and some re-

TABLE 22–1.	Life-threatening causes of delirium—WWHHHHHIMPS

Withdrawal (from alcohol, benzodiazepines, etc.)

Wernicke's encephalopathy

Hypoxia

Hypoglycemia

Hypertensive urgency or emergency

Hyper- or hypothermia

Hypoperfusion/hypotension

Intracerebral hemorrhage

Meningitis/encephalitis

Poisoning

Status epilepticus

searchers are inventing bedside devices in the hope of finding a convenient way to assess for delirium physiologically (Oh et al. 2017; van der Kooi et al. 2015). Because the EEG in dementia also shows diminished alpha activity and increased slow waves, it can be difficult to differentiate dementia from delirium on EEG.

CT and MRI may be warranted, depending on the history and findings from the neurological examination. Brain MRI is more sensitive than CT for identifying brain lesions (e.g., primary tumors, metastases, embolic strokes, leukoencephalopathy, chronic white matter damage) and posterior fossa lesions; it should be considered if a basic workup is negative.

Treatments of Neuropsychiatric Syndromes in Delirium

Pharmacological Treatments

While the definitive treatment of most forms of delirium is correction of the underlying medical cause, the neuropsychiatric symptoms of delirium can be managed with medications. There is also some research investigating pharmacological prevention of delirium in intensive care unit (ICU) settings (Serafim et al. 2015). Even after the underlying cause of delirium has been corrected, symptoms of delirium can persist for a long time, especially in elderly patients who have aging-related volume loss at baseline (Inouye et al. 2014).

Antipsychotics.   FGAs and SGAs can be used to treat psychotic symptoms and agitation. In the hospital setting, antipsychotics can be administered orally, intravenously, or intramuscularly. The FGA haloperidol, if given intravenously, has a much lower risk of causing extrapyramidal side effects and can thus be a good as-needed medication for symptom management in hyperactive delirium. Haloperidol has also been used as a continuous infusion for some patients, but there is less evidence to support this dosing (Wang et al. 2012). Haloperidol can prolong the QT interval and increase the risk of torsades de pointes. If intravenous haloperidol is used, the patient should receive careful cardiac monitoring, which is standard practice in ICUs but not on general medical wards. Close attention must be paid to electrolyte repletion. Haloperidol may be less sedating than many of the SGAs and can be a helpful medication scheduled throughout the day without causing sleepiness. Chlorpromazine, another FGA, is also available in oral and intramuscular forms. It can be extremely sedating, which is helpful for patients with hyperactive delirium. However, chlorpromazine can cause hypotension and should be avoided in patients with low blood pressure.

In comparison with FGAs, SGAs have a better overall safety profile in elderly adults with delirium (Kishi et al. 2016) but still carry significant risks. Because of the risk of stroke and death associated with antipsychotic use in the elderly, these medications should be used only if the patient's agitation or psychotic symptoms have failed to respond to other classes of medications or nonpharmacological interventions and are so severe that they are causing harm to the patient or endangering others (Reus et al. 2016). The SGAs quetiapine, olanzapine, and risperidone all may be used in the management of behavioral symptoms. In comparison with haloperidol, quetiapine and olanzapine are more sedating, which can be a helpful side effect for a patient with insomnia, agitation, or psychosis. As previously noted, clinicians should be extra cautious in using antipsychotics in patients with dementia associated with Parkinson's disease or Lewy body disease. The dopamine antagonism of antipsychotics can worsen motor symptoms in these diseases. Low-dosage quetiapine is the safest option in these patients (Walker et al. 2015).

Benzodiazepines for delirium tremens.   Treatment of delirium tremens usually requires intravenous administration of rapid-acting benzodiazepines at dosages high enough to maintain light sedation until alcohol withdrawal is completed (Mayo-Smith et al. 2004). Care requires a monitored setting, close attention to volume status, electrolyte repletion, and treatment for other medical disorders.

Antidepressants.   Trazodone, a serotonin antagonist and reuptake inhibitor, is an antidepressant with strong histaminergic properties that make it helpful for treating agitation, insomnia, and depressive symptoms associated with delirium, although there is little research on its use in delirium (Okamoto et al. 1999). Mirtazapine is an atypical antidepressant that antagonizes certain adrenergic, serotonergic, and histaminergic receptors. When given at nighttime, mirtazapine can help delirious patients with insomnia. It can also increase appetite in patients with hypoactive or mixed delirium with abulia. There is no particular role for SSRIs in treating delirium. Tricyclic antidepressants and monoamine oxidase inhibitors should be avoided, because these medications can precipitate or worsen delirium.

Mood stabilizers.   Valproic acid is an adjunct for treating labile mood, agitation, and hyperactivity in delirium. One study of patients ages 40–70 years in the ICU found that valproic acid reduced symptoms within 48 hours (Gagnon et al. 2017). There are several case reports on its use for management of behavioral symptoms in delirium, also showing efficacy with minimal significant side effects (Bourgeois et al. 2005). Valproic acid is metabolized by the liver and should be used with caution in patients with hepatic disease. Liver function tests should be monitored during initial titration, as should the complete blood count because of the risk of thrombocytopenia.

Stimulants.   Methylphenidate has been shown to be effective in cancer patients with hypoactive delirium. It improves cognitive function and increases patient activity so that they are more awake and better able to participate in care (Gagnon et al.

2005). Judicious use of methylphenidate at low dosages and with careful monitoring of behavior can promote wakefulness and activity, leading to increased appetite. Short-acting methylphenidate can be given at an initial dose of 2.5 mg. This can be increased, depending on efficacy and tolerability, and given up to two times daily.

Melatonin. Beyond its use in assisting with sleep-wake cycle regulation, melatonin is thought to be neuroprotective and potentially helpful in the prevention of delirium. Limited evidence suggested that low-dosage melatonin might be protective against delirium in elderly hospitalized patients (Al-Aama et al. 2011), but systematic reviews of the literature concluded that it provided no benefit (Siddiqi et al. 2016; Walker and Gales 2017).

Nonpharmacological (Including Behavioral) Treatments

Nonpharmacological strategies should be used in all elderly hospitalized patients to prevent delirium and lessen delirium symptoms. These strategies are widely accepted as the most effective approach for combating delirium (Inouye et al. 2014). The Hospital Elder Life Program (HELP) is one of the most widely used approaches. It involves frequent reorientation, promotion of sleep (opening shades and turning on lights during the day, minimizing nighttime noise and interruptions), early mobilization and stimulation (e.g., participating in physical and occupational therapy, coloring), maintenance of adequate nutrition and hydration, minimizing use of psychoactive drugs, and maximizing access to glasses and hearing aids so that patients can fully engage with their environment (Inouye et al. 2006).

Conclusion

As research into neurocognitive disorders expands, we are gaining an understanding of the neurobiological processes that drive these conditions. So far, however, definitive biomarkers remain elusive, and management is focused primarily on alleviation of neuropsychiatric symptoms. As the knowledge base grows, there is likely to be a rapid expansion and evolution of diagnostic tools and treatment options for these conditions. In the meantime, as we await such advancements, a thorough assessment and characterization of the clinical presentation—combined with cautious, targeted psychopharmacology directed at specific symptoms with constant ongoing evaluation and adjustment—represents the best standard of care, and this approach is likely to remain the foundation of care even after more is learned about these conditions.

References

Abraha I, Rimland JM, Trotta FM, et al: Systematic review of systematic reviews of non-pharmacological interventions to treat behavioural disturbances in older patients with dementia. The SENATOR-OnTop series. BMJ Open 7(3):e012759, 2017 28302633

Aizenstein HJ, Baskys A, Boldrini M, et al: Vascular depression consensus report—a critical update. BMC Med 14(1):161, 2016 27806704

Al-Aama T, Brymer C, Gutmanis I, et al: Melatonin decreases delirium in elderly patients: a randomized, placebo-controlled trial. Int J Geriatr Psychiatry 26(7):687–694, 2011 20845391

Alzheimer's Association: Interim Results From the IDEAS Study Reported at AAIC 2017 in London. Presented at the Alzheimer's Association International Conference, London, July 2017. Available at: https://www.ideas-study.org/2017/07/20/interim-results-from-the-ideas-study-reported-at-aaic-2017-in-london/. Accessed November 25, 2017.

American Geriatrics Society 2015 Beers Criteria Update Expert Panel: American Geriatrics Society 2015 updated Beers criteria for potentially inappropriate medication use in older adults. J Am Geriatr Soc 63(11):2227–2246, 2015 26446832

American Psychiatric Association: Diagnostic and Statistical Manual of Mental Disorders, 3rd Edition, Revised. Washington, DC, American Psychiatric Association, 1987

American Psychiatric Association: Diagnostic and Statistical Manual of Mental Disorders, 5th Edition. Arlington, VA, American Psychiatric Association, 2013

Auger RR, Burgess HJ, Emens JS, et al: Clinical practice guideline for the treatment of intrinsic circadian rhythm sleep-wake disorders: advanced sleep-wake phase disorder (ASWPD), delayed sleep-wake phase disorder (DSWPD), non-24-hour sleep-wake rhythm disorder (N24SWD), and irregular sleep-wake rhythm disorder (ISWRD). An update for 2015: an American Academy of Sleep Medicine clinical practice guideline. J Clin Sleep Med 11(10):1199–1236, 2015 26414986

Bang J, Spina S, Miller BL: Frontotemporal dementia. Lancet 386(10004):1672–1682, 2015 26595641

Baumgart M, Snyder HM, Carrillo MC, et al: Summary of the evidence on modifiable risk factors for cognitive decline and dementia: a population-based perspective. Alzheimers Dement 11(6):718–726, 2015 26045020

Bédard M, Molloy DW, Pedlar D, et al: 1997 IPA/Bayer Research Awards in Psychogeriatrics. Associations between dysfunctional behaviors, gender, and burden in spousal caregivers of cognitively impaired older adults. Int Psychogeriatr 9(3):277–290, 1997 9513028

Bourgeois JA, Koike AK, Simmons JE, et al: Adjunctive valproic acid for delirium and/or agitation on a consultation-liaison service: a report of six cases. J Neuropsychiatry Clin Neurosci 17(2):232–238, 2005 15939979

Bradford A, Kunik ME, Schulz P, et al: Missed and delayed diagnosis of dementia in primary care: prevalence and contributing factors. Alzheimer Dis Assoc Disord 23(4):306–314, 2009 19568149

Broen MP, Leentjens AF, Köhler S, et al: Trajectories of recovery in depressed Parkinson's disease patients treated with paroxetine or venlafaxine. Parkinsonism Relat Disord 23:80–85, 2016 26739248

Buoli M, Serati M, Caldiroli A, et al: Pharmacological management of psychiatric symptoms in frontotemporal dementia: a systematic review. J Geriatr Psychiatry Neurol 30(3):162–169, 2017 28351199

Camargos EF, Pandolfi MB, Freitas MPD, et al: Trazodone for the treatment of sleep disorders in dementia: an open-label, observational and review study. Arq Neuropsiquiatria 69(1):44–49, 2011 21359422

Castello MA, Jeppson JD, Soriano S: Moving beyond anti-amyloid therapy for the prevention and treatment of Alzheimer's disease. BMC Neurol 14(1):169, 2014 25179671

Chou R, Selph S, Dana T, et al: Screening for HIV: Systematic Review to Update the U.S. Preventive Services Task Force Recommendation. Evidence Synthesis No. 95. AHRQ Publication No. 12-05173-EF-1. Rockville, MD, Agency for Healthcare Research and Quality, November 2012. Available at: https://www.ncbi.nlm.nih.gov/books/NBK114872/. Accessed May 12, 2019.

Cipriani G, Lucetti C, Danti S, et al: Sleep disturbances and dementia. Psychogeriatrics 15(1):65–74, 2015 25515641

Cohen-Mansfield J: Conceptualization of agitation: results based on the Cohen-Mansfield Agitation Inventory and the Agitation Behavior Mapping Instrument. Int Psychogeriatr 8 (suppl 3):309–315; discussion 351–354. 1996 9154580

Combs BL, Cox AG: Update on the treatment of Parkinson's disease psychosis: role of pimavanserin. Neuropsychiatr Dis Treat 13:737–744, 2017 28331324

Cummings JL: Depression in vascular dementia. Hillside J Clin Psychiatry 10(2):209–231, 1988 3224947

Cummings JL: Behavioral and psychiatric symptoms associated with Huntington's disease. Adv Neurol 65:179–186, 1995 7872139

Cummings JL: The Neuropsychiatric Inventory: assessing psychopathology in dementia patients. Neurology 48 (5 suppl 6):S10–S16, 1997 9153155

Devanand DP, Strickler JG, Huey ED, et al: Lithium Treatment for Agitation in Alzheimer's disease (Lit-AD): clinical rationale and study design. Contemp Clin Trials 71:33–39, 2018 29859917

Dichgans M, Leys D: Vascular cognitive impairment. Circ Res 120(3):573–591, 2017 28154105

Doody RS, Thomas RG, Farlow M, et al: Phase 3 trials of solanezumab for mild-to-moderate Alzheimer's disease. N Engl J Med 370(4):311–321, 2014 24450890

Dyer SM, Harrison SL, Laver K, et al: An overview of systematic reviews of pharmacological and non-pharmacological interventions for the treatment of behavioral and psychological symptoms of dementia. Int Psychogeriatr 30(3):295–309, 2018 29143695

Emre M, Aarsland D, Brown R, et al: Clinical diagnostic criteria for dementia associated with Parkinson's disease. Mov Disord 22(12):1689–1707; quiz 1837, 2007 17542011

First MB: DSM-5 Handbook of Differential Diagnosis. Washington, DC, American Psychiatric Publishing, 2014

Flannery AH, Oyler DR, Weinhouse GL: The impact of interventions to improve sleep on delirium in the ICU: a systematic review and research framework. Crit Care Med 44(12):2231–2240, 2016 27509391

Fochtmann LJ: The American Psychiatric Association Practice Guideline on the Use of Antipsychotics to Treat Agitation or Psychosis in Patients With Dementia. Arlington, VA, American Psychiatric Association, 2016

Gagnon B, Low G, Schreier G: Methylphenidate hydrochloride improves cognitive function in patients with advanced cancer and hypoactive delirium: a prospective clinical study. J Psychiatry Neurosci 30(2):100–107, 2005 15798785

Gagnon DJ, Fontaine GV, Smith KE, et al: Valproate for agitation in critically ill patients: a retrospective study. J Crit Care 37:119–125, 2017 27693975

González-Salvador MT, Arango C, Lyketsos CG, et al: The stress and psychological morbidity of the Alzheimer patient caregiver. Int J Geriatr Psychiatry 14(9):701–710, 1999 10479740

Green RC, Cupples LA, Go R, et al: Risk of dementia among white and African American relatives of patients with Alzheimer disease. JAMA 287(3):329–336, 2002 11790212

Grover S, Sharma A, Aggarwal M, et al: Comparison of symptoms of delirium across various motoric subtypes. Psychiatry Clin Neurosci 68(4):283–291, 2014 24372977

Gutzmann H, Qazi A: Depression associated with dementia. Z Gerontol Geriatr 48(4):305–311, 2015 25962363

Hebert LE, Weuve J, Scherr PA, et al: Alzheimer disease in the United States (2010–2050) estimated using the 2010 census. Neurology 80(19):1778–1783, 2013 23390181

Hegeman JM, Kok RM, van der Mast RC, et al: Phenomenology of depression in older compared with younger adults: meta-analysis. Br J Psychiatry 200(4):275–281, 2012 22474233

Herscovitch P: Amyloid imaging coverage with evidence development and the IDEAS study. J Nucl Med 56(5):20N, 2015 25934680

Huang H-C, Chen Y-T, Chen P-Y, et al: Reminiscence therapy improves cognitive functions and reduces depressive symptoms in elderly people with dementia: a meta-analysis of randomized controlled trials. J Am Med Dir Assoc 16(12):1087–1094, 2015 26341034

Hurd MD, Martorell P, Delavande A, et al: Monetary costs of dementia in the United States. N Engl J Med 368(14):1326–1334, 2013 23550670

Inouye SK, Baker DI, Fugal P, et al: Dissemination of the hospital elder life program: implementation, adaptation, and successes. J Am Geriatr Soc 54(10):1492–1499, 2006 17038065

Inouye SK, Westendorp RG, Saczynski JS: Delirium in elderly people. Lancet 383(9920):911–922, 2014 23992774

Kishi T, Hirota T, Matsunaga S, et al: Antipsychotic medications for the treatment of delirium: a systematic review and meta-analysis of randomised controlled trials. J Neurol Neurosurg Psychiatry 87(7):767–774, 2016 26341326

Knopman DS, DeKosky ST, Cummings JL, et al: Practice parameter: diagnosis of dementia (an evidence-based review). Report of the Quality Standards Subcommittee of the American Academy of Neurology. Neurology 56(9):1143–1153, 2001 11342678

Koponen H, Partanen J, Pääkkönen A, et al: EEG spectral analysis in delirium. J Neurol Neurosurg Psychiatry 52(8):980–985, 1989 2795067

Li HC, Wang HH, Lu CY, et al: The effect of music therapy on reducing depression in people with dementia: a systematic review and meta-analysis. Geriatr Nurs 40(5):510–516, 2019 31056209

Livingston G, Kelly L, Lewis-Holmes E, et al: Non-pharmacological interventions for agitation in dementia: systematic review of randomised controlled trials. Br J Psychiatry 205(6):436–442, 2014 25452601

Lonergan E, Luxenberg J: Valproate preparations for agitation in dementia. Cochrane Database Syst Rev (3):CD003945, 2009 19588348

Loy CT, Schofield PR, Turner AM, et al: Genetics of dementia. Lancet 383(9919):828–840, 2014 23927914

Magni E, Binetti G, Bianchetti A, et al: Risk of mortality and institutionalization in demented patients with delusions. J Geriatr Psychiatry Neurol 9(3):123–126, 1996 8873875

Mayo-Smith MF, Beecher LH, Fischer TL, et al: Management of alcohol withdrawal delirium. An evidence-based practice guideline. Arch Intern Med 164(13):1405–1412, 2004 15249349

McCurry SM, Logsdon RG, Teri L, et al: Characteristics of sleep disturbance in community-dwelling Alzheimer's disease patients. J Geriatr Psychiatry Neurol 12(2):53–59, 1999 10483925

McKeith IG, Boeve BF, Dickson DW, et al: Diagnosis and management of dementia with Lewy bodies: fourth consensus report of the Dementia with Lewy Bodies (DLB) Consortium. Neurology 89(1):88–100, 2017 28592453

Meagher DJ, Moran M, Raju B, et al: Motor symptoms in 100 patients with delirium versus control subjects: comparison of subtyping methods. Psychosomatics 49(4):300–308, 2008 18621935

Meagher DJ, Leonard M, Donnelly S, et al: A longitudinal study of motor subtypes in delirium: relationship with other phenomenology, etiology, medication exposure and prognosis. J Psychosom Res 71(6):395–403, 2011 22118382

Morandi A, Di Santo SG, Cherubini A, et al: Clinical features associated with delirium motor subtypes in older inpatients: results of a multicenter study. Am J Geriatr Psychiatry 25(10):1064–1071, 2017 28579352

O'Brien JT, Thomas A: Vascular dementia. Lancet 386(10004):1698–1706, 2015 26595643

Oh ES, Fong TG, Hshieh TT, et al: Delirium in older persons: advances in diagnosis and treatment. JAMA 318(12):1161–1174, 2017 28973626

Okamoto Y, Matsuoka Y, Sasaki T, et al: Trazodone in the treatment of delirium. J Clin Psychopharmacol 19(3):280–282, 1999 10350040

Olney NT, Spina S, Miller BL: Frontotemporal dementia. Neurol Clin 35(2):339–374, 2017 28410663

Ownby RL, Crocco E, Acevedo A, et al: Depression and risk for Alzheimer disease: systematic review, meta-analysis, and metaregression analysis. Arch Gen Psychiatry 63(5):530–538, 2006 16651510

Pagan F, Torres-Yaghi Y, Altshuler M: The diagnosis and natural history of Huntington disease. Handb Clin Neurol 144:63–67, 2017 28947126

Pedersen SKA, Andersen PN, Lugo RG, et al: Effects of music on agitation in dementia: a meta-analysis. Front Psychol 8:742, 2017 28559865

Rabins PV, Rovner B, Rummans MW, et al: Guideline watch for the practice guideline for the treatment of patients with Alzheimer's disease and other dementias. APA Guideline Watch, October 2014. Available at: https://psychiatryonline.org/pb/assets/raw/sitewide/practice_guidelines/guidelines/alzheimerwatch.pdf. Accessed April 6, 2019.

Reus VI, Fochtmann LJ, Eyler AE, et al: The American Psychiatric Association practice guideline on the use of antipsychotics to treat agitation or psychosis in patients with dementia. Am J Psychiatry 173(5):543–546, 2016 27133416

Rohrer JD, Guerreiro R, Vandrovcova J, et al: The heritability and genetics of frontotemporal lobar degeneration. Neurology 73(18):1451–1456, 2009 19884572

Ropacki SA, Jeste DV: Epidemiology of and risk factors for psychosis of Alzheimer's disease: a review of 55 studies published from 1990 to 2003. Am J Psychiatry 162(11):2022–2030, 2005 16263838

Rosen J, Burgio L, Kollar M, et al: The Pittsburgh Agitation Scale: a user-friendly instrument for rating agitation in dementia patients. Am J Geriatr Psychiatry 2(1):52–59, 1994 28531073

Sachdev P, Kalaria R, O'Brien J, et al: Diagnostic criteria for vascular cognitive disorders: a VASCOG statement. Alzheimer Dis Assoc Disord 28(3):206–218, 2014 24632990

Salloway S, Sperling R, Fox NC, et al: Two phase 3 trials of bapineuzumab in mild-to-moderate Alzheimer's disease. N Engl J Med 370(4):322–333, 2014 24450891

Santa Cruz MR, Hidalgo PC, Lee MS, et al: Buspirone for the treatment of dementia with behavioral disturbance. Int Psychogeriatr 29(5):859–862, 2017 28124634

Serafim RB, Bozza FA, Soares M, et al: Pharmacologic prevention and treatment of delirium in intensive care patients: a systematic review. J Crit Care 30(4):799–807, 2015 25957498

Shin H-Y, Han HJ, Shin D-J, et al: Sleep problems associated with behavioral and psychological symptoms as well as cognitive functions in Alzheimer's disease. J Clin Neurol 10(3):203–209, 2014 25045372

Siddiqi N, Harrison JK, Clegg A, et al: Interventions for preventing delirium in hospitalised non-ICU patients. Cochrane Database Syst Rev (3):CD005563, 2016 26967259

Tabrizi SJ, Scahill RI, Owen G, et al: Predictors of phenotypic progression and disease onset in premanifest and early stage Huntington's disease in the TRACK-HD study: analysis of 36-month observational data. Lancet Neurol 12(7):637–649, 2013 23664844

van der Kooi AW, Zaal IJ, Klijn FA, et al: Delirium detection using EEG: what and how to measure. Chest 147(1):94–101, 2015 25166725

Vasilevskis EE, Han JH, Hughes CG, et al: Epidemiology and risk factors for delirium across hospital settings. Best Pract Res Clin Anaesthesiol 26(3):277–287, 2012 23040281

Walker CK, Gales MA: Melatonin receptor agonists for delirium prevention. Ann Pharmacother 51(1):72–78, 2017 27539735

Walker Z, Possin KL, Boeve BF, et al: Lewy body dementias. Lancet 386(10004):1683–1697, 2015 26595642

Wang EHZ, Mabasa VH, Loh GW, et al: Haloperidol dosing strategies in the treatment of delirium in the critically ill. Neurocrit Care 16(1):170–183, 2012 22038577

Wang J, Yu J-T, Wang H-F, et al: Pharmacological treatment of neuropsychiatric symptoms in Alzheimer's disease: a systematic review and meta-analysis. J Neurol Neurosurg Psychiatry 86(1):101–109, 2015 24876182

Weinhouse GL, Schwab RJ, Watson PL, et al: Bench-to-bedside review: delirium in ICU patients—importance of sleep deprivation. Crit Care 13(6):234, 2009 20053301

Woodward MR, Harper DG, Stolyar A, et al: Dronabinol for the treatment of agitation and aggressive behavior in acutely hospitalized severely demented patients with noncognitive behavioral symptoms. Am J Geriatr Psychiatry 22(4):415–419, 2014 23597932

Yeh Y-C, Ouyang W-C: Mood stabilizers for the treatment of behavioral and psychological symptoms of dementia: an update review. Kaohsiung J Med Sci 28(4):185–193, 2012 22453066

Yohanna D, Cifu AS: Antipsychotics to treat agitation or psychosis in patients with dementia. JAMA 318(11):1057–1058, 2017 28975291

PART IV

Conditions and Syndromes
at the Medical–Psychiatric
Boundary

CHAPTER 23

Chronic Pain

Robert M. McCarron, D.O.

Samir J. Sheth, M.D.

Charles De Mesa, D.O., M.P.H.

Michelle Burke Parish, Ph.D., M.A.

Both physical pain and mental health–related disorders are widely prevalent and collectively account for the patient conditions most frequently seen by primary care providers. These conditions present a complex challenge for both patients and providers, generate high utilization of medical services, and cause increased morbidity. Patients with these complicated conditions often present with largely unexplained physical complaints that may take the form of conditions such as fibromyalgia, irritable bowel syndrome, complex regional pain syndrome, or pelvic floor dysfunction, among others. In this chapter, we emphasize the importance of recognizing and understanding the interface between chronic pain management and psychiatric disorders and provide some practice pointers for diagnosis and treatment of common chronic pain conditions.

Chronic Pain: An Overview

Pain, both physical and emotional, is the number one reason that people seek medical attention. According to the Institute of Medicine (2011), nearly 100 million Americans suffer from chronic pain. This number is greater than the number of Americans with heart disease, cancer, and diabetes combined (Gaskin and Richard 2012). In 2012, 25.3 million adults (11.2%) reported having experienced pain every day for the preceding 3 months, and those with more severe pain had worse overall health, utilized more health care, and had more disability than those with less severe pain (Nahin 2015).

The International Association for the Study of Pain defines *pain* as "an unpleasant sensory and *emotional* experience associated with actual or potential tissue damage, or described in terms of such damage" (Merskey and Bogduk 1994, p. 210 [emphasis added]). Implicit in this definition is the fact that pain is rarely a purely physiological phenomenon. Although chronic pain is widely acknowledged as a biopsychosocial phenomenon, its psychological and social dimensions are often inadequately addressed and routinely unrecognized clinically (American Psychiatric Association 2013; Bair et al. 2003; Dersh et al. 2002b). This circumstance endures despite an established body of literature demonstrating the relationship of chronic pain to numerous psychosocial factors, including depression, stress, anxiety, and posttraumatic stress disorder (PTSD) (Dersh et al. 2002b; Grant et al. 2004; Hahn 2001; Hahn et al. 1994). Thus, there is a need for physicians and other clinicians to learn how to recognize, promptly refer, and even assist in the treatment of common pain disorders, which are frequently comorbid with psychiatric conditions.

Unfortunately, standard care for some chronic pain conditions increasingly relies on diagnostic tests and treatment options that have not been well validated in terms of safety or effectiveness, and abuse of pain medication has become a major public health concern (Jackson and Kroenke 1999). Since 2003, opioid analgesics have been involved in more overdose deaths than heroin and cocaine combined. For every unintentional overdose death related to an opioid analgesic, 9 people are admitted for substance abuse treatment, 161 people report drug abuse or dependence, and 461 people report nonmedical uses of opioid analgesics (Centers for Disease Control Prevention 2012). Chronic pain is a complex biopsychosocial phenomenon with significant costs to our society in terms of both personal suffering and economic burden. The Institute of Medicine (2011) estimated the annual economic burden of chronic pain in medical costs and lost productivity to be more than $600 billion dollars, an amount that exceeds the cost of each of the nation's priority health conditions (McWilliams et al. 2003). Integrated, evidence-based care that incorporates the psychosocial components of chronic pain is urgently needed, given the dual epidemics of chronic pain and abuse of certain pain medications that our country faces. Psychiatrists are well positioned to use their general medical and psychotherapeutic skills to help treat common chronic pain conditions.

Chronic Pain and Psychiatry Comorbidity

Patients with chronic pain conditions are disproportionately burdened by comorbid psychiatric conditions. An estimated 40%–50% of patients with chronic pain conditions have a comorbid mood disorder, and an estimated 35% have a comorbid anxiety disorder (McWilliams et al. 2003). Major depressive disorder, dysthymia, generalized anxiety disorder, agoraphobia, panic disorder, social phobia, PTSD, and substance use disorders are each more prevalent among people who are receiving treatment for chronic pain conditions than among those who are not (Demyttenaere et al. 2007). Table 23–1 presents the odds ratios for comorbidity of selected DSM-IV (American Psychiatric Association 1994) mental disorders among community-dwelling adults with low back or neck pain compared with those without such pain.

Comorbid psychiatric conditions often complicate the management of chronic pain conditions. For example, among individuals with chronic pain, comorbid depression and anxiety are associated with poorer treatment outcomes, more pain complaints,

TABLE 23–1. **Likelihood of comorbid psychopathology among adults with versus without chronic neck or low back pain**

DSM-IV diagnosis	OR (95% CI) of comorbidity[a]
Major depressive episode	2.8 (2.3, 3.5)
Dysthymia	3.7 (2.8, 5.0)
Generalized anxiety disorder	3.0 (2.3, 3.9)
Agoraphobia or panic disorder	2.1 (1.6, 2.7)
Social phobia	1.9 (1.5, 2.3)
Posttraumatic stress disorder	2.8 (2.3, 3.5)
Alcohol abuse or dependence	1.8 (1.4, 2.5)

[a]Odds ratio (95% confidence interval) for presence of a psychiatric diagnosis in individuals with low back or neck pain compared with individuals without such pain.
Source. Data from Demyttenaere et al. 2007.

greater pain intensity, longer duration of pain, and greater likelihood of nonrecovery (Bair et al. 2003, 2008).

Somatic symptom and related disorders also are commonly comorbid with chronic pain. However, because of frequently changing diagnostic categorization of these disorders and disagreements over diagnostic validity, reliable estimates of the prevalence of these disorders are not available (Dersh et al. 2002b). With the advent of the *with predominant pain* specifier in the fifth edition of the *Diagnostic and Statistical Manual of Mental Disorders* (DSM-5; American Psychiatric Association 2013), the somatic symptom disorder diagnosis has become more inclusive and likely will be appropriate for a significant percentage of chronic pain patients.

Personality disorders are present in an estimated 31%–81% of chronic pain patients, whereas only 10%–15% of the general American population is thought to have a personality disorder (Grant et al. 2004). Patients with personality disorders who have multiple, mainly unexplained, or treatment-refractory somatic complaints often are labeled "difficult patients" by their providers (Hahn 2001; Hahn et al. 1994). Encounters with such patients are estimated to compose 10%–20% of primary care visits (Hahn et al. 1994; Jackson and Kroenke 1999). Lack of clinician training in the management of patients with personality disorders and multiple somatic complaints can lead to provider burnout and worse patient outcomes. This situation illustrates the importance of team-based care, which incorporates psychiatric assessment and treatment within the primary care setting.

From a theoretical standpoint, the diathesis-stress model is used most often to explain how chronic pain can lead to the development or worsening of comorbid mental disorders (Dersh et al. 2002a). This model posits that each individual has preexisting, semidormant characteristics that if activated and aggravated by the stress of chronic pain may eventually result in psychopathology. For example, a patient who sustains an injury and experiences functional impairment may lose his or her job or become unable to maintain close relationships, and may subsequently develop depression. Consistent with this model, most studies suggest that in people with chronic pain and a comorbid mental disorder, the mental disorder (especially if a depressive disorder) occurred after the chronic pain, rather than the other way around

(Fishbain et al. 1998). If the development of personality disorders could also be explained by the diathesis-stress model, that would raise concern that what is diagnosed as a personality disorder may in reality be an overrepresentation of maladaptive coping mechanisms in a patient with chronic pain (Monti et al. 1998).

Among patients with chronic pain and psychiatric comorbidity, suicide is a devastating potential outcome. Mental disorders have long been known to constitute independent risk factors for suicidal ideation, attempted suicide, and completed suicide (Kessler et al. 2005). Among psychiatric disorders, major depressive disorder is the most common single diagnosis and anxiety disorders the most common diagnostic category associated with suicidal ideation, attempted suicide, and completed suicide (Kessler et al. 1999, 2005).

A growing body of literature has established that chronic pain conditions also constitute independent risk factors for suicidal behavior. Migraines, back problems, and abdominal pain have been the most frequently researched chronic pain conditions associated with suicidal ideation and attempted suicide. A large epidemiological study using the Canadian Community Health Survey found migraine and back problems to be independently associated with suicidal ideation and suicide attempts (Ratcliffe et al. 2008). Comorbidity with multiple psychiatric diagnoses and chronic pain conditions only strengthens the association and the risk of danger to self. However, not all chronic pain conditions have shown an association with suicidal ideation and suicide attempts. Fibromyalgia and arthritis, for example, do not appear to be independently associated with suicidal ideation or attempted suicide.

The following subsections provide an overview of some of the most frequently encountered chronic pain complaints or syndromes in primary care or mental health treatment facilities: fibromyalgia syndrome (FMS), complex regional pain syndrome (CRPS; formerly known as reflex sympathetic dystrophy), and headache. This information will aid the reader in understanding how to recognize, diagnose, and work with primary and specialty care teams to treat these often-complex pain conditions. In particular, psychotherapy, especially cognitive-behavioral therapy (CBT) and other brief psychotherapies, can be used in both psychiatric and general medical settings to help improve patients' overall function and decrease the perception of pain. Psychiatrists are generally more skilled in early recognition of frequently encountered psychiatric conditions, such as mood and anxiety disorders, which are commonly comorbid with FMS, CRPS, and headache as well as with other chronic pain conditions.

Fibromyalgia Syndrome

FMS is present in 1%–8% of the general population (Clauw 2009; Macfarlane et al. 2017). It is a disorder characterized mainly by chronic widespread pain; patients with FMS often presents with sleep disturbances, headaches, abdominal pain, or depression (Clauw 2009). For years, the diagnosis of fibromyalgia required the presence of "tender points" in at least 11 of 18 designated locations throughout the body. Although these diagnostic criteria were designed mainly for research purposes, they eventually were widely adopted for clinical use (Clauw 2009; Gerwin 2005), and as a consequence of their emphasis on tender points, FMS became a disease almost exclusive to females. In 2010, the requirement for tender points was removed, and as a result, the prevalence of males with FMS greatly increased (Clauw 2009; Wolfe et al.

2010). In addition to requiring the presence of widespread pain, the new diagnostic criteria added a symptom severity scale and required that clinicians rule out other disorders, such as rheumatoid arthritis or systemic lupus erythematosus (SLE) (Clauw 2009), that also can lead to chronic widespread pain. Although it has been nearly a decade since the criteria were revised, many clinicians continue to rely on a tender point examination to diagnose FMS.

When conducting the differential diagnosis for FMS, clinicians should consider any other condition that can cause widespread pain (e.g., rheumatoid arthritis, SLE) as well as myofascial pain syndrome. In order to diagnose conditions such as rheumatoid arthritis and SLE, clinicians should conduct a thorough physical examination, complemented by laboratory testing. In the case of myofascial pain syndrome, diagnosis is based mainly on the presence of trigger points on physical examination. It is common for clinicians to confuse tender points with trigger points. Tender points are located at tendons, ligaments, and joint capsules and produce excessive pain when palpated with 4 kg of pressure (enough pressure to make nail beds blanch). In contrast, trigger points are taut bands of muscle in the muscle belly that produce a characteristic referred pain pattern (Vázquez-Delgado et al. 2010).

Treatment of FMS requires a multimodal approach. The first step, which is often overlooked, is to ensure that the patient understands the diagnosis of FMS and the key features of FMS, such as abnormal pain and sensory processing (Macfarlane et al. 2017). Understanding the diagnosis will help the patient to realize the impact of the disorder and the rationale for the multimodal approach. It is then important for the clinician to understand the severity of the syndrome in each patient so that an individualized treatment plan can be developed.

All patients with FMS should be enrolled in a low-impact exercise program. In patients with significant psychological issues, such as pain-related depressive symptoms or catastrophizing, treatment should begin with CBT. In patients with significant pain or sleep-related complaints, the clinician should consider prescribing amitriptyline or pregabalin (Macfarlane et al. 2017). Many other therapies have been used, with varying evidence in terms of efficacy. However, in general, therapy should be guided by a careful consideration of the risks and benefits of each treatment offered. Modalities such as acupuncture, tai chi, and yoga are safe and potentially very effective and should be among the first interventions considered, whereas opioids have very limited long-term efficacy in patients with FMS and carry significant risks (Macfarlane et al. 2017); therefore, opioids should be used sparingly, and only in patients for whom multiple therapies have been unsuccessful. Overall, FMS can be very difficult to treat, but engaging patients in a therapy program that emphasizes both pharmacological and nonpharmacological therapies helps to mitigate pain and leads to improvements in function and quality of life. Psychiatrists and behavioral health care providers should screen for and address common comorbid conditions, such as mood, anxiety, and substance use disorders.

Complex Regional Pain Syndrome

CRPS is a syndrome characterized by extreme pain associated with atypical temperature, vasomotor, and trophic changes. CRPS is divided into type 1 (formerly known as *reflex sympathetic dystrophy*) and type 2 (formerly known as *causalgia*). The main distinction between the two subtypes is that in type 2, an identifiable nerve has been in-jured; however, treatment is the same for both types. CRPS has an overall estimated incidence of 26 cases per 100,000 person-years (Goebel 2011), which is greater than that of multiple sclerosis (4 cases per 100,000 person-years) but less than that of rheu-matoid arthritis (30 cases per 100,000 person-years). The syndrome is more common in females and in middle-aged and older patients. It is rare in pediatric patients (Borchers and Gershwin 2014; Goebel 2011).

CRPS occurs most often after surgical procedures, especially joint operations, but can also occur after simple injuries and even spontaneously (Goebel 2011; Poree et al. 2013). CRPS can be a debilitating disorder; over time, approximately 30% of cases re-solve, 54% persist with stable symptoms, and 16% worsen (Bruehl 2015; Marinus et al. 2011).

CRPS is characterized by allodynia and hyperalgesia combined with edema; color changes; hair, nail, or skin changes; weakness; dystonia; and temperature changes in the affected extremity. To properly diagnose CRPS, clinicians must use the "Budapest criteria" (Harden et al. 2010), which categorize symptoms by sensory, sudomotor/ edema, motor/trophic, and vasomotor changes at the time of physical examination as well as by patient-reported symptoms over the preceding week (Harden et al. 2013). CRPS is purely a clinical diagnosis; no imaging or laboratory tests can confirm the diagnosis. Despite this, it is important to order diagnostic radiological examinations as well as laboratory tests to ensure that other potential causes of the patient's symp-toms are ruled out.

The exact cause of CRPS is unknown. Possible contributing factors include genetic predisposition, exaggerated peripheral inflammatory response, paradoxical decrease in sympathetic outflow, enhanced sensitivity to catecholamines by way of upregula-tion of adrenergic receptors in the periphery combined with sprouting of adrenergic receptors on nociceptive fibers, and diminished representation in the somatosensory cortex of the affected limb (Bruehl 2010, 2015).

Early identification and treatment can often improve outcomes. The cornerstone of treatment for CRPS is physical therapy along with desensitization therapy. Medica-tions or interventional therapies are used to decrease pain so that patients can partic-ipate in meaningful physical therapy. Toward that end, treatments include topical compounding medications, psychological modalities such as CBT and biofeedback, sympathetic blocks, neuropathic pain medications, intravenous ketamine infusions, and spinal cord stimulation. As with many conditions, it is important to employ a stepwise approach that minimizes risks and maximizes benefits, and therefore, inter-ventions that are less invasive should be considered first. Overall, the use of a bal-anced multimodal approach can provide the patient with improved outcomes in pain, function, and quality of life (Bruehl 2015).

Headache

According to the World Health Organization (2016), 50% of the general population have recurrent headaches during any given year. Headache disorders are a public health concern given the socioeconomic burden directly due to health care costs and indirectly due to missed workdays or reduced competence (Rasmussen 1999). Most patients with headache initially present for treatment in the primary care setting, so it is essential to make the correct diagnosis and develop an appropriate plan of care. Headaches fall into two categories: primary and secondary. By definition, a primary headache is due to the headache itself, whereas a secondary headache is due to a demonstrable disease or underlying structural abnormality. Ninety percent of headaches seen in clinical practice are primary headaches (Rasmussen et al. 1991). Because secondary headaches are rare and pose significant risks, they must be effectively ruled out.

Primary Headache Disorders

The three types of primary headache are migraine, tension-type, and trigeminal autonomic cephalgias (TACs), which include cluster headaches (Headache Classification Committee of the International Headache Society 2004, 2013). Tension-type headache (TTH) is the most prevalent headache type, affecting 60%–80% of the population (Ahmed 2012). However, in the outpatient setting, migraine is far more common than TTH or cluster headache because it is disabling enough for an individual to seek medical attention (Lipton et al. 2003).

Migraine

Migraines are unilateral, pulsating, moderately to severely intense headaches that are aggravated by physical activity. Diagnostic criteria for migraine without aura from the *International Classification of Headache Disorders*, 3rd Edition (ICHD-3; Headache Classification Committee of the International Headache Society 2013), are as follows:

A. At least five attacks fulfilling criteria B–D
B. Headache attacks last 4–72 hours (untreated or unsuccessfully treated)
C. Headache has at least two of the following four characteristics:

1. Unilateral location
2. Pulsating quality
3. Moderate or severe pain intensity
4. Aggravation by or causing avoidance of routine physical activity

D. During headache at least one of the following:

1. Nausea and/or vomiting
2. Photophobia and phonophobia

E. Not better accounted for by another ICHD-3 diagnosis

Treatment strategies focus on improving functioning and reducing the number of headache days. The best approach with migraine is to individualize the treatment on the basis of the patient's unique symptoms. Treatment should include both medication management and nonpharmacological strategies. For migraine prophylaxis, treatments with strong evidence for chronic migraine include topiramate and onabotulinumtoxinA (Chiang et al. 2016), although there are other medications for episodic migraine. First-line agents belong to three broad classes: antihypertensives, antiepileptics, and antidepressants (Garza and Schwedt 2010). If first-line agents are ineffective, triptans and ergots can successfully relieve pain. Nonpharmacological options include CBT, physical therapy, biofeedback, and mindfulness training as a form of relaxation therapy (Saper et al. 2005). Neurostimulation devices are another potential option.

Tension-Type Headaches

TTHs are recurrent episodes of bilateral head pain lasting minutes to weeks. Pain is mild to moderate in intensity with a pressing or tightening quality. TTH may be distinguished from migraine by location (generally bilateral), absence of associated nausea or vomiting, and symptoms that typically *do not* worsen with physical activity. Pain relievers such as naproxen, ibuprofen, or acetaminophen are effective but should not be used repeatedly, because they may contribute to medication-overuse headaches. Preventive medications for TTH include tricyclic antidepressants and other antidepressants, such as venlafaxine.

Trigeminal Autonomic Cephalgias

TACs are primary headaches characterized by unilateral pain in the trigeminal distribution associated with ipsilateral cranial autonomic features. These include cluster headaches, paroxysmal hemicrania, hemicrania continua, and short-lasting unilateral neuralgiform headache with conjunctival injection and tearing or with cranial autonomic features. Cluster headache is characterized by attacks of severe orbital, supraorbital, or temporal pain, accompanied by autonomic phenomena or restlessness or agitation (Teckchandani and Barad 2017). Cluster headaches occur in cyclic patterns or clusters and are one of the most painful types of headache. Individuals with cluster headache commonly experience nighttime awakening by an intense pain in or around one eye on one side of the head (Lenaerts 2009). Ipsilateral autonomic symptoms, including conjunctival injection, eyelid closure, lacrimation, and rhinorrhea, may be present (May 2003).

Rapid symptomatic relief may be achieved with oxygen inhalation or subcutaneous sumatriptan. Prophylaxis includes verapamil or a short course of corticosteroids. In severe and refractory cases, surgical options (e.g., deep brain stimulation) can be used, but only following careful evaluation (Clauw 2014).

Secondary Headaches

Secondary headaches may be caused by conditions such as trauma, brain tumors, intracranial hypertension or hypotension, temporal arteritis, subarachnoid hemorrhage, substance use or withdrawal, or underlying systemic disease (Rasmussen et al. 1991). The physical examination for primary headaches will be essentially normal in comparison with that for secondary headaches. Identification of red flags is essential for the appropriate workup, management, and treatment of the conditions causing these headaches. Red flags in the physical examination include systemic and neurological symptoms and signs; new-onset headache after age 50 years; sudden "thunderclap" headache; or a significant change in the frequency, severity, or type of headache (Detsky et al. 2006; Dodick 2002).

Conclusion

Chronic pain is common and is frequently comorbid with psychiatric conditions. Physicians and other clinicians are on the front lines working with patients who have both physical and emotional pain. CBT and motivational interviewing can help augment the general medical treatment of chronic pain. Psychiatrists are well positioned to detect early symptoms of fibromyalgia, headache, and CRPS so that functional improvement can be optimized.

Diagnosing headache requires careful attention to history, examination, and prior treatments. Exclusion of secondary headaches is imperative. Treatment strategies should be exhausted before declaring failure. A multimodal approach is beneficial, with an emphasis on diminishing pain intensity and enhancing quality of life.

References

Ahmed F: Headache disorders: differentiating and managing the common subtypes. Br J Pain 6(3):124–132, 2012 26516483

American Psychiatric Association: Diagnostic and Statistical Manual of Mental Disorders, 4th Edition. Washington, DC, American Psychiatric Association, 1994

American Psychiatric Association: Diagnostic and Statistical Manual of Mental Disorders, 5th Edition. Arlington, VA, American Psychiatric Association, 2013

Bair MJ, Robinson RL, Katon W, et al: Depression and pain comorbidity: a literature review. Arch Intern Med 163(20):2433–2445, 2003 14609780

Bair MJ, Wu J, Damush TM, et al: Association of depression and anxiety alone and in combination with chronic musculoskeletal pain in primary care patients. Psychosom Med 70(8):890–897, 2008 18799425

Borchers AT, Gershwin ME: Complex regional pain syndrome: a comprehensive and critical review. Autoimmun Rev 13(3):242–265, 2014 24161450

Bruehl S: An update on the pathophysiology of complex regional pain syndrome. Anesthesiology 113(3):713–725, 2010 20693883

Bruehl S: Complex regional pain syndrome. BMJ 351:h2730, 2015 26224572

Centers for Disease Control Prevention: CDC grand rounds: prescription drug overdoses—a U.S. epidemic. MMWR Morb Mortal Wkly Rep 61(1):10–13, 2012 22237030

Chiang CC, Schwedt TJ, Wang SJ, et al: Treatment of medication-overuse headache: a systematic review. Cephalalgia 36(4):371–386, 2016 26122645

Clauw DJ: Fibromyalgia: an overview. Am J Med 122 (12 suppl):S3–S13, 2009 19962494

Clauw DJ: Fibromyalgia: a clinical review. JAMA 311(15):1547–1555, 2014 24737367

Demyttenaere K, Bruffaerts R, Lee S, et al: Mental disorders among persons with chronic back or neck pain: results from the World Mental Health Surveys. Pain 129(3):332–342, 2007 17350169

Dersh J, Polatin PB, Gatchel RJ: Chronic pain and psychopathology: research findings and theoretical considerations. Psychosom Med 64(5):773–786, 2002a 12271108

Dersh J, Gatchel RJ, Polatin P, et al: Prevalence of psychiatric disorders in patients with chronic work-related musculoskeletal pain disability. J Occup Environ Med 44(5):459–468, 2002b 12024691

Detsky ME, McDonald DR, Baerlocher MO, et al: Does this patient with headache have a migraine or need neuroimaging? JAMA 296(10):1274–1283, 2006 16968852

Dodick DW: Thunderclap headache. J Neurol Neurosurg Psychiatry 72(1):6–11, 2002 11784817

Fishbain DA, Cutler BR, Rosomoff HL: Comorbidity between psychiatric disorders and chronic pain. Current Review of Pain 2(1):1–10, 1998. Available at: https://link.springer.com/article/10.1007/s11916-998-0057-7. Accessed May 10, 2019.

Garza I, Schwedt TJ: Diagnosis and management of chronic daily headache. Semin Neurol 30(2):154–166, 2010 20352585

Gaskin DJ, Richard P: The economic costs of pain in the United States. J Pain 13(8):715–724, 2012 22607834

Gerwin RD: A review of myofascial pain and fibromyalgia—factors that promote their persistence. Acupunct Med 23(3):121–134, 2005 16259310

Goebel A: Complex regional pain syndrome in adults. Rheumatology (Oxford) 50(10):1739–1750, 2011 21712368

Grant BF, Hasin DS, Stinson FS, et al: Prevalence, correlates, and disability of personality disorders in the United States: results from the national epidemiologic survey on alcohol and related conditions. J Clin Psychiatry 65(7):948–958, 2004 15291684

Hahn SR: Physical symptoms and physician-experienced difficulty in the physician-patient relationship. Ann Intern Med 134 (9 Pt 2):897–904, 2001 11346326

Hahn SR, Thompson KS, Wills TA, et al: The difficult doctor-patient relationship: somatization, personality and psychopathology. J Clin Epidemiol 47(6):647–657, 1994 7722577

Harden RN, Bruehl S, Perez RS, et al: Validation of proposed diagnostic criteria (the "Budapest Criteria") for Complex Regional Pain Syndrome. Pain 150(2):268–274, 2010 20493633

Harden RN, Oaklander AL, Burton AW, et al; Reflex Sympathetic Dystrophy Syndrome Association: Complex regional pain syndrome: practical diagnostic and treatment guidelines, 4th edition. Pain Med 14(2):180–229, 2013 23331950

Headache Classification Committee of the International Headache Society: The International Classification of Headache Disorders, 2nd edition. Cephalalgia 24 (suppl 1):9–160, 2004 14979299

Headache Classification Committee of the International Headache Society: The International Classification of Headache Disorders, 3rd edition (beta version). Cephalalgia 33(9):629–808, 2013 23771276

Institute of Medicine: Relieving Pain in America: A Blueprint for Transforming Prevention, Care, Education, and Research. Washington, DC, National Academies Press, 2011

Jackson JL, Kroenke K: Difficult patient encounters in the ambulatory clinic: clinical predictors and outcomes. Arch Intern Med 159(10):1069–1075, 1999 10335683

Kessler RC, Borges G, Walters EE: Prevalence of and risk factors for lifetime suicide attempts in the National Comorbidity Survey. Arch Gen Psychiatry 56(7):617–626, 1999 10401507

Kessler RC, Berglund P, Borges G, et al: Trends in suicide ideation, plans, gestures, and attempts in the United States, 1990–1992 to 2001–2003. JAMA 293(20):2487–2495, 2005 15914749

Lenaerts M: Headache, in Atlas of Clinical Neurology, 3rd Edition. Edited by Rosenberg RN. Philadelphia, PA, Current Medicine Group, 2009, pp 56–57

Lipton RB, Dodick D, Sadovsky R, et al: A self-administered screener for migraine in primary care: the ID Migraine validation study. Neurology 61(3):375–382, 2003 12913201

Macfarlane GJ, Kronisch C, Atzeni F, et al: EULAR recommendations for management of fibromyalgia. Ann Rheum Dis 76(12):e54, 2017 28476880

Marinus J, Moseley GL, Birklein F, et al: Clinical features and pathophysiology of complex regional pain syndrome. Lancet Neurol 10(7):637–648, 2011 21683929

May A: Headaches with (ipsilateral) autonomic symptoms. J Neurol 250(11):1273–1278, 2003 14648142

McWilliams LA, Cox BJ, Enns MW: Mood and anxiety disorders associated with chronic pain: an examination in a nationally representative sample. Pain 106(1–2):127–133, 2003 14581119

Merskey H, Bogduk N: Classification of Chronic Pain: Description of Pain Syndromes and Definitions of Pain Terms, 2nd Edition. Seattle, WA, IASP Press, 1994

Monti DA, Herring CL, Schwartzman RJ, et al: Personality assessment of patients with complex regional pain syndrome type I. Clin J Pain 14(4):295–302, 1998 9874007

Nahin RL: Estimates of pain prevalence and severity in adults: United States, 2012. J Pain 16(8):769–780, 2015 26028573

Poree L, Krames E, Pope J, et al: Spinal cord stimulation as treatment for complex regional pain syndrome should be considered earlier than last resort therapy. Neuromodulation 16(2):125–141, 2013 23441988

Rasmussen BK: Epidemiology and socio-economic impact of headache. Cephalalgia 19 (suppl 25):20–23, 1999 10668114

Rasmussen BK, Jensen R, Schroll M, et al: Epidemiology of headache in a general population—a prevalence study. J Clin Epidemiol 44(11):1147–1157, 1991 1941010

Ratcliffe GE, Enns MW, Belik S-L, et al: Chronic pain conditions and suicidal ideation and suicide attempts: an epidemiologic perspective. Clin J Pain 24(3):204–210, 2008 18287825

Saper JR, Dodick D, Gladstone JP: Management of chronic daily headache: challenges in clinical practice. Headache 45 (suppl 1):S74–S85, 2005 15833093

Teckchandani S, Barad M: Treatment strategies for the opioid-dependent patient. Curr Pain Headache Rep 21(11):45, 2017 28932964

Vázquez-Delgado E, Cascos-Romero J, Gay-Escoda C: Myofascial pain associated to trigger points: a literature review part 2: differential diagnosis and treatment. Med Oral Patol Oral Cir Bucal 15(4):e639–e643, 2010 20173729

Wolfe F, Clauw DJ, Fitzcharles MA, et al: The American College of Rheumatology preliminary diagnostic criteria for fibromyalgia and measurement of symptom severity. Arthritis Care Res (Hoboken) 62(5):600–610, 2010 20461783

World Health Organization: Headache disorders. Geneva, Switzerland, World Health Organization, 8 April 2016. Available at: https://www.who.int/news-room/fact-sheets/detail/headache-disorders. Accessed June 12, 2019.

CHAPTER 24

Insomnia

Karl Doghramji, M.D.

Insomnia is one of the most commonly encountered conditions in clinical settings. It is accompanied by a variety of psychiatric, medical, and neurological conditions. Identification of these comorbidities is the first step in the effective management of insomnia. Once comorbidities are identified, treatment can be specifically tailored to the patient.

Prevalence

Large community-based demographic studies indicate that insomnia is one of the most commonly encountered maladies in clinical medicine; after pain, it represents the second most commonly expressed complaint (Mahowald et al. 1997). An astounding 35% of the adult population experiences insomnia during the course of a single year (Mellinger et al. 1985), and half of those who experience insomnia report the problem as severe. Studies also indicate that 20% of adults are dissatisfied with their sleep or take medication for sleeping difficulties (Ohayon 1996). Insomnia is an emerging problem in children and adolescents; an estimated 4% of children complain of insomnia at least three times weekly over the course of a year (Zhang et al. 2009). The risk of insomnia is greatest in certain populations (e.g., persons with poor mental and physical health; those who misuse recreational substances), further compounding the impairments associated with these conditions. Other at-risk populations include women, in whom the prevalence of insomnia peaks during pregnancy and the perimenopausal and postmenopausal years; seniors, in whom insomnia afflicts more than one-third of the population ages 65 years and older; individuals with nontraditional occupational schedules, such as shift workers; individuals of lower socioeconomic status; divorced, widowed, or single individuals; and people who live in settings that are not conducive to sound sleep, such as noisy environments (Doghramji et al. 2009).

Impact

Compared with individuals without sleep complaints, patients with insomnia report greater difficulty in coping with and accomplishing tasks, complain of greater impairment in mood, and experience greater breaches in interpersonal relationships and psychosocial upheaval. They also exhibit greater cognitive deficits, especially when responding to challenging reaction time tasks (Ancoli-Israel and Roth 1999; Espie et al. 2000; Hauri 1997). Insomnia is also associated with heightened rates of work-related impairment and absenteeism (Kuppermann et al. 1995). Emerging evidence links persistent insomnia to a heightened risk of development of new cardiovascular and metabolic abnormalities, such as hypertension, heart failure, and glucose intolerance (Lanfranchi et al. 2009; Laugsand et al. 2014; Vgontzas et al. 2009a, 2009b). Longitudinal studies link insomnia to premature mortality. A community-based prospective cohort study of 3,430 adult subjects, with a median follow-up period of nearly 16 years, reported that the relative risk for all-cause death in adults with insomnia was considerably elevated (Chien et al. 2010). Mortality rose in proportion to the severity of the disorder; in severe insomnia, the relative risk was 1.70.

Pathophysiology

Some of the earliest attempts to explain the causes of insomnia can be attributed to Sigmund Freud, who suggested that insomnia represents a failure of dream work (Freud 1900/1986). Freud hypothesized that successful dream work is necessary for the preservation of sleep; however, in insomnia, unconscious wishes that are aversive and conflict-laden become activated. Dream work was viewed to be unsuccessful because of the intensity of the anxiety caused by the underlying conflict, resulting in the awakening of the dreamer and the complaint of insomnia.

Later psychological formulations focusing on cognitive and behavioral principles theorized that patients with insomnia are predisposed to have an exaggerated emotional reaction to everyday stressors, requiring less activation to achieve high levels of arousal, which, in turn, leads to disturbed sleep. Insomniac individuals also harbor distorted beliefs about sleep itself, including the belief that poor sleep is inevitable and that the lack of a full night's sleep will inevitably lead to disastrous health consequences. These beliefs, in turn, can induce further emotional and cognitive arousal. Such catastrophizing is exacerbated by many nights of poor sleep, which can foment cognitive rumination and worry about not falling asleep and about the potential for disastrous next-day consequences of sleeplessness. Therefore, such a cycle of apprehension and worry can perpetuate insomnia and make future sleep even less likely. Individuals with insomnia are prone to excessive cognitive monitoring at bedtime, which can further perpetuate insomnia; these individuals carefully monitor mental and bodily sensations as well as external cues such as the bedroom clock and environmental noises (Yang et al. 2006). The repeated experience of poor sleep also promotes an association between sleeplessness and both presleep activities and the sleep setting. Once these connections are established, the bedtime rituals and environment become contextual cues for arousal rather than for sleep.

In parallel with technological refinements in the assessment of neurophysiological function, research into sleep has focused on the state of physiological and psychological hyperarousal, or an overly active arousal system, during both sleep and wakefulness. Findings from sleep electroencephalography research now indicate that in comparison with healthy control subjects, individuals with chronic insomnia show reductions in low-frequency delta power (typical of deep, non–rapid eye movement [NREM] sleep) across the night, particularly during the first part of the night, and increases in high-frequency beta power across the entire night (Merica et al. 1998). Single-photon emission computed tomography (SPECT) and positron emission tomography (PET) scans reveal increases in global glucose metabolic rates during both wakefulness and sleep in insomniac patients compared with healthy control subjects. In addition, PET scans show that the usual sleep-related decline in metabolism in brain stem arousal centers is attenuated in patients with insomnia compared with healthy subjects (Nofzinger et al. 2004). Studies suggest that the changes noted in the central nervous system are paralleled throughout peripheral physiological and metabolic systems. In comparison with healthy subjects, people with insomnia exhibit an increase in heart rate, a decrease in beat-to-beat variability (Bonnet and Arand 1998), and an increase in whole-body metabolic rate (Bonnet and Arand 1998).

Research over the past decade has implicated the circadian system in the genesis of insomnia, pointing to irregularities in the circadian control of sleep/wakefulness, melatonin, cortisol, core body temperature, and, presumably, other endogenous rhythms. A mutation in the human clock gene *Per2* is associated with advanced sleep phase disorder, and a functional polymorphism in *Per3* is associated with delayed sleep phase disorder. Advanced sleep phase disorder and delayed sleep phase disorder are associated with terminal and initiation insomnia, respectively (Hamet and Tremblay 2006).

Diagnosis

Evolving views regarding insomnia are reflected in the fifth edition of the *Diagnostic and Statistical Manual of Mental Disorders* (DSM-5; American Psychiatric Association 2013) (Table 24–1). In the previous edition, DSM-IV-TR (American Psychiatric Association 2000), insomnia appeared as a diagnostic entity in four separate forms: primary insomnia; insomnia related to another mental disorder; sleep disorder due to a general medical condition, insomnia type; and substance-induced sleep disorder, insomnia type.

Insomnia has traditionally been subdivided into two broad categories: primary insomnia and secondary insomnia. Thus, insomnia was presumed to represent either an independent disorder or one that was secondary to other medical or psychiatric disorders. Inherent in this view is the notion of one-way causality.

A National Institutes of Health (2005) State of the Science Conference challenged the primary/secondary distinction in light of observations that psychiatric, medical, and other sleep disorders and insomnia can assume potentially independent, yet mutually interactive, temporal courses. The conference recommended use of the term *comorbid insomnia* for those instances in which insomnia occurs in the context of other medical and psychiatric disorders. In addition, Edinger et al. (2004) used goodness-of-fit ratings with insomnia patients and concluded that the category of primary in-

---

TABLE 24–1.   **DSM-5 diagnostic criteria for insomnia disorder**

A. A predominant complaint of dissatisfaction with sleep quantity or quality, associated with one (or more) of the following symptoms:

    1. Difficulty initiating sleep. (In children, this may manifest as difficulty initiating sleep without caregiver intervention.)

    2. Difficulty maintaining sleep, characterized by frequent awakenings or problems returning to sleep after awakenings. (In children, this may manifest as difficulty returning to sleep without caregiver intervention.)

    3. Early-morning awakening with inability to return to sleep.

B. The sleep disturbance causes clinically significant distress or impairment in social, occupational, educational, academic, behavioral, or other important areas of functioning.

C. The sleep difficulty occurs at least 3 nights per week.

D. The sleep difficulty is present for at least 3 months.

E. The sleep difficulty occurs despite adequate opportunity for sleep.

F. The insomnia is not better explained by and does not occur exclusively during the course of another sleep-wake disorder (e.g., narcolepsy, a breathing-related sleep disorder, a circadian rhythm sleep-wake disorder, a parasomnia).

G. The insomnia is not attributable to the physiological effects of a substance (e.g., a drug of abuse, a medication).

H. Coexisting mental disorders and medical conditions do not adequately explain the predominant complaint of insomnia.

Specify if:

With non–sleep disorder mental comorbidity, including substance use disorders

With other medical comorbidity

With other sleep disorder

Coding note: The code 307.42 (F51.01) applies to all three specifiers. Code also the relevant associated mental disorder, medical condition, or other sleep disorder immediately after the code for insomnia disorder in order to indicate the association.

Specify if:

Episodic: Symptoms last at least 1 month but less than 3 months.

Persistent: Symptoms last 3 months or longer.

Recurrent: Two (or more) episodes within the space of 1 year.

Note: Acute and short-term insomnia (i.e., symptoms lasting less than 3 months but otherwise meeting all criteria with regard to frequency, intensity, distress, and/or impairment) should be coded as an other specified insomnia disorder.

Source.   Reprinted from American Psychiatric Association: *Diagnostic and Statistical Manual of Mental Disorders,* 5th Edition, Arlington, VA, American Psychiatric Association, 2013, pp. 362–363. Copyright © 2013, American Psychiatric Association. Used with permission.

---

somnia has marginal reliability and validity. These views are reflected in DSM-5, in which the diagnosis of primary insomnia is eliminated in favor of *insomnia disorder,* and secondary insomnia conditions are eliminated altogether in favor of insomnia disorder with concurrent specification of clinically comorbid medical and psychiatric conditions. Other criteria for DSM-5 insomnia disorder (see Table 24–1) include minimum frequency and duration criteria. Finally, the provision of an "adequate opportunity for sleep" is important in distinguishing insomnia from sleep deprivation or restriction. In sleep deprivation/restriction, sleep is curtailed because of externally induced or self-imposed reductions in the opportunity for sleep, whereas in insomnia, sleep is impaired in quality or quantity despite adequate opportunity to obtain it.

Medical Comorbidities

Population studies suggest that comorbid medical and psychiatric conditions abound in insomnia patients; around 40% of these comorbid conditions fall within the realm of psychiatric disorders (excluding insomnia disorder), the most common of which are mood, anxiety, and substance use disorders (Ford and Kamerow 1989; Taylor et al. 2007). Notably, however, a significant proportion of persons with insomnia have nonpsychiatric comorbidities. Community-based studies of people with insomnia indicate that medical comorbidities abound in this population. In a survey of 772 adults ages 20–98 years, individuals with chronic insomnia reported more of the following than did those without insomnia: heart disease (21.9% vs. 9.5%), high blood pressure (43.1% vs. 18.7%), neurological disease (7.3% vs. 1.2%), breathing problems (24.8% vs. 5.7%), urinary problems (19.7% vs. 9.5%), chronic pain (50.4% vs. 18.2%), and gastrointestinal problems (33.6% vs. 9.2%) (Taylor et al. 2007). Conversely, people with the following medical problems reported more chronic insomnia than did people without those medical problems: heart disease (44.1% vs. 22.8%), cancer (41.4% vs. 24.6%), high blood pressure (44.0% vs. 19.3%), neurological disease (66.7% vs. 24.3%), breathing problems (59.6% vs. 21.4%), urinary problems (41.5% vs. 23.3%), chronic pain (48.6% vs. 17.2%), and gastrointestinal problems (55.4% vs. 20.0%).

Budhiraja et al. (2011) surveyed 3,282 adults ages 18–65 years, a subset of whom underwent polysomnography, and determined that insomnia was 2.2 times as likely to occur in individuals with preexisting medical disorders as in those without such disorders. These medical disorders included heart disease, hypertension, diabetes, stomach ulcers, arthritis, migraine, asthma, chronic obstructive pulmonary disease, neurological problems, and menstrual problems. The prevalence of insomnia increased as the number of comorbid medical conditions increased (Budhiraja et al. 2011). Table 24–2 lists some of the medical disorders that are commonly comorbid with insomnia disorders, as well as their defining symptoms (Doghramji et al. 2009).

Insomnia can be caused by a variety of medications, including anticholinergics, antihypertensives, antineoplastics, central nervous system stimulants, hormones, antidepressants, and antipsychotics. Withdrawal from sedating agents may also result in insomnia (Doghramji and Doghramji 2006; Doghramji and Jangro 2016).

Evaluation of Medical Comorbidities

Because medical and psychiatric comorbidities are so common in people with insomnia, a rational approach to the evaluation of insomnia prioritizes the identification of these comorbid conditions so that those presumed to contribute to the insomnia disorder can be directly managed. Key elements of this evaluation include a systematically derived history, a physical examination, and judicious use of diagnostic screening instruments and symptom rating scales.

TABLE 24–2. **Hallmark symptoms of nonpsychiatric conditions commonly comorbid with insomnia disorder**

Disorder	Hallmark symptoms
Impaired sleep hygiene	Violation of one or more of the key recommendations for optimal sleep hygiene
Restless legs syndrome	Irresistible urge to move the extremities Limb paresthesias Onset of symptoms during periods of rest and in the evening or at bedtime Relief of symptoms with movement
Periodic limb movement disorder	Repetitive involuntary movements of the extremities during sleep or just prior to falling asleep
Obstructive sleep apnea	Snoring Breathing pauses during sleep Choking Gasping Morning dry mouth
Chronic obstructive pulmonary disease	Dyspnea on exertion
Heart failure	Paroxysmal nocturnal dyspnea Orthopnea
Gastroesophageal reflux	Epigastric pain or burning Laryngospasm Acid taste in mouth Sudden nocturnal awakenings
Prostatic hypertrophy	Nocturia
Nocturnal seizures	Thrashing in bed Loss of bladder or bowel control
Rapid eye movement sleep behavior disorder	Repeated episodes of arousal during sleep with vocalization or complex motor behaviors, often with vivid dreaming
Delayed sleep phase disorder	Inability to fall asleep at desired time Inability to awaken at desired time
Advanced sleep phase disorder	Inability to stay awake until the desired bedtime Inability to remain asleep until the desired awakening time
Shift work disorder	Excessive sleepiness or insomnia associated with a recurring work schedule that overlaps with the usual time for sleep

Source. Adapted from Table 2 (p. 446) in Doghramji K, Grewal R, Markov D: "Evaluation and Management of Insomnia in the Psychiatric Setting." *Focus: The Journal of Lifelong Learning in Psychiatry* 7(4):441–454, 2009. Copyright © 2009, American Psychiatric Association. Used with permission.

History

Table 24–3 outlines the essential elements of the history for evaluation of insomnia (Doghramji et al. 2009).

The nocturnal pattern of insomnia can help distinguish among various diagnostic possibilities; for example, delayed sleep phase disorder is characterized by difficulty falling asleep, whereas advanced sleep phase disorder is characterized by early bedtimes and early-morning awakenings. Awareness of the nocturnal pattern of insomnia can also be useful in determining treatment choice, because longer-acting hypnotic agents may be better suited for midnocturnal awakenings and early-morning insomnia.

The duration and frequency of symptoms are important for identifying the degree of impairment. Insomnias of longer duration and greater frequency are thought to have a greater impact on daytime functioning and therefore may require earlier and more aggressive treatment. Symptom inventories can assist in dimensional assessment or quantification of the severity of insomnia; although many instruments are available, the Insomnia Severity Index (ISI; Bastien et al. 2001) is one of the few that have been subjected to empirical validation. The ISI takes into account subjective symptoms and consequences of insomnia and the degree of concern or distress caused by the disturbance. It is also a useful clinical and research tool for measuring treatment response and outcome.

Precipitants of the insomnia complaint can identify etiology and guide management. Common precipitants include job loss, shift work or travel across time zones, relationship breakups or bereavement, onset of medical and psychiatric illness, and introduction of new medications or changes in dosages and times of administration of existing medications. Following the onset of insomnia, perpetuating factors can transform it into a chronic disorder. Such factors include poor sleep hygiene and anticipatory anxiety experienced around bedtime. Similarly, patients' attitudes toward their insomnia can have an important influence on their ability to sleep. In particular, the presence of dysfunctional beliefs and attitudes about sleep, as well as of sleep-related anxiety that builds as bedtime approaches and persists during bedtime hours, provides the clinician with important insights into the role these processes play in perpetuating or exacerbating the insomnia. Therefore, information should be solicited about the dysfunctional cognitions of the insomniac patient (e.g., catastrophic attributions regarding the effects of insomnia), the time of day that the person first begins to worry about sleep, and the state of mind of the person during time awake during the night (Yang et al. 2006).

An assessment of daytime symptoms is also useful in understanding the impact of insomnia on the individual's functioning. Reduction in daytime impairment is an important measure of treatment efficacy. Sleep-related habits and the behaviors in which the patient engages during the few hours prior to bedtime, during bedtime hours, and just after morning awakening can cause or significantly intensify existing insomnia. Although these factors are seldom the sole cause of an insomnia complaint, ignorance of or inattention to these habits and behaviors can lead to failure in other treatment modalities.

Daytime habits and behaviors that can adversely affect nocturnal sleep include engaging in intense exercise and taxing work-related activities too close to bedtime, and eating meals and ingesting excessive fluids within 2–3 hours of bedtime (Stepanski

TABLE 24–3.   **Essential elements of the sleep-wake history in the evaluation of insomnia**

1. Nature of the complaint of insomnia
   a. Nocturnal pattern (initial, middle, terminal)
   b. Duration (acute, long term)
   c. Frequency (nightly, weekly, monthly, etc.)
   d. Precipitants (e.g., illnesses, shift work, medications, substances)
   e. Perpetuating factors (e.g., learned/conditioned response, hyperarousal, sleep hygiene habits)
2. Daytime symptoms
   a. Fatigue
   b. Irritability
   c. Anergia
   d. Memory impairment
   e. Mental slowing
3. Habits and behaviors related to sleep and the sleep environment that aggravate insomnia
   a. Caffeine and alcohol prior to bedtime
   b. Nicotine (both smoking and cessation)
   c. Large meals or excessive fluid intake within 3 hours of bedtime
   d. Exercising within 3 hours of bedtime
   e. Using the bed for nonsleep activities (work, telephone, Internet)
   f. Staying in bed while awake for extended periods of time
   g. Activating behaviors up to the point of bedtime
   h. Excessive worrying at bedtime
   i. Clock watching prior to sleep onset or during nocturnal awakenings
   j. Exposure to bright light prior to bedtime or during awakenings
   k. Keeping the bedroom too hot or too cold
   l. Noise
   m. Behaviors of a bed partner (e.g., snoring, leg movements)
4. Daytime habits and behaviors that aggravate insomnia
   a. Prolonged bed rest, inactivity, and excessive napping
   b. Insufficient light exposure
   c. Frequent travel and shift work
5. Patterns of sleep and wakefulness
   a. Bedtime
   b. Sleep latency (time to fall asleep after lights out)
   c. Nocturnal awakenings (number and duration)
   d. Time of final morning awakening
   e. Rising time (i.e., time out of bed)
   f. Number, time, and duration of daytime naps
   g. Daytime symptoms, including levels of sleepiness and fatigue over the course of the day

and Wyatt 2003). Long periods of daytime bed rest, inactivity, and excessive napping can foment circadian rhythm disturbances and aggravate insomnia. Exposure to bright light can be helpful in establishing circadian cycling—and, conversely, lack of sufficient light exposure during the morning hours can disrupt sleep timing. Frequent travel and shift work also can disrupt sleep and contribute to both insomnia and daytime sleepiness. It is useful to be aware of the patient's preferred social and occupational activities, because this information can be helpful in devising a daily structure that promotes consistent sleep scheduling.

Patterns of sleep and wakefulness should be clarified during the initial and follow-up visits. These patterns can also be assessed by using patient-completed sleep logs or diaries that track sleep-wake patterns over time. Notably, sleep logs and diaries are particularly valuable and may be more useful than subjective summaries in documenting clinically relevant patterns. People with insomnia tend to underestimate their total sleep time and to overestimate their sleep onset latency (i.e., how long it takes them to fall asleep), possibly because of a preferential bias toward recalling particularly bad nights of insomnia that may not reflect the average longitudinal course of their complaints (Carskadon et al. 1976).

Ideally, individuals should retire to and emerge from bed at consistent times every day, including on weekends. The time spent in bed between retiring and falling asleep should preferably be less than 20 minutes, and individuals should get out of bed soon after waking up in the morning. In people with healthy sleep, nighttime awakenings are typically limited to one or two, and time spent in bed following awakening is kept to a minimum (i.e., less than 15 minutes). Individuals with insomnia can show considerable divergence from these norms, and patterns may emerge that suggest specific underlying causes of insomnia that can help guide treatment. It is useful to ascertain details for each of these sleep schedule parameters, not only over an "average" day but also over sequential days, because such a temporal record may demonstrate variability in sleep patterns over time that can, in turn, contribute to poor sleep. An assessment of variability among workdays or schooldays, weekends, and vacations can also be useful. Insomniac patients characteristically do not rigorously maintain sleep-wake schedules, and introducing such regularity into their lives is one of the primary elements of sleep hygiene education and other cognitive-behavioral techniques.

Clinicians should specifically question patients about hallmark symptoms of the various disorders, as described in Table 24–2. For example, the STOP-Bang Scoring Model (Chung et al. 2008) is a validated inventory that succinctly summarizes the hallmark symptoms (including historical findings) of obstructive sleep apnea (OSA) and can be used to identify individuals who are at high risk for the disorder. A "Yes" answer to three or more questions denotes a high risk for OSA. Collateral information from bed partners can be useful in obtaining details about sleep behaviors of which the patient may not be aware, such as snoring, breathing pauses during sleep, or limb movements, as well as the patient's daily habits, such as frequent napping. The history should include information on past medical illnesses and procedures, prescribed medications, and substance use. Family history is relevant because some sleep disorders can have a hereditary component; for example, 50% of patients with primary restless legs syndrome (RLS) have a positive family history (Montplaisir et al. 2005). A social and occupational history is likewise important, because life experiences can contribute to irregular sleep-wake habits.

Physical Examination

Although a physical examination is not routinely performed in psychiatric practice, it is essential in the evaluation of insomnia. A neck circumference of 16 inches or greater in women and 17 inches or greater in men is associated with an increased risk for OSA (Millman et al. 1995), as is obesity with fat distribution around the neck or midriff. Other contributors to OSA include nasal obstruction, mandibular hypoplasia, retrognathia, tonsillar hyperplasia, enlarged tongue, elongated and edematous uvula and soft palate, diminished pharyngeal patency, and redundant pharyngeal mucosa (American Academy of Sleep Medicine 2014). The Mallampati Airway Classification (Nuckton et al. 2006) is used in assessing pharyngeal patency. During assessment, the patient is asked to open his or her mouth as wide as possible, while protruding the tongue as far as possible. The patient is instructed to refrain from emitting sounds during the assessment. On the basis of the structures visible in the oropharynx with maximal mouth opening, the patient is assigned a Mallampati score of I through IV, as follows: Class I: soft palate and entire uvula visible; Class II: soft palate and portion of uvula visible; Class III: soft palate visible (may include base of uvula); Class IV: soft palate not visible. On average, for every 1-point increase in the Mallampati score, the odds of having OSA increases more than twofold (Nuckton et al. 2006).

The chest should be examined for expiratory wheezes and kyphoscoliosis, conditions that are indicative of asthma and restrictive lung disease, respectively, and can be associated with the complaint of insomnia. Signs of heart failure, such as rales and peripheral edema, should be noted; heart failure can cause abnormalities of breathing during sleep, which in turn can be associated with the complaint of frequent nocturnal awakenings and unrefreshing sleep. A basic neurological examination can determine whether a neurological disorder is present; for example, evidence of increased resting muscle tone, cogwheel rigidity, and tremor can indicate the presence of Parkinson's disease. A mental status examination should be performed if a psychiatric disorder is suspected (Vaughn and O'Neill 2005).

Diagnostic Testing

The utility of serum laboratory tests in the evaluation of insomnia has not been systematically explored. It seems reasonable to consider ordering general serum laboratory tests, including thyroid function studies, if they have not been performed in the preceding 6 months to 1 year. RLS is more common in iron-deficient states and conditions associated with iron deficiency, such as pregnancy and anemia (Sun et al. 1998). The level of serum ferritin, even in the absence of anemia, is inversely correlated with severity of RLS symptoms, and a level of 50 µg/L or lower predicts positive response in reduction of RLS symptoms following iron supplementation.

Actigraphy is an ambulatory technology that uses small, wristwatch-like devices to record movement. It assumes that lack of movement is equivalent to sleep and therefore is not useful for measuring exact sleep times. However, it can be useful for the assessment of sleep-wake patterns when such information is not reliably available by other means (e.g., sleep logs). Actigraphy also can be appropriate for use in documenting changes in sleep patterns over prolonged periods—information that is important in the diagnosis of circadian rhythm disorders. Finally, this technology can be used in the assessment of treatment adherence (e.g., by showing whether a person with insomnia is following sleep hygiene recommendations, such as curtailing time in bed and regularizing wake-up times) and of treatment efficacy (e.g., by showing changes in insomnia patterns following behavioral treatment) (Morgenthaler et al. 2007). A variety of consumer sleep monitors are available (e.g., Fitbit, Sleeptracker), although these devices have not yet been validated for use in medical settings (Russo et al. 2015).

Polysomnography is the technique of monitoring multiple physiological measures during sleep, including brain waves, eye movements, heart rate, respirations, oxyhemoglobin saturation, and muscle tone and activity. Video recording identifies abnormal movements during sleep. This testing is typically performed in a sleep laboratory, although home testing is gaining popularity. Referral for polysomnography is appropriate if the insomnia evaluation raises suspicion for OSA, periodic limb movement disorder (PLMD), parasomnias such as rapid eye movement (REM) sleep behavior disorder, or paroxysmal arousals or other sleep disruptions thought to be seizure related. Consultation with a sleep medicine specialist may be helpful if the office-based evaluation is not fruitful or if the patient does not respond as expected to treatment of the presumed disorder.

Treatment

Treatment of specific medical comorbidities is the first step in the management of insomnia. Treatment options for selected comorbid medical conditions seen with insomnia are shown in Table 24–4. Various studies have indicated that management of these comorbidities diminishes insomnia burden. For example, one study found that treatment of comorbid OSA with positive airway pressure devices resulted in a significant reduction of insomnia symptoms in 78.6% (44 of 56) patients (Mendes and dos Santos 2015). On the other hand, direct management of insomnia with sedatives may impair respiration during sleep in sleep-related breathing disorders.

Treatment of RLS with dopaminergic agents has been associated with insomnia reduction (Estivill and de la Fuente 1999). Insomnia can be directly managed with hypnotic medications, but this approach runs the risk of introducing safety concerns, because many patients with insomnia are already taking multiple medications or have complex cardiopulmonary issues that may be intensified by sedating agents. Although cognitive-behavioral therapy does have a safety advantage over medications, it may be less effective when complex medical factors are fueling a patient's insomnia.

Disturbed sleep is a common symptom of gastroesophageal reflux, possibly related to the finding that esophageal clearance of refluxate is markedly prolonged during sleep and requires an arousal for termination of the reflux episode. Disturbed sleep in the form of arousals and awakenings is thought to serve a protective function for the esophagus because it facilitates esophageal acid clearance; however, it is also associated with insomnia and daytime fatigue (Dickman et al. 2007). In fact, patients with primary sleep disorders can exhibit prominent nocturnal acid reflux without symptoms of daytime acid reflux (Herdman et al. 2013). Treatment of insomnia directly in the gastroesophageal reflux patient can result in a reduction of the arousal response to nocturnal acid exposure, increased esophageal acid exposure, and increased risk for complicated disease (Gagliardi et al. 2009).

TABLE 24–4. **Treatment options for selected medical comorbidities in insomnia disorder**

Obstructive sleep apnea
Weight loss
Avoidance of CNS suppressants
Continuous positive airway pressure
Oral appliances
Upper airway surgery
Body positioning appliances

Restless legs syndrome
Alpha-2 delta ligands
Dopaminergic agents

Gastroesophageal reflux
Proton pump inhibitors
H$_2$-receptor blockers

Shift work disorder
Bedtime melatonin
Judicious use of caffeine
Wake-promoting agents prior to night shift
Bright light therapy

Medication-induced insomnia
Dosage alteration
Change in medication administration time
Medication change

Note. CNS=central nervous system.

Conclusion

When confronted with a clinical complaint of insomnia, clinicians should adhere to the following guidelines:

1. Conduct a systematic evaluation to search for comorbidities.
2. Perform physical and mental status examinations.
3. Use instruments such as sleep logs and insomnia severity scales to establish the diagnosis and to monitor treatment.
4. Order diagnostic studies such as blood tests and polysomnography when the office-based evaluation is inconclusive.
5. Whenever possible, treat medical and psychiatric comorbidities first, including with cognitive-behavioral therapy.

References

American Academy of Sleep Medicine: International Classification of Sleep Disorders: A Diagnostic and Coding Manual, 3rd Edition. Darien, IL, American Academy of Sleep Medicine, 2014
American Psychiatric Association: Diagnostic and Statistical Manual of Mental Disorders, 4th Edition. Washington, DC, American Psychiatric Association, 1994
American Psychiatric Association: Diagnostic and Statistical Manual of Mental Disorders, 4th Edition, Text Revision. Washington, DC, American Psychiatric Association, 2000
American Psychiatric Association: Diagnostic and Statistical Manual of Mental Disorders, 5th Edition. Arlington, VA, American Psychiatric Association, 2013

Ancoli-Israel S, Roth T: Characteristics of insomnia in the United States: results of the 1991 National Sleep Foundation Survey, I. Sleep 22 (suppl 2):S347–S353, 1999 10394606

Bastien CH, Vallières A, Morin CM: Validation of the Insomnia Severity Index as an outcome measure for insomnia research. Sleep Med 2(4):297–307, 2001 11438246

Bonnet MH, Arand DL: Heart rate variability in insomniacs and matched normal sleepers. Psychosom Med 60(5):610–615, 1998 9773766

Bonnet MH, Arand DL: Hyperarousal and insomnia: state of the science. Sleep Med Rev 14(1):9–15, 2010 19640748

Budhiraja R, Roth T, Hudgel DW, et al: Prevalence and polysomnographic correlates of insomnia comorbid with medical disorders. Sleep (Basel) 34(7):859–867, 2011 21731135

Carskadon MA, Dement WC, Mitler MM, et al: Self-reports versus sleep laboratory findings in 122 drug-free subjects with complaints of chronic insomnia. Am J Psychiatry 133(12):1382–1388, 1976 185919

Chien KL, Chen PC, Hsu HC, et al: Habitual sleep duration and insomnia and the risk of cardiovascular events and all-cause death: report from a community-based cohort. Sleep 33(2):177–184, 2010 20175401

Chung F, Yegneswaran B, Liao P, et al: STOP questionnaire: a tool to screen patients for obstructive sleep apnea. Anesthesiology 108(5):812–821, 2008 18431116

Dickman R, Green C, Fass SS, et al: Relationships between sleep quality and pH monitoring findings in persons with gastroesophageal reflux disease. J Clin Sleep Med 3(5):505–513, 2007 17803014

Doghramji K, Doghramji P: Clinical Management of Insomnia. West Islip, NY, Professional Communications, 2006

Doghramji K, Jangro WC: Adverse effects of psychotropic medications on sleep. Sleep Med Clin 11(4):503–514, 2016 28118873

Doghramji K, Grewal R, Markov D: Evaluation and management of insomnia in the psychiatric setting. Focus: The Journal of Lifelong Learning in Psychiatry 7(4):441–454, 2009. Available at: https://doi.org/10.1176/foc.7.4.foc441. Accessed May 10, 2019.

Edinger JD, Bonnet MH, Bootzin RR, et al: Derivation of research diagnostic criteria for insomnia: report of an American Academy of Sleep Medicine Work Group. Sleep 27(8):1567–1596, 2004 15683149

Espie CA, Inglis SJ, Harvey L, et al: Insomniacs' attributions. psychometric properties of the dysfunctional beliefs and attitudes about sleep scale and the sleep disturbance questionnaire. J Psychosom Res 48(2):141–148, 2000 10719130

Estivill E, de la Fuente V: The efficacy of ropinirole in the treatment of chronic insomnia secondary to restless legs syndrome: polysomnography data. Rev Neurol 29(9):805–807, 1999 10696651

Ford DE, Kamerow DB: Epidemiologic study of sleep disturbances and psychiatric disorders. An opportunity for prevention? JAMA 262(11):1479–1484, 1989 2769898

Freud S: The interpretation of dreams (1900), in The Standard Edition of the Complete Psychological Works of Sigmund Freud, Vols 4 and 5. Translated and edited by Strachey J. London, Hogarth Press, 1986, pp 1–715

Gagliardi GS, Shah AP, Goldstein M, et al: Effect of zolpidem on the sleep arousal response to nocturnal esophageal acid exposure. Clin Gastroenterol Hepatol 7(9):948–952, 2009 19426833

Hamet P, Tremblay J: Genetics of the sleep-wake cycle and its disorders. Metabolism 55 (10 suppl 2):S7–S12, 2006 16979429

Hauri PJ: Can we mix behavioral therapy with hypnotics when treating insomniacs? Sleep 20(12):1111–1118, 1997 9493920

Herdman C, Marzio DH, Shah P, et al: Sleep disorders and the prevalence of asymptomatic nocturnal acid and non-acid reflux. Ann Gastroenterol 26(3):220–225, 2013 24714269

Kuppermann M, Lubeck DP, Mazonson PD, et al: Sleep problems and their correlates in a working population. J Gen Intern Med 10(1):25–32, 1995 7699483

Lanfranchi PA, Pennestri MH, Fradette L, et al: Nighttime blood pressure in normotensive subjects with chronic insomnia: implications for cardiovascular risk. Sleep 32(6):760–766, 2009 19544752

Laugsand LE, Strand LB, Platou C, et al: Insomnia and the risk of incident heart failure: a population study. Eur Heart J 35(21):1382–1393, 2014 23462728

Mahowald MW, Kader G, Schenck CH: Clinical categories of sleep disorders I. Academy of Neurology CONTINUUM: Lifelong Learning in Neurology 3(4):35–65, 1997. Available at: https://journals.lww.com/continuum/toc/1997/03040. Accessed May 10, 2019.

Mellinger GD, Balter MB, Uhlenhuth EH: Insomnia and its treatment. Prevalence and correlates. Arch Gen Psychiatry 42(3):225–232, 1985 2858188

Mendes MS, dos Santos JM: Insomnia as an expression of obstructive sleep apnea syndrome—the effect of treatment with nocturnal ventilatory support. Rev Port Pneumol (2006) 21(4):203–208, 2015 25926264

Merica H, Blois R, Gaillard JM: Spectral characteristics of sleep EEG in chronic insomnia. Eur J Neurosci 10(5):1826–1834, 1998 9751153

Millman RP, Carlisle CC, McGarvey ST, et al: Body fat distribution and sleep apnea severity in women. Chest 107(2):362–366, 1995 7842762

Montplaisir J, Allen RP, Walters AS, Ferini-Strambi L: Restless legs syndrome and periodic limb movements during sleep, in Principles and Practice of Sleep Medicine, 4th Edition. Edited by Kryger MH, Roth T, Dement WC. Philadelphia, PA, Elsevier/Saunders, 2005, pp 839–852

Morgenthaler T, Alessi C, Friedman L, et al: Practice parameters for the use of actigraphy in the assessment of sleep and sleep disorders: an update for 2007. Sleep 30(4):519–529, 2007 17520797

National Institutes of Health: National Institutes of Health state of the science conference statement on manifestations and management of chronic insomnia in adults, June 13–15, 2005. Sleep 28(9):1049–1057, 2005 16268373

Nofzinger EA, Buysse DJ, Germain A, et al: Functional neuroimaging evidence for hyperarousal in insomnia. Am J Psychiatry 161(11):2126–2128, 2004 15514418

Nuckton TJ, Glidden DV, Browner WS, et al: Physical examination: Mallampati score as an independent predictor of obstructive sleep apnea. Sleep 29(7):903–908, 2006 16895257

Ohayon M: Epidemiological study on insomnia in the general population. Sleep 19 (3 suppl):S7–S15, 1996 8723370

Russo K, Goparaju B, Bianchi MT: Consumer sleep monitors: is there a baby in the bathwater? Nat Sci Sleep 7:147–157, 2015 26604847

Stepanski EJ, Wyatt JK: Use of sleep hygiene in the treatment of insomnia. Sleep Med Rev 7(3):215–225, 2003 12927121

Sun ER, Chen CA, Ho G, et al: Iron and the restless legs syndrome. Sleep 21(4):371–377, 1998 9646381

Taylor DJ, Mallory LJ, Lichstein KL, et al: Comorbidity of chronic insomnia with medical problems. Sleep 30(2):213–218, 2007 17326547

Vaughn BV, O'Neill FD: Cardinal manifestations of sleep disorders, in Principles and Practice of Sleep Medicine, 4th Edition. Edited by Kryger MH, Roth T, Dement WC. Philadelphia, PA, Elsevier/Saunders, 2005, pp 594–601

Vgontzas AN, Liao D, Bixler EO, et al: Insomnia with objective short sleep duration is associated with a high risk for hypertension. Sleep 32(4):491–497, 2009a 19413143

Vgontzas AN, Liao D, Pejovic S, et al: Insomnia with objective short sleep duration is associated with type 2 diabetes: a population-based study. Diabetes Care 32(11):1980–1985, 2009b 19641160

Yang CM, Spielman AJ, Glovinsky P: Nonpharmacologic strategies in the management of insomnia. Psychiatr Clin North Am 29(4):895–919, 2006 17118274

Zhang J, Li AM, Kong AP, et al: A community-based study of insomnia in Hong Kong Chinese children: prevalence, risk factors and familial aggregation. Sleep Med 10(9):1040–1046, 2009 19410511

CHAPTER 25

Somatic Symptom and Related Disorders

Anna L. Dickerman, M.D.

Philip R. Muskin, M.D., M.A.

Somatic symptom and related disorders (SSRDs) are a group of psychiatric illnesses in which patients experience bodily symptoms along with associated abnormal thoughts, feelings, and behaviors that cause clinically significant distress and functional impairment. Patients with SSRDs typically first present in medical settings. They experience themselves as having a medical disorder or (in the case of one disorder) create symptoms that make them appear to have a medical disorder. SSRDs account for significant medical and psychiatric morbidity and increased costs due to greater chronicity of symptoms, increased health care utilization, and higher rates of disability. Patients with SSRDs can be among the most challenging for psychiatric and nonpsychiatric clinicians alike. Evidence-based treatments exist for these illnesses. Timely recognition and appropriate referral may significantly improve outcomes. It behooves all clinicians—in particular, those working in the medical setting, who often encounter these patients before psychiatrists do—to be familiar with these complex conditions.

This chapter and the disorders we discuss are different from others in this textbook. Unlike patients who have psychiatric disorders that may be due to a medical disorder, patients with SSRDs have symptoms that they believe indicate a medical condition despite evidence to the contrary, or they have a disproportionate response to medical symptoms. Although most patients do not wish to be ill, some of the patients with SSRDs wish to be treated as though they were ill, or at least as though they had symptoms that impair their functioning. In this chapter, we focus on the various diagnoses in the fifth edition of the *Diagnostic and Statistical Manual of Mental Disorders* (DSM-5; American Psychiatric Association 2013), along with the changes in diagnostic criteria in this new edition of DSM. We provide an overview of the different types of SSRDs, their epidemiology and pathophysiology, and treatment strategies.

Somatic Symptom and Related Disorders in DSM-5

The DSM-IV somatoform disorders underwent significant changes in DSM-5. Table 25–1 presents a summary of these changes.

There were several problematic issues with the DSM-IV criteria for SSRDs (formerly referred to as *somatoform disorders*) (American Psychiatric Association 1994). Clinicians underdiagnosed these illnesses because of confusion about terminology. The DSM-IV diagnostic criteria were particularly challenging for nonpsychiatric clinicians. Furthermore, the hallmark of somatoform disorders in DSM-IV was the absence of a medical explanation for the somatic symptoms. Requiring the absence of a medical explanation resulted in a problematic mind-body dualism that does not conform well to actual clinical experience. Conditions that are medically "unexplained" are not necessarily psychogenic in origin; for example, fibromyalgia and chronic fatigue syndrome are not considered to be psychiatric illnesses. Having a medically unexplained symptom is not in itself sufficient to warrant a psychiatric diagnosis; indeed, many patients in general medical practice have symptoms that are medically unexplained. Conversely, it is possible to have a documented medical condition and still have what could be construed as a particularly intense psychological response to physical symptoms. Patients with SSRDs *may or may not have a comorbid diagnosed medical condition.* The distinctive characteristic of these disorders has been shifted away from the somatic symptoms or their underlying etiology per se and is now focused on the maladaptive way in which the patient presents and interprets symptoms.

The terminology of SSRDs in DSM-5 reduces the number of disorders and subcategories to minimize problematic overlap and diagnostic confusion. SSRDs are defined on the basis of *positive* psychiatric symptoms rather than the *absence* of medical explanation for symptoms. Diagnosis of SSRDs no longer requires an exhaustive workup necessitating that the clinician exclude any physiologically based medical condition. The notable exceptions to this new rule are conversion disorder (functional neurological symptom disorder) and pseudocyesis. DSM-5 also eliminated the use of numerous symptom requirements that existed in the diagnostic criteria in DSM-IV, particularly for what was then known as "somatization disorder." A large body of research has shown that the relationship between somatic symptoms and psychopathology exists along a spectrum that was not adequately reflected by these symptom-count prerequisites.

The DSM-IV diagnosis of body dysmorphic disorder was moved to a new chapter on obsessive-compulsive disorder and related illnesses in DSM-5. A large body of research has established pathophysiological connections between obsessive-compulsive illness and body dysmorphia that have considerable implications for treatment. Body dysmorphic disorder is thus no longer considered an SSRD. Somatization disorder, undifferentiated somatoform disorder, hypochondriasis, and pain disorder (all diagnoses in DSM-IV) have been removed and in some cases incorporated into the

TABLE 25–1. **DSM-IV somatoform disorders and new DSM-5 somatic symptom and related disorders**

DSM-IV somatoform disorders	DSM-5 somatic symptom and related disorders
Somatization disorder Undifferentiated somatoform disorder	Somatic symptom disorder[a] (DSM-5 pp. 311–315)
Hypochondriasis	Illness anxiety disorder[b] (DSM-5 pp. 315–318)
Conversion disorder	Conversion disorder (functional neurological symptom disorder) (DSM-5 pp. 318–321)
Pain disorder	— (Removed from chapter)[c]
— Psychological factors affecting medical condition (appeared in DSM-IV chapter "Other Conditions That May Be a Focus of Clinical Attention")	Psychological factors affecting other medical conditions (DSM-5 pp. 322–324)
— Factitious disorder (appeared in DSM-IV chapter "Factitious Disorders")	Factitious disorder imposed on self (DSM-5 pp. 324–326)
— Factitious disorder by proxy (appeared in DSM-IV chapter "Criteria Sets and Axes Provided for Further Study")	Factitious disorder imposed on another (DSM-5 pp. 324–326)
Body dysmorphic disorder	— (Moved to the new chapter "Obsessive-Compulsive and Related Disorders" [DSM-5 pp. 242–247])
Somatoform disorder not otherwise specified	Other specified somatic symptom and related disorder (DSM-5 p. 327) Unspecified somatic symptom and related disorder (DSM-5 p. 327)

[a]According to DSM-5, there is not a direct correspondence between DSM-IV somatization disorder and DSM-5 somatic symptom disorder; per "Highlights of Changes From DSM-IV to DSM-5" (p. 813) in DSM-5 Appendix, "Individuals previously diagnosed with somatization disorder will usually have symptoms that meet DSM-5 criteria for somatic symptom disorder, but only if they have the maladaptive thoughts, feelings, and behaviors that define the disorder, in addition to their somatic symptoms."

[b]According to DSM-5, there is not a direct correspondence between DSM-IV hypochondriasis and DSM-5 illness anxiety disorder; per "Diagnostic Features" subsection under the DSM-5 diagnostic criteria for illness anxiety disorder (p. 315), "Most individuals with hypochondriasis are now classified as having somatic symptom disorder; however, in a minority of cases, the diagnosis of illness anxiety disorder applies instead." Clarification on the "minority of cases" for which a diagnosis of illness anxiety disorder would apply is provided in the "Highlights of Changes From DSM-IV to DSM-5" (p. 813): "Individuals who have high health anxiety *but no somatic symptoms* would receive a DSM-5 diagnosis of illness anxiety disorder (unless their health anxiety was better explained by a primary anxiety disorder, such as generalized anxiety disorder)."

[c]Per "Highlights of Changes From DSM-IV to DSM-5" (p. 813) in DSM-5 Appendix, "Some individuals with chronic pain would be appropriately diagnosed as having somatic symptom disorder, with predominant pain. For others, psychological factors affecting other medical conditions or an adjustment disorder would be more appropriate."

Source. American Psychiatric Association 1994, 2013.

two central SSRD diagnoses in DSM-5: somatic symptom disorder (SSD) and illness anxiety disorder (IAD). Factitious disorder is now considered an SSRD in DSM-5, because individuals with this disorder often present with somatic symptoms in general medical settings. Psychological factors affecting other medical conditions (PFAOMC), which in DSM-IV appeared in the chapter "Other Conditions That May Be a Focus of Clinical Attention"), is now grouped with the SSRDs in DSM-5. The PFAOMC diagnosis is quite prevalent in medical and surgical patients. It is hoped that the revised DSM-5 criteria will help reduce stigmatization of patients with distressing somatic and psychological symptoms as well as improve diagnostic accuracy across various medical disciplines.

Table 25–2 summarizes the hallmark features of the DSM-5 SSRDs.

Somatic Symptom Disorder

SSD is defined as an illness in which patients experience at least 6 months of one or more distressing somatic symptoms in addition to maladaptive thoughts, feelings, and behaviors related to these symptoms (American Psychiatric Association 2013). These maladaptive associated features may include disproportionate distress or persistent thoughts about symptoms, an abnormally high level of anxiety about symptoms, and excessive time and energy devoted to the symptoms.

People who previously had a diagnosis of somatization disorder will meet criteria for SSD only if their somatic symptoms are accompanied by the maladaptive thoughts, feelings, and behaviors that characterize this new diagnosis (see Table 25–1). There is no diagnosis in DSM-5 that correlates to the DSM-IV diagnosis of somatization disorder. This diagnosis is still valid in ICD-10 (World Health Organization 1992).

Case 1

A 50-year-old woman (married with a teenage daughter) reports chronic abdominal pain. Extensive workup is unrevealing. She continues to go to work daily but finds herself so exhausted at the end of the day from her pain that she goes to bed immediately when she returns home, unable to participate in any of the family's activities. When reassured by her internist and instructed to return for follow-up in 6 months, her pain increases and she seeks out a new physician.

The new physician recommends that the patient see a psychiatrist, in conjunction with continued regular visits with him for primary care follow-up. The psychiatrist diagnoses her condition as somatic symptom disorder, with predominant pain, and also diagnoses a comorbid depressive disorder. The patient improves with duloxetine treatment and cognitive-behavioral therapy (CBT), as well as continued interdisciplinary follow-up.

Epidemiology

The prevalence of SSD is approximately 5%–7% in the general adult population (Rief et al. 2011). Females report distressing somatic symptoms more frequently than do males. Initial symptoms can begin at any age but usually appear by early adulthood.

Certain demographic factors are associated with a more severe clinical course, including female gender and older age. In elderly individuals, SSD is more likely to go unrecognized because of comorbid medical illness. The physical complaints of older

TABLE 25–2. **Clinical characteristics of DSM-5 somatic symptom and related disorders**

Somatic symptom disorder
One or more distressing somatic symptoms (including pain)
Maladaptive thoughts/feelings/behaviors related to the symptom(s)
Lasts at least 6 months

Illness anxiety disorder
Preoccupation with having or acquiring a serious illness
Somatic symptoms *mild or absent*
High level of health anxiety disproportionate to actual physical illness or risk of illness
Lasts at least 6 months

Psychological factors affecting other medical conditions
Psychological or behavioral symptoms that adversely impact an underlying medical or neurological condition (either by interference with treatment, by constituting additional health risks, or by adversely impacting underlying pathophysiology)

Conversion disorder (functional neurological symptom disorder)
One or more symptoms of altered voluntary motor or sensory functions that cause significant distress or impairment
Symptom(s) incompatible with recognized neurological or medical condition

Factitious disorder
Falsified physical or psychological signs/symptoms via *identified deception*
Patient presents him- or herself (or his or her relative) as ill, impaired, or injured
Deceptive behavior in the *absence of obvious external reward*

Source. American Psychiatric Association 2013.

patients may also be misattributed to "normal aging" or "understandable" concerns about the aging process and increasing medical comorbidity and may not be taken seriously as indications for a full workup. SSD occurs more frequently in individuals with lower educational attainment and socioeconomic status. Such persons have more severe illness and worse outcomes. Demographic factors that adversely affect clinical course include unemployment, a history of childhood physical or sexual abuse or other adversity, medical and psychiatric comorbidity, and external factors that reinforce the illness (e.g., disability payments).

Pathophysiology and Etiology

As is the case for most psychiatric illnesses, there are biological, psychological, and social factors that contribute to the development of SSD. Biological risk factors include genetic propensity toward a heightened sensitivity to pain and other physical sensations. An emerging literature suggests a potential role for psychoneuroimmune mechanisms of somatic symptom amplification. Proinflammatory cytokines are known to be involved in the production of *illness behavior* (defined as an adaptive and motivational reaction to disease that may include lethargy, depression, anorexia, energy conservation, fever, anhedonia, cognitive impairment, hyperalgesia, and decreased social interaction); chronic activation or sensitization of the brain cytokine system may result in nonspecific somatic symptoms and chronic pain (Dantzer 2009). Some researchers have hypothesized that immunological mechanisms in the setting of infectious triggers may contribute to the development of SSRDs (Dimsdale and Dantzer 2007; Rief and Barsky 2005). Functional neuroimaging studies have demonstrated aberrant cortical and limbic activity that may have an impact on conscious processing of mild or chronically painful stimuli (Gündel et al. 2008; Stoeter et al. 2007).

Psychosocial risk factors for SSD include early childhood trauma such as physical, sexual, or emotional abuse or neglect. Social learning mechanisms such as the attention gained from physical illness or the lack of reinforcement of nonsomatic (emotional) expressions of distress also may also contribute to the occurrence of SSD. Intrinsic temperamental factors such as alexithymia (difficulty identifying inner emotional states) and neuroticism (high levels of negative affect) may correlate with a higher risk of developing SSD (Costa 1987; Costa and McCrae 1987; Russo et al. 1997; Sifneos 1973; Vassend 1994). Difficulties in communication resulting from intellectual, emotional, or social limitations can predispose an individual to bodily expression of distress.

Differential Diagnosis and Comorbidity

Patients with psychiatric illness often present with somatic symptoms. Patients with major depressive disorder may experience prominent fatigue, and patients with anxiety disorders may experience tachycardia or abdominal pain. Usually, the cardinal feature of these illnesses is a pronounced mood disturbance accompanied by numerous other physical and mental symptoms, whereas the distress in SSRDs emanates predominantly from the physical symptoms themselves. Mood and anxiety disorders frequently co-occur with SSRDs. Depressive disorders are common in patients with SSD, particularly in the elderly. Patients with SSD are at risk of developing secondary substance use disorders.

Medical comorbidity is common among patients with SSD, which may further complicate the diagnosis. Iatrogenically created symptoms may be subsequently mislabeled as psychogenic. Common complications of SSD include iatrogenic harm from invasive procedures or dependence on habit-forming prescribed medications such as opioid analgesics. Greater medical and psychiatric comorbidity is typically associated with greater severity of illness, greater degree of distress, and greater functional impairment.

Cultural factors are crucial when considering the diagnosis of SSD; many cultural syndromes manifest with prominent physical symptoms. Differences in medical care across cultures also can affect the presentation and course of SSRDs. The ways in which individuals recognize and respond to bodily sensations are influenced by numerous interactions that occur within a given social and cultural context, which in turn affect the way in which individuals perceive illness and seek medical attention.

Treatment

SSD is difficult to treat, and the literature does not suggest a single superior treatment approach. It is recommended that the patient form a stable relationship with a primary care physician who regularly and reliably follows up on a predetermined, scheduled basis. In their interactions with patients with suspected SSD, clinicians should maintain an empathic approach to help put the patient at ease and, when possible, to facilitate recommended practices regarding psychiatric referral and follow-up. Objectively corroborated problems should be judiciously investigated; however, unnecessarily extensive diagnostic testing should be avoided, because such testing may inadvertently reinforce the development of new somatic symptoms or even cause iatrogenic harm. The therapeutic focus should shift from "cure" to symptom management. In the case of SSD with predominant pain, use of potentially addictive analgesics should be avoided as much as possible.

Early psychiatric intervention is likely to improve outcomes for patients with SSD; greater chronicity of undiagnosed somatization is correlated with worse outcomes and makes subsequent mental health treatment more challenging. An interdisciplinary team approach to the patient is crucial; close collaboration between the psychiatrist or other mental health care practitioner and the general medical care provider can help minimize errors of diagnostic omission in either domain. Frequent communication between treatment disciplines helps to maximize consistency and reduce the likelihood of the patient's feeling dismissed or abandoned.

When discussing a suspected diagnosis of SSD with a patient, the clinician may emphasize that stress can generate physical symptoms without the patient's awareness. Providing education about the illness and giving patients a list of psychiatric diagnostic criteria is helpful in legitimizing and validating their complaints by giving them a genuine diagnosis. Developing a relationship with the patient's family also may be helpful for understanding and managing the greater social context in which somatic symptoms tend to occur.

Various treatments are successful for SSRDs. Psychotherapy is the mainstay of treatment for somatizing patients; such approaches include CBT (Allen and Woolfolk 2010; Kroenke 2007) and psychodynamic psychotherapy (Abbass et al. 2009).

Data suggest that pharmacotherapy can be helpful in the management of SSRD (Somashekar et al. 2013). Serotonergic antidepressants are moderately effective in reducing the intensity of functional somatic symptoms. Medications are helpful, especially in treating comorbid depressive and anxiety disorders. Agents commonly used for neuropathic pain (e.g., serotonin-norepinephrine reuptake inhibitors, tricyclic antidepressants, certain anticonvulsants) may be helpful. The mechanism of action of these agents has not been fully elucidated, but recent research findings suggest potential modulation of psychoneuroimmune pathophysiology (Bai et al. 2014; Dahl et al. 2014).

When treating patients with SSD, it is important to consider the reinforcing role of secondary gain in maintaining symptoms. Although patients with SSD clearly suffer, they may also obtain relief from certain social, personal, and professional responsibilities as a result of their illness. Any successful treatment of SSD will seek as much as possible to eradicate these reinforcing agents and to help reduce the possibility of further iatrogenic harm.

Illness Anxiety Disorder

IAD is characterized by a preoccupation with having or acquiring a serious medical illness (American Psychiatric Association 2013). In this condition, bodily complaints and symptoms are often absent or mild. The hallmark of IAD is distress that is focused not on the physical symptoms themselves, but rather on the individual's anxiety about the meaning or significance of these symptoms. Patients with IAD have a high level of health anxiety that is disproportionate to the severity of their actual physical illness or risk of illness. They may engage in excessive health-related behaviors, including frequently checking their bodies for signs of illness or compulsively re-searching diseases on the Internet. Medical reassurance or negative diagnostic tests are unlikely to alleviate these patients' excessive concerns.

Among people who previously had a DSM-IV hypochondriasis diagnosis, most will meet criteria for DSM-5 SSD; however, for individuals with high health anxiety but no somatic symptoms, the diagnosis of DSM-5 IAD will apply instead (see Table 25–1).

Case 2

A 35-year-old man finds what he thinks is a lump on his testicle. He has a strong family history of testicular cancer. He requests an emergency appointment with his internist, who does not detect a mass on physical examination. Ultrasound of the patient's testi-cle shows no pathology, and relevant tumor marker levels are within normal limits. De-spite these reassuring findings, the man continues to fear that he has testicular cancer, examines himself repeatedly, and calls his physician's office weekly regarding his con-cerns that he might have testicular cancer.

The physician refers the patient to a psychiatrist, along with continued regular med-ical follow-up. The patient improves with sertraline treatment and CBT.

Epidemiology

Estimates of the prevalence of IAD are based on epidemiological studies of the DSM-IV diagnosis of hypochondriasis. These community surveys and population-based samples demonstrate a 1- to 2-year prevalence of health anxiety or disease conviction ranging from 1.3% to 10% (Noyes et al. 2005; Rief et al. 2001). In ambulatory medical populations, the prevalence rates are between 3% and 8% (Barsky et al. 1990; Gureje et al. 1997). Illness anxiety is equally prevalent in males and females.

IAD is a chronic/relapsing condition that begins in early to middle adulthood. In the general population, health-related anxiety—often focused on cognitive deficits—increases with age. In medical settings, no significant age differences have been found between those with low and those with high levels of illness anxiety.

Pathophysiology and Etiology

There are biological and psychosocial components to the development of IAD. A his-tory of childhood abuse or neglect or serious childhood illness is a risk factor for the development of IAD in adulthood. Major life stressors or illnesses are factors that may trigger the development of IAD.

Differential Diagnosis and Comorbidity

When evaluating the patient with illness anxiety, it is important to consider the pres-ence of underlying medical disease. Anxiety related to health is a normal response to being diagnosed with a major medical illness. In order to make a diagnosis of IAD, symptoms must be *disproportionate* to the underlying physical disease. The patient must have severe and continuous anxiety that causes significant distress for a mini-mum of 6 months.

Major mood and anxiety disorders are other differential diagnostic considerations. Depressed patients can become preoccupied with concerns about their body and health, and patients with IAD may develop depression; this comorbidity may make it difficult to tease apart which of the two disorders is the primary psychiatric diagnosis. What distinguishes IAD from depressive and anxiety disorders is the patient's narrowed and persistent focus on health-related anxiety. Patients with psychosis who have somatic delusions typically have other symptoms of psychosis, such as hallucinations or disorganized thinking. *Delusions* are fixed, false beliefs that are held with a degree of conviction and intensity that is not typically seen in IAD. Patients with psychotic delusions are not able to be dissuaded from their concerns, whereas patients with IAD are usually able to accept the possibility that they may not be as sick as they fear. Somatic delusions in psychosis are often more bizarre or striking (e.g., delusions of complete bodily decay) than the fears associated with IAD.

IAD is a new diagnosis; therefore, exact rates of comorbidities are not yet known. Prior research on hypochondriasis suggests that comorbidity is high, with as many as two-thirds of patients having at least one other major mental disorder (Barsky et al. 1992; Noyes et al. 1994). Patients with significant illness anxiety are particularly likely to have comorbid depressive and anxiety disorders. Other common comorbid conditions include SSD and personality disorders.

Treatment

The treatment of IAD has not been thoroughly researched. Patients referred early for psychiatric evaluation tend to have a better prognosis compared with those who receive only medical assessment and treatment. Psychiatric referral should be presented as a supplement to, rather than an alternative or replacement for, ongoing medical care and evaluation. Regularly scheduled, supportive treatment visits with a consistent primary care physician are helpful.

Evidence suggests that serotonergic antidepressants may be effective for SSRDs characterized by predominant illness anxiety (Fallon et al. 2008; Greeven et al. 2007). Therapeutic dosages may need to be higher than those used to treat depressive and anxiety disorders. CBT may be a particularly effective form of psychotherapy (Barsky and Ahern 2004; Greeven et al. 2007), with 12-month response rates as high as 57%.

Conversion Disorder (Functional Neurological Symptom Disorder)

Patients with conversion disorder exhibit one or more symptoms of altered voluntary motor or sensory functions that cause significant distress or functional impairment. DSM-5 specifies that *conversion disorder symptoms must be incompatible with recognized medical or neurological conditions.* The diagnosis should not be made simply because clinical test findings are normal or because the symptom is "bizarre." Functional neurological symptoms may be acute or chronic and may affect multiple sensory or motor modalities. The diagnosis of conversion disorder in DSM-5 does *not* require that a psychological stressor precede the development of symptoms. The decision to remove this requirement was made by experts in the field in recognition of the fact that it is not always possible to identify an antecedent stressor in conversion disorder. Nevertheless, it is important to make the diagnosis as quickly as possible in order to minimize morbidity and iatrogenic complications. The change in the diagnostic criteria is not meant to imply that psychological factors are not present or important for the patient and the symptoms.

The conventional psychodynamic model of conversion posits that patients with conversion disorder unconsciously transmute their psychic distress into physical symptoms. It can be difficult to eliminate definitively the possibility of conscious feigning when initially encountering a patient with conversion disorder. Thus, the new diagnostic criteria for conversion disorder no longer require a definitive judgment that the symptoms are unconsciously produced.

Case 3

A 33-year-old married woman is admitted after a sudden loss of function of her right arm. She smokes one pack of cigarettes daily, is overweight, and is taking oral contraceptives. The loss of function in her arm occurred during an argument with her ex-husband at a point when (she admitted) she felt as if "I could just hit him." Neuroimaging shows no evidence of infarct or hemorrhage. When hypnotized by the psychiatric consultant, she is able to lift her right arm; however, her arm becomes limp when she is out of the trance state.

The psychiatric consultant provides brief bedside therapy geared toward psychoeducation and support around the patient's diagnosis, as well as positive encouragement about her prognosis. The consultant explores the patient's relationship with her husband and refers her for further psychotherapy on discharge.

Presentation and Epidemiology

Transient conversion symptoms are common, but the precise prevalence of diagnosed conversion disorder is unknown. This is partly because the diagnosis usually requires assessment in secondary care, where it is found in approximately 5% of referrals to neurology clinics (Stone et al. 2010). The incidence of individual persistent conversion symptoms is estimated to be 2–5 cases per 100,000 per year (Reuber 2008).

Onset of conversion disorder usually occurs in early adulthood. The disorder is approximately two to three times more common in females (American Psychiatric Association 2013). Conversion disorder is also more frequently seen in individuals of lower socioeconomic status and with relatively less education. As with the other SSRDs, psychiatric comorbidity (e.g., depressive, anxiety, and personality disorders; posttraumatic stress disorder; impairment of psychosocial functioning) is high. Although conversion symptoms can be short lived, it is not unusual for symptoms to recur in the same individual; 1-year relapse rates can be as high as 20%–25% (Perez et al. 2012).

There is great variation in the degree of symptom severity among patients with conversion disorder. Good prognostic factors include acute onset, short duration of symptoms, presence of an identifiable stressor at symptom onset, short interval between onset and referral to treatment, higher intelligence, and willingness to accept that the illness has a psychological component. A comorbid personality disorder is a poor prognostic indicator, as is comorbid SSD. The more long-standing the conversion symptoms, the more difficult it becomes to treat the disorder. Symptom chronicity may evolve from the accumulation of associated benefits over time (e.g., secondary gain). Comorbid psychiatric and medical illness is also associated with worse outcomes.

Pathophysiology and Etiology

A personal or family history of neurological disease is a risk factor for the development of conversion symptoms. For example, individuals with epilepsy are more likely than individuals in the general population to develop psychogenic nonepileptic seizures (PNES); approximately 10% of patients with epilepsy have comorbid PNES (LaFrance and Benbadis 2002). Maladaptive coping styles and personality traits, as well as difficulties in identifying and expressing emotion (alexithymia), may predispose an individual to develop conversion symptoms.

In comparison with healthy volunteers, patients with PNES have been found to have higher basal cortisol levels, a marker of an overall greater stress level that is unrelated to seizure frequency, physical activity, or acute psychological stress (Bakvis et al. 2010). When patients with PNES were compared with patients with complex partial seizures, they demonstrated statistically significant preictal heart rate elevations and postictal heart rate reductions compared with baseline measurements before the seizure or nonepileptic seizure (Reinsberger et al. 2012).

Environmental factors such as childhood abuse or neglect and other stressful or traumatic life events are associated with the development of conversion disorder. Dissociation, a commonly seen psychological response to trauma, also has been described in patients with conversion disorder, particularly those with PNES (Goldstein et al. 2000). Researchers have hypothesized that similar psychological processes underlie conversion disorder and dissociative disorders, despite the descriptive differences between the two conditions (Harden 1997). Any clinician treating patients with conversion disorder should be aware of the potential role that past trauma plays in this illness and should be sensitive to the therapeutic implications of this role for the management of a traumatized patient (particularly as it relates to forming a stable treatment alliance).

Neuroimaging studies comparing patients with conversion disorder and patients who consciously feign symptoms show different patterns of brain activation and deactivation in the two groups (Stone et al. 2007). Although there is no commonly accepted theory about the functional neuroanatomy of conversion disorder, available evidence suggests that the illness may represent a *functional unawareness syndrome* (Perez et al. 2012) involving networks responsible for the processing of emotion and affect. Several studies have established the presence of abnormal limbic-motor connectivity in conversion disorder (Halligan et al. 2000; Marshall et al. 1997; Spence et al. 2000; Voon et al. 2010; Vuilleumier et al. 2001; Ward et al. 2003).

Differential Diagnosis and Comorbidity

A diagnosis of conversion disorder should be made only after a thorough neurological assessment that includes a detailed history and examination and relevant imaging or other studies. Conversion disorder can be differentiated from neurological illness by its incompatibility with known features of neurological disease, including incompatibility with known neuroanatomy; however, as with the other SSRDs, actual physical illness and conversion disorder (or other apparent psychological contributions to symptoms) are not mutually exclusive. Overt evidence of deliberate feigning or exaggeration of symptoms suggests factitious disorder or malingering. It is important to note that some patients present with a history that is so obviously inconsistent with a purely organic etiology that the physician may end the diagnostic evaluation prematurely, concluding that the patient's symptoms are purely psychiatric.

Case 4

A 45-year-old woman is admitted to Neurology with acute cognitive deficits. She is confused, disoriented, and unable to give any history. She was found on the street, outside her truck, which was parked but still running. She had asked a passerby to call her partner on his cell phone, because she could not figure out how to make the call herself. On the seat of the truck was an empty bottle of narcotic analgesics. When the woman's partner arrives at the hospital, she reports that the patient had left their house the previous evening, a hot summer night, following an argument. The partner further notes that all of the jewelry customarily worn by the patient is gone, as is her wallet. Neurology requests a psychiatric consultation to rule out conversion disorder, because the woman shows no overt neurological symptoms except for the confusion. The consultant, suspecting that the patient had been assaulted and that her subsequent confusion might be part of a conversion reaction to the assault, recommends that the patient be seen by Gynecology. However, before that can be done, the consultant receives the results of the patient's brain magnetic resonance imaging (MRI) scan, which show bilateral hippocampal injury. The neuroradiologist reports that only carbon monoxide poisoning could cause this finding. The attempt to reconstruct the events of the past 12 hours leads to the conclusion that the exhaust from the truck had been pulled into the cabin by the air conditioning, rendering the patient unconscious. Whoever had robbed the patient of her jewelry, wallet, and analgesic medication must have seen her unconscious in the cabin. The robbery inadvertently saved her life by opening the truck door. However, the patient's cognitive deficits do not resolve, and she requires placement in a skilled nursing facility.

Treatment

Effective treatment of conversion disorder begins with empathic and positive communication of the diagnosis. To prevent embarrassment, clinicians should avoid making any comments that suggest to patients that there is nothing biologically wrong with them. It is helpful to inform patients that although they are clearly experiencing real symptoms that are distressing and disruptive, they are expected to recover. Patients should be told that there is no need to be exposed to unnecessary medications or studies, but treatment focusing on managing the emotional issues and distress associated with the symptoms is very important for ultimate improvement. This type of phrasing can help engage the patient in a dialogue about any stress associated with the symptoms. Although the psychological conflict producing the symptoms may seem obvious to the physician, delicacy is required in presenting an interpretation of the proposed etiology to the patient. The most common precipitants of conversion symptoms are aggressive and/or sexual thoughts that are unacceptable to the patient; if the patient could easily cope with such thoughts, then the symptoms would not be manifested.

Despite the illness burden of conversion disorder and the therapeutic challenges inherent in its management, empirical data on effective treatment strategies are lacking. The majority of evidence for the treatment of conversion disorder is in the form of uncontrolled case series and reports. In general, the cornerstone of management for conversion disorder has been psychotherapy of various kinds. Psychotherapy of patients with conversion disorder should be geared toward helping the individual develop more adaptive coping strategies to deal with emotional conflicts and more effective ways of communicating distress. CBT offers this kind of help (Speckens et al. 1995). Psychoanalytic approaches to conversion disorder also can be quite effective (Hinson et al. 2006).

In addition to psychotherapy, there are studies of small sample sizes with preliminary findings suggesting possible efficacy for hypnosis (Moene et al. 2002, 2003), behavioral therapy and rehabilitation, physical therapy, and paradoxical intention therapy (having the patient intentionally engage in the unwanted behavior or conversion symptoms). These treatments can be potentially face-saving for the patient because they are based on a physical model of recovery, and they may be particularly helpful for patients who have difficulty engaging in psychotherapy.

In the absence of any comorbid psychiatric conditions such as depressive or anxiety disorders, there is little clinical evidence to support the use of pharmacotherapy. Some success has been reported with antidepressants and antipsychotics; however, treatment with antipsychotics is problematic, given these agents' potential for inducing or exacerbating movement disorders in patients who may already have psychogenic movement disorders.

Factitious Disorder

Unlike the other SSRDs, factitious disorder involves *intentional falsification of physical or psychological symptoms or induction of injury or disease.* The individual is aware of the deception and presents as ill, injured, or impaired. A subtype of factitious disorder involves the presentation of someone else close to the patient as ill, injured, or impaired. This subtype was called *factitious disorder by proxy* in DSM-IV and is now referred to as *factitious disorder imposed on another* in DSM-5. Patients with factitious disorder may present with single or recurrent episodes. Munchausen syndrome, which is not a psychiatric diagnosis, is a particularly chronic and intractable form of factitious disorder, as is its variant when imposed on another, Munchausen by proxy.

Unlike the malingering patient, a person with factitious disorder exhibits deceptive behavior *in the absence of any obvious external reward.* The traditional model of this illness is based on the idea that patients seek primary gain via assumption of the sick role; however, DSM-5 does not specifically list primary gain as a diagnostic criterion, because it is often not possible to infer a patient's motivation reliably early on in the disease course.

Common clinical characteristics of factitious disorder include a history of numerous prior medical evaluations and treatments, particularly hospitalizations, operations, and other invasive procedures. Other features that suggest the diagnosis include a dramatic or inconsistent history that is vague or variable in its detail, inconsistent physical findings, inexplicable laboratory results, use of highly medicalized jargon, minimization of the presence of scars from prior invasive procedures, or confabulation of details when attempts are made to corroborate history. Patients may also demonstrate remission of symptoms when they believe no one is observing them. The classic example of a patient with factitious disorder is someone who, when confronted by health care professionals, migrates to different treatment settings in order to avoid discovery of the psychopathology.

Case 5

A 48-year-old woman is admitted for fever and polymicrobial bacteremia. She reports a history of a rare immunodeficiency. At points during her admission, nursing staff observe her manipulating her lines. She requires high-dose opiates for pain control. Efforts to obtain records from outside hospitals produce a history of similar behavior with suspicion for self-induced illness. When confronted, the patient becomes angry, calls Patient Services, and threatens to sue the doctors.

The psychiatric consultation service is asked to see the patient, and the consultant diagnoses factitious disorder. The patient demands to sign out against medical advice and is deemed to have capacity to do so.

Epidemiology

Because of the level of deception in patients with factitious disorder, exact estimates of prevalence are unknown. In the general hospital setting, approximately 1% of individuals meet criteria for the disorder, but rates may be higher in specialized treatment settings (Reich and Gottfried 1983; Sansone et al. 1997). The typical course of factitious disorder involves recurrent, intermittent episodes throughout life. Patients usually present during adulthood. Factitious disorder is more common in women, but its course is often more severe and refractory in men.

Pathophysiology and Etiology

Patients with factitious disorder may first present for care following a hospitalization for a medical condition or mental disorder. In factitious disorder imposed on another, the initial presentation often follows the child's or dependent party's hospitalization. Risk factors for the disorder include a history of childhood abuse, disturbed parental relationships or emotional deprivation, early life illness or extended hospitalizations, and exposure to or employment in a medical setting.

Several psychodynamic as well as cognitive, social learning, and behavioral theories have been proposed to explain the development of factitious disorder. Neurobiological findings from functional imaging studies have been inconsistent.

Differential Diagnosis and Comorbidity

The major differential diagnostic consideration in factitious disorder is malingering. Patients may have features or elements of both conditions—that is, a patient may be unconsciously motivated to complain of pain while enjoying access to opiates.

Many clinicians have difficulty differentiating between the somatic symptoms of factitious disorder and those of conversion disorder. The hallmark of factitious disorder is deliberate deception or fabrication of symptoms. In conversion disorder, patients do not intentionally produce symptoms.

Patients with factitious disorder who injure themselves do so specifically in order to assume the sick role. They are not attempting to kill themselves or to obtain affective or emotional release from the self-injury. This difference in motivation distinguishes their self-harming behavior from the self-harming behaviors of patients with mood or personality disorders. Patients with factitious disorder may have comorbid personality disorders and frequently have comorbid substance use disorders.

Treatment

Factitious disorder is one of the most difficult psychiatric illnesses to treat. Not surprisingly, clinicians often have strong negative emotional reactions to patients who falsify symptoms. Care providers may feel exploited or humiliated, and may be angry with the patient as a result. When treating patients with factitious disorder, it is important that care providers remember that these individuals are in fact quite ill, but not in the way that they present themselves as being. These patients are at significant risk of self-inflicted injury or death. If a diagnosis of factitious disorder is suspected, it is often helpful—and in fact it may be necessary—to confer with hospital administrative and legal services.

An additional therapeutic challenge is the fact that patients often abruptly flee from care once they are confronted about the false nature of their symptoms; other responses include denial or threats of litigation. There is a dearth of comparative literature examining the efficacy of various treatment approaches. In general, it is recommended that treatment be collaborative, involving interdisciplinary team meetings and communication among providers to coordinate efforts and manage negative emotions. Psychodynamic and behavioral approaches have been used to treat the disorder. Pharmacotherapy has a role in treating specific comorbid symptoms, such as mood or psychotic disorders, if present.

Psychological Factors Affecting Other Medical Conditions

PFAOMC is a very common condition. This diagnosis is included in the SSRD chapter because of its usual appearance in primary care and other medical settings. Psychological or behavioral symptoms may include psychological distress, dysfunctional patterns of interpersonal interaction, and maladaptive coping strategies such as denial or poor adherence to treatment. These thoughts, feelings, and behaviors can have an adverse impact on known medical conditions in a variety of ways. A common example of a PFAOMC is denial of the significance of physical symptoms, which may in turn lead to delay in seeking medical intervention.

There may be a temporal relationship between psychological factors and development or exacerbation of a medical condition, as in the example of a depressed patient with diabetes mellitus who begins to neglect glucose control. Psychological factors may also interfere with treatment of a medical condition. Patients with a history of trauma may be particularly sensitive to certain invasive procedures and become resistant to medical workups. Psychological factors can constitute additional health risks or adversely influence underlying pathophysiology. A hypoxic patient with pulmonary disease who subsequently develops anxiety will experience vasoconstriction secondary to release of catecholamines, resulting in further reduction of oxygen delivery to tissues and a positive feedback loop contributing to exacerbation of both hypoxia and anxiety.

Case 6

A 58-year-old man admitted after a syncopal episode is found to be in atrial fibrillation, with a rapid ventricular rate. He initially states that he has been taking all of his medications regularly; however, his serum digoxin level is undetectable. When confronted with this information, the man admits that he stopped his medication because "drugs are for weak people."

The primary team requests a psychiatric consultation to rule out depression leading to nonadherence. The consultant diagnosis the patient with PFAOMC, and performs brief bedside therapy exploring the patient's personal life narrative around illness and themes of masculinity. The patient discloses a history of seeing his father suffer from chronic illness and being told by his mother that his father was "weak." The patient also reveals a fear of sexual side effects due to medication.

Epidemiology

The exact prevalence of PFAOMC is unknown; however, private insurance billing data from the United States indicate that this diagnosis is made more commonly than SSD (Levenson 2011). Psychological factors may have impacts on a medical illness at any point during the life cycle. Denial of medical illness is not currently a diagnosable disorder in DSM-5, but it is commonly seen in clinical settings.

Differential Diagnosis and Comorbidity

By definition, the diagnosis of PFAOMC necessitates the presence of a comorbid medical illness along with a psychological symptom or behavior. The hallmark of PFAOMC is the directionality of psychological factors adversely affecting underlying medical or neurological disease. Conversely, when psychiatric symptoms develop predominantly in response to the stressor of medical illness, a diagnosis of adjustment disorder is more appropriate. In actual clinical practice, psychological syndromes often co-occur with medical illness in a mutually exacerbating fashion, making it difficult to determine the exact direction of causality. If the symptoms leading to aggravation of medical illness are best explained by another mental illness, such as major depressive disorder, then it is that condition that should be diagnosed, rather than PFAOMC.

Conclusion

SSRDs are a costly group of psychiatric illnesses that cause much suffering on the part of the patient and frequent frustration on the part of the clinician. In this chapter, we reviewed major recent findings on epidemiology and pathophysiology specific to each of the SSRDs. Fortunately, a variety of evidence-based therapeutic modalities are available for some of these disabling disorders. Treatment should be focused on understanding and treating the dysfunctional thoughts, feelings, and behaviors related to the somatic symptoms, as opposed to attempting to completely eliminate the symptoms themselves. Invasive workups should be initiated with caution. Early recognition of these disorders and appropriate referral by general medical practitioners remain the initial crucial steps in facilitating treatment and may significantly improve outcomes. Ongoing medical follow-up is important to prevent feelings of abandonment and to ensure that relevant organic illness has not been missed.

References

Abbass A, Kisely S, Kroenke K: Short-term psychodynamic psychotherapy for somatic disorders: systematic review and meta-analysis of clinical trials. Psychother Psychosom 78(5):265–274, 2009 19602915

Allen LA, Woolfolk RL: Cognitive behavioral therapy for somatoform disorders. Psychiatr Clin North Am 33(3):579–593, 2010 20599134

American Psychiatric Association: Diagnostic and Statistical Manual of Mental Disorders, 4th Edition. Washington, DC, American Psychiatric Association, 1994

American Psychiatric Association: Diagnostic and Statistical Manual of Mental Disorders, 5th Edition. Arlington, VA, American Psychiatric Association, 2013

Bai YM, Chiou WF, Su TP, et al: Pro-inflammatory cytokine associated with somatic and pain symptoms in depression. J Affect Disord 155:28–34, 2014 24176538

Bakvis P, Spinhoven P, Giltay EJ, et al: Basal hypercortisolism and trauma in patients with psychogenic nonepileptic seizures. Epilepsia 51(5):752–759, 2010 19889016

Barsky AJ, Ahern DK: Cognitive behavior therapy for hypochondriasis: a randomized controlled trial. JAMA 291(12):1464–1470, 2004 15039413

Barsky AJ, Wyshak G, Klerman GL, Latham KS: The prevalence of hypochondriasis in medical outpatients. Soc Psychiatry Psychiatr Epidemiol 25(2):89–94, 1990 2336583

Barsky AJ, Wyshak G, Klerman GL: Psychiatric comorbidity in DSM-III-R hypochondriasis. Arch Gen Psychiatry 49(2):101–108, 1992 1550462

Costa PT Jr: Influence of the normal personality dimension of neuroticism on chest pain symptoms and coronary artery disease. Am J Cardiol 60(18):20J–26J, 1987 3321965

Costa PT Jr, McCrae RR: Neuroticism, somatic complaints, and disease: is the bark worse than the bite? J Pers 55(2):299–316, 1987 3612472

Dahl J, Ormstad H, Aass HC, et al: The plasma levels of various cytokines are increased during ongoing depression and are reduced to normal levels after recovery. Psychoneuroendocrinology 45:77–86, 2014 24845179

Dantzer R: Cytokine, sickness behavior, and depression. Immunol Allergy Clin North Am 29(2):247–264, 2009 19389580

Dimsdale JE, Dantzer R: A biological substrate for somatoform disorders: importance of pathophysiology. Psychosom Med 69(9):850–854, 2007 18040093

Fallon BA, Petkova E, Skritskaya N, et al: A double-masked, placebo-controlled study of fluoxetine for hypochondriasis. J Clin Psychopharmacol 28(6):638–645, 2008 19011432

Goldstein LH, Drew C, Mellers J, et al: Dissociation, hypnotizability, coping styles and health locus of control: characteristics of pseudoseizure patients. Seizure 9(5):314–322, 2000 10933985

Greeven A, van Balkom AJ, Visser S, et al: Cognitive behavior therapy and paroxetine in the treatment of hypochondriasis: a randomized controlled trial. Am J Psychiatry 164(1):91–99, 2007 17202549

Gündel H, Valet M, Sorg C, et al: Altered cerebral response to noxious heat stimulation in patients with somatoform pain disorder. Pain 137(2):413–421, 2008 18022320

Gureje O, Üstün TB, Simon GE: The syndrome of hypochondriasis: a cross-national study in primary care. Psychol Med 27(5):1001–1010, 1997 9300506

Halligan PW, Athwal BS, Oakley DA, et al: Imaging hypnotic paralysis: implications for conversion hysteria. Lancet 355(9208):986–987, 2000 10768440

Harden CL: Pseudoseizures and dissociative disorders: a common mechanism involving traumatic experiences. Seizure 6(2):151–155, 1997 9153729

Hinson VK, Weinstein S, Bernard B, et al: Single-blind clinical trial of psychotherapy for treatment of psychogenic movement disorders. Parkinsonism Relat Disord 12(3):177–180, 2006 16364676

Kroenke K: Efficacy of treatment for somatoform disorders: a review of randomized controlled trials. Psychosom Med 69(9):881–888, 2007 18040099

LaFrance WC, Benbadis SR: How many patients with psychogenic nonepileptic seizures also have epilepsy? Neurology 58(6):990; author reply 990–991, 2002 11914432

Levenson JL: The somatoform disorders: 6 characters in search of an author. Psychiatr Clin North Am 34(3):515–524, 2011 21889676

Marshall JC, Halligan PW, Fink GR, et al: The functional anatomy of a hysterical paralysis. Cognition 64(1):B1–B8, 1997 9342933

Moene FC, Spinhoven P, Hoogduin KA, et al: A randomised controlled clinical trial on the additional effect of hypnosis in a comprehensive treatment programme for in-patients with conversion disorder of the motor type. Psychother Psychosom 71(2):66–76, 2002 11844942

Moene FC, Spinhoven P, Hoogduin KA, et al: A randomized controlled clinical trial of a hypnosis-based treatment for patients with conversion disorder, motor type. Int J Clin Exp Hypn 51(1):29–50, 2003 12825917

Noyes R Jr, Kathol RG, Fisher MM, et al: Psychiatric comorbidity among patients with hypochondriasis. Gen Hosp Psychiatry 16(2):78–87, 1994 8039697

Noyes R Jr, Carney CP, Hillis SL, et al: Prevalence and correlates of illness worry in the general population. Psychosomatics 46(6):529–539, 2005 16288132

Perez DL, Barsky AJ, Daffner K, et al: Motor and somatosensory conversion disorder: a functional unawareness syndrome? J Neuropsychiatry Clin Neurosci 24(2):141–151, 2012 22772662

Reich P, Gottfried LA: Factitious disorders in a teaching hospital. Ann Intern Med 99(2):240–247, 1983 6881779

Reinsberger C, Perez DL, Murphy MM, et al: Pre- and postictal, not ictal, heart rate distinguishes complex partial and psychogenic nonepileptic seizures. Epilepsy Behav 23(1):68–70, 2012 22100065

Reuber M: Psychogenic nonepileptic seizures: answers and questions. Epilepsy Behav 12(4):622–635, 2008 18164250

Rief W, Barsky AJ: Psychobiological perspectives on somatoform disorders. Psychoneuroendocrinology 30(10):996–1002, 2005 15958280

Rief W, Hessel A, Braehler E: Somatization symptoms and hypochondriacal features in the general population. Psychosom Med 63(4):595–602, 2001 11485113

Rief W, Mewes R, Martin A, et al: Evaluating new proposals for the psychiatric classification of patients with multiple somatic symptoms. Psychosom Med 73(9):760–768, 2011 22048838

Russo J, Katon W, Lin E, et al: Neuroticism and extraversion as predictors of health outcomes in depressed primary care patients. Psychosomatics 38(4):339–348, 1997 9217404

Sansone RA, Wiederman MW, Sansone LA, Mehnert-Kay S: Sabotaging one's own medical care. Prevalence in a primary care setting. Arch Fam Med 6(6):583–586, 1997 9371054

Sifneos PE: The prevalence of "alexithymic" characteristics in psychosomatic patients. Psychother Psychosom 22(2):255–262, 1973 4770536

Somashekar B, Jainer A, Wuntakal B: Psychopharmacotherapy of somatic symptoms disorders. Int Rev Psychiatry 25(1):107–115, 2013 23383672

Speckens AE, van Hemert AM, Spinhoven P, et al: Cognitive behavioural therapy for medically unexplained physical symptoms: a randomised controlled trial. BMJ 311(7016):1328–1332, 1995 7496281

Spence SA, Crimlisk HL, Cope H, et al: Discrete neurophysiological correlates in prefrontal cortex during hysterical and feigned disorder of movement (letter). Lancet 355(9211):1243–1244, 2000 10770312

Stoeter P, Bauermann T, Nickel R, et al: Cerebral activation in patients with somatoform pain disorder exposed to pain and stress: an fMRI study. Neuroimage 36(2):418–430, 2007 17428684

Stone J, Zeman A, Simonotto E, et al: FMRI in patients with motor conversion symptoms and controls with simulated weakness. Psychosom Med 69(9):961–969, 2007 17991812

Stone J, Warlow C, Sharpe M: The symptom of functional weakness: a controlled study of 107 patients. Brain 133(Pt 5):1537–1551, 2010 20395262

Vassend O: Negative affectivity, subjective somatic complaints, and objective health indicators. Mind and body still separated? in International Review of Health Psychology. Edited by Maes S, Leventhal H, Johnston M. London, Wiley, 1994, pp 97–118

Voon V, Brezing C, Gallea C, et al: Emotional stimuli and motor conversion disorder. Brain 133(Pt 5):1526–1536, 2010 20371508

Vuilleumier P, Chicherio C, Assal F, et al: Functional neuroanatomical correlates of hysterical sensorimotor loss. Brain 124(Pt 6):1077–1090, 2001 11353724

Ward NS, Oakley DA, Frackowiak RS, et al: Differential brain activations during intentionally simulated and subjectively experienced paralysis. Cogn Neuropsychiatry 8(4):295–312, 2003 16571568

World Health Organization: International Statistical Classification of Diseases and Related Health Problems, 10th Revision. Geneva, World Health Organization, 1992

Index

*Page numbers printed in **boldface** type refer to tables or figures.*

Aβ hypothesis, for Alzheimer's disease, 630–631
Abnormal Involuntary Movement Scale, 24–25
Abstraction, and executive functions, **46**
Abulia, and delirium, 641
Acamprosate, 595
Acne, and psychoactive drugs, 437
Acromegaly, 216–218
ACTH. *See* Adrenocorticotropic hormone
Actigraphy, and insomnia, 672
Activated charcoal
    alcohol intoxication and, **114**
    anticholinergic toxicity and, 100
Activities of daily living
    executive functioning in neurological disorders and, 344
    fetal alcohol syndrome and, 493
Acute confusional state, and systemic lupus erythematosus, 235
Acute intermittent porphyria (AIP), 509
Acute stress disorder, 182–183
Acyclovir, 267, 508
Adaptive immune system, 230
Adaptive pacing therapy (APT), and chronic fatigue syndrome, 281
Addenbrooke's Cognitive Examination–Revised (ACE-R), 32, 41, 43
Addison's disease. *See* Adrenal insufficiency
Adjustment disorders, in patients with renal disease, 325–326
Adolescents. *See also* Age; Children
    cannabis use in, 615, 616
    eating disorders in, 196, 197
    treatment of opioid disorders in, 606
Adrenal insufficiency, 222–224, 506, **581**
Adrenocorticotropic hormone (ACTH), and multiple sclerosis, 362.
    See also Cushing's syndrome

Advanced sleep phase disorder, 665, **668**
Affective bias, in diagnosis, 7
African Americans
    end-stage renal disease and, 319
    sarcoidosis and, 249
    systemic lupus erythematosus and, 232
Age, as risk factor for mood symptoms during perimenopause, **467.**
    See also Adolescents; Age at onset; Children; Older adults
Agency for Healthcare Research and Quality (AHRQ), 596–597
Age at onset
    of Huntington's disease
    of multiple sclerosis, 512
    of obsessive-compulsive disorder, 576
Aggression
    medical etiologies of, **484**
    neurological disorders and, 348
Aggression Questionnaire (AQ), 348
Agitation
    alcohol abuse and, **111**
    Alzheimer's disease and, 547
    anticholinergic toxicity and, **98,** 100
    delirium and, 640
    dementia and, 633–634, 637
    hallucinogens and, **116**
    serotonin syndrome and, 94
    stimulant use disorder and, 619–620
Agnosia, 44
AIDS, 274, 276, 552. *See also* HIV
Akinetic mutism, 529–530
Albuterol, 568
Alcohol, and alcohol use disorder.
    See also Alcohol withdrawal syndrome; Fetal alcohol syndrome; Substance abuse
    dermatological conditions and, **428**
    drug-induced liver injury and, 145

Alcohol, and alcohol use disorder
(*continued*)
generalized anxiety disorder and, 572
inpatient medical setting and, 588–596
irritable bowel syndrome and, 293
multiple sclerosis and, 360
psychiatric symptoms of, 109, **110–113,**
512, 514–515
pulmonary infections and, 269
testosterone deficiency and, 210
Alcoholic cerebellar degeneration, **111**
Alcoholic hallucinosis, **110, 111,** 595
Alcoholic hepatitis, 306, 307
Alcoholic withdrawal syndrome (AWS), **110,**
514–515, 590
Alcohol Use Disorders Identification Test
(AUDIT), 589–590
ALDEN tool (algorithm of drug causality for
epidermal necrolysis), 437
Aldosterone, 221
Alemtuzumab, 363
Alexander, Franz, 570
Allopregnanolone, 448
Alpha-lipoic acid, 363
Alprazolam, **96**
Altered mental status, and alcohol use
disorders, 595
Alternating sequences, and writing, **46**
Aluminum, **131–132**
Alzheimer's disease
depression and, 547, 634
Down syndrome and, 486
etiology and pathogenesis of, 630–631
memory and, 42
mood disorders and, 547
neuroimaging findings in, 63, **64,** 66–67
psychotic symptoms and, 509–510, 633
Amanita muscaria (fly agaric), **125**
Amantadine, **91, 96,** 532, 534
American Academy of Pediatrics, 454
American Association for Emergency
Psychiatry (AAEP), 8, **9**
American Association of Endocrine
Surgeons, 205
American College of Obstetricians and
Gynecologists, 453–454, 599
American College of Rheumatology (ACR),
6, 232, 235
American Diabetes Association, 198
American Heart Association, 181, 183
American Psychiatric Association, 637

American Society of Addiction Medicine, 607
American Society of Clinical Oncology, 402
Amiodarone, 186
Amitriptyline, 240, 300, 366
Ammonia, and liver disease, 307
Amphetamines. *See also* Stimulants
cardiovascular events and, 620
psychiatric symptoms caused by, 104,
105–106
serotonin syndrome and, **92**
Amyloid PET, **64,** 67
Anabolic steroids, 128, **129,** 210
Analytic reasoning, and diagnosis, 4, 5–6
Anatomic analytic reasoning, 5, 6
Androgen Excess and PCOS (AE-PCOS)
Society, 207
Anemia, **581**
Angelman syndrome, 487–489
Anger, in patients with heart disease, 180
Angina pectoris, **581**
Anisotropy, and diffusion-weighted
imaging, 58
Anomia, 44
Anorexia nervosa, and choking phobia, 574.
See also Eating disorders
Anterograde memory, 41
Antiandrogen agents, and polycystic ovary
syndrome, **208**
Antibiotics. *See also* Penicillin
drug-drug interactions with
psychotropics, **271**
infectious diseases and, 283
mood disorders and, **555**
psychiatric side effects of, **271**
Anticholinergic agents, 87, 514.
See also Antihistamines
Anticholinergic toxicity, 95, **96,** 97, **98–99,**
100, **101**
Anticipatory nausea and vomiting (ANV),
and chemotherapy, 403
Anticonvulsants
alcohol withdrawal and, 593
centrally mediated abdominal pain
syndrome and, 297
drug-drug interactions and, 357, **358**
pregnancy and, 457–458
Antidepressants.
See also Selective serotonin reuptake
inhibitors; Tricyclic antidepressants
cardiovascular effects of in heart disease
patients, 184–185

chemotherapeutic agents and, 410
delirium and, 643
dementia and, 637
drug-induced liver injury and, 144–145, **146**
epilepsy and, 355
essential tremor and, 386
inflammatory bowel disease and, 303
mood disorders and, 554
neurological disorders and, 342
Parkinson's disease and, 384
pheochromocytoma and, 216
poststroke depression and, 352–353
renal disease and, 321, 323–324
systemic lupus erythematosus and, 237
torsades de pointes and, **150**
Antiepileptic drugs (AEDs), 357, **358**
Antigliadin antibodies (AGA), 304
Antiglutamatergic agents, and catatonia, 533–534
Antihypertensive agents, and depressive or manic states, **555**
Antihistamines
anticholinergic toxicity and, 95, **97, 98–99**
dementia and, 638
insomnia and, 461
neuropsychiatric side effects of, **439**
serotonin syndrome and, **92**
Antimycobacterial drugs, 270, **271**
Anti-NMDAR encephalitis
catatonia and, 527
electroencephalography and, 79
neuropsychiatric manifestations of, 250–254, 379–380, 464
ovarian teratomas and, 251, 379, 409, 464, 503
paraneoplastic syndromes and, 409
psychotic symptoms and, 409, 503–505
Antipsychotics
Alzheimer's disease and, 509–510
anticholinergic toxicity and, 95, **96, 98–99**
anti-NMDAR encephalitis and, 252, 254, 504
cancer and, 405
cannabinoids and, 611
cardiac effects of, 182, 185
catatonia and, 526, 534, 535
chemotherapeutic agents and, 410
delirium and, 330–331, 502, 642–643
delusional infestation and, 282, 283

dementia and, 637
dermatological conditions and, 430
diabetes mellitus and, 198
drug-induced liver injury and, 145, **146**
drug-induced long QT syndrome and, 149
drug-induced orthostatic hypotension and, 152, **154**
electroencephalographic abnormalities and, **71,** 75
electrolyte abnormalities due to, **143**
epilepsy and, 355–356
gastrointestinal disorders and, 295
HIV and, 507
hyperprolactinemia and, 213, 214
neuroleptic malignant syndrome and, 86, 90
neurosyphilis and, 507
Parkinson's disease and, 384
pregnancy and, 458–459, 464
stimulant use disorder and, 619–620
sudden cardiac death and, 148
systemic lupus erythematosus and, 237, 502
torsades de pointes and, **150**
Wilson's disease and, 508–509
Antiretroviral therapy (ART), and HIV, 272, 507.
See also Combined antiretroviral therapy
Antisaccide task, and neurological examination, 20
Antiviral drugs, psychiatric side effects of, **271**
Anxiety. *See also* Anxiety disorders
acromegaly and, 218
cardiovascular disease and, 180–181, 548
dermatological conditions and, 422–423
diabetes mellitus and, 196–197
frequency of in medical settings, 563
gastrointestinal disorders and, 292
Hashimoto's thyroiditis and, 245, 246
inflammatory bowel disease and, 301, 553
liver disease and, 307–308
multiple sclerosis and, 361
Parkinson's disease and, 384
rheumatoid arthritis and, 238–239
sarcoidosis and, 249, 250
scleroderma and, 244
Sjogren's syndrome and, 241–242
thyroid disorders and, 202

Anxiety disorders.
    See also Anxiety; Generalized anxiety
    disorder; Illness anxiety disorder
    cancer and, 401
    DSM-5 and classification of, 563
    epilepsy and, 354
    menopause and, 468
    migraine and, 367
    prevalence of in women, 447
    renal disease and, 324–325
    systemic lupus erythematosus and, 234
    treatment of in general medical setting,
        580–582
Anxiolytics.
    See also Benzodiazepines; Buspirone
    dementia and, 638
    drug-induced liver injury and, **147**
    pregnancy and, 459–460
    torsades de pointes and, **150**
Aortic dissection, and Turner syndrome, 487
Apathetic hyperthyroidism, 202, 248, 550
Apathy
    Alzheimer's disease and, 547
    neurological disorders and, 345–346, 384
Apathy Evaluation Scale (AES), 346
Aphasia, and cognitive assessment, 32, **40**
Apraxia, 24, 43–44
Aprosody, 40
Areca nut (betel), **127**
Aripiprazole, 153, 535
Arizona Center for Education and Research
    on Therapeutics (AZCERT), 148
Aromatase inhibitors, **208,** 209
Arousal, and insomnia, 664–665.
    See also Cognition
Arrhythmias, and psychiatric symptoms due
    to cardiovascular disorders, 178, **179**
Arsenic, 128, **131**
Arthritis Self-Management Program, 240
Ascorbic acid, and vitamin C deficiency, 137
Asenapine, 153
Asparaginase, **411**
Aspiration pneumonia, 269
Aspirin, 331
Associative learning, and anxiety in cancer
    patients, 401
Asthma, 567–568, 672
Ataxia, and cerebellar dysfunction, 22
Ataxia-telangiectasia, **18**
Atherosclerosis, and cognitive disorders,
    183

Atomoxetine, **151**
Atrial myxoma, 178–179
Attention, and tests of cognitive functions,
    32, 35–37
Attention-deficit/hyperactivity disorder
    (ADHD), 235, 460, 490, 491
Auditory extinction, and neurological
    examination, 23
Aura, and migraine, 365, 368
Autism spectrum disorder
    celiac disease and, 305
    Down syndrome and, 486
    epilepsy and, 354
    fragile X syndrome and, 485
    gastrointestinal issues in, 311–312
    medical etiologies of, **483**
    neurocutaneous syndromes and, 490, 491
    Prader-Willi syndrome and, 488
    prenatal exposure to SSRIs and, 456
Autoimmune disorders, and autoimmunity,
    230, 502
Autoimmune encephalitis, **28,** 79, 377–381
Autoimmune thyroiditis.
    See Hashimoto's thyroiditis
Automatic thoughts, and anxiety disorders,
    582
Automatisms, and epilepsy, **356**
Ayahuasca, **125**

Babesiosis, 279
Babinski reflex, 22
Back pain, and comorbid psychopathology,
    571–573, **653,** 654
Backward digit span, 37–38
Baclofen, 526
Bacterial pneumonia, 268–269
BAL, and alcohol abuse, **111**
Balance, and neurological examination,
    23–24
Barbiturates, and alcohol withdrawal
    syndrome, 593
Basal ganglia, diseases of, 511–512
Bear-Fedio questionnaire, 348
Beck Anxiety Inventory, 325
Beck Depression Inventory, 177, 237, 240,
    323, 399
Bedside cognitive examination, 31–45
Behavior. *See* Aggression; Agitation; Apathy;
    Compulsive behaviors; Disruptive
    behavior disorders; Illness behavior;
    Self-harming behavior

Behavioral interventions
for dementia in older adults, 638–639
for insomnia, 327
for psychosomatic symptoms in cancer patients, 403
for psychotic symptoms in Alzheimer's disease, 509
Behavioral variant frontotemporal dementia (bvFTD), 67, 632, 633
Benzodiazepines
alcohol withdrawal and, 591–593
anticholinergic toxicity and, **96, 101**
anxiety disorders and, 581–582
catatonia and, 532–533
chemotherapy and, 403
delirium tremens and, 643
dementia and, 638
dermatological conditions and, 423
insomnia and, 327
neuroleptic malignant syndrome and, **91,** 535
Parkinson's disease and, 384, 386
pregnancy and, 459–460
renal disease and, 325
serotonin syndrome and, 536
stimulant use disorder and, 619
withdrawal from use of, **113**
Benzoyl peroxide, 437
Bevacizumab, **411**
Bicarbonate, and laboratory testing for toxicological conditions, **167**
Biliary cirrhosis, 311
Biopsychosocial analytic reasoning, 6
Bipolar disorder
essential tremor and, 386
frontotemporal dementia and, 546
Hashimoto's thyroiditis and, 245
inflammation and, 231
menopause and, 467
menstrual cycle and, 449
migraine and, 366, 367
multiple sclerosis and, 360, 362, 548
postpartum psychosis and, 462, 463
pregnancy and, 454
rheumatoid arthritis and, 239
sarcoidosis and, 249
secondary to neurological disorders, 342
systemic lupus erythematosus and, 234
thyroid disorders and, 202
Blood-brain barrier, and chemotherapeutic agents, **407**

Blood-injection-injury phobia, 573–574
Blood pressure, and cerebral palsy, 485. *See also* Hypotension
Body dysmorphic disorder, **427,** 430–431
Body language, 40
Bone density, and cerebral palsy, 485
Borderline personality disorder, and dermatological conditions, **429,** 435
Borrelia burgdorferi, 279
Boston Collaborative Drug Surveillance Program, 235
Botulinum toxin, and migraine, 366
Bovine spongiform encephalopathy, 508
Bowel disorders, 291
Brain. *See also* Blood-brain barrier; Brain tumors; Traumatic brain injury
conditions treated by neurosurgery, 368–371
physical examination and abnormal development of, 16–17
relationship between gastrointestinal tract and, 289
Brain-gut axis, and gastrointestinal disorders, 292, 301
Brain tumors, 342, 370, 408–409, 510, 543–544
Breast cancer, 399, 404, 406, 410
Breathalyzer testing, **111**
Brexanolone, 462
Brief Aggression Questionnaire (BAQ), 348
Brief interventions, for substance use disorders, 600, 609
Bright Futures guidelines, 454
Bright light therapy, and premenstrual mood disorders, 452. *See also* Light therapy
Broca's aphasia, **40**
Bromocriptine, **91,** 535
Budapest criteria, for complex regional pain syndrome, 656
Buprenorphine, **151,** 602, 604, 606, 607
Bupropion
chemotherapeutic agents and, 410, 412
depression in cancer patients and, 400
drug-drug interactions and, 186
inflammatory bowel disease and, 303
liver disease and, 309–310
renal disease and, 321
tobacco-related disorders and, 610
Bush-Francis Catatonia Rating Scale (BFCRS), **27,** 524, **525**
Buspirone, **92,** 294, 325, 638

Cadmium, 128, **130**

Caffeine, 610

CAGE Questions Adapted to Include Drug Use (CAGE-AID), 599–600

Caine criteria, and Wernicke's encephalopathy, 594

Calciphylaxis, 331

Calcitonin gene-related peptide (CGRP) antagonists, 366

Calcium, levels of, **167,** 205, 452

Calculation, and bedside cognitive examination, 45

Callosal dysfunction, 23

Canadian Community Health Survey (CCHS), 301, 654

Cancellation tasks, 36

Cancer. *See also* Breast cancer; Chemotherapy; Lung cancer; Pancreatic cancer
    anxiety disorders and, 401
    cognitive changes after chemotherapy for, 371–373
    depression and, 397–400
    mania and, 400–401
    marijuana use and, 613, 616
    mood disorders and, 553
    neurocognitive and neuropsychiatric complications of, 404–410
    posttraumatic stress disorder and, 401
    psychiatric sequelae of treatment for brain lesions, 370
    psychosomatic symptoms and, 402–404
    stem cell transplantation and, 407–408

Cannabinoid(s) (CBDs), 104, **107–108,** 403.
    See also Marijuana; Synthetic cannabinoids

Cannabinoid hyperemesis syndrome (CHS), 616–617

Cannabis use disorder (CUD), and medical conditions, **589,** 611–617.
    See also Marijuana

Carbamazepine
    anticholinergic toxicity and, **96**
    dementia and, 637
    drug-induced hyponatremia and, 142, **143**
    drug-induced liver injury and, 145, **147, 164**
    laboratory testing for toxicological complications of, **164**

Carbidopa-levodopa, and neuroleptic malignant syndrome, **91**

Carcinoid syndrome, **581**

Carcinomatous meningitis, 408

Cardiac testing, for complications or conditions associated with psychiatric illness, **164**

Cardiff Acne Disability Index, 423

Cardiovascular disease
    cardiac effects of medications for psychiatric problems in patients with, 184–186
    as cause of anxiety and panic attacks, **565**
    drug-drug interactions and, 186
    left ventricular assist devices and, 188
    mood disorders and, 549, **555**
    psychiatric disorders in patients with, 179–184
    psychiatric symptoms caused by, 175–179
    stimulant use disorder and, 620

Caregivers, of patients with dementia, 630

Carmustine, **411**

Carotid bruits, auscultation for, 17

Case examples
    of conversion disorder, 686, 688
    of dermatological conditions, 420, 421–422, 424, 436, 437
    of factitious disorder, 690
    of illness anxiety disorder, 684
    of psychological factors affecting other medical conditions, 691–692
    of somatic symptom disorder, 680
    of strategies to reduce misdiagnosis of psychiatric symptoms caused by medical conditions, 11–12

Catastrophizing
    generalized anxiety disorder and, 571
    insomnia and, 664

Catatonia
    anti-NMDAR encephalitis and, 252
    diagnosis of, 531
    differential diagnosis of, 529–531
    etiology of, 524–529
    limbic encephalitis and, 79
    neurological examination and, 26, **27**
    pathophysiology of, 531–532
    phenomenology of, 523–524
    prognosis and complications of, 534
    related syndromes, 534–537
    subtypes of, 524
    treatment of, 532–534

Cathinones, 104, **105–106**

Causalgia, 655–656

Ceftriaxone, 279

Celiac disease, 304–306

Cellulitis, 577

Center for Epidemiologic Studies Depression scale, 249, 399

Center for Neurologic Study–Lability Scale, 346–347

Centers for Disease Control and Prevention (CDC), 269, 272, 275, 277, 278, 373, 461, 606

Centrally mediated abdominal pain syndrome (CAPS), 295–298

Central nervous system
catatonia and infections of, 526–527
HIV and, 274
lumbar puncture and infections of, 78
systemic lupus erythematosus and, **233**
tuberculosis and, 270, **271**

Cerebellar ataxia, and gait, 24

Cerebellar lesions, 22, 409

Cerebellar tremor, **25**

Cerebral aneurysm, 370

Cerebral angiography, 59–60

Cerebral autosomal dominant arteriopathy with subcortical infarcts and leukoencephalopathy (CADASIL), 631

Cerebral palsy, 484–485

Cerebrospinal fluid (CSF)
limbic encephalitis and antibodies in, 79
lumbar puncture and, 76, **77**
multiple sclerosis and, 361
Venereal Disease Research Laboratory testing of, 278, 279

Cerebrovascular disease, 545

Chasteberry (*Vitex agnus-castus*), 452

Chemotherapy
cognitive changes associated with, 371–373, 405–407
depression and mania associated with, **555**
gastrointestinal irritation and, 403

Child-Pugh score, and liver functioning, 309

Children. *See also* Infants
anti-NMDAR encephalitis in, 252
diabetes mellitus in, 196
gastrointestinal issues in autism spectrum disorder and, 311
heavy metal exposure and, **130, 133, 135**
insomnia in, 663
obsessive-compulsive disorder in, 576
stimulants and psychotic symptoms in, 513
zinc deficiency in, 141

Chlamydia pneumoniae, 268

Chlorambucil, **411**

Chlorpromazine
delirium and, 643
drug-induced liver injury and, 145, **146**
drug-induced long QT syndrome and, **152**
drug-induced orthostatic hypotension and, 153, **154**
serotonin toxicity and, 95
torsades de pointes and, **150**

Choking, and specific phobia, 574

Cholecalciferol, 141

Cholinesterase inhibitors, and dementia, 636–637.
See also Donepezil

Chorea, and Huntington's disease, 633

Choreoathetoid movements, 24

Chromosomal abnormalities, and psychotic symptoms, 505

Chronic idiopathic pruritus, 432, 433

Chronic kidney disease (CKD), 319

Chronic obstructive pulmonary disease (COPD), 566–568, **581**, 608, **668**

Chronic pain. *See* Pain

Chronic traumatic encephalopathy (CTE), 375–377, 544, 545

Circadian system, and insomnia, 665

Circumlocution, **40**

Cisplatin, **411**

Citalopram
agitation in patients with dementia and, 637
cardiovascular effects of in heart disease patients, 184
depression in patients with coronary disease, 182
gastrointestinal disorders and, 294
torsades de pointes and, **150**

Clanging, **40**

Claustrophobia, and MRI scanning, 59, 401

Clinical Antipsychotic Trials of Intervention Effectiveness (CATIE), 153, **154**

Clinical Institute Withdrawal Assessment for Alcohol–revised version (CIWA-Ar), 590, 592

Clinically isolated syndrome (CIS), and multiple sclerosis, 359

Clinical Opioid Withdrawal Scale (COWS), 602, 603

Clock Drawing Test, 33, 344, 370, 372

Clomiphene, **208,** 209

Clomipramine, 431
Clonidine, 298, 300, 593, 603
Clorazepate, **96**
Clozapine
    anticholinergic toxicity and, **96**
    catatonia and, 526, 532, 535
    dementia in older adults and, 637
    drug-drug interactions with antibiotics,
        283
    drug-induced long QT syndrome and,
        152, 164
    drug-induced orthostatic hypotension
        and, 153, **154**
    electroencephalographic abnormalities
        and, 75
    laboratory testing for toxicological
        complications of, **165**
    Parkinson's disease and, 385
    pulmonary infections and, 269
    tobacco-related disorders and, 610
Cluster headaches, 657, 658
Cobalamin deficiency, 139–140, 551
Cocaine
    cardiovascular toxicity of, 620
    prevalence of use, 617
    psychotic symptoms and, 104, **105–106,**
        513
    street and slang names for, 618
Coccidioidomycosis, 378
Co-cyprindiol, **439**
Cognition, dysfunctions and impairments of.
        See also Bedside cognitive examination;
        Cognitive disorders; Executive
        functions; Metacognition
    alcohol abuse and, **110**
    anti-NMDAR encephalitis and, 252
    cancer and neurocognitive complications,
        404–410
    chemotherapy and changes in, 371–373,
        405–407
    dementia and, 635–636
    Graves' disease and, 247
    hepatitis and, 307
    hierarchy of, 32
    Huntington's disease and, 633
    hyperparathyroidism and, 205
    inflammatory bowel disease and, 302
    multiple sclerosis and, 361–362
    neurocutaneous syndromes and, 491
    Parkinson's disease and, 384
    rheumatoid arthritis and, 239

Sjogren's syndrome and, 242
    systemic lupus erythematosus and,
        232–233
    tests of individual domains, 34–45
    thyroid disorders and, 246
    vitamin deficiencies and, 551
Cognitive-behavioral therapy (CBT)
    anger in patients with heart disease and,
        180
    anxiety disorders and, 582
    cannabis use disorder and, 616
    chronic fatigue syndrome and, 281
    depression in diabetes mellitus, 197
    depression during menopause, 468
    depression in patients with coronary
        disease, 182
    dermatological conditions and, 423
    fibromyalgia syndrome and, 655
    gastrointestinal disorders and, 295
    illness anxiety disorder and, 433, 685
    inflammatory bowel disease and, 303
    rheumatoid arthritis and, 240
    systemic lupus erythematosus and, 237
    web-based for psychosomatic symptoms
        in cancer patients, 403
Cognitive disorders. *See also* Cognition;
        Neurocognitive disorders
    cardiovascular disease and, 183
    neuroimaging findings and, 62–69
Cognitive estimations, and executive
        functions, **46**
Cognitive examination.
        See Bedside cognitive examination
Cognitive forcing strategy (CFS), and
        diagnosis, 5, 9–10, **11**
Cognitive monitoring, and insomnia, 664
Cognitive psychology, and diagnosis, 4, 7
Cohen-Mansfield Agitation Inventory, 634
Collateral information, and patient history.
        See also Family history
    dermatological conditions and, 425
    insomnia and, 671
Columbia-Suicide Severity Rating Scale,
        439
Coma
    anticholinergic toxicity and, **98**
    cognitive domains and, 34
Combined antiretroviral therapy (cART),
        273–274, 275, 382–383
Community-acquired pneumonia (CAP),
        268

Comorbidity, of psychiatric and/or medical disorders. *See also* Medical conditions; Multimorbidity; Psychiatric disorders
  chronic pain and, 652–658
  Down syndrome and, **487**
  illness anxiety disorder and, 684
  inflammatory diseases and, 231
  insomnia and, 665, 667, **668**
  irritable bowel syndrome and, 291
  Klinefelter syndrome and, 486–487
  multiple sclerosis and, 364
  neurocutaneous syndromes and, 491
  neurodevelopmental disorders and, 482
  obsessive-compulsive disorder and, 576
  of panic disorder and chronic obstructive pulmonary disease, 567
  Prader-Willi syndrome and, 488
  sarcoidosis and, 249
  somatic symptom disorder and, 682
  22q11.2 deletion syndrome and, 490
Complex motor sequencing, and executive functions, **46**
Complex regional pain syndrome (CRPS), 655–656
Composite International Diagnostic Interview (CIDI), 234
Comprehension, and language function, 38–39
Compulsions, definition of, 575
Compulsive behaviors, and postpartum obsessive-compulsive disorder
Computed tomography (CT)
  advantage and limitations of, **54**
  background and history of, 53
  clinical applications of, 56
  delirium and, 642
  dementia and, 635
  common neurological disorders and, **70**
  iodinated contrast and, 56–57
  traumatic brain injury and, 373, 374
Concentration, and tests of cognitive domains, 35
Concussions, and mood disorders, 544. *See also* Postconcussion syndrome
Confidence ratings, of physicians on diagnostic accuracy, 10
Confirmation bias, and causes of diagnostic errors, 8
Confrontational naming, 39
Confusion Assessment Method (CAM), 330, 641

Congestive heart failure, **581**
Conn's syndrome, 220
Conotruncal cardiac defects, and 22q11.2 deletion syndrome, 490
Consciousness, disturbance of, and anticholinergic toxicity, **98.** *See also* Catatonia; Cognition; Coma
Consultations. *See also* Referrals
  management of alcohol withdrawal syndrome and, 591
  psychiatric symptoms in dermatological patients and, 441
Contamination, and obsessive-compulsive disorder, 577
Contested illnesses, neuropsychiatric presentations of, 280–283
Contraceptives, and premenstrual exacerbation of depressive disorder, 452
Conversion disorder, 530, **679, 681,** 685–689, 690
Coordination, and neurological examination, 22
Coping mechanisms, and personality disorders, 184
Copper metabolism, disorders of, **132,** 508
Coronary artery bypass surgery, 183
Coronary artery disease (CAD), 176
Coronary heart disease, 608
Cortical sensory testing, 23
Cortisol, and Cushing's syndrome, 218, 219, 220
Corticosteroids
  adrenal insufficiency and, 223, 224
  anti-NMDAR encephalitis and, 253
  dermatological conditions and, **439**
  Hashimoto's encephalitis and, 246
  mood disorders and, 554
  multiple sclerosis and, 362
  psychotic symptoms and, 235, 513
  rheumatoid arthritis and, **240**
  sarcoidosis and, 250
  Sjogren's syndrome and, 242
  systemic lupus erythematosus and, 235–236, **237**
Costs. *See* Economics
Counseling, and heart transplantation, 188
Countertransference. *See also* Transference
  dermatological conditions and, 440–441
  emotional factors in diagnosis and, 7
CRAFFT Screening Test, 599
Cranial irradiation, and brain metastases, 408

Cranial nerves, and neurological
    examination, 18–21
Creatine kinase, and laboratory testing for
    toxicological conditions, **170**
Creatinine, and laboratory testing for
    toxicological conditions, **167**
Creutzfeldt-Jakob disease, 508
Criminal justice system, and substance use
    disorders, 599
Criteria-based analytic reasoning, 5–6
Crohn's disease, 301, 302, 553
Cryptococcosis, 274–275
Culture, and cultural factors
    psychological and social aspects of
        women's mental health and, 469–470
    somatic symptom disorder and, 682
Cushing's syndrome, 218–220, 409–410, 506,
    550–551, **581**
Cutaneous signs, and physical examination,
    17, **18**
Cyclophosphamide, **411**
Cyclosporine A, **240**
Cyclothymia, and multiple sclerosis, 362
Cyproheptadine, 95, 536
Cysticercosis, 378
Cytarabine, **411**
Cytochrome P450 isoenzymes, and drug-
    drug interactions, 186, **187, 412**
Cytokines, and immune system, 229, 230
Cytomegalovirus encephalitis, 274

Da Costa, Jacob Mendes, 290
Damocles syndrome, 325
Dantrolene, 90, **91**, 536
Dapsone, **439**
Death. *See* Mortality; Sudden cardiac death
Decision-making, and neurosurgery, 371
Deep vein thrombosis, and catatonia, 534
Defense mechanisms, and denial, 440
Dehydroepiandrosterone (DHEA), and
    adrenal insufficiency, 224
Delayed sleep phase disorder, 665, **668**
Delirious mania, 536–537
Delirium
    alcohol withdrawal syndrome and, 514–515
    anticholinergic toxicity and, **98**
    cancer and, 404–405
    cardiac surgery and, 183
    catatonia and, 528–529, 531
    definition of, 639
    depression in cancer patients and, 399

differential diagnosis of dementia and,
    635–636
hallucinogens and, **115**
hepatic encephalopathy and, 310
laboratory findings in, 641–642
major subtypes of, 639–640
medical conditions and, 501–502
neuroleptic malignant syndrome and, 86
as neuropsychiatric emergency, **28**
neuropsychiatric presentations in,
    640–641
renal disease and, 329–331
sepsis-associated as emergency, 267
stem cell transplantation and, 408
systemic lupus erythematosus and, 235
thyroid disorders and, 202
treatment of neuropsychiatric syndromes
    in, 642–644
Delirium tremens (DTs)
    benzodiazepines for, 643
    management of alcohol withdrawal
        syndrome and, **112,** 590
    as medical emergency, 594
    prevalence of in patients hospitalized for
        alcohol withdrawal, **110**
    psychotic symptoms and, 595
Delusion(s)
    dementia with Lewy bodies and, 510
    dermatological conditions and, 438–439
    illness anxiety disorder and, 685
    multiple sclerosis and, 512
    postpartum psychosis and, 463
Delusional infestation, 282–283
Delusional parasitosis, 426, 430
Dementia. *See also* Alzheimer's disease;
    Dementia with Lewy bodies;
    Frontotemporal dementia; Huntington's
    disease; Parkinson's disease dementia;
    Vascular dementia
    definition of, 629
    Down syndrome and, 486
    etiology and pathogenesis of, 632
    laboratory findings in, 635–636
    major subtypes of, 630–633
    neuroimaging findings in, 62–69
    neuropsychiatric presentations of,
        633–635
    semantic memory and, 42
    systemic lupus erythematosus and, 233
    treatment of neuropsychiatric syndromes
        in, 636–639

Dementia care mapping, 639
Dementia with Lewy bodies (DLB)
    hallucinations and, 633
    memory patterns and, 42
    neuroimaging findings in, **65,** 68–69
    psychotic symptoms and, 510, 632
Demoralization, and renal disease, 323
Demyelinating disease, and neurological
    examination, 26, **27**
Denial, and psychiatric symptoms in
    dermatological patients, 440–441
Department of Health and Human Services,
    597
Depersonalization/derealization, and
    epilepsy, **356**
Depression. *See also* Major depressive
    disorder; Mood disorders; Postpartum
    depression; Poststroke depression;
    Vascular depression
    acromegaly and, 218
    adrenal insufficiency and, 223–224
    Alzheimer's disease and, 547, 634
    biliary diseases and, 311
    cancer and, 311, 397–400, 553
    cardiovascular disease and, 181–182, 349
    celiac disease and, 305
    cerebral palsy and, 485
    chemotherapy and, 372
    Cushing's syndrome and, 220, 551
    delirium and, 641
    dementia and, 634
    dermatological conditions and, 422–423
    diabetes mellitus and, 196
    epilepsy and, 354, **355,** 548–549
    folic acid deficiencies and, 138
    gastroparesis and, 300
    Hashimoto's thyroiditis and, 246
    HIV and, 276, 552
    Huntington's disease and, 546, 634
    illness anxiety disorder and, 684–685
    inflammation and, 230–231
    inflammatory bowel disease and,
        301–302, 553
    liver disease and, 307–308
    medications associated with, **555**
    menopause and, 466, 468
    multiple sclerosis and, 360, 361, 548
    neurological disorders and, 346, 350
    Parkinson's disease and, 384, 386, 546
    pregnancy and, 453, 464
    renal disease and, 320, 332

rheumatoid arthritis and, 238
sarcoidosis and, 249, 250
scleroderma and, 244
Sjogren's syndrome and, 241–242
systemic lupus erythematosus and,
    233–234
testosterone deficiency and, 211–212
thyroid disorders and, 201, 202, 203, 245,
    550
traumatic brain injury and, 544
vitamin deficiencies and, 128, 137
zinc deficiency and, 141
Dermatitis artefacta, 433–434
Dermatological conditions.
    See also Neurocutaneous syndromes
    biological interaction between stress and
        skin, 420–421
    case examples of, 420, 421–422, 424, 436,
        437
    countertransference and, 440–441
    management strategies for in primary
        care setting, 422–424
    as manifestations of psychiatric disorders,
        424–435
    neuropsychiatric consequences of
        medications for, **439**
    obsessive-compulsive disorder and,
        576–577, 578
    in patients with delusions or limited
        insight, 438–439
    prevalence of psychiatric disorders in
        patients with, 419
    psychological impact of, 421–422
    psychopharmacotherapy and, 435–438
Dermatology Life Quality Index, 423
Descriptive analytic reasoning, 5–6
Desensitization therapy, for complex
    regional pain syndrome, 656
Designer drugs, 618
Desipramine, **96**
Detoxification, and opioids, 602, 606
Dexmedetomidine, 593
Dextroamphetamine, 618
Dextromethorphan, **92,** 117
Diabetes mellitus, 193–197
Diagnosis. *See also* Bedside cognitive
    examination; Differential diagnosis;
    Electroencephalography; Laboratory
    tests; Misdiagnosis; Neuroimaging;
    Neurological examination
    of alcohol use disorders, 589

Diagnosis *(continued)*
  analytic and nonanalytic reasoning in, 4–6
  of cannabis use disorder, 614
  of catatonia, 531
  cognitive psychology approaches to, 4, 7
  confidence ratings on accuracy of, 10
  definition of, 4
  of insomnia, 665–667
  of major depressive disorder in cancer
    patients, 399
  medical causes of psychiatric illness and,
    7–8
  mixed physical and psychiatric
    symptomatology in, **8**
  of neurodevelopmental disorders, 483
  of neuroleptic malignant syndrome,
    86–87, **88–89**
  neuropsychiatric disorders and, 6–7
  of opioid use disorder, 600
  of personality disorders, 184
  of premenstrual dysphoric disorder, **451**
  of serotonin syndrome, 92–93, **94**
  of somatic symptom and related
    disorders, 678–680
  of stimulant use disorder, 618–619
  of tobacco-related disorders, 608–609
  of valproic acid-induced
    hyperammonemic encephalopathy,
    102
Diagnostic verification CFS, 10, **11**
Dialysis, and renal disease, 320, 321–322, 327,
    329, 331, 332–333
Diathesis-stress model, for chronic pain and
    comorbid psychiatric disorders, 653–654
Diazepam, 593
Diet. *See also* Lifestyle modifications;
    Nutrition; Vitamin deficiencies
  diabetes mellitus and, 195
  gastrointestinal disorders and, 295
  premenstrual mood disorder and, 452
Differential diagnosis.
    See also Diagnosis; Misdiagnosis
  of anxiety symptoms in cancer patients,
    401
  of catatonia, 529–531
  of conversion disorder, 687–688
  of delirium, 635–636, 641, **642**
  of dementia, 635–636
  of factitious disorder, 690
  of fibromyalgia syndrome, 655
  of illness anxiety disorder, 684–685

  of neurodevelopmental disorders,
    482–483
  of neuroleptic malignant syndrome, 87
  psychiatric conditions in HIV/AIDS and,
    273
  of psychological factors affecting other
    medical conditions, 692
  of serotonin syndrome, 93
  of somatic symptom disorder, 682
  of valproic acid-induced
    hyperammonemic encephalopathy,
    102
Diffuse body pain, and posttraumatic stress
    disorder, 579–580
Diffuse encephalopathies, **71, 72**
Diffusion tensor imaging (DTI), and cancer
    patients, 406
Diffusion-weighted MRI imaging, **54, 58**–59
Digit span, and tests of working memory,
    37–38
Dihydrocodeine, 605
Diltiazem, 186
Disease-modifying antirheumatic drugs
    (DMARDs), 238, 240
Disease-modifying therapies, for multiple
    sclerosis, 359, 362–364
Disorders of gut-brain interaction.
    See Functional gastrointestinal disorders
Disruptive behavior disorders, and Prader-
    Willi syndrome, 488
Disseminated intravascular coagulation
    (DIC), and neuroleptic malignant
    syndrome, 87
Dissociation, and conversion disorder, 687
Dissociative anesthetics, 117, **121–123**
Disulfiram, 526, 595–596
DMT (N,N-dimethyltryptamine), and
    psychiatric symptoms, **115**, 515
Docetaxel, **411**
Donepezil
  cognitive changes after chemotherapy
    and, 372
  dementia and, 636
  drug-drug interactions and, 186
  HIV and, 383
  torsades de pointes and, **151**
Dopamine agonists, 214, 347
Dorsal stream, and language function, 38
Dorsolateral frontal meningiomas, 371
Double-check, of diagnosis made through
    nonanalytic reasoning, 5

Double simultaneous stimulation test, 23
Down syndrome, 485–486, **487**
Dronabinol, 612, 638
Drug Abuse Screening Test (DAST-10), 598, 600
Drug Addiction Treatment Act in 2000, 607
Drug-drug interactions
    antibiotics and, **271,** 283
    antiviral medications and, **271,** 274
    cardiovascular disease and, 186
    drugs with primary psychiatric or primary neurological indications and, 341
    mood disorders and, 556
    psychiatric medications and agents used in cancer treatment, 410, **411–412,** 412
Drug-induced electrolyte abnormalities, 142, **143,** 144
Drug-induced hyponatremia, 142, **143,** 144
Drug-induced liver injury (DILI), 144–145, **146–147,** 148
Drug-induced long QT syndrome, 148–149, 152, **164, 167**
Drug-induced orthostatic hypotension, 152–153, **154**
Drug resistance, and tuberculosis, 269, 270
Drug testing, for toxicological complications or conditions associated with psychiatric illness, **164–166**
DSM-I, and classification of disorders, 6
DSM-III, and criteria-based diagnosis, 6
DSM-IV
    alcohol use disorders and, 589
    diagnostic criteria for panic disorder and, 566
    psychiatric terminology for neuropsychiatric symptoms and, 232
    somatic symptom and related disorders and, 678, **679**
DSM-IV-TR, and insomnia, 665
DSM-5 (American Psychiatric Association 2013)
    alcohol use disorders and, 589
    analytic reasoning and diagnostic model of, 6
    cannabis use disorder and, 614
    catatonia and, 524, 528
    classification of anxiety disorders and, 563
    conversion disorder and, 685
    definition of anxiety and, 234
    delirium and, 235, 528

    delusional disorders and, 426
    dementia and, 629
    factitious disorder and, 689
    fetal alcohol syndrome and, 493
    generalized anxiety disorder and, 569–570
    insomnia and, 665, **666**
    major depressive disorder and, 399
    mood disorders and, 541
    obsessive-compulsive disorders and, 575
    postconcussion syndrome and, 374
    posttraumatic stress disorder and, 578
    premenstrual dysphoric disorder and, 450, **451**
    somatic symptom disorders and, 653, 678
    specific phobia and, 573
    stimulant use disorder and, 618
    tobacco-related disorders and, 609
    vascular dementia and, 631
Dual-stream language-processing networks, 38
Duodenal ulcers, 298
Dysarthria patterns, and neurological examination, 21
Dysdiadochokinesia, 22
Dyskinesia, and neurological examination, 25
Dysmetria, 22
Dysmorphic features, and neurological examination, 17, **18,** 482, **483**
Dyspepsia, 290–291, 293, 294
Dysphagia, 21, 290, 292–293, 574
Dysphoria, and cancer, 553
Dyspraxia, 43–44
Dysthymia, and Parkinson's disease, 384
Dystonias, and neurological examination, 25–26

Eastern equine encephalitis, 267–268, 378
Eating disorders
    diabetes mellitus and, 196
    inflammatory bowel disease and, 302
    irritable bowel syndrome and, 293
    specific phobia and, 574
    women's mental health and, 447
Ebola, 268
Ebstein's cardiac malformation, 457
Ecchymosis, and Cushing's syndrome, 219
Echolalia, **40**
Economics
    costs related to chronic pain, 652
    costs related to dementia, 630
    impact of wage gap on women, 469

Edinburgh Postnatal Depression Scale
  (EPDS), 454, 462
Education.
  See Psychoeducation; Self-education
Efavirenz, 274
Ego-dystonic thoughts, and postpartum
  obsessive-compulsive disorder, 463
Ehrlichiosis, 279
Electrocardiogram (ECG), **99**, 149
Electroconvulsive therapy (ECT)
  anti-NMDAR encephalitis and, 254
  catatonia and, 533
  epilepsy and, 357, 359
  neuroleptic malignant syndrome and,
    90
  Parkinson's disease and, 384
Electroencephalography (EEG)
  anti-NMDAR encephalitis and, 251, 253,
    504
  antipsychotics and, 75
  chronic traumatic encephalopathy and,
    376, 377
  delirium and, 641–642
  encephalitis and, 381
  Hashimoto's encephalitis and, 246
  history and background of, 69–70
  indications for, **52**
  limbic encephalitides and, 78–79, **80**
  laboratory testing for toxicological
    conditions and, **164**
  psychotic symptoms and, 500
  traumatic brain injury and, 375
Electrolytes, and laboratory testing for
  toxicological conditions, **167–168**
Emergency. *See also* Emergency department
  catatonia as, 26, **28**
  delirious mania as, 537
  delirium tremens as, 594
  infectious diseases and, 266–268
  neuroleptic malignant syndrome as, **28,**
    87
  neuropsychiatric forms of, **28**
  PCP/ketamine intoxication as, **122**
  postpartum psychosis as, 453, 462
  serotonin syndrome as, **28,** 92
Emergency department (ED).
  See also Hospitalization
  chest pain related to panic disorder and,
    176
  migraines and, 365
  opioid intoxication and, 601

psychiatric symptoms in dermatological
    patients and, 439
  stimulant use disorder and, 620
  substance use disorders and, 588
  traumatic brain injury and, 373
Encephalitis, and encephalopathies.
  See also Anti-NMDAR encephalitis;
    Autoimmune encephalitis; Hashimoto's
    encephalitis; Herpes simplex
    encephalitis; Infectious encephalitis;
    Limbic encephalitis; Toxic encephalitis;
    Viral encephalitis
  catatonia and, 527
  electroencephalography and diagnosis of,
    71, 72, 73
  as emergency, 267–268
  Hashimoto's thyroiditis and, 200
  psychiatric symptoms of, 377–381
Endicott criteria, for depression in medically
  ill, 399, **400**
End-of-life planning, and renal disease, 332
Endocrine disorders. *See also* Acromegaly;
  Adrenal insufficiency; Cushing's
  syndrome; Diabetes mellitus;
  Hyperparathyroidism;
  Hyperprolactinemia;
  Pheochromocytoma; Polycystic ovary
  syndrome; Primary aldosteronism;
  Testosterone deficiency; Thyroid
  disorders
  catatonia and, 528
  as causes of anxiety and panic attacks, **565**
  laboratory testing for toxicological
    conditions and, **168–169**
  mood disorders and, 550–551
  psychosis and, **501**
Endocrine Society, 141
Endotoxin, and alcoholic hepatitis, 307
End-stage renal disease (ESRD), 319, 332–333
Engel, George, 6
Environmental autonomy, and executive
  functions, **46**
Environmental exposures, and
  neuropsychiatric toxidromes, 128,
    130–136
Environmental Protection Agency, 128
Ephedra species, **126**
Epidemics. *See also* Pandemics
  of infectious diseases, 268, **284**
  of opioid use, 652
Epidemiology. *See* Prevalence

Epigastric pain syndrome, 290–291
Epilepsy. *See also* Temporal lobe epilepsy
 cerebral palsy and, 484–485
 conversion disorder and, 687
 depression and, 354, **355,** 548–549
 definition of as neurological disorder, 339
 mood disorders and, 548–549
 neurocutaneous syndromes and, 490
 psychiatric issues in patients with,
  353–359
 psychosis and, 511
 stigma and, 341
Episodic memory dysfunction, 42
Epstein-Barr virus (EBV), 281
Epworth Sleepiness Scale, 34
Erectile dysfunction, and renal disease, 329
Erethism, **136**
Ergocalciferol, 141
Erythrocyte transketolase activity (ETKA),
 139
Escitalopram, **150,** 178, 182
Esophageal disorders, 290, 294
Essential tremor, **25,** 383–384, 385–386
Estrogen, 448
Etoposide, **411**
Euphoria sclerotica, 548
European League Against Rheumatism
 (EULAR), 236
Excessive daytime sleepiness, 327, 488
Excited catatonia, 524, 537
Excoriation disorder, **427,** 431–432, 488
Executive functions
 bedside cognitive examination and, 45, **46**
 fetal alcohol syndrome and, 493
 neurological disorders and, 344
 tests of cognitive domains and, 36, 37
Executive Interview Test, 344, 370
Exercise, and exercise programs
 cancer patients and, 402–403
 fibromyalgia syndrome and, 655
Exposure and response prevention, for
 obsessive-compulsive disorder, 577
Extreme delta brush activity, and EEG, 79

Face2Gene.com, 17
Facial sensation, and neurological
 examination, 20–21
Factitious disorder. *See also* Malingering
 cardiovascular symptoms and, **177**
 case example of, 690
 catatonia and, 530

clinical characteristics of, **681,** 689
 dermatological conditions and, **428,**
  433–434
 differential diagnosis and comorbidity,
  690
 epidemiology of, 690
 treatment of, 691
Family history.
  See also Collateral information
 of head size, 16–17
 of insomnia, 671
 of substance use disorders, 599
Fatigue
 cancer patients and, 399, 402–403
 cerebral palsy and, 485
 chronic fatigue syndrome and, 281
 gastroparesis and, 300
 multiple sclerosis and, 364
 neurological disorders and, 345
 poststroke depression and, 352
 sarcoidosis and, 249–250
Fatigue Severity Scale, 345
FDG-PET, **64,** 66–67, 68
Fear
 epilepsy and, **356**
 worry in generalized anxiety disorder as
  distinct from, 569
Fentanyl, 332, 601
Fetal alcohol syndrome, and fetal alcohol
  spectrum disorder (FASD), 492–493
Fibromyalgia syndrome, 654–655
Fingolimod, 363
Firearms, suicide risk and access to, 350
"5 A's" (ask, advise, assess, assist, arrange)
  model, and tobacco use disorders, 609
5-hydroxyindoleacetic acid (5-HIAA), 76
Fixed-dosage approach, to management of
  alcohol withdrawal, 592–593
Flashbacks, and hallucinogens, **116**
Florida Obsessive-Compulsive Inventory,
 577
Fludrocortisone, 153, 223
Fluency, and assessment of language, 39
5-Fluorouracil, **411**
Fluoxetine, 182, 450
Fluphenazine, **96,** 152
Focus, and tests of cognitive domains, 35
Folic acid deficiency, 138, **170**
Follicle-stimulating hormone (FSH), 211
Food and Drug Administration (FDA), 346,
 438, 455, 459, 610

4 *Ps* Plus questionnaire, 599
Fragile X syndrome, 485
Freud, Sigmund, 664–665
Frontal Assessment Battery, 32, 45, **46**
Frontal lobe(s), and cerebral lesions, 408–409
Frontal lobe epilepsy (FLE), **71,** 73, 75
Frontotemporal dementia, **64,** 67–68, 510,
     546–547, 632–633
Functional Assessment of Cancer Therapy—
     Cognitive Function, 372
Functional Assessment of Chronic Illness
     Therapy–Fatigue (FACIT-F), 402
Functional gastrointestinal disorders,
     290–295
Functional magnetic resonance imaging
     (fMRI), 60, **61**
Functional neuroimaging modalities, 60–62
Functional unawareness syndrome, 687
Fungal meningitis, 378
Fyn activation, and Alzheimer's disease, 630

Gabapentin, 328
Gadolinium contrast, and MRI, **55,** 59
Gait
     Angelman syndrome and, 488, 489
     neurological examination and, 23–24
Galactorrhea, 213
Galantamine, 636
Gamma-hydroxybutyrate (GHB), 117,
     118–120
Gastric ulcers, 298
Gastroduodenal disorders, 290–291
Gastroenterological diseases.
     See also Celiac disease; Functional
     gastrointestinal disorders;
     Gastrointestinal abnormalities;
     Gastrointestinal pain disorders;
     Inflammatory bowel disease; Liver;
     Lymphocytic colitis
     autism spectrum disorder and, 311–312
     generalized anxiety disorder and, 293,
     302, 305
     pancreatic and biliary diseases, 310–311
     primary disorders of, 298–300
     relationship between brain and
     gastrointestinal tract, 289
Gastroesophageal reflux, **668,** 673, **674**
Gastrointestinal abnormalities, and
     anticholinergic toxicity, **98**
Gastrointestinal pain disorders, 295–298
Gastroparesis, 299–300

Gegenhalten, and catatonia, 22, 524, 530
Gemcitabine, **411**
Generalized anxiety disorder (GAD).
     See also Anxiety disorders
     cardiovascular symptoms and, 177
     diabetes mellitus and, 196
     gastrointestinal disorders and, 293, 302,
        305
     in general medical setting, 569–573
     Graves' disease and, 247
     Hashimoto's thyroiditis and, 245
     neurological disorders and, 343
     rheumatoid arthritis and, 238–239
     sarcoidosis and, 249
Generalized Anxiety Disorder 7-item
     (GAD-7) scale, 422, 572
Genetic factors, and genetic disorders
     in Alzheimer's disease, 631
     catatonia and, 527
     in frontotemporal dementia, 632
     in gastrointestinal disorders, 292
     in mood disorders, 398, 542–543
     in pheochromocytoma, 215
     psychosis and, **501**
     vascular dementia as, 631
Gerstmann's syndrome, 45
Geschwind syndrome, 347–349
Glasgow Coma Scale (GCS), 34, **35,** 103, 373
Glatiramer, 363
Global aphasia, **40**
Global functions, tests of, 32–33
Glomerular filtration rate (GFR), 319
Glucocorticoids, 438, 506
Gluten sensitivity, and celiac disease, 304–306
Gnosis, 44
Graded exercise therapy (GET), and chronic
     fatigue syndrome, 281
Graft-versus-host disease, 408
Graves' disease, 200, 247–248, 569
Growth hormone, and acromegaly, 216, 217
Gynecomastia, 213

Habit-reversal therapy, and dermatological
     conditions, 431
Hallucinations
     alcohol use disorders and, **110,** 595
     anticholinergic toxicity and, **98**
     dementia with Lewy bodies and, 510, 633
     epilepsy and, **356**
     postpartum psychosis and, 463
     stimulant abuse and, 104

Hallucinogens
    plants as, 117, **124–127**
    psychiatric symptoms caused by, 109,
        115–116, 515, 516
Haloperidol
    anticholinergic toxicity and, **96**
    cardiac effects of, **150, 152,** 153, **154,** 185
    delirium and, 642–643
Hamilton Anxiety Scale, 325
Hamilton Rating Scale for Depression, 177,
    323
HAND. *See* HIV-associated neurocognitive
    disorder
Hand-washing compulsion, and obsessive-
    compulsive disorder, 576–577
Hashimoto's encephalitis, 246, 502–503
Hashimoto's thyroiditis, 199, 200, 244–247,
    379, 380
Headaches, 365, 378, 571, 656–658.
    See also Migraine
Head size, and abnormal brain development,
    16–17
Health care. *See also* Hospitalization; Medical
        complications; Medical conditions;
        Physical examination
    blood-injection-injury phobia and,
        573–574
    categorization of patients as either
        "neurological" or "psychiatric,"
        340–341
    frequency of anxiety in, 563
    management of dermatological
        conditions in primary care setting,
        422–424
    prevalence of substance abuse disorders
        in, 587
    quality of for patients with comorbid
        medical and psychiatric disorders,
        425
    treatment of anxiety disorders in, 580–582
Hearing, and neurological examination, 21
Heartburn, 290, 292
Heart failure, 179, **668,** 672
Heart transplantation, 187–188
Heavy metals, 128, **130–136**
Helicobacter pylori, 298–299
Hematin, 509
Hematological disorders, as cause of anxiety
    and panic attacks, **565**
Hematological testing, and laboratory tests
    for toxicological conditions, **169**

Hematopoietic stem cell transplantation
    (HSCT), 407–408
Hemianesthesia, and malingering, 26
Hemochromatosis, 308, 310
Hemodialysis, 321, 322
Hemoglobin, and laboratory testing for
    toxicological conditions, **168**
Hepatic encephalopathy, 307, 308–309
Hepatitis B virus (HBV), 276–277, **280**
Hepatitis C virus (HCV), 276–277, **280,** 306,
    307, 606
Hepatitis serology, **170**
Herbs and herbal remedies.
    See Plant(s); St. John's wort
Hereditary hemochromatosis, 306–307
Heroin, 605
Herpes simplex encephalitis (HSE), **28,** 378,
    379, 507
Herpes simplex virus (HSV), 267, 507
HIV
    cognitive impairment and, 636
    life cycle and treatment of, 272–274
    mood disorders and, 551–552
    opioid use disorder and, 606
    opportunistic infections and, 274–275
    prevention of, 275–276
    psychiatric complications of, 276,
        382–383, 506–507
    screening for, **280**
HIV-associated dementia, 507
HIV-associated neurocognitive disorder
    (HAND), 276, 382–383, 636
HIV Care Continuum initiative, 275
Homeostasis, and immune system, 229
Hoover's sign, and neurological
    examination, 26
Hormonal therapy
    for depression during perimenopause,
        468
    for premenstrual dysphoric disorder,
        451–452
Hospital Anxiety and Depression Scale
    (HADS), 237, 240, 325, 349, 399, 422
Hospital Elder Life Program (HELP), 644
Hospitalization.
    See also Emergency department;
        Health care; Intensive care unit
    related to opioid misuse and dependence,
        597
    tobacco-related disorders and, 608
Hostility, in patients with heart disease, 180

Hot flashes, and menopause, 466, 467
HPA axis, and gastrointestinal disorders, 291–292
Human granulocytic anaplasmosis, 279
Hunter Serotonin Toxicity Criteria set, 92, **93**, 536
Huntington's disease, 511–512, 546, 633, 634
Hydrocortisone, and adrenal insufficiency, 223
Hydrogen-1 MRS, 62
Hydroxyurea, **411**
Hyperactive delirium, 639–640
Hyperammonemia, and valproic acid–induced hyperammonemic encephalopathy, 100
Hyperarousal, and tests of cognitive domains, 34
Hypercalcemia, and lithium, **143**, **167**
Hypercortisolism, 506
Hyperemesis gravidarum, 464–465
Hyperglycemia, and diabetes mellitus, 195
Hyperhidrosis, 438
Hyperkinetic movements, 24
Hypernatremia, and lithium, **143**
Hyperparathyroidism, **167**, 204–206
Hyperprolactinemia, 212–214
Hypertension, and primary aldosteronism, 221
Hyperthermia
    anticholinergic toxicity and, **98**
    MDMA and GHB, **118**
    neuroleptic malignant syndrome and, 87
    serotonin syndrome and, 95
Hyperthyroidism. *See also* Thyroid disorders
    anxiety and, **581**
    diagnostic and laboratory tests for, **202**
    Graves' disease and, 247
    lithium and, **169**
    manifestations of, 199
    mood disorders and, 550
    panic disorder and, 568–569
    psychiatric symptoms of, 201–202, 505–506
Hypnotherapy, and gastrointestinal disorders, 295
Hypoactive delirium, 640
Hypoalbuminemia, 321
Hypocalcemia, and 22q11.2 deletion syndrome, 490
Hypochondriasis, 684
Hypoglycemia, and diabetes mellitus, 196–197, 197–198

Hypogonadism, 210, 213, 329
Hypokinesis, and neurological examination, 26
Hypomagnesemia, 595
Hypomania, 362, 542.
    See also Mania
Hypomania Checklist–32–Revised, 367
Hyponatremia
    cancer patients and, 410
    drug-induced, 142, **143**, 144
    laboratory tests for, **168**
    psychotic symptoms and, 506
Hypopituitarism, and acromegaly, 218
Hypotension, and anticholinergic toxicity, **99**.
    See also Drug-induced orthostatic hypotension
Hypothyroidism. *See also* Thyroid disorders
    diagnostic and laboratory tests for, **202**
    lithium and, **168**
    manifestations of, 199, 245
    mood disorders and, 550
    psychiatric symptoms and, 201, 246, 505
Hypoventilation, and sedating drugs, **167**
Hypoxemia, 327

ICD-10, and postconcussion syndrome, 374
Ictal psychiatric symptoms, and epilepsy, 354
Ideational apraxia, 44
Ideomotor apraxia, 44
Ifosfamide, **411**
Illness anxiety disorder
    cardiovascular disease and, 176–177
    case example of, 684
    clinical characteristics of, **681**, 683–684
    dermatological manifestations of, **427**
    differential diagnosis and comorbidity, 684–685
    DSM-5 and classification of, **679**
    epidemiology of, 684
    treatment of, 433, 685
Illness behavior, and somatic symptom disorder, 681
Illness scripts, 5
Iloperidone, 153
"Imaging Dementia—Evidence for Amyloid Scanning" (IDEAS) study, 635
Immune system. *See also* Autoimmune disorders; Immunotherapy; Infections
    contested diseases and, 281
    depressive and manic states, 543
    inflammation and, 229–230

Immunosuppressants, **411,** 502

Immunotherapy, and anti-NMDAR encephalitis, 253–254, 504

Impulsive-compulsive syndrome, of Parkinson's disease, 347, 385

Incidence rate ratio (IRR), of autoimmune disorders to psychiatric illness, 283

Indoleamine 2,3-dioxygenase (IDO), 231

Infants, and prenatal exposure to psychoactive drugs, 456–460. *See also* Children; Fetal alcohol syndrome; Pregnancy

Infections, and infectious diseases. *See also* Hepatitis B virus; Hepatitis C virus; HIV; Syphilis; Tick-borne diseases aggressive behavior and, **484** contested illnesses, 280–283 emergencies and, 266–268 epidemiological linkage of to psychiatric illness, 283 laboratory testing for toxicological conditions and, **170** lumbar puncture and central nervous system, 78 mood disorders and, 551–552 obsessive-compulsive disorder in children and, 576 psychosis and, **501,** 506–508 pulmonary infections, 268–272 roles for psychiatrists, **284** of skin, **422** substance use disorders and, 599 web-based resources on, **266**

Infectious Disease Society of America, 282

Infectious encephalitis, 377, 378

Inflammation, and inflammatory diseases. *See also* Encephalitis; Graves' disease; Hashimoto's thyroiditis; Inflammatory bowel disease; Rheumatoid arthritis; Sarcoidosis; Scleroderma; Sjogren's syndrome; Systemic lupus erythematosus depressive or manic states and, 543 dermatological conditions and stress, 421, **422** immune system and, 229–230 mood disorders and, 552–553 psychiatric disorders and, 230–231

Inflammatory bowel disease (IBD), 300–303, **304,** 553

Infliximab, 230, 231

Influenza, 269

Informed consent, and neurosurgery, 371

Innate immune system, 229–230

Insight, dermatological conditions in patients with limited, 438–439

Insomnia. *See also* Sleep and sleep disorders delirium and, 641 dementia and, 634–635 diagnosis of, 665–667 generalized anxiety disorder and, 572 impact of, 664 medical comorbidities and, 667–673 pathophysiology of, 664–665 posttraumatic stress disorder and, 579 pregnancy and treatment of, 461 prevalence of, 663 renal disease and, 327 treatment of, 673, **674**

Insomnia Severity Index (ISI), 669

Institute of Medicine, 281, 651, 652

Integrase inhibitors, 273, 274

Intellectual disability, 484–485, 490

Intelligence quotient (IQ), and Klinefelter syndrome, 486

Intensive care unit (ICU). *See also* Hospitalization alcohol-related disorders and, 588–596 tobacco-related disorders and, 608, 610

Interferon (IFN), **240,** 277, 309, **411,** 514

Interferon-γ release assays (IGRAs), 270

Interictal personality, of temporal lobe epilepsy, 347–349

Interictal psychosis, 511

International Agency for Research on Cancer, 128

International Association for the Study of Pain, 651–652

International Classification of Headache Disorders, 3rd Edition (ICHD-3), 657

International Cognition and Cancer Task Force (ICCTF), 406

International Expert Consensus (IEC) diagnostic criteria, for catatonia, 534

International Lyme and Associated Diseases Society, 282

Internet-based self-management, and rheumatoid arthritis, 240

Internuclear ophthalmoplegia, 20

Intestinal microbiome, and gastrointestinal disorders, 289, 292, 301, 311

Intoxication
  alcohol and, **114**
  cannabis use disorder and, 614–615
  dissociative anesthetics and, 117
  MDMA and GHB, **118, 120**
  opioids and, 601
  PCP/ketamine and, **122, 123**
  sedative-hypnotics and, **113, 114**
  stimulants and, 619
Intracranial hemorrhage, and computed
  tomography, 56
Intravenous (IV) hydration, for neuroleptic
  malignant syndrome, 87
Involuntary movements, and neurological
  examination, 24–26
Iodinated contrast, and computed
  tomography, **54,** 56–57
Irritable bowel syndrome (IBS), 291, 293, 294,
  295
Ischemia, and coronary artery disease, 178
Isoniazid, 270
Isotretinoin, 438, **439**
Itch-scratch cycle, and dermatological
  conditions, 421

Jaw jerk, and facial sensation, 20
Jimsonweed (*Datura stramonium*), **126**

Keratoconjunctivitis sicca, and Sjogren's
  syndrome, 241
Ketamine, 117, **121–123**
Khat/qat, **127**
Kidney injury, and drug toxicity, **167**
Klebsiella, 269
Klinefelter syndrome, 486–487
Korsakoff syndrome, **111,** 139, 513, 594, 595
Kratom (*Mitragyna speciosa*), **124,** 606–607

Laboratory tests
  alcohol use disorders and, 590, 591
  anticholinergic toxicity and, **100**
  catatonia and, 531
  delirium and, 641–642
  dementia and, 635–636
  hyperparathyroidism and, 205
  hyperprolactinemia and, 213
  insomnia and, 672–673
  medical etiologies of anxiety and, **581**
  neuroleptic malignant syndrome and,
    87, **89**
  new-onset psychosis and, 500, **501**

  opioid use disorders and, 600
  pheochromocytoma and, 215
  sarcoidosis and, 250
  serotonin syndrome and, 93, **94**
  testosterone deficiency and, 211
  thyroid disorders and, **202**
  toxicological complications and
    conditions associated with
    psychiatric illness, **164–171**
  valproic acid-induced hyperammonemic
    encephalopathy and, **103**
Lactation, and psychotropic medications,
  465–466
Lactulose, and valproic acid-induced
  hyperammonemic encephalopathy,
  103
Lamotrigine, **166,** 437, 457–458
Language, and language deficits
  Angelman syndrome and, 489
  bedside cognitive examination and,
    38–39, **40**
  Turner syndrome and, 487
Latent autoimmune diabetes in adults
  (LADA), 194
Latent tuberculosis infection (LTBI),
  269–270
LBD. *See* Dementia with Lewy bodies
Lead, 128, **132–134**
Learning disorders, 491
Left ventricular assist devices (LVADs), and
  cardiovascular disease, 188
Legalization, of marijuana, 613, 614
Legionella spp., 268
Leptomeningeal disease, 408
Leukoencephalopathy, 407
Leuprolide, **411**
Levothyroxine, 199
Lewy bodies.
    See Dementia with Lewy bodies
Lexical fluency, and executive functions, **46**
Lidocaine patches, 331
Lifestyle modifications.
    See also Diet; Exercise
  depression in patients with renal disease
    and, 323
  dermatological conditions and, 424
  polycystic ovary syndrome and, **208**
  premenstrual mood disorders and, 452
Light therapy, for sleep-related disorders in
  older adults, 638.
    See also Bright light therapy

Limbic encephalitis. *See also* Paraneoplastic
limbic encephalitis
catatonia and, 531
mood disorders and, 552–553
neurodiagnostic testing and, **71,** 76, 78–79,
80
NMDAR-associated, 409
psychiatric symptoms of, 250–251
Limb-kinetic apraxia, **44**
Line bisection task, 36
Linezolid, **92**
Listeria monocytogenes, 267
Listeriosis, 267
Lithium
behavioral symptoms of dementia and, 638
cardiac effects of, **151,** 186
drug-induced orthostatic hypotension
and, 153
hypernatremia and, **143,** 144
laboratory testing for toxicological
complications of, **165, 168**
mania in cancer patients and, 400–401
pregnancy and, 457
psoriasis and, 437–438
thyroid function and, **168,** 203–204
Liver, and liver diseases
assessment for preexisting disease of, 145
benzodiazepines and, 591
clinical presentation of, 307–308
diagnosis of, 308–309
drug-induced injury to, 144–145, **146–147,**
148
etiology of, 307
function tests, **111, 171**
subtypes and defining criteria of, 306–307
treatment of, 309–310
Locked-in syndrome, 529, **530**
Long QT syndrome, drug-induced, 148–149,
152
Lorazepam, **91,** 325, 532–533, 594
LSD (lysergic acid diethylamide), and
psychiatric symptoms, **116,** 515
Lumbar puncture
background and history of, 76
central nervous system infections and, 78
contraindications to, 76
indications for, **52**
limbic encephalitides and, 78–79, **80**
Lung cancer, 404, 409
Lurasidone, 153
Luria three-step test, **46**

Luteinizing hormone (LH), 209, 211
Lyme disease, 279, **280,** 281–282
Lymphocytic colitis, 303
Lysergic acid amide (LSA), **126**

Macrocephaly, 16–17
Macrocytic anemia, 551
Magnesium
chronic alcohol use and depletion of, 595
laboratory testing for toxicological
conditions, **167**
Magnetic resonance imaging (MRI)
advantages and limitations of, **54–55,** 57–58
Alzheimer's disease and, 63, **64,** 66
anti-NMDAR encephalitis and, 253, 504
background and history of, 57
brain tumors and, 408
cancer patients and phobias related to
repeated, 401
cognitive changes after chemotherapy
and, 372
common neurological disorders and, **70**
delirium and, 642
dementia and, 635
diffusion-weighted imaging, **54,** 58–59
encephalitis and, 381
gadolinium contrast and, **55,** 59
indications for, **52**
leukoencephalopathy and, 407
limbic encephalitis and, 79, **80**
multiple sclerosis and, 361
psychotic symptoms and, 500
stress associated with, 59
susceptibility-weighted imaging, **55,** 59
systemic lupus erythematosus and, 236
T1- and T2-weighted sequences, **54,** 58
T2-weighted fluid-attenuated inversion
recovery (T2-FLAIR), **54,** 58, **70**
traumatic brain injury and, 374, 375, 376,
377
Magnetic resonance spectroscopy, 61–62
Major depressive disorder (MDD).
See also Depression
cancer patients with, 398
cardiovascular symptoms and, 177
coronary disease and, 181
dermatological conditions and, 423
diabetes mellitus and, 196
Graves' disease and, 247
menopause and, 466
migraine and, 366

Major depressive disorder (MDD)
   (continued)
   neurological disorders and, 343
   Parkinson's disease and, 385
   prevalence of in women, 447
   renal disease and, 322–324
   sarcoidosis and, 249
   suicidal ideation and, 654
   systemic lupus erythematosus and,
     233–234
Malignant hyperthermia, 529, **530**
Malingering
   cardiovascular symptoms and, **177**
   catatonia and, 530
   factitious disorder versus, 689, 690
   neurological examination and, 26
Mallampati Airway Classification, 672
Management.
   See also Prevention; Treatment
   of alcohol withdrawal, **592**
   of anticholinergic toxicity, 95, 97, 100
   of depression and anxiety in patients with
     dermatological conditions, 422–424
   of drug-induced liver injury, 145, 148
   of drug-induced long QT syndrome, 149,
     152
   of drug-induced orthostatic hypotension,
     153
   of pain in patients with renal disease,
     331–332
   of psychiatric symptoms caused by
     substance abuse, **120, 123, 129**
Manganese, **130**
Mania. *See also* Bipolar disorder;
   Delirious mania
   adrenal insufficiency and, 224
   cancer patients and, 400–401, 553
   cardiovascular conditions and, 549
   Cushing's syndrome and, 220, 551
   definition of episode, 542
   epilepsy and, 549
   Graves' disease and, 248
   HIV and, 276, 552
   medications associated with, **555,** 556
   misdiagnosis of, 548
   secondary to brain lesions, 342
   thyroid disorders and, 202, 550
   traumatic brain injury and, 544–545
   vascular disease and stroke, 545
Manitoba IBD Epidemiology Database, 302
Mantoux tuberculin skin test, 270

Marijuana, and psychiatric symptoms,
   107–108, 515.
     See also Cannabinoid(s); Cannabis use
     disorder
"Matchbox sign," and delusional parasitosis,
   426
Maternity leave, impact of on maternal and
   child health, 470
Maturity-onset diabetes of the young
   (MODY), 194
MCI. *See* Mild cognitive impairment
MDMA. *See* 3,4-
   Methylenedioxymethamphetamine
Medical clearance criteria, for discharge of
   medical patient to psychiatric facility,
   9, 10
Medical complications. *See also* Comorbidity;
   Medical conditions
   of alcohol abuse, **113**
   of MDMA and GHB, **118–119**
   of mercury exposure, **136**
   of PCP/ketamine, **123**
   of sedative-hypnotic abuse, **113**
   of serotonin syndrome, 536
Medical conditions. *See also* Cancer;
   Cardiovascular disease; Comorbidity;
   Dermatological conditions; Diabetes
   mellitus; Endocrine disorders;
   Gastroenterological diseases; Health
   care; Infections; Inflammation; Medical
   complications; Neurological disorders;
   Physical examination; Renal disease
   cannabis-related disorders and, 611–617
   case example of misdiagnosis of
     psychiatric symptoms caused by,
     11–12
   catatonia caused by, 524–526
   diagnosis of psychiatric illness caused by,
     7–8
   generalized anxiety disorder and, 569–573
   insomnia and, 667–673
   lead exposure and, **133, 134**
   mood disorders caused by, 543–553
   neurological plus psychiatric symptoms
     from, 341
   obsessive-compulsive disorder and,
     575–578
   opioid-related disorders and, 596–607
   panic disorder and, 564–569
   posttraumatic stress disorder and,
     578–580

psychosis caused by, **501,** 501–513
social anxiety disorder and, 574–575
somatic symptom disorder and, 682
specific phobia and, 573–574
stimulant-related disorders and, 617–620
tobacco-related disorders and, 607–611
Medical marijuana, 611, 613
Medications. *See also* Antibiotics;
    Anticonvulsants; Antihistamines; Drug-
    drug interactions; Hormonal therapy;
    Opioids; Psychoactive drugs; Side effects
    brain tumors and, 510
    cannabinoids and, 611
    catatonia and, 526, **527**
    as cause of anxiety and panic attacks, **565**
    heart disease and psychiatric symptoms
        due to, 179
    insomnia and, 667, **674**
    mood disorders associated with, 554, **555**
    neuropsychiatric consequences of
        dermatological, **439**
    psychotic symptoms and, **501,** 510,
        513–516
    tobacco-related disorders and, 609
    tremor and toxicity of, **25**
Meiosis, and anticholinergic toxicity, **98**
Melatonin, 326, 327, 405, 638, 644
Memantine, 298, 532, 534
Memory, and bedside cognitive examination,
    40–42.
    See also Short-term memory; Working
    memory
Meningioma, 371
Meningitis, 78, 267
Meningoencephalitis, 377–381
Menopause, and psychiatric symptoms, 452,
    466–468
Menstrual cycle, psychiatric disorders
    associated with, 449–452
Mental Health Parity and Addiction Equity
    Act of 2008, 588
Mercury, 128, **135**
Metabolic disorders
    encephalopathies as, 70, 72
    psychosis and, **501,** 508–509
    tremor and, **25**
Metacognition, and neurological disorders,
    344–345, 382, 383
Metformin, 195, 198, **208,** 209
Methadone, **97, 151,** 602–603, 604–605, 606
Methamphetamine, 513–514, 617, 620

Methimazole, 203
Methotrexate, **240, 411, 439**
Methylene blue, **92**
Methylenedioxymethamphetamine
    (MDMA), **92,** 117, **118–120,** 618
Methylphenidate, 618, 643–644
Microdeletion syndromes, 487–490
Microglia, and immune system, 229–230
Middle East respiratory syndrome, 268
Midodrine, 153
Migraine
    bipolar disorder and, 342
    chronic pain and, 654, 657
    generalized anxiety disorder and, 571
    neurological symptoms and psychiatric
        comorbidity, 365–368
Mild cognitive impairment (MCI), 62, 63,
    276, 547
Mild traumatic brain injury, 373
Mindfulness-based stress reduction (MBSR),
    240
Mini-Cog, 33
Minimata disease, **135**
Mini-Mental State Examination (MMSE), 32,
    39, 41, 43, 44, 330, 344
Minocycline, **439**
Mirtazapine
    centrally mediated abdominal pain
        syndrome and, 297
    delirium and, 643
    dementia and, 637
    depression in cancer patients and, 400
    gastrointestinal disorders and, 294, 299, 300
    liver disease and, 310
    renal disease and, 324
    thyroid disorders and, 203
Misdiagnosis.
    See also Diagnosis; Differential diagnosis
    case example of psychiatric symptoms
        caused by medical condition and,
        11–12
    of catatonia, 524
    contested illnesses and, 281
    controversy on incidence of medical in
        patients with psychiatric symptoms, 7
    of mania, 548
    of panic disorder, 566
    of postpartum obsessive-compulsive
        disorder, 464
    psychiatric symptoms of medical
        disorders and, 3

Misdiagnosis *(continued)*
of pulmonary infections as depression, 269
stimulant-induced psychoses and, 104
strategies for minimizing medical, 8–10
theory-based strategy to reduce, 10–12
Mitochondrial encephalopathy with lactic acidosis and stroke-like episodes (MELAS), 631
Mixed delirium, 640
Modified Mini-Mental State Examination, 32
Monitoring, of anticholinergic toxicity, 97. *See also* Cognitive monitoring
Monitoring the Future study, 613–614
Monoamine oxidase inhibitors (MAOIs)
cardiovascular effects of in heart disease patients, 184–185
drug-induced orthostatic hypotension and, 152
pheochromocytoma and, 216
pregnancy and, 457
serotonin syndrome and, 90, **92,** 535, 536
Month of the year backward test, 36
Montreal Cognitive Assessment (MoCA), 32, 39, 41, 43, 344, 372
Mood Disorder Questionnaire (MDQ), 367, 454
Mood disorders. *See also* Depression
definition of abnormal mood states, 541–542
genetic factors in, 542–543
medical conditions as causes of, 543–553
medications associated with, 554, **555**
migraine and, 367
principles of treatment for, 554, 556
systemic lupus erythematosus and, 233–234
Mood-stabilizing agents. *See also* Carbamazepine; Lithium; Valproate
abnormal mood states and, 556
anticholinergic toxicity and, **96**
delirium and, 643
dementia and, 637–638
drug-induced liver injury and, 145, **147**
pregnancy and, 453, 457–458
torsades de pointes and, **151**
Moraxella, 268
Morgellons disease, 426
Morphine, 332
Mortality. *See also* Sudden cardiac death
Angelman syndrome and, 489

antipsychotics for elderly patients with dementia, 509
depression in cancer patients and, 398
depression in patients with coronary disease and, 182
diagnosis of cancer and, 553
encephalitis and, 267
maternity leave and rate of for infants, 470
neuroleptic malignant syndrome and, 90
opioid overdoses and, 597
Prader-Willi syndrome and, 488
pulmonary infections and, 268
tobacco-related disorders and, 607–608, 611
Turner syndrome and, 487
Motivational enhancement therapy, for substance use disorders, 616, 620
Motor functions, and neurological examination, 21–22
Motor vehicle collisions, and cannabis intoxication, 615
Movement disorders, and anti-NMDAR encephalitis, 251. *See also* Parkinson's disease
Multidrug resistance (MDR), and tuberculosis, 270
Multimorbidity, and cerebral palsy, 485
Multiple endocrine neoplasia type 2 (MEN-2), 568
Multiple sclerosis, 26, **27,** 359–364, 512, 547–548
Munchausen syndrome, 689
Muscle rigidity, and neuroleptic malignant syndrome, 86, **88,** 93
Music therapy, for dementia in older adults, 638
Mutism, and catatonia, 524
Mycobacterium, 270
Mycoplasma pneumoniae, 268
Myocardial infarction, 180
Myocarditis, **164**
Myoclonus, and serotonin syndrome, 93
Myofascial pain syndrome, 655
Myoglobinuria, and neuroleptic malignant syndrome, 87
Myxedema, 199, 200, 201, 505

Nabilone, 612
Naloxone, 602, 604
Naltrexone, 596, 601, 605
Naming ability, and language, 38
Narcotic bowel syndrome (NBS), 296–298

Narcotics Anonymous, 606
National Comorbidity Survey, 367
National Comprehensive Cancer Network
    (NCCN), 402
National Health Interview Survey, 608–609
National Health and Nutrition Examination
    Survey, 141
National HIV/AIDS Strategy, 275
National Institute on Drug Abuse single-item
    drug use screen (NIDA-1), 598, 599, 600
National Institute of Neurological Disorders
    and Stroke-Association Internationale
    pour la Recherché et l'Enseignement en
    Neurosciences (NINDS-AIREN), 68
National Institutes of Health (NIH), 207, 613,
    665
National Population Health Survey (NPHS),
    301
National Survey on Drug Use and Health,
    468, 614
Nausea, anticipatory in cancer patients, 403
Nefazodone, 186
Neisseria meningitidis, 267
NEO Five-Factor Inventory, 348
Neologism, **40**
Neonatal adaptation syndrome, 456
Neoplasms, and mood disorders, 543–544
Nephrogenic diabetes insipidus, 144
Neural tube defects, 458
Neurasthenia, and mercury exposure, **135**
Neurobehavioral disorder associated with
    prenatal alcohol exposure, 493
Neurocognitive disorders, and psychotic
    symptoms, 509–511.
    See also Cognitive disorders; Delirium;
    Dementia
Neurocognitive profile, and Klinefelter
    syndrome, 486
Neurocognitive testing, and psychiatric
    complications of HIV, 276
Neurocutaneous syndromes, 17, **18**, 490–491
Neurodegenerative disorders, 546–547
Neurodevelopmental disorders.
    See also Cerebral palsy; Down
    syndrome; Fetal alcohol syndrome;
    Fragile X syndrome; Klinefelter
    syndrome; Microdeletion syndromes;
    Neurocutaneous syndromes; Nonverbal
    learning disorder; Turner syndrome
    classification of, 481–482
    diagnosis of, 481, 482, **483**

differential diagnosis of, 482–483
    medical etiologies of aggressive behavior
        and, **484**
Neurodevelopmental signs (soft signs),
    17–18, **19**
Neurodiagnostic testing.
    See Electroencephalography; Lumbar
    puncture; Neuroimaging
Neuroendocrine conditions, and psychotic
    symptoms, 505–506
Neurofibrillary tangles, and chronic
    traumatic encephalopathy, 376
Neurofibromatosis type I, **18**, 491, 568
Neuroimaging.
    See also Computed tomography;
    Magnetic resonance imaging
    findings in dementia and neurocognitive
        disorders, 62–69, 635
    functional modalities of, 60–62
    indications for, **52**
    limbic encephalitides and, 78–79, **80**
    structural modalities of, 53–60
Neuro-immuno-cutaneous system, and
    dermatological conditions, 420
Neuroleptic malignant syndrome
    catatonia and, 534–535
    clinical presentation and diagnosis of,
        86–87, **88–89**
    differential diagnosis of, 87, 93
    as emergency, **28**, 87
    epidemiology of and risk factors for, 86
    treatment of, 87, 90, **91**
Neurological disorders.
    See also Chronic traumatic
        encephalopathy; Encephalitis; Epilepsy;
        HIV; Migraine; Multiple sclerosis;
        Neurodevelopmental disorders;
        Neurological examination; Neurosurgery;
        Parkinson's disease; Stroke; Temporal
        lobe epilepsy; Traumatic brain injury
    aggressive behavior and, **484**
    apathy and, 345–346
    bidirectional relationship between
        psychiatric disorders and, 351
    brain conditions treated by neurosurgery,
        368–371
    catatonia and, 526–527, **528**
    categorization of patients as "psychiatric"
        or "neurological," 340–341
    definition of, 339
    depression and, 350

Neurological disorders *(continued)*
  executive function and, 344
  fatigue and, 345
  metacognition and, 344–345
  mood disorders and, 543–549
  pain and, 349
  pseudobulbar affect and, 346–347
  psychiatric symptoms of, 340, 343
  psychotic symptoms and, **501**
  stigma of, 341
  suicide risk and, 350–351
Neurological Disorders Depression Inventory
  for Epilepsy (NDDI-E), 348, 349
Neurological examination.
    See also Neuropsychiatric examination;
    Neuropsychological testing; Physical
    examination
  coordination and, 22
  cranial nerves and, 18–21
  demyelinating disease and, 26, **27**
  embellishment and malingering, 26
  gait and balance, 23–24
  involuntary movements and, 24–26
  motor function and reflexes, 21–22
  neurodevelopmental signs and, 17–18,
    19
  neuropsychiatric formulation and,
    28–29
  physical examination and, 15–17
  rating scales for, **17**
  sensation and, 23
Neuropsychiatric disorders, diagnosis of, 6–7.
    See also Neurological disorders
Neuropsychiatric examination, basic toolkit
  for, **16**
Neuropsychiatric formulation, and
  neurological examination, 28–29
Neuropsychiatric Inventory (NPI), 348, 634
Neuropsychiatric toxidromes.
    See also Neuroleptic malignant
    syndrome; Serotonin syndrome
  anticholinergic toxicity, 95–103
  definition of, 85
  drugs of abuse and, 103–128, **129**
  environmental exposures to heavy
    metals, 128, **130–136**
  laboratory tests for, **164–171**
  micronutrient deficiencies and, 128,
    137–142
  valproic acid-induced hyperammonemic
    encephalopathy, 100, 102–103

Neuropsychological testing, and cognitive
  deficits in Sjogren's syndrome, 243.
    See also Neurological examination
Neurosarcoidosis, 249
Neurosurgery, and brain conditions, 368–371
Neurosyphilis, **170**, 278–279, 507.
    See also Syphilis
Niacin, 137–138, 595
Nicotinamide, 138
Nicotine. *See* Tobacco-related disorders
Nicotine Anonymous, 609
Nicotine replacement treatment (NRT), 608,
  610
Nightmares, and posttraumatic stress
  disorder, 579
NMDAR-associated psychiatric illness, 380.
    See also Anti-NMDAR encephalitis
NMS-like syndromes, 86
Nocturnal seizures, **668**
Noise, and stress from MRI scanning, 59
Nonalcoholic steatohepatitis, 306, 308, 310
Nonanalytic reasoning, and diagnosis, 4–5
Nonconvulsive status epilepticus (NCSE),
  71, 73, 75
Nonlateralizing neurological signs, 18, **19**
Nonsteroidal anti-inflammatory drugs
  (NSAIDs)
  combined with triptans for migraine, 365
  for depressive and manic states, **555**
  posttraumatic stress disorder and, 580
  psychiatric side effects of, **240**
  renal disease and, 331
  rheumatoid arthritis and, 238, **240**
Nonverbal learning disorder (NVLD),
  491–492
Nortriptyline, 465
Nutmeg (*Myristica fragrans*), **124**
Nutrition. *See also* Diet; Vitamin deficiencies
  as cause of anxiety and panic attacks, **565**
  choking phobia and, 574
  laboratory testing for toxicological
    conditions and, **170**
  micronutrient deficiencies and, 128,
    137–142
  neurological disorders and, 343

Obesity
  Cushing's syndrome and, 218, 219
  insomnia and, 672
  Prader-Willi syndrome and, 488
Obsessions, definition of, 575

Obsessive-compulsive disorder
dermatological conditions and, **427,** 430
in general medical setting, 575–578
Hashimoto's thyroiditis and, 245
postpartum period and, 463–464
Prader-Willi syndrome and, 488
systemic lupus erythematosus and, 234
tics and, 24
Obsessive Compulsive Inventory–Revised, 577
Obstructive sleep apnea (OSA)
cardiovascular disease and, 183
cognitive domains and, 34
insomnia and, **668,** 671, 672, **674**
physical examination and, 17
renal disease and, 327–328
Obtundation, and cognitive domain, 34
Ocrelizumab, 363
Ocular motility, and neurological examination, 19
Olanzapine
anticholinergic toxicity and, **96**
delirium and, 643
drug-induced long QT syndrome and, **152**
drug-induced orthostatic hypotension and, 153, **154**
EEG abnormalities and, 75
Parkinson's disease and, 385
Older adults.
See also Age; Alzheimer's disease
antipsychotic use in, 637, 643
avoidance of benzodiazepines for, 638
insomnia in, 663
pharmacokinetics and treatment of dementia in, 636
phenomenology of depression in, 634
psychotic side effects of anticholinergic medications in, 514
somatic symptom disorder in, 680–681
vascular depression in, 545
vitamin deficiencies and psychiatric symptoms in, 551
Olfaction, loss of as sign of neurodegenerative disease, 18–19
"Ophelia syndrome," 379
Ophthalmopathy, and Graves' disease, 247
Opioid(s). *See also* Opioid use disorders
cannabis use by pain patients and, 612–613
epidemic and overdose deaths from, 652
fibromyalgia syndrome and, 655
inflammatory bowel disease and, 302

mood disorders and, **555**
narcotic bowel syndrome and, 296–298
overdoses of, 597, 601
posttraumatic stress disorder and, 580
psychiatric symptoms and, 104
renal disease and, 331, 332
serotonin syndrome and, **92**
Opioid use disorders, medical conditions associated with, **589,** 596–607
Opportunistic infections, and HIV, 274–275
Optic nerve, and neurological examination, 19
Optokinetic nystagmus (OKN), 20
Oral reflexes, 22
Orbital groove meningiomas, 371
Organ transplantation, and renal disease, 320, 326
Orientation, and tests of cognitive domains, 34–35
Orthostatic hypotension, **581**
Osteoporosis, and Cushing's syndrome, 219
Ostomy surgery, psychological adjustment after, 312
Ovarian teratoma, 251, 379, 409, 464, 503
Oxcarbazepine, and drug-induced hyponatremia, 142, **143**

Paclitaxel, **411**
Pain
aggressive behavior and, **484**
buprenorphine and, 607
cerebral palsy and, 485
definition of chronic, 651–652
gastrointestinal disorders and, 295–298
generalized anxiety disorder and, 571
neurological disorders and, 349
opioid use disorders and, 599
poststroke depression and, 352
posttraumatic stress disorder and, 579–580
psychiatric comorbidity and, 652–658
renal disease and management of, 331–332
Palilalia, **40**
Palmomental reflex, 22
Pancreatic cancer, 310–311
Pandemics, of influenza, 269
Panic attacks
definition of panic disorder and, 564
gastrointestinal symptoms and, 293
medical causes of, **565**
pheochromocytoma and, 215
specific phobia and, 574

Panic disorder
    cardiovascular symptoms and, 176, **177**
    celiac disease and, 305
    gastrointestinal disorders and, 293
    in general medical setting, 564–569
    Hashimoto's thyroiditis and, 245
    inflammatory bowel disease and, 302
    renal disease and, 326
    sarcoidosis and, 249
    scleroderma and, 244
    systemic lupus erythematosus and, 234
Paraneoplastic limbic encephalitis (PLE), 79,
    409–410, 503, 553.
        See also Limbic encephalitis
Paranoid delusions, 640
Paraparetic gait, 24
Paraphasia, **40**
Parathyroidectomy, 205
Parietal lobe lesions, 409
Parkinsonism
    differential diagnosis of catatonia and,
        530
    gait examination and, 23, 24
    tremor and, **25**
Parkinson's disease
    dementia and, 632
    depression and, 384, 386, 546
    hypokinesis and, 26
    impulsive-compulsive syndrome of, 347
    mood disorders and, 546
    motor disorders and tremor, 383, 384–385
    psychosis and, 511
Paroxetine
    anticholinergic toxicity and, **96**
    inflammatory bowel disease and, 303
    lactation and, 465
    premenstrual mood disorders and, 450
    renal disease and, 321
Paroxysmal nocturnal dyspnea (PND), 566
Paroxysmal supraventricular tachycardia
    (PSVT), 178, 564–566
Pathological laughing and crying (PLC), and
    multiple sclerosis, 548
Pathophysiological analytic reasoning, 5, 6
Patient Health Questionnaire (PHQ-9), 323,
    342, 374, 422, 454, 462
Patient history. *See also* Collateral
    information; Family history
    causes of diagnostic errors and, 7
    infectious diseases and, 266
    insomnia and, 669–671

neurological disorders and, 342, 343
    new-onset psychotic symptoms and, 499
Patient Protection and Affordable Care Act
    of 2010, 588
Pediatric autoimmune neuropsychiatric
    disorders associated with streptococcal
    infections (PANDAS), 282, 576
Peduncular hallucinosis, 510
Pellagra, 137–138
Pembrolizumab, **411**
Pemetrexed, **411**
Penicillin, 278–279, 507
Peptic ulcer disease, 298–299
Periodic catatonia, 524
Periodic limb movement disorder (PLMD),
    328, **668**
Peritoneal dialysis, 321–322
Perphenazine, **96, 153, 154**
Persistent pulmonary hypertension of the
    newborn (PPHN), 456
Personality disorders
    cardiovascular disease and, 183–184
    chronic pain and, 653
    conversion disorder and, 686
    dermatological conditions and, **429,**
        434–435
    systemic lupus erythematosus and, 235
Pessimism, in patients with dermatological
    conditions, 441
Peyote/mescaline, **124**
Phencyclidine (PCP), 117, **121–123,** 515
Phenelzine, 303
Pheochromocytoma, 214–216, 568, **581**
Phobias, and cancer treatment, 401.
        See also Social phobia; Specific phobia
Phosphodiesterase-5 inhibitors, 186, 329
Physical examination.
        See also Neurological examination
    causes of diagnostic errors and, 7
    dermatological conditions and
        comprehensive, 424–425
    generalized anxiety disorder and, 572–573
    insomnia and, 672
    neurological examination and, 15–17
    new-onset psychotic symptoms and,
        499–500, **501**
Physical manifestations, of obsessive-
    compulsive disorder, 576–577
Physical therapy, for complex regional pain
    syndrome, 656
Physiological tremor, **25**

Physostigmine, **101**
Pimavanserin, 385, 511, 637
Pimozide, **150,** 430
Pittsburgh Agitation Scale, 634
Pittsburgh Sleep Quality Index, 374
Place orientation, testing of, 35
Plant(s), as hallucinogens, 117, **124–127**
Plantar reflex, 21–22
Platelet count, and laboratory testing for toxicological conditions, **169**
Pneumonia, 268–269
Pollution, and heavy metal exposure, 128
Polycystic ovary syndrome (PCOS), 206–209
Polypharmacy, and anticholinergic medications, 514
Polysomnography, and insomnia, 326, 673
Porphyria, 438
Positron emission tomography (PET), 60–61, **64, 80,** 635
Post-Concussion Symptom Scale, 374
Postconcussion syndrome, 374
Posterior dominant rhythm (PDR), and EEG, 72
Posterior reversible encephalopathy syndrome (PRES), 408
Postictal psychosis, 511
Postinfectious syndromes, and contested illnesses, 281–282
Postpartum blues, 462
Postpartum depression, 461–462, 463–464
Postpartum obsessive-compulsive disorder, 463–464
Postpartum period, psychiatric disorders during, 453, 461–465
Postpartum psychosis, 453, 454, 462–463
Postprandial distress syndrome, 291
Poststroke depression (PSD), 351–353
Posttraumatic stress disorder (PTSD)
    cancer and, 401
    cardiovascular disease and, 182–183
    gastrointestinal disorders and, 293
    in general medical settings, 578–580
    inflammatory bowel disease and, 302
    MDMA and, 117
    migraine and, 367
    multiple sclerosis and, 364
    prevalence of in women, 447
    scleroderma and, 244
    traumatic brain injury and, 373
Potassium, and laboratory testing for toxicological conditions, **167**

Potentially lateralizing neurological signs, 18, **19**
Powassen virus, 279
Prader-Willi syndrome (PWS), 487, 488, 527
Pramipexole, 328
Praxis, and bedside cognitive examination, 43–44
Prediction of Alcohol Withdrawal Severity Scale (PAWSS), 591
Prednisone, 400
Preeclampsia, 464
Preexposure prophylaxis, and HIV prevention, 275
Pregnancy. *See also* Lactation
    alcohol use disorders and, 596, **597**
    adrenal insufficiency and, 223
    hyperprolactinemia and, 212
    insomnia during, 461
    opioid use disorders and, 606
    psychiatric disorders during, 452–454
    psychoactive drugs during, 455–460
    substance abuse and, 469, 599
Prehension behavior, and executive functions, **46**
Premenstrual dysphoric disorder (PMDD), 449–452
Premenstrual exacerbation of a depressive disorder (PME-DD), 449–452
Premenstrual syndrome (PMS), 449–452, **467**
Prevalence
    of cigarette smoking, 607
    of dementia, 630
    of depression in cancer patients, 397–398
    of depression in patients with heart disease, 181
    of depression during pregnancy, 453
    of diabetes mellitus, 194
    of end-stage renal disease, 319
    of illness anxiety disorder, 684
    of insomnia, 663
    of mood and anxiety disorders in women, 447
    of multiple sclerosis, 360–361
    of obsessive-compulsive disorder, 575
    of panic disorder, 564, 567
    of personality disorders, 434
    of postpartum obsessive-compulsive disorder, 463
    of posttraumatic stress disorder, 578
    of psychiatric disorders in patients with dermatological conditions, 419

Prevalence *(continued)*
   of psychiatric disorders in patients with
      renal disease, 322
   of psychiatric symptoms in patients with
      systemic lupus erythematosus, 232,
      235
   of somatic symptom disorder, 680
   of substance use disorders in medical
      setting, 587
Prevention
   of delirium in patients with renal disease,
      330
   of drug-induced liver injury, 145
   of HIV, 275–276
   of infectious diseases, **284**
   of relapses in treatment of opioid
      disorders, 603–604
   of tuberculosis, 272
Primary aldosteronism, 220–222
Primary gastrointestinal diseases, 298–300
Primary progressive aphasia (PPA), 67,
   632–633
Primary progressive multiple sclerosis
   (PPMS), 359
Primidone, 386
Primitive reflexes, 22
Probabilistic analytic reasoning, 6
Problem-solving psychotherapy, for
   depression in patients with coronary
   disease, 182
Procarbazine, **411**
Processing speed, and tests of cognitive
   domains, 35
Prochlorperazine, **96**
Prodopaminergic agents, and obsessive-
   compulsive behavior, 576
Progressive multifocal leukoencephalopathy
   (PML), 275
Prolactin, and laboratory testing for
   toxicological conditions, **169.**
   See also Hyperprolactinemia
Propranolol, 248, 366, 386, 593
Propylthiouracil, 203
Prosody, and assessment of language,
   39–40
Prostatic hypertrophy, **668**
Proteinuria, 321
Proverb interpretation, and executive
   functions, **46**
Pruritus, 421, 432
Pseudobulbar affect, 346–347, 362

Pseudobulbar palsy, and neurological
   examination, 21
Pseudodysphagia, 574
Psilocybin, **126**
Psoralen ultraviolet A and ultraviolet B, **439**
Psoriasis, and lithium, 437–438
pSS. *See* Sjogren's syndrome
Psychiatric disorders.
   See also Anxiety disorders; Autism
      spectrum disorder; Bipolar disorder;
      Comorbidity; Major depressive
      disorder; Obsessive-compulsive
      disorder; Panic disorder; Personality
      disorders; Posttraumatic stress disorder;
      Psychiatric symptoms; Psychotic
      disorders; Somatic symptom disorder
   bidirectional relationship between
      neurological disorders and, 351
   chronic pain and, 652–658
   definition of, 339
   dermatological manifestations of, 424–435
   diabetes mellitus and, 193–194
   diagnosis of medical causes of, 7–8
   epidemiological linkage of infections to,
      283
   fetal alcohol syndrome and, 493
   inflammation and, 230
   liver disease and, 308
   in patients with heart disease, 179–184
   postpartum period and, 461–465
   Prader-Willi syndrome and, 488
   pregnancy and, 452–461
   prevalence of in patients with
      dermatological conditions, 419
   pubertal transition and menarche,
      448–449
   substance use disorders and, 599
   tobacco-related disorders and, 608
Psychiatric symptoms.
   See also Psychiatric disorders;
    Psychological symptoms; Psychosis
   acromegaly and, 218
   adrenal insufficiency and, 223–224
   Alzheimer's disease and, 547
   anti-NMDAR encephalitis and, 252–254,
      504
   cardiovascular disease and, 175–179
   case example of misdiagnosis of medical
      condition and, 11–12
   contested illnesses and, 280–283
   Cushing's syndrome and, 220

dermatological conditions and, 420–424, 438

diabetes mellitus and, 196

encephalitis and, 377–381

Graves' disease and, 247–248

Hashimoto's thyroiditis and, 245–247

HIV and, **273,** 276

hyperparathyroidism and, 205

hyperprolactinemia and, 214

limbic encephalitis and, 250–251

menopause and, 466–468

neurological disorders and, 340, 343

pheochromocytoma and, 216

polycystic ovary syndrome and, 207, 209

pregnancy and new-onset, 464

primary aldosteronism and, 222

rheumatoid arthritis and, 238–241

sarcoidosis and, 249

scleroderma and, 244

Sjogren's syndrome and, 241–243

substance abuse and, 103–128, **129**

systemic lupus erythematosus and, 232–237

testosterone deficiency and, 211–212

thyroid disorders and, 201–202

22q11.2 deletion syndrome and, 489

vitamin B deficiencies and, 137, 140

Psychiatrists. *See also* Consultations; Countertransference; Referrals; Transference

infectious diseases and roles for, 268, **284**

long-term management of psychiatric comorbidities of multiple sclerosis, 364

prevention of HIV and, 275–276

roles for in disaster preparedness, 268

roles for in neurosurgery, 368–369

tuberculosis prevention and, 272

Psychoactive drugs. *See also* Antidepressants; Antipsychotics; Anxiolytics; Benzodiazepines; Drug-drug interactions; Medications; Monoamine oxidase inhibitors; Mood-stabilizing agents; Sedative-hypnotics; Selective serotonin reuptake inhibitors; Serotonin-norepinephrine reuptake inhibitors; Side effects; Stimulants

anticholinergic toxicity and, 100, **101**

cancer patients and, 401

delirium and, 642–644

dementia and, 636–638

dermatological conditions and, 435–438

diabetes mellitus and, 198

epileptic patients with current or past psychiatric comorbidity, 354–355, 357

lactation and breast-feeding, 465–466

liver disease and, 309, **310**

lymphocytic colitis and, 303

menopause and psychiatric symptoms, 468

neuroleptic malignant syndrome and, 90, **91**

peptic ulcer disorder and, 299

pregnancy and, 455–461

renal disease and dosing of, 321

serotonin syndrome and, 95

thyroid disorders and, 203

Psychoeducation, and dermatological conditions, 424

Psychogenic nonepileptic seizures (PNES), **71,** 75, 353, 687

Psychogenic polydipsia, 144

Psychogenic tremor, **25**

Psychological factors affecting other medical conditions (PFAOMC), **679,** 680, **681,** 691–692

Psychological symptoms, of cannabis withdrawal, 615

Psychology

impact of dermatological conditions on, 420, 421–422, 423–424

social and cultural aspects of women's mental health and, 469–470

Psychopharmacology. *See* Psychoactive drugs

Psychosis, and psychotic symptoms. *See also* Psychotic disorders

anti-NMDAR encephalitis and, 252

cannabis use disorder and, 615

Cushing's syndrome and, 220

delirium and, 640

dementia and, 633

diabetes mellitus and, 197

encephalitis and, 379, 380

epilepsy and, **355**

hallucinogens and, **115, 116**

liver disease and, 308

marijuana-induced, 104

medical conditions as cause of, **501,** 501–513

medical evaluation of new-onset, 499–500, **501**

Psychosis, and psychotic symptoms
    (*continued*)
    multiple sclerosis and, 360, 362
    Parkinson's disease and, 385
    systemic lupus erythematosus and,
        234–235, 237
    stimulant-induced, 104
    thyroid disorders and, 201, 202
Psychosocial assessment, and diagnosis of
    centrally mediated abdominal pain
    syndrome, 297
Psychosocial interventions
    for cannabis use disorder, 616
    for depression in cancer patients, 400
    for opioid disorders, 605–606
    for tobacco-related disorders, 609
Psychosomatic symptoms, in cancer patients,
    402–404
Psychotherapy. *See also* Cognitive-behavioral
    therapy; Motivational enhancement
    therapy; Psychosocial interventions;
    Supportive-expressive psychotherapy
    anxiety disorders and, 582
    conversion disorder and, 688–689
    dermatological conditions and, 423, 436
    obsessive-compulsive disorder and, 577
    organ transplantation and, 326
    poststroke depression and, 352
    somatic symptom disorder and, 683
Psychotic disorders. *See also* Postpartum
    psychosis; Psychosis; Schizophrenia
    cardiovascular disease and, 182
    dermatological conditions and, 426, **427,**
        430
Ptosis, and neurological examination, 20
Puberty, psychiatric disorders associated
    with in women, 448–449
Public health. *See also* Epidemics
    postpartum depression and, 461
    tobacco-related disorders and, 611
Pull test, for postural instability, 23, 24
Pulmonary infections, 268–272
Pupillary diameters, and neurological
    examination, 19, **20**

QT prolongation. *See also* Drug-induced long
    QT syndrome
    anticholinergic toxicity and, **99**
    antipsychotics and, 185
    drugs used in cancer treatment and, **412**
Quality of life (QOL) assessment tools, 423

Questionnaire for Impulsive-Compulsive
    Disorders in Parkinson's Disease
    (QUIP), 347, 385
Quetiapine
    anticholinergic toxicity and, **96**
    delirium and, 643
    dementia and, 637
    drug-induced long QT syndrome and, **152**
    drug-induced orthostatic hypotension
        and, 153, **154**
    EEG abnormalities and, 75
    gastrointestinal disorders and, 295, 298
    Parkinson's disease and, 385
    pregnancy and, 458
Quick Inventory of Depressive
    Symptomatology—Self Report, 323

Rapid eye movement sleep behavior
    disorder, **668**
Rating scales, for neurological issues, **17,** 343,
    348.
    See also Screening
Receptive aprosodia, 40
Referrals. *See also* Consultations
    dermatological conditions and, 423, 439
    illness anxiety disorder and, 685
    obsessive-compulsive disorder and, 577
Reflection-based cognitive forcing strategy,
    10
Reflexes, and neurological examination,
    21–22
Reflex sympathetic dystrophy, 655–656
Relapses
    of multiple sclerosis, 359, 362, 364
    treatment of opioid disorders and,
        603–604, 607
Relapsing-remitting multiple sclerosis
    (RRMS), 359, 360
Reminiscence therapy, for dementia, 639
Renal disease. *See also* Dialysis
    delirium and, 329–331
    frequency of psychiatric diagnoses in
        patients with, 319
    mood and affective disorders, 322–328
    pain management and, 331–332
    physical and psychosocial challenges for
        patients with, 320–321
    psychiatric medications and, 321
    sexual dysfunction and, 328–329
    treatment nonadherence and suicide,
        332–333

Renal function testing, for toxicological complications and conditions, **167–168**

Repetition aprosodia, 40

Respiratory acidosis, **167**

Respiratory depression, and anticholinergic toxicity, **99**

Respiratory diseases, as cause of anxiety and panic attacks, **565**

Respiratory infections, and catatonia, 534

Restless legs syndrome (RLS), 328, **668**, 673, **674**

Retrograde memory, 41

Rheumatoid arthritis, 238–241, 655

Ribavirin, 309

Rifampin, and rifapentine, 270

Rinné test, and hearing, 21

Risperidone, 75, **152**, 153, **154**

Rituximab, 363, **411**

Rivastigmine, 186, 636–637

Rivermead Post-Concussion Symptoms Questionnaire, 374

Rocky Mountain spotted fever, 279

Romberg's test, and balance, 23, 24

Rome IV criteria, for functional gastrointestinal disorders, 290

Rotterdam criteria, for polycystic ovary syndrome, 207

Roussel Uclaf Causality Assessment Method (RUCAM) criteria, 144, **146–147**

Saccadic intrusions, and neurological examination, 19

St. John's wort, and serotonin syndrome, **92**

Salford Psoriasis Index, 423

Salvia, **124**

Sarcoidosis, 248–250

Schizophrenia
    autoimmune disorders and severe infections, 231
    cardiovascular disease and, 182
    celiac disease and, 305
    dermatological conditions and, **427**
    diabetes mellitus and, 197
    irritable bowel syndrome and, 293
    NMDAR hypofunction and, 504
    obsessive-compulsive disorder and, 576
    pregnancy and, 453
    substance abuse and misdiagnosis of, 104
    22q11.2 deletion syndrome and, 489
    velocardiofacial syndrome and, 505

Scientific method, and diagnosis, 4

Scleroderma, 243–244

Sclerosing cholangitis, 311

Screening. *See also* Rating scales
    for alcohol use disorders, 589–590
    algorithm to identity patients with psychiatric symptoms of medical disease, 9
    bedside cognitive examination and, 33–34
    for cannabis use disorder, 614
    for depression and anxiety in patients with dermatological conditions, 422–423
    for depression in patients with renal disease, 323
    global cognitive assessment and, 32
    for HIV, 272, 277, **280**
    for opioid use disorders, 598–600
    of pregnant and postpartum women, 453–454, 462
    for suicidal ideation in patients with renal disease, 333
    for syphilis, **280**
    for trauma exposure, 580

Script theory, and diagnosis, 4–5

Scurvy, 128, 137

Seasonal influenza, 269

Seborrheic dermatitis, 438

Secondary gain, and somatic symptom disorder, 683

Secondary headaches, 657, 658

Secondary progressive multiple sclerosis (SPMS), 359

Secondary syphilis, 378

Second opinions, and diagnostic accuracy, 11

Sedative-hypnotics, 109, **113–114**, 461

Seizures. *See also* Epilepsy; Psychogenic nonepileptic seizures
    alcohol use disorders and, 594, 595
    catatonia and, 530
    electroencephalography and, 70, 72–73, **74**, 75
    fragile X syndrome and, 485
    psychotic symptoms and, 511

Selective serotonin reuptake inhibitors (SSRIs)
    anticholinergic toxicity and, **96**
    anxiety disorders in general medical setting, 581
    anxiety in heart disease patients and, 181
    cardiovascular effects of in heart disease patients, 184

Selective serotonin reuptake inhibitors
(SSRIs) *(continued)*
chemotherapeutic agents and, 410, 412
dementia and, 637
dermatological conditions and, 423
drug-induced hyponatremia and, 142, **143**
gastrointestinal disorders and, 294
inflammatory bowel disease and, 303
liver disease and, 309
menopause and, 468
mood disorders and, 554
peptic ulcer disorder and, 299
pregnancy and, 455–457
premenstrual mood disorders and, 450–451
renal disease and, 324
rheumatoid arthritis and, 240–241
serotonin syndrome and, 90, **92**
systemic lupus erythematosus and, 237
Self-education, and posttraumatic stress
disorder, 579
Self-harming behavior
borderline personality disorder and, 435
dermatological conditions and, 440
factitious disorder and, 690
Semantic memory, and bedside cognitive
examination, 42–43
Semantic variant of primary progressive
aphasia, 633
Sensation, and neurological examination,
23, 26
Sensory ataxia, and gait, 24
Sepsis, as emergency, 266–267
Serious mental illness (SMI), and diabetes
mellitus, 197
Serotonergic system, and estrogen, 448
Serotonin-norepinephrine reuptake
inhibitors (SNRIs)
cancer medications and, 412
centrally mediated abdominal pain
syndrome and, 297
dementia and, 637
depression in cancer patients and, 400
dermatological conditions and, 423
electrolyte abnormalities due to, **143**
gastrointestinal disorders and, 294
menopause and, 468
mood disorders and, 554
pregnancy and, 457
serotonin syndrome and, **92**
Serotonin receptor agonists, and migraine,
365

Serotonin syndrome
catatonia and, 535–536
clinical presentation and diagnosis of,
92–93, **94**
as emergency, **28,** 92
psychopharmacology and, 90, **92, 99**
Sertraline
for depression in patients with coronary
disease, 182
lactation and, 465
lymphocytic colitis and, 303
for premenstrual mood disorders, 450
rheumatoid arthritis and, 240
Set shifting and response inhibition, and
executive functions, **46**
Severe acute respiratory syndrome, 268
Severity Measure for Panic Disorder, 326
Sexual dysfunction
cardiovascular disease and, 183
hyperprolactinemia and, 214
Parkinson's disease and, 384
renal disease and, 328–329
Sexually transmitted diseases, 279.
See also Syphilis
SGA. *See* Antipsychotics
Shared psychotic disorder, 430
Shift work disorder, **668, 674**
Short-term memory, compared to working
memory, 37
Sialorrhea, and anticholinergic toxicity, **98**
Sibutramine, and serotonin syndrome, **92**
Sick role, and factitious skin disorder, 433
Side effects, of medications.
See also Neuroleptic malignant
syndrome; Serotonin syndrome
aggressive behavior as form of, **484**
antibiotics and psychiatric symptoms as,
271
antidepressant-associated in patients with
renal disease, 324
antiviral medications and psychiatric
symptoms as, **271**
corticosteroids and severe psychiatric
symptoms as, 554
medications for chronic obstructive
pulmonary disorder and, 568
neuropsychiatric consequences of
dermatological drugs, **439**
rheumatoid arthritis and psychiatric
symptoms as, **240**
Sildenafil, 329

Silent myocardial ischemia, 178, **179**

Simvastatin, 363

Single-photon emission computed tomography (SPECT), **61, 62, 64, 65,** 69

Siponimod, 363

Sitophobia, 574

Sjogren's syndrome (pSS), 241–243

Skindex, 423

Sleep and sleep disorders. *See also* Insomnia
Angelman syndrome and, 489
breast feeding and disruption of, 465–466
cancer and, 403–404
logs or diaries of, 671
menopause and, 467
neurological disorders and, 343
renal disease and, 326–328
tests of cognitive domains and, 34

SMART Recovery, 606

Smoking cessation therapy, 608, 609

Social issues, and cultural aspects of women's mental health, 469–470

Social phobia (social anxiety disorder)
celiac disease and, 305
in general medical setting, 574–575
Graves' disease and, 247
inflammatory bowel disease and, 302
scleroderma and, 244
systemic lupus erythematosus and, 234

Social support, and depression in patients with renal disease, 323.
See also Psychosocial interventions; Support groups

Social work, and consultation for alcohol withdrawal syndrome, 591

Sodium levels
laboratory testing for toxicological conditions, **167**
syndrome of inappropriate antidiuretic hormone secretion and, 410

Soft signs, neurological, 17–18, **19,** 482, **483**

Somatic symptom disorder (SSD)
cardiovascular disease and, 175–177
case example of, 680
chronic pain and, 653
conversion disorder and, 686
dermatological conditions and, **427,** 432–433
differential diagnosis and comorbidity in, 682
epidemiology of, 680–681
generalized anxiety disorder and, 570

multiple sclerosis and, 360
pathophysiology and etiology of, 681–682
posttraumatic stress disorder and, 579
treatment of, 682–683

Somatic symptom and related disorders (SSRDs), 677, 678, **679,** 680.
See also Conversion disorder; Factitious disorder; Illness anxiety disorder; Psychological factors affecting other medical conditions; Somatic symptom disorder

Somatosensory extinction, and neurological examination, 23

Somnolence.
See also Excessive daytime sleepiness
anticholinergic toxicity and, **98**
cognitive functions and, 34

Spanish flu pandemic (1918), 269

Specific phobia, 234, 573–574

Speech, and language, 38

Spinal accessory nerve, and neurological examination, 21

Spontaneous smile, and symmetrical smile, 20–21

Stages of Reproductive Aging Workshop (STRAW) criteria, 466

States, and legalization of marijuana, 613, 614

Status epilepticus, as emergency, **28**

Steatosis, 306

Stein-Leventhal syndrome.
See Polycystic ovary syndrome

Stem cell transplantation, 407–408

Sternbach criteria, and serotonin syndrome, 92, **93,** 536

Steroids, and mania in cancer patients, 400.
See also Corticosteroids

Stevens-Johnsons syndrome (SJS), 437

Stigma
dermatological conditions and, 421
neurological disorders and, 341

Stimulant(s). *See also* Amphetamines; Cocaine; Methamphetamine
cancer patients and, 400, 403, 405
cardiac effects of, 185–186
delirium and, 643–644
HIV-associated neurocognitive disorder and, 383
overdoses of, 619
pregnancy and, 460
psychiatric symptoms caused by, 104, **105–106,** 513–514

Stimulant-related disorders, 617–620
STOP-Bang Scoring Model, 671
Streptococcus pneumoniae, 267, 268
Stress. *See also* Acute stress disorder
    caregivers of patients with dementia and,
        630
    dermatological conditions and, 420–421,
        422
    kidney transplantation and, 320
    MRI scanning and, 59
    multiple sclerosis and, 364
    patients with heart disease and, 179–180
    peptic ulcer disease and, 298
    rheumatoid arthritis and, 239
Stroke
    pain and, 349
    psychiatric disorders and, 351–353
    vascular dementia and, 631
Structural MRI, and frontotemporal lobar
        degeneration, 68
Structured Clinical Interview for DSM-IV
        Axis I Disorders, 367
Stupor, and cognitive functions, 34
Sturge-Weber syndrome, **18**
Subarachnoid hemorrhage, 370
Subdural hematoma, 370–371
Substance abuse, and substance abuse
        disorders. *See also* Alcohol abuse;
        Cannabis; Cocaine; Hallucinogens;
        Intoxication; Withdrawal
    catatonia and, 526, **527**
    as cause of anxiety and panic attacks, **565**
    dermatological conditions and, **428**
    family history of, 599
    HIV and, 272, 506–507
    inflammatory bowel disease and, 302
    neuropsychiatric toxidromes and,
        103–128, **129**
    peptic ulcer disease and, 298
    posttraumatic stress disorder and, 579
    prevalence of in medical settings, 587
    specific drugs associated with initiation
        of, **612**
    tobacco-related disorders and relapse of,
        608
    women and, 468–469
Sudden cardiac death, and antipsychotics, 148
Suicide, and suicidal ideation
    cerebrospinal fluids and risk of, 76
    chronic pain and, 654
    Cushing's syndrome and, 220

    depression and anxiety in patients with
        dermatological conditions, 422
    dermatological conditions and, 431, 438,
        439
    epilepsy and, 357
    Huntington's disease and, 546, 634
    left ventricular assist devices and, 188
    migraine and, 367
    multiple sclerosis and, 364
    neurological disorders and, 350–351
    Parkinson's disease and, 384
    postpartum psychosis and, 463
    poststroke depression and, 352
    renal disease and, 323, 332–333
    systemic lupus erythematosus and, 234
    traumatic brain injury and, 545
Sulfasalazine, **240**
Sundowning, and delirium, 330
Support groups, and tobacco-related
        disorders, 609.
    See also Social support
Supportive-expressive psychotherapy, for
        depression in cancer patients, 400
Supportive therapy
    for neuroleptic malignant syndrome, 87
    for opioid disorders, 603, 605–606
    for serotonin syndrome, 94
Supranuclear gaze, and neurological
        examination, 20, 26
Surgeon General, U.S., 609
Surgery, and surgical treatment for epilepsy,
        357.
    See also Neurosurgery
Susceptibility-weighted MRI imaging, **55,** 59
Sydenham's chorea, 282
Sympathomimetics, and
        pheochromocytoma, 216
Symptom-triggered approach, to
        management of alcohol withdrawal, 592
Syndrome of inappropriate antidiuretic
        hormone (SIADH), 144, 410
Synthetic cannabinoids, **107–108,** 515–516, 616
Synthetic cathinones ("bath salts"), 515, 618
Syphilis, **270,** 278–279, **280,** 507, 636.
    See also Neurosyphilis
Systemic lupus erythematosus (SLE),
        232–241, 502, 526, 553, 655

T-ACE brief screening tool, for alcohol use
        disorder in pregnancy, 596, **597**
Tachyarrhythmias, 564–566, **581**

Tacrolimus, **240**, 526

Takotsubo cardiomyopathy, 180, 215

Tamoxifen, 410, **411**

Telescoping, and substance abuse, 468

Temporal lobe(s), and brain tumors, 409

Temporal lobe epilepsy (TLE), **71**, 73, **74**, 347–349, 549

Temporal lobe meningiomas, 371

Tension-type headaches (TTH), 657, 658

Testicular cancer, 616

Testosterone, and testosterone deficiency, 128, 209–212, 329

Tetrabenazine, **151**

Tetrahydrocannabinol (THC), 515, 611–612

Thiamine deficiency, 138–139, 512–513, 594–595

Thiazolidinediones, **208**, 209

Thinking, and thoughts.
    See also Catastrophizing
    anxiety disorders and automatic, 582
    epilepsy and, **356**
    postpartum obsessive-compulsive disorder and ego-dystonic, 463

Thioridazine, **96**, **150**, **152**, 185

Three-words/three-shapes test, 43

Thyroid disorders. *See also* Hashimoto's thyroiditis; Hyperthyroidism; Hypothyroidism
    celiac disease and, 305
    clinical presentations of, 200
    etiology of, 199–200
    interactions of psychoactive drugs in, 203
    laboratory testing for toxicological conditions and, **168–169**
    lithium and, 203–204
    mood disorders and, 550
    neuropsychiatric presentations in, 201–202
    panic disorder and, 569
    subclinical manifestations of, 198–199
    subtypes of, 199
    treatment of, 201, 202–203

Thyroid function tests, and Hashimoto's thyroiditis, 246–247

Thyrotoxicosis, 199, 200, 202, 505–506

Tick-borne diseases, 279, **280**, 380

Tics, and neurological examination, 24

Time orientation, and cognitive testing, 35

Timolol, 366

Tinnitus Handicap Inventory, 374

Tobacco-related disorders, 607–611

Tolerance, to opioid use, 600–601

Topiramate, 366, 386

Torsades de pointes (TdP), drug-induced, 148–149, **150–151**, 152, **167**, 185

Tourette syndrome, 24

Toxic encephalopathies, and EEG, 70, 72

Toxicity, and complications or conditions associated with psychiatric illness. *See* Neuropsychiatric toxidromes

Toxoplasmosis, 274

Tracers, and positron emission tomography, 61

Trail Making Test, 32, 36

Tramadol, 331–332

Transcobalamin II deficiency, 140

Transcranial direct current stimulation (tDCS), and epilepsy, 359

Transference, and emotional factors in diagnosis, 7

Trastuzumab, **411**

Trauma, and conversion disorder, 687. *See also* Posttraumatic stress disorder

Trauma intensive care units (TICUs), and substance use disorders, 588, 589, 599

Traumatic brain injury (TBI)
    catatonia and, 526
    chronic traumatic encephalopathy and history of, 376–377
    late neurological effects of, 373–375
    mania and, 544–545
    posttraumatic stress disorder and, 578

Trazodone, 637, 643

Treatment.
    See also Behavioral interventions; Electroconvulsive therapy; Management; Prevention; Psychoactive drugs; Psychosocial interventions; Psychotherapy; Supportive therapy
    of acromegaly, 217–218
    of adrenal insufficiency, 223, 224
    of alcohol use disorders, 590–596
    of anxiety disorders in general medical setting, 580–582
    of cannabis use disorder, 616
    cardiovascular effects of for psychiatric problems in heart disease patients, 184–186
    of catatonia, 532–534
    of centrally mediated abdominal pain syndrome and narcotic bowel syndrome, 297–298

Treatment (continued)
    of conversion disorder, 688–689
    of Cushing's syndrome, 220
    of dementia, 636–639
    of depression in cancer patients, 399–400
    of diabetes mellitus and neuropsychiatric
        symptoms, 195, 197–198
    of factitious disorder, 691
    of fibromyalgia syndrome, 655
    of folic acid deficiency, 138
    of gastrointestinal disorders, 294–295
    of hyperparathyroidism, 205
    of hyperprolactinemia, 213–214
    of illness anxiety disorder, 685
    of infectious diseases, 283
    of insomnia, 673, 674
    of mood disorders, 554, 556
    of multiple sclerosis, 359–360, 362–364
    of neuroleptic malignant syndrome, 87,
        90, 91
    of obsessive-compulsive disorder,
        577–578
    of opioid use disorders, 601–607
    of pheochromocytoma, 215–216
    of polycystic ovary syndrome, 207, 208,
        209
    of primary aldosteronism, 221–222
    renal disease and nonadherence to,
        332–333
    of serotonin syndrome, 94–95
    of somatic symptom disorder, 682–683
    of stimulant use disorder, 619–620
    of systemic lupus erythematosus, 237
    of testosterone deficiency, 211, 212
    of thyroid disorders, 201, 202–203
    of tobacco-related disorders, 609–610
    of valproic acid-induced hyperammonemic
        encephalopathy, 102–103
    of vitamin deficiencies, 137, 138, 139, 140,
        141
    of zinc deficiency, 142
Tremor
    neurological examination and, 24, 25
    panic disorder and, 568–569
    Parkinson's disease and, 383, 384–386
Treponema pallidum, 278
Trichotillomania, 427, 431
Tricyclic antidepressants (TCAs)
    anticholinergic toxicity and, 95, 96, 98–99,
        100

cardiovascular effects of in heart disease
    patients, 184
centrally mediated abdominal pain
    syndrome and, 297
depression in cancer patients and, 400
drug-induced liver injury and, 144
drug-induced orthostatic hypotension
    and, 152
electrolyte abnormalities due to, 143
epilepsy and, 355
esophageal disorders and, 294
inflammatory bowel disease and, 303
laboratory testing for toxicological
    complications of, 166
pregnancy and, 457
renal disease and, 321, 324
serotonin syndrome and, 92
Trifluoperazine, 96
Trigeminal autonomic cephalalgias (TACs),
    657, 658
Triphasic waves, and EEG, 72
Triptans, and migraine, 365
Troponin, 164
Tryptophan, and celiac disease, 305
T2-weighted fluid-attenuated inversion
    recovery (T2-FLAIR), 54, 58, 70
Tuberculosis, 269–272
Tuberculous meningitis, 378
Tuberous sclerosis, 18, 490–491
Turner syndrome, 487
TWEAK brief screening tool, for alcohol use
    disorder in pregnancy, 596, 597
22q11.2 deletion syndrome, 489–490, 505
Type 1 (T1DM) and Type 2 (T2DM), as
    subtypes of diabetes mellitus, 194

Ulcerative colitis, 301, 553
Underdiagnosis. See Misdiagnosis
Unilateral thalamotomy, and essential
    tremor, 386
United Nations, 469
U.S. Institute of Medicine, 141
U.S. Preventive Services Task Force, 141, 200,
    636
U.S. Renal Data System survey, 332–333
Urea nitrogen, and laboratory testing for
    toxicological conditions, 167
Uremia, 320, 323
Urinalysis, and laboratory testing for
    toxicological conditions, 168

Urinary abnormalities, and anticholinergic toxicity, **98**
Urine testing, and alcohol abuse, **111**

Vaccines, and infectious diseases, 269
Valbenazine, **151**
Valproate
    dementia and, 637–638
    drug-induced liver injury and, 145, **147**, 310
    electrolyte abnormalities and, **143**
    laboratory testing for toxicological complications of, **165–166**
    migraine and, 366
Valproic acid, 458, 643
Valproic acid–induced hyperammonemic encephalopathy (VHE), 100, 102–103
Varenicline, 610
Vascular dementia (VaD), **64–65**, 68, 631–632, 634
Vascular depression, and vascular mania, 545, 634
Vasomotor symptoms, of menopause, 466
Vasovagal syncope, 574
Vegetative states, and catatonia, 529
Velocardiofacial syndrome (VCFS), 505
Venereal Disease Research Laboratory (VDRL) testing, 278, 279, 507, 636
Venlafaxine
    dementia and, 637
    drug-induced hyponatremia and, 142
    pregnancy and, 457
    renal disease and, 321
    serotonin syndrome and, 90
Ventral stream, and language function, 38
Verbal Trail Making Test, **46**
Vestibulo-ocular reflex, 20
Veterans Affairs Medical Center, 567
Video EEG, 70, 75
Vigilance, and tests of cognitive domains, 35
Vinca alkaloids, **411**
Viral encephalitis, 380
Viral hepatitis, **171**
Viral infections, of skin, **422**
Visceral hypersensitivity, and gastrointestinal disorders, 292, 300
Visual acuity, and neurological examination, 19, **20**
Visual extinction, and neurological examination, 23

Visual field testing, and symptom embellishment, 26
Visuospatial ability, and bedside cognitive examination, 43
Vitamin deficiencies. *See also* Diet; Nutrition
    catatonia and, 528
    cobalamin deficiency and, 139–140
    mood disorders and, 551
    pellagra and, 137 138
    psychotic symptoms and, 512–513
    scurvy and, 128, 137
    vitamin D and, 140–141
Voice, and language, 38
Vomiting, and anticipatory nausea in cancer patients, 403
Von Hippel–Lindau (VHL) disease, 215, 568

Wage gap, and gender, 469
Wakefulness, and cognitive domains, 34
Web-based resources
    cognitive-behavioral therapy programs for cancer patients, 403
    dermatological conditions and online apps, 424
    for infectious diseases, **266**
    self-management for rheumatoid arthritis and, 240
Weber test, for hearing, 21
Wechsler Intelligence Scale for Children, 491
Wernicke-Korsakoff syndrome, 138–139, 512–513
Wernicke's aphasia, **40**
Wernicke's encephalopathy, **110–112**, 526, 594, 595
Western equine encephalitis, 378
West Haven criteria, and hepatic encephalopathy, 308, **309**
West Nile virus (WNV), 267
Wheezing, and panic disorder, 566–568
White blood cell count, and laboratory testing for toxicological conditions, **169**
White matter hyperintensities (WMH), 545
Wide Range Achievement Test, 491
Wilson's disease, **25**, 307, 308, 310, 508–509
Withdrawal.
    See also Alcohol withdrawal syndrome
    benzodiazepines and, **113**
    cannabis use disorder and, 615
    catatonia and, **527**
    hallucinogens and, **116**